Pediatric Surgery

VOLUME 1

PEDIATRIC SURGERY

edited by

WILLIAM T. MUSTARD, M.D., F.R.C.S.(C), F.A.C.S.

Associate Professor of Surgery, University of Toronto
Chief of Cardiovascular Surgery, Hospital for Sick Children, Toronto

MARK M. RAVITCH, B.A., M.D., F.A.C.S.

Professor of Surgery, The University of Pittsburgh School of Medicine
Surgeon-in-Chief, Montefiore Hospital, Pittsburgh

WILLIAM H. SNYDER, JR., M.D., F.A.C.S.

Clinical Professor of Surgery, University of Southern California School of Medicine
Head of the Department of Surgery, Childrens Hospital of Los Angeles

KENNETH J. WELCH, A.B., M.D., F.A.C.S.

Clinical Associate in Surgery, Harvard Medical School; Associate in Surgery,
Children's Hospital Medical Center, Boston; Honorary Consultant,
Harvard Surgical Unit, Boston City Hospital; Surgeon, Newton-Wellesley Hospital

CLIFFORD D. BENSON, B.S., M.D., F.A.C.S.

Adjunct Professor of Surgery, Wayne State University Medical School
Senior Pediatric Surgeon, Children's Hospital of Michigan; Surgeon, Harper Hospital

Volume **1** *Second Edition*

35 EAST WACKER DRIVE • CHICAGO
YEAR BOOK MEDICAL PUBLISHERS • INC.

First Edition, June 1962

Second Edition, December 1969

Library of Congress Catalog Card Number: 71-75015
8151-6251-0

Foreword

THESE TWO NEW VOLUMES, the second edition of PEDIATRIC SURGERY, picture great progress in the surgical care of infants and children. One can't help but marvel at the phenomenal growth of children's surgery in the 25 years since it has been recognized as a specialty.

Why is a second edition of PEDIATRIC SURGERY, written so few years after the first, essential? For the simple reason that much has been learned during this time and needs to be presented to the medical profession. Eighty specialists in various branches of children's surgery have contributed to this new two-volume edition. Many of the chapters have been rewritten, and 31 new chapters and sections are presented.

The tremendous amount of time and energy spent by all these outstanding authors in putting into writing their knowledge and that of confreres all over the world deserves the reward of close reading by all who care for children. Pediatricians, and generalists above all, should have these books at hand as a guide to the best treatment of surgical problems arising in their practices. When, for geographic or other reasons, a trained pediatric surgeon is not available for an emergency surgical problem, and a surgeon who is a specialist in his field of adult surgery is called upon, he will be well directed by the guideposts to be found in these volumes.

Helpless little children and infants tragically born with serious deformities ask that the surgeon chosen to operate upon them exercise the best judgment in deciding what to do, that he use skilled techniques, and that he provide postoperative care suitable to this tender age.

The great satisfaction of successfully operating upon an infant lies in attaining a 70-year cure.

Read these books—don't just let them showfully decorate your bookshelf.

WILLIS J. POTTS*

---

*Deceased May 6, 1968.

Preface to the Second Edition

THE WARM RECEPTION accorded to the First Edition has been gratifying, and has imposed upon the editors the obligation of maintaining high standards in the preparation of the Second Edition. A completely new edition was undertaken because in the rapidly developing field of pediatric surgery it was obvious that most sections and chapters would be extensively rewritten, and because there was a substantial amount of totally new material under separate chapter headings which we believed required inclusion. Several of the subjects have been reassigned, generally because in the interval the new author has made distinguished contributions in the area. While we were anxious to avoid increasing the size of the volumes, the necessity for including a substantial amount of entirely new material has made some increase unavoidable.

Subjects new to the Second Edition, or for the first time accorded full chapter status, are Genetic Considerations, Inhalation Therapy, Chemotherapy of Solid Tumors, Birth Trauma, Physical Abuse During Childhood (The Battered-Child Syndrome), Tetanus and Gas Gangrene, The Salivary Glands, Cysts and Sinuses of the Neck, New Diagnostic Methods in Congenital Heart Disease, Congenital Complete Heart Block, Acquired Heart Disease, Surgery in Patients with Disorders of the Clotting Mechanism, Gastrointestinal Polyps, Renal Homotransplantation, Abdominal Musculature Deficiency Syndrome, Cloacal Exstrophy, and Urinary Diversion. Subjects now elevated to separate section status within existing chapters are Preoperative and Postoperative Care of Infants and Children, Abnormal Tracheobronchial Communications, Aortico—Left Ventricular Tunnel, Double Outlet from Right Ventricle, Single Ventricle, Persistent Truncus Arteriosus, Aortic Origin of Right Pulmonary Artery, Congenital Mitral Insufficiency, Ebstein's Anomaly, Hyperbaric Oxygenation, Fetal Ascites, Perforation of the Colon in the Newborn, Gangrene of the Extremities. Chapters and sections assigned to new contributors are Torticollis, Reconstruction of the Esophagus, Congenital Anomalies and Tumors of the Liver, Cholecystitis and Cholelithiasis, Choledochal Cyst, Ulcerative Colitis, Recurring Urinary Tract Infections, Renovascular Hypertension, Intersex, and The Female Genital Tract. Absence of the subchapter on Sacrococcygeal Teratoma from the Second Edition is regrettable and is due to editorial oversight.

The editors are grateful to the contributors for their continued support and cooperation. The allocation of areas of principal editorial responsibility is unchanged. The volumes continue to be a collective effort, as reflected by the alphabetical change in the listing of the editors for the present edition. Doctor Ravitch functioned as Chairman of the Board. Our secretaries, Rita Macklin, Therese Fox, Beryl Sharkey, Nancy Jane Robinson, and Helen Keller have put in long and arduous hours in typing and retyping the manuscripts. We are grateful to them for their patient and sustained efforts.

The style and arrangement of the book have not been altered except that the addition of many new illustrations and the removal of some of the old ones suggested the advisability of numbering the illustrations separately in each chapter.

It is a pleasure to express our warm appreciation to the staff of Year Book Medical Publishers for their unfailing support and wise counsel, and for the extraordinarily high level of performance with respect to the accuracy of the text, clarity of the illustrations, layout of the pages, and format of the volumes.

THE EDITORS

Preface to the First Edition

PEDIATRIC SURGERY today is one of the most vigorously growing fields in surgery. The establishment of chairs, divisions, and departments of pediatric surgery in university centers attests to an increasing awareness of the special problems in this field. Several societies have been founded to promote knowledge in this area, and special sections exist in others. Two journals are devoted entirely to pediatric surgery, a third has a special department and others publish special issues concerned with its problems.

In June of 1959, an editorial board was formed to enroll the services of recognized authorities in writing a complete textbook of pediatric surgery that would reflect the best thoughts of men from representative institutions, covering a wide geographic area in the United States, Canada and England. As in any branch of surgery, during a period of rapid development and experimentation, much of the material is new, and much of it is as yet unpublished elsewhere in any form.

Our colleagues in many countries are contributing importantly to the growth of pediatric surgical knowledge. They will find repeated references to their published material. We regret that we could not enlist the services of many worthwhile contributors from Australia, Scandinavia, and Continental Europe.

This project was conceived to meet the need for a comprehensive work on pediatric surgery presented from as broad a point of view as possible. There was agreement that all aspects of pediatric surgery would be covered, although, in order to limit the work to a reasonable size, it was necessary to restrict the space allotted to such specialty fields as ophthalmology, otolaryngology, orthopedics, and neurosurgery. The heaviest concentration is in the traditional fields of general, thoracic and urologic surgery.

Particular emphasis has been laid on appropriate treatment of the physiologic, anatomic, and embryologic aspects of specific surgical problems. Because we feel that the current state of knowledge is best understood in the light of its development, we have prefaced many subjects with an historical résumé.

Contributors have been urged to express their own feelings clearly on controversial points, to draw particularly on their own experience, and, in addition, to evaluate and comment upon the work of others. To this end, we have encouraged extensive bibliographic lists, with annotations in the text. Particular attention has been paid to the illustrations and the publishers have been generous concerning the number included.

Our contributors have been cooperative, prompt, and patient with our editorial suggestions, and we are grateful to them. Some duplication of coverage will necessarily occur in a multiauthor textbook, and we think this not undesirable. Differences of opinion are expressed in some areas, and such differences will be found to exist. In details of treatment, and in other matters, in a variety of aspects of pediatric surgery, the editors do not hold uniform opinions

—nor do the contributors. It was felt important only that an individual contribution present a valid and supportable point of view and a satisfactory method of treatment.

It is hoped that the various sections are developed in a manner systematic enough to make them useful to the student or house officer interested in the field of pediatric surgery, that the presentations are broad enough and sufficiently free from surgical minutiae to be useful to the pediatrician, and yet detailed enough to convey to the informed general surgeon each author's assessment of current knowledge in his field and his own recommendations.

We have felt strongly that the value of this presentation would be increased in direct proportion to the briefness of time between the preparation of the manuscript and publication. In a multiauthor work, a good deal of time is necessarily expended in the transmission of manuscripts from authors to editors, in circulation among editors, and resubmission to authors for consideration of joint editorial suggestions. Six months were spent by the editorial board in organizing the form of the work, the division of subject matter, the manner of presentation, the division of editorial responsibilities, and the assignment of subjects to the editors and contributors. The actual writing, editing, and publication have been accomplished in less than two years.

The editorial board has functioned in a coordinated effort. While the editors were individually responsible for given Parts, each contributed Sections to Parts for which others were editorially responsible. Every chapter has been reviewed by several members of the board. The distribution of a model chapter, prepared by Doctor Mustard, greatly simplified the problem of achieving uniformity. Doctor Welch served as chairman of the board and was editorially responsible for PART I: *General*, PART II: *Head and Neck*, and PART V: *Genitourinary System*. Doctors Mustard and Ravitch were responsible for PART III: *The Thorax*, Doctor Mustard for PART VI: *Integument and Musculoskeletal System*, and Doctor Ravitch for PART VII: *Nervous System*. Doctors Benson and Snyder prepared PART IV: *Abdomen*. The selection of contributors was a joint editorial effort. Mrs. Muriel McL. Miller was responsible for the uniform pen and ink illustration concept.

We wish to acknowledge our gratitude to our secretaries, Mrs. Ralph Conjour, Miss June Gerkens, Mrs. Grace Crabbe, Mrs. Josephine Dyer, and Miss Linda Morse, for their tolerance and patience, and their willingness to type and retype manuscripts at a rapid pace and make early publication a reality.

We are grateful also to the staff of Year Book Medical Publishers for their enthusiasm and cooperation. The many meetings of the editorial board have been made possible through their generous support.

THE EDITORS

List of Contributors

ABLE, LUKE W., M.D.: Clinical Associate Professor of Surgery, Baylor University College of Medicine; Surgeon-in-Chief, Texas Children's Hospital, Houston, Tex.

ALBARRACIN, AURORA, M.D.: Fellow in Hematology, Children's Hospital, Columbus, Ohio

ARONSON, NEAL I., M.D.: Assistant Professor of Neurological Surgery, Johns Hopkins University School of Medicine, Baltimore

BAFFES, THOMAS G., M.D., F.A.C.S.: Associate, Department of Surgery, Northwestern University Medical School; Attending Surgeon, Children's Memorial Hospital, Chicago

BAHNSON, HENRY T., M.D.: George Vance Foster Professor of Medicine, and Chairman, Department of Surgery, University of Pittsburgh School of Medicine

BEARDMORE, HARVEY E., B.Sc., M.D., C.M., F.R.C.S.(C), F.A.C.S., F.A.A.P.(S): Assistant Professor of Surgery, McGill University; Associate Surgeon, The Montreal Children's Hospital, Montreal

BENSON, CLIFFORD D., M.D., F.A.C.S.: Clinical Professor of Surgery, Wayne State University Medical School; Senior Pediatric Surgeon, Children's Hospital of Michigan; Surgeon, Harper Hospital, Detroit

BERNHARD, WILLIAM F., M.D.: Senior Associate in Cardiovascular Surgery, and Director, Surgical Research Laboratory, Children's Hospital Medical Center; Associate Clinical Professor of Surgery, Harvard Medical School, Boston

BILL, ALEXANDER H., Jr., M.D.: Chief of Surgical Services, Children's Orthopedic Hospital and Medical Center; Clinical Associate Professor of Surgery, University of Washington School of Medicine, Seattle

BIRSNER, JOHN W., M.D.: Senior Attending Radiologist, Kern General Hospital, Bakersfield, Calif.

BOLES, E. THOMAS, Jr., M.D.: Associate Professor of Surgery, Ohio State University College of Medicine; Attending Staff, Children's and University Hospitals, Columbus

BORDLEY, JOHN E., M.D.: Emeritus Professor of Otolaryngology and Otology, Johns Hopkins University School of Medicine; Formerly, Otolaryngologist-in-Charge, The Johns Hopkins Hospital, Baltimore

BRAYTON, DONALD, M.D.: Clinical Professor of Surgery, University of California School of Medicine, Los Angeles

BROWN, JAMES BARRETT, M.D., F.A.C.S.: Professor Emeritus, Washington University School of Medicine, St. Louis, Mo.

CATLIN, FRANCIS I., M.D.: Associate Professor of Otolaryngology, Johns Hopkins University School of Medicine; Otolaryngologist, The Johns Hopkins Hospital, Baltimore

CHAFFIN, LAWRENCE, M.D.: Emeritus Clinical Professor of Surgery, University of Southern California School of Medicine, Los Angeles

CHISHOLM, TAGUE C., M.D., F.A.C.S.: Clinical Professor of Surgery, University of Minnesota Medical School; Chief of Pediatric Surgery, Hennepin County General Hospital, Minneapolis

CLATWORTHY, H. WILLIAM, Jr., M.D.: Professor and Director, Division of Pediatric Surgery, Ohio State University College of Medicine, Columbus

CONN, ALAN W., M.D., F.R.C.P.(C), F.A.C.A.: Assistant Professor, Department of Anaesthesia, University of Toronto; Anaesthetist-in-Chief, Hospital for Sick Children, Toronto

COOLEY, DENTON A., M.D., F.A.C.S.: Physician-in-Chief and Director, Texas Heart Institute, Houston

COTTON, BURT, M.D.: Associate Clinical Professor, Department of Surgery, University of California School of Medicine, Los Angeles; Senior Active Staff, Huntington Memorial Hospital, Pasadena, Calif.

CRAWFORD, JOHN S., M.D., C.M., D.O.M.S. (Eng): Professor of Ophthalmology, University of Toronto; Chief of Ophthalmology, Hospital for Sick Children, Toronto

CRESSON, SAMUEL LUKENS, M.D., F.A.C.S., F.A.A.P.(S): Professor of Clinical Surgery, and Chief of the Division of Pediatric Surgery, Temple University School of Medicine; Surgeon-in-Chief, St. Christopher's Hospital for Children, Philadelphia

CROCKER, DEAN, M.D., C.M.: Director, Department of Respiratory Therapy, Children's Hospital Medical Center; Clinical Associate in Anesthesia, Harvard Medical School, Boston

DAMMANN, J. FRANCIS, Jr., M.D.: Professor of Surgical Cardiology and Pediatrics, University of Virginia School of Medicine, Charlottesville

DIBBINS, ALBERT W., M.D.: Assistant Professor of Pediatric Surgery, University of Pittsburgh School of Medicine

EHRENPREIS, Th., M.D., F.A.A.P.: Associate Professor of Pediatric Surgery, Karolinska Institutet, University of Stockholm; Head of the Department of Pediatric Surgery, Karolinska Sjukhuset, Stockholm, Sweden

ERAKLIS, ANGELO J., M.D., F.A.C.S.: Associate in Surgery and Director of Surgical Out-Patient Department, Children's Hospital Medical Center; Assistant Professor of Surgery, Harvard Medical School, Boston

EVANS, AUDREY E., M.D.: Associate Professor of Pediatrics, University of Pennsylvania School of Medicine; Head, Pediatric Oncology, Children's Hospital, Philadelphia

FARMER, ALFRED WELLS, M.B.E., M.B., M.D., F.R.C.S.(C): Professor of Surgery, University of Toronto; Surgeon-in-Chief, Sunnybrook Hospital; Consultant, Hospital for Sick Children, Toronto

FERGUSON, COLIN C., M.D., F.R.C.S.(C), F.A.C.S.: Professor and Head, Department of Surgery, University of Manitoba; Surgeon-in-Chief, Children's Hospital of Winnipeg

FISHER, JOHN H., M.D., M.S.: Associate Professor of Surgery (Pediatrics), Tufts University School of Medicine; Chief of Pediatric Surgical Service, New England Medical Center Hospitals, Boston

FRYER, MINOT P., M.D.: Professor of Surgery, Washington University School of Medicine, St. Louis, Mo.

GREANEY, EDWARD M., Jr., M.D.: Assistant Clinical Professor of Surgery, University of Southern California School of Medicine, Los Angeles; Attending Surgeon, Childrens Hospital of Los Angeles

GRUNDY, BETTY L. B., M.D.: Director, Inhalation Therapy, and Anesthesiologist, St. Luke's Hospital, Saginaw, Mich.

HAIGHT, CAMERON, M.D., F.A.C.S.: Professor of Surgery, University of Michigan Medical School; Surgeon-in-Charge, Section of Thoracic Surgery, University Hospital, Ann Arbor

HALLMAN, GRADY L., M.D., F.A.C.S.: Associate Professor of Surgery, Baylor University College of Medicine; Attending Cardiovascular Surgeon, St. Luke's Episcopal Hospital; Consultant Cardiovascular Surgeon, Texas Children's Hospital, Houston

HASTINGS, NEWLIN, M.D.: Instructor in Surgery, University of Southern California School of Medicine; Attending Surgeon, Childrens Hospital of Los Angeles

HAYS, DANIEL M., M.D.: Associate Professor of Surgery, University of Southern California School of Medicine; Attending Surgeon, Childrens Hospital of Los Angeles

HENDREN, W. HARDY, M.D.: Surgical Chairman, Children's Service, and Associate Visiting Surgeon, Massachusetts General Hospital; Assistant Clinical Professor of Surgery, Harvard Medical School, Boston

HIGHTOWER, BILLY M., M.D.: Instructor, Department of Surgery, University of Alabama Medical Center, Birmingham

HINMAN, FRANK, Jr., M.D.: Clinical Professor of Urology, University of California School of Medicine; Chief of Urology, San Francisco General and Children's Hospitals, San Francisco

HOLINGER, PAUL H., M.D.: Professor of Bronchoesophagology, Department of Otolaryngology, University of Illinois College of Medicine; Attending Bronchologist, Presbyterian-St. Luke's, Children's Memorial, and Research and Educational Hospitals, Chicago

HUME, DAVID M., M.D.: Stuart McGuire Professor and Chairman, Department of Surgery, Medical College of Virginia, Richmond

HUMPHREYS, GEORGE H., II, M.D., Med.Sc.D.: Valentine Moss Professor of Surgery, Columbia University College of Physicians and Surgeons; Attending Surgeon and Director, Surgical Service, Presbyterian Hospital, New York

JONES, PETER G., M.S.(Melb), F.R.C.S.(Eng), F.R.A.C.S., F.A.C.S.: Surgeon, Royal Children's Hospital; Instructor of Surgery, University of Melbourne

KIDD, B. S. LANGFORD, M.D., F.R.C.P.(Eng): Associate Professor of Pediatrics, University of Toronto School of Medicine; Physician-in-Charge, Cardiovascular Laboratory, Hospital for Sick Children, Toronto

KIESEWETTER, WILLIAM B., M.D.: Professor of Pediatric Surgery, University of Pittsburgh School of Medicine; Surgeon-in-Chief, Children's Hospital of Pittsburgh

KIRKLIN, JOHN W., M.D.: Professor and Chairman, Department of Surgery, University of Alabama Medical Center; Surgeon-in-Chief, University Hospitals and Clinics, Birmingham

LATTIMER, JOHN K., M.D., Sc.D.: Professor and Chairman, Department of Urology, Columbia University College of Physicians and Surgeons; Director, Squier Urologic Clinic; Director, Urology Service, Babies Hospital; Director of Urology, Francis Delafield Hospital, New York

LINDSAY, WILLIAM KERR, M.D., B.Sc.(Med.), F.R.C.S.(C), F.A.C.S.: Associate Professor, Department of Surgery, University of Toronto; Chief, Division of Plastic Surgery, Department of Surgery, and Chairman, Maxillo-facial Clinic, Hospital for Sick Children, Toronto

LLOYD, JAMES R., M.D.: Instructor in Surgery, Wayne State University Medical School; Associate Surgeon, Children's Hospital of Michigan and Harper Hospital, Detroit

LYNN, HUGH B., M.D.: Associate Professor of Surgery, Mayo Graduate School of Medicine, University of Minnesota; Section of Pediatric Surgery, Mayo Clinic, Rochester, Minn.

McPARLAND, FELIX A., M.D.: Clinical Instructor in Pediatric Surgery, University of Minnesota Medical School; Attending Pediatric Surgeon, Minneapolis General Hospital

McQUEEN, J. DONALD, M.D.: Associate Professor of Neurological Surgery, Johns Hopkins University School of Medicine; Neurosurgeon-in-Charge, Baltimore City Hospitals

MARTIN, LESTER W., M.D.: Associate Professor of Surgery, University of Cincinnati College of Medicine; Director of Pediatric Surgery, Children's Hospital, Cincinnati

MELICOW, MEYER M., M.D.: Given Professor Emeritus in Uropathology, and Special Lecturer in Uropathology, Columbia University College of Physicians and Surgeons;

Consultant in Uropathology, Francis Delafield, Harlem and St. Albans Naval Hospitals, New York

MINOR, CHARLES L., M.D., F.A.C.S., F.A.A.P.: Associate in Pediatric Surgery, University of Pennsylvania School of Medicine; Associate Surgeon, Children's Hospital of Philadelphia; Assistant in Pediatric Surgery, Wilmington Medical Center and St. Francis Hospital, Wilmington, Del.

MORGAN, A. LLOYD, M.B., M.D.: Assistant Professor of Ophthalmology, University of Toronto; Chief of Ophthalmology, Hospital for Sick Children, Toronto

MORSE, THOMAS S., M.D.: Associate Professor of Surgery, Ohio State University College of Medicine; Attending Surgeon, Children's Hospital, Columbus

MULLER, WILLIAM H., Jr., M.D.: Stephen H. Watts Professor and Chairman, Department of Surgery; Surgeon-in-Chief, University of Virginia Hospital, University of Virginia Medical Center, Charlottesville

MUSTARD, WILLIAM T., M.B.E., M.D., M.S.(TOR), F.R.C.S.(C), F.A.C.S., F.A.C.C.: Associate Professor of Surgery, University of Toronto; Chief of Cardiovascular Surgery, Hospital for Sick Children, Toronto

NEWTON, WILLIAM A., M.D.: Professor of Pathology and Pediatrics, Ohio State University College of Medicine, Columbus

PICKETT, LAWRENCE K., M.D., F.A.C.S., F.A.A.P.: Professor of Surgery and Pediatrics, Yale University School of Medicine; Attendant in Surgery, Yale-New Haven Medical Center, New Haven, Conn.

PILLING, GEORGE P., IV, M.D., F.A.C.S., F.A.A.P.(S): Associate Professor of Clinical Surgery, Temple University School of Medicine; Associate Attending Surgeon, St. Christopher's Hospital for Children, Philadelphia

POLLOCK, WILLIAM F., M.D.: Associate Clinical Professor of Surgery, University of California School of Medicine, Los Angeles; Attending Surgeon, Childrens Hospital of Los Angeles

RAVITCH, MARK M., B.A., M.D., F.A.C.S.: Professor of Surgery, The University of Pittsburgh School of Medicine; Surgeon-in-Chief, Montefiore Hospital, Pittsburgh

REED, JOSEPH O., M.D.: Clinical Assistant Professor of Radiology, Wayne State University Medical School; Radiologist-in-Chief, Children's Hospital of Michigan, Detroit

RICKHAM, P. P., M.D., M.S., F.R.C.S., D.C.H.: Senior Consultant Paediatric Surgeon, Alder Hay Children's Hospital, Liverpool; Director of Paediatric Surgical Studies, University of Liverpool

RIKER, WILLIAM L., M.D., F.A.C.S.: Associate Professor of Surgery, Northwestern University Medical School; Attending Surgeon and Associate Surgeon-in-Chief, Children's Memorial Hospital, Chicago

RUSH, BENJAMIN F., Jr., M.D.: Professor and Chairman, Department of Surgery, New Jersey College of Medicine, Newark

SABISTON, DAVID C., Jr., M.D.: Professor and Chairman, Department of Surgery, Duke University Medical Center, Durham, N. C.

SALTER, ROBERT BRUCE, M.D., M.S., F.R.C.S.(C), F.A.C.S.: Professor of Surgery, University of Toronto; Surgeon-in-Chief and Senior Orthopaedic Surgeon, Hospital for Sick Children, Toronto

SANTULLI, THOMAS V., M.D.: Professor of Surgery, Columbia University College of Physicians and Surgeons; Chief of the Pediatric Surgical Service, Babies Hospital, New York

SCHUSTER, SAMUEL R., M.D.: Senior Associate in Surgery, Children's Hospital Medical Center; Assistant Clinical Professor of Surgery, Harvard Medical School, Boston

SCOTT, H. WILLIAM, Jr., M.D., F.A.C.S.: Chairman, Department of Surgery, Vanderbilt University School of Medicine; Surgeon-in-Chief, Vanderbilt University Hospital, Nashville, Tenn.

SCOTT, WILLIAM W., Ph.D., M.D.: Professor of Urology, Johns Hopkins University School of Medicine; Urologist-in-Charge, Johns Hopkins Hospital, Baltimore

SHUMACKER, HARRIS B., Jr., M.D.: Professor of Surgery, Indiana University School of Medicine, Indianapolis

SIEBER, WILLIAM K., M.D.: Clinical Assistant Professor of Surgery, University of Pittsburgh School of Medicine; Senior Staff, Department of Surgery, Children's Hospital of Pittsburgh

SLOAN, HERBERT E., M.D., F.A.C.S., F.A.A.P.: Professor of Surgery, University of Michigan Medical Center, Ann Arbor

SMITH, BLANCA, M.D., Ph.D.: Associate Professor of Surgery, Ohio State University Medical School; Attending Surgeon, Children's Hospital, Columbus

SMITH, ROBERT M., M.D.: Director of Anesthesiology, Children's Hospital Medical Center; Associate Clinical Professor of Anesthesia, Harvard Medical School, Boston

SNYDER, WILLIAM H., Jr., M.D., F.A.C.S.: Emeritus Professor of Surgery, University of Southern California School of Medicine; Formerly, Surgeon-in-Chief, Childrens Hospital of Los Angeles; Senior Attending Surgeon, Los Angeles County-University of Southern California Medical Center, Los Angeles

SPENCER, BERNARD J., M.D., F.A.C.S.: Clinical Assistant Professor of Pediatric Surgery, University of Minnesota Medical School; Attending Pediatric Surgeon, Minneapolis General Hospital

SPENCER, FRANK COLE, M.D.: Chairman and George David Steward Professor, Department of Surgery, New York University Medical Center, New York

SPENCER, ROWENA, M.D.: Clinical Associate Professor, Department of Surgery, Tulane University School of Medicine, New Orleans, La.

STERN, AARON M., B.A., M.D., F.A.A.P.: Professor of Pediatrics and Communicable Diseases, University of Michigan Medical School, Ann Arbor

THOMPSON, J. S., M.A., M.D.: Professor and Chairman, Department of Anatomy, University of Toronto

THOMPSON, MARGARET W., Ph.D.: Associate Professor of Paediatrics, University of Toronto; Geneticist, Hospital for Sick Children, Toronto

TRUMP, DAVID S., M.D., E.A.A.P., F.A.C.S.: Associate Surgeon, St. Joseph's Hospital, Good Samaritan Hospital and Maricopa County Hospital, Phoenix

TRUSLER, GEORGE A., M.D., M.S., F.R.C.S.(C), F.A.C.S.: Associate, Department of Surgery, University of Toronto; Assistant Surgeon, Hospital for Sick Children, Toronto

UDVARHELYI, GEORGE B., M.D., F.A.C.S.: Professor of Neurosurgery, and Associate Professor of Radiology (Neuroradiology), Johns Hopkins University School of Medicine, Baltimore

USON, AURELIO C., M.D.: Associate in Urology, Columbia University College of Physicians and Surgeons; Assistant Urologist, Presbyterian Hospital, Harkness Pavilion and Babies Hospital, New York

VATHAYANON, SATHAPORN, B.S., M.D., F.A.C.S.: Instructor in Surgery, University of Michigan Medical School, Ann Arbor

WADE, JOHN C., M.D.: Fellow in Urology, Johns Hopkins University School of Medicine; Resident in Urology, Johns Hopkins Hospital, Baltimore

WALKER, A. EARL, M.D.: Professor of Neurological Surgery, Johns Hopkins University School of Medicine, Baltimore

WATERSTON, DAVID J., M.B.E., F.R.C.S.: Consultant Paediatric Surgeon, Hospital for Sick Children, Great Ormond Street, London

WELCH, KENNETH J., A.B., M.D., F.A.C.S.: Clinical Associate in Surgery, Harvard Medical School; Associate in Surgery, Children's Hospital Medical Center, Boston; Honorary Consultant, Harvard Surgical Unit, Boston City Hospital; Surgeon, Newton-Wellesley Hospital, Newton, Mass.

WILLIAMS, D. INNES, M.D., M.Chir., F.R.C.S.: Urologist, Hospital for Sick Children, Great Ormond Street, and St. Peter's and St. Paul's Hospitals, London; Senior Lecturer in Urology, Institute of Child Health and Institute of Urology, University of London

WILLIAMS, G. MELVILLE, M.D.: Professor of Surgery and Director of Surgical Research Laboratory, Medical College of Virginia, Richmond

WILSON, HARWELL, M.D.: Professor and Chairman, Department of Surgery, University of Tennessee College of Medicine; Surgeon-in-Chief, City of Memphis Hospitals

WOOLLEY, PAUL V., Jr., M.D.: Professor and Chairman, Department of Pediatrics, Wayne State University Medical School; Pediatrician-in-Chief, Children's Hospital of Michigan, Detroit

Table of Contents

VOLUME 1

PART I
General

PART II
Head and Neck

PART II
Head and
Neck

PART III
The Thorax and Cardiovascular System

SECTION ONE

SECTION TWO

PART III
The Thorax
and
Cardiovascular
System

PART III

The Thorax
and
Cardiovascular
System

PART IV
Abdomen

PART IV
Abdomen

VOLUME 2 (PARTIAL CONTENTS)

PART I

General

Introduction

HISTORY.—Until relatively recently, the surgery of infants and children has been considered simply a part of surgery, with some presumed differences owing to the size of the patients. Nevertheless, the special nature of the surgical problems of childhood has been recognized for a good many years. In 1860, J. Cooper Forster, Surgeon to Guy's Hospital and to the Royal Infirmary for Children, published *The Surgical Diseases of Children* (Fig. 1), a volume of 348 pages.[7] In his words, "The absence of any other work in the English language devoted to this subject" stimulated the effort. In the same year, A. W. Johnson delivered a course of lectures on *The Surgery of Childhood* at the Hospital for Sick Children, Great Ormond Street, London. In 1863, the Lettsomian Lectures on Surgical Pediatrics were established by the Council of the Medical Society of London, in the belief that "the interests of its members might be promoted, and the profession benefited by having their attention drawn from the broad field of general surgery to the . . . diseases of childhood." The lectures were given by Thomas Bryant and subsequently were published.[3] In 1868, Timothy Holmes, "to supply an admitted want in our surgical literature," published *The Surgical Treatment of Diseases of Infancy and Childhood*, a book of 687 pages.[12] In France, M. P. Guersant, Surgeon to the Hôpital des Enfants Malades, in Paris, delivered lectures on the surgery of children from 1840 to 1860, published as *Notices*, eventually translated by R. J. Dunglison of Philadelphia in 1873.[11] The children's hospitals of London and Paris for several years remained unique in providing a separate surgical program. In the year that Holmes published his textbook of pediatric surgery, the Children's Hospital of Boston was founded, modeled its charter after that of the Hospital for Sick Children, Great Ormond Street, and soon developed an independent surgical program with a major interest in skeletal disease. Simultaneously, other institutions for the care of children sprang up in response to the immediate success of the new specialty of pediatrics. S. W. Kelley,[13] President of the Association of American Teachers of the Diseases of Children, in 1909 published the first textbook in North America on surgical diseases of children. In the 1920's there emerged the pediatric surgeon, who devoted a substantial effort to work within a children's hospital. Barrington-Ward of London, Coe of Seattle, Ladd of Boston, Penberthy of Detroit, and Fraser of Edinburgh were among the earliest to concentrate their interests in this way. The books of Barrington-Ward[1] and of Fraser,[8] and particularly of Ladd and Gross[14] in English, Ombrédanne's work in French,[17] and the more extensive and encyclopedic publication of Drachter and Gossmann in German (Fig. 2)[4] were important contributions and stimuli to the new field.

More recently, the books of Gross,[10] of Potts,[18] and of Swenson,[19] in the United States, of Grob,[9] in Switzerland, Oberniedermayr[16] in Germany, Mason Brown,[14] Nixon and O'Donnell,[15] and White and Dennison[20] in Great Britain, and Fèvre[6] and Duhamel[5] in France have enriched the growing literature of pediatric surgery, together with an increasing number of monographs on special problems and facets. Some of these books are already in second and third editions.

Pediatric Surgery

A true specialty grows in response to need. Ladd[14] in 1941 hoped that "an appropriate number of men in each community would take a particular interest in this field, and give it the attention which it rightfully deserves."

A field of surgery defined solely by the age of its patients must obviously cut across the lines of the usual disciplinary divisions of surgery. As the constitution of the editorial board and the composition of the contributors to this volume indicate, it is our feeling that the cardinal emphasis should be on the need that pediatric surgery, of any special kind, be performed by individuals with a special interest, a special experience, and a special understanding of the problems involved, whatever their nominal specialty designation.

One can no longer shrug off errors of diagnosis, technique, and management in these young patients. Particularly with patients in the first year of life there has often been a tendency for the surgeon to anticipate failure, and for his medical colleagues to be consoling when this occurs. This misdirected charity would not be offered, and would not be accepted, by the conscientious surgeon who loses a patient in the prime of life with a straightforward surgical problem, yet there have often been few evident pangs of conscience over the death of a neonate who succumbed unnecessarily to complications following operation upon any of the major correctable anomalies. The varying incidence of surgical conditions in children and in adults, the varying response of children to the same lesions, the rarity of some conditions, and the occurrence, in the newborn, of lesions incompatible with life, unless corrected, and therefore not seen in later years, all plead for management by those specially interested in these problems and specially prepared to meet them.

The Child, the Hospital, and the Surgeon

A good deal has been written and said about the response of children to the hospital, and it is fashionable among some parents to inquire about the emotional trauma to the child involved in a necessary hospitalization. The fact is that children adjust remarkably well, and in a well-run pediatric surgical

THE

SURGICAL DISEASES

OF

CHILDREN.

BY

J. COOPER FORSTER,

FELLOW OF THE ROYAL COLLEGE OF SURGEONS; BACHELOR OF MEDICINE
OF THE UNIVERSITY OF LONDON;
ASSISTANT-SURGEON TO, AND LECTURER ON ANATOMY AT, GUY'S
HOSPITAL; AND
SURGEON TO THE ROYAL INFIRMARY FOR CHILDREN, ETC.

LONDON:
JOHN W. PARKER AND SON, WEST STRAND.
1860.

Fig. 1.——Title page of book by J. Cooper Forster.[7]

CHIRURGIE DES KINDESALTERS

VON

PROF. DR. R. DRACHTER
LEITER DER CHIRURGISCHEN ABTEILUNG
DER UNIVERSITÄTSKINDERKLINIK, MÜNCHEN
UND
DR. J. R. GOSSMANN
ASSISTENZARZT DER ABTEILUNG

3., VÖLLIG UMGEARBEITETE UND VERMEHRTE AUFLAGE

MIT 714 TEXTFIGUREN

1 9 3 0
VERLAG VON F. C. W. VOGEL IN LEIPZIG

Fig. 2.——Title page of book by Drachter and Gossmann.[4]

service, with understanding nurses, play teachers, and attendants, and with physicians and house staff who welcome the obligation of caring for children, hospitalization can be an interesting experience for the child. It has been our observation that well-adjusted children who come from emotionally stable homes, and who have trust and confidence in their parents, and whose parents have trust and confidence in the hospital and the physician, accept hospitalization in the context of this calm atmosphere and suffer no significant emotional distress. Per contra, children from tense, disturbed homes, with parents who are fearful of the hospital and of operation, and distrustful of physicians, sense the prevailing atmosphere and respond accordingly. The surgeon must be particularly aware of this difference and, if anything, devote more attention to calm explanations in children of the latter sort. Absolute honesty and patient firmness are the keystones of a productive relationship with young patients. The child who has been hurt when told he would not be, or who has suddenly received a treatment which he had been told would not be given, will not soon forgive or trust his betrayer.

Ordinarily it is of help to have the mother of a newly admitted child spend a few hours in the hospital with the child, to smooth out the transition from home to hospital. Details of the child's likes and dislikes, habits, and food preferences constitute useful knowledge for the nursing staff.

Opinions, prejudices, and practices vary in regard to the role of the parent, once the patient has been admitted to the hospital. On busy ward services it is not likely that arrangements can be made for parents

to "room in" with children, or even to be with them except for relatively short visiting periods. Even with special accommodations, it must be recognized that some children are unduly disturbed by the presence of overconcerned parents. Physicians must realize that a child's exposure to mismanagement in the home for a lifetime, be it a brief one, cannot be corrected during a week or two of hospitalization, but there are times when a display of calm firmness by the physician is accepted with relief by parent and child, both glad to accept a truce in the battle for supremacy between them. It is important, furthermore, to consider that the child's future care and welfare will be determined in part by the reaction of the parent to the hospitalization, and to see that undue trauma is not visited upon the parent, just as we are obviously careful to protect the child. Warmth, understanding, patience, and, above all, common sense, make for success in the handling of young patients. A mother can frequently feed or soothe a sick child who is recalcitrant with strangers, however kind. Other mothers are so disturbed that their alarm is contagious. In such instances, the mothers are well advised to remove themselves from the situation. There is no need for absolute rules. A willingness to deal with infants and children is meaningless without an equal willingness to deal with their parents.

With older children, the policy of honesty and of explanation of all that transpires begins before admission to the hospital, either in emergency or nonemergency situations. This honesty need not be carried too far. It is enough to assure the child that he is going to the hospital to get well and that he will be put to sleep for the corrective procedure, and that when he wakes up he will have some discomfort, described as need be. From this point on no more need be said, except in answer to direct questions. Great care should be taken in answering questions lest the implication of answers be misunderstood. In the circumstances of elective admission to the hospital, the shorter the period of such preparation the better. There is nothing to be gained by announcing an impending operation days or weeks in advance; indeed, in many instances this may be harmful.

The trip to the operating room of a conscious child suddenly strapped to a stretcher, and wheeled through long corridors away from obviously tearful parents, may be a harrowing experience. Proper sedation and the provision of a familiar nurse or physician to accompany him to the operating room are important factors in allaying the child's apprehension. With adequate sedation, the child should have little or no recollection of the trip to the operating room or of the induction.

Children are capable of great fantasies in their interpretation of what constitutes an operation, or even of casual remarks over the telephone in their presence concerning another patient, the conversation being mistakenly taken as applying to themselves. These fantasies may deal with fear of mutilation and may carry particular concern about facial features, locomotion, and the genitourinary apparatus. Surgical procedures relating to these should be explained at the child's level, and in a way to inspire the necessary confidence and reassurance that all will be well. Detailed analysis of a forthcoming operation should be avoided, and can be adequately substituted for by the obvious evidence of the surgeon's personal interest in the child, and his reassurances, in a simple, truthful discussion of the problem with the child. Once a relationship of trust and friendship is established, the rest is easy.

The surgeon does well to spend whatever time is required to gain the confidence of his patient. With infants, this may imply no more than a slow, easy, and deliberate approach. With older children, this may require a little time spent in conversation, which can be utilized gradually under cover of continued conversation, in beginning the peripheral portions of the examination, taking of the pulse, palpation of the joints, search for glands, gentle palpation of the neck, or abdomen, as the case may be.

From the standpoint of the availability of the history from the patient, the practice of pediatrics has been likened to that of veterinary medicine. This may be true in infants, but older children frequently are capable of giving a history and may well provide details which escape their parents or which have been incorrectly interpreted by them. The manner in which a child gives a history may suggest a functional complaint or, on the contrary, the bona fides of the symptoms. In most instances it is preferable to have the parents give their version of the history in the presence of the child, rather than to have the child left alone, and suspicious of dealings between parent and surgeon. Children vary. The stable, trustful child will readily accept the statement that the doctor wishes to talk to the mother alone, whether this be before or after the examination. With a tense, apprehensive child it is best to arrange for such discussions privately, without obviously excluding the child.

The "routine" physical examination has little place in the examination of children. Portions of the examination which may be uncomfortable or painful, as in examination of the throat or of the ears in infants, or alarmingly strange, such as rectal examination in an older child, should be deferred until the end of the examination. In the child with an acute abdominal emergency, almost all of the physical examination should be completed before the abdomen is directly examined and palpated. Along the way, valuable information can be obtained from the manner in which the child breathes, moves about on the examination table, and from his general behavior. By the same token, once attention is directed to the abdomen, the last area to examine is that which it is expected will be most painful. Thus, in examination for appendicitis, one starts at the left lower quadrant, passes to the left upper quadrant, to the right upper quadrant, and finally to the right lower quadrant, and one repeats this several times, progressing from a light, stroking palpation, which is little more than a caress, to as firm a pressure as is required to elicit any signs.

We have long dispensed with bandages after operation except where necessary to absorb the secretions of drained wounds. At most, merely an aerosol plastic spray is applied. Fortunately, children generally seem to have the good sense not to play with their wounds and sutures, and it is well to spare their tender skins the insult of adhesive strapping, the principal objection to the strapping being that it obscures so much of the patient from examination. Subcuticular sutures, where practicable, eliminate the need for removing sutures, and are one more contribution to the patient's comfort. Smaller children in particular do not generally indulge in more physical activity after operation than is good for them. Having due regard for the special circumstances of certain operations, restraints generally are not necessary, and older children may be allowed up and about whenever they wish. When catheters or drainage tubes are in place, they must be so securely taped as to be tamperproof in the smaller children, or restraints must be resorted to.

In the smaller infants, airway obstructions may arise so quickly, and result in disaster so rapidly, that it is essential to provide expert special nursing around the clock for a number of days after operation, depending upon the child and the procedure. It makes little sense to marshal highly qualified skills for a concerted operative effort upon an infant who must fight his way in the hours after operation only "looked in on" by the busy ward nurse. These tiny patients, with their feeble coughs, must be turned frequently and suctioned often.

The organism of children of any age is strong enough to withstand the most massive procedures if the children have been properly prepared for operation, if the proper operation is properly performed, and if the care given the patient after the operation is as expert as that accorded in the operating room.

BIBLIOGRAPHY

1. Barrington-Ward, L. E.: *Abdominal Surgery of Children* (London: Oxford University Press. 1928).
2. Brown, J. J. Mason (ed.): *Surgery of Childhood* (Baltimore: Williams & Wilkins Company, 1963).
3. Bryant, T.: *Surgical Diseases of Children* (London: Churchill & Sons, 1863).
4. Drachter, R., and Gossmann, J. R.: *Chirurgie des Kindesalters* (Leipzig: F. C. W. Vogel, 1930).
5. Duhamel, B.: *Chirurgie du Nouveau-né et du Nourrisson* (Paris: Masson & Cie, 1953).
6. Fèvre, M.: *Chirurgie Infantile d'Urgence* (Paris: Masson & Cie, 1958).
7. Forster, J. C.: *The Surgical Diseases of Children* (London: John W. Parker & Son, 1860).
8. Fraser, J.: *Surgery of Childhood* (London: Edward Arnold, 1926).
9. Grob, M.: *Lehrbuch der Kinderchirurgie* (Stuttgart: Georg Thieme Verlag, 1957).
10. Gross, R. E.: *Surgery of Infancy and Childhood* (Philadelphia: W. B. Saunders Company, 1953).
11. Guersant, M. P.: *Surgical Diseases of Infants and Children*, translated by R. J. Dunglison (Philadelphia: Henry C. Lea, 1873).
12. Holmes, T.: *Surgical Treatment of the Diseases of Infancy and Childhood* (London: Longmans, Green, Reader & Dyer, 1868).
13. Kelley, S. W.: *Surgical Diseases of Children: A Modern Treatise on Pediatric Surgery* (New York: E. B. Treat & Co., 1909).
14. Ladd, W. E., and Gross, R. E.: *Abdominal Surgery in Infancy and Childhood* (Philadelphia: W. B. Sanders Company, 1941).
15. Nixon, H. H., and O'Donnell, B.: *The Essentials of Pediatric Surgery* (London: J. B. Lippincott Company, 1961).
16. Oberniedermayr, A.: *Lehrbuch der Chirurgie und Orthopädie des Kindesalters* (Berlin: Springer-Verlag, 1959).
17. Ombrédanne, L.: *Précis Clinique et Opératoire de Chirurgie Infantile* (2d ed.; Paris: Masson & Cie, 1925).
18. Potts, W. J.: *The Surgeon and The Child* (Philadelphia: W. B. Saunders Company, 1959).
19. Swenson, O.: *Pediatric Surgery* (New York: Appleton-Century-Crofts, Inc., 1958).
20. White, M., and Dennison, W. M.: *Surgery in Infancy and Childhood* (Baltimore: Williams & Wilkins Company, 1958).

THE EDITORS

1

Genetic Considerations

THE REMARKABLE GROWTH OF MEDICAL GENETICS has a number of important implications for pediatric surgery. Not only can genetics contribute usefully to the surgeon's understanding of basic mechanisms of disease, but it can also be of highly practical assistance in diagnosis, prognosis and genetic counseling, in the recognition and management of such surgical problems as coagulation defects and unusual drug reactions and in the selection of compatible donors for tissue and organ transplantation. When the phenotype of a genetically determined trait has been fully characterized, a knowledge of genetics can even help the surgeon to know what anomalies to look for in patients with that trait.

Medical genetics may be said to have its origin in the work of the pediatrician Garrod, whose studies of the disorders he called "inborn errors of metabolism"[14] laid the foundation of human biochemical genetics, with its basic concept that *one gene has one primary effect*. The primary effect of a gene is the specification of the amino acid sequence of an enzyme or other protein. A gene mutation results in the synthesis of a polypeptide chain in which there is a substitution of one amino acid for another at some one point. Though the biochemical difference between the direct products of normal and of mutant genes is slight, the clinical consequences of the difference may be extensive.

General references to medical aspects of genetics include those of McKusick,[19] Sutton[33] and Thompson and Thompson.[34]

Classification of Genetic Diseases

Gene mutation is not the only mechanism by which genetic disorders can arise. Three categories of genetic disease are recognized, on the basis of the nature of the defect present in the genetic information:

1. *Single-gene traits*, determined by an abnormal (mutant) gene or pair of genes at a single locus.

Each gene has a specific position on a specific chromosome, which is its *locus*; genes occupying the same locus on members of a pair of homologous chromosomes are *alleles* of one another. If both alleles of a pair are alike, the individual is *homozygous* at that locus; if the alleles are different, the individual is *heterozygous*. If a single abnormal gene, part-nered by a normal allele, determines a clinical disorder, the disorder is said to show *dominant* inheritance; if it is expressed only when both alleles are abnormal, inheritance is *recessive*.

2. *Multifactorial traits*, in which the genetic determinants are many genes at different loci, each with a minor effect. Though these genes are not individually deleterious, their combined action may produce an abnormality.

3. *Chromosomal aberrations*, in which an abnormality of chromosome number or structure (abnormal karyotype) is associated with a relatively well-defined syndrome of congenital malformations.

GENETIC HETEROGENEITY

It may be difficult or impossible to determine from the clinical findings the actual genetic basis of a patient's condition. This is because different basic genetic defects can produce similar findings. Despite this genetic heterogeneity, it is important to bear in mind that two patients have an identical disorder only if the genetic basis of the disorder is precisely the same in both.

Consider a child with cleft lip and palate. This structural defect can be produced by one of several single mutant genes, by multiple genes with a "threshold effect" (see later), or by a chromosomal aberration (D trisomy). Prenatal environmental factors are also known to be important in some cases. The value of surgical repair is usually much higher in cleft lip and palate of single-gene or multifactorial etiology than in cases associated with D trisomy, because in D trisomy there are usually several severe malformations and the prognosis is poor. On the other hand, the risk that a later child of the same parents will be similarly affected is high (25% or even 50%) if a single gene is involved, lower (about 5%) if the condition is multifactorial, and usually very low if it is caused by a chromosomal aberration. One can sometimes distinguish between the possible genetic mechanisms on the basis of a detailed family history and a chromosome analysis. However, if one has a good clinical description of the patient's abnormality, the problem of identifying its genetic basis may often be solved.

TABLE 1-1.—SOME AUTOSOMAL DOMINANT TRAITS OF SURGICAL INTEREST*

†Achondroplasia
†Acoustic neuroma
†Acrocephalosyndactyly, several
  types
†Angioneurotic edema
†Aniridia
  Ankylosing spondylitis
  Anus, imperforate
†Aortic stenosis, supravalvular
  Atrial septal defect
  Arms, malformation of
†Basal cell nevus syndrome
†Branchial cleft anomalies,
  including branchial cysts
  Cancer: rare "cancer families"
†Cataract, several forms
†Charcot-Marie-Tooth peroneal
  atrophy
†Cleft lip, "lip pits" type

†Cleidocranial dysostosis
  Clubfoot
  Craniofacial dysostosis
†Dentinogenesis imperfecta
  Dupuytren's contracture
  Ectopia lentis
  Ectrodactyly
†Ehlers-Danlos syndrome
  Epiphyseal dysostosis
†Glaucoma, juvenile
  Hernia
†Keloids
  Legg-Calvé-Perthes disease
†Mandibulofacial dysostosis
†Marfan syndrome
†Metaphyseal dysostosis
†Muscular dystrophy, facioscapulo-
  humeral type
†Myotonic dystrophy

†Neurofibromatosis
†Osteogenesis imperfecta
  Patent ductus arteriosus
  Pheochromocytoma
†Polycystic kidneys
†Polydactyly
†Polyposis, intestinal (often pre-
  malignant)
†Porphyria, acute intermittent
†Precocious puberty
†Ptosis
†Retinoblastoma
†Spastic paraplegia
†Spherocytosis
†Split-hand deformity
†Spondyloepiphyseal dysplasia
†Symphalangism
†Syndactyly
†Von Willebrand's syndrome

*Extracted from McKusick.[21] It is important to note that many of the traits listed may also have other patterns of inheritance, or nongenetic etiology.
†This type of inheritance is regarded as definitely established.

For example, it helps to know that cleft lip associated with "lip pits" (fistulas or cysts of the lower lip) is inherited as an autosomal dominant and that the cleft lip of D trisomy is part of a well-defined syndrome of developmental anomalies.

Single-gene Inheritance

A large number of conditions of surgical significance are determined by single genes (or paired genes at a single locus). These traits show simple patterns of inheritance, the particular pattern depending on whether the gene responsible is autosomal or X-linked and whether the trait is dominant (clinically evident in heterozygotes) or recessive (expressed only in homozygotes).

McKusick[21] has enumerated nearly 1,500 single-gene traits, with brief descriptions and key references. Some conditions of obvious surgical significance, selected from McKusick's catalogs, are listed in Table 1-1 (autosomal dominants), Table 1-2 (autosomal recessives) and Table 1-3 (X-linked traits, both dominant and recessive). It should be noted that only those traits marked with a dagger (†) are regarded as *proved* to be inherited as stated. Even then, the reader can be misled if he is not alert to the fact that the appearance of a certain trait on such a list means only that it *has* shown the stated type of inheritance, not that it invariably or even usually does; in other words, genetic heterogeneity must constantly be kept in mind.

HOW TO RECOGNIZE PATTERNS OF SINGLE-GENE INHERITANCE

If one has a good clinical description of a trait and an adequate family history, it may be quite easy to recognize the pattern of inheritance.

If the disorder appears in every generation, af-

TABLE 1-2.—SOME AUTOSOMAL RECESSIVE TRAITS OF SURGICAL INTEREST*

†Adrenal hyperplasia
†Agammaglobulinemia
†Cataract, several forms
  Choanal atresia
  Coagulation factor deficiencies V,
  VII and X
  Cystinosis
†Cystinuria
  Diaphyseal dysplasia
†Dysautonomia
  Ectrodactyly
†Ellis-van Creveld syndrome
†Glaucoma, juvenile
†Goitrous cretinism, familial

  Hirschsprung's disease, long
  segment
†Keratoconus
†Mediterranean fever, familial
†Mucopolysaccharidosis (Hurler's
  syndrome)
  Multiple myeloma
†Muscular atrophy
†Muscular dystrophy, limb-girdle
  type
  Myasthenia gravis
†Nephrosis, congenital
†Osteogenesis imperfecta congenita
  Osteoporosis, juvenile

†Pernicious anemia, juvenile
†Pituitary dwarfism
†Polycystic kidney
†Retinitis pigmentosa
†Sickle cell anemia
  Situs inversus viscerum
†Suxamethonium sensitivity
†Thalassemia major
†Thrombasthenia
  Wilms' tumor
†Wilson's disease
†Xeroderma pigmentosum

*Extracted from McKusick.[21] It is important to note that many of the traits listed may also have other patterns of inheritance, or nongenetic etiology.
†This type of inheritance is regarded as definitely established.

TABLE 1-3.— SOME X-LINKED TRAITS OF SURGICAL INTEREST*

†Agammaglobulinemia	†Hypophosphatemia
†Anemia, hypochromic	†Lowe's oculocerebrorenal syndrome
†Angiokeratoma (Fabry's disease)	†Mucopolysaccharidosis, one form
Anus, imperforate	†Muscular dystrophy
†Cataract, some types	Duchenne type
†Charcot-Marie-Tooth peroneal atro-phy	Becker type
	Dreifuss type
†Diabetes insipidus, nephrogenic	†Spondyloepiphyseal dysplasia, one type
†Glucose-6-phosphate dehydrogenase variants	Testicular feminization (may be au-tosomal dominant)
†Hemophilia A (factor VIII deficiency)	†Thrombocytopenia
†Hemophilia B (factor IX deficiency)	
†Hydrocephaly	

*Extracted from McKusick.[21] It is important to note that many of the traits listed may also have other patterns of inheritance, or nongenetic etiology.
†This type of inheritance is regarded as definitely established.

---

fecting about half the sibs and offspring of affected persons, and the sex ratio is approximately even, the disorder is probably dominant. If it ever shows male-to-male transmission, it is not X-linked (because males transmit the Y, not the X, to their sons), so it must be an *autosomal* dominant. If all of the daughters but none of the sons of affected males are affected, it is probably an *X-linked* dominant.

If the disorder appears only within a single sibship, and nowhere else within a family tree, it is probably an autosomal recessive. If the parents of the affected sibs are consanguineous, the case for autosomal recessive inheritance is strengthened. With recessive inheritance, approximately a quarter of the sibs of propositi are affected.

If far more males than females are affected and affected males within a kindred are related through females, the trait is probably an X-linked recessive. This pattern of inheritance is the easiest one to recognize, because the trait may be seen to skip a generation from an affected man to half of his daughters' sons.

COMPLICATIONS IN GENETIC PATTERNS

Single-gene transmission can be obscured by many factors. Expression of a trait may vary in different family members from mild to severe and may even be so mild as to escape clinical diagnosis. A trait is said to show *failure of penetrance* if it sometimes fails to appear in individuals having the appropriate genotype, as in many pedigrees of malformations of the hand. It is said to show *variable expressivity* if it is always expressed, but not always with equal severity (epiloia, osteogenesis imperfecta). *Age of onset* of clinical symptoms may vary widely in different family members (diabetes mellitus, myotonic dystrophy). *Sex* may affect the recognition of the trait, even when the gene concerned is on an autosome (adrenal hyperplasia). New *mutation*, especially of autosomal dominant or X-linked recessive genes, may lead to the

observation of kindreds in which only the propositus is affected; perhaps 80% of all cases of achondroplasia and 50% of all boys with Duchenne muscular dystrophy have no affected relatives. *Small family size* may, by chance, be responsible for the occurrence of only a single affected member in a family.

Multifactorial Inheritance

There are many clinical disorders which, though showing a tendency to aggregate in families, neither follow any regular pattern of genetic transmission nor are associated with an abnormal karyotype. These disorders affect far more individuals than do single-gene and chromosomal disorders combined and include many congenital malformations amenable to surgical treatment. Their type of inheritance is multifactorial, that is, determined by the concerted action of genes at several or many loci, each with a small effect. This type of inheritance is particularly resistant to genetic analysis. Traits determined by multiple factors behave genetically as though they are based on an underlying continuous variation but are sharply differentiated into two categories, normal and defective, by a threshold.

A detailed account of multifactorial inheritance is beyond the scope of this discussion. Useful recent reviews of this topic as applied to congenital malformations have been provided by Carter,[8] Fraser,[12] Fraser Roberts[13] and Newcombe.[25]

A number of congenital malformations for which multifactorial inheritance has been postulated or convincingly demonstrated are listed in Table 1-4. It is important to note, however, that other genetic mechanisms have also been implicated in the etiology of several of the disorders listed. Cleft lip and palate was briefly discussed earlier. Congenital malformations of the heart are common in chromosomal syndromes and are being reported with increasing frequency within family groups in patterns suggestive of single-gene inheritance,[20,26] probably because the suc-

TABLE 1-4.—Congenital Malformations with
Multifactorial Inheritance[*]

Central nervous system malformations
  Anencephaly
  Hydrocephaly
  Meningocele
  Spina bifida
Cleft lip with or without cleft palate
Cleft palate without cleft lip
Clubfoot
  Talipes equinovarus
  Talipes calcaneovalgus
  Metatarsus varus
Congenital dislocation of the hip
Congenital malformations of the heart
Exomphalos
Indirect inguinal hernia
Pyloric stenosis
Situs inversus viscerum

[*]It is important to note that some of these disorders are also inherited
by other genetic mechanisms, or may have nongenetic etiology.

cess of surgeons in ameliorating many heart defects allows patients who would formerly have had short life spans to survive and reproduce. The genetic heterogeneity of these and other congenital malformations further complicates their genetic analysis.

The multifactorial traits listed in Table 4 have several characteristics in common: (1) The sex ratio may be abnormal, varying from about one male to two females for anencephaly to five males to one female for pyloric stenosis. (2) The trait is not always concordant in monozygotic twins. (3) No simple pattern of genetic transmission is evident. (4) The incidence in first-degree relatives (parents, sibs and children) of affected individuals is about 5% or, very approximately, 50 times the incidence in the general population. (5) The frequency of the trait in second- and third-degree relatives is much lower than in first-degree relatives. This is in contrast to autosomal dominant inheritance with reduced penetrance, in which the risk falls only by one-half with each more distant degree of relationship.

Since the development of a surgical technique for the treatment of pyloric stenosis by Ramstedt[28] in the second decade of this century, many children who would formerly have succumbed to pyloric stenosis in infancy have lived to reproduce, and study of the genetic transmission of this disorder has become feasible.[7] Carter's[7] observations provide a genetic model of multifactorial inheritance with a threshold effect. The frequency of pyloric stenosis per thousand births is five for males and only one for females. Consequently, affected girls have genotypes more "extreme" than those of affected boys, and, though males are more likely to be affected, relatives of affected girls are more likely to have pyloric stenosis than are relatives of affected boys. The risks for sibs and offspring, expressed as multiples of population risks for the same sex, are as follows:

Male relatives of male patients   × 10
Female relatives of male patients   × 25
Male relatives of female patients   × 35
Female relatives of female patients × 80

Wynne-Davies[35] has described rather similar observations in a genetic study of talipes equinovarus; again, there is a preponderance of affected males but a greater risk in relatives of affected females.

Chromosomal Aberrations

The impetus given to medical genetics by the discovery of sex chromatin[4] and of the chromosomal basis of mongolism,[17] Klinefelter's syndrome[16] and Turner's syndrome[11] can hardly be over-rated. Although previously it had been suspected that chromosomal aberrations might underlie certain syndromes in which multiple congenital anomalies occurred, the frequency and variety of the chromosomal aberrations now known to exist in man was quite unexpected. Chromosomal abnormalities occur with an estimated frequency of 0.25–0.40% of live births and with a much higher frequency in children born to mothers late in their child-bearing years. Among abortuses, the rate is very much higher; 22% of a series of 200 spontaneous abortions have been found to be chromosomally abnormal.[6]

The 46 chromosomes of a human somatic cell are made up of 22 pairs of autosomes and a pair of sex chromosomes (XX in females, XY in males) (Fig. 1-1). One of the two X chromosomes of the female is condensed and genetically inactive, appearing in interphase as the sex chromatin.[18] Aberrations of the chromosomes may be either numerical or structural. Individuals with other than the normal chromosome number are *aneuploids*. The most frequent type of aneuploidy is *trisomy*, the presence of a whole extra chromosome, either an autosome or a sex chromosome. Absence of one chromosome (monosomy) is less frequent; the XO type of Turner's syndrome is the only well-documented example. Structural aberrations are of several main types: *translocation, deletion, inversion, duplication. Ring chromosomes* have undergone a deletion at each end, with rejoining of the broken ends. *Isochromosomes* have two identical arms. A chromosomal aberration may be present in all cells of the body, or in only a portion of them (*mosaicism*).

The clinical significance of chromosomal aberrations is low in proportion to their over-all frequency, chiefly because the developmental confusion induced by a chromosomal abnormality is too deep-seated and diverse to be readily amenable to treatment. Nevertheless chromosomal defects underlie many problems of malformation, infertility, intersex and repeated abortion. Among the many useful reviews of

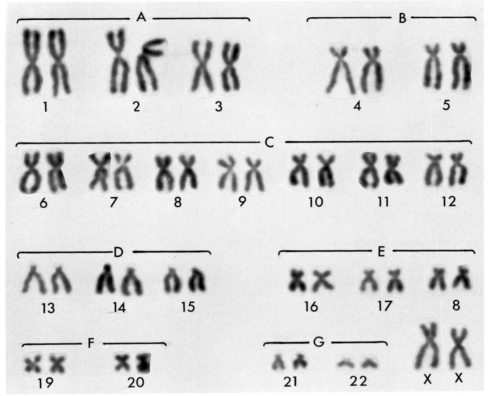

Fig. 1-1.—Karotype (chromosome set) of a normal female, arranged according to the standard classification (*Chicago Conference: Standardization in Human Cytogenetics.* Birth Defects Original Article Series, Vol. II, no. 2. New York, N.Y.: The National Foundation, 1966).

chromosomal abnormalities are those of Bartalos and Baramki,[5] Miller,[22] Mittwoch,[23] Moore[24] and Smith.[30]

TECHNIQUES

SEX CHROMATIN.—The simple and rapid buccal smear technique for the examination of sex chromatin is widely used. The buccal mucosa is scraped gently, and the scrapings are spread thinly on a slide, fixed immediately in Papanicolaou's fixative and stained. The sex chromatin is seen in female cells as a small, densely stained mass lying close against the nuclear membrane.

The number of sex chromatin masses is always one less than the number of X chromosomes per cell, and the size is abnormal in individuals with an X chromosome of abnormal size and structure. Thus the sex chromatin gives a clue to the patient's X-chromosome constitution but gives no information, of course, about the Y chromosome or any autosome.

CHROMOSOMES.—Chromosomes are most conveniently studied in leukocyte cultures, in which cells are stimulated to divide by phytohemagglutinin, arrested in mitosis by colchicine, treated with hypotonic solution to swell and separate the chromatids, spread on slides, fixed and stained. Photographic enlargement of good chromosome spreads facilitates accurate karyotyping.

Biopsy specimens of other tissues, especially skin, have advantages in that they may be cultured for long periods and are more likely than leukocyte cultures to show mosaicism.

CLINICAL USES OF SEX CHROMATIN

Because abnormalities of the sex chromosomes usually do not cause symptoms until puberty, they may remain undiagnosed throughout the pediatric age range unless sex chromatin studies are made. Sex chromatin studies are particularly helpful in the following types of patients:

1. Turner's syndrome, in which the chromosome constitution is usually XO. The patient appears to be a normal female of below average height, but the buccal smears are chromatin-negative, as are those of normal males. Webbing of the neck and peripheral

edema are the most obvious signs of this condition in infancy. Among the malformations present in these patients are coarctation of the aorta, cataracts and renal anomalies.

2. Klinefelter's syndrome, in which the chromosome constitution is usually XXY and the buccal smears are chromatin-positive even though the phenotype is that of a normal male. The patients are taller than average and often subnormal in intelligence but usually show no abnormalities in the pediatric age range. After puberty, gynecomastia is the chief finding of surgical significance.

3. Testicular feminization. Patients with this disorder have a normal XY karyotype, but the phenotype may be that of a normal female, ambiguous or of a normal male with development of gynecomastia at puberty. Here, sex-chromatin studies can help to decide on the appropriate sex of up-bringing. As the disorder is genetically determined, sex-chromatin studies in sisters and the female maternal relatives of known patients are also indicated. Half of the cases recognized in the pediatric age range in an Edinburgh study came under observation because of inguinal hernias, which contained testes.[15]

4. Abnormal or ambiguous external genitalia. In these children, sex-chromatin studies are a requisite part of the determination of sex assignment and most appropriate surgical procedure. The three types of congenital adrenal hyperplasia, all inherited as autosomal recessives, or maternal androgens, exogenous or endogenous, are the most common causes of abnormality of external genitalia in XX children.

In all cases in which there is disparity between sex chromatin and phenotype, complete karyotyping should be performed.

Indications for Chromosome Analysis

In consequence of the great activity of the past several years in the field of descriptive cytogenetics, several different syndromes associated with chromosomal aberrations are now well recognized. In addition to patients with these syndromes, the best known of which are listed briefly in Table 1-5, other patients with undiagnosed disorders of sexual development or certain congenital malformations may be suitable subjects for chromosome analysis. Many infants with multiple congenital anomalies have been studied with few positive findings. On the other hand, in a recent series of 105 children with syndactyly, an anomaly not typically seen in chromosomal syndromes, five patients with abnormal karyotypes were observed: a prepubertal boy with previously undiagnosed XXY Klinefelter's syndrome, a short girl with previously undiagnosed XO Turner's syndrome, two with known trisomy 21, and a boy with 45 chromosomes including a familial D/D translocation.[9] These observations point up the difficulty of selection of appropriate cases for chromosome study. The karyo-

TABLE 1-5.—Surgical Aspects of Common Chromosomal Aberrations[*]

Condition	Typical Karyotype	Anomalies Significant in Pediatric Surgery†
Turner's syndrome (gonadal dysgenesis)	XO	Coarctation of aorta Renal anomalies Cataracts
Klinefelter's syndrome	XXY	Gynecomastia at puberty
Mongolism (Down's syndrome)	Trisomy 21	Tracheoesophageal fistula Duodenal atresia Umbilical hernia Aganglionic megacolon Cardiac anomalies (atrioventricular communis, ventricular septal defect, patent ductus, tetralogy of Fallot) Cystic ovaries
Trisomy 18	Trisomy 18	Multiple and severe
D trisomy	Trisomy of a chromosome in the D group	Multiple and severe
Cri du chat syndrome	Deletion of short arm of chromosome 4	Not yet described

[*]Based on Bartalos and Baramki,[5] Smith[30] and personal observations, unpublished.
†These anomalies are variable in occurrence and do not appear in all patients.

types found in the three common autosomal trisomy syndromes are shown in Figures 1-2 (trisomy 21), 1-3 (trisomy 18), and 1-4 (D trisomy).

Dermatoglyphics.—Many children with chromosome anomalies have unusual dermatoglyphics (patterns of the ridged skin of the digits, palms and soles) in consequence of disturbed limb growth produced by the abnormal chromosomal constitution. In some disorders, especially mongolism, the patterns are so stereotyped that they have diagnostic value. Abnormal dermatoglyphics, including the presence of a single palmar crease (simian crease), may signal that a specific chromosomal defect is present.[27] Several disorders in which no chromosomal aberration has been demonstrated also have characteristic dermatoglyphics.

Transplantation

Perhaps the most exciting surgical advance of recent years has been the development of techniques for the grafting of organs and tissues in man. The success of this endeavor must be credited to the joint efforts of laboratory workers concerned with the many biologic problems that can be illuminated by transplantation research and of surgeons concerned with clinical applications. The barriers to success in

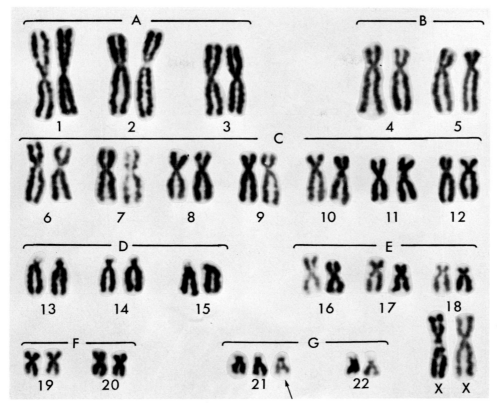

Fig. 1-2.—Karyotype of a female with trisomy 21 (Down's syndrome, mongolism). The extra chromosome 21 (**arrow**) may also be present as a translocation to another G-group chromosome, or to a D-group chromosome. Surgical lesions in this disorder are listed in Table 1-5. About 3% of cases treated for tracheoesophageal fistula and esophageal atresia and 2% of patients with Hirschsprung's disease have Down's syndrome. Cardiac lesions treated surgically in 33 Down's syndrome patients at the Hospital for Sick Children include: aortic valve stenosis 1, atrioseptal defect (secundum) 1, atrioseptal defect (ostium primum) 1, atrioventricular communis 10, persistent patent ductus arteriosus 5, tetralogy of Fallot 9, ventricular septal defect 6.

human tissue and organ transplantation are genetic rather than surgical in nature, and the contributions of surgeons have done much to broaden our knowledge of the genetics of transplantation. At the same time, transplantation research has made it mandatory for surgeons to have at their command some understanding of the principles of genetics.

The central problem of transplantation is homograft (allograft) rejection, the reaction of the host by which a graft is rejected if histocompatibility antigens present in the donor tissue differ from those of the host. In clinical practice, homograft rejection can to some extent be circumvented by the use of immunosuppressive agents. A more effective approach to securing graft persistence has been sought through studies of the genetics of histocompatibility and application of the findings to the selection of compatible donor-host combinations.

The antigens that determine graft compatibility in man and experimental animals are on the cell membrane and may be components of it. They have the property of inciting an immune response when transplanted to a host which lacks those particular antigens. Histocompatibility antigens are the end-products of the action of genes, which are in turn known as histocompatibility genes. The allelic genes at any one histocompatibility locus are codominant; in other words, in heterozygotes, both alleles of a pair are expressed as antigens.

GENETICS OF TRANSPLANTATION IN THE MOUSE

The principles of transplantation genetics were first established with the use of inbred strains of mice. Several useful reviews of transplantation genetics are available, of which the most recent and authoritative is that of Snell and Stimpfling.[31] Inbred mice, developed by brother-sister mating for at least

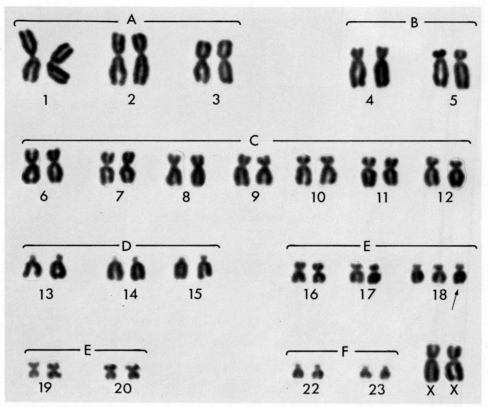

Fig. 1-3.—Karyotype of a female with trisomy 18. The extra chromosome is indicated by an arrow. The common surgical lesions seen in this anomaly are ventricular septal defect and patent ductus arteriosus. Prognosis is poor; only 25% of patients live past the age of 3 months.

20 generations, have two chief characteristics: members of any one strain are *genetically identical* and *homozygous at all loci* (with the rather rare exception of loci at which a new mutation has recently occurred). Consequently, grafts between members of an inbred strain survive; but grafts between members of different inbred strains are rejected, because they carry different histocompatibility antigens. With some minor exceptions, animals of the F_1 generation (first-generation hybrids between two different inbred strains) accept grafts from members of their own generation and from either parent strain, because F_1 animals have all of the histocompatibility antigens of each parent. Most but not all members of the F_2 or subsequent generations cannot accept grafts from either parent strain, because through segregation and recombination of histocompatibility alleles they are very unlikely to have *all* of the histocompatibility alleles of both parent stocks.

Further analysis of the histocompatibility alleles of the mouse was made possible by the development by Snell of coisogenic lines, that is, lines of mice identical at all loci except a single histocompatibility locus.

With the use of these animals, it has been shown that there are probably 15 or more different histocompatibility loci (*H* loci), some of which have numerous alleles. It is also known that these loci are not all of equal importance in determining tissue compatibility, some being "strong" and others "weak"; in fact, difference at a single locus, the *H-2* locus, is far more important than any other histocompatibility difference as a barrier to transplantation. Moreover, the concentration of histocompatibility antigens varies greatly from tissue to tissue.

DONOR SELECTION IN MAN

The survival or rejection of homografts, in man as in the mouse, is determined largely by the degree of antigenic similarity or disparity between donor and host. This is why identical twins and first-degree relatives are at present the donors of choice. Although the genetic material of man cannot be manipulated like that of the mouse, in recent years several techniques have been developed for the estimation of histocompatibility antigens in man. One such technique is the

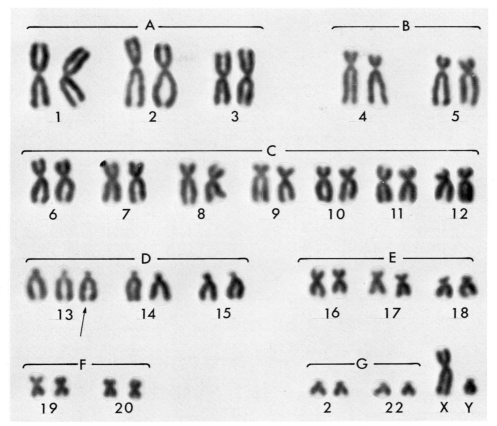

Fig. 1-4.—Karyotype of a male with D trisomy. The extra chromosome is indicated by an arrow. These children usually die in early infancy, and gross cerebral defects are frequently seen at autopsy. Among survivors, the chief lesion of surgical significance is cleft palate, usually with cleft lip.

mixed leukocyte culture (MLC) test, first described by Bain and Lowenstein.[3] The principle of the MLC test is that mixtures of leukocytes from two genetically unrelated donors mutually stimulate one another in culture to undergo transformation and mitosis, whereas no such stimulatory effect is seen when leukocytes from genetically identical individuals (monozygotic twins) are cultured together. This "matching" technique has been improved by the use of mitomycin C to inhibit DNA synthesis in the leukocytes of one of the donors while allowing them to stimulate mitosis in the cells of the other donor, thus enabling measurement of "one-way" stimulation.[2] Another technique makes use of suitable antisera, such as those of certain multiparous women (whose repeated pregnancies have enabled them to form a variety of antibodies) or of subjects specifically immunized against leukocytes or skin grafts, to allow the "typing" of individual antigens. The closer the antigenic similarity of two individuals, as shown by either of these tests, the more probable it is that a homograft from one to the other will show prolonged survival.

Evidence has accumulated that in man there is probably only one major histocompatibility locus, HL-A (formerly called the Hu-1 locus[1]). Many different alleles at this locus are postulated, on the basis of one-way MLC tests within families and between unrelated individuals. If the "one-locus, many alleles" hypothesis is proved, there should be at least a 25% chance that a graft to a patient from one of his sibs would be accepted. Minor histocompatibility loci may also exist in man,[10, 29] but the HL-A locus appears to be much the most important. Renal homograft survival seems better when donor and recipient are compatible at the HL-A locus than when they are not.[32]

Cells of dizygotic twins, even when typing shows them to be disparate, fail to stimulate in the MLC test. This might be the basis for the observation that grafts from dizygotic twins show better survival in their co-twins than do grafts from ordinary sibs.

Complete characterization of the human histocompatibility genes is an important area of further research, with significance both for genetics and for clinical transplantation surgery.

REFERENCES

1. Bach, F. H., and Amos, D. B.: Hu-1: Major histocompatibility locus in man, Science 156:1506, 1967.
2. Bach, F. H., and Voynow, N. K.: One-way stimulation in mixed leukocyte cultures, Science 153:545, 1966.
3. Bain, B., and Lowenstein, L.: Genetic studies on the mixed leukocyte reaction, Science 145:1315, 1964.
4. Barr, M. L., and Bertram, E. G.: A morphological distinction between neurones of the male and female and the behaviour of the nucleolar satellite during accelerated nucleoprotein synthesis, Nature (London) 163:676, 1949.
5. Bartalos, M., and Baramki, T. A.: *Medical Cytogenetics* (Baltimore: Williams & Wilkins Company, 1967).
6. Carr, D. H.: Chromosome studies in spontaneous abortions, Obst. & Gynec. 26:308, 1965.
7. Carter, C. O.: The Genetics of Common Malformations, in Fishbein, M. (ed.): *Papers and Discussions Presented at the Second International Conference on Congenital Malformations* (New York: International Medical Congress, 1964).
8. Carter, C. O.: The Inheritance of Common Congenital Malformations, in Steinberg, A. G., and Bearn, A. G. (ed.): *Progress in Medical Genetics* (New York: Grune & Stratton, Inc., 1965), Vol. IV.
9. Conen, P. E.; Thomson, H. G., and Hampole, M. K.: Personal communication.
10. Dausset, J., *et al.*: Leucocyte groups and their importance in transplantation, Transplantation 5:323, 1967.
11. Ford, C. E., *et al.*: The chromosomes of a patient showing both mongolism and the Klinefelter syndrome, Lancet 1:709, 1959.
12. Fraser, F. C.: Genetics and Congenital Malformations, in Steinberg, A. G. (ed.): *Progress in Medical Genetics* (New York: Grune & Stratton, Inc., 1961), Vol. I.
13. Fraser Roberts, J. A.: Multifactorial Inheritance and Human Disease, in Steinberg, A. G., and Bearn, A. G., (ed.): *Progress in Medical Genetics* (New York: Grune & Stratton, Inc., 1964), Vol. III.
14. Garrod, A. E.: The Croonian Lectures on inborn errors of metabolism, Lancet 2:1, 73, 142 and 214, 1908.
15. Harnden, D. G.: Sex chromosome abnormalities in children, J. Pediat. Surg. 1:218, 1966.
16. Jacobs, P. A., and Strong, J. A.: A case of human intersexuality having a possible XXY sex-determining mechanism, Nature (London) 183:302, 1959.
17. Lejeune, J.; Gautier, M., and Turpin, R.: Étude des chromosomes somatiques de neuf enfants mongoliens, Compt. rend. Acad. sc. 248:1721, 1959.
18. Lyon, M. F.: Sex chromatin and gene action in the mammalian X-chromosome, Am. J. Human Genet. 14:135, 1962.
19. McKusick, V. A.: *Human Genetics* (Englewood Cliffs, N.J.: Prentice-Hall, Inc., 1964).
20. McKusick, V. A.: A genetical view of cardiovascular disease, Circulation 30:326, 1964.
21. McKusick, V. A.: *Mendelian Inheritance in Man* (Baltimore: Johns Hopkins Press, 1966).
22. Miller, O. J.: The sex chromosome anomalies, Am. J. Obst. & Gynec. 90:1078, 1964.
23. Mittwoch, U.: *Sex Chromosomes* (New York: Academic Press, Inc., 1967).
24. Moore, K. L. (ed.): *The Sex Chromatin* (Philadelphia: W. B. Saunders Company, 1966).
25. Newcombe, H. B.: Epidemiological Studies: Discussion, in Fishbein, M. (ed.): *Congenital Malformations: Papers and Discussions Presented at the Second International Conference on Congenital Malformations* (New York: International Medical Congress, 1964).
26. Nora, J. J., and Meyer, T. C.: Familial nature of congenital heart disease, Pediatrics 37:329, 1966.
27. Penrose, L. S.: Finger-prints, palms and chromosomes, Nature (London) 197:933, 1963.
28. Ramstedt, C.: Zur Operation der angeborenen Pylorusstenose, Med. Klin. 8:1702, 1912.
29. Simonsen, M.: Immunogenetic speculations on human kidney transplants, Transplantation 4:354, 1966.
30. Smith, D. W.: Autosomal abnormalities, Am. J. Obst. & Gynec. 90:1055, 1964.
31. Snell, G. H., and Stimpfling, J. H.: Genetics of tissue transplantation, in Green, E. L. (ed.): *Biology of the Laboratory Mouse* (2nd ed.; New York: McGraw-Hill Book Company, 1966).
32. Stickel, D. L., *et al.*: Cited by Bach and Amos.[1]
33. Sutton, H. E.: *An Introduction to Human Genetics* (New York: Holt, Rinehart and Winston, Inc., 1965).
34. Thompson, J. S., and Thompson, M. W.: *Genetics in Medicine* (Philadelphia: W. B. Saunders Company, 1966).
35. Wynne-Davies, R.: Family studies and the cause of congenital club foot, J. Bone & Joint Surg. 46:445, 1964.

M. W. THOMPSON
J. S. THOMPSON

2

Anesthesia

WHEN DEALING WITH infants and children, the anesthesiologist is concerned before the operation with the elimination of fear and anxiety, during operation with the control of pain, the provision of a satisfactory working field for the surgeon and maintenance of the safety of the patient, and following operation with protection and supervision throughout the early period of recovery. The variety of agents and techniques now at the disposal of the pediatric anesthesiologist has introduced technical improvements, but basic understanding of the psychologic, pathologic and physiologic characteristics of the infant and child remains the key to successful anesthetic management of these young patients.

Characteristic Response of Infants and Children to Anesthesia

A definite pattern of response is shown by infants and children undergoing anesthesia. It is one of rapid change and variability, the response being more marked, the younger the patients. If exposed to unusual conditions, these small subjects will show rapid fatigue and severe complications. Yet if the basic needs are fulfilled, even newborn infants will tolerate prolonged surgical procedures. The pediatric patient shows a number of features which differentiate him from the adolescent and adult.

Anatomic differences are first to be noticed. The discrepancy in size is obvious and, among other things, necessitates a large variety of anesthetic apparatus. Differences in proportion are also important. An infant's large head, short neck, narrow chest, horizontal ribs and weak shoulder girdle present the anesthesiologist with problems in maintaining adequate ventilation. The greater proportional surface area of the infant has a significant effect on the regulation of body temperature and also is responsible for greater oxygen requirement and more rapid fluid exchange than in the older child.

The *psychologic aspect* of the child's nature is an outstanding feature that differentiates him from the adult. Through infancy, and sometimes well into childhood, the patient's emotional reactions may be entirely uncontrolled and must be considered an essential part of the over-all problem. Neglect of this aspect can lead to important complications both during and after operation.

Physiologic factors which characterize the child pertain to general metabolism and to most of the organ systems as well. The elevated metabolic activity of the infant and young child calls for greater oxygen supply and entails more rapid onset of hypoxia if the demands are not fulfilled.

The incomplete development of the nervous system in the small infant is responsible for the poor control of many body systems and underlies much of the variability typical of this age group. Throughout early life, respiration is easily deranged. Owing to the combined effects of anatomic disadvantages, poor control and easy fatigability, the young child is in constant danger of respiratory obstruction or depression regardless of the extent of the operation.

The cardiovascular system shows more stability than the nervous system. Although blood pressure in the newborn baby is low and variable (60–85 mm Hg systolic) and the pulse rate often reaches 200/minute under anesthesia, the heart is strong, tolerates stressful procedures and shows remarkable powers of recovery. Yet the danger of operative shock is relatively great in these small patients because of the difficulty in estimating blood loss and the paucity of physiologic signs by which one can judge the adequacy of circulating blood volume.

Although liver function does not attain maximal development until an infant is several months old, this is not evident in clinical experience. Agents such as procaine and the relaxant succinylcholine which are metabolized by the liver have been given the newborn without prolonged or enhanced effect.

The kidneys are functionally immature at birth, excrete solids inefficiently and do not tolerate sodium excess. Fluid metabolism in the infant and child shows a rapidly changing pattern and is of major importance to anesthesiologist and surgeon. The newborn infant has an increased total body water, but during the first days of life he loses fluid and takes little or none in return. Thereafter, there is a rapid increase of fluid metabolism until a maximum is reached during the first and second years of life, when the child may be handling three to five times as much per pound of body weight as the adult. The problems of fluid replacement are discussed later.

Control of body temperature is notoriously poor in infants and children.[13] Heat production is impeded by feeding problems in immature or ill patients, and heat loss is affected by the disproportionately large surface area and the lack or excess of protective body fat. Whereas the young infant frequently suffers severe loss of body heat, the older child more often has dangerous hyperthermic reactions during anesthesia.

The response of endocrine function in the child undergoing operation is not well understood, but certainly it is important. Ketosteroid production is thought to be low or nonexistent at birth, but for several days the infant is maintained by steroids received from the mother. From the end of the first week until the onset of steroid production in the third or fourth week of life, the infant shows a low reaction to stress, as measured by eosinophil response. This may have direct bearing on his tolerance to major operative procedures. Once past early infancy, the child is thought to show normal endocrine responses. Thyroid function is undoubtedly increased, as evident from the general acceleration of all metabolic activity.

Pathologic features that characterize the pediatric patient include typical lesions that are encountered as well as the child's reaction to disease. The striking anomalies found in newborn infants present some of the most unusual pathology found in the civilized world today. Infants bearing encephaloceles or sacrococcygeal teratomas, premature infants with intestinal atresia and conjoined twins represent but a few of the conditions to be dealt with in this age group.

The child's *response to disease* is still another variable that must be considered. The newborn infant shows a remarkably ill-defined reaction to overwhelming infection, with slight change of temperature or white cell count, whereas the response of the older infant and young child is quite the opposite, revealing extremes of temperature elevation, prostration and leukocytosis.

Finally, the *pharmacologic response* must be considered in anesthetic management of infants and children. Changes in uptake, distribution, metabolism or excretion are seen in relation to several drugs, with resultant change in the degree of expected response, or the appearance of side effects and toxicity. Relaxants have altered potency in the pediatric period, and drugs such as chloramphenicol have caused death because of failure of normal rate of metabolism.

Preparation and Preoperative Sedation

PREPARATION

A child should be intelligently prepared for his operation from a psychologic point of view. All children who are old enough to comprehend should be made to understand that they are going to the hospital and should be told in general terms that they will have an operation. (If they are to awaken later with a leg in a cast or a bandage over their eyes, this should be explained to them; probably the best time is shortly before the operation.) All children must be told the truth. Usually the child will consider the information briefly, ask one or more questions, then return to matters of more immediate interest. He should not be troubled by lengthy explanations and boring details. When a nervous child shows undue apprehension, time and care may be taken to reassure him. Booklets and stories about children going to the hospital are an especially useful means of showing young patients what to expect.

On admission to the hospital, care is taken by all personnel to help the child adjust to his new surroundings. Although psychiatrists stress that separation from the parents is quite traumatic, normal children appear to tolerate this if nurses and doctors show them a reasonable amount of kindness, if other children are near and if television is available.

A child should be admitted a day or more before operation to enable him to get accustomed to his surroundings and to allow ample time for a suitable work-up. The anesthesiologist visits the child at least once before the operation to learn about his personal and medical problems and to gain his confidence. The time needed and effort expended vary greatly according to the individual child.

The well-adjusted child who knows he is to have an operation but continues to chase his friends around the ward does not need psychotherapy. Instead, time should be spent in dealing with the 5-year-old who is returning for her tenth burn dressing and is understandably apprehensive or with the small boy who lies with his head in his mother's lap, both of them weeping and full of fear.

In checking the patient from the medical standpoint, the anesthesiologist first examines the history and makes sure that the work-up is adequate to justify acceptance of the risk. In the history, the anesthesiologist obviously must learn the diagnosis and pertinent facts. If there is a tumor, he should know its size and location, the type of incision planned, the operative position intended and similar details. When indicated, x-ray films and reports of other examinations should be reviewed. It is also important to learn about previous operations and anesthetic history, as well as to look for special complicating factors such as drug sensitivities, allergies and therapy with steroids, adrenolytic agents or rauwolfia alkaloids which may alter the patient's response to anesthesia.

Laboratory findings deserve careful scrutiny. Patients of all ages should have routine urinalysis and blood counts performed before operation. Since the hemoglobin and hematocrit vary considerably during the first years of life (Fig. 2-1), it is difficult to decide what should be termed the minimal preoperative requirement. A hemoglobin level of 10 Gm/100 ml has been accepted for all ages, but this allows much

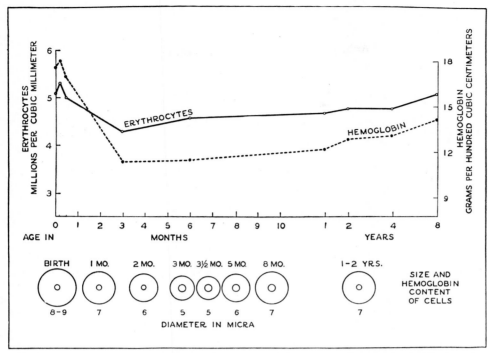

Fig. 2-1. — Normal values of erythrocytes and hemoglobin of different ages. (From Blackfan and Diamond[3].)

variation from the normal in early infancy and little margin in the 3-month-old infant. It would certainly be reasonable to elevate this standard to 12 Gm/100 ml in infants under 1 month old. One hesitates, however, to lower the standard below 10 Gm in infants 1–9 months old, since it is not known whether the lower average is due to physiologic or to unphysiologic cause. In any event, it is usually more important to look for the cause of a low hemoglobin level in a patient than to postpone the operation.

Important *physical findings* should be reviewed and checked by the anesthesiologist, especially if they involve the cardiovascular and respiratory systems. The anesthesiologist must check the nose, mouth, throat and chest of all patients in order to note previously unsuspected respiratory infection or contagious disease. Signs of upper respiratory infection denote increased anesthetic risk. *The decision to cancel operation is sometimes difficult to make, but is indicated if there is fever above 100 F by rectum, mucopurulent nasal discharge, injected pharynx, swollen cervical nodes or altered breath sounds.* Leukocytosis and x-ray evidence are further contraindications to anesthesia, but their absence does not justify undertaking the operation in the face of other significant signs.

Preoperative orders, written the night before surgery should include restriction of oral intake, preoperative sedation and pertinent special procedures. Young infants may be given their 2 A.M. feeding and then be scheduled for early operation to minimize the interruption of fluid intake. Children may have fluids until midnight. Enemas are no longer considered essential and are ordered only when specifically indicated.

Preoperative Medication

Preoperative medication is ordered to reduce vagal responses, control salivation and prevent fear and excitement. Many agents and combinations can be used that have relatively similar effects. Anticholinergic agents for prevention of an excess of secretions and reduction of vagal activity include atropine, scopolamine, bellafoline, methantheline (Banthine) and oxyphenonium (Antrenyl). Scopolamine and atropine are most widely used, scopolamine being characterized by better drying effect plus cortical depression, though with occasional disorientation, while atropine has greater vagolytic effect and does not cause excitement.

Barbiturates have long served as satisfactory sedative hypnotics. Recently a host of tranquilizing nonbarbiturates have appeared in confusing numbers. As yet, none has shown a definite superiority to the barbiturates, and pentobarbital (Nembutal) is still the most popular hypnotic for preoperative use.

The need for a narcotic in a routine preoperative medication for adults has been questioned, but agents

TABLE 2-1.—PREOPERATIVE MEDICATION FOR INFANTS AND CHILDREN*

AGE	Av. Wt. Lb	PENTOBARBITAL (NEMBUTAL) Mg	Gr	MORPHINE Mg	Gr	ATROPINE OR SCOPOLAMINE Mg	Gr
Newborn	7	. . . . . .	. . .	. . . .		0.1	1/600
6 mo.	16	30 p.r.	1/2	. . . .		0.2	1/300
1 yr.	21	50 p.r.	3/4	1.0	1/60	0.2	1/300
2 yr.	27	60 p.r.	1	1.5	1/40	0.3	1/200
4 yr.	35	90 p.r.	1½	2.0	1/30	0.3	1/200
6 yr.	45	100 p.r.	1½	3.0	1/20	0.4	1/150
8 yr.	55	100 p.os	2	4.0	1/15	0.4	1/150
10 yr.	65	100 p.os	2	5.0	1/12	0.4	1/150
12 yr.	85	100 p.os	2	6.0	1/10	0.6	1/100

1. This chart is a guide only, to be followed for average, well-developed patients. Reductions must be made in medication for subnormal patients.

2. Atropine is to be given to all patients who are to receive anesthesia.

3. Patients receiving Avertin should have atropine but no morphine or barbiturate.

4. No morphine or barbiturate is to be given to patients under 6 months of age.

5. Nembutal is to be given by rectum to children under 8 years of age.

6. For rectal use, Nembutal is to be dissolved in 10 cc of water and administered with syringe and catheter, at least 90 minutes before operation, or may be given in the form of a suppository.

7. Morphine and atropine are to be given intramuscularly 45 minutes before operation.

8. Before ether, cyclopropane or Pentothal anesthesia, give Nembutal, morphine and atropine as suggested by chart.

9. Approximate dosage: barbiturate 2–2.5 mg/lb of body weight; morphine 0.5–0.75 mg/year of age.

*From Smith.[15]

such as morphine and meperidine (Demerol) have an excellent pacifying effect on children and are advocated if used sparingly. Every anesthesiologist has his favorite agents, each of which must be ordered with a specific patient in mind. For an average patient who has no underlying disease or deficiency, a guide may be used from which to start. Suggested dosages are shown in Table 2-1. Here it will be noted that atropine is started at birth, pentobarbital added when the child is 6 months old and morphine at 1 year.

Infants between 1 and 3 years of age usually are most difficult to control either by personalized attention or by combinations of sedatives. In this age group, and in older children with special emotional problems, tribromoethanol (Avertin) 80 mg/kg or thiopental (Pentothal) 30 mg/kg by rectum will quickly induce a deep narcosis and may be used to great advantage. When either of these agents is used, other preoperative sedatives are omitted.

Choice of Anesthetic Agents, Techniques and Equipment

There are many agents and methods that can be employed for children, and the choice depends on a number of factors. The safety of the child comes first, then the operating needs of the surgeon, the experience and ability of the anesthesiologist, the preference of the patient, and so on. Ether remains a useful agent but no longer claims the commanding position it held so long in pediatric anesthesia. It appears probable that all explosive agents will be replaced by nonflammable ones, thereby definitely eliminating one serious hazard. Since this can now be done without impairing the quality of anesthesia, it seems a desirable goal.

The preference for general inhalation anesthesia for infants and children is still widespread in this country and is based on the safety, simplicity and adaptability that it entails. Intravenous agents are favored for pediatric work by some experts, proving that this is possible, but this view has not been generally accepted. The advantages and limitations of several agents will be discussed briefly.

ETHER, C_2H_5-O-C_2H_5.—For years, ether held first place as the agent of choice for pediatric anesthesia. Due to its stimulating effect on respiration, excellent relaxation and wide adaptability, it was a reliable agent known to almost every anesthetist. Introduction of agents that are nonexplosive, less irritating, and more rapidly expelled has reduced the advantage of ether, which now is used rarely in many hospitals, and in some not at all.

DIVINYL ETHER (VINETHENE), C_2H_3-O-C_2H_3.—This agent is less irritating than ether and has a remarkably rapid effect, but it is toxic if given for more than 30–45 minutes. It has been used chiefly for induction of anesthesia, but overdosage often causes a convulsive response. It has been largely replaced by nonexplosive, nonirritant agents.

NITROUS OXIDE, N_2O.—This odorless nontoxic gas is excellent for induction of general anesthesia and may be used as a supplement to intravenous agents or may be used alone for minor procedures not requiring relaxation.

CYCLOPROPANE, C_3H_6.—This sweet-smelling, inflammable anesthetic gas should be administered by means of closed or semiclosed apparatus. Its advantage lies in pleasant, rapid induction and easy controllability with quick recovery. Although it has been replaced to a great extent by halothane, it is still often used for sick patients, small infants and patients in hypovolemic shock.

HALOTHANE (FLUOTHANE), $CFl_3CBrClH$.—A potent, nonflammable agent, halothane combines rapid controllability with freedom from respiratory tract irritation and nausea.[4] It is widely adaptable and is used in North America for 90% of pediatric anesthesia. Hepatoxicity is rarely seen but cannot be ruled out, and repeated use of halothane may be contraindicated.[1]

METHOXYFLURANE (PENTHRANE), $CHCl_2CF_2OCH_3$. —This agent is highly soluble in blood, and induction and recovery are prolonged. It gives better analgesia and relaxation than halothane and has been reported on favorably for short outpatient procedures. Nausea may be troublesome.[8]

FLUROXENE (FLUROMAR) $CF_3CH_2OC_2H_3$.—This is a less potent agent than the foregoing, with moderate analgesic and slight relaxant quality. Its use may be advantageous in poor cardiac risks.

INTRAVENOUS AGENTS. — *Thiopental* (Pentothal) still dominates the intravenous agents and may be used for induction of anesthesia in many pediatric cases. It is especially useful when a child already has an infusion in place before operation and when a child resists inhalation induction and has an easily available vein.

Methohexital (Brevital) has relatively similar effects. It is an oxibarbiturate rather than a thiobarbiturate, and its elimination is slightly more rapid. Both thiopental and methohexital may be used by rectal route for induction of anesthesia.

Two intravenous agents have been added to the armamentarium which are of quite different nature. A phencyclodine agent, Ketalar (Parke, Davis[5]), provides marked analgesia with minimal respiratory depression and little loss of the protective gag reflex. This has been especially valuable in burn graft procedures. Also, *Propanedid,*[17] a congener of eugenol, has truly rapid metabolic breakdown, which makes it of value for short outpatient operations. This type of agent has caused vascular irritation and requires further evaluation.

MUSCLE RELAXANTS. — The use of muscle relaxants in pediatric anesthesia has been most popular in England. Rees[11] and his associates have promoted the use of muscle relaxants and endotracheal intubation for all pediatric anesthesia, and although this practice has not been universally accepted, the experience of this group has been highly informative.

Succinylcholine (Anectine) a short-acting relaxant, is used chiefly for periods of brief relaxation, as for endotracheal intubation or the relief of vocal cord spasm, whereas *gallamine* and *d-tubocurarine* are used for muscular relaxation during prolonged opera-

tions. Succinylcholine, being vagotonic, may induce severe bradycardia if patients are not protected by atropine. Gallamine and d-tubocurarine have few side effects, but all involve the danger of hypoxia if ventilatory support is inadequate. The action of gallamine and d-tubocurarine should be reversed by use of neostigmine after completion of operation.

LOCAL ANESTHETIC AGENTS. — There is a definite place for these agents in pediatric anesthesia. In the newborn period, many of the abdominal procedures may be performed safely and with satisfaction under local infiltration. Local block anesthesia is useful for reduction of simple fractures in older children, and in selected cases, spinal and epidural anesthesia can be employed. For emergency procedures, when children are suspected of having eaten recently, local anesthesia has its greatest value. In such cases, one must bear in mind the danger of overadministration. When lidocaine (Xylocaine) is used, a dosage of 5 mg/lb probably should be considered the maximum.

TECHNIQUES FOR ADMINISTRATION OF GENERAL ANESTHESIA

The past 10 years have seen striking changes in the techniques used in pediatric anesthesia. Even before ether lost its place of importance, the open-drop method had virtually disappeared, and in its place has come a variety of closed, semiclosed and non-rebreathing techniques. To-and-fro and infant circle systems (Fig. 2-2) have been used for administration of cyclopropane and ether to small patients, but these in turn have given way to a great extent to non-rebreathing systems which eliminate problems of carbon dioxide accumulation and valve resistance, and at the same time afford greatest accuracy in con-

Fig. 2-2 (left). — The Bloomquist infant circle absorption apparatus. (From Smith[15].)

Fig. 2-3 (right). — The non-rebreathing technique with adapted T-piece.

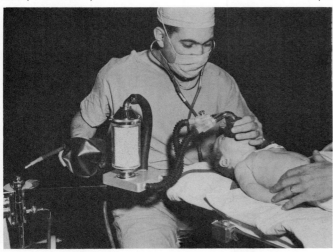

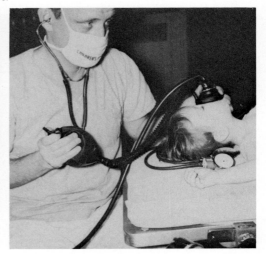

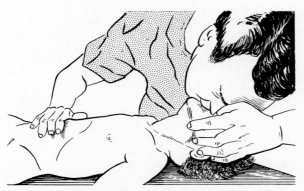

Fig. 2-4. — Mouth-to-mouth resuscitation. Care must be taken to extend neck, support chin and prevent gastric distention.

trolling the concentration of anesthetic mixtures. At present, the T-piece non-rebreathing system (Fig. 2-3) is being used as the most suitable apparatus for children weighing less than 35 lb, while adult circle systems are employed for larger patients. With non-rebreathing apparatus, one disadvantage is that the high flow of dry gases causes considerable loss of body heat and moisture unless care is taken to provide additional humidification.

ENDOTRACHEAL INTUBATION. — The question of endotracheal intubation in infants and children has caused some dispute not only between surgeons and anesthesiologists but among anesthesiologists themselves. With judgment, gentleness and clean apparatus, however, intubation is accomplished safely, and the cause for disagreement has largely disappeared.

Some pediatric anesthesiologists believe that all infants and children are best served by intubation, and they accomplish it successfully. Since an occasional mishap will befall any routine procedure, it may be preferable for those less experienced in pediatric anesthesia to intubate only when intubation is definitely indicated. Indications include intracranial and intrathoracic procedures, operations in the prone position and the presence of intestinal obstruction or full stomach. Intubation is also preferable for surgery around the face, mouth, neck and in the upper abdomen. Routine intubation for herniorrhaphy or for simple orthopedic or plastic procedures on patients in the supine position certainly is not mandatory, and justification will be determined by local conditions.

Regarding the dangers of intubation, there has probably been greatest concern about intubation of small infants, such as those undergoing repair of tracheoesophageal fistula. Bachman[2] has found that these infants are remarkably free from postintubation sequelae and that actually it is the relatively obese 1- to 2-year-old child who is more likely to have postoperative vocal cord edema.

EQUIPMENT

Details of anesthesia apparatus are not of great concern to the surgeon. It is occasionally necessary, however, for a surgeon to resuscitate a child on the ward, and familiarity with endotracheal apparatus at such times will be life-saving. Although mouth-to-mouth methods are excellent (Fig. 2-4), a bag-and-mask combination should be available in the operating room and on the ward at all times, as well as a laryngo-

Fig. 2-5 (left). — Laryngoscope with Wis-Hipple, Flagg no. 2 and Macintosh no. 3 blades.

Fig. 2-6 (right). — Intubation of the trachea is most easily performed when the patient's head is elevated and extended.

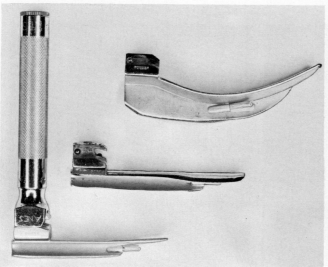

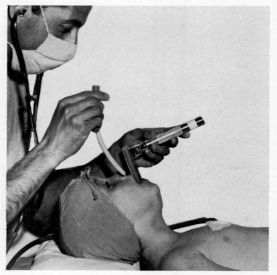

scope, endotracheal tubes and suction appliances of suitable sizes.

To meet the requirements of all age groups, a laryngoscope with at least three different blades should be available. A combination such as the Wis-Hipple infant blade, the straight Flagg no. 2 and the curved Macintosh no. 3 blade (Fig. 2-5) is recommended. Endotracheal tubes should include all sizes from 12 to 32 F., sizes 12–24 being without cuff.

Where an endotracheal tube is to be passed, the proper position of the patient is extremely important. The head should not be hyperextended, for this angulates the trachea. The head is elevated on a pillow, and the chin pulled forward, thus creating a uniformly curved trachea (Fig. 2-6) and offering excellent exposure.

Induction and Maintenance of General Anesthesia

Induction involves many perils and usually represents the most trying phase of the entire anesthetic procedure. It is well for the surgeon to bear this in mind and allow the anesthesiologist ample time to assemble his equipment, get assistance and coax the patient to sleep.

Although the small infant does not show signs of fear, induction under volatile agents causes irritation and breath-holding, and cyclopropane may induce respiratory obstruction, retraction and hypoxia.

To gain adequate depth of anesthesia for endotracheal intubation also takes time. Attempts to intubate before relaxation is achieved will lead to vocal cord spasm and will result in prolongation of the preoperative phase. A moderately slow induction that provides gradual physiologic transition from the awake state to loss of reflexes and into surgical anesthesia has many advantages and usually is worth the time required.

During induction, it is important for the surgical team to speak softly and to refrain from moving the child, examining him or starting to prepare him for operation prematurely. At this stage, the patient is easily startled, and a smooth induction may suddenly be turned into chaos.

When the child is sufficiently anesthetized, the operative site is washed and draped. As the surgeon is about to make the first incision, he should call this to the attention of the anesthesiologist. This is not a fetish, nor a matter of pride on the part of the anesthesiologist, but serves a real purpose. The anesthesiologist has been trying to do many things throughout the induction and may not be ready to cope with the new problems which begin with operation. At the beginning of every operation, the whole team should be alerted and be allowed to start together if they are to act in harmony throughout the procedure.

During maintenance of anesthesia, the anesthesiologist must support and protect the patient, yet provide the surgeon with the best possible operating conditions. Usually these two objectives do not conflict. Occasionally, however, retraction of a lung, manipulation of the heart or abnormal body positioning on the operating table definitely interferes with normal physiologic function, and a reasonable compromise will be necessary.

In the case of small patients, the anesthesiologist is more occupied with supporting the infant than with keeping him asleep. Special attention must be given to preserving body temperature and to guarding against excessive weight of drapes, instruments or hands on the child's body. As in all major pediatric operations, blood replacement involves many difficult problems, which usually are shared by surgeon and anesthesiologist.

The required depth of anesthesia will depend on the operation. A child need not be kept completely relaxed at all times, but merely deep enough to bear the procedure. Many infants will tolerate major surgery while they lie moving their arms and legs.

With children, it is more difficult than with adults to follow the signs of anesthetic level and physiologic function. Depth and rhythm of respiration give essential information, and blood pressure and the volume of heart sounds also must be followed attentively. Complicated monitoring devices have been advocated, but their use does not seem practical in small infants. A simple stethoscope, strapped to the infant's chest, a special infant-size blood pressure cuff and a

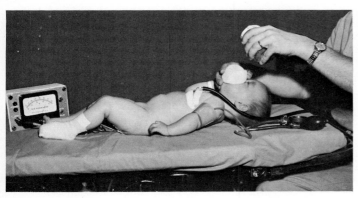

Fig. 2-7.—Stethoscope, blood pressure cuff and thermometer are the most valuable monitors available for pediatric anesthesia.

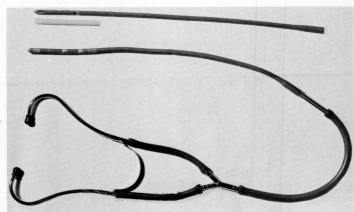

Fig. 2-8.—To make an esophageal stethoscope, three or four extra holes are cut toward the end of a urethral catheter, then covered by a thin tubular rubber dam. The catheter is then joined to a binaural earpiece.

device for measuring rectal temperature give real assistance and should be considered standard equipment (Fig. 2-7) When the left side of the chest is to be operated on, a stethoscope placed in the right axillary line is quite satisfactory in small patients. An esophageal stethoscope (Fig. 2-8) is used in large patients or when operations involve the entire chest, as in the case of severe burns or complex injuries involving both pleural cavities.

Anesthesia for Infants

Operations on small infants pose many problems not encountered in older patients, and the mortality in this group is higher than in any other until the ninth decade is reached. Prematurity, anomalies incompatible with life and poor resistance to infection contribute to the mortality, but anesthetic and surgical management play contributing roles.

Conditions causing the most serious problems during the newborn period are intestinal obstruction, tracheoesophageal fistula, diaphragmatic hernia and omphalocele, plus a variety of tumors and abnormal growths such as teratoma, meningocele and cystic hygroma. Intestinal obstruction may be caused by a variety of lesions, including intestinal atresia, tumors and meconium ileus. These lesions are frequently seen in premature infants. If a tumor is to be excised or if the distention will be relieved by operation, and closure is not expected to be a problem, the entire operation probably can be performed under local infiltration. In such cases, the anesthesiologist stands by fully equipped but usually provides only supportive care. Measures are taken to conserve the infant's body heat by warming the operating room, using a heating pad or wrapping the limbs in sheet wadding. A cut-down infusion is established, a rectal thermistor electrode is inserted, blood pressure cuff (see Fig. 2-7) and precordial stethoscope are applied, the limbs are restrained with cloth tape, and the operation is undertaken. During the procedure, oxygen is administered, and if the infant is restless, a 50% mixture of nitrous oxide and oxygen may be blown over his face or a sugared brandy nipple given him to suck. The anesthesiologist follows signs of cardiovascular tone and administers fluids as needed. Cyclopropane may be used during closure of the abdomen if momentary relaxation is requested. General anesthesia may be necessary in these infants if abdominal relaxation is needed for closure of a distended abdomen, as may be the case in a patient with meconium ileus.

In strong mature infants requiring abdominal operation at birth, general anesthesia throughout is preferable. Here, endotracheal anesthesia usually is indicated. Intubation in newborn infants may be performed without anesthesia but is facilitated by intramuscular use of succinylcholine. Induction is then accomplished rapidly by addition of halothane or cyclopropane and oxygen and maintained with to-and-fro, circle or non-rebreathing systems. We prefer to use halothane and nitrous oxide by non-rebreathing technique.

Infants with *tracheoesophageal fistula and esophageal atresia* often are premature and have complicating conditions such as pneumonia or cardiac defects. Gastrostomy is performed on admission, under local anesthesia, to relieve distention and prevent regurgitation. Ligation of fistula and esophageal anastomosis is performed in 12–24 hours, after the infant has been adequately prepared. General anesthesia with endotracheal intubation is mandatory, but the choice of cyclopropane, halothane or of relaxants plus nitrous oxide depends largely on experience and personal preference.

Repair of *omphalocele* and diaphragmatic hernia have been two great problems shared by anesthetist and surgeon, inasmuch as both have involved difficult wound closure and the threat of severe or total suppression of respiration. The staged omphalocele closure developed by Schuster[12] has diminished the danger and has obviated the need to interfere with the infant's ventilatory exchange. *Diaphragmatic hernia* remains a major problem. Although the closure is less apt to be under severe pressure, the unexpanded lung and resultant respiratory insufficiency have caused many deaths. Some believe that no attempt should be made to expand the "rudimentary" lung, but it often appears that this lung is expanded by the day after operation, and the child is much improved. It seems possible that a gentle attempt to expand the lung at operation might be rewarding.

Regardless of the technique used, respiratory exchange may be critically limited for 2 or 3 days. As yet, no mechanical apparatus has been found sufficiently reliable to cope with this problem, and manual assistance, provided from time to time with a bag and mask, probably is most dependable.

In operations involving excision of large masses, such as *teratoma* and *cystic hygroma*, surgical shock is a major hazard. The signs of shock are poorly defined in infants, and blood loss is difficult to estimate. Blood pressure can be followed if infant-size cuffs are used. The volume of the pulse and the intensity of heart sounds are extremely important. With severe blood loss, whether gradual or sudden, the peripheral pulse fades and disappears; next, the heart sounds become faint and then inaudible. Proper blood replacement is followed by prompt reappearance of pulse and heart sounds unless other complications occur.

Pyloromyotomy and herniorrhaphy are probably the commonest operations in infants who have passed the neonatal period. Infants with pyloric stenosis may be extremely dehydrated and alkalotic and even after adequate fluid and electrolytic therapy present increased anesthetic risk. Consequently the procedure is best carried out under halothane or cyclopropane anesthesia or under local infiltration. In infants who have pyloric obstruction, there is danger of regurgitating retained gastric contents unless the stomach is kept empty. For this reason, a 10 or 12 F. catheter with several holes must be passed into the infant's stomach before induction of anesthesia and frequent aspiration carried out until the operation is completed. Endotracheal intubation is indicated if curds or barium are found in the stomach.

For *herniorrhaphy* on a normal infant, the anesthesiologist has a wide choice of agents and methods. It seems preferable, however, to avoid complicated techniques unless there is special indication for them. In usual conditions, halothane is adequate and endotracheal intubation is unnecessary.

Infants who present the most serious anesthetic problems are those with congenital cardiac lesions. These are discussed below.

Anesthesia for Thoracic Surgery in Children

Thoracic surgery in children now includes (1) procedures on lungs and chest wall, (2) operations on great vessels and heart without by-pass and (3) open-heart procedures. Anesthetic procedures for all thoracic operations share certain common requirements, including need of ventilatory control, light anesthesia without relaxation and exacting management of blood replacement. In addition, the age and condition of the patient and the pathology of each lesion pose problems that must be treated on an individual and highly selective basis.

Preparation is extremely important in patients facing thoracic procedures. These operations are rarely urgent, and there is little excuse for subjecting any patient to such a hazardous procedure if he has any trace of respiratory infection or other lesion that can be corrected, even though it requires last-minute cancellation of operation or a delay of several weeks.

OPERATIONS ON LUNG AND CHEST WALL. — Anesthesia for lobectomy or pneumonectomy can be induced with any of the general anesthetic agents so long as a light steady plane can be provided and an air-tight system maintained. Purulent secretions must be reduced to a minimum by preoperative therapy, but ample provision must be made for clearing the airway during operation. Fluothane has definite advantages here because it does not stimulate secretory activity.

Correction of pectus excavatum may require a large wound, but if the deformity is not great, the operation involves little risk and blood replacement may not be required. Two special considerations have proved important. (1) It is always possible for the surgeon to open either pleural cavity; consequently it is advisable to monitor each lung with an individual stethoscope. (2) Due to malformation of the thorax, the maintenance of adequate ventilation is especially difficult, and respiratory acidosis and hyperthermia may develop in spite of special care. A successful outcome depends more on attention to these factors than on the agent chosen.

OPERATIONS ON GREAT VESSELS AND HEART WITHOUT BY-PASS. — Vascular ring deformities usually are diagnosed during infancy, and the anesthesiologist faces the problems met in all infants plus the problem of low tracheal obstruction. Mild sedation helps quiet the child before operation. The chief difficulty lies in airway management. Endotracheal intubation is definitely indicated but entails special problems. If the end of the tube is inserted beyond the low tracheal constriction, it may pass the carina and enter one bronchus. To prevent occlusion of the other bronchus, multiple holes should be cut in the end of the endotracheal tube (Fig. 2-9). Passage of the tube through the tracheal constriction may cause irritation and further narrowing of the lumen during the early recovery period. It may be wise, therefore, to keep the tip of the tube just above the constriction if possible. A moderate amount of postoperative respiratory obstruction is seen in many cases, since the deformed tracheal rings do not immediately assume normal shape.

Division or ligation of patent ductus usually is performed on children with strong active hearts and can

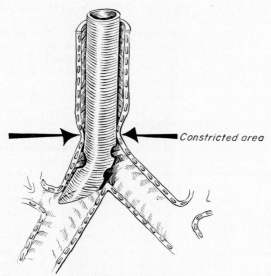

Constricted area

Fig. 2-9.—Anesthesia for vascular ring surgery may require passage of endotracheal tube through constricted area, and result in endobronchial intubation. Perforation of the endotracheal tube will prevent obstruction of opposite bronchus.

be accomplished under any general anesthesia with endotracheal intubation. When the situation is complicated by pulmonary hypertension, cardiac failure or reversal of shunt, the risk is much increased.

The anesthetic agent must be chosen and administered in a manner to minimize cardiac irritation and avoid further increase of pulmonary artery pressure. Hypoxia, deep anesthesia, tracheal obstruction or irritation and vascular overload accentuate pulmonary hypertension and must be eliminated at all costs.

In most circumstances, coarctation of the aorta is seen in healthy adolescents who tolerate anesthesia well. Blood replacement is the chief problem, because of the large wound involved and the collateral circulation through the chest wall. Before application of the aortic clamps, it is preferable to have the blood pressure at not more than 150 mm Hg systolic in order to prevent excessive pressure elevation. The pressure may be controlled if halothane or ether is the anesthetic agent, although some prefer to use such ganglionic blocking agents as hexamethonium or Arfonad. On completion of the anastomosis, the clamps are released slowly while the anesthesiologist continually monitors blood pressure, and blood is administered as needed.

Infants with coarctation present much more serious problems, for they usually have enlarged, failing hearts plus the usual disadvantages of extreme youth. Light cyclopropane anesthesia has been used with success, with care being taken to avoid depression of cardiac activity and to replace blood with accuracy.

Blalock and Potts procedures for tetralogy of Fallot involve poor-risk patients in whom both hypoxia and low blood pressure are major hazards. Oxygenation is improved by preoperative sedation and by assisting ventilation during operation, but is imperiled while the pulmonary artery is ligated. Hypotension has been countered by using two cut-down infusions, one for blood or plasma, the other for a drip infusion consisting of 500 mg of calcium gluconate and 5 mg of phenylephrine (Neosynephrine) in 125 cc of 5% glucose. Cyclopropane by endotracheal intubation is the anesthetic most widely used for these operations. It is especially important to maintain blood pressure following a Blalock procedure in order to keep blood flowing actively through the new shunt.

OPEN-HEART PROCEDURES.—Extracorporeal circulation is necessary for most intracardiac procedures, including repair of atrial septal defects, aortic stenosis, pulmonary stenosis, ventricular septal defects, tetralogy of Fallot, total anomalous pulmonary venous drainage and transposition of great vessels, unless these are being performed under hyperbaric oxygenation. Most of these patients are considered poor operative risks, and all precautions are taken. Patients are nursed into their best possible condition, they are re-examined to confirm the diagnosis, and digitalis dosage is regulated to provide maximal support. Atropine, pentobarbital and morphine are ordered in suitably reduced dosages to be effective but not depressing. The actual pump-oxygenator combination may be any one of a wide variety of combinations involving bubble, film or membrane oxygenators, and sigma motor or rotary (De Bakey) type pumps. Anesthetic requirements are relatively simple, and the same techniques may be employed for most patients regardless of the lesion or type of by-pass machine employed. The anesthetic agent should not cause cardiac depression, should be nonexplosive and should provide a means for controlling the patient while the lungs are not functioning. The two most popular methods consist of (1) relaxant-nitrous oxide combination with thiopental supplement, and (2) halothane. The first combination is easily administered, using succinylcholine or d-tubocurarine by intermittent intravenous injection and nitrous oxide-oxygen by inhalation. During by-pass, patients tend to awaken, but may be controlled by addition of thiopental to the blood passing through the pump.

Monitoring consists of arterial blood pressure measurement by pneumatic duff; check on venous pressure; use of the external or esophageal stethoscope and rectal and esophageal thermistors, and electrocardiography. During by-pass, the anesthetist keeps mild pressure on the breathing bag (5–10 cm H_2O) and watches for vascular congestion of the head and pupillary dilation. The major problems in patients undergoing by-pass procedures appear after completion of by-pass and consist of hypotension, heart block and continued bleeding. Pulmonary hypertension, seen with both atrial and ventricular septal defects, is the great underlying pathologic problem determining the outcome in many patients.

The postoperative phase is usually the most critical period for open-heart surgery, and surgeon, anesthetist and cardiologist must work together actively. Patients who have severe cardiac disease or have had extensive or prolonged repair usually should be supported by a mechanical ventilator for 1 or 2 days until cardiorespiratory function has proved adequate.[6] Use of a cardiac pacemaker and inotropic stimulants such as isoproterenol is often of critical importance here.

Diagnostic cardiovascular procedures.—Right heart catheterization requires even sedation lasting 1–2 hours without use of additional oxygen. A number of general and basal anesthetic agents, sedatives and narcotics have been employed to meet this demand, and several combinations have been reported on favorably. One of the simplest and most effective is that of Davenport,[7] who uses meperidine (Demerol) and pentobarbital (Nembutal), each in dosage of 2 mg/lb of body weight.

The combination of phenothiazine, meperidine and chlorpromazine, recommended by Code Smith et al.[14] has been very satisfactory. The solution is:

Phenothiazine	50 mg	2 cc
Meperidine	200 mg	4 cc
Chlorpromazine	50 mg	2 cc
		8 cc solution

The basic dose is 1 cc/20 lb of body weight for noncyanotic patients, and is reduced to 0.7 cc/20 lb for children with the cyanotic forms of congenital cardiac disease.

Anesthesia for General Surgery and Plastic Procedures

Intra-abdominal operations.—A variety of anesthetic agents and techniques may be used for infants and children undergoing operations within the abdomen, although the choice will vary somewhat with the operation and the age and condition of the patient. In most children, general anesthesia usually is the most successful from the standpoint of both the surgeon and the patient, although spinal anesthesia often is useful in children of 8–12 years or older.

In elective operations in good-risk patients, the child is sedated with atropine, pentobarbital and morphine. In children weighing under 35 lb, a T-piece non-rebreathing system is usually employed; closed circle adult equipment is used for larger children. Nitrous oxide and halothane are suitable for most abdominal procedures. If halothane has been employed previously, one's next choice would be a pentothal induction with d-tubocurarine and nitrous oxide. Ether is certainly not to be condemned, but it is not popular because of the explosive hazard. In small

infants, or in children in poor general condition, cyclopropane is often chosen, administered by closed circle technique. Penthrane is chosen for abdominal procedures because of the relaxation it induces, but this advantage is not usually critical in pediatric work. Operations on the liver, stomach, spleen or kidney usually require operative manipulation near the diaphragm and may necessitate positions that interfere with ventilation. For this reason, endotracheal intubation is indicated. Also, a catheter with several holes should be passed into the stomach. As will be mentioned in the discussion of emergency procedures, spinal anesthesia is most useful when older children are brought to the hospital for unscheduled operations, especially when they have eaten recently.

It should be noted that excision of large abdominal tumors such as neuroblastoma and Wilms' tumor (Fig. 2-10) and operations on the liver often involve excessive blood loss and in addition require considerable operative manipulation. These two factors together have often led to profound shock and have made it obvious that special precautions should be taken. Before operation, ample quantities of whole blood should be prepared. It has been especially helpful to have fresh blood, to buffer it to pH 7.4 and to warm it before use. Two cut-down infusions are established, and it is important to have these in the arms, to ensure continuous flow in case of inferior vena caval injury or obstruction during operation. Tris buffer is used for alkalinization of the blood. A pint of blood at pH 6.8 usually requires approximately 1,200 mg of Tris for correction to 7.4, but it is advisable to titrate this by blood gas analysis. When plasma is being used for volume replacement, it is even more important to correct the pH to normal.

If marked blood loss is encountered during an operation, the surgeon should be ready to halt until the child's condition has stabilized. When a patient is in danger of shock, it is a dangerous error to plunge ahead for the sake of finishing quickly. Invariably this takes longer than expected, and the final insult may be dealt in these precarious moments.

Operations on the bladder or kidney require general anesthesia. Intubation is indicated if the child is to be in the lateral position, since breathing will be limited and ventilatory assistance is required. A nonrebreathing apparatus is suitable for children under 4–6 years, a circle system for older children. As previously mentioned, excision of an embryoma or Wilms' tumor involves maximal risk of blood loss and operative shock and requires utmost precautions. It is especially important to monitor temperatures during genitourinary procedures.

Plastic operations.—Cleft lip may be repaired in the neonatal period, but some surgeons prefer to wait until the infant is a month old. In either case, anesthetic management involves definite airway problems. Anatomic distortion interferes with the infant's

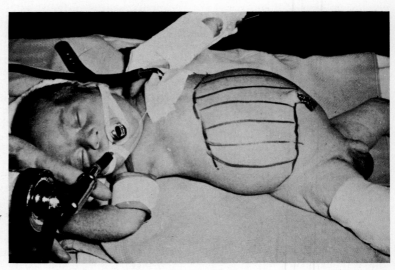

Fig. 2-10.—Children with Wilms' tumor and liver masses present greatest danger of massive hemorrhage.

respiration both while awake and during induction. Endotracheal intubation is indicated to provide airway control, but exposure of the glottis is complicated by difficulty in positioning the laryngoscope. To overcome this problem, it may be helpful to block the cleft with a sponge.

For maintenance of anesthesia, halothane may be administered by the Ayre non-rebreathing technique. A light plane with nitrous oxide supplementation will enable the infant to awaken at the end of the procedure.

Cleft palate is repaired when the child is about a year old. Here, endotracheal intubation is advocated, again with a non-rebreathing system. In repair of either lip or palate, the surgeon and anesthesiologist must make sure that blood does not enter the trachea by running down along the outside of the tube. Careful auscultation of the chest is necessary both during and at the end of the operation.

The treatment of burns, whether considered in the realm of general or plastic surgery, poses special problems in anesthesia. Immediate treatment of severe burns consists chiefly of fluid therapy. A light general anesthesia that has minimal effect on the liver and kidneys is advised. Nitrous oxide supplemented with light cyclopropane using a circle system with high oxygen administration is satisfactory. Blood must be replaced liberally.

Continued therapy of burns usually requires many return trips to the operating room for dressing and grafting. These children must be treated with much understanding, for they certainly suffer. Continued encouragement between operations is helpful, and such attention on the part of the anesthesiologist will enable the child to meet a friend each time he returns for operation. Sedation must be adequate but not depressing to liver or kidneys, and the anesthetic agent should be pleasant, easily excreted and cause

no upsetting after-effects. Halothane has been employed for repeated burn dressings in numerous children, and its use appears to be justified provided no postoperative fever or jaundice is noted.

The Poor-Risk Patient

When patients are anemic or have other remediable conditions, preoperative therapy can restore them to acceptable condition. Children with advanced malignancy, cardiac defects or ventilatory limitation occasionally require operation and represent definitely increased risks. Operations may be performed only if actually necessary and only when such children have been brought to the best possible condition that time allows. Individualized preoperative care will enable the anesthesiologist to omit most sedative agents and to use a light plane of anesthesia with high oxygen flow. In very weak patients, nitrous oxide and oxygen may suffice even for abdominal procedures. Cyclopropane has been useful in most poor-risk infants and children, affording analgesia and relaxation with minimal metabolic disturbance and rapid recovery. Before any anesthesia is started in a poor-risk patient, an intravenous infusion should be established, and atropine, relaxants and calcium should be ready for use at any moment. It is an excellent rule to have two anesthesiologists on hand for any operation involving an increased risk.

Minor and Emergency Operations

ELECTIVE OPERATIONS.—Many simple procedures involving one or two sutures can be performed under local infiltration anesthesia in the surgeon's office. In such instances a child should be given the benefit of a narcotic to help control his fear and lessen the discomfort. Nerve blocks of finger, wrist or arm are adequate for more extensive procedures in outpatient clinics. Hypnosis, whether used as supplement or as principal agent, is of very real benefit and may give further assistance in this area.

Circumcision, excision of skin lesions and similar procedures may require general anesthesia of short duration, but this is given only if the patient has not eaten and has had proper sedation. All patients receive a drying agent and those over a year old receive a narcotic. There must be suction available and complete resuscitative equipment at hand before any general anesthesia is begun. Nitrous oxide and halothane are well adapted for short operations. It is preferable not to use endotracheal intubation when children are operated on as outpatients, for subglottic edema might develop and become a real danger. All patients must be allowed to regain full consciousness and neuromuscular control before being discharged.

EMERGENCY PROCEDURES. — Some of the most tragic errors in medicine occur in the management of healthy children who enter the hospital for "emergency" surgery. These are the children who have a fractured wrist or abdominal pain and are rushed to the operating room in spite of having just eaten three apples and a hamburger sandwich. Anesthesia, vomiting, aspiration and death follow in rapid succession and throughout the United States account for a large and entirely unnecessary mortality each year.

There are few conditions that require "emergency" treatment. When possible, the term should be avoided since it invites errors of haste and omission, often converting a minor accident into a major catastrophe.

In most situations, children who require treatment of injury or acute lesions are in no immediate danger, and time can be allowed for obtaining a regular history and physical examination as well as blood examination and urinalysis. These measures will reveal the presence of drug sensitivity, diabetes or other conditions that might otherwise have been overlooked.

Unscheduled procedures present two special problems for the anesthesiologist: calming of the frightened, injured child, and management of the full stomach. An excited child may become more upset if given pentobarbital for sedation. Best results in children 1–5 years old are gained with rectal administration of tribromoethanol (Avertin) 80 mg/kg or thiopental 30 mg/kg, either of which will provide basal anesthesia and induce sleep in 7–8 minutes. Older children usually are more manageable and are quieted by morphine and pentobarbital. General anesthesia should not be forced on excited, resisting children.

Many methods have been suggested for handling patients with a full stomach. A wait for a specified number of hours is not reliable. Attempts to wash out the stomach or make the patient vomit are more upsetting than effective. The policy that has been safe, practical and effective has been (1) to use local anes-thesia when possible, or (2) if general anesthesia is required, either to use nitrous oxide-oxygen without abolishing the gag reflex or else to induce general anesthesia with cyclopropane or halothane, and insert an endotracheal tube. The tube will protect the trachea in case of vomiting and *must be left in place until the patient is actually awake*, moving his extremities, opening his eyes and ready to talk.

A few situations may arise which actually require immediate treatment. These include respiratory obstruction, head injury and hemorrhage. Among children, the danger of acute respiratory obstruction is definitely increased. Although tracheostomy may be performed, it is preferable to avoid it as an "emergency" measure and instead, to pass an endotracheal tube or bronchoscope first to establish an airway and then perform the tracheostomy without haste.

Complications of Anesthesia

The nature of anesthetic complications has changed considerably during recent years. Ether was associated with active respiration and increased secretions, resulting in irregular, gasping ventilation, aspiration of secretions and vomiting. With the change to halogenated agents, relaxants and endotracheal intubation, respiration is intentionally depressed or paralyzed and is taken over by the anesthesiologist so that stridor, gasping and secretions are virtually eliminated, leaving ventilatory depression as the only significant respiratory complication.

Newer anesthetic agents may induce stimulation of vagus nerve and myocardial depression. Cyclopropane, halothane and succinylcholine may cause severe bradycardia unless the patient is well atropinized. Both cyclopropane and halothane sensitize the myocardium to catecholamines, and use of epinephrine involves danger of inducing ventricular fibrillation. Another disadvantage shared by halothane and cyclopropane is a tendency to cause wild thrashing excitement during the patient's awakening. Although the patients have no memory of this, it is certainly disturbing to those for some distance around them, and the active motions can disrupt wounds and displace newly approximated bone fragments.

Ether convulsions are rarely seen now, but abnormal temperature responses have been of real concern. Small infants rapidly lose body heat,[13] with resultant respiratory depression, atelectasis or pneumonia and retarded awakening. Zealous efforts to warm such infants may lead to severe burns which, in some instances, have proved fatal.

Hyperthermia has been a far greater problem than cooling. This has occurred in older children who have entered the hospital with peritonitis and whose temperatures have soared to 106–108 F during operation. It has also occurred in apparently normal children and adults, in a somewhat unique syndrome recently termed malignant hyperthermia.[9] In this, patients have shown a prolonged myotonic response to succinylcholine and less frequently to halothane and have subsequently developed high temperatures with fatal result. Over 30 such cases have been documented.

The problem of liver toxicity with halogenated drugs, and with halothane in particular, continues to harass anesthetists, surgeons and especially patients. In spite of the fact that an examination of 800,000 cases of halothane anesthesia by a special committee of the National Research Council[16] failed to disclose definite evidence that halothane was more dangerous than any other anesthetic agent, individual instances of suspected liver toxicity appear too frequently to allow one any real peace of mind. It had been thought that children were relatively safe from this type of hepatitis, but an 11-year-old girl recently died at our hospital of massive hepatic necrosis following three halothane anesthetics, and similar cases have been encountered in this area.

Although halothane has been administered hundreds of thousands of times, it seems probable that the combination of stress, enzyme depression, hypoxia and halothane might initiate a form of sensitivity which would have serious implications on subsequent exposure to the agent.

REFERENCES

1. Babior, B. M., and Davidson, C. S.: Postoperative massive liver necrosis, New England J. Med. 276:645, 1967.
2. Bachman, L.: Personal communication.
3. Blackfan, K. D., and Diamond, L. K.: *Atlas of the Blood* (New York: Commonwealth Fund, 1944).
4. Brennan, H. J.; Hunter, A. R., and Johnstone, M.: Halothane, a clinical assessment, Lancet 2:453, 1957.
5. Corssen, G., and Domino, E. F.: Dissociative anesthesia: Further pharmacologic studies and first clinical experience with phencyclidine derivative CI-581, Anesth. & Analg. 45:29, 1966.
6. Dammann, J. F., Jr., *et al.*: The management of the severely ill patient after open-heart surgery, J. Thoracic & Cardiovas. Surg. 45:80, 1963.
7. Davenport, H. T.: Personal communication.
8. Davenport, H. T., and Quan, P.: Methoxyflurane anesthesia in pediatrics, Canad. M. A. J. 91:1291, 1964.
9. Hogg, S., and Renwick, W.: Hyperpyrexia during anesthesia, Canad. Anaesth. Soc. J. 13:429, 1966.
10. Nyhan, W. L., and Lamport, F.: Response of the fetus and newborn to drugs, Anesthesiology 26:487, 1966.
11. Rees, G. J.: Paediatric anaesthesia, Brit. J. Anaesth. 32:132, 1960.
12. Schuster, S. S.: New method for staged repair of large omphaloceles, Surg., Gynec. & Obst. 125:837, 1967.
13. Silverman, W. A.; Sinclair, J. C., and Scopes, J. W.: Regulation of body temperature in pediatric surgery, J. Pediat. Surg. 1:321, 1966.
14. Smith, C.; Rowe, R. D., and Vlad, P.: Sedation of children for cardiac catheterization with an ataractic mixture, Canad. Anesth. Soc. J. 5:35, 1958.
15. Smith, R. M.: *Anesthesia for Infants and Children* (3rd ed.; St. Louis: C. V. Mosby Company, 1968).
16. Subcommittee on the National Halothane Study of the Committee on Anesthesia, National Academy of Sciences-National Research Council: Summary of the National Halothane Study: Possible association between halothane anesthesia and postoperative hepatic necrosis, J.A.M.A. 197:775, 1966.
17. Zindler, M. (ed.): Intravenous anaesthesia for outpatients, Acta anaesth. scandinav., supp. XVII, 1964.

R. M. SMITH

Drawings by
MURIEL MCLATCHIE MILLER

3

Inhalation Therapy

HISTORY.—There are numerous early reports of resuscitative efforts by artificial ventilation, beginning with the Biblical account of successful mouth-to-mouth ventilatory resuscitation applied by the prophet Elijah. Supplemental oxygen was first used by Priestly on himself and two mice in 1774. Shortly thereafter, oxygen inhalations became fashionable treatment for many ailments. Sir Thomas Beddoes is usually credited with founding inhalation therapy by his establishment of the Pneumatic Institute at Clifford, England, in 1798, for the therapy of a variety of diseases by placing the patient in a "factitious atmosphere."[10] By 1926, an external respirator was developed by Thunberg which used high negative and positive pressures. This was soon modified by Drinker, who designed the tank respirators still in use.[8] The BLB (Boothby, Lovelace and Bulbulian) mask and positive pressure assisted ventilation were developed in 1938, partly for the military advantage of allowing aviators to reach higher altitudes than had previously been possible. Subsequently, intermittent positive pressure ventilators were developed for clinical use in patients, although as late as 1952 some 200 medical students were employed to ventilate victims of the polio epidemic in Copenhagen by manual compression of a bag.[15]

Special Problems in the Pediatric Patient

In recent years, respiratory therapy for adults has become well established.[3,21] There may be, however, special problems associated with pediatric respiratory care because of the peculiar physiology, pathology and surgical problems of the young patient.

PHYSIOLOGIC CONSIDERATIONS. – Although an older child may differ from the adult mostly in size, the infant and especially the newborn have many physiologic characteristics that differentiate them clearly from the adult and require special consideration. The infant or newborn has small respiratory volumes and perhaps a relatively large deadspace; he is capable of generating less total force than an older patient. Airway diameters are very small, so that even minimal obstruction by edema, secretions or small artificial airways may be critical. Infants and children have more rapid respiratory rates and a greater frequency of sighing than adults. They are particularly susceptible to temperature changes and may either gain or lose heat via the respiratory tract. Large amounts of fluids also may be gained or lost via the respiratory tract.

PATHOLOGIC CONSIDERATIONS. – The pathologic conditions which may be encountered in the pediatric age group include a wide variety of congenital anomalies which may require surgical correction and present unusual postoperative problems. Of particular interest are the numerous cardiovascular abnormalities and the other conditions involving the chest, such as congenital cystic lung, tracheoesophageal fistula and diaphragmatic hernia. Most patients with these conditions require some of the services provided by a respiratory therapy department. The department will also be called on to assist in the care of patients with respiratory distress syndrome of the newborn, spasmodic asthma, cystic fibrosis, laryngotracheobronchitis, pneumonia and various other forms of respiratory tract disease. Children with neurologic or neuromuscular disorders, such as poliomyelitis, tetanus, Guillain-Barré syndrome and dermatomyositis, may require ventilatory support, as may patients with a variety of neurosurgical problems. Intoxications are not uncommon in children, and the patient unconscious from whatever cause requires special respiratory care. Chemical and mechanical injuries of the lungs may present challenging problems, as exemplified by the child with smoke inhalation and a large burn or the child with a crushed chest and numerous accompanying traumatic injuries. Children with severe scoliosis have abnormal pulmonary function on this basis alone and may have even greater impairment due to an underlying disease such as poliomyelitis.

SURGICAL CONSIDERATIONS. – The pediatric patient who comes for surgery is often a potential candidate for respiratory therapy. Respiratory function may be disordered by anesthesia and by the surgical procedure itself. Patients may be loath to breathe deeply or cough in the presence of pain and fear. Physiologic shunting and physiologic deadspace are increased in the postoperative period because of abnormal ventilation-perfusion relationships.[12] Children are especially susceptible to traumatic laryngotracheobronchitis or stridor after endotracheal intubation or other airway manipulation. Major difficulties can often be averted by appropriate prophylactic measures. Any patient with a previous respiratory problem will require special care, and this should begin in the preoperative period.

REQUIREMENTS FOR SPECIAL EQUIPMENT. – A pediatric respiratory therapy service must supply special equipment to satisfy the requirements of the pediatric patient. Several sizes of airways, endotracheal tubes, laryngoscopes and masks are needed. Ventilators must be able to deliver accurately very small volumes at rapid rates. Deadspace in apparatus can be a formidable problem when ordinary connecting tubing may have a volume greater than the tidal volume of a newborn. Resistance may also be a critical factor in assisting ventilation in infants and children.

Patient Services in Pediatric Inhalation Therapy

What services will be offered to the pediatric patient by a respiratory therapy department?

OXYGEN

METHODS OF APPLICATION. – Oxygen is given by various means. A concentration approaching 100% oxygen may be achieved by using a well-fitting face mask with a reservoir bag. A face tent with high-flow oxygen (10 liters/minute) may provide 50% oxygen, and a well-placed nasopharyngeal catheter, 40% oxygen. Nasal cannulas, or "prongs," are capable of delivering a maximal inspired oxygen concentration of only 25–30%. Oxygen insufflated by funnel could probably achieve 50% inspired oxygen if meticulously applied.

Tents find a wide use in pediatrics, and besides supplying oxygen, they are of great value for humidification, "air conditioning" and partial physical and psychologic isolation of the patient. Flow into a tent must always be greater than the patient's minute ventilation if carbon dioxide accumulation is to be avoided. If oxygen flows are no greater than this, peak-inspired oxygen concentrations will be in the range of 45% and, when the tent is frequently opened, less than 30%. However, if three or four oxygen ports are used at extremely high flows (in the range of 6.0 liters/minute from each port), 75% inspired oxygen can be maintained even with fairly frequent opening of the tent. Incubators and intermittent positive pressure ventilators, particularly the volume control ventilators, can usually provide any desired concentration of oxygen.

OXYGEN TOXICITY.—Oxygen should be used with the same caution as any other agent that is potentially toxic in large doses. High concentrations of oxygen for prolonged periods have been known for many years to cause central nervous system and pulmonary damage, but full clinical attention has only recently been drawn to these complications of oxygen therapy. The first measurable change of pulmonary function is a 15–20% fall of vital capacity, which occurs in normal volunteers breathing 100% oxygen after 18–24 hours.[4] Diffusing capacity is decreased with continued oxygen breathing, and there may be an increase in the alveolar-arterial oxygen gradient.

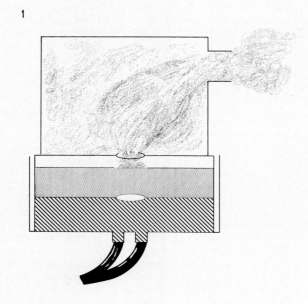

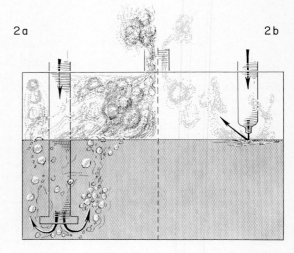

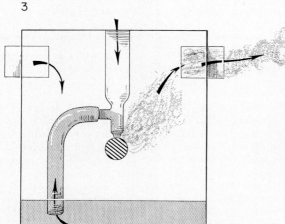

Fig. 3-1.—Types of humidifiers: **1**. ultrasonic: ultrahigh frequency sound waves at 2.5 megacycles strike a thin layer of water on a plastic diaphragm, vibrate and break up the water into particle sizes of $1_u \rightarrow 5_u$. **2a**, bubble: humidification is produced by forcing a gas through water to pick up moisture; the humidified gas is then delivered to the patient. **2b**, jet: humidification occurs when a gas is blown across the top of a liquid where it picks up the vapor moisture, which is then delivered to the patient. **3**, Venturi: humidification is produced when gas picks up moisture from the capillary tube of the reservoir and breaks it into very fine mist, which is then delivered to the patient.

Atelectasis is frequent,[9] possibly in part due to a decreased activity of surfactant. Thus both physical damage to lung structure and biochemical damage to cells occur. Frank pulmonary oxygen toxicity has been described as beginning with an exudative process (edema and congestion with or without hyaline membranes) which leads to a later proliferative phase.[18,19] In spite of these complications, high inspired oxygen concentrations will be necessary on occasion. Oxygen should be given in a quantity sufficient to maintain normal arterial oxygenation, as estimated by serial measurements of the arterial partial pressure of oxygen. Oxygen concentrations of less than 40% may be considered safe for long periods. There is some evidence that even 10% nitrogen may have a specific protective effect against pulmonary oxygen toxicity.[9] Whenever oxygen is used, the inspired concentration should be monitored at regular intervals. This can be done easily and quickly at the bedside with a paramagnetic oxygen analyzer.

HUMIDIFICATION

Humidification (addition of water vapor to a gas) and nebulization (production of a particulate mist) may be even more important in a pediatric hospital than oxygen. Heated rooms in winter often have a relative humidity at 20 or 25C of 10% or less. As the humidity in the alveoli is 100% at 37C, and contains 53 mg of water/liter, the patient's upper airways must supply large amounts of water vapor to the inspired air. Secretions may become dried and difficult or impossible to remove; the bronchi may even develop a lining of crusts, leading to severe respiratory distress. The magnitude of this problem is greatly increased if the upper airways are by-passed by means of tracheostomy or an endotracheal tube. In the normal situation, air inside the trachea is 100% saturated with water vapor at 32–35C, the nose normally warming and humidifying inspired air. When the upper airways are passed by, their functions must be performed artificially. Adequate humidification for endotracheal tube or tracheostomy requires the delivery of a mist or heated vapor so that relative humidity will be 100%, or more if desired, at body temperature. Fifty-three mg of water vapor must be added to every liter of dry gas if the partial pressure of water vapor is to be maintained at its normal alveolar level of 42 mm Hg.

A relative "body humidity" (i.e., relative humidity at an alveolar temperature of 37C) of 50% can be achieved in a fog room or in large "high humidity" oxygen tents. Ordinary bubble humidifiers, which give 100% relative humidity at room temperature, will have a humidity of as low as 20% when heated to 37C without further addition of water vapor (Fig 3-1, 2a). Sidestream nebulizers used on pressure-controlled intermittent positive pressure breathing machines such as the Bird ventilator can deliver only 16% body humidity (Fig. 3-1, 3), whereas mainstream nebulizers (Fig. 1 2b) on these machines can deliver 70% body humidity and, if heated, greater than 100% body humidity.[21] The ultrasonic nebulizer delivers up to 6 cc of water/minute as a dense mist[2] (Fig 3-1, 1). Volume-controlled ventilators are usually equipped with heated nebulizers.

In addition to the maintenance of normal physiology in a healthy chest, addition of water vapor and mist to inspired air has a marked therapeutic effect in many respiratory disorders. This treatment often produces dramatic results in laryngotracheobronchitis. In diseases such as cystic fibrosis and pulmonary infection, liquefaction of secretions by nebulized water or saline allows their removal to an extent which would not otherwise be possible.

Total body fluid balance is significantly influenced by the amount of fluid gained or lost via the respiratory tract.[14] For instance, if inspired air has 100% humidity at 37C, that part of the insensible loss which normally is used in humidifying inspired air will be retained. With the use of heated nebulizers, and particularly ultrasonic nebulizers, a patient may receive such large amounts of fluid that his circulation is overloaded. Temperature regulation may also be affected; the temperature of heated nebulizers should be constantly monitored to prevent overheating.

NEBULIZATION

Delivery of aqueous mist or nebulized medications to the peripheral areas of the lung depends on droplet size and mist density as well as other factors such as flow rates of carrier gases. Technical problems have made meaningful measurements of the ideal droplet size difficult; but most workers agree that the range of $1-10 \mu$ seems best, with 3μ often cited as optimal particle size for peripheral deposition in the lung. In-line and sidestream nebulizers as well as ultrasonic nebulizers produce a large proportion of droplets near this size.[21,2] The droplet may grow as it is cooled in tubing and become smaller or evaporate entirely on rewarming in the larger airways, although some stabilization of droplets has been achieved by addition of salt or propylene glycol to aerosols. Large droplets often impact or settle out on the walls of tubing or large airways, and very small droplets may reach peripheral areas but be exhaled without settling. To achieve maximal peripheral deposition, breathing should be slow and the breath held momentarily on deep inspiration. Intermittent positive pressure breathing is of great assistance in achieving these conditions in the pediatric patient who might not be capable of so performing spontaneously.

INTERMITTENT POSITIVE PRESSURE BREATHING

Intermittent positive pressure breathing treatments are often required in the pediatric patient to assist in

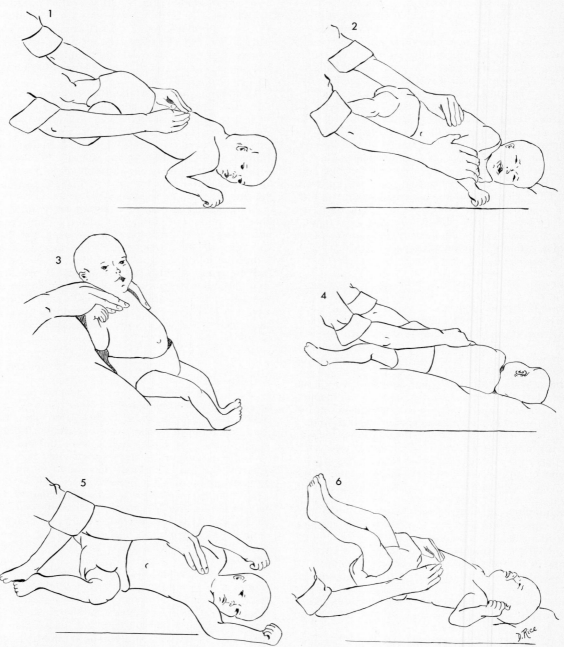

Fig. 3-2.—Postural drainage, clapping and vibrating. **1**, posterior basal segments, right and left. **2**, right lateral basal segments. **3**, upper lobes, anterior segments. **4**, lingula, left upper lobe.

5, right lateral and medial segments. **6**, anterior basal segment of right lung; anterior medial basal segment of left lung.

deep breathing as well as to deliver nebulized water and drugs. A mask, mouthpiece or endotracheal tube may be used, and prophylactic intermittent positive pressure breathing therapy is often given to surgical patients who seem likely victims of atelectasis or other pulmonary problems in the postoperative period.[20] The stomach may occasionally be distended with air when these treatments are given with mask or mouthpiece. Deep breaths may be given manually with a self-inflating or anesthesia-type bag as well as with intermittent positive pressure breathing machines.

CHEST PHYSIOTHERAPY

Chest physiotherapy is an essential part of over-all respiratory care. It is often provided by the physical therapy service or by the general nursing staff, but more or less responsibility for this may fall to the respiratory therapy service. A "stir-up regimen," with turning and deep breathing, is part of routine care in a good recovery room. Some patients may need endotracheal suctioning, vibrations, percussion and postural drainage to rid them of secretions (Fig. 3-2). Breathing exercises should be taught preoperatively to patients who are to undergo thoracic or abdominal surgery, if age and understanding permit.

ARTIFICIAL VENTILATION

Patients with actual or impending respiratory failure require artificial ventilation.[17]

INDICATIONS.—Downes *et al.*[7] have offered the following criteria for children in status asthmaticus, any three of which they deem adequate to diagnose respiratory failure: (1) inspiratory retractions or gasping; (2) markedly decreased or absent inspiratory breath sounds; (3) generalized muscular weakness; (4) decreased level of consciousness; (5) cyanosis with inspired oxygen concentration of 40% (6) arterial partial pressure of carbon dioxide greater than 65 mm Hg. In general, artificial ventilation is indicated when the patient is unable to maintain acceptable arterial oxygenation and prevent progressive respiratory or hypoxic metabolic acidosis or when the work of breathing makes demands beyond the patient's capacities.[6]

METHODS.—Rocking beds can provide some ventilatory assistance but now need be mentioned only in a historical sense. Tank respirators (Fig. 3-3) are used much less now than in the past, but they may still offer certain advantages in patients with compliant chests and lungs who are able to co-operate, to handle their own secretions and somehow to manage the large quantity of air that may be drawn into their stomachs. Past victims of poliomyelitis with impaired ventilatory reserve who are already familiar with tank respirators and may need assistance briefly, as postoperatively, are probably the best candidates for this type of therapy. Cuirass respirators find even less use than tank respirators. The chief theoretical advantage of external positive-negative pressure respirators over ventilators which apply positive pressure to an airway is that the use of an endotracheal or tracheostomy tube may be avoided if not otherwise indicated.

The great majority of ventilatory assistance is furnished by machines which provide positive pressure to the airway. These may be volume-controlled,[11] a set

Fig. 3-3.—Emerson tank respirator. **1,** hand operation handle. **2,** connecting rod. **3,** hand operation lever. **4,** respiration rate adjustment. **5,** negative pressure adjustment. **6,** auxiliary electric outlets. **7,** motor switch. **8,** light switch. **9,** positive pressure adjustment. **10,** tilting jack valve. **11,** tilting jack handle. **12,** head-rest adjustment. **13,** bed height adjustments. **14,** socket for intravenous rod. **15,** pressure gauge **16,** instruction panel. **17,** alarm. **18,** dome pressure gauge. **19,** intravenous tube opening and stopper. **20,** mirror and book-rest supports. **21,** collar clamp ring. **22,** head-end closing clamps.

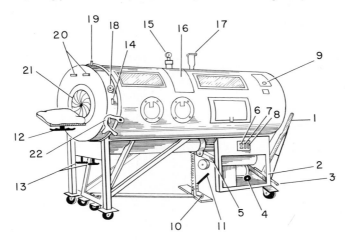

volume being delivered regardless of pressures required, or pressure-controlled,[13] the inspiratory phase ceasing when a certain airway pressure is reached regardless of volume delivered to the patient. Constant-volume ventilators are indicated for patients with changing compliance, as those with severe pneumonia or contused lungs, so that an adequate minute ventilation will be reliably delivered even though pressures required for delivery change markedly. Pressure-cycled machines find their best use when it is desirable to have the patient initiate each breath. A constant-volume ventilator allowing patient initiation of inspiration has recently been introduced but is not yet widely used. Both pressure-cycled and volume-controlled ventilators can satisfactorily deliver the small volumes at rapid rates that may be required by the pediatric patient. Volume ventilators in current use are capable of overcoming the deadspace problem even in newborns by using slightly increased minute volumes in a one-way circle with a Y-connector at the airway. Pressure-controlled ventilators have been adapted to reduce deadspace by using small circles with valves near the patient and constantly clearing the lines in the circle by means of a small Venturi-generated negative pressure.[1] These circles are available in two sizes, for infants and for children. The negative pressure clearance of the circle also makes the system sensitive enough for patient-initiated assisted ventilation even in a newborn infant.

STERILIZATION OF EQUIPMENT

Ventilators and other equipment used in respiratory care may infect already debilitated patients unless stringent precautions are taken. Most apparatus requires sterilization as well as thorough physical cleaning before use by a second patient. Equipment used for several days on one patient should be re-sterilized daily, and regular cultures should be taken from ventilators and nebulizers. Though high-pressure steam sterilization is effective, it damages many materials in current use. For many years, articles which did not withstand steam sterilization could only be chemically treated. Liquid germicides include mercurials, phenolic compounds, quaternary ammonium compounds, chlorine compounds, iodine and iodophors, alcohols, formaldehyde and gluteraldehyde.[22] Gluteraldehyde destroys tubercle bacilli, viruses and spores; it does not usually damage plastic, rubber or metals. Now, most airway equipment, tubings, instruments and even ventilators can be best sterilized by ethylene oxide, which penetrates cellophane and polyethylene wrappers[16] (Fig. 3-4). Ten per cent ethylene oxide in 90% carbon dioxide is not flammable. Four hours' exposure at 130C produces effective sterilization, but equipment must be aired 48 hours before use because of the vesicant action of ethylene oxide. Although the process is time-consuming, it makes possible adequate sterilization of virtually all equipment. Most steam sterilizers can be converted for ethylene oxide sterilization.

EQUIPMENT FOR RESUSCITATION

The respiratory therapy department often maintains emergency resuscitative equipment throughout the hospital. The particular items to be provided should be decided on by a member or group of the medical staff, and also the number of kits and their locations. Kits should be replenished and inspected at regular intervals as well as after each use, and should not be used except in emergencies. Oxygen and suction should be available at each location chosen for emergency equipment.

OTHER SERVICES

Maintenance of miscellaneous types of equipment such as hypothermia machines and blankets, Isolettes and suction equipment often falls to the respiratory therapy department. Facilities for blood gas determinations, essential in the management of patients on respirators, must be provided.

Education in Inhalation Therapy

A definite responsibility in respiratory care which may be overlooked is that of teaching. Inhalation therapists have usually received on-the-job training, though some consideration has been given to a junior college program.[5] Standards for inhalation therapy schools have been set forth by the Council on Medical Education and Hospitals of the American Medical Association. The American Association of Inhalation Therapists now examines and registers qualified personnel. Continuing education is essential for inhalation therapists, nursing personnel and physicians, particularly regarding the capabilities and limitations of available equipment.

The question of education for lay personnel in resuscitative methods arises, as well as the even more controversial question of how much should be done in caring for the patient, routinely and in case of emergency, by non-physician paramedical personnel such as the inhalation therapist.[23] Answers to these problems will probably become apparent only with the continued evolution of over-all medical care.

REFERENCES

1. Ahlegren, E. W., and Stephen, C. R.: Mechanical ventilation of the infant, Anesthesiology 27:692, 1966.
2. Andrews, A. H. (ed.): *Proceedings of the First Conference on Clinical Applications of the Ultrasonic Nebulizer* (Somerset, Pa.: The DeVilbiss Company, 1966).
3. Bendixen, H. H., *et al.: Respiratory Care* (St. Louis: C. V. Mosby Company, 1965).
4. Caldwell, P. R. B., *et al.*: Changes in lung volume, diffusion capacity, and blood gases in men breathing oxygen,

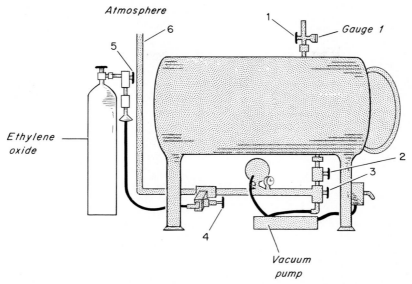

Fig. 3-4.—Ethylene oxide sterilizer. Sterilization takes place after air is removed from the chamber of the autoclave and ethylene oxide is allowed to enter and remain for 6 hours. After sterilization is completed, ethylene oxide is removed by a vacuum process and atmospheric air then enters.

J. Appl. Physiol. 21:1477, 1966.

5. Collins, V. J., *et al.*: Guide book for an approved school of inhalation therapy, Inhal. Therap. 10:16, 1965.
6. Damman, J. F., Jr.: Indications for tracheostomy, Ann. New York Acad. Sc. 121:849, 1965.
7. Downes, J. J., *et al.*: Diagnosis and treatment: Advances in the management of status asthmaticus in children, Pediatrics 38:286, 1966.
8. Drinker, P., and Shaw, L.: An apparatus for the prolonged administration of artificial respiration, J. Clin. Invest. 7:229, 1929.
9. DuBois, A. B., *et al.*: Pulmonary atelectasis in subjects breathing oxygen at sea level or at simulated altitude, J. Appl. Physiol. 21:828, 1966.
10. Eisenbert, L.: History of inhalation therapy equipment, Internat. Anesth. Clin. 4:549, 1966.
11. Engstrom, C. G.: The clinical application of prolonged controlled ventilation, Acta anaesth. scandinav., suppl. XIII, 1963.
12. Hedley-Whyte, J.; Laver, M. B., and Bendixen, H. H.: Effect of changes in tidal ventilation on physiologic shunting, Am. J. Physiol. 206:891, 1964.
13. Herzog, H.: Pressure-cycled ventilators, Ann. New York Acad. Sc. 121:751, 1965.
14. Herzog, P.; Norlander, O. P., and Engstrom, C. G.: Ultrasonic generation of aerosol for the humidification of inspired gas during volume-controlled ventilation, Acta anaesth. scandinav. 8:79, 1964.
15. Lassen, H. C. A.: Preliminary report on the 1952 epidemic of poliomyelitis in Copenhagen with special reference to the treatment of acute respiratory insufficiency, Lancet 1:37, 1953.
16. Lloyd, R. S.: Ethylene oxide sterilization of medical and surgical supplies, J. Hosp. Res. 1:1, 1963.
17. Mushin, W. W.; Rendell-Baker, L., and Thompson, P. W.: *Automatic Ventilation of the Lungs* (Springfield, Ill.: Charles C Thomas, Publisher, 1959).
18. Nash, G.; Blennerhasset, J. B., and Pontoppidan, H.: Pulmonary lesions associated with oxygen therapy and artificial ventilation, New England J. Med. 276:367, 1967.
19. Northway, W. H.; Rosan, R. C., and Porter, D. Y.: Pulmonary disease following respiratory therapy, New England J. Med. 276:357, 1967.
20. Pierce, E. C., Jr., and Vandam, L. D.: Intermittent positive pressure breathing, Anesthesiology 23:478, 1962.
21. Safar, P. (ed.): *Respiratory Therapy* (Philadelphia: F. A. Davis Company, 1965).
22. Spaulding, E. H.: Chemical disinfection in the hospital, J. Hosp. Res. 3:1, 1965.
23. Stead, E. A.: Conserving costly talents—providing physicians new assistants, J.A.M.A. 198:1108, 1966.

DEAN CROCKER
BETTY L. B. GRUNDY
Drawings by
D. RICE *and*
PAMELA BERGLUND

4

Preoperative and Postoperative Care

Neonates

THE PREOPERATIVE AND POSTOPERATIVE care of infants differs in many important respects from that of adults. Special consideration must be given to nursing care, the management of psychologic adjustments or maladjustments in hospital and the medical complications which arise after operations. These differences are particularly pronounced in infants, especially newborns. This discussion deals therefore primarily with the managment of infants and more particularly with infants during the first 4 weeks of life (neonates). It is in the care of these small babies that most mistakes have been made in the past. Many surgeons who occasionally operate on small infants know very little about their nursing care, normal physiologic reactions, intravenous therapy, feeding and other problems. They are frequently only too glad to leave these matters to the pediatricians and thus become, as William Ladd has aptly said, "surgical technicians." Unfortunately, the pediatrician is not always the ideal person to look after pre- and postoperative management. He is a specialist in medical pediatrics and often not very familiar with problems encountered before and after operation. A surgeon who wants to operate on small infants should acquaint himself with current thoughts on pre- and postoperative management. Any skilled surgeon may be able to operate on an infant, but whether this child lives or dies often depends mainly on what happens to him before and after operation.

Lack of space forbids a lengthy discussion on the various views held by pediatric surgeons on pre- and postoperative care. This discussion is based on the experience gained during the past 14 years in the Neonatal Surgical Unit at Alder Hey Children's Hospital, Liverpool, where more than two and a half thousand newborn infants were admitted during this period. The management of older infants is discussed only when it differs markedly from that of neonates. This account must be brief and tends therefore to be dogmatic. It is fully realized that different methods have proved equally successful elsewhere and that in working in different climates with different patient material, other methods may be more advisable. Be that as it may, the methods which we have found moderately successful, and the lessons which we have learned from the many mistakes we have made, may be of some value to those who want to practice this difficult but fascinating branch of surgery.

Management of Neonates during Transport

The large team of pediatric specialists, surgeons, physicians, anesthesiologists, pathologists, radiologists, biochemists, nurses and others necessary for dealing satisfactorily with newborn infants subjected to operation will usually be available only in a few centers.[46] In England and even more in the United States, transporting these infants safely over considerable distances is therefore very important.[5, 20] As approximately two children per thousand live births require urgent surgery,[37] the size of the problem is not inconsiderable.

Infants travel well even over long distances, provided certain precautions are taken.[40] During transport they should be nursed flat, lying on their sides. In those with suspected intestinal obstruction, a soft rubber nasogastric catheter no. 3 or 4 F. should be passed and aspirated with a syringe at 10-minute intervals. Should vomiting or respiratory obstruction occur in spite of these precautions, the accompanying nurse must have some simple but efficient apparatus, such as a mucus extractor, for aspirating the mouth and pharynx. Oxygen must always be available and may have to be administered by tube and funnel.

Care should be taken to prevent heat loss during transport, especially during the cold seasons, by using well-protected carry-cots or bassinets and by supplying extra warmth with hot water bottles. The latter must be kept at a distance from the child to prevent scalding. Premature infants should be transported in a portable incubator. The incubator used in our region (Fig. 4-1) is heated electrically from the car battery and the temperature remains constant at 85 F. Oxygen can be given; automatic control prevents concentrations of oxygen over 30%. A special device allows humidification of the atmosphere up to 80 or 90%. Heat loss of the infant by radiation is largely pre-

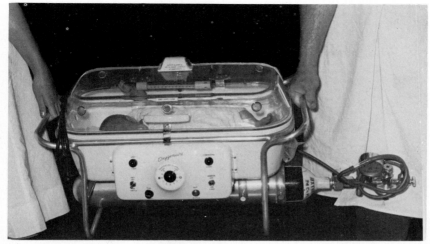

Fig. 4-1. — Light weight of the portable incubator allows it to be carried with ease. Control panel and oxygen cylinder are attached beneath the incubator.

vented by using an incubator with a double skin of Perspex.

Infants with large diaphragmatic hernias that cause marked respiratory distress may not survive transport unless an endotracheal tube is passed and positive pressure ventilation carried out during transport.

Management and Prevention of Infections

Only infants born in maternity hospitals and therefore known to be free from infection are admitted to the main neonatal surgical ward. Infants born at home or where there is some suspicion of contact with infection are admitted to isolation cubicles. As all infants are nursed postoperatively with a slightly positive pressure inside the incubator, air will flow out when the incubators are opened, and there is, therefore, little chance for air-borne infection to enter. All medical and nursing personnel wear masks and gowns and the hands are washed before handling each baby. On admission, babies are powdered with Zac baby powder that contains hexachlorophene, and powdering is repeated daily.

ANTIBIOTICS AND ANTISEPTICS. — On admission and for 5 days after operation, the infant is routinely given parenteral injections of streptomycin 25 mg/lb of body weight, and calcium penicillin 125,000 units daily.

If infections occur, specific antibiotics are given after culturing the organism and testing for drug sensitivity. The administration of broad-spectrum antibiotics by mouth to reduce the pathogenic intestinal flora is not encouraged because a few infants have died of fulminating staphylococcic enteritis

following oral medication with broad-spectrum antibiotics.

Thrush is routinely treated with 1% watery solution of gentian violet or nystatin paint made from a suspension containing 25,000 units/cc.

VITAMINS. — Every infant receives an injection of 1 mg of vitamin K on admission. Once the child is on oral feeding, 25 mg of ascorbic acid is given orally twice a day.

Management of Vomiting and Ileus

The most common cause of death in infants during the preoperative and postoperative periods is vomiting and aspiration of vomitus. An infant who suddenly collapses and becomes gray or cyanosed with signs of respiratory embarrassment has almost certainly vomited and aspirated some vomitus, whether or not there is external evidence of vomiting. Unless the air passages are immediately cleared, the infant will probably die. The management of vomiting infants is twofold: prevention and emergency treatment.

PREVENTION. — Infants admitted with a history of vomiting or with a suspected intestinal obstruction have a no. 10 F. soft rubber catheter passed through the nostril into the stomach and aspiration carried out with a syringe. The catheter is then connected to a continuous suction device. A low-powered electric suction pump is used. The pump may produce such a strong negative pressure that the gastric mucosa will be sucked into the catheter opening, causing blockage of the catheter and bleeding from the mucosa. The negative pressure must therefore be reduced by incorporating into the circuit a bottle partly filled with water (Fig. 4-2). A long straight glass tube dips into

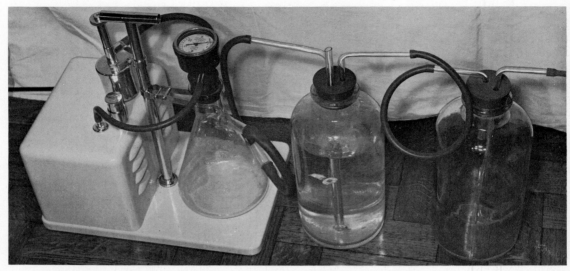

Fig. 4-2.—Continuous gastric suction apparatus. On the left is the small electric sucker. The bottle on the right receives the aspirated material. The center bottle controls the negative pressure. Air bubbles are rising from the lower end of the glass tube dipping into the water.

the water for a variable distance and the negative suction pressure causes air to be sucked through the tube into the bottle; air bubbles will be seen coming out of the lower end of the tube dipping into the water. By varying the length of the tube beneath the water level, the strength of the negative pressure can be altered. In our practice, a negative pressure of 8 in. has been found to be most suitable for newborn babies.

In spite of these precautions, the catheter may block, and a nurse must aspirate it by syringe at half-hourly or hourly intervals. Color, consistency and amount of the aspirated fluid must be recorded.

EMERGENCY TREATMENT.—It occasionally happens that the infant vomits in spite of all preventive de-

Fig. 4-3.—Emergency tray, with laryngoscope, endotracheal catheter and connectors, thin rubber catheters for sucking out trachea and bronchi, and rubber bag connected to an Ayre T-piece.

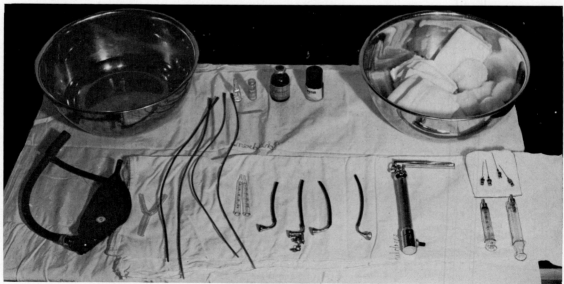

vices. He must therefore be observed constantly, and a powerful electric sucker must be available for aspirating mouth and pharynx at a moments's notice. An emergency tray with laryngoscopes, sterile endotracheal and suction tubes as well as syringes, appropriate drugs and other aids always stands in the ward (Fig. 4-3), and an anesthesiologist experienced in intubating small infants is on call in the hospital day and night.

Infants with ileus must be put on constant gastric suction at a negative pressure of 8 in. of water supplemented by hourly hand aspiration. In the majority of cases this will reduce abdominal distention to a remarkable degree, even if the obstruction is low in the intestine, and we have not found it necessary to resort to intestinal suction tubes.[49] Abdominal distention is a dangerous condition. The newborn infant uses only the diaphragm for respiration, and abdominal distention will markedly interfere with respiratory excursions. Infants should therefore be nursed with the head end of the cot or incubator slightly elevated to allow gravity to counteract the pressure exerted by the abdominal contents on the diaphragm. Although it has been shown that nursing in high concentrations of oxygen will improve abdominal distention, the dangers of high oxygen concentrations to the eyes of newborn infants[26] militate against concentrations in excess of 30%.

Control of Body Temperature

The body temperature of newborn infants readily falls. This is especially true for premature infants whose body temperature often tends to fluctuate with the environmental temperature.[47] The relatively larger body surface area and the high metabolic rate and small amount of subcutanious fat allow heat to be lost much more rapidly from newborn infants than from adults.

During the pre- and postoperative periods, body temperature must frequently be determined. This is facilitated by using an electric thermometer with an anal lead, thereby allowing frequent temperature readings to be taken without the risk of exhausting the infant by repeated handling (Fig. 4-4).

By varying the temperature inside the incubator, the body temperature of the infant can be satisfactorily controlled, allowing him to be nursed naked and simplifying nursing supervision. All newborn infants admitted to the Neonatal Surgical Unit are nursed in special surgical incubators.[45] These incubators are so constructed that all nursing procedures, the taking of blood samples, setting up of intravenous drips, and so on, can be carried out without removing the infant from the incubator (Fig. 4-5). The incubators have their own oxygen supply and drip stands attached, and the child can be transported in them from the ward to the operating table and vice versa.

Full-term infants are kept at a constant incubator temperature of 85 F. When nursing premature infants, the temperature has frequently to be raised to 90 F or even 95 F in order to keep their body temperature above 95 F. To protect these infants from sudden heat loss when the incubator is opened, they are placed in a special hot room during the immediate postoperative period. This room is air-conditioned with constant temperature of 80–85 F and humidity of 90% (Fig. 4-6).

Infants lose heat not only by convection but also by evaporation and radiation, so the ambient temperature is not the only environmental condition which must be controlled. Loss of body heat can be very

Fig. 4-4 (left).—Infant nursed postoperatively in surgical incubator, showing temperature taken with an electric thermometer and anal lead, gastric aspiration via nasogastric tube, and scalp vein drip. Large sliding doors at the front of the incubator allow easy access to the infant.

Fig. 4-5 (right).—Intravenous infusion being set up by cutting down on the internal saphenous vein in front of the right internal malleolus while the infant lies in the incubator.

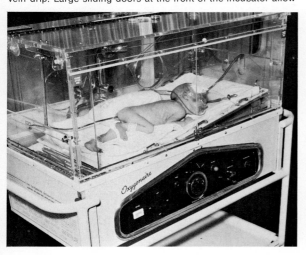

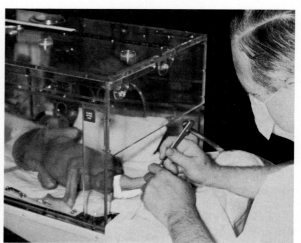

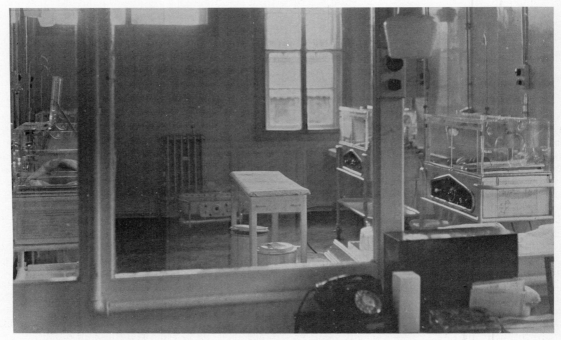

Fig. 4-6. — Hot room with incubators. Large window allows constant inspection from the nurses' duty room.

considerable, especially when the incubator stands near a cold surface, such as an outside window. Additional protection can be given against heat loss by radiation by surrounding the incubator with a double skin of Perspex or by nursing the infant in the incubator under a curved Perspex screen.

In older infants, the temperature control center is more mature, but even infants of some months of age may have their temperature-regulating center temporarily disturbed by dehydration, toxemia or other conditions. During the postoperative phase, their temperature should therefore be constantly watched, as sudden hyperpyrexia and collapse are not uncommon. Facilities for tepid sponging and fanning must always be at hand. If these simple methods do not bring the temperature down quickly, a very rapid drop of the body temperature can be effected by repeated injections of 10 ml of ice-cold saline into the stomach through a stomach tube, leaving the saline in situ for 2 minutes before aspirating it again. Care must be taken that the temperature does not drop too far.

EFFECTS OF PROLONGED EXPOSURE OF THE NEWBORN TO COLD. — If a newborn infant is exposed to cold for a prolonged period, his body temperature will be lowered. The carbon dioxide contents of the extracellular fluid will be decreased and the acidity increased. The metabolic rate will be increased and the depletion of energy stores will be accelerated. Acidosis, hyperkalaemia and hypoglycaemia will develop.

SCLEREMA NEONATORUM. — Newborn infants under-going major operation not infrequently develop sclerema neonatorum. This dreaded complication is especially common in premature infants but may affect any newborn child. The subcutaneous fat solidifies, encasing the body in a rigid shell.[24] The thighs, abdomen and chest especially are involved. The condition is often fatal since it interferes with respiratory excursions in an already gravely ill infant. Although it has been commonly assumed that sclerema is closely connected to a drop of the infant's body temperature, investigations carried out in our Unit[25] have shown no relationship between sclerema and low body temperature. Its true etiology remains undiscovered.

The milder degrees of sclerema tend to disappear spontaneously if the patient's general condition improves. Many therapeutic measures have been suggested, such as elevation of the environmental temperature and administration of glucose and cortisone.[57] Series of one or two "cures" have been published, although it is quite possible that these patients may have improved spontaneously. Severe cases of sclerema appear to be invariably fatal, even if one uses the three methods outlined above.

Management of Radiographic and Diagnostic Aids

It has been mentioned already that newborn infants who are ill and have to undergo a major operation tolerate handling very poorly. This fact is especially important when considering radiography which

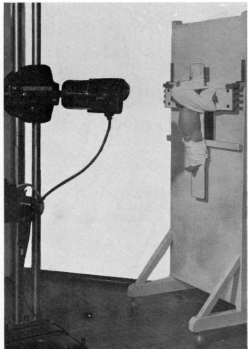

Fig. 4-7. — Mobile roentgen screen. The infant is bandaged to the crucifix, and the head also bandaged to it to prevent its falling forward.

Fig. 4-8. — The drawer beneath the tray on which the baby is nursed is drawn out and the x-ray plate put in position.

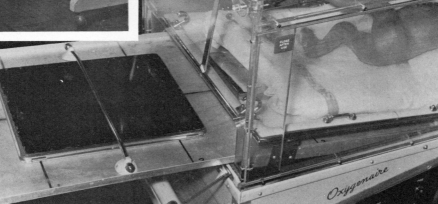

must be carried out preoperatively in most cases.

The danger of radiation to infants is well known, even when small dosages are administered.[9] Fortunately, practically all cases of obstruction of the alimentary tract require only one x-ray film for diagnosis, provided this picture includes both chest and abdomen and is taken in the anteroposterior view with the patient upright. Contrast medium is rarely needed.

It is of great importance that these infants not be sent to the radiology department to mingle with older children from whom they may contract infections. All roentgenograms are taken in our Unit with a portable x-ray machine permanently situated in the ward. Holding the infants in an upright position during roentgenography will expose the nurses to an undue amount of radiation. To avoid this danger and still obtain satisfactory pictures, a screen for suspending the infant should be used.[35] The screen used in our Unit[42] consists of a mobile lead shield. The infant is bandaged on a crucifix and suspended in front of the screen with a cassette fixed behind (Fig. 4-7).

Postoperatively, radiography usually is limited to the diagnosis of chest complications. The surgical incubators have facilities for radiography to be carried out while the infant lies in the incubator (Fig. 4-8), thus avoiding further exposure to sepsis.

Management of Respiratory Complications

The newborn infant's lung capacity is very limited and barely enough for normal requirements. The slightest interference with respiration may therefore result in respiratory distress. The danger of abdominal distention interfering with respiration has already been mentioned.

Many of these infants are admitted with such lung complications as pulmonary collapse and pneumonia caused by aspiration of mucus (as in esophageal atresia) or vomitus (as in intestinal obstruction). It is not surprising, therefore, that lung complications are of frequent postoperative occurrence.

Postoperative pulmonary collapse is especially common in grossly premature infants. Often they have an imperfectly developed cough and swallowing reflex and may aspirate saliva and mucus.

It has already been mentioned that the infants are nursed with the head end of the incubator tray slightly elevated. They lie on their sides and are turned from side to side every 2 hours to facilitate adequate aeration of both lungs. The greatest single factor in the prevention of lung complications is exposure to an atmosphere of 100% humidity. This will tend to liquefy the sticky mucus in the air passages and facilitate expectoration. The humidity in the incubator can be raised to about 80%. A special water vaporizer is incorporated which will increase the atmospheric humidity to 100%.

Because of respiratory difficulties, many infants need to be placed in an oxygen-enriched atmosphere. The relationship between too high an oxygen concentration and retrolental fibroplasia has already been mentioned.[26] It must be stressed that it is not the oxygen concentration in the surrounding atmosphere which matters but the concentration in the infant's blood. If the infant is still dangerously cyanosed when nursed in a 30% concentration of oxygen, we do not hesitate to increase the oxygen concentration until the cyanosis disappears. So far, we have not seen retrolental fibroplasia resulting from this policy.

If pulmonary collapse occurs, the infant is nursed with the collapsed side uppermost and is only turned onto the other side for 10 minutes every 2 hours. This simple maneuver, coupled with gentle tapping of the affected side of the chest, will in most cases shift the mucus plug blocking the bronchus. Only infrequently is it necessary to resort to endotracheal intubation and toilet. Bronchoscopy is very rarely required, mainly with collapse of the left lung, when catheters passed through the endotracheal tube will not enter the left main bronchus. Infants who have had lung collapse and had their air passages cleared may not resume spontaneous respiration for prolonged periods. Positive pressure ventilation may then have to be instituted, using one of the many mechanical respirators suitable for newborn infants.

Special care must be taken when nursing infants with tracheostomy. They must be placed in an atmosphere of 100% humidity and constantly observed, as the small tubes employed may easily become blocked with mucus. Soft rubber catheters of appropriate size

and a powerful electric sucker must be at hand. These catheters should be kept in sterile solution.

Fluid Therapy

Intravenous Infusion

If an infant is unable to take adequate amounts of fluid by mouth, parenteral therapy must be instituted. Fluids formerly were administered by such methods as colonic irrigation, subcutaneous and intramarrow infusions. These methods are now out of date as it is impossible to supply adequate amounts of water, salts and proteins by these routes. Furthermore, intramarrow infusions carry a great risk of infection. In the past, reluctance to employ the intravenous route was due to the technical difficulties related to the tiny veins of small infants. Undoubtedly it is more difficult to set up intravenous infusions in infants than in adults, but with experience and a meticulous technique it is possible to keep infants on infusions for prolonged periods. Although, in general, infants do not suffer from prolonged postoperative ileus, it may occur when the intestinal lumen has been opened either before or during the operation. Parenteral fluid therapy may thus be necessary for many days. We have had to keep newborn infants on continuous intravenous infusions for periods of up to 30 days.

Two methods of intravenous infusion are employed: the cut-down, where a cannula is inserted into a vein which is surgically exposed, and percutaneous venipuncture. We cut down only once, just before operation, to allow for the transfusion of large amounts of blood if required, and to protect against dislodgment of the cannula from the vein on transport to and from the operating room. The infusion usually can be allowed to run for 48 hours or more. All subsequent infusions are given through needles inserted into a scalp vein. Scalp vein infusions can be repeated many times if each infusion is not allowed to run for more than 24 hours. In older infants with more subcutaneous fat, scalp veins are often difficult to see, and it is then better to insert a needle into a vein on the dorsum of the wrist or ankle.

Cut-down. — The foot, leg and thigh are strapped to a padded right-angled splint (Fig. 4-9, *A*) and the internal saphenous vein is exposed in front of the internal malleolus through a small horizontal incision. The distal end of the vein is ligated and the ligature used for traction on the vein (Fig. 4-9, *B*). A 0000 catgut ligature is then passed beneath the proximal segment of the vein and a small transverse incision into the vein is made with a pair of sharp scissors or a fine triangular blade. A no. 4 polyethylene catheter cut obliquely (in premature infants a no. 3 catheter may be all that is feasible) is then introduced for a distance of at least 1 in. up the vein and the proximal ligature is tied firmly around the vein and the catheter (Fig. 4-9, *C*). The wound is then closed. The seg-

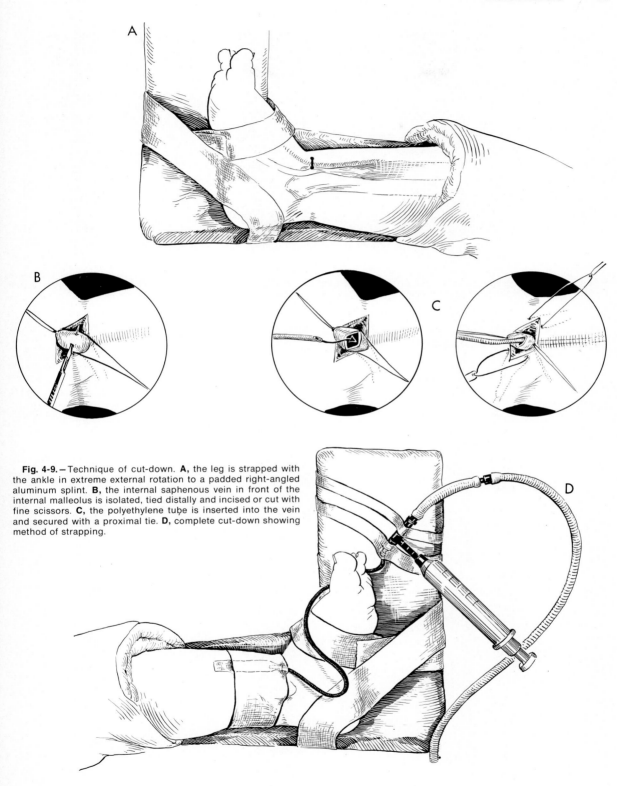

Fig. 4-9.—Technique of cut-down. **A,** the leg is strapped with the ankle in extreme external rotation to a padded right-angled aluminum splint. **B,** the internal saphenous vein in front of the internal malleolus is isolated, tied distally and incised or cut with fine scissors. **C,** the polyethylene tube is inserted into the vein and secured with a proximal tie. **D,** complete cut-down showing method of strapping.

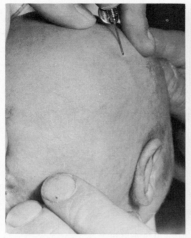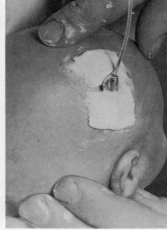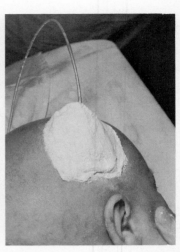

Fig. 4-10. — Technique of scalp infusion. **Left,** needle is placed alongside a scalp vein before piercing the skin. Note immobilization of the head by an assistant. **Center,** after the vein is entered, plaster of paris strips are built up to support the needle. **Right,** finished plaster of paris cap fixes the needle securely to the scalp.

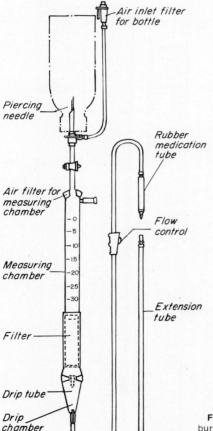

Air inlet filter for bottle

Piercing needle

Rubber medication tube

Air filter for measuring chamber

Flow control

—0
—5
—10
—15
—20
—25
—30

Measuring chamber

Extension tube

Filter

Drip tube

Drip chamber

Fig. 4-11. — Disposable plastic infusion set incorporating a buret graduated in cubic centimeters.

ment of the isolated vein markedly contracts with manipulation, and it often appears impossible to insert a polyethylene tube of several times its apparent diameter, but patience and a little gentle pressure will usually allow insertion of the tube.

Insertion of scalp vein needle. — The baby's head is shaved and an assistant holds it firmly between his hands. The special scalp vein needle with a length of polyethylene tube attached is then gently inserted through the skin just alongside a scalp vein and about 1 cm away from a bifurcation (Fig. 4-10). The vein is then punctured and the needle inserted along the vein for a distance of 0.5–1 cm. If the lumen of the vein has been entered, blood often flows back through the needle and the attached polyethylene tube. If this does not happen, 0.5 cc of saline may be injected down the tube in order to see whether it flows into the vein or raises a subcutaneous wheal. The needle is then fixed by winding 10-cm-long strips of plaster of paris bandage around the needle to form a plaster cap which will fix the needle securely to the scalp (Fig. 4-10).

Whether a cut-down procedure or a scalp vein needle is used, the polyethylene tube is connected to a three-way tap. This is connected on one side to a 2-cc syringe and on the other to the infusion-giving set. This three-way tap and attached syringe are of great importance. They permit accurate control of the infusion rate, yet allow rapid administration of large quantities of blood into the infant's vein if necessary.

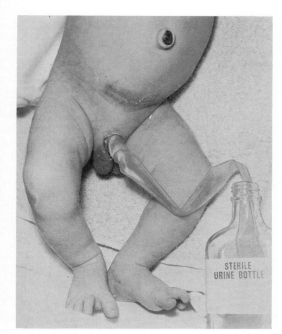

Fig. 4-12.—Collection of urine from male infant by means of Paul's tubing strapped to the penis.

To measure the slow rate of infusion accurately, a measuring buret graduated into cubic centimeters is incorporated into the drip set either as a separate glass buret[39] or incorporated in a plastic disposable set which we now employ (Fig. 4-11).

CHARTING.—Whenever intravenous therapy is employed, it is of the greatest importance to chart fluid intake and output accurately. The rate of infusion must be recorded hourly as cubic centimeters per hour, and as drops per minute, and the nature of the infused fluid must also be charted.

It is equally important to record the infant's output. In females, it is impossible to collect the urine with any reasonable accuracy, and one must rely on the observations of an experienced nurse about the number of wet diapers per day. In males, urine can be collected relatively simply by fixing a thin piece of Paul's colostomy tubing round the penis and connecting it to a bottle (Fig. 4-12). The gastric aspirations must also be collected and their nature and volume charted. The information collected is recorded on a fluid intake and output chart.

INTRAVENOUS WATER AND ELECTROLYTE REPLACEMENT

Contrary to what is often thought, disturbances of fluid and electrolyte balance are much less common during infancy than in adult life.[54] If they do occur, however, they may be very serious. Unfortunately, we know very little about the normal metabolism of newborn infants and even less about their metabolic response to surgical trauma. An enormous amount of research has been done on these subjects and many contradictory and conflicting reports have been published. It is therefore understandable that many surgeons dealing with small infants are somewhat confused about intravenous therapy. Nevertheless it is certain that unless the surgeon has a good understanding of the problems involved in pre- and postoperative fluid and electrolyte therapy in infancy, he will not get consistently satisfactory results. It is impossible to give a detailed description of the many views and theories which have been formulated and the description of the therapeutic methods, and the discussion must therefore be somewhat dogmatic. It must be emphasized that in a discussion of replacement therapy, only a very rough guide can be given and that every case must be considered separately on the basis of the individual clinical and biochemical findings. The methods outlined below are based on our experience with parenteral fluid replacement therapy in over a thousand newborn infants undergoing surgery during the past 14 years, on all of whom routine serial blood chemistry estimations had been performed. Experience has also been drawn from a small number of selected infants on whom metabolic balance studies and other special investigations were carried out. Over half of these infants were operated on for intestinal obstruction.

WATER BALANCE AND REQUIREMENTS.—The total body water forms a considerably higher proportion in newborn infants than in adults, estimates varying from 70.2 to 83%.[19,21,16] The extracellular fluid volume is also relatively greater and constitutes about 40% of the body weight at birth.[18] As the body surface of an infant is relatively much larger and the respiratory rate higher than in adults, it is not surprising that the insensible water loss is relatively greater.[28] The efficiency of the neonatal kidneys to excrete water once was thought to be much less in neonates than in adults, but recent investigations have shown that the neonatal kidney is a remarkably efficient organ. When urinary excretion is compared on the basis of total body water, infants excrete urine as rapidly and as diluted as adults, although they cannot excrete within 4 hours the whole of a test dose of water given by mouth, as do adults.[28]

FLUID REPLACEMENT.—In the past, when confronted with the problem of intravenous fluid replacement in infants, pediatricians all over the world have accepted the time-honored basic figure of $2\frac{1}{2}$ oz/lb of body weight per day (165 cc/kg) for normal infants. In practice, much greater amounts of fluid have been given when dealing with older infants suffering from infective enteritis, pyloric stenosis and similar conditions.[11, 14] Fluid requirements of the newborn infant are both absolutely and relatively much smaller than those of older babies. For practical purposes, it can be assumed that a newborn infant weighing 3.5 kg will lose 90 cc/day as insensible water loss and a further 30–100 cc as urine per day. In other words, water will have to be replaced only at a rate of between 130 and 190 cc a day.[54] These normal fluid requirements are still further reduced by operative trauma,[40] although this response is not as conspicuous in newborn infants as that seen in adults following operation.[2, 10] Even more important is the fact that if infants are nursed in incubators in an atmosphere approaching 100% humidity, the insensible water loss is cut down by half,[34] or to almost 14 cc/kg of body weight per day.

Pediatric surgeons, remembering how infants used to be drowned by excessive postoperative intravenous therapy, have therefore tended to follow Gross's advice[23] to keep newborn infants on the dry side following operation. Fluid balance tests carried out during the postoperative period have confirmed the clinical impression that this treatment is correct.[41,55] In recent years, opposition to this view has been expressed by some pediatricians who routinely give much greater water loads to their newborn infants postoperatively without producing water intoxication in the majority.[29,30,58] As mentioned before, the neonatal kidney is a remarkably efficient organ and will stand overloading with water without ill effect in most although not in all cases. There is, however, little doubt that it is unwise to rely on the kidney of the newborn to withstand therapeutic assaults.

Finally, it should be mentioned that some recent investigations seem to suggest that sclerema neonatorum may be more likely to occur in infants who receive fluid replacement of only 20 cc/kg/day during the postoperative period.[25]

INTRAVENOUS FLUID THERAPY

NEWBORN INFANTS. — In the absence of dehydration and abnormal fluid losses from the gastrointestinal tract through vomiting and gastric suction, fluid replacement should not exceed 40 cc/kg of body weight per day during the early postoperative period.[41] These figures pertain to infants under 1 week of age. With increasing urinary output during the second week of life, fluid replacement must be increased. Clinical estimation of the state of hydration is most important in order to judge whether fluid replacement is adequate. The well-known signs of dehydration in infancy—a sunken fontanel, dry mucous membranes and a dry, inelastic skin—are noticeable only when 6% of the body water has already been lost.[12]

Urinary output gives a good indication of the state of hydration. It is normally 20–30 cc during the second and third day of life, rising to 120–150 cc by the seventh day.[50]

Of the laboratory investigations, the blood urea concentration is perhaps the most useful one for evaluating the state of hydration. An abnormally high blood urea level is observed frequently in newborn

infants and may be due to a variety of reasons,[3, 6, 27] but a normal concentration indicates that the infant is adequately hydrated. A falling blood urea concentration in an infant with abnormally high values indicates that fluid replacement is adequate.

Abnormal fluid losses from the gastrointestinal tract must be accurately measured, charted and replaced. When calculating such fluid loss, one must remember that in low intestinal obstruction a considerable amount of fluid may lie trapped in the lumen of the intestine and therefore be lost from the body fluid compartments.[36]

OLDER INFANTS. — In older infants, the conventional 2½ oz/lb of body weight (165 cc/kg) should be given, but it must be remembered that during the first 1 or 2 postoperative days they may suffer from considerable suppression of urinary excretion, and correspondingly smaller quantities should therefore be infused. In dehydrated infants, 100 cc/lb of body weight per day can be given with safety (220 cc/kg of body weight). Gastrointestinal fluid losses have to be meticulously replaced.

NITROGEN AND ELECTROLYTE BALANCE AND REQUIREMENTS

PHYSIOLOGY. — The normal infant is not just a miniature adult. He is growing rapidly and therefore he retains nitrogen to a remarkable degree for synthesis of tissue proteins. Potassium is retained to an even greater degree, considerably in excess of what would be expected from the potassium-nitrogen ratio in normal tissues.[53] The infant is supposed to have some difficulty in excreting sodium and potassium, but if there is adequate diuresis, even the neonatal kidney can manage the excretion of electrolytes surprisingly well. There is some limitation, however, to electrolyte excretion if large quantities are given by intravenous infusion.

NITROGEN REPLACEMENT. — Operation increases nitrogen breakdown and the urinary nitrogen excretion increases. As in adults, the increased urinary nitrogen excretion in infants is not greater than that found when the patient is starved. As most of these infants are not fed for several days following the operation, it is not surprising that the nitrogen loss is considerable.

Nitrogen can be administered intravenously either in the form of amino acids or protein hydrolysates or in the form of human plasma. On the whole, we prefer plasma infusions, as they do not cause thrombosis of the veins[29] commonly seen with some amino acid preparations, and supply all the necessary proteins. We have seen no infants with homologous serum hepatitis following plasma infusion. If adults are given plasma infusions, it appears to take several days before the body is able to break down the plasma proteins and utilize them.[1] Newborn infants do not seem to have this difficulty.[41] Postoperatively, the plasma protein concentration of infants falls rapidly, and, as in adults, the plasma volume decreases before the protein concentration drops.[30] Plasma infusions are therefore of the greatest use during the pre- and postoperative phases.

In newborn infants undergoing gastrointestinal operations, it is our practice to give daily between 50 and 100 cc of plasma diluted with an equal amount of 5% glucose solution (in order to halve the electrolyte concentration) from the second postoperative day onward.

In older infants who are dehydrated because of vomiting (e.g., cases of neglected pyloric stenosis), the first 40 cc of the 100 cc/lb of body weight of fluid replacement (see above) should be given in the form of diluted plasma during the first 6 hours of treatment, in order to restore their plasma volume to normal proportions and stimulate urinary excretion.

Once there is adequate nitrogen intake by mouth, marked nitrogen retention occurs in all infants to provide sufficient protein for growth.

The blood urea concentration in infants is less constant than in adults. Slight dehydration, fever or trauma tends to cause a marked rise of the blood urea. For this reason, an elevated blood urea value need not have the same serious prognosis as in adults. On the other hand, a normal reading always indicates that the infant is adequately hydrated. Postmature large infants delivered after a difficult labor show increased destruction of their body proteins during the first 48 hours after birth and often have an elevated blood urea.[28] These infants tolerate operative trauma badly and it is well to determine if the blood urea is markedly elevated before operation.

SODIUM AND CHLORIDE REPLACEMENTS: ALKALOSIS AND ACIDOSIS.—It is now generally accepted that if large amounts of saline are administered by intravenous infusion to infants, their kidneys have difficulty in dealing with the sudden load and there is less complete diuresis than in adults. Postoperative sodium and chloride retention is common, and it is therefore inadvisable to infuse large quantities of normal saline into young infants during the postoperative phase. This is especially true in newborn infants, who excrete very little sodium and potassium during the first days of life.

In infants who have no loss of gastrointestinal secretions by vomiting or gastric suction, it is usually not necessary to administer any sodium and chloride during the first 2 or 3 days of intravenous therapy, and 5% glucose solution is all that need be given.

The gastrointestinal juices of young infants contain nearly as much sodium and chloride as those of adults. Prolonged vomiting or continuous gastric suction will therefore result in loss of ions. The stomach contents of newborn infants exhibit a very acid reaction at birth but become practically neutral within the first week of life. Gastric suction will remove an excess of chloride ions over sodium ions and will tend to produce alkalosis. It often takes a number

of days of continuous gastric suction in infants before alkalosis develops. This delay in the development of alkalosis may be related to the fact that normal newborn infants often tend to develop acidosis with high plasma chloride levels.[1, 8, 14] If gastric suction must be prolonged for more than a week, alkalosis invariably results.

It is obvious that infants who are subjected to prolonged postoperative gastric suction must have the sodium and chloride replaced. We use 0.18% sodium chloride and 4.3% glucose solution for these cases. If laboratory and clinical studies indicate that further quantities of sodium and chlorides are needed, we do not hesitate to infuse 0.43% saline and 2.5% glucose solution, and very occasionally we have used small amounts of normal saline. This is rarely necessary since a considerable amount of saline is routinely administered when giving daily infusions of plasma (see above). Infants with prolonged gastrointestinal suction often develop alkalosis in spite of adequate sodium, chloride and potassium replacement, and treatment then becomes very difficult. These children tend to develop tetany and convulsions.[48] Theoretically, the alkalosis could be overcome by infusion of one-sixth molar ammonium chloride. Of this solution, 1 cc/kg of body weight should lower the alkali reserve by 0.43 mEq/liter.[15] In practice, we have found that ammonium chloride is not very effective in lowering the alkali reserve, probably due to the fact that most of these children have been subjected to extensive operative trauma, intestinal obstruction, prolonged gastric aspiration and intravenous infusions. They suffer from a depression of liver function and therefore have difficulty in breaking down the ammonia radical.[41] A much more satisfactory preparation for this purpose is a solution of Lysinmonochlorhydrate (1,000 ml containing 28.29 Gm Lysinmonochlorhydrate = 155 mval C).

Fortunately, we have rarely seen severe alkolosis leading to convulsions. It seems that adequate fluid and electrolyte replacement can prevent this dangerous complication to a large extent.

Severe acidosis is very rare in infancy and is practically seen only in infants with gross renal damage. If the acidosis reaches dangerous levels, it can be controlled by intravenous infusion of sodium lactate solution. Thus 4.4 cc of one-sixth molar solution of sodium lactate will lower the alkali reserve by 1 mEq/kg of body weight in a hypothetical case. A more efficient means of combating acidosis is the intravenous administration of bicarbonate solution.

It has been argued by some investigators that the changes in electrolyte equilibrium following prolonged suction in infants are so profound that it is impossible to maintain the equilibrium by intravenous therapy alone. It has been suggested that attempts should be made to replace the sucked-out gastrointestinal juices by feeding them back into the intestine via jejunostomy or ileostomy.[55] Although this is theoretically correct, we have usually found it perfectly feasible to maintain electrolyte balance by using suitable intravenous fluid and electrolyte replacements. We do not think that the added dangers and complications of enterostomies in newborn infants are justified.

POTASSIUM REPLACEMENT.—In recent years, interest has centered on the excessive excretion of potassium following surgical trauma. It has been known for some time that in potassium depletion the loss is mainly intracellular,[13] that surgery causes an increased potassium output,[4] that the potassium leaving the cell is replaced by sodium entering the cell even if there is no intake of sodium[17, 32] and that the increased potassium excretion is only partly derived from tissue breakdown[7] but mainly from intracellular fluids passing out of the cell through the intact cell membrane.[56]

When studying potassium loss following operation, one should remember that in normal newborn infants the plasma concentration is often considerably elevated and can range up to 9.8 mEq/liters.[46] It must also be realized that infants retain potassium three to four times in excess of that needed for protein synthesis.[53]

Moore and Ball[33] showed that after operation in adults, the ratio of excreted potassium to nitrogen is considerably in excess of that in lean muscle tissue; that is, more potassium is excreted than can be accounted for by tissue breakdown due to starvation.

In older infants, especially following operation necessitating prolonged drainage of gastrointestinal fluid (which contains considerable amounts of potassium), potassium must be replaced intravenously.

In newborn infants, the problem is somewhat different. Not only do they excrete very little potassium in the urine during the first few days of life, but following operation the potassium diuresis is much less marked than that in older infants, children and adults, and the potassium-nitrogen ratio in the urine is the same as that for lean muscle tissue; that is, there is no potassium shift.[41]

It follows that in newborn infants who have no marked loss of gastrointestinal fluid before and after operation, it is unnecessary to give any potassium during the first 3 or 4 postoperative days. When there is marked loss, this must be replaced, and it should be remembered that the gastric aspirations in newborn infants contain nearly as much potassium as those of adults.[41] We have found that apart from the diluted daily plasma infusions referred to above, daily infusions of 50–100 cc of Darrow's solution (containing 35.7 mEq/liter of potassium chloride) is usually sufficient in newborn infants.

In older infants, especially in those who are already dehydrated from prolonged vomiting, as infants suffering from pyloric stenosis, the regimen must be different.

These infants receive 100 cc/lb of body weight dur-

ing the first 24 hours. During the first 6 hours, 40 cc/lb of body weight is given as diluted plasma to re-expand the blood volume; during the following 12 hours, 40 cc of Darrow's solution per lb of body weight is given, and during the last 6 hours, 20 cc/lb of body weight of 0.18% saline and 5% glucose solution is administered. This regimen, first devised for infants suffering from gastroenteritis, has also proved valuable in infants suffering from dehydration due to preoperative vomiting.

CALCIUM AND MAGNESIUM REPLACEMENT.—It is usually not necessary to give calcium parenterally to neonates during the first postoperative days. Once the infant is given milk feedings, he will receive a satisfactory oral calcium intake. If gastric suction has to be employed for many days or if there is profuse diarrhea, it is necessary to watch the plasma calcium concentration closely and if necessary to give a 10% solution of calcium gluconate intravenously if the plasma calcium level sinks too low or if tetany develops.

Magnesium loss during the postoperative period is usually not excessive. In infants with very large intestinal losses by ileostomy or fecal fistulas or in infants whose proximal jejunum has been resected, serious magnesium losses may develop, with epileptiform convulsions and tetany. Surgeons must therefore be aware of this possibility and perform repeated plasma magnesium estimations in patients at risk. The prevention of magnesium deficiency in such patients by the daily administration of 4 mEq of magnesium chloride or acetate should be considered.

LABORATORY CONTROL.—The above rules are only a very rough guide to intravenous fluid and electrolyte therapy. It must be stressed that each infant should be assessed and treated individually. Clinical evaluation of the patient is by far the most important guide to therapy. Occasionally, a few laboratory data are helpful. We have found that daily estimations of plasma proteins, blood urea, plasma chlorides, sodium, potassium and alkali reserve are all that is needed. These estimations are of value only if they can be performed speedily and accurately, using micromethods necessitating less than a total of 1 cc of blood obtained from a heel stab.

INTRAVENOUS CALORIC INTAKE.—During the first 2 weeks of life, infants do not reach the normal caloric intake of 80 calories/kg of body weight. Caloric replacement is therefore not of great importance. If infants are kept on intravenous therapy for prolonged periods and are unable to take food by mouth, the caloric intake becomes a great problem. The few calories given by plasma and 5% glucose infusions will be of little practical importance. We have found that 10% glucose[23] or invert sugar[51] infusions are useful but tend to thrombose the infant's veins when given at the slow drip rates which we employ. Intravenous infusion of fat emulsion (Lipomul) using 15% cottonseed oil emulsion combined with 4% glucose solution, providing 1,350 calories/liter, is now manufactured commercially. Our experience with this emulsion in newborn infants has been very satisfactory. In infants needing prolonged gastric suction and intravenous infusions, 90–100 cc of the infusion has been given daily, in some cases for up to a week. Clinically, all of these infants did very well and there have been no serious reactions. A considerable degree of lipemia was occasionally observed if the emulsion was given for more than 3 consecutive days, but this usually disappeared within a day after emulsion infusion had been stopped. We were, however, unable to demonstrate an increased nitrogen retention in these infants, which has been observed in adults.[52]

Blood Transfusions: Blood Replacement

Newborn infants have a high hemoglobin concentration, often up to 20 Gm/100 ml. This drops rapidly during the first 2 weeks of life as physiologic hemolysis occurs. Later, the speed of hemolysis is greatly diminished, but in England, infants 3 months of age rarely have a hemoglobin concentration of more than 10 Gm/100 ml.

In spite of the initial high hemoglobin concentration in newborn infants, blood loss at operation should be meticulously measured and replaced. Of the various methods for blood loss estimations,[38] many are not accurate enough when operating on small infants. We have found the electrocalorimetric method to be satisfactory. The drapes and sponges of the operation are washed in 10 liters of water to which a small amount of ammonia and detergent is added, and the determination is made on this water. It is our practice to transfuse 10–20 cc more blood than was estimated to be lost during a given operative procedure.

When massive blood transfusions have to be given, there is danger of citrate intoxication. This can be prevented by the intravenous administration of 10% calcium gluconate solution. In a neonate weighing 3.5 kg, 50 mg of calcium gluconate should be given with every 100 ml of blood transfused.

The hemoglobin concentration must be watched postoperatively. If it falls below 12 Gm/100 ml, small replacement transfusions should be given.

Special Problems of Intravenous Therapy in Premature Infants

In these babies, the water requirements are relatively and absolutely less than in full-term newborn infants. It has been the practice of many pediatricians to give no fluids for the first 3 or 4 days of life, and it has been shown that infants treated in this way lose about the same amount of weight as those who have been fed.[22] Many premature babies have considerable generalized edema, and injudicious intravenous therapy may aggravate the condition. It is therefore our practice to give no infusions during the first 2 postoperative days unless considerable amounts are lost by gastric aspiration. Thereafter, the fluid lost by aspiration is replaced and a further 3–5 cc/hour, according to the weight of the child, is added.[39]

The kidneys of premature infants have more difficulty in excreting sodium and chloride than those of full-term infants, and in general nothing but 5 or 10% glucose infusions are given postoperatively unless the losses caused by vomiting and aspiration have to be replaced. There is little potassium loss after operation and no potassium shift. Administration of potassium intravenously is therefore not necessary unless there are large continuous potassium losses from the gastrointestinal tract.

The initial hemoglobin concentration of premature infants is very high, but the concentration falls rapidly and many of these infants tend to become anemic. Repeated small blood transfusions during the postoperative period are often necessary to keep the blood volume and hematocrit within normal range.

Feeding

Oral feeding. — It will be seen from the foregoing discussion that there are considerable dangers and difficulties connected with intravenous alimentation in infants. The sooner these infants can be put on oral feeding the better. Once the infant is on milk feeding, metabolic disturbances usually disappear within 24 hours, quite apart from the fact that it is only thus possible to provide a really satisfactory caloric intake. Unfortunately, many infants having gastrointestinal tract surgery suffer from paralytic ileus for some time. The frequency and danger of vomiting in infancy have already been discussed.

Oral feeding should proceed very slowly and carefully and, once started, the dangers of aspiration of vomitus must always be kept in mind.

The continuous gastric suction is first stopped and two-hourly aspiration of the gastric catheter by hand is instituted. If the aspirated material is colorless and amounts of not more than 5 cc are obtained every 2 hours, two-hourly feeding is commenced and the indwelling gastric tube is removed. For the first 24 hours, a glucose and water solution is given. We start with 1 dram and slowly increase the amount so that after 24 hours, 1 oz is given at two-hourly intervals to full-term infants, and 4–6 drams, according to the weight of the infant, to premature babies. Before each feeding, a stomach tube is passed and the stomach is aspirated. If the aspiration material increases to above 10 cc, feeding is stopped for 4 hours, and then a smaller feeding is given. As the fluid intake by mouth increases, the amount given by intravenous infusion is diminished. After 24 hours, expressed breast milk diluted with an equal amount of 5% glucose solution is offered in quantities of 1–1¼ oz every 2 hours. Stomach aspirations are carried out

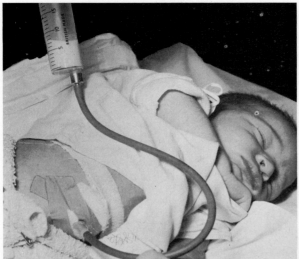

◀ **Fig. 4-13.** — Infant fed by gastrostomy tube. Note the low level of reservoir suspended above the infant.

Fig. 4-14. — Infant fed by continuous intragastric drip. The left limb of the Y-shaped glass tube is connected to the milk bottle. The rubber tube connected to the right upper limb of the Y-shaped glass tube is suspended by a strip of adhesive tape 10 cm. above the abdomen. This prevents the pressure in the system from rising above 10 cm ▼ of water.

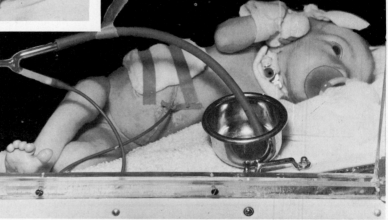

only at four-hourly intervals, and if all goes well are discontinued after 48 hours. On the third day, undiluted breast milk is given, and on the fourth day the infant is put on six feedings of milk every 3 hours, using 2½ oz/lb of body weight.

If breast milk is not available, diluted evaporated milk may be used. It will often be observed that infants will start gaining weight satisfactorily only when it is possible to give 3 or 3½ oz, and in premature infants 4 or 4½ oz, of milk/lb of body weight during the latter part of the postoperative period.

FEEDING BY GAVAGE. — Babies who are unable to swallow for anatomic reasons or because of prematurity may have to be fed by stomach tube. We have found indwelling soft plastic tubes size 3 or 4 F. most satisfactory. The tubes are passed through the nose into the stomach and fixed to the upper lip and nose with ¼-in.-wide adhesive tape. After each milk feeding, the tube is irrigated with water. The tape is connected to the barrel of a 20-cc syringe suspended not higher than 4 in. above the infant. No higher pressure must ever be used.

Great care is taken to prevent mouth infections when feeding by indwelling catheters. The mouth is painted every 2 hours with glycerin and a 1:500 solution of Bradosol.

FEEDING BY GASTROSTOMY. — The feeding regimen is similar to that by gavage. The gastrostomy tube is connected to the barrel of a 20 cc syringe suspended not higher than 4 in. above the infant (Fig. 4-13). When the child is crying, stomach contents frequently are pushed up into the reservoir. This does not matter. Occasionally it has been necessary to employ continuous intragastric milk drips. The drip must then be so constructed that the pressure inside the system cannot rise above 4 in. of water (Fig. 4-14).

ORAL FEEDING IN OLDER INFANTS. — Following operation on older infants, gastric suction can be stopped earlier and the feedings can be increased much quicker than in neonates. In children operated on for pyloric stenosis, no stomach tube is left in situ, and feeding is commenced 4 hours after operation. Alternating milk and 5% glucose solution feedings are given at two-hour intervals, starting with 1 dram, gradually increasing to 1 oz after 14 hours and 1½ oz after 24 hours. During the second 24-hour period, alternating feedings of 5% glucose solution and milk are given every 2 hours in quantities of 1½ oz.

During the third 24-hour period, normal feedings of 3–4 oz, according to body weight, are given at 3-hour intervals.

REFERENCES

1. Albright, F.; Forbes, A. B., and Reifenstein, E. J., Jr.: The fate of plasma protein administered intravenously, Tr. A. Am. Physicians 59:221, 1946.
2. Ariel, I. M.: Effects of water load administered to patients during immediate postoperative period, Arch. Surg. 62:303, 1951.
3. Barnett, H. L., and Vesterdal, J.: The physiologic and clinical significance of immaturity of kidney function in young infants, J. Pediat. 42:98, 1953.
4. Berry, R. E. L.; Iob, V., and Campbell, K. N.: Potassium metabolism in immediate postoperative period, Arch. Surg. 57:470, 1948.
5. Bishop, H. L.: Safe transportation of newborn infants for emergency surgery, J.A.M.A. 165:1230, 1957.
6. Black, D. A. K.; McCance, R. A., and Young, W.F.: Study of dehydration by means of balance experiment, J. Physiol. 102:406, 1944.
7. Blixenkrone-Møller, N.: Potassium metabolism in connection with operations, Acta chir. scandinav. 97:300, 1949.
8. Branning, W. S.: Acid-base balance of premature infants, J. Clin. Invest. 21:101, 1942.
9. British Faculty of Radiologists' Report on Dangers of Radiation, 1960.
10. Coller, F. A., et al.: Postoperative salt intolerance, Ann. Surg. 119:533, 1944.
11. Danowski, T.S., et al.: Electrolyte and nitrogen balance in infants following the cessation of vomiting, Pediatrics 5:57, 1950.
12. Darrow, D. C.: The pharmacopeia and the physician treatment of dehydration acidosis and alkalosis, J.A.M.A. 114:655, 1940.
13. Darrow, D. C.: Body fluid physiology, New England J. Med. 233:91, 1945.
14. Darrow, D. C.: Retention of electrolyte during recovery from severe dehydration due to diarrhea, J. Pediat. 23:515, 1946.
15. Doxiadis, S. A.; Goldfinch, M. K., and Holt, K. S.: Alkalosis in infants: Treatment by intravenous infusion of ammonium chloride, Lancet 2:801, 1953.
16. Edelman, I. S., et al.: Further observation on total body water, Surg., Gynec. & Obst. 95:1, 1952.
17. Elkinton, J. R.; Winkler, A. W., and Danowski, T. S.: Transfer of cell sodium and potassium in experimental and clinical conditions, J. Clin. Invest, 27:74, 1948.
18. Fellers, F. X., et al.: Change in thiocyanide and sodium space during growth, Pediatrics 3:622, 1949.
19. Flexner, L. B., et al.: Estimation of extracellular and total body water in newborn human infants with radioactive sodium and deuterium oxide, J. Pediat. 30:413, 1947.
20. Forshall, I., and Rickham, P. P.: Neonatal intestinal obstruction, Brit. M. J. 1:782, 1953.
21. Friis-Hansen, B. J., et al.: Total body water in children, Pediatrics 7:321, 1951.
22. Gaisford, W., and Schofield, S.: Prolongation of initial starvation period in premature infants, Brit. M. J. 1:1404, 1950.
23. Gross, R. E.: Surgery of Infancy and Childhood (Philadelphia: W. B. Saunders Company, 1953).
24. Hughes, W. E., and Hammond, M. L.: Sclerema neonatorum, J. Pediat. 32:676, 1948.
25. Hyde, G.: Sclerema and Neonatal Surgery. Lecture delivered at the 7th Annual Meeting, British Association of Paediatric Surgeons, 1960.
26. Kinsey, V. E.: Retrolental fibroplasia, Arch. Ophth. 56:481, 1956.
27. McCance, R. A., and Widdowson, E. M.: Blood urea in first nine days of life, Lancet 1:787, 1947.
28. McCance, R. A.; Naylor, N. J. B., and Widdowson, E. M.: Response of infants to large doses of water, Arch. Dis. Childhood 29:104, 1954.
29. McCrory, W. W.: Discussion on the response of the newborn to major surgery, Am. J. Dis. Child. 96:475, 1958.
30. MacLean, E. C., and Paulsen, E. P.: The response of the newborn to major surgery, Am. J. Dis. Child. 96:473, 1958.
31. Madden, S. C. et al.: Blood plasma protein production and utilization, J. Exper. Med. 71:283, 1940.
32. Miller, H. C., and Darrow, D. C.: Relation of muscle electrolyte and alteration in serum potassium, Am. J. Physiol. 130:74, 1940.
33. Moore, F. D., and Ball, M. R.: *Metabolic Response to Surgery* (Springfield, Ill.: Charles C. Thomas, Publisher, 1952).
34. O'Brien, D.; Hansen, J. D. L., and Smith, C. A.: Effects of supersaturated atmosphere on insensible water loss in newborn infants, Pediatrics 13:126, 1954.
35. Potts, W. J.: Respiratory emergencies in the newborn, Ann. Roy. Coll. Surgeons England 23:275, 1958.
36. Randall, H. T.: Water and electrolyte balance in surgery, S. Clin. North America 32:445, 1952.
37. Rickham, P. P.: Neonatal surgery, Lancet 1:332, 1952.
38. Rickham, P. P.: Investigation of blood loss during operations on newborn infants, Arch. Dis. Childhood 29:304, 1954.
39. Rickham, P. P.: Surgery of premature infants, Arch. Dis. Childhood 32:508, 1957.
40. Rickham, P. P.: Surgery of newborn infants, Brit. J. Clin. Pract. 11:816, 1957.
41. Rickham, P. P.: *The Metabolic Response to Neonatal Surgery* (Cambridge, Mass.: Harvard University Press, 1957).
42. Rickham, P. P.: Protective screen for neonatal radiography, Brit. M. J. 1:716, 1959.
43. Rickham, P. P.: A burette for intravenous infusion in infants, Lancet 1:556, 1959.
44. Rickham, P. P., and Hall, E. J.: Unpublished data.
45. Rickham, P. P., and Jenkins, J. M.: Incubators for infants undergoing surgery, Arch. Dis. Childhood 35:71, 1960.
46. Rickham, P. P., and Mason, H. R.: New neonatal surgical unit, Hospital 45:605, 1959.
47. Smith, C. A.: *Physiology of the Newborn Infant* (2nd ed.; Oxford: Blackwell Scientific Publications, 1951).
48. Stephens, L. H.: Neonatal Homeostasis. Lecture delivered at the 7th Annual Meeting of the British Association of Paediatric Surgeons, 1960.
49. Swenson, O.: *Pediatric Surgery* (New York: Appleton-Century-Crofts, Inc., 1958).
50. Thomson, J.: Observations on urine of the newborn infant, Arch. Dis. Childhood 19:169, 1944.
51. Todd, R. McL.: Some observations on the use of fructose and invert sugar in infants, Proc. Roy. Soc. Med. 46:1066, 1953.
52. Upjohn, H. L.; Creditor, M. C., and Levenson, S. M.: Metabolic studies of intravenous fat emulsion in normal and malnourished patients, Metabolism 6:607, 1957.
53. Wallace, W., quoted by Moore and Ball.[33]
54. Wilkinson, A. W.: *Body Fluids in Surgery* (Edinburgh: E. & S. Livingstone, Ltd., 1960).
55. Wilkinson, A. W.: Neonatal Homeostasis. Lecture deliv-

ered at the 7th Annual Meeting of the British Association of Paediatric Surgeons, 1960.

56. Wilkinson, A. W., *et al.*: Excretion of potassium after partial gastrectomy, Lancet 1:533, 1950.

57. Wickes, I. G.: Sclerema neonatorum: Recovery with cortisone, Arch. Dis. Childhood 31:419, 1956.

58. Young, W. F., *et al.*: Parenteral fluid therapy for children undergoing major abdominal surgery, Brit. J. Surg. 47:261, 1959.

P. P. RICKHAM

Infants and Children

THE IMPROVEMENT IN SURGICAL RESULTS in the past 25 years has been largely the consequence of advances in preoperative evaluation, intraoperative support and postoperative care. Their foundations have been good clinical judgment, sound clinical research and the transfer of knowledge gained in the surgical laboratory to the clinical setting. Unfortunately, the metabolic surgeons of these decades have concentrated on the neonate and on the adult, leaving the older infant and child somewhat in limbo. These groups are neither exactly overgrown neonates nor undersized adults, but are in a dynamic, rapidly growing equilibrium somewhere between. Their responses to surgical stress are both qualitatively and quantitatively relatively unknown. For this reason, much of the discussion here is theoretical, conjectural and an extension of data from other ages. It represents an attempt to find a system which will provide consistently sound preoperative and postoperative care for the older infant and child.

Metabolic Response to Injury

The consequences of surgical trauma have been well defined in adults. They are characterized by tissue breakdown, the release of intracellular components, mobilization of energy stores, the production of adrenal cortical and medullary hormones, the release of antidiuretic hormone and changes in renal function. Some of the responses of the older infant and child are quite similar; others appear to be quite different.

RELEASE OF INTRACELLULAR COMPONENTS

The classic adult response to trauma is an increase of urinary nitrogen excretion and of the urinary potassium-nitrogen ratio.[22] In marked contrast, nitrogen excretion of infants under 2 years of age is diminished and of older children is unchanged in the postoperative period after moderate surgical stress.[29] The levels of nitrogen excretion are similar to those of children of the same age undergoing starvation.[9, 29] Although there is a negative nitrogen balance be-cause of lack of nitrogen intake, there is not the apparent increase in protein catabolism seen in older ages. Only under severe surgical stress is urinary nitrogen excretion increased in the older infant and child. No quantitative studies of potassium-nitrogen ratios are available for comparison.

It has been shown experimentally that the negative nitrogen balance may be reduced by increasing the caloric intake through carbohydrates. In practice, it is difficult in the adult, the older infant or the child to provide an adequate number of calories to produce a positive nitrogen balance. Neither glucose nor fructose alone has a significant protein-sparing effect.

On the other hand, infants and children can be kept in positive nitrogen balance postoperatively by providing protein hydrolysates intravenously. Hydrolysate alone, without the provision of additional calories as carbohydrate, will produce the positive balance; increased positivity may be obtained by administering a hexose sugar. This effect is apparently related to the protein-sparing effect of the total caloric intake of the hexose-hydrolysate mixture; this will be discussed later in more detail.

MOBILIZATION OF ENERGY STORES

The finding of decreased nitrogen excretion in the older infant and child raises interesting speculations about the basic surgical metabolism of these age groups.

Postoperatively, the carbohydrates provide a small pool of energy which is readily available but rapidly exhausted. It can be supplemented by the transformation of liver glycogen, but this source of energy is no greater in the young than in the adult. The burning of protein is a relatively inefficient source of energy. One gram of nitrogen in the urine represents the addition of approximately 20 calories to the total metabolism.[22] The decrease of urinary nitrogen excretion in the older infant and child would seem to indicate that there may be a basic protein-sparing type of postoperative metabolism.

The other major source of energy is the storage triglycerides available from the fat tissues. These triglycerides are metabolized to glycerol phosphate and free fatty acid, producing the two carbon fragments available for utilization in the Krebs cycle. Many stimuli trigger the release of free fatty acids, including the catecholamines. The levels of plasma free fatty acids are considered to be an indicator of the response to stress.[30] Studies of infants undergoing herniorrhaphy have disclosed a significant rise of the plasma free fatty acid levels in the absence of any significant elevation of the catecholamine level. Although this may be interpreted as an adequate response to stress, it may also indicate that the younger age groups preferentially resort to this type of metabolism in the face of surgical trauma. Further elucidation of the basic energy factors is urgently needed.

Adrenocortical Hormones

An increase of cortisol production and 17-hydroxycorticosteroids in the urine is characteristic of the response to injury. This has been well quantitated in the adult but has been observed only in a qualitative fashion in the older infant and child.[22] The changes in protein metabolism speculated on above may reflect the changes in the quantitative production of adrenal hormones in these age groups.

The other cortical hormone, aldosterone, is secreted in response to a large number of stimuli; ACTH, reduction of volume and the renin-angiotensin system are the major known determinants.[35] Aldosterone secretion rates have been studied in normal subjects from the age of 1 week to adulthood.[33] After approximately 7 days of age, resting aldosterone levels are comparable to those of the adult. Older infants and children show the typical adult responses to sodium restriction. Elevated levels have been observed in an infant at birth whose mother had been receiving a thiazide diuretic during the latter portion of her pregnancy.[10,33] Thus it would seem that after 1 week of age, an active feedback system for the secretion of aldosterone exists. That this is true may be inferred from the finding of markedly decreased urinary sodium concentrations in both older infants and children undergoing moderate to severe surgical stress.[10,28] The major stimulus to aldosterone secretion is volume reduction in these age groups, as in the adult; this may be seen in the studies cited in the section on renal function, demonstrating that the dehydrated child shows marked sodium and water retention in the postoperative period.

Antidiuretic Hormone

Antidiuretic hormone (ADH) has classically been supposed to be primarily under the control of the tonicity of the body fluids, but it has become apparent that volume reduction as well as surgical manipulation plays a significant part in its release.[35] Antidiuretic hormone levels prior to the induction of anesthesia in adults are elevated and are rapidly corrected by the infusion of fluids and the restoration of volume.[23] Visceral traction during intraoperative manipulations may greatly increase ADH levels, but the pattern is one of a gradual rise to a stable plateau two to three times that of the preoperative level, with a gradual decrease beginning 6–12 hours postoperatively.

Because the infant has a concentrating defect which prevents him from producing markedly hypertonic urine in response to dehydration, it had been felt that the ADH responses were abnormal.[21] It is now known that the ADH level in umbilical cord blood is greatly increased in response to birth trauma and that, within the first week of life, ADH concentrations rise progressively to reach approximate adult levels at the end of the first month.[16] At 3 months of age, infants undergoing elective or emergency surgical procedures may show a 30-fold increase of plasma ADH concentration.

Changes in Renal Function

Under the stress of trauma, characteristic changes occur in renal tubular function in adults.[22] There is a depression of free water clearance and a fixation of urinary osmolality at approximately 750 milliosmols (mOsm) per liter. In addition, the urinary sodium concentration is conspicuously diminished and the tubular reabsorption of sodium and bicarbonate is increased. The result of these changes is a reduced urinary volume with a low sodium content. These changes are a response to the reduction of volume which occurs with moderate trauma and are designed to maintain the volume of the internal fluids at the expense of tonicity.[35]

Although the older child has been known to exhibit similar changes, the infant and the younger child have been thought to respond more as does the neonate, without excessive retention of either sodium or water in the intraoperative and postoperative periods. The basis of these assumptions is a set of paired studies relating to the effect of surgery on the postoperative excretion of water and sodium.[9,25] In these studies, the initial observations on children between 2½ weeks and 12½ years of age suggested that there was a good correlation between intake of fluids in the operative and immediate postoperative periods and the urine volume. In those children whose urine volume was decreased, urinary osmolality was increased, indicating good renal function but dehydration. None of the children could be demonstrated to have a significant decrease of glomerular filtration rate postoperatively, as measured by inulin clearances. It therefore appeared that the urinary volume postoperatively was primarily dependent on the hydration of the child at the time of surgery. In infants who were dehydrated preoperatively, intraoperatively and postoperatively and who had a relatively standard weight loss of 30 Gm/M²/hour, there was a marked decrease in the ability to excrete a water load in the postoperative period. In contrast, infants who were provided with fluid during surgery and who had no significant weight loss prior to water loading showed no diminution of the ability to excrete a postoperative water load.

Two other groups of infants were studied by subjecting them to hypertonic sodium loads in the postoperative period. There was no impairment of the ability of the well-hydrated infants and younger children to excrete a sodium load after mild surgical trauma; controlled dehydration preoperatively, intraoperatively and postoperatively, however, greatly decreased their ability to excrete a postoperative sodium load.[25]

The disparity between these observations in infants and children and the classic adult renal response to trauma can be explained. Most, if not all, of the operative renal mechanisms are now thought to be designed to maintain volume. If volume is adequately maintained, it would seem that much of the sodium and water retention characteristic of the stress response might be obviated. The lack of weight loss during the intraoperative and postoperative periods in the children studied would indicate that the volumes both of total body water and of effective extracellular fluid had been adequately maintained. In a majority of the studies in these circumstances and in those of relatively mild trauma, the classic adult changes in renal function might not be expected to occur.

Our own studies indicate that in moderate to severe surgical trauma, the standard practice of providing either glucose water alone or glucose water with a small amount of electrolytes regularly results in decreased urinary volume, decreased sodium excretion and the classic production of mild hyponatremia.[10,28] This persists until the postoperative diuresis begins. This response is seen as early as 4–6 weeks of age. Its severity is related to the restoration of volume and replacement of sodium for the sequestration which occurs in moderate to severe surgical trauma.

Fluids and Electrolytes
CHANGING COMPOSITION

The premature or newborn infant has a body composition quite different from that of his older counterpart or the adult. At birth, 80% of the body weight is water, and approximately one half of this is extracellular water. These volumes progressively decline over the first 6–12 months. At the end of this time, the total body water is 60% of the weight and the extracellular water approximately 30% of the total weight. A major portion of this change is probably provided by a decrease of water content of the skin, which, in the young infant, is approximately 20% of the body mass and contains 30% of the total extracellular water.[21]

This process of change in water distribution and in concentration of intracellular and extracellular solute is achieved initially by the excretion of a dilute urine. The newborn is unable to obtain a concentration of greater than 800 mOsm/liter, although the older infant and the adult are easily able to concentrate from 1,200 to 1,400 mOsm/liter. Although there appears to be no primary renal defect in the younger infant, it has been concluded that his "osmostat" has been set at a different level to allow him to change his body composition gradually as he grows. It also allows him to maintain normal body composition in the face of diets which provide excess amounts of expendable water. In such circumstances, the provision of excess solute produces both weight gain and the expansion of extracellular fluid. In addition, since the younger infant in many ways resembles a perfect sphere, with his area and volume related as the square and cube, his water turn-over is extremely rapid and dehydration occurs in a short period of time. Thus in the calculation of maintenance fluids for a child, adequate water must be provided to meet this rapid turn-over. It must also take into account his ability to excrete only a relatively dilute urine, as well as provide solute loads which are not excessive.

MAINTENANCE NEEDS

FLUIDS.—In an effort to find a system which is applicable to all extremes of age, that of Holliday and Segar[14,15] has been adopted. This relates the need for water to the caloric expenditures in normal activity ranges. In this way, water losses are computed on the basis of metabolic energy expended. Since the hospitalized child is neither at full activity nor at basal caloric levels, the values in between are used. They are also related to weight, as seen in Table 4-1. Thus the child weighing from 0 to 10 kg is assumed to expend 100 calories for every kilogram of body weight, and the 5-kg child will have a basic total expenditure of 500 calories for a 24-hour period. Similarly, the child over 10 kg requires at least 1,000 calories, plus 50 calories for every kilogram between 10 and 20 kg. Over 20 kg, 20 calories per kilogram are added to the 1,500-calorie basic expenditure.

Once the caloric needs are estimated on the basis of the weight formula, 100 ml of water is provided for every 100 calories as the fluid requirement of the individual for 24 hours.

This is a flexible system which allows calculation in all weight ranges up to and including the adult scale. In comparison with the surface-area system for computing fluids, the major discrepancy lies in the area from 6 to 15 kg, the fluid volumes being 30–40% higher than those computed on the basis of surface area. The reason for this is that energy expenditure is higher per unit of surface area for those of this inter-

TABLE 4-1.—CALORIC EXPENDITURES AND WATER REQUIREMENTS BY WEIGHT*

1–10 kg	100 calories/kg
11–20 kg	1,000 calories + 50 calories/kg
20+ kg	1,500 calories + 20 calories/kg

*Basic: 100 ml of water for each 100 calories.

mediate weight than for the infant, the older child and the adult.

The provision of 100 ml of fluid per 100 calories metabolized may also be shown to be applicable by calculating insensible fluid loss and volume necessary for solute excretion.[21] Insensible loss at all ages, measured in a comfortable environment at a resting level, is approximately 45 ml/100 calories of energy expenditure. Urinary water loss is considered to be a function of solute excretion. Solute concentration of the urine may vary from 75 to 1,200 mOsm/liter in the older child, with the previously noted ceiling of 800 mOsm/liter in the younger infant. It is apparent that at the extremes of these dilution and concentration ranges, 1 mOsm of solute may be excreted in either 0.8 ml of water at maximal concentration or 13.5 ml of water at maximal dilution. Studies of infants equilibrated on glucose water for 5 days show that the average excretion in the midportion of the period is 15 mOsm/100 calories of expenditure per day. The minimal excretion rate is 10 mOsm/100 calories. If a solution is provided for parenteral maintenance therapy which contains 5–10 mEq of a cation, 10–20 mOsm/100 calories per day is added to the solute load. For example, a solution of 5% dextrose in hypotonic saline generates a solute load of from 25 to 35 mOsm/100 calories per day. If, in the maintenance fluids, 50 ml of water/100 calories is provided for excretion of this solute load, an adequate volume is made available that enables the infant and child to excrete urine well within the normal osmolar range. In addition to the water provided with maintenance fluids, 10–15 ml of endogenous water is produced, providing a total of about 115 ml/100 calories per day. This is similar to the solute load of 40 mOsm/100 calories which a diet of whole milk provides.

ELECTROLYTES.—Along with adequate water to meet insensible losses and solute excretion requirements, electrolytes should be provided in the maintenance fluids. Minimal electrolyte concentrations per 24 hours are: 3 mEq of sodium/100 calories; 2 mEq of chloride/100 calories, and 2 mEq of potassium/100 calories. Although this solution is easily calculated and mixed, in actual practice 5% dextrose in 0.2% saline as a basic solution will provide the sodium requirements of this formula. Potassium must be added to the basic fluids at the recommended concentrations. An alternative solution is a mixture of two-thirds 5% dextrose in water and one-third 5% dextrose in lactated Ringer's solution, again with potassium added.

CALORIES.—The provision of 3–5 Gm of glucose/kg of body weight is probably sufficient through the pediatric age range. Although there is not an absolute protein-sparing effect of glucose during fasting, provision of calories at this level is usually sufficient to diminish cellular protein metabolism and reduce the nitrogen and organic acids requiring excretion as a solute load.

REPLACEMENT SOLUTIONS.—Two solutions are used for replacement of loss by nasogastric drainage. Under 6 months of age, one-half 5% dextrose in water and one-half 5% dextrose in saline is given in volumes equal to the loss. If the amount of drainage is excessive, 1 mEq of potassium is added to each 100 ml. Over 6 months of age, two-thirds 5% dextrose in saline and one-third 5% dextrose in water with 1.5–2 mEq of potassium/100 ml is administered.

Abnormal losses of small bowel content and ileostomy drainage may be adequately replaced by lactated Ringer's solution with 15 mEq of potassium added to each liter.

ADMINISTRATION OF SOLUTIONS.—We find it convenient to divide fluid administration into 8-hour compartments: 8 A.M. to 4 P.M., 4 P.M. to midnight, midnight to 8 A.M. The total daily requirement is calculated and distributed evenly over these periods. Thus a 6-kg child who receives 600 ml of 5% dextrose in 0.2% saline and 12 mEq of potassium as daily maintenance will receive 200 ml of 5% dextrose in 0.2% saline with 4 mEq of potassium chloride every 8 hours.

When replacement solutions must be added, for example, to compensate for nasogastric drainage, the volume from the preceding 8-hour period is administered during the next 8 hours. If there are deficits in electrolytes or acid-base balance and corrections are being made, the clinical and metabolic situation may be reassessed every 8 hours and appropriate steps taken.

PREOPERATIVE CORRECTION OF DEHYDRATION

THEORETICAL BASIS.—Although the strict definition of dehydration is the loss of body water, pure water loss exists only rarely in the clinical setting, and the common types of dehydration seen in pediatric surgery are accompanied not only by the loss of body water but by the loss of electrolyte as well.

Dehydration is estimated on the basis of body weight alone. It is conveniently described as "mild" when a 5% dehydration exists, "moderate" when a 10% dehydration exists, and "severe" when a 15% or greater dehydration exists. On a clinical basis, any child who appears to be dehydrated may be assumed to be a minimum of 5% dehydrated. A child with a 10% dehydration has a depressed fontanel, dry mucous membranes and sunken eyes. The skin has lost turgor and remains briefly tented when pinched between the fingers. The child may be lethargic and usually responds poorly to stimulation. The severely dehydrated child may present a variety of clinical signs. All of those described for the moderately dehydrated child are accentuated, particularly the dark and sunken appearance of the eyes and the striking decrease of responsiveness. In many cases, there is frank clinical shock, with pale skin and mucous membranes and generalized peripheral vasoconstriction.

PRACTICAL CONSIDERATIONS.—In addition to providing corrective fluids and electrolytes for the dehy-

TABLE 4-2.—FLUID AND ELECTROLYTE
DEFECTS IN DEHYDRATION

DEHYDRATION, %	WATER, ml/kg	NA	CL mEq/kg	K
5	50	5	5	3
10	100	10	10	6
15	150	15	15	9

dration already present, maintenance fluids must be given for the period during which the defect will be corrected. A convenient estimate of fluids and electrolytes necessary to correct isotonic dehydration is given in Table 4-2. Assume, as an example, that a 5-kg child is 10% dehydrated. The calculations for repletion of his fluid and electrolyte losses are given in Table 4-3. Maintenance fluids, calculated at 100 ml/100 calories, amount to 500 ml. Maintenance sodium is 15 mEq, maintenance potassium 10 mEq. The 10% dehydration is equated as a 10% loss of body weight. This is 500 Gm, or 500 ml of fluid. Thus 100 ml of fluid per kilogram of weight will be needed to repair the deficit. In addition, a deficit of 10 mEq of sodium and of 6 mEq of potassium per kilogram must be replaced. Adding together the maintenance and dehydration requirements, one obtains a corrective solution consisting of 1,000 ml of 5% dextrose in water, 65 mEq of sodium and 40 mEq of potassium. This solution might be approximated by mixing one-half 5% dextrose in water and one-half 5% dextrose in lactated Ringer's solution with potassium added. It could also be achieved by mixing one-half 5% dextrose in water and one-half 5% dextrose in saline. Either solution is adequate for the purpose, although the dextrose and lactated Ringer's is particularly applicable in the treatment of dehydration due to diarrhea. Dextrose and saline are used in the treatment of dehydration due to vomiting, as will be pointed out later.

In moderate 10% dehydration, correction may be obtained in 15–20 hours without danger of overloading. An adequate rate of fluid replacement is 10 ml/kg/hour, which will correct a 10% dehydration in 20 hours and a 5% dehydration in 15 hours.

The child with severe 15% dehydration presents a much more critical problem. The loss of electrolytes is major, and replacement is best started with a solution of either sodium chloride or lactated Ringer's, de-

TABLE 4-3.—REPLACEMENT THERAPY IN DEHYDRATION

Example: 5-kg child: 10% dehydration
Basic calories: 500/24 hr

	WATER, ml	NA, mEq	CL, mEq	K, mEq
Maintenance	500	15	10	10
Dehydration	500	50	50	30
Total	1,000	65	60	40

pending on the primary disease. In this situation, a dextrose-containing solution is not used. Both 5% dextrose in saline and 5% dextrose in lactated Ringer's are hyperosmolar solutions. An essentially isosmolar solution is produced during infusion by the metabolism of the glucose. Rapid rates of infusion of a hyperosmolar solution in these circumstances will result in an osmotic diuresis because the glucose is not adequately metabolized and exceeds the transfer maximum of the tubules. Coincident with the osmotic diuresis due to the sugar, there will be a significant loss of electrolyte, defeating the therapeutic aim. With dehydration of 15% or more, approximately 25% of the calculated fluid and electrolyte is given within the first 4 hours, or 20 ml/kg/hour, until the first urine is produced.

Although the calculated requirements in moderate to severe dehydration may indicate the need for a solution containing greater than 40 mEq of potassium/liter, this concentration is never exceeded. In actual practice, no potassium is added to the first infusions in dehydration until urine has been produced.

In addition to needing fluid and electrolyte solutions, the severely dehydrated child may require colloid infusion as well. Protracted diarrhea and vomiting with inadequate oral intake often produce a state of nutritional deficiency. Children with significant protein depletion may present periorbital or lower extremity edema on the initial examination, or this may become evident as initial hydration is completed. A minimum of 25 cc of plasma/kg may be given as an initial dose for expansion of extracellular volume. A solution of 4% serum albumin in lactated Ringer's at the same volume may be substituted for plasma.

It must be remembered that the formulas given here are only reasonable approximations of the deficits which may occur in dehydration. Initial studies of blood chemistry and, if possible, acid-base measurements should be made; corrections of outstanding deficits in electrolytes and acid-base balance must be made independently of the other calculations. The best guides to the improving status of the child are his clinical appearance, rate of weight gain and his urinary output.

INTRAOPERATIVE AND POSTOPERATIVE NEEDS

THEORETICAL BASIS.—The fluid volumes and electrolyte requirements outlined above have been found to be satisfactory for the maintenance of the young infant and the older infant and child subjected only to mild surgical trauma. Reviews of postoperative fluid balance in our own patients, however, reveal a relatively consistent pattern of mild hyponatremia accompanied by varying degrees of oliguria.[10] Studies of sodium balance indicated that the child over 4 or 5 kg in weight and over 5–6 months of age subjected to significant surgical trauma manifested maximal stress response in terms of sodium retention.[28] An unexplained deficit (in the range of 3–7 mEq/kg) between the sodium administered and that excreted could be demonstrated. Studies of adults suggested that sodium sequestration occurred in a physiologic third space and that the provision of sodium during the intra- and postoperative periods in increased amounts had beneficial effects on both homeostasis and urine volume. Increased amounts of sodium and of fluids were administered to older infants and children during the intraoperative period, the maintenance sodium was increased in the postoperative fluids, and the volume was maintained constant, as described earlier, in the discussion of the water needs. These pilot studies showed that the older infant and child undergoing major surgery benefit from maintenance of volume with sodium-containing fluids.[21] There is minimal depression of serum sodium level, and only rarely is there significant oliguria in the postoperative period.

On the basis of what is known of renal function, it would seem that adequate amounts of sodium must be available to the renal tubules to assure proper functioning of the "countercurrent system."[21] The sequestration of sodium and fluid into a third space decreases the effective circulating volume. The resulting reduction of the glomerular filtration rate in turn reduces the fluid volume and solute load reaching the loop of Henle. Removal of sodium in the loop from the small volume of fluid effectively increases the osmotic gradient within the medulla. The secretion of ADH, triggered by reduction of the effective circulating volume, increases the permeability of the collecting systems to water, and a major portion of the water from the small volume of urine passes into the hypertonic medulla. Volume reduction, neurohypophyseal stimulation and reduction of renal flow all stimulate the release of significant amounts of aldosterone. This results in further retention of sodium by absorption from the distal tubule in an effort to augment the depleted stores.

In ways not well understood, the provision of both increased fluids and increased sodium serves to minimize the acute changes in hormonal production and to re-establish the renal tubular flow. Adequate urine volumes with sodium concentrations markedly above what may be normally expected are then produced. The administration of only glucose water or a hypotonic sodium solution only aggravates the pre-existing defect. Some of the ability of sodium solutions to correct this hormonally induced chain of events is, in all probability, due to simple augmentation of effective volume. The provision of solute within the renal tubules, even in the presence of ADH, increases urine volume significantly. A secondary effect of this is improved homeostasis in terms of acid-base balance: by the normal mechanisms, sodium is then available within the tubule for exchange with hydrogen ions.

PRACTICAL CONSIDERATIONS. – The problem in the young infant, and to a lesser degree in the older infant, is to provide adequate solute and volume to accomplish these ends without overwhelming the ability of the stress-modified kidney to excrete the load. It is our feeling that in children up to 5 kg weight or 3–4 months of age, intraoperative volume support should be maintained by the administration of one-half 5% dextrose in water and one-half 5% dextrose in lactated Ringer's at the rate of 10 cc/kg/hour. This will provide good homeostasis. Maintenance fluids in the postoperative period should consist of either 5% dextrose in 0.2% saline or a mixture of two-thirds 5% dextrose in water and one-third 5% dextrose in lactated Ringer's. Appropriate amounts of potassium, as outlined earlier, should be added on the first postoperative day after urinary output is adequate. These recommendations do not apply to the neonate in the first 30 days of life or to the child who is still physiologically premature on clinical grounds even at 8–10 weeks of age. In the face of acute peritonitis from perforation or bacterial contamination, we have not hesitated to use 5% albumin solutions in lactated Ringer's, or plasma, for replacement of the volume deficit.

For the child between 6 and 20 kg undergoing major surgery, one-half 5% dextrose in water and one-half 5% dextrose in lactated Ringer's at 10 ml/kg/hour for the first 2 hours, and at 5 ml/kg/hour for the remainder of the procedure is sufficient. Postoperative maintenance consists of one-half 5% dextrose in water and one-half 5% dextrose in lactated Ringer's in volumes described in the foregoing section.

Children over 20 kg are maintained on 5% dextrose

TABLE 4-4. – INTRAOPERATIVE AND POSTOPERATIVE FLUID WITH
MODERATE TO SEVERE TRAUMA*

	OPERATIVE	POSTOPERATIVE	
2.5–5 kg	½ D5W – ½ D5RL 10 ml/kg/hr	D5/0.2% NaCl *or* 2/3 D5W – 1/3 D5RL	+ potassium
6–20 kg	½ D5W – ½ D5RL 10 ml/kg/hr × 2 hr; 5 ml/kg/hr thereafter	½ D5W – ½ D5RL	+ potassium
20+ kg	D5RL 5 ml/kg/hr	D5RL	+ potassium

*D5W = 5% dextrose in water. D5/0.2% NaCl = 5% dextrose in 0.2% saline. D5RL = 5% dextrose in lactated Ringer's.

in lactated Ringer's at 5 ml/kg/hour during surgery. Postoperatively, 5% dextrose in lactated Ringer's is given in the volumes indicated in Table 1. These recommendations are summarized in Table 4-4.

This fluid regimen for moderate to severe trauma produces a mild postoperative metabolic alkalosis which, combined with the aldosterone secretion and the sodium loading, will cause hypokalemia unless potassium is added to the maintenance fluids. Nevertheless we believe that more adequate homeostasis is achieved by the regimen than is provided either by moderate amounts of a hypotonic electrolyte solution or by small amounts of a nonelectrolyte-containing dextrose solution.

Acid-Base Balance

Appreciation of the profound physiologic disturbances that accompany major changes in the acid-base equilibrium in the postoperative period has been one of the most significant advances in surgical care of the child. At the same time, it has been one of the most confusing to the clinician. Part of the confusion results from conspicuous divergence of old and new nomenclature. Further confusion has resulted because of continuing debates on the interpretation of acid-base data. Nevertheless the basic knowledge of the normal and the abnormal that is available allows intelligent care of the infant and child.

DEFINITIONS AND MEASUREMENTS

The concepts of acid-base balance rest on the definitions of acid and base. Older literature is replete with discussions of "fixed base" and "fixed acid," equating the major cations (Na, K, Mg, Ca) with the former and the major anion (Cl) with the latter. These are truly neither acids nor bases as the system is now defined. Major changes in acid-base equilibrium may lead to secondary changes in distribution of anion and cations, but these do not function as an integral portion of the acid-base buffer system.

An *acid* is defined as a hydrogen ion or proton donor. A *base* is defined as a hydrogen ion or proton acceptor. *Acid-base balance* is thought of and explained in terms of the hydrogen ion concentration of the medium and the regulation of buffer concentrations of the medium. These buffer systems consist of weak acids and their conjugate bases. In man, carbonic acid, phosphoric acid and the acid groups of the protein molecules form the major buffer systems.

For practical purposes, discussions of acid-base balance center on measurements of hydrogen ion concentration and variations in the carbonic acid and bicarbonate ion concentrations—pH, Pco_2 and bicarbonate, respectively.

Traditionally, the plasma pH, the blood or plasma Pco_2 and the plasma bicarbonate concentration are measured. These three values, with an accurate clinical assessment, provide information regarding the acid-base status of the individual. Fortunately for the patient, and perhaps unfortunately for the clinician, no single parameter changes by itself. Compensation occurs in an effort to maintain homeostasis. Thus, if Pco_2 rises because of respiratory difficulties, reabsorption of bicarbonate by the kidney is increased to maintain a nearly normal pH. Conversely, the addition of acid or hydrogen ion to the body with a fall of pH and consumption of buffers results in hyperventilation and a decrease of Pco_2. Situations arise clinically in which there is a chronic, steady state of acidosis or alkalosis, or a mixture of two disease processes such as respiratory acidosis and metabolic acidosis. It is in the latter circumstances that efforts have been made to define and describe the metabolic component of the acid-base equilibrium for clinical purposes.

Astrup[3] and Siggaard-Andersen and Engel[27] have developed a widely used and generally applicable system for estimation of the acid-base status.[3, 27] Although great controversy exists as to the exact validity of the system, the intelligent use of the values derived and a knowledge of the inherent problems allow it to be applied to most clinical situations.[24] The pH, Pco_2 and a pair of values known as "standard bicarbonate concentration" and "base excess" are estimated by this method. A whole blood sample is equilibrated with carbon dioxide under a high and under a low partial pressure. The pH of the samples after equilibration is measured and the result is plotted on a logarithmic pH graph. By measurement of the true pH of the original sample, the Pco_2 can be extrapolated, and values for the standard bicarbonate and the base excess are read from a nomogram. The standard bicarbonate is designed to obviate the problems inherent in the estimation of carbon dioxide-combining power and in the plasma bicarbonate measurement when the Pco_2 is greatly elevated. *Standard bicarbonate* is defined as the bicarbonate concentration in the plasma from whole blood equilibrated to a Pco_2 of 40 mm Hg at 37 C. A value is also derived which is termed the *base excess*; this represents the base concentration of the whole blood at a pH of 7.4, a Pco_2 of 40 mm and a temperature of 37 C. By the terms of the definition, a loss of base or a negative base excess represents the addition of hydrogen ion, indicating acidosis; excessive accumulation of base or a positive base excess represents loss of hydrogen ion, indicating alkalosis. The buffer system of whole blood is composed of plasma and red cell bicarbonate, hemoglobin proteins, plasma proteins, and plasma and red cell phosphate buffers. Base excess, a measure of the buffering capacity of the whole blood, may not exactly parallel the standard bicarbonate concentrations. However, except in the face of severe anemia or hypoproteinemia, their direction of change and magnitude of change are roughly similar.

As with any system, this one has flaws. Total reliance on the numbers obtained without regard to the clinical situation may lead to serious difficulties. Part of the controversy which exists results from the fact that the CO_2 titration curves of whole blood in vitro and in vivo differ.[6] During in vitro titration, as the PCO_2 increases, the production of carbonic acid increases. The whole blood buffers remove the hydrogen ion, and the bicarbonate of the system rises in an amount equal to the decrease of the other buffers. Therefore no decrease of whole blood buffer base is detected, and, by definition, base excess is zero. In the body, the situation is different. As PCO_2 rises and carbonic acid is produced, body buffers outside the bicarbonate system again take up the newly produced hydrogen ion of the carbonic acid. However, the bicarbonate does not remain in the circulating volume but diffuses into the interstitial space. Similarly, the bicarbonate produced by buffering within the cells diffuses into the interstitial space and the entire area acts as a large bicarbonate "sink." Therefore, in vivo, a rising PCO_2 will not produce an equal rise of the plasma bicarbonate concentration.[34]

When a blood sample from a patient with a high PCO_2 is titrated by the Astrup system and compared with the in vitro titration curve, the whole blood buffer base will be decreased. By definition, a negative base excess will exist, although true metabolic acidosis is not present. If these limitations of the system are known and remembered, the Astrup measurements provide a reasonable method for rapidly estimating the approximate acid-base status of the individual using a very small volume of blood.[34] In situations of pure "metabolic acidosis," the values are relatively reliable. The warning of Schwartz and Relman[26] that all data must be interpreted physiologically should be heeded at all times.

ACID-BASE VALUES FOR NORMAL INFANTS AND CHILDREN

A large group of infants from 3 months to 2 years of age has been studied by the Astrup technique.[1] The measurements were performed on arterialized heel blood. The basic pattern, in contrast to that of the adult, shows a normal pH but a decrease of both bicarbonate and PCO_2. There is a corresponding decrease of the base excess. The most attractive explanation is that the diet of the child is the cause of the abnormality. The diet in this age range contains two to three times as much protein as that of the adult. The high protein intake causes an increase of catabolic hydrogen ion production. This hydrogen ion is then excreted either as a titratable acid or as ammonia in the urine. The fact that the primary reduction appears to be in the metabolic component may indicate that some of the excess hydrogen ion production is buffered at the expense of the body bicarbonate. This hypothesis is rendered even more attractive by the observation that the decreases of bicarbonate or total

CO_2 are greater in children given cow's milk than in those receiving breast milk; the hydrogen ion production of the child fed cow's milk is greater than that of the child who is breast fed.

This might seem to place the infant and younger child at a mild disadvantage, but it has not been our experience that these children are more apt to succumb to the effects of acidosis in the postoperative period. However, it may be that the minimal metabolic alkalosis usually seen in the postoperative period is a reflection of this basic difference from the adult population.

CLINICAL DISTURBANCES OF ACID-BASE EQUILIBRIUM

METABOLIC ACIDOSIS.—Metabolic acidosis is the abnormality which most frequently confronts the surgeon. Theoretically, it may be induced by the addition of acids to the intracellular and extracellular surroundings or by the primary loss of bicarbonate buffer. Primary loss of bicarbonate almost never occurs except in the child with a bicarbonate-losing nephropathy. The common pattern of metabolic acidosis is most often the result of dehydration, volume reduction and hypoperfusion.[22]

Adequate treatment of metabolic acidosis is adequate treatment of the cause. In the low perfusion states attendant on volume reduction, two mechanisms are operative. Cellular hypoxia causes a shift from aerobic to anaerobic metabolism and the production of acid metabolites such as lactic acid, with consequent consumption of body bicarbonate stores. As pH falls, increased depth and rate of respiration drives down the PCO_2, and an initial respiratory compensation for the metabolic acidosis occurs. However, this is limited in extent, and major compensation must take place by the renal excretion of increased amounts of hydrogen ion and increased reabsorption of bicarbonate. As volume depletion and hypoperfusion continue, the lowering of glomerular filtration rate and renal plasma flow reduces the ability of the kidney to secrete hydrogen ion and reabsorb bicarbonate.

Although the picture just described is primarily that seen in shocklike states, it is not uncommon in the younger child who is severely dehydrated as the result of diarrhea. Although it has been traditionally accepted that the acidosis of diarrhea is primarily due to the loss of bicarbonate, examinations of the titratable acidity and CO_2 content of diarrheal stools have failed to confirm this.[31] The simple loss of fluids, reduction of circulating volume, increasing cation loss as diarrhea progresses, and an increase of protein catabolism are sufficient to produce the acidosis.

Therapy.—The treatment of metabolic acidosis is primarily the treatment of volume reduction and hypoperfusion. The degree of dehydration is estimated, and fluids and colloid are administered as described in the preceding section. In severe depletion and shock, a central venous pressure line established through the upper extremity into the superior vena cava is an invaluable aid in the assessment of fluid therapy. An initial set of blood gases and electrolytes is drawn. The necessary calculations for fluid and electrolyte replacement are made, and a rapid infusion of lactated Ringer's is started. If the initial pH is less than 7.3, bicarbonate is given according to the following formula:

$$\frac{\text{(weight in kg} \times 0.3)}{\text{extracellular space}} \times \frac{\text{base excess}}{\text{mEq/L of whole}} = \text{mEq bicarbonate}$$
$$\text{in L} \qquad \text{blood base deficit}$$

It is in these circumstances that we have found the Astrup system to be of the greatest use. Although base excess is not an exact number, it will at least provide a guide to initial therapy. If acidosis is severe enough to depress the pH below 7.1, bicarbonate is given according to the following formula:

$$\frac{\text{(weight in kg} \times 0.6)}{\text{total body water}} \times \frac{\text{base excess}}{\text{mEq/L of whole}} = \text{mEq bicarbonate}$$
$$\text{in L} \qquad \text{blood base deficit}$$

It will be seen that the formulas are similar, but that the calculation of total space for bicarbonate distribution is twice as large in the patient whose pH is more severely reduced. The rationale is that in extracellular acidosis of this degree, a major portion of the intracellular buffers has been used up and the volume of distribution requiring buffering is more likely to approximate that of body water than that of the extracellular space.

There are several theoretical disadvantages to the use of bicarbonate to combat acidosis initially. A major reduction of intracellular pH occurs before extracellular fluid is affected. It would be preferable to use a substance which penetrates cells rapidly. Bicarbonate will not do so. About 6 hours is required for a significant amount of bicarbonate to reach the intracellular space, and the half-life of the bicarbonate in the body is approximately 12 hours. There has been considerable interest in the use of tromethamine (THAM) in the treatment of metabolic acidosis.[2] We have had little experience with this drug. Because of the problems of hypoglycemia and the depression of Pco_2 which may necessitate the use of a respirator, we have preferred to use bicarbonate. In very small infants in whom the amount of sodium to be administered was a significant problem and in children who had combined respiratory and metabolic acidosis and were already on a respirator, THAM has been used.

In most cases, initial treatment is followed by reevaluation of the acid-base status in 2–3 hours. If significant clinical and metabolic improvement has occurred, treatment is continued with intravenous fluids, and further buffering is withheld unless the pH remains severely depressed. We repeat that the treatment of the underlying cause, the restitution of general circulatory perfusion and the restoration of maximal renal function are the most significant aspects of treatment of metabolic acidosis in the child.

RESPIRATORY ACIDOSIS. – Fortunately, the patient with chronic respiratory acidosis is infrequently seen in pediatric surgery. Acute episodes of respiratory acidosis usually occur only in the immediate postoperative period and, in our experience, are most satisfactorily treated with intermittent positive pressure ventilation. By this means, the basic defect (e.g., pneumonia, overdosage of drugs or chest trauma) has been remedied. We have made no effort to treat younger infants with elevated Pco_2 in the postoperative period with THAM alone.

METABOLIC ALKALOSIS. – The lesion which produces metabolic alkalosis most frequently in the pediatric surgical environment is pyloric stenosis. A brief review of the pathogenesis of the underlying metabolic defects will illustrate the complicated nature of the acid-base equilibrium and the cation-anion exchanges.[19]

The prolonged vomiting which occurs with upper gastrointestinal obstruction results in the loss of a large amount of hydrogen ion and the depletion of effective extracellular volume. Production of the hydrogen ion in the gastric juice is accompanied by an equal production of bicarbonate, which is transferred to the plasma. The loss of gastric juice causes a fall of the hydrogen ion concentration, a loss of chloride and both a relative and a total increase of bicarbonate. This produces metabolic alkalosis with elevated pH, increased plasma bicarbonate values, a positive base excess and, in the early stages, a mild increase of Pco_2. The last is the result of an initial response to the alkalosis. A far greater response is the secretion of bicarbonate by the kidney, a preferential reabsorption of chloride and the exchange of sodium and potassium in the tubule for hydrogen ion, producing an initial mild decrease of serum sodium and potassium content. As the vomiting continues, potassium is shifted into the renal tubular cell as a result of the extracellular alkalosis. It has been suggested that this is the initial cause of increased potassium excretion in the urine. As urinary potassium losses continue, potassium is removed from the intracellular space to compensate for the decrease of plasma concentration. For every three potassium ions which leave the intracellular space, two sodium ions and one hydrogen ion enter it, producing the paradoxical situation of extracellular alkalosis and intracellular acidosis. Moreover, these shifts further aggravate both the alkalosis and the hypokalemia. If they continue unchecked, the intracellular depletion of potassium will disrupt the membrane integrity in the renal tubular cells and, in the face of alkalosis, a "paradoxical" acid urine will be excreted.

The correction of metabolic alkalosis involves three steps: correction of volume deficits, provision of potassium, and provision of chloride. As in other metabolic disturbances of acid-base equilibrium, dehydration is initially corrected, using the calculations described earlier. Because it has been demonstrated that long-standing alkalosis is inadequately corrected unless sufficient chloride is provided, the initial fluids used for hydration are sodium chloride in the severely dehydrated child and one-half 5% dextrose in water and one-half 5% dextrose in sodium chloride in the moderately dehydrated child. The pH, blood gases and electrolytes are estimated and any outstanding deficits corrected. After the establishment of adequate urine output and approximately 12 hours of therapy, electrolytes, pH and blood gases are used as a guide to further treatment. It should be emphasized that it is impossible to provide enough potassium in the first 24 hours to replenish the total body stores. Nevertheless, as soon as urine is obtained, potassium chloride is administered at a maximal rate. If "paradoxical aciduria" is present, the change to an alkaline urine as potassium and chloride are given is an adequate index of correction.

RESPIRATORY ALKALOSIS.—Respiratory alkalosis is known to occur with a shunting from atelectasis, with peritonitis and in patients being maintained on artificial ventilation. There is considerable interest in the derangements which may be produced by alkalosis.[12, 20, 34] Alkalosis produces a shift of the oxyhemoglobin dissociation curve to the left so that, at any given Po_2, hemoglobin saturation is increased; but during the passage of blood through the tissues, dissociation is inhibited and less oxygen is available for cellular metabolism. Accompanying this hypoxia is an increase of production of lactic acid. This is apparently mediated both by the decreased delivery of O_2 and by a reduction of the Pco_2 interfering with carbohydrate metabolism.

Patients maintained in a state of respiratory alkalosis for an extended period have a gradual decrease of bicarbonate, probably as a result of the processes enumerated above. The greatest danger occurs as the alkalosis ends. This is often seen after the abrupt cessation of intermittent positive pressure ventilation. In the face of decreased respiratory reserve, inadequate clinical assessment and insufficient monitoring, Pco_2 rapidly rises and causes a severe, mixed respiratory and metabolic acidosis within a short time. It is our practice to monitor children who have been receiving respiratory assistance carefully as this assistance is discontinued. They are changed from intermittent positive pressure ventilation with an endotracheal tube in place to a heated, high-oxygen-flow mist attached to the endotracheal tube without assistance. If acid-base equilibrium returns to normal with cessation of the respiratory alkalosis, the oxygen is discontinued and the endotracheal tube finally removed.

The other clinical situation in which respiratory alkalosis has proved to be a problem is in the digitalized patient receiving controlled or assisted ventilation. Although hypokalemia, in itself, will not produce alkalosis, respiratory alkalosis will cause a significant hypokalemia. In the digitalized patient who is alkalotic and hypokalemic, transitory, but occasionally serious, cardiac arrhythmias have been observed. These have responded to restoration of the potassium concentrations to normal and adjustments of the artificial ventilation to decrease the degree of respiratory alkalosis.

Blood, Colloids and Protein Hydrolysates

BLOOD

Blood is usually available in one of two forms: as whole blood, preserved in a variety of fashions, or as packed red blood cells. Although it has been the practice for a number of years to give whole blood transfusions whenever anemia is a clinical problem, the trend is toward a more selective use of whole blood and packed red blood cells.[32]

Whole blood has its greatest usefulness in replacing losses due to acute bleeding or when anemia is accompanied by a decrease of circulating blood volume. Packed red blood cells with an average hematocrit of 70% are used most often in preoperative transfusion to correct chronic anemias when a normal or expanded circulating volume already exists; this is particularly true in the child with cardiac disease or borderline congestive heart failure. Various secondary gains may also be noted from the use of packed cells. These include a decrease of transfusion reactions due to plasma factors and a reduction of the amount of sodium administered in the preservative.

Safe transfusion volumes are 10 ml of whole blood and 20 ml of packed cells per kilogram. No untoward reactions due to overloading have been seen at these volumes. It is preferable to use blood that is as fresh as possible because of several of the problems to be discussed.

Studies of the toxicity of banked blood have centered on the problems of acidosis, citrate intoxication and elevated potassium levels.[4] Most of the blood available is collected in an acid-citrate-dextrose (ACD) solution as a preservative. Since the solution is acid, the pH of the blood, which approximates 7.2 initially, gradually decreases over the 3 weeks of storage; commonly accepted pH values for banked blood 2–3 weeks old range from 6.5 to 6.7. The decrease of pH is attributable to three factors: the acidity of the preservative solution; the change of the dextrose of the buffer to lactic acid, and a rise of Pco_2 as the plasma and cellular buffers release CO_2 after reacting with the hydrogen ion of the preservative mixture. Increased carbon dioxide tension ranges from 130 to 180 mm Hg are found in banked blood 2–3 weeks of age.[17] Under general anesthesia, adequate ventilation is possible and there is no hazard. However, in the face of massive transfusions with respiratory depression or significant pulmonary disease, the elevation of Pco_2 may be a factor in the production of acidosis. Because of the low pH and the accumulation of citrate and lactate in the banked blood, the initial result of any large transfusion is a fall of the recipient's pH. However, as the lactate and citrate are metabolized and as the products are redistributed, pH returns to normal.

Except in cases of shock, in which the general metabolism of the recipient is impaired, the transformation of citrate into bicarbonate usually results in mild metabolic alkalosis.

If citrate intoxication is, by definition, myocardial depression and hypocalcemia from excessive administration of citrate, there has been some question as to whether or not it truly exists in the clinical setting.[7] It has been adequately demonstrated that perfusion of the isolated heart with ACD blood at pH 7.1 effectively reduces ventricular contraction by 50%. The intravenous infusion of sodium citrate into anesthetized animals will also result in cardiac standstill at serum citrate concentrations varying from 50 to 190 mg/100 ml. Concentrations in this range have been measured in the face of rapid transfusion in adult man. The fact that many of the experimentally induced effects of cardiac depression are not seen in massive transfusion in man is the outstanding evidence against true citrate intoxication.

In most instances, the hypocalcemia of excessive citrate administration is neutralized by the rapid mobilization of calcium from bone. Experimentally, elevations of serum total calcium in the range of 5 mg/100 ml above normal have been seen during citrate infusions in nephrectomized animals. With intact renal function, massive calciuria results. If calcium is administered routinely during transfusion, overdosage of calcium is more likely than is a beneficial effect. However, in the face of massive transfusion, that is, replacement of more than 50% of the blood volume, the administration of modest amounts of calcium salts would seem to be indicated. This can be effectively done by using 0.1 Gm of calcium gluconate/100 ml of blood.

Storage of blood at low temperatures releases potassium from the red cells into the plasma. ACD blood at the end of 2–3 weeks of storage may contain potassium in concentrations of 15–20 mEq/liter. Fortunately, as blood is rewarmed, some of the ability of the red cell membrane to maintain intracellular potassium levels returns and potassium goes back into the cell. Although it has been classically supposed that elevations of serum potassium cause pronounced changes of myocardial function, this has not been proved experimentally; until ventricular fibrillation occurs at exceedingly high potassium levels in the experimental animal, there is little myocardial change. However, potassium elevations will potentiate the myocardial effects of calcium, and the effect of the two, in massive transfusions of banked blood, may be synergistic.

Varying opinions have been expressed regarding the buffering and warming of blood prior to administration.[5, 17] Considering only massive transfusions in adults, the mortality rate for patients receiving 10–19 units of blood was lowered from 18 to 2.5% by warming and buffering. In patients receiving more than 20 units, the mortality was reduced from 47 to 8% by the same procedures.[18] Other studies have indicated that the incidence of cardiac arrest decreased from 58 to 6.8% with the warming of blood alone.

Although there are no adequate studies in children, it seems reasonable to buffer the ACD blood with THAM and to bring the blood to body temperature by interposing a warming coil between the blood pack and the patient. In addition, blood as fresh as possible should be utilized in smaller children.

Colloids

When volume expansion alone is required, without correction of anemia, either plasma or albumin may be administered intravenously. Although plasma has the advantage of not requiring reconstitution, it presents, theoretically, a risk of hepatitis and its use has been condemned for this reason. On the other hand, the use of a 4 or 5% albumin solution in lactated Ringer's carries no risk of hepatitis and has approximately the same effect on volume expansion as equal volumes of plasma. The practice of using concentrated serum albumin alone for expansion of volume is not sound. The administration of albumin for volume expansion presupposes that there is sufficient interstitial fluid to provide the increase of vascular volume which is desired. This is usually not the case, and administration of albumin alone results only in further depletion of the interstitial and intracellular stores.

Plasma and albumin given intravenously will provide protein building blocks necessary for maintenance and for growth when oral feeding is not possible.[13] Puppies maintained on intravenously administered plasma as their only source of protein or on protein hydrolysates are able to maintain a growth rate equal to that of their litter mates. The half-life of transfused plasma or albumin is approximately 15 days, and replacements and administration of these components to provide protein intake should be based on this turn-over rate.[13] Patients who have a significant protein loss from wound surface or from diarrhea will require more frequent infusions.

Protein Hydrolysates

We have favored the use of protein hydrolysates over extended periods to provide adequate protein intake in children unable to maintain sufficient oral alimentation.[29] The ability to maintain the child postoperatively in positive nitrogen balance by the use of protein hydrolysates has been repeatedly demonstrated. The ability to maintain a positive balance is apparently related to the total caloric intake as well as to simple provision of protein.[9, 11] At an intake level of 25 calories/kg, there is no significant nitrogen retention. Above 50 calories/kg, positive nitrogen balance is almost invariably achieved unless there are abnormal protein losses. Children given 40 calories/kg with no protein intake will show a negative nitrogen balance.[9] If caloric intake is maintained at 40 calories and 100 mg of nitrogen per kilogram as protein hydrolysate is added, the rate of nitrogen excretion is increased, but two thirds of the children will show a positive nitrogen balance. When the protein hydrolysate administration is discontinued, a steady nitrogen excretion rate occurs, indicating that the amino acids are probably being incorporated into the total pool. Tagged studies show that the hydrolysate is not retained in the vascular volume or deaminated to urea or excreted immediately as amino nitrogen. These observations indicate that the amino acids provided are being used for protein synthesis.

REFERENCES

1. Albert, M. S., and Winters, R. W.: Acid base equilibrium of blood in normal infants, Pediatrics 37:728, 1966.
2. Proceedings of the Conference on the Uses of Amine Buffers, Ann. New York Acad. Sc. 92:333, 1961.
3. Astrup, P., et al: The acid base metabolism: A new approach, Lancet 1:1035, 1960.
4. Baue, A. E.; Hermann, G., and Shaw, R.: A study of blood bank toxicity, Surg., Gynec. & Obst. 113:40, 1961.
5. Boyan, C. P.: Cold or warmed blood for massive transfusions? Ann. Surg. 160:282, 1964.
6. Brackett, N. C., Jr.; Cohen, J. J., and Schwartz, W. B.: Carbon dioxide titration curve of normal man, New England J. Med. 272:6, 1964.
7. Bunker, J. P.: Metabolic effects of blood transfusion, Anesthesiology 27:446, 1966.
8. Calcagno, P. L.; Rubin, M. I., and Singh, W. S. A.: The influence of surgery on renal function in infancy: I. The effect of surgery on the postoperative renal excretion of water—the effect of dehydration, Pediatrics 16:619, 1955.
9. Calcagno, P. L.; Rubin, M. I., and Mukherji, P. K.: Utilization of parenterally administered nitrogen by infants receiving suboptimal calories, Pediatrics 16:619, 1955.
10. Dibbins, A. W. Unpublished data.
11. Dudrick, S. J.; Wilmore, D. W., and Vars, H. M.: Long term parenteral nutrition with growth in puppies and positive nitrogen balance in patients, S. Forum 18:356, 1967.
12. Flemma, R. J., and Young, W. G., Jr.: The effects of mechanical ventilation and respiratory alkalosis in postoperative surgical patients, Surgery 56:36, 1964.
13. Gitlin, D.: Some concepts of plasma protein metabolism A.D. 1956, Pediatrics 19:657, 1957.
14. Holliday, M. A., and Segar, C.: *Parenteral Fluid Therapy* (Indianapolis: Indiana University Medical Center Press, 1956).
15. Holliday, M. A., and Segar, C.: The maintenance need for water in parenteral fluid therapy, Pediatrics 19:823, 1957.
16. Hoppenstein, J. M.; Miltenberger, F., and Moran, W. H., Jr.: ADH blood levels in infants from birth to 3 months of age, S. Forum 18:292, 1967.
17. Howland, W. S., and Schweizer, O.: Increased carbon dioxide tension as a factor in the acidity of bank blood, Surg., Gynec. & Obst. 115:599, 1962.
18. Howland, W. S.; Schweizer, O., and Boyan, C. P.: The effect of buffering on the mortality of massive blood replacement, Surg., Gynec. & Obst. 121:771, 1965.
19. LeQuesne, L. P.: Body fluid disturbances resulting from pyloric dysfunction, Surg., Gynec. & Obst. 113:1, 1961.
20. Lyons, J. H., and Moore, F. D.: Post-traumatic alkalosis: Incidence and pathophysiology of alkalosis in surgery, Surgery 60:93, 1966.
21. Metcoff, J.: Renal regulation of body fluids, Pediat. Clin. North America 11:833, 1964.
22. Moore, F. D.: *Metabolic Care of the Surgical Patient* (Philadelphia: W. B. Saunders Company, 1959).
23. Moran, W. H., Jr., et al.: The relation of antidiuretic hormone secretion to surgical stress, Surgery 56:99, 1964.
24. Nahas, G. G.: Further light on acid base debate, Anesthesiology 27:6, 1965.
25. Rubin, M. I., et al: The influence of surgery on renal function in infancy and childhood: II. The effect of surgery on the renal excretion of sodium, Pediatrics 22:923, 1958.
26. Schwartz, W. B., and Relman, A. S.: A critique of the parameters used in acid base disorders, New England J. Med. 268:1382, 1963.
27. Siggaard-Andersen, O., and Engel, K.: A new acid base nomogram: An improved method for the calculation of blood acid base data, Scandinav. J. Clin. & Lab. Invest. 12:177, 1960.
28. Sukarochana, K.: Unpublished data.
29. Sukarochana, K., et al: Postoperative protein metabolism in pediatric surgery, Surg., Gynec. & Obst. 121:79, 1965.
30. Talbert, J. L., et al: Assessment of the infant's response to stress, Surgery 61:626, 1967.
31. Teree, T. M., et al: Stool losses and acidosis in diarrheal disease of infancy, Pediatrics 36:704, 1965.
32. Vogel, J. M., and Vogel, P.: Transfusion of blood components, Anesthesiology 27:363, 1966.
33. Weldon, V. V.; Kowarski, A., and Migeon, C. J.: Aldosterone secretion rates in normal subjects from infancy to adulthood, Pediatrics 39:713, 1967.
34. Winters, R. W.: Studies of acid-base disturbances, Pediatrics 39:700, 1967.
35. Zimmerman, B.: Pituitary and adrenal function in relation to surgery, S. Clin. North America 45:299, 1965.

A.. W. Dibbins
W. B. Kiesewetter

5

Drugs and Antibacterial Agents

Few drugs are necessary in the treatment of surgically ill infants and children. When employed, they should be used for their specific therapeutic action, as for sedation before and after operation, for reduction of fever and for the control of infection.

The preferred route of administration often cannot be used because of the child's failure to co-operate or the nature of the illness. Oral administration is less likely to be accurate, since the dosage administered may not be the same as that actually ingested. The sublingual route requires co-operation and is of little value except in older children. Rectal administration is occasionally a good substitute, but absorption is variable and uncertain. Rectally administered doses usually are double the oral dose. Most potent drugs are given subcutaneously, intramuscularly or intravenously. Drug dosages may be calculated on the basis of age, surface area or body weight. Drug dosage most commonly is stated in milligrams per kilogram or grains per pound of body weight, including a maximum amount of drug not to be exceeded. To use any empiric system of reference in calculating dosages of untried drugs in infants and children may be dangerous. Safe and effective dosage of some drugs differs from that which would be calculated, due perhaps to immaturity of metabolic processes and renal function in infants and very young children.

Evaluation of drug effects may be difficult because the infant or young child is unable to say how he feels, and the usual objective indications of drug effect and toxicity, such as pulse rate, blood pressure, respiratory rate and mental status may be unreliable or obscured by illness.

Sedative and narcotic drugs are among those most commonly employed in pediatric surgery. They are used to quiet the apprehensive child, to secure adequate preoperative medication, to provide basal sedation for local anesthesia, as in minor emergency room procedures, to control convulsions and to diminish pain. Their use to control pain is rarely necessary in children under 4–5 years of age. The barbiturates in the form of phenobarbital, Seconal and Nembutal are generally used. Codeine is prescribed rarely because its action is uncertain and other drugs such as meperidine (Demerol) are more effective. Since meperidine is available in ampule form, small doses can be safely administered. It is less effective in relieving pain than morphine. Intravenously administered meperidine in a concentration as small as 0.5–1 mg/1 cc provides controlled basal sedation without respiratory depression for such procedures as bronchoscopy and bronchography.[31] This is safe even in small infants, provided the solution is well diluted and the drug is given very slowly. Morphine remains the most predictable and efficient drug for severe pain and deep sedation and for specific therapy of acute cyanotic episodes in congenital heart disease. Its usefulness is to some extent impaired by the inconvenience of preparation of the small doses which are necessary. In Table 5-1 is presented a simple and practical method of preparation used at the Children's Hospital of Pittsburgh.[31]

TABLE 5-1.— DILUTION AND PREPARATION OF SMALL DOSES OF MORPHINE*

To Make ms gr	ms mg	Dissolve and Mix Well	In	Discard	Inject
1/8	8	Tab. gr 1/8 (8 mg)	1 cc	–	1 cc
–	6	"	1.3 cc	0.3 cc	"
1/12	5	"	1.6 cc	0.6 cc	"
1/16	4	"	2 cc	1 cc	"
–	3	"	2.7 cc	1.7 cc	"
1/24	2.5	"	3 cc	2 cc	"
1/32	2.0	"	4 cc	3 cc	"
–	1.5	"	5.3 cc	4.3 cc	"
1/48	–	"	6 cc	5 cc	"
1/64	1.0	"	8 cc	7 cc	"
1/72	–	"	9 cc	8 cc	"
–	0.8	"	10 cc	9 cc	"
1/96	–	"	12 cc	11 cc	"
–	0.6	"	13 cc	12 cc	"
1/112	–	"	14 cc	13 cc	"
–	0.5	"	16 cc	15 cc	"
1/144	–	"	18 cc	17 cc	"
–	0.4	"	20 cc	19 cc	"
–	0.3	"	27 cc	26 cc	"
1/240	0.25	"	30 cc	29 cc	"
1/320	0.2	"	40 cc	39 cc	"
–	0.15	"	53 cc	52 cc	"
1/480	–	"	60 cc	59 cc	"

*Equipment required: 1 10-cc syringe,
1 2-cc syringe,
1 sterile medicine cup,
1 tablet 1/8 gr morphine.

Corticosteroids in Pediatric Surgery

Adrenal corticosteroid administration is essential in pediatric surgical patients with congenital adrenal hyperplasia or adrenal insufficiency from any cause. In idiopathic Addison's disease or total surgical absence of the adrenal gland, the patient requires mineralocorticoids in addition to cortisone. A daily dose of 1–2 mg of DOCA intramuscularly fulfills this requirement.

Corticosteroids are helpful in the care of children with terminal malignancy and may be valuable in serious infections such as septicemia with shock. Their use as cholagogues and as a therapeutic diagnostic test in biliary tract obstruction has been disappointing. Other drugs are more effective in treating operative and postoperative shock, except when adrenal insufficiency plays a role. Administration of corticosteroids is indicated pre- and postoperatively when surgery in the area of the hypothalamus and the hypophysis is contemplated.[47]

Adrenal corticosteroids are administered to suppress host immune mechanisms in organ transplant surgery. They are used systemically and locally with varying success in the management of patients with ulcerative colitis and regional enteritis.

By their powerful anti-inflammatory action, these drugs may prevent or control postintubation laryngeal edema. A single massive intramuscular dose (4 mg of dexamethasone up to, and 8 mg beyond, the age of 1 year) prophylactically or therapeutically has at times made tracheostomy unnecessary.[14]

The administration of adrenosteroid drugs has been mandatory when a patient who has received appreciable amounts of steroid drugs during the preceding year requires surgery.[30] Serious problems occurred when this precaution was neglected in patients who underwent surgery as long as 2 years after they had completed intensive, prolonged adrenosteroid therapy.[39] Re-evaluation of adrenal and adrenal-pituitary axis recovery following prolonged suppressive therapy indicates that recovery, even after massive short-term therapy, is rapid and complete. After suppression for 1 year or more, adrenal activity is revived within 48 hours, although complete recovery may take as long as 5 months and may, rarely, never be completed. No tests are available, however, to evaluate the ability of the adrenal to respond to severe stress. There is little objective evidence to support the generally accepted assumption that there is a real risk of adrenal failure in patients undergoing surgery after corticosteroid therapy. Adrenal cortical insufficiency has not been documented in such patients. When catastrophes have occurred, recovery with steroid administration and autopsy evidence of adrenal atrophy do not appear to be conclusive proof of adrenal failure.[12] Although the ability of the adrenal glands to respond may be questioned, it seems wise to continue the use of a regimen of adrenal corticosteroid replacement in such patients who undergo surgery.

An effective routine in the care of children who have been receiving steroids is to give 100 mg of cortisone acetate intramuscularly 24 hours before surgery. Fluids given prior to the induction of anesthesia, during surgery and in the immediate postoperative period should contain 100 mg of hydrocortisone in each 250 cc of fluid. On the day of surgery, 50 mg of cortisone acetate is given intramuscularly. When feeding is resumed, steroids are given orally, the dosage being rapidly reduced and discontinued within 5–7 days. When continuing administration is necessary, the dose is diminished until the maintenance dose is reached. In general, an excess of steroids is administered for coverage during surgery, since no ill effects follow short-term administration of excessively large doses of these drugs.

The steroids commonly used in children are cortisone, hydrocortisone, prednisone and dexamethasone. Adrenocorticotropic hormone (ACTH), although formerly in vogue to prevent adrenal suppression, has few indications. Intermittent long-term use of these drugs is now advocated to avoid undesirable side effects such as Cushingoid appearance and osteoporosis.[23]

Long-term steroid administration can be associated with deleterious side effects.[17] Reduction of linear growth is a well-documented danger.[49] Although this has been ascribed to interference with production of pituitary growth hormone, the actual mechanism of this phenomenon remains controversial. Osteoporosis may result in painful and crippling compression fractures of the dorsal and lumbar vertebrae. The induction of pituitary as well as adrenal insufficiency is well documented.

So-called steroid ulcers of the stomach and duodenum, interference with wound healing and increased susceptibility to infection are well-known effects of even short-term corticosteroid therapy.

Antibacterial Drugs

Material for culture should be collected before antimicrobial therapy is started. Cultures taken after therapy is instituted may be unreliable and may not even represent the actual infecting organism. Arguments have been advanced in favor of withholding antibiotic therapy until laboratory reports are available,[18] but in acute surgical situations, delay can be disastrous. Therapy should be started promptly, with the clinical impression guiding initial therapy until the bacteriologic report is available.[16] In the rare instances of generalized infection whose nature and origin are obscure, broad-spectrum antibiotic therapy is begun and the indicated antibiotic substituted when the organism has been identified.

SENSITIVITY STUDIES.—Because susceptibility of strains of bacteria of the same species to an antibiotic varies, in vitro sensitivity tests are used in the selection of the appropriate agent. Sensitivity studies have become a routine part of clinical bacteriologic practice. The most accurate method involves serial dilution of the drug in subcultures of the organism. This technique is time-consuming. A more rapid method employs filter paper disks of standard sizes impregnated with various antibiotics in standard concentrations. The disks are placed on agar plates inoculated with the organism. Sterile zones surround the disks. The results of this test are readily available and helpful, but must be evaluated with the knowledge that certain inaccuracies may be found. Because standard disk concentrations of antibiotic are used, a report of resistance of the organism to a specific drug using the standard concentration may be misleading. Sensitivity is expressed as millimeters of clearing around the disk in the culture medium, implying a quantitative value. Such an interpretation is not valid, because the extent of clearing depends on many variables, one of which is diffusion rate. Because of rapid diffusion, chloramphenicol appears to be more effective than the serial dilution test or clinical trial would indicate. The organism should be considered to be sensitive or resistant to the drug in question, but quantitative values should not necessarily be inferred. Sensitivity tests may be done either as primary procedures, using the original material inoculated on agar plates on which appropriate filter paper disks have been placed, or with organisms obtained from subcultures. Primary testing allows a rapid report and probably reflects accurately the bacterial sensitivity as it exists in the infection. Mixed infections with bacteria in various proportions subjected to subculturing may undergo changes in sensitivity.

The significance of sensitivity testing has been questioned. Although there is general agreement that these tests are valuable, their correlation with clinical response has not been adequately studied. Available reports[7,37] do indicate a high correlation. Sensitivity tests should be evaluated with the awareness that discrepancies between laboratory and clinical response can and do occur and that bacteria in living tissues are often more sensitive to antibacterials than in in vitro testing. In the final analysis, clinical trial is the only sure way of testing the effectiveness of the specific agent in a given individual with a specific infecting organism.

DEVELOPMENT OF DRUG RESISTANCE.—The emergence of resistant strains of the organism during therapy poses a major problem. Some individuals among bacterial populations are sensitive and others are resistant to specific antibacterials. Therapy eliminates the sensitive ones, allowing resistant individuals to flourish. Mutants of increased resistance appear. Resistance may be acquired slowly and in a steplike fashion, as in the case of penicillin acting on staphylococci, most of which are sensitive and the population relatively homogeneous, or resistance may develop rapidly and explosively, as in the resistance of tubercle bacilli to streptomycin. Both the antibiotic and the organism influence the rate of development of resistance.

To combat the ever-present problem of the emergence of resistant strains of bacteria, new antibiotics are periodically introduced, combinations of agents are recommended, and the use of specific antibiotics is restricted. Emphasis has been placed on the restriction of use of specific antibiotics to established indications and to their use in proper dosage. Barber et al.[3] have shown that antibiotic resistance in hospital infections can be reversed by such a controlled plan of antibiotic administration. By virtually eliminating the use of penicillin, restricting the use of other antibiotics to established indications and using two antibiotics in combination, penicillin-resistant organisms were reduced from 70 to 30%, and penicillin-sensitive strains increased from 12 to 48% of the infections encountered during their 2-year study.

COMBINED DRUG THERAPY.—Antimicrobial therapy with a single drug sometimes fails because of the early appearance of resistant bacterial mutants. This may be circumvented by using a second drug. The simultaneous use of two independently acting agents allows the destruction or suppression of resistant bacterial mutants and is the underlying principle of combined drug therapy. When prolonged therapy may be necessary, particularly when gram-negative enteric organisms are involved, multiple antibacterials may prevent the emergence of resistant strains. Nonetheless, the use of fixed combinations should be condemned.[15] Particularly is this true of penicillin and streptomycin in pediatric patients. Such preparations, sponsored by drug houses, have encouraged indiscriminate drug therapy and have tended to discourage the use of adequate bacteriologic studies in the control of infections. Fixed combinations may employ excessive amounts of one agent and inadequate amounts of the other. By individualizing the dose of each antibiotic, one can take into account the sensitivity of the organism and the diffusibility of the agent into the site of infection. Each drug in a combination must be used in its individual therapeutic dosage. Drug combinations are selected which tend to minimize the development of resistant strains, avoiding possible incompatibility and using synergistic combinations when possible. Drugs between which there is cross-resistance such as tetracycline, oxytetracycline and chlortetracycline, or erythromycin and carbomycin, do not effectively prevent the emergence of resistant strains of organisms. Cross-resistance between chloramphenicol and erythromycin has been demonstrated.[3] It has been shown in vitro that penicillin and the broad-spectrum agents tetracycline and chloramphenicol can be mutually antagonistic.[26] This laboratory observation is not clinically valid, since the combination of these drugs is often effective clinically.[38]

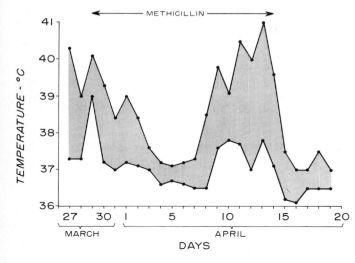

Fig. 5-1. — Drug fever due to methicillin given a 6-year-old girl for staphylococcic septicemia, with positive blood culture and pelvic abscess. Daily high and low rectal temperatures are recorded. Note prompt fall of temperature, with the patient afebrile, by the 5th day of treatment. Fever recurred the 10th day, but temperature promptly fell to normal when the drug was discontinued.

Another advantage of combined therapy depends on the variations and distribution of different agents within the body. The disadvantages and dangers of combined therapy include the use of powerful agents, each of which has toxic effects, the increased risk of sensitization, and the reduction of normal bacterial populations.

DANGERS OF ANTIBACTERIAL DRUG THERAPY. — Hazards of antibacterial therapy center on the toxicity of the drugs themselves, the changes brought about in normal bacterial flora and the development of sensitivity reactions to the drug.[20] Many of these agents are in themselves pharmacologically active and are capable of injuring various organ systems. Vomiting and diarrhea occur most commonly during therapy with the tetracyclines, chloramphenicol and erythromycin. Streptomycin may cause vestibular nerve palsy, and dihydrostreptomycin is toxic to the auditory nerve, causing deafness. Chloramphenicol has been associated with aplastic anemia and bone marrow depression with sulfonamide administration. Drug rash can occur with any of these agents but is more commonly due to sulfonamides, streptomycin and penicillin. Fever may occur with any of these drugs characteristically after 5 days of treatment, leading to diagnostic and therapeutic dilemmas (Fig. 5-1). Skin reactions

Fig. 5-2. — Gram-stained smear of feces from 3-week-old infant with diarrhea beginning 5 days after repair of jejunal atresia. Penicillin-streptomycin and tetracycline were given postoperatively. Cultures of feces revealed no pathogens. Smear shows gram-positive staphylococci. Recovery followed administration of novobiocin.

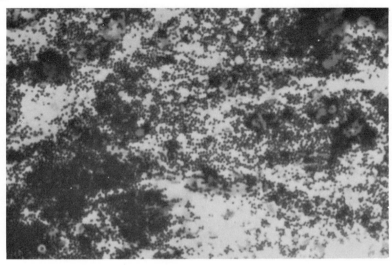

may progress to exfoliative dermatitis and be fatal. Photosensitivity has been reported with Declomycin. Bacitracin and polymyxin are known to be nephrotoxic, causing proteinuria, urinary casts and elevation of the blood urea nitrogen level. This damage seems always to be reversible.[27] Renal tubular blockage by sulfonamide crystals is a well-known hazard. It may be lessened by using three forms of sulfonamide simultaneously, as in the triple sulfa preparations, or by using the more soluble sulfisoxazole.

Hypersensitivity reactions may accompany prolonged or repeated administration of such drugs. These reactions may be mild or life-threatening in severity. Such reactions are uncommon in infants but are increasingly frequent as adolescence is approached. Penicillin is the commonest offender, causing reactions resembling serum sickness with urticaria and, in the most violent form, sudden death from anaphylactoid shock. Treatment of such reactions has been facilitated by the use of steroid drugs and penicillinase.[50] Before any of these drugs are administered, direct questioning regarding sensitivity to antibiotics should be part of the carefully taken history.

The destruction of the normally occurring bacterial population by broad-spectrum antibacterials allows rapid multiplication of other organisms, pathogens and nonpathogens alike, which are resistant to the agent being used. Prolonged penicillin administration, especially by the oral route, often results in monilial vaginitis and stomatitis (thrush). Thrush may extend to the trachea and bronchi, resulting in terminal moniliasis. Resistant staphylococci multiplying in the alimentary tract can cause diarrhea which may proceed to fatal enterocolitis. Postoperative diagnosis of this entity in the infant can be difficult, since stool cultures may fail to grow the infecting organism. Gram-staining of a smear of the feces (Fig. 5-2) will often provide objective evidence of the responsible organism. In debilitated infants, *Pseudomonas aeruginosa* and *Proteus vulgaris* may flourish, resulting in generalized terminal untreatable infection.

A further hazard of therapy is related to repeated intramuscular and intravenous injections. Injection into the sciatic nerve has caused permanent nerve damage[40] and can be prevented. The deltoid region of the upper arm and the anterolateral aspect of the thigh (Fig. 5-3) are safe sites for injection. Tetracycline drugs are especially prone to cause phlebitis when given intravenously. It has been suggested[29] that the anticoagulant nature of many of these drugs

Fig. 5-3.—Proper injection site for intramuscular administration of drugs and antibacterial agents. The anterolateral aspect of the midthigh is preferred rather than the upper outer quadrant of the buttock because of the threat of sciatic palsy. In infants, a 1-inch needle should be used, making it impossible to pith the femoral artery or sciatic nerve.

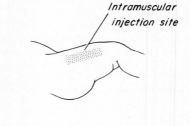

Intramuscular injection site

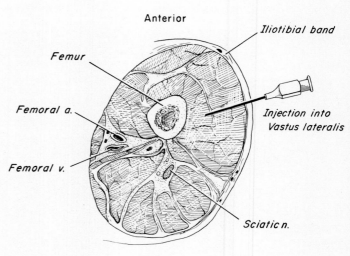

Anterior

Iliotibial band

Femur

Femoral a.

Femoral v.

Injection into Vastus lateralis

Sciatic n.

Posterior

TABLE 5-2. – ANTIMICROBIAL DRUGS USED IN PEDIATRIC SURGERY

DRUG	DOSAGE	ORGANISMS EFFECTIVE AGAINST	TOXICITY	USE
Cephalothin	50 – 100 mg/kg/24 hr, q 4 – 6 hr; IM or IV only	Gram-positive cocci; gram-negatives resistant except *P. mirabilis*, salmonella and shigella.	Rash; urticaria; neutropenia.	A penicillin substitute for resistant staph. infection and penicillin-sensitive patients.
Penicillin G	25,000 – 50,000 U/kg/24 hr, q 4 – 6 hr; 0, IM, IV or SC	Gram-positive cocci; enterococci.	Rash; urticaria; fever; anaphylactoid serum sickness (*rare* in young children).	The single most useful antibiotic for gram-positive organisms and enterococci.
Ampicillin	50 – 200 mg/kg/24 hr, q 4 – 6 hr; IV or IM	Gram-positive cocci; many gram-negatives, as *H. influenzae*, gonococci, meningococci, *P. mirabilis* and some strains of *E. coli*, shigella and salmonella.	Skin rashes; urticaria; GI disturbances; eosinophilia.	With kanamycin for sepsis in children over 6 months; effective in certain GU infections. Destroyed by penicillinase. Not a penicillin substitute. Used only when laboratory confirms a susceptible organism.
Methicillin	100 mg/kg/24 hr, q 4 – 6 hr; IV or IM	Penicillin spectrum plus most penicillin-resistant staphylococci.	Penicillin allergies; bone marrow.	Effective against most staphylococci.
Penicillin V	25,000 – 50,000 U/kg/24 hr, q 6 hr; orally	Same as penicillin G.	Same as Penicillin G.	The effective orally administered penicillin.
Kanamycin	15 mg/kg/24 hr, q 12 hr; IM	Bactericidal against many gram-negative and -positive organisms Streptococci, pneumococci, and clostridia are resistant.	Nephrotoxic (negligible in infancy); neurotoxic (8th nerve).	With penicillin provides initial therapy in infants and young children. Urinary tract infections when renal damage minimal. For gram-negative coverage when pseudomonas not the identified organism.
Streptomycin	40 mg/kg/24 hr, q 12 hr; IM	Most gram-negative acid-fast (TB).	Neurotoxic (vestibular); nephrotoxic.	Tuberculosis. Second best to kanamycin because resistance to it develops rapidly. Pulmonary resection and esophageal surgery.
Neomycin	50 – 100 mg/kg/24 hr, q 6 hr; orally	Gram-negative.	Ototoxic; nephrotoxic.	Preoperative "sterilization" of bowel for colon surgery. For pathogenic *E. coli* infections (resistant strains now increasingly common).
Polymyxin B	4 mg/kg/24 hr, q 6 hr; IM or IV	*Ps. aeruginosa.*	Nephrotoxic; neurotoxic.	Pseudomonas infections, sepsis, empyema, meningitis. May be used intrapleurally and intrathecally.
Polymyxin E (Colistin)	8 mg/kg/24 hr over age 1 yr	*Ps. aeruginosa.*	Neurotoxic; nephrotoxic.	Pseudomonas infections, sepsis, empyema, meningitis. May be used intrapleurally and intrathecally.
Tetracyclines: Tetracycline Chlortetracycline Methacycline Oxytetracycline	25 – 50 mg/kg/24 hr, q 6 hr; orally	Broad spectrum – a bacteriostatic drug vs. large viruses and agent of atypical pneumonia sensitive. Many strains of beta-hemolytic strep and enteric organisms are resistant.	Discolors teeth, promotes caries. Growth inhibition of prematures. Pseudo tumor cerebri. Nausea and emesis.	Prophylaxis in cystic fibrosis of pancreas (meconium ileus PO). Widely used for nonhospitalized patients.
Erythromycin	25 – 40 mg/kg/24 hr, orally 10 mg/kg/24 hr, IM	Bacteriostatic range similar to penicillin, plus neisseria, *H. influenzae* and diphtheroids.	Hypersensitivity; jaundice rarely.	Penicillin substitute. For oral use in outpatients.
Chloramphenicol	50 – 100 mg/kg/24 hr	Bacteriostatic. Broad-spectrum gram-positive and -negative except pseudomonas and proteus.	Gray syndrome in infants. Hematologica depression (aplastic anemia).	Urinary tract and eye infections; salmonella infections. A dangerous drug.
Succinyl sulfathiazole (Sulfasuxidine)	0.25 Gm/kg/24 hr, q 4 hr; orally	Gram-negative organisms.	Not absorbed.	Preparing bowel for colon surgery.
Salicylazo-sulfapyridine (Azulfidine)	150 mg/kg/24 hr, q 4 hr, orally			Ulcerative colitis.
Sulfisoxazole (Gantrisin)	150 mg/kg/24 hr	Bacteriostatic.	Fever; skin eruptions.	Urinary tract infections.
Isoniazid	15 mg/kg/24 hr, q 6 – 8 hr; orally	Tubercle bacilli.		Tuberculosis (cervical adenitis).
Nitrofurantoin (Furadantin)	6 mg/kg/24 hr, q 6 hr; orally			Urinary tract infections.

NOTE: Bacitracin, Vancomycin and Ristocetin are rarely used since newer penicillins are available.

is partly responsible for the troublesome ecchymoses occasionally encountered with repeated intramuscular administration.

DISCONTINUING ANTIBACTERIAL THERAPY. — In general, antibacterial therapy should be discontinued 48–72 hours after all clinical evidence of infection has subsided. This rule cannot be applied, however, in infants with serious staphylococcic infection. In such instances, therapy must be continued for at least 1 or 2 weeks after all clinical evidence of infection has subsided. In some circumstances, continuous prophylactic and therapeutic antibiotic administration is essential, as in cystic fibrosis of the pancreas. Special conditions may require prolonged treatment, as in nonsurgical urinary tract infections, for which less than 3 months of therapy is considered inadequate by some.[35]

DRUGS IN CURRENT USE. — Antimicrobial agents are designated as bactericidal drugs, which kill susceptible organisms, or as bacteriostatic drugs, which inhibit multiplication of sensitive organisms. In different circumstances and in increased concentrations, a bacteriostatic drug may be bactericidal.[27] The important difference in their action is that bacteriostatic action is reversible, whereas bactericidal action is not. Antimicrobials are most effective during the stage of multiplication of bacteria. This observation implies that their effect depends on interference with bacterial metabolism. The bactericidal action of antimicrobials can be antagonized by any factor which would reduce the relative number of multiplying bacteria. Thus the prior administration of a bacteriostatic drug or the simultaneous administration of bacteriostatic and bactericidal drugs could theoretically be antagonistic. It seems unlikely that the experimental conditions under which antagonism of antibacterials has been observed would be encountered clinically. There is little evidence to suggest that antagonism may be of clinical significance.[25] Current practice advocates the use of a bactericidal drug in preference to a bacteriostatic one for primary treatment and the avoidance of combining bacteriostatic and bactericidal drugs.[33]

The antibiotics in current use may be grouped according to their effective spectrum of antibacterial activity (Table 5-2). Penicillin is most effective against gram-positive but shows little activity against gram-negative organisms. Cephalothin, erythromycin and bacitracin, like penicillin, are effective against gram-positive bacteria but are relatively ineffective against gram-negative organisms. The so-called broad-spectrum antibiotics, which include the tetracycline group and chloramphenicol, are effective against both gram-negative and gram-positive bacteria. The tetracyclines are also effective against rickettsia and larger viruses. Streptomycin, kanamycin and polymyxin form a third group, showing activity against gram-negative organisms and the tubercle bacillus. Antibacterials effective against fungi are nystatin and amphotercin.

The sulfonamides and the nitrofurans are chemotherapeutic agents. The sulfonamides in current use include sulfadiazine, sulfisoxazole (Gantrisin), sulfasuxidine and sulfathalidine. They are useful in the treatment of urinary tract infections and in preparation of the bowel for surgery. Nitrofurantoin (Furadantin) is used in the treatment of urinary tract infections.

PROPHYLACTIC PRE- AND POSTOPERATIVE USE OF ANTIBACTERIAL DRUGS

There is no evidence that the incidence of postoperative infections is reduced when antibacterial drugs are used prophylactically in clean surgical procedures. Rather do controlled studies indicate a greater incidence of major and minor infections.[5,34,46] Furthermore, when infection occurs, clinical detection may be difficult because the classic symptoms and signs of infection are masked. Resistant bacteria tend to flourish, and superinfection may become a problem. For these reasons, antibacterial drugs should not be used in clean surgical procedures.

There are, however, some clear indications for prophylactic administration of antibacterial drugs. In patients with congenital heart disease, crystalline and procaine penicillin given parenterally 1–1½ hours preoperatively and followed postoperatively by penicillin orally for 2 days will provide protection against bacterial endocarditis. Erythromycin and tetracycline are less valuable substitutes.

Rationale for the preoperative administration of antibacterial drugs is suggested by experimental evidence which indicated that the administration of an antimicrobial agent prior to the time of contamination, by producing a high level of drug in the tissues at the time of contamination, may significantly reduce the incidence and severity of infection postoperatively.[6, 11]

Antibacterial drugs are administered to all newborn infants undergoing surgery. They are indicated because of the hazard of postoperative pneumonia[21] and because of the nature of most procedures carried out in neonatal infants. It is general practice to give penicillin and streptomycin for 5–7 days postoperatively to infants undergoing primary esophageal anastomosis for esophageal atresia. Resection of the small intestine, intestinal anastomosis and colostomy done in the first few days of life require antibacterial coverage. Antibacterials should be continued prophylactically after the infant with surgically treated meconium ileus is discharged from the hospital. The tetracycline drugs are effective for this purpose.

Infants with ruptured meningoceles should receive antibiotics both before and after surgery. In infants and children with compound skull fractures, manifested by bleeding from the ear or nasopharynx or blood in the spinal fluid, prophylactic antibacterial therapy is indicated. Prophylactic therapy against pneumonia in the comatose patient is valueless.[36] The likelihood of fungous overgrowth and superinfection makes this practice hazardous.

Pulmonary resection involves transection of the bronchus and consequent pleural contamination. Prophylactic penicillin therapy is indicated.

In trauma associated with gross contamination of surrounding tissue, as in compound fractures, thoracic wounds with pleural soiling and abdominal wounds with injury to the bowel, the use of antibacterial drugs is a routine part of surgical management.

When prophylactic therapy is indicated in infants under 18 months of age, penicillin combined with kanamycin given intramuscularly every 12 hours is used. Kanamycin has replaced streptomycin for this purpose in premature and newly born infants. Its wider spectrum and the slow development of resistance to it by sensitive organisms make kanamycin a superior choice. Toxicity is low in this age group. If therapy is necessary beyond 7–10 days, another agent, preferably one indicated by bacteriologic sensitivity tests, is substituted.

Elective surgery should not be done in the presence of respiratory infection or unexplained fever. The practice of administering penicillin to allow elective surgery under these conditions should be condemned.[5] There is indication, however, for the use of antimicrobials to combat bacterial infections in children who require emergency surgery.

ANTIBACTERIALS IN PREPARATION OF THE BOWEL FOR COLON SURGERY.—Postoperative infection after colon operations is more common than after procedures at any other surgical site. It is logical to believe that any means of preventing such infections would be a boon to the surgeon and patient alike. Many, but not all, surgeons agree that it is wise to reduce the bacterial flora of the colon before elective surgery. Evaluation of the influence of antibiotic preparation of the bowel on complications after colon surgery has shown no significant advantage when antibiotics have been used, except in patients whose anastomosis is extraperitoneal.[24] Simple mechanical cleansing with enemas and purgatives, when permissible, will drastically reduce the bacterial content of the colon. Unless the colon can be relieved of impactions and adequately emptied, antibacterial drugs are not effective in controlling bacterial growth. Penicillin, streptomycin and the tetracyclines allow overgrowth of resistant organisms and can lead to superinfection with resulting staphylococcic enterocolitis. Neomycin is generally used for preoperative sterilization of the colon.[8] Less than 3% of the orally administered drug is absorbed from the intestinal tract,[1] and the bacterial flora is significantly reduced after 24 hours of its administration. Such reduction persists for 5–7 days.

After this period, organisms rapidly replace the bacterial vacuum. Since yeast overgrowth occurs rapidly and may be troublesome, nystatin or amphotericin has been recommended in combination with neomycin.[10] Although staphylococci resistant to neomycin have not been encountered, staphylococcic enterocolitis has been reported following its administration. Irrigation of the bowel lumen at surgery with solutions of neomycin is contraindicated. Spillage of neomycin into the peritoneal cavity has resulted in respiratory failure and death.[13]

The oral administration of kanamycin has been recommended for preoperative preparation of the colon. Its action is essentially similar to that of neomycin for this specific purpose. Among the sulfonamide drugs, sulfazuxidine and sulfathalidine provide effective preparation of the bowel but must be given for 5 days. Since bacterial synthesis of vitamin K is interfered with when such sulfonamides are used, vitamin K should be administered intramuscularly.

Bacterial decomposition of intraluminal blood contributes to ammonia intoxication and hepatic coma in the presence of bleeding esophageal varices. Sterilization of the bowel contents may therefore be indicated in management of the patient with bleeding esophageal varices due to portal hypertension. Preoperative bowel sterilization may be used for colonic surgery for megacolon, imperforate anus and colonic transplants. In Table 5-3 is a suggested routine of bowel sterilization for colonic surgery.

It is the opinion of some pediatric surgeons[21, 45] and many general surgeons[24] that to prevent postoperative infections, reliance should be placed on thorough mechanical cleansing of the colon with purgatives and enemas rather than on antimicrobial drugs to prepare the colon for surgery.

URINARY TRACT INFECTIONS.—Urine cultures repeated at specified intervals are essential in the antimicrobial management of urinary tract infections. Initial therapy should be continued for a minimum of 10–14 days. Urologic investigation is indicated when acute primary urinary tract infection does not re-

---

TABLE 5-3.—ROUTINE OF BOWEL PREPARATION FOR ELECTIVE COLON SURGERY

1. Liquid diet.
2. Castor oil, 1 oz (30 cc) under age 2 years; 2 oz (60 cc) over age 2 years.
3. Saline enema the night of admission.
   Cleansing enemas (using saline, Colase or hydrogen peroxide diluted 1:4 in saline) as indicated to remove residual feces completely the evening prior to surgery.
4. Neomycin 50 mg/lb of body weight (100 mg/kg) per day divided into 6 doses administered every 4 hr and continued for 24 but no more than 48 hr preoperatively.
5. Penicillin and streptomycin parenterally, 5–7 days postoperatively.
CAUTION: Neomycin may be absorbed in toxic quantities in ulcerative colitis.

TABLE 5-4.—Dosages of Antimicrobial Drugs in Premature and Newborn Infants*

Drug	Dosage	Remarks
Penicillin G	60,000 U/kg/24 hr, q 12 hr; IM or IV	First choice for gram-positive organisms.
Ampicillin	20 mg/kg/24 hr, q 12 hr; IM or IV (50 mg/kg/q 6–8 hr)†	Not often used in this age group. Urinary tract infection and a penicillin substitute.
Methicillin	40 mg/kg/24 hr, q 6 hr; IM or IV (250–300 mg/kg/24 hr)†	Not often used in this age group. For penicillin-resistant staph. infections.
Erythromycin	25–40 mg/kg/24 hr, q 6 hr; orally 10 mg/kg/24 hr, q 12 hr; IM or IV	A second choice drug substitute for penicillin.
Kanamycin	15 mg/kg/24 hr, q 12 hr; IM	12 days only. The drug choice for gram-negative enteric organism coverage.
Streptomycin	20–30 mg/kg/24 hr, q 12 hr	10 days only. Kanamycin preferable.
Polymyxin B	2.5–3 mg/kg/24 hr, q 6 hr; IM or IV	7 days only. Nephro- and neurotoxic. Only drug effective against pseudomonas infections.
Polymyxin E (Colistin)	8 mg/kg/hr; orally 1.5–5 mg/kg/24 hr, q 6–12 hr; IM	7 days only. Nephro- and neurotoxic. Only drug effective against pseudomonas infections.
Nystatin	400,000 U/24 hr, q 6 hr; orally Topically, q 6 hr	For thrush and yeast overgrowth.

Contraindicated agents
    Sulfonamides: Dangerous up to 2 months of age.
    Chloramphenicol: Dangerous up to 1 month of age.
    Fixed combinations of drugs are dangerous (see text).

*Precise dosage is not available for many of these drugs. Doses given here are on recommendation of Committee on the Control of Infectious Diseases, 1966, American Academy of Pediatrics, and McCracken and Eichenwald.[33]
†McCracken and Eichenwald.[33]

spond to antimicrobial therapy within a few days, when the urinary tract infection is recurrent and when such infection occurs in infants under 1 year of age.

Prophylactic antimicrobial therapy is indicated in association with surgery of the urinary tract that requires the insertion of indwelling tubes or catheters. Nitrofurantoin (Furadantin) and sulfisoxazole (Gantrisin) are useful in this respect and may be given safely for long periods.[32,44]

Currently, Gantrisin and ampicillin are the most commonly primarily prescribed drugs for urinary tract infections. Kanamycin, the polymyxins and, rarely, chloramphenicol are used.

ANTIBIOTICS IN PREMATURE INFANTS.—Since control of infection has been largely responsible for the lowered mortality in premature nurseries in recent years, it would seem logical to believe that here is an indication for prophylactic antibacterial drug administration in the routine care of premature infants. It has been pointed out that infection is difficult to detect in the premature and that perhaps routine prophylactic antibiotic therapy with penicillin and streptomycin may actually be therapeutic more often than prophylactic (Table 5-4). Reports conflict, however,

concerning the value of routine penicillin and streptomycin prophylaxis in the premature infant.[42] Recent reports indicate that chloramphenicol is a dangerous drug and may cause death in premature infants when given in standard doses.[9] Since metabolic processes of the premature are inadequately developed and renal function is immature, dosages of all drugs must be modified in treating premature infants. Chloramphenicol is conjugated to the glucuronide form and also excreted by the kidney. Glucuronide formation in the premature may be faulty, leading to an accumulation of the drug, high serum values and vasomotor collapse described as the gray syndrome. Chloramphenicol should be used only when no other agent can be substituted for the treatment of the specific infection. When used, the administered dosage should not exceed 25 mg/kg of body weight per day. Sulfonamides likewise are not efficiently detoxified for excretion, and their use in premature infants is contraindicated. Their use in the presence of jaundice leads to kernicterus by competing with bilirubin for protein binding.[42]

The drugs most often used for premature infants are the penicillins, kanamycin, polymyxin and nystatin.

BURNS.—Controversy continues concerning the

advisability of routine prophylactic antibiotic treatment of all major burns. The administration of antibiotics to patients recently burned is indicated when the burns are contaminated or extensive. In these circumstances, penicillin is recommended for the first 48 hours. Usually the drug is not given until the first major change of dressing; strict isolation and careful asepsis are employed to prevent infection. Bacteremia and septicemia tend to occur when the first major dressing is done, and huge doses of penicillin 24 hours before and after dressing the burn are preventive. Cultures determine the antibiotic to be used to cover subsequent procedures. Local application of antibiotics to burns is not advised. Pseudomonas sepsis remains a major problem in extensive burns. Gentamicin is the most effective available therapeutic drug.[43]

SPECIAL PROBLEMS IN PEDIATRIC SURGERY.—*Cervical adenitis* is a common infection that is usually responsive to the tetracycline drugs and even more responsive to penicillin. Occasionally, the infection progresses to suppuration, and incision and drainage become necessary. At times, the adenitis will become a ligneous fixed mass, moderately tender and unchanging for weeks despite intelligently directed antibiotic therapy. This static situation is best resolved by discontinuing all antibiotics and awaiting either absorption or, what is less likely, suppuration.

The patient with a *ruptured acute appendix and peritonitis* is treated with penicillin and streptomycin or with tetracycline or with chloramphenicol. It is wise to discontinue all antibiotics at least 48 hours prior to discharge to eliminate the possibility of a quiescent intra-abdominal or incisional abscess. A rectal examination 24 hours before discharge from the hospital is wise. In patients in whom no definite source of fever following surgery can be found, discontinuation of all antibiotics will allow the site of the infection to become obvious.

Staphylococcic infections are a serious source of morbidity and mortality. The relative frequency of various organisms recovered from superficial abscesses among patients at the Children's Hospital of Pittsburgh during various years is shown in Table 5-5.[41] These data document the clinical impression that with the introduction of penicillin the pneumococcus practically disappeared as the cause of abscesses; a gradual reduction of streptococcic infec-

tions occurred, and the staphylococcus continued to be the most common organism responsible for such abscesses. Until recently, penicillin provided effective treatment in most instances, but the problem has become compounded by the emergence of penicillin- and tetracycline-resistant strains of staphylococci. Furunculosis, mastitis and adenitis, progressing to septicemia, pneumonia and empyema, are common. A number of agents are available to combat these serious infections. Methicillin, kanamycin, chloramphenicol, bacitracin and cephalothin are powerful effective agents. Since these are toxic and require laboratory controls, their use should be reserved for hospitalized patients. The solution of the problem of staphylococcic infection is not so simple that it can be answered by a listing of drugs. The age of the patient, sources of infection, reinfection, changes in resistance of the organism and changes in the infant's resistance determine the course of the disease. Relatively fewer serious staphylococcic infections have been seen in the past 2 years.

Initial treatment of *osteomyelitis* consists of the administration of large doses of penicillin combined with emergency drainage of abscesses, infected joints and areas of early bone involvement. Cultures taken at operation indicate the appropriate antibiotic, which is then continued in lesser dosage for at least 1 month after hospitalization. Reliance on antibiotic therapy alone sometimes delays necessary surgery and results in irreversible damage with crippling deformities. The incidence of crippling deformities secondary to osteomyelitis has not appreciably declined with the introduction of antibiotics.[41]

Generalized infections due to Pseudomonas pyocyaneus and proteus organisms are usually untreatable. Polymyxin B and Colistin may have a remarkable effect when infections due to these organisms are localized. Local instillation into the pleural space in empyema may bring about dramatic recovery. Parenterally administered polymyxin is poorly tolerated in doses above 2.5 mg/kg of body weight per 24 hours. Since optimal serum concentrations are not consistently obtained even after the administration of the maximal tolerated doses, combined therapy with tetracycline, streptomycin or any other indicated antibacterial is necessary to control pseudomonas infections.[2] Novobiocin in combination with other indicated drugs is the most effective agent available in the treatment of proteus infections.

TABLE 5-5.—ORGANISMS CULTURED FROM SUPERFICIAL ABSCESSES

ORGANISMS	1934	1941	1950	1957	1966
Staphylococcus	43	43	60	66.5	65
Streptococcus	30	24	14	6.4	4
Mixed streptococcus and staphylococcus	0	21	12	8.6	7
Coliform	20	2.5	14	18.5	23
Diplococcus	7	9.5	0	0	1

REFERENCES

1. A.M.A. Council on Pharmacy and Chemistry: Neomycin sulfate, J.A.M.A. 154:338, 1954.
2. Asay, L. D., and Koch, R.: Pseudomonas infections in infants and children, New England J. Med. 262:1062, 1960.
3. Barber, M., *et al.*: Reversal of antibiotic resistance in hospital staphylococcal infection, Brit. M. J. 1:11, 1960.
4. Barnes, J., *et al.*: Prophylactic postoperative antibiotics, Arch. Surg. 79:190, 1959.

5. Bernard, H. R., and Cole, W. R.: The role of antimicrobial agents in the care of the pediatric surgical patient, South. M. J. 54:1303, 1961.

6. Bernard, H. R., and Cole, W. R.: Prophylaxis of surgical infection: Effect of prophylactic antimicrobial drugs on incidence of infection following potentially contaminated operations, Surgery 56:151, 1964.

7. Broom, N. H., et al.: A correlation of the results of disk antibiotic sensitivity tests and the clinical course of sixty-nine patients with acute bacterial meningitis, Antibiotics & Chemother. 3:409, 1953.

8. Bronsther, R.: Sterilization of the bowel in infants and children, Am. J. Surg. 98:605, 1959.

9. Burns, L. E., et al.: Fatal circulatory collapse in infants receiving chloramphenicol, New England J. Med. 261:1318, 1959.

10. Cohen, I., Jr.: Antimicrobial therapy for surgical gastrointestinal diseases, Pediat. Clin. North America 8:1251, 1961.

11. Cole, W. R., et al.: Chemoprophylaxis with penicillin, Arch. Surg. 94:182, 1967.

12. Cope, C. L.: The adrenal cortex in internal medicine, Brit. M. J. 2:847, 1966.

13. Daremus, W. P.: Respiratory arrest following intraperitoneal use of neomycin, Ann. Surg. 149:546, 1959.

14. Deming, M. V.: Steroid and antihistaminic therapy for postintubation subglottic edema in infants and children, Anesthesiology 22:933, 1961.

15. Editorial: Antibiotics in fixed combination, New England J. Med. 262:225, 1960.

16. Editorial: Choice of antimicrobial drugs when infecting organisms have not been identified, M. Lett. Drugs Therap. 8:57, 1966.

17. Good, R. A., Vernier, R. L., and Smith, R. T.; Serious untoward reactions to therapy with cortisone and adrenocorticotropin in pediatric practice: I and II, Pediatrics 19:95 and 272, 1957.

18. Gould, J. C.: The laboratory control of antibiotic therapy, Brit. M. Bull. 16:29, 1960.

19. Graber, A. L., et al.: Natural history of pituitary adrenal recovery following long term suppression with corticosteroids, J. Clin. Endocrinol. 25:11, 1965.

20. Gray, H. G., III: Antibiotic sensitivity reactions in children, North Carolina M. J. 26:49, 1965.

21. Gross, R. E.; Textbook of Pediatric Surgery (Philadelphia: W. B. Saunders Company, 1952).

22. Halzel, A.: Drug toxicity in children, Practitioner 194:98, 1965.

23. Harter, J. G.; Reddy, W. J., and Thorn, G. W.: Studies on an intermittent corticosteroid dosage regimen, New England J. Med. 269:591, 1963.

24. Herter, F. P., and Slanetz, C. A., Jr.: Influence of antibiotic preparation of the bowel on complications after colon resection, Am. J. Surg. 113:165, 1967.

25. Hodes, H. L.: Antibiotic prophylaxis, Pediatrics 24:126, 1959.

26. Jawetz, E., and Gunnison, J. B.: Studies on antibiotic synergism and antagonism, Antibiotics & Chemother. 11:243, 1952.

27. Kempe, C. H.: A rational approach to antibiotic therapy of childhood infections, Postgrad. Med. 24:325, 1958.

28. Kerr, A., Jr.: Bacterial endocarditis—Revisited, Mod. Concepts Cardiovas. Dis. 33:831, 1964.

29. Kurkguoglu, M., and McElfresh, A. E.: An anticoagulant property of antibiotics from streptomyces species, New England J. Med. 260:929, 1960.

30. LaFemine, A. A., et al.: The adrenocortical response in surgical patients, Am. Surgeon 146:26, 1957.

31. Marcey, J.: Personal communication.

32. Marshall, M., and Johnson, S. H., III: Use of nitrofurantoin in chronic and recurrent urinary tract infection in children, J.A.M.A. 169:919, 1959.

33. McCracken, G. H., and Eichenwald, H. F.: Antimicrobial therapy in infancy and childhood, Pediat. Clin. North America 13:231, 1966.

34. McKittrick, L. S., and Wheelock, F. C.: The routine use of antibiotics in elective abdominal surgery, Surg., Gynec. & Obst. 99:376, 1954.

35. Normand, I. C. S., and Smellie, J. M.: Prolonged maintenance chemotherapy in the management of urinary infection in childhood, Brit. M. J. 1:1023, 1965.

36. Petersdorf, R. G., et al.: A study of antibiotic prophylaxis in unconscious patients, New England J. Med. 257:1001, 1957.

37. Rodger, K. C., et al.: Antibiotic therapy: Correlation of clinical results with laboratory sensitivity tests, Canad. M.A.J. 74:605, 1956.

38. Ross, S.: Penicillin: Applied pharmacology, Pediat. Clin. North America 3:259, 1956.

39. Salassa, R. M., et al.: Postoperative adrenal cortical insufficiency; occurrence in patients previously ʋreated with cortisone, J.A.M.A. 152:1509, 1953.

40. Scheinberg, L., and Allensworth, M.: Sciatic neuropathy in infants related to antibiotic injections, Pediatrics 19:261, 1957.

41. Sieber, W. K., and Ferguson, A. B.: Surgical and orthopedic aspects of infections in newly born and young infants, Pediatrics 24:145, 1959.

42. Silverman, W. A., et al.: A difference in mortality rate and incidence of kernicterus among premature infants allotted to two prophylactic antibacterial regimens, Pediatrics 18:614, 1956.

43. Stone, H. H.: Review of pseudomonas sepsis in thermal burns: Verdoglobin determination and gentamicin therapy, Ann. Surg. 163:297, 1966.

44. Stanfeld, J. M.: Relapses of urinary tract infections in children, Brit. M. J. 1:635, 1966.

45. Swensen, O.: Pediatric Surgery (New York: Appleton-Century-Crofts, Inc., 1958).

46. Tachdjian, M. O., and Compere, E. L.: Postoperative wound infections in orthopedic surgery: Evaluation of prophylactic antibiotics, J. Internat. Coll. Surgeons 28:797, 1959.

47. Troen, P., and Rynearson, E. H.: An evaluation of the prophylactic use of cortisone for pituitary operations, J. Clin. Endocrinol. 16:737, 1946.

48. Tronzo, R. G., and Dowling, J. J.: Acute hematogenous osteomyelitis of children in era of broad spectrum antibiotics, Clin. Orthop. 22:108, 1962.

49. Van Metre, T. E., Jr.; Niermann, W. A., and Rosen, J. J.: Comparison of growth suppression effect of cortisone, prednisone, and other adrenal cortical hormones, J. Allergy 31:531–542, 1960.

50. Westerman, G., et al.: Adverse reactions to penicillin: A review of treatment, J.A.M.A. 198:193, 1966.

WILLIAM K. SIEBER

Drawings by
PAMELA BERGLUND (Figure 5–3)

6

Chemotherapy of Solid Tumors

HISTORY.—The first chemicals used with effect in the treatment of cancer were the alkylating agents. Sulfur mustard, first synthesized in 1854, was noted to have vesicant properties in 1887. In World War I, mustard gas was used as a chemical warfare agent with devastating results. Initially, the vesicant action on skin, eyes and respiratory tract was thought to be the primary toxic effect, but Krumbhaar and Krumbhaar made the pertinent observation that other effects included leukopenia, bone marrow aplasia, lymphoid depletion and gastrointestinal ulceration. Between the two World Wars, the effect of nitrogen mustard was investigated extensively, and Goodman and Gilman noted regression of transplanted lymphosarcoma in mice treated with nitrogen mustard. The first clinical trial with nitrogen mustard, at Yale in 1942, produced dramatic results in a patient with a far-advanced malignant lymphoma.

The next major step was the observation by Farber, in 1947, of an "acceleration" effect of folic acid on the leukemic process seen in the bone marrow. In children with acute leukemia, treatment of 4-aminopteroyl glutamic acid, Aminopterin, a folic acid antagonist, resulted in complete hematologic remissions. Adrenocorticosteroids and ACTH were the next drugs used with good effect in the treatment of leukemia. Since then, thousands of agents have been tested in an attempt to control cancer by affecting its growth, its ability to metastasize, its implantation in remote sites, or all three. Many of these agents are effective in causing cure of cancer in laboratory animals, but relatively few have been effective in human beings.

Aims of Chemotherapy

The growing emphasis in the past 15 years on the combined approach to the child with cancer, including operation, chemotherapy and irradiation, has been a major factor in producing the gratifying improvement in survival. At this stage of development in the field of cancer chemotherapy, there are only two situations in which a chemical alone appears to have cured cancer. Metastatic choriocarcinoma in women can be cured in approximately 50% of cases following treatment with Methotrexate, and when the same disease becomes resistant to Methotrexate, vincristine also appears to produce cures. The second example is in children with Burkitt's lymphoma, found principally in certain geographic areas of Africa. In a group of these children, with large lymphosarcomatous masses of the jaw and cervical nodes treated with one or two large doses of Cytoxan, a proportion were living and well several years later. In choriocarcinoma, it is possible to invoke the existence of a host

immune response as aiding the chemotherapy, since genetic material from the father is incorporated in the tumor. There is some evidence from the geographic distribution of Burkitt's lymphoma that it has a viral etiology, and this also suggests the possibility of an immune response. At all events, these are special and unusual tumors, and the success of chemotherapy in them has no parallel in the common solid tumors of childhood.

Children differ from adults in two ways: they are afflicted with other types of tumors, and their response to chemotherapy is not the same. On the whole, they are able to tolerate relatively larger amounts of drugs than adults, possibly because of their active bone marrow. Also, some tumors which in adults are more differentiated and considered resistant to treatment, such as rhabdomyosarcoma, prove to be very sensitive in childhood.

The drug doses given below are calculated on the basis of weight and are appropriate for small children. When used for large children or adults, they should be recalculated for surface area.

Mode of Action of Chemotherapeutic Agents

The knowledge about the various ways in which chemical agents can inhibit cellular growth and metabolism has been gained from experiments in tissue culture, animal and bacterial models and also in man. The mechanism of the differential sensitivity that exists between malignant and most normal cells is not clear. Originally, it was thought that malignant cells grew and divided more rapidly than their normal counterparts and were more vulnerable because of their increased requirements. However, more and more evidence is being accumulated to show that some malignant cells have an increased resting phase, and the over-all turn-over time is indeed much longer than that of normal cells. Perhaps when the essential genetic, molecular and biochemical differences characteristic of malignant transformation are understood, the reason for the differential response to chemotherapy will become obvious, and more specific therapeutic agents will be evolved.

The cell is a complex structure with a nucleus and

ribosomes for protein synthesis, and there are many sites where normal function could be interrupted. The DNA of the nucleus is composed of four purine and pyrimidine bases and their attached deoxyribose sugar, all held together in the double helix by phosphate and hydrogen bonds. These chains of nucleic acids in DNA must grow and replicate and also act as templates for messenger RNA synthesis. DNA synthesis, in theory, could be affected in various ways: (1) The whole chain could be affected physically by heat, light, sound or x-radiation, causing breakage. (2) Physical agents such as x-rays could cause abnormal linkage of the base pairs which might induce incorrect reading of the code or dissociation from the regulator genes. (3) Purine and pyrimidine analogues can be substituted into both DNA and RNA chains, again interrupting the sequence and possibly causing false coding. (4) Alterations of the sugar of the nucleoside could inhibit DNA or RNA function. (5) Purine and pyrimidine analogues could give fraudulent feedback inhibition, shutting off the synthesis of the correct compound. (6) Modifications of the enzymes and coenzymes involved in synthesis of purine or pyrimidine or of DNA and RNA polymerase could alter replication. (7) Some agents, such as actinomycin D, are known to bind to DNA, blocking messenger RNA. (8) Messenger, transfer and ribosomal RNA could be altered by abnormalities in purine and pyrimidine metabolism in a manner similar to DNA. (9) The transfer of amino acids to the ribosomes can be affected by inhibition of the activator enzyme or by alteration and reduction in the number of amino acids. (10) Folic acid antagonists, such as Methotrexate, can interfere with amino acid synthesis by inhibition of folic acid metabolism, essential in de novo synthesis of some amino acids. (11) Formed protein in the cell, such as enzymes, can be attacked chemotherapeutically, thereby inhibiting activity.

The anticancer drugs for the most part appear to function not by active differential destruction of malignant cells but by interrupting cell metabolism in one of the various ways mentioned above. An exception to this is the effect of steroids on malignant lymphocytes, in which actual cell lysis appears to occur.

Specific Agents: Mode of Action, Dose and Toxicity

Table 6-1 shows the classes of agents effective in the chemotherapy of cancer in man.

ANTIMETABOLITES

Historically, analogues of nucleic acid and coenzymes have been classed together as antimetabolites. However, now that more is known about the method of action of all the compounds in use, one could say that any one of the agents used is directed against the metabolism of a cell and in that sense is an antimetabolite.

METHOTREXATE. — A folic acid antagonist, Methotrexate closely resembles the reduced form of folic acid, folinic acid, in having additions of an amino and a methyl group in the N4 and 10 positions. It competes for the enzyme folic reductase and inhibits the conversion of folic to tetrahydrofolic acid. The latter compound is essential for the transfer of 1-carbon fragments in many biochemical reactions, such as the conversion of deoxyuridylic to thymidylic acid, and also the synthesis of the amino acids serine and histidine.

The therapeutic indications are acute childhood leukemia and choriocarcinoma. It has been used, with varying effectiveness, as an intra-arterial infusion for solid tumors with the simultaneous intermittent intramuscular administration of the antidote, citrovorum factor, to protect tissues, especially bone marrow, in the noninfused area.

Dose. — Methotrexate can be given by mouth and by injection. Its action, though toxic, is predictable, and it is not a difficult agent to use despite its toxicity. The conventional oral dose is 0.1 mg/kg/day. In recent modifications of this regimen, much larger amounts, up to 3 mg/kg, are given at more widely spaced intervals such as every 4–14 days. It is usually given intravenously when such large amounts are used, but it can be given intramuscularly.

Toxicity. — Signs of toxicity are disturbance of the gastrointestinal tract, with oral ulcerations and diarrhea, and bone marrow depression. Rarely, skin rashes and alopecia are encountered. After prolonged use, a megaloblastic anemia can occur. Renal clearance is one of the main factors influencing toxicity, and difficulties can occur in the presence of unsuspected renal impairment. The agent should be discontinued in the presence of oral ulceration, diarrhea, white blood cell count below 3,000 and platelet count less than 75,000/cu mm.

6-MERCAPTOPURINE. — There are several purine antagonists, the one in commonest use being 6-mercaptopurine (6-MP). Structurally, 6-MP is an analogue of hypoxanthine with an SH group in the 6 position. In the body, it is converted to the ribonucleotide derivative and competes for enzymes involved in the synthesis of inosinic acid, forming thioinosinic acid. The latter compound inhibits the formation of adenylic acid and guanylic acid. Mercaptopurine also inhibits the biosynthesis of purines from small molecule precursors, possibly by means of a pseudofeedback inhibition of the formation of inosinic acid.

The main value of this compound is in the treatment of leukemia. It has shown disappointing results in the treatment of other forms of cancer.

Dose. — Mercaptopurine is usually given daily by mouth, in a dose of 2.5 mg/kg. Modifications of this dose, with larger amounts given less frequently, do not seem to have improved its therapeutic effectiveness.

Toxicity. — The first sign of toxicity is usually gin-

TABLE 6-1.—CANCER CHEMOTHERAPEUTIC AGENTS

AGENT	THERAPEUTIC INDICATION	DOSE	TOXICITY
Antimetabolites			
Methotrexate	Acute leukemia, choriocarcinoma	0.1 mg/kg/day, orally; larger doses given systemically	Oral ulceration, GI, bone marrow depression
6-Mercaptopurine	Acute leukemia	2.5 mg/kg/day, orally	Bone marrow depression
5-Fluorouracil	Ca of liver and GI tract	15 mg/kg/day × 5 IV	Nausea, stomatitis, bone marrow depression
Cytosine arabinoside	Acute leukemia	Not established	Nausea, bone marrow depression
Alkylating agents			
Nitrogen mustard	Neuroblastoma, lymphoma	0.2 mg/kg/day × 2 IV	Nausea, GI, bone marrow depression
Chlorambucil	Lymphoma	0.1 mg/kg/day, orally	Lymphoid suppression
Myleran	Chronic myeloid leukemia	2–6 mg/day, orally	Myeloid suppression
Cytoxan	Acute leukemia, neuroblastoma, lymphoma	3 mg/kg/day, orally	Bone marrow suppression, alopecia, cystitis
Antibiotics			
Actinomycin D	Wilms', x-ray potentiation	15 μg/kg/day × 5 IV	Bone marrow suppression, nausea, GI
Daunomycin	Acute leukemia, neuroblastoma	Not established	Bone marrow suppression
Mitomycin C	Chronic myeloid leukemia, lymphoma	Not established.	Bone marrow suppression
Streptonigrin	Lymphoma	Not established	Bone marrow suppression
Mithromycin	CNS tumors	Not established	Bone marrow suppression
Plant alkaloids			
Vincristine	Acute leukemia, neuroblastoma, lymphoma	1–2 mg/M²/week, IV	Neurotoxicity, bone marrow suppression, alopecia
Vinblastine	Lymphoma	0.1 mg/kg/week, IV	Bone marrow suppression
Hormones			
Prednisone	Acute leukemia, lymphoma	2 mg/kg/day, orally	Fluid and salt retention
Miscellaneous			
L-Asparaginase	Lymphocytic leukemia, lymphoma	Not established	Not established

givitis; this stomatitis is a little different from the mouth ulcerations seen early following administration of Methotrexate. Diarrhea is rare. Depression of the bone marrow may be the earliest manifestation, with leukopenia, thrombocytopenia and anemia. This depression can be prolonged, and therapy should be interrupted if the white blood cell count falls below 2,500 and platelet count below 75,000/cu mm. Liver damage can also occur, and liver enzymes should be checked if there are symptoms suggestive of liver disease.

5-FLUOROURACIL AND 5-FLUORODEOXYURIDINE.—It has been shown that the fluorine analogues of uracil and uridine inhibit thymidylate synthetase, interfering with the incorporation of formate into the methyl group of thiamine; probably this is the principal locus of antitumor activity. Also, they are incorporated extensively into RNA and are thought to interfere with the reading of the genetic code. These two agents have not been very effective in the treatment of tumors of childhood, although some observers report promising results in the treatment of carcinoma of the stomach and colon in adults. Some beneficial effect has been noticed in primary carcinoma of the liver in children.

Dose.—Both agents are given by intravenous or intra-arterial routes. The dose for 5-fluorouracil is 15 mg/kg/day for 5 days followed by 7 mg/kg every other day until leukopenia or gastrointestinal toxicity develops. 5-Fluorodeoxyuridine can be given in twice this amount, with 30 mg/kg/day for 5 days, followed by 15 mg/kg/day every other day.

Toxicity.—Like other antimetabolites, these agents cause gastrointestinal disturbances, with stomatitis, nausea and diarrhea. Bone marrow depression also occurs.

CYTOSINE ARABINOSIDE.—Cytosine arabinoside is a little different from the usual purine and pyrimidine antimetabolites in that the modification is on the sugar of cytosine. This altered compound competitively inhibits the conversion of cytidine ribotide to the deoxyribotide and is itself incorporated into both DNA and RNA. Its main therapeutic effect is probably by fraudulent feedback inhibition. It is a recent addition to the group, and although it has been effective in the treatment of leukemia, particularly the acute myeloid type, it has had little trial in the treatment of solid tumors. This drug is still in the investigational stages, and the dose and administration schedule has not been standardized.

ALKYLATING AGENTS

The alkylating agents are all modifications of the original sulfur mustard used as a chemical warfare agent in World War I. They are powerful electrophilic compounds that react with (alkylate) neutrophilic substances and also combine with the phosphate, amino, sulfhydryl, hydroxyl and carboxyl groups in nucleic acids and in proteins. These agents have two or more alkylating groups which cause cross-linking of DNA, linkage of DNA to protein and of protein to protein. The capacity of mustards to inhibit DNA synthesis exceeds their ability to impair the production of RNA, and this differential capability appears to extend even to viral nucleic acids. The specific loci of the reactions are not known. Cellular inhibition occurs in the premitotic stage, causing nuclear damage and chromosomal clumping. The alkylating agents are termed "radiomimetic" drugs because they have an effect on chromosomes grossly similar to that of irradiation, though the mechanism of action may well be different. A great variation exists between the sensitivity of cells of different types, lymphocytes being particularly sensitive. This class of compounds is most effective in the treatment of tumors of lymphoid origin.

NITROGEN MUSTARD.—This is the most effective and most toxic of the alkylating agents. It is of value in the treatment of neuroblastoma, lymphosarcoma and Hodgkin's disease. It is unstable in solution and rapidly inactivated in the blood stream. It is locally toxic and must be given intravenously, since local tissue necrosis occurs when the chemical leaks outside the vein.

Dose.—The dose in children is 0.2 mg/kg on 2 or 3 consecutive days, in courses at intervals not less than every 6–8 weeks.

Toxicity.—Vomiting and depression of hemopoiesis are the chief signs of toxicity. Troublesome vomiting can be overcome by agents such as the chlorpromazine derivatives. It is often helpful to give the drug at night while the patient is under sedation with barbiturates, administering it into the tubing of a previously established infusion.

CHLORAMBUCIL (PHENYLBUTYRIC ACID).—This compound was synthesized in an attempt to find an agent that could be absorbed from the alimentary tract and also have a wider therapeutic ratio than nitrogen mustard. It is a useful drug in the treatment of lymphomas when a slow, sustained activity is desired.

Dose.—The dose is 0.1 mg/kg daily by mouth.

Toxicity.—During prolonged treatment, a careful watch should be kept on the peripheral white cell count, particular note being made of the total lymphocyte count because these are the cells first affected by this agent.

MYLERAN (BUSULFAN).—This alkylating agent for oral administration was found to act selectively on rat myeloid cells. It is probably the most effective agent for the treatment of human chronic myeloid leukemia.

CYTOXAN (CYCLOPHOSPHAMIDE).—Cytoxan, first studied clinically in Germany, is relatively inactive and requires enzyme activation to break the cyclic ring. It was hoped that the increased amount of this activating enzyme found in tumor tissue would lead to a corresponding differential sensitivity between normal and malignant cells. Unfortunately, a considerable quantity of this enzyme is found in the liver, which limits the amount of the compound that can be given. However, it is a very effective alkylating agent in the treatment of neuroblastoma, lymphoma and, less consistently, soft tissue sarcomas and Ewing's sarcoma. It is the only alkylating agent that has induced remissions in acute leukemia.

Dose.—The dose is 2–3 mg/kg/day by mouth. An alternative is the intravenous route, with injections of up to 10 mg/kg being given daily or weekly until leukopenia develops, with a white blood cell count of 2,000/cu mm. Unless a very rapid response is required, the large intravenous dose schedule does not seem to be more beneficial than the daily oral dose.

Toxicity.—The toxic side-effects are on hemopoiesis, bladder mucosa and growth of hair. The effect on the marrow is usually not prolonged, and when the white cell count falls below 2,000, interruption of treatment for about a week is usually sufficient for recovery to take place. Alopecia occurs in some patients following large doses and can be a distressing complication, particularly in the older child, although the hair will regrow. Wigs these days are inexpensive and should be recommended for girls afflicted with alopecia. Hemorrhagic cystitis can sometimes be prevented by making sure that a large amount of fluid is taken at the time of each dose. Treatment should be interrupted if this complication occurs.

ANTIBIOTICS

The large amount of screening of microbiologic filtrates for antimicrobial therapy has also led to their testing in many cancer systems. The results are encouraging, although only a few have been found to be effective against malignant disease in man.

ACTINOMYCIN D.—The actinomycins were discovered by Waksman in 1940, but it was not until 1952 that their carcinolytic effect was noted by Hackmann. These antibiotics are found in the filtrate of *Bacillus subtilis* and have been studied extensively. Actinomycin D has been isolated, and its chemical structure is known. It consists of a 3-ring phenoxazone chromophore group with 2 peptide chains. Differences in the amino acids and their sequence on the peptide chains give various modifications coded by letters of the alphabet, e.g., actinomycin C and F. The mode of action of actinomycin D appears to be attachment of the amino group to the hydroxyl group of guanine in DNA, preventing the transcription of the DNA code by messenger RNA. Thus it inhibits DNA-dependent RNA synthesis. This inhibiting effect acts, however, on the DNA of all cells, so the reason for a differential effect on malignant cells is not obvious. Clinically and in animals, actinomycin D enhances radiation effects in normal as well as neoplastic tissues. This fact has to be borne in mind when the two are given in combination. The agent is effective in the treatment of Wilms' tumor, soft tissue sarcomas and Ewing's sarcoma. It has not proved useful for treatment of neuroblastoma or the lymphomas.

Dose.—The dose is usually 15 μg/kg/day for 5 days to a total of 75 μg/kg/course and a maximum single injection of 500 μg. It is given intravenously daily or every other day. It is safe to repeat the course in 2–3 months.

Toxicity.—The compound is toxic locally, and a severe tissue reaction can be produced if the antibiotic is extravasated outside the vein. Other signs of toxicity are nausea, vomiting, stomatitis, diarrhea in severe cases, alopecia and depression of the bone marrow, particularly of platelet formation. It is our practice to interrupt therapy if the platelet count falls below 100,000 and to start again when there is some evidence of recovery. Treatment should be interrupted immediately at the first sign of diarrhea. Cumulative toxicity can occur, so that subsequent courses are sometimes more toxic than the original one. The potentiation of x-rays by actinomycin D increases the radiation effects, so that skin erythema and so on occur at a lower dose range than when x-rays are given alone.

DAUNOMYCIN.—Daunomycin was isolated from *Streptomyces pencetius* and has a structural formula similar to the anthracyclines. It is a glycosidic compound with an aglycone chromatophore link to an amino sugar. It inhibits cellular RNA synthesis and DNA-dependent RNA synthesis, apparently by complexing with DNA. The initial clinical trials have not yet been completed, and the dose range and side effects are not fully known. It appears to be effective in the treatment of lymphomas and neuroblastoma.

MITOMYCIN C.—Most of the work on mitomycin C, a product of *Streptomyces caespitosus*, has been carried out in Japan. Clinical trials in this country have been disappointing in most malignancies, although it is of some help in the treatment of chronic myeloid leukemia. In Japan, regression of carcinoma of the stomach has been reported. A safe therapeutic dose range has not been established.

STREPTONIGRIN.—This antibiotic, structurally similar to mitomycin C, is derived from *Streptomyces flocculus*. It causes a decrease of adenosine triphosphate and protein synthesis in intact cells, and strand breakage of DNA. It has no effect on ribosomal protein synthesis. It has little effect on childhood malignant disease, but it has been effective in some patients with lymphomas and is quite often used in the treatment of mycosis fungoides.

MITHROMYCIN.—Mithromycin, another antibiotic derived from streptomyces, was noted to affect the central nervous system, causing drowsiness and confusion. It was therefore tried in the treatment of brain tumors with some benefit. It has also been effective in the treatment of testicular tumors. It inhibits the synthesis of RNA and has little effect on DNA.

Dose.—Dose has not yet been standardized, but 25 and 50 μg/kg have been given daily until toxic signs developed.

Toxicity.—Toxicity is manifested by nausea and vomiting. Other manifestations are liver disturbance with elevated enzyme and decreased prothrombin values and bone marrow depression causing thrombocytopenia.

PLANT ALKALOIDS

The four alkaloids obtained from *Vinca rosea Linn* are similar chemically. They are asymmetrical dimeric compounds with the empiric formula approximately $C_{40}H_{56-58}O_9N_4$. They appear to inhibit mitosis at the metaphase stage, possibly by affecting the spindles. In isolated cell systems, they appear to have no effect on respiration or on nucleic acid or protein synthesis.

VINCRISTINE.—This is the vinca alkaloid most commonly used in the treatment of solid tumors such as neuroblastoma, Wilms' tumor and lymphomas. It has also been effective in the treatment of acute childhood leukemia.

Dose.—The dose is 0.05 mg/kg or 1–2 mg/M² of body surface. It is given intravenously, usually once weekly. It is probably better given in interrupted courses of 4–8 weeks, with a rest period of a month, to prevent serious toxicity.

Toxicity.—There are several undesirable side-effects, mainly on the nervous system. Peripheral neuritis, leading to loss of deep tendon reflexes and actual paresis, and generalized convulsions have been encountered. It causes bone marrow depression, particularly on the red cell series, with red cell arrest.

Alopecia occurs in about 50% of patients, but the hair regrows 1 or 2 months after cessation of treatment. Severe constipation, myalgia and irritability are additional troublesome complications. Measures should be taken to prevent constipation; Colace can be given. The mother should be instructed to give milk of magnesia if a bowel movement does not occur for 2 days.

VINBLASTINE.—This alkaloid is easier to use and less toxic than vincristine, but it has a smaller spectrum of activity. It is helpful in the long-term treatment of lymphoma, particularly Hodgkin's disease.

Dose.—Intravenous injections of 0.1 mg/kg are given once weekly, with gradual increase to 0.25 mg/kg/week.

Toxicity.—Toxicity is similar to that of vincristine except that the nervous system is less affected. Myelotoxicity is perhaps more pronounced with leukopenia, a major problem.

HORMONES

The biochemical effects of hormones on cellular metabolism are numerous, though which of these effects has the antineoplastic action is not known. Cortisone affects oxidative phosphorylation through increased permeability of mitochondrial membranes, and this may be the site of its inhibiting effect. Sex hormones inhibit the growth of tumors with certain hormonal patterns, though the manner of inhibition is not clear. In childhood malignancies, hormones are used mainly in the treatment of leukemia and have some value in the treatment of lymphosarcomatous masses. Prednisone, the corticosteroid usually chosen, is given as 1 or 2 mg/kg/day by mouth divided into three or four doses. Salt retention and hypertension are managed usually by dietary salt limitation and diuretics.

ENZYMES

L-ASPARAGINASE.—This enzyme breaks down the amino acid asparaginine. It has been found in guinea pig serum and in cultures of *Escherichia coli*. Most normal cells are able to synthesize asparaginine de novo, but others are dependent on external sources. In vitro testing has demonstrated that some malignant lymphocytes are asparaginine-dependent.

Treatment of patients and laboratory animals with such cell types by asparaginase has produced dramatic responses, including complete remission of acute leukemia. The supply of this compound is so limited that only very preliminary studies have been possible. This offers a new and exciting approach to the treatment of cancer because of the exquisitely selective action on asparaginine-dependent malignant cells.

Initial Investigation of the Child with Cancer

Once the presence of a malignant tumor is suspected in a child, the further investigations and pos-sible course of treatment should be discussed by those who will be involved in the management. The people concerned are the pediatrician interested in chemotherapy, the radiotherapist and the surgeon. Much time can be saved and useful information obtained if the detailed work-up necessary for such a child is planned by all those concerned.

The *history* should include not only the standard information but data regarding bodily functions, obtained by direct questions. Thus the frequency, consistency and color of the stools may reveal the chronic diarrhea sometimes associated with neuroblastoma. Information regarding the color of the urine may suggest the presence of blood or bile.

The detailed *physical examination* should include note of the regional lymph nodes draining the area suspected of having a tumor and the blood pressure, because some abdominal tumors can cause hypertension by compression of the renal artery or sudden distention of the capsule after hemorrhage.

The *laboratory investigation* should include a complete blood cell count, including platelets; some malignant tumors cause thrombocytopenia in the same manner as giant hemangiomas. Bone marrow should be aspirated in patients suspected of having a lymphoma or neuroblastoma or any tumor when there is pronounced unexplained anemia. Investigation of the urine should include a comment on the presence or absence of red cells, and a 24-hour urine collection should be analyzed for total catecholamine content and for the degradation products of norepinephrine. As this investigation takes time, a spot test for vanylmandelic acid, which is often positive in patients with neuroblastoma and can be carried out without delay, is worth while as a screening test. X-ray examination should include a chest study, skeletal survey and, with flank and abdominal tumors, an intravenous pyelogram, combined with an inferior venacavagram. The contrast medium is introduced into an ankle vein so that the inferior cavagram is obtained simultaneously with the pyelogram. Lymphangiography is of great value in patients with nonleukemic varieties of lymphoma and in selected patients with tumors of other types. Guidance of the radiologist should be sought regarding more specialized studies, such as angiography and laminagraphy.

Selection of Appropriate Chemotherapy

In considering indications for chemotherapy, one must bear in mind that none of the agents used for the treatment of cancer is benign. They all carry varying degrees of risk to the patient. Also, the addition of chemotherapy to radiotherapy may alter the radiosensibility of normal tissues, decreasing the margin of safety. In the decision as to the best chemotherapy, one must take into account a variety of factors. The tumor type is of obvious importance. What is the prognosis if complete removal can be accomplished? The extent of the disease and the age of the patient affect the prognosis. For example, the very small baby with neuroblastoma metastatic to the liver or skin, dreadful as this manifestation may seem, has an excellent outlook, and probably no chemotherapy is indicated. "Hopelessness" by older criteria must be reviewed in the light of the known chemotherapeutic effect on some tumors. For example, actinomycin D is known to affect Wilms' tumors. Widespread disease does not necessarily mean a hopeless prognosis, and a child with pulmonary metastases from a Wilms tumor still has a very good chance of being cured. The value of prophylactic chemotherapy has been questioned and the point raised as to whether this suppresses the development of metastases or simply postpones their appearance. When actinomycin D is given prophylactically to children with Wilms' tumor, late metastases do not seem to occur and the metastatic rate appears to be diminished. It seems reasonable to suppose that if a chemical can affect visible metastases, it should also affect microscopic disease or perhaps provide unfavorable conditions for the implantation of malignant cells. The combination of chemotherapy with x-ray therapy appears to have improved survival by increasing the sensitivity of the tumor, but it also produces a combined toxicity, so that the amount of radiation delivered must be recalculated, to prevent damage to normal structures.

Chemotherapy of Specific Tumors

WILMS' TUMOR

In the past 10 years, treatment of children with this tumor of the kidney has become one of the most rewarding efforts made by the pediatric oncologist. In the 1950's, the combination of aggressive operation and radiotherapy had improved the survival rate to better than 40%.[11] With the addition of actinomycin D, the survival has doubled, and there are now small series with reported survival rates of over 90%.[9] It is possible that actinomycin D is only in part responsible for this great improvement in survival. Meticulous follow-up and aggressive treatment of metastases have also had considerable influence. Farber[7] suggested that actinomycin D given routinely, at spaced intervals, to apparently disease-free children could prevent the development of metastases after removal of the tumor and postoperative irradiation of the bed. Data are accumulating to substantiate this point.

From our own experience, as well as the studies cited above, we believe that chemotherapy is indicated in the treatment of Wilms' tumors and that the agent of choice is actinomycin D. At the time of operation, once the diagnosis is confirmed, it is our custom to start a course of actinomycin D. This is given intravenously, with either 15 μg/kg for five injections or 10 μg/kg for seven injections, making a total of

70–75 μg/kg/course. If a large x-ray treatment field is required, the more prolonged course should be chosen since it more readily allows for interruption of drug therapy should signs of toxicity, most often thrombocytopenia, develop. At present it is conventional to add radiotherapy to the tumor bed, even following removal of an encapsulated tumor. Any pulmonary metastases present should be treated at the same time. Children will tolerate radiation to the whole chest and abdomen in a single shaped field combined with actinomycin D, without excessive toxicity. Following the primary course of actinomycin D, subsequent courses should be given at intervals of 3 months. In our hands, a safe schedule has been five daily intravenous injections of 15 μg/kg/day every 3 months for 18 months.

The follow-up of these children is important, and a chest x-ray series should be taken every 3 months. Pulmonary metastases will be seen early, and treatment can be instituted at once with the combination of radiation and actinomycin D. Long-term cures have resulted from such treatment.[8]

The Southwest Chemotherapy Group has had considerable experience with the use of vincristine, both for primary treatment of Wilms' tumor and for metastases.[20,21] It is their belief that it is as good as actinomycin D, and a study is under way to evaluate the relative effectiveness of these two compounds when given separately or combined. Certainly, vincristine should be used whenever metastases do not appear to be responding to actinomycin D. Vincristine is given by a weekly intravenous injection, with 1–2 mg per square meter per injection.

The alkylating agents and antimetabolites have been a disappointment in the treatment of Wilms' tumor. The excellent results with the two agents just discussed have not encouraged further clinical investigation of other compounds but rather have led to studies to determine how better to use these, which are known to be active.

NEUROBLASTOMA

The results of treatment of this tumor, one of the commonest neoplasms in childhood, remain disappointing. Although neuroblastoma is initially responsive to chemotherapy, the response is short-lived, and the over-all survival has been little improved. However, patient survival is not the only aim of chemotherapy, and the morbidity can be considerably decreased by the use of drugs. There are instances in which the combination of x-ray and chemotherapy has decreased the tumor in size and infiltration sufficiently so that it could be removed, with ultimate survival of the patient. There are also patients on record with metastatic disease in whom chemotherapy appears to have played the major role in the cure of their disease.[14] In a large series reported by Lingley et al.,[15] the over-all survival of patients with neuroblastoma at the Babies Hospital in New York was 35%, which is an improvement on the previous survival of 25%.[10] This improvement may well be the result of vigorous combined therapy. The most important factor influencing the poor prognosis of patients with neuroblastoma is the presence of metastases in 70% at the time of diagnosis.

The most effective preparations for the treatment of neuroblastoma are the alkylating agents, in particular, nitrogen mustard and Cytoxan. At the time of operation for a primary tumor, it is our practice to give two daily injections of nitrogen mustard, the total dose being 0.4 mg/kg. Because the number of patients with metastases is so high with this tumor, we follow this initial treatment with a course of Cytoxan given orally for 1–2 years, even when the primary tumor is apparently completely removed. An exception to this rule is the child under 1 year with no x-ray or histologic evidence of metastases, in whom a localized tumor had been removed. Such a child has a particularly good prognosis, and the addition of chemotherapy does not appear to have improved the results obtained with x-rays and surgery alone.[19] Cytoxan is easily administered by mouth, and toxicity, if it occurs, is usually short-lived.

The excellent results reported by James *et al.*[12] with a combination of Cytoxan and vincristine in children with metastatic neuroblastoma have not been duplicated by others.[2] The choice of treatment for metastatic neuroblastoma is a course of Cytoxan given intravenously until mild toxicity develops, followed by maintenance doses of Cytoxan by mouth. If the response is poor, vincristine should be added to the regimen.

Antibiotics such as actinomycin D and daunomycin have been used in a limited number of cases, but the results reported are too inconstant to evaluate. In Bodian's hands[1] vitamin B_{12} gave good results, particularly in infants under 1 year of age. The experience of other investigators with this treatment has not been encouraging.[18]

SOFT TISSUE SARCOMAS

Soft tissue sarcomas can be grouped together for treatment purposes. They include the hemangio-endotheliosarcoma, rhabdomyosarcoma and the poorly differentiated embryonal sarcoma. Treatment for the primary tumor is resolutely undertaken, with widespread excision. In children, the undifferentiated tumors respond to irradiation and chemotherapy, unlike the situation in adults, in whom the neoplasms tend to be more mature and are therefore often radioresistant. Treatment with actinomycin D and x-ray therapy to the regional lymph nodes should be given if there is any suspicion that the tumor has spread outside the primary area; lymphangiography is an important confirming aid. Unfortunately, even more distant metastases appear in the lungs and bones soon after excision of the primary lesion. The prognosis is so poor after simple excision that it seems reasonable to add chemotherapy to the long-term management of such patients. "Prophylactic" courses of chemotherapy can be restricted to relatively short periods, such as 9 months, because metastases occur most often before the twelfth month. Combined courses of actinomycin D and vincristine may be tried if the patient can be followed closely. Cytoxan has been shown to be effective in metastatic rhabdomyosarcoma and can also be used prophylactically. In this case, toxicity is more easily controlled and the patient need be seen less frequently.

There is no consistently effective regimen known for treatment of metastatic soft tissue sarcomas. If the metastatic spread appears to be limited and can be encompassed in a circumscribed x-ray therapy field, radiation combined with actinomycin D is the treatment of choice. Neither local recurrence nor regional lymph node spread necessarily has a fatal prognosis and both should be treated as vigorously as the primary lesion.[4] The correct agent or combination of agents has not been established for this tumor although, like neuroblastoma, it is temporarily responsive to chemotherapy. Individual patients have responded to Cytoxan,[17] vincristine[22] and mitomycin.[6]

LYMPHOMA

In this category of diseases are included Hodgkin's disease, lymphosarcoma, reticulum cell sarcoma and giant follicle lymphoma. The treatment of lymphomatous diseases is unsettled, and there is continuous debate as to the relative value of surgery, radiotherapy and chemotherapy. The course of the disease varies greatly from patient to patient, making it difficult to find comparable groups for evaluation of the results of therapy. Most authorities agree, however, that the bulwark of treatment in cases of localized disease lies in radiotherapy given in adequate dosage.

HODGKIN'S DISEASE.—Chemotherapy has a place in the management of widespread Hodgkin's disease, seen in stages III and IV, and because of its simplicity often offers the best means of palliation, though it does little to alter the long-term survival. The alkylating agents have proved value in the management of widespread Hodgkin's disease, and in a severely ill patient, nitrogen mustard is the treatment of choice. When the symptoms are not so acute or long-term maintenance is desired, chlorambucil is given orally. The plant alkaloids, and particularly vinblastine, have caused long-term remission in patients with Hodgkin's disease.

LYMPHOSARCOMA.—Localized lymphosarcoma, particularly in the cervical region and the gastrointestinal tract, can be cured by excision, radiation, or combination of the two. Unfortunately, in childhood this tumor frequently becomes widespread, involving numerous lymph nodes and the bone marrow. Then the treatment is essentially the same as that for leukemia.

I think there is little evidence that prophylactic chemotherapy during the lymphosarcomatous phase has prevented the development of leukemia. The alkylating agents, the antimetabolites (in particular Methotrexate) and the plant alkaloid vincristine have all produced dramatic responses in patients with lymphosarcoma. Although this tumor reacts well to chemotherapy, the response unfortunately is usually transient. The superior mediastinal syndrome, due to compression by lymphoma, is sufficiently life-threatening to justify initiation of treatment without a tissue diagnosis. A malignant tumor is practically the only cause of rapidly progressive superior mediastinal compression in childhood. The dangers of the syndrome far outweigh those of the treatment advocated, which is small increments of radiotherapy and large doses of cortisone.[5] If the mediastinal mass is due to lymphosarcoma, the response will be dramatic; I have seen a large mass, appearing to occupy half the chest, disappear completely in 48 hours.

Ewing's Tumor

The choice of treatment for the primary tumor lies between operation and adequate radiotherapy. Since high-dose radiotherapy can control the primary tumor, widespread removal is better reserved for such sites as the rib, where surgery can be performed without significant sacrifice of function and radiotherapy is difficult to administer in adequate volume-dose without producing disabling pneumonitis. When radiation is chosen for primary treatment, it is our practice to add a course of actinomycin D.

Ewing's tumor is virtually unique among the solid tumors in childhood in that metastases may first be discerned 5 years or longer after the time of diagnosis. In spite of the poor prognosis, an occasional child with metastases to lung or bone can be retrieved by aggressive combined chemo- and radiotherapy. The value of prophylactic chemotherapy has not been proved, and difficulties are encountered because it must be given for a long period of time, in view of the late manifestations of metastases. Metastatic Ewing's tumor is quite sensitive to treatment with a number of chemical agents, but the effect is usually short-lived. Chemotherapy should be tried when there is widespread disease, because it will often alleviate symptoms even if survival is not significantly prolonged. I have seen a dramatic response to a combination of Cytoxan and vincristine in a patient with advanced disease involving multiple sites, including the bone marrow. There was complete alleviation of symptoms and clearing of the bone marrow, which lasted some months. The combination of actinomycin D, Methotrexate and chlorambucil has also been effective on occasion. X-ray therapy should be tried to relieve painful or disfiguring masses. Two or three doses of 250 rads each will often give prompt and prolonged relief.

Osteogenic Sarcoma

Although there are occasional reports of metastatic osteogenic sarcoma responding to various forms of chemotherapy, no consistent response has been noted, and chemotherapy probably has added little to the treatment of this highly malignant tumor.

Central Nervous System Tumors

The difficulties of operating in such vital areas and the fact that metastases rarely occur outside the craniospinal axis make the central nervous system tumors especially challenging to the oncologist. Combined treatment regimens might have real contributions to make. One could predict that local removal of the bulk of the tumor and injection of an effective chemical into the tumor bed or regional blood supply with or without postoperative irradiation would improve the control of these tumors. Alas, this promise has not so far been fulfilled. One problem is created by the "blood-brain barrier" that exists to many chemotherapeutic agents, though this is partly negated by the tumor blood supply.

Three routes of administering chemotherapy for brain tumors have been tried: (1) systemically, (2) into the regional blood supply, and (3) intrathecally. Mithromycin has been given systemically in a small series of patients with medulloblastoma with encouraging results, though not cures.[13] Antimetabolites, alkylating agents and hydrogen peroxide have been infused into the carotid artery with occasional response in undifferentiated tumors. Newton and Sayens[16] treated 23 children with brain tumors with intrathecal injections of Methotrexate, achieving a subjective response in 20 and objective response in 7. D'Angio et al.[3] have developed a regimen using both internal and external sources of radiation, with preliminary teletherapy followed by radioactive gold given intrathecally. This is designed to deliver a high dose to a very small depth so that the tolerance of the brain and spinal cord to radiation is not exceeded. It is particularly useful in tumors with known tendency to seed via the cerebrospinal fluid. Initial encouraging results have been reported.

REFERENCES

1. Bodian, M.: Neuroblastoma, Arch. Dis. Childhood 38:606, 1963.
2. Children's Cancer Study Group A: J.A.M.A. (in press).
3. D'Angio, G. J., et al.: Intrathecal radioisotopes for the treatment of brain tumors, Clin. Neurosurg. 15:288, 1968.
4. D'Angio, G. J., and Teft, M.: Radiation therapy in the management of children with gynecologic cancers, Ann. New York Acad. Sc. 142:675, 1967.
5. D'Angio, G. J.; Mitus, A., and Evans, A. E.: The superior mediastinal syndrome in children with cancer, Am. J. Roentgenol. 93:537, 1965.
6. Evans, A. E.: Mitomycin C, Cancer Chemotherap. Rep. 14:1, 1961.

7. Farber, S.: Chemotherapy in the treatment of leukemia and Wilms' tumor, J.A.M.A. 198:826, 1966.
8. Farber, S.; D'Angio, G. J., and Evans, A. E.: The treatment of children with disseminated Wilms' tumor by actinomycin D and roentgen therapy, Am. J. Dis. Child. 100:795, 1960.
9. Fernbach, D. J., and Martyn, D. T.: The role of dactinomycin in the improved survival of children with Wilms' tumor, J.A.M.A. 195:1005, 1966.
10. Gross, R. E.; Farber, S., and Martin, L. W.: Neuroblastoma sympatheticum: A study and report of 217 cases, Pediatrics 23:1179, 1960.
11. Gross, R. E., and Neuhauser, E. B. D.: Treatment of mixed tumors of the kidney in childhood, Pediatrics 6:843, 1950.
12. James, D. H., Jr., *et al.*: Combination chemotherapy of childhood neurobastoma, J.A.M.A. 194:123, 1965.
13. Kennedy, B. J.; Brown, J. H., and Yarbro, J. W.: Mithromycin therapy for primary glioblastomas, Cancer Chemotherap. Rep. 48:59, 1965.
14. Konkras, S. B., and Newton, W. A., Jr.: Cyclophosphamide therapy of childhood neuroblastoma, Cancer Chemotherap. Rep. 12:39, 1961.

15. Lingley, J. F., *et al.*: Neuroblastoma, management and survival, New England J. Med. 277:1227, 1967.
16. Newton, W. A., Jr., and Sayens, M. P.: Intrathecal methotrexate therapy of brain tumors of childhood, Proc. Cancer Res. 6:48, 1965.
17. Pinkel, D.: Cyclophosphamide in children with cancer, Cancer 15:42, 1962.
18. Sawitsky, A., and Desposito, F.: A survey of American experience with vitamin B_{12} therapy of neuroblastoma, J. Pediat. 67:99, 1965.
19. Schneider, K. M.; Becker, J. M., and Krasna, I. H.: Neonatal neuroblastoma, Pediatrics 36:359, 1965.
20. Sutow, W. W., and Sullivan, M. P.: Vincristine in the primary treatment of Wilms' tumor, Texas J. Med. 61:794, 1965.
21. Sutow, W. W., *et al.*: Vincristine in the treatment of children with metastatic Wilms' tumor, Pediatrics 32:880, 1963.
22. Sutow, W. W.: Vincristine sulphate therapy in children with metastatic soft tissue sarcoma, Pediatrics 38:465, 1966.

A. E. EVANS

7

Birth Trauma

TRAUMA OF THE NEWBORN is chiefly that of actual birth injury and is caused by the forces encountered by the infant during passage through the birth canal and during delivery and the immediate postpartum period. Many forms of birth trauma are so rare that an individual physician may never see them in a lifetime of practice. For example, Dr. Arthur H. Parmelee, with his experience of a lifetime at Children's Hospital of Chicago and then in Los Angeles, stated that he had never seen a rupture of the spleen in a newborn except at autopsy.[30] Table 7-1 gives the neonatal mortality rates per 100,000 live births in the United States in 1965.[23]

Traumatic injury to the large or postmature baby occurs more frequently than to the small or premature infant. The incidence of traumatic injury to infants weighing over 2,500 Gm at birth is twice that of infants with birth weight of 1,000 Gm or less. [31a,31b]

Other factors affecting the rate of birth injuries are the fetal position and presentation and the disproportion between the size of the infant and that of the mother's pelvis. Injury rate among breech extractions appears to be the highest, lower in spontaneous breech deliveries and still less in cephalic deliveries without obstetric complications. Delivery by cesarean section carries the least risk of injury to the infant.

Injuries to the infant during birth fall into the following categories: skin and subcutaneous tissues, head, skeletal and nerve injuries, and internal injuries.

TABLE 7-1.— NEONATAL MORTALITY (PER 100,000 LIVE BIRTHS) IN THE UNITED STATES (1965)

Birth injuries	205
Accidents	12
Respiratory obstruction	5
Miscellaneous (accid.)	7

Skin and Subcutaneous Tissues

Trauma to the skin and subcutaneous tissues is so common and usually so benign as to be considered a normal accompaniment of delivery. The chief danger is the possibility of infection or of extravasation of blood in the case of a blood dyscrasia.

Marks, abrasions and lacerations of superficial tissues may occur when forceps are used. Injuries to ears, eyes, nose, genitalia, extremities, head and trunk have all been reported. Fat necrosis of the cheek resulting from pressure of forceps may require surgical excision.

Traumatic effects may develop in the eye from pressure at the pelvic outlet. Transitory conjunctival edema and minor hemorrhage are common; rarely, there may be damage to the cornea or dislocation of the lens. Retinal hemorrhages are more commonly present than is generally realized, with a reported incidence as high as 24% with regular deliveries and 40% with vacuum extraction,[17] although they are usually transitory and have little or no clinical significance.[35]

The vacuum extractor can cause excoriations and edema, seen in about half of the infants delivered by this means. If a vacuum is applied to the presenting part for 30 minutes or longer at a negative pressure of 0.8 kg/cm[2], tissue necrosis will usually result. Slough of the necrotic tissue eventually ensues, and infection and, later, cicatricial alopecia have been reported.[14]

Head and Cranial Nerves

Caput succedaneum is the commonest soft tissue injury found in head presentations. It is a soft diffuse swelling over the presenting part of the head, commonest in the parietal and occipital regions. Left alone, it subsides in a few days. It sometimes must be differentiated from cephalhematoma, which is a collection of blood between the periosteum and the bone. Cephalhematoma occurs in 1–5% of cephalic deliveries and, of course, much less frequently in other presentations. Cephalhematoma is limited by the suture lines to one area of calvarial bone and appears as a soft tissue swelling a day or two after birth and disappears spontaneously in 2–3 weeks. Occasionally, such a hematoma fails to reabsorb and may even calcify. Treatment of cephalhematoma is unnecessary. No incision is advised, for it may lead to infection.

Fractures of the skull have been found in as many as 25% of newborn infants with cephalhematoma.[4] Because of the low calcium content of the calvarium, considerable molding is possible and even an apparent "depressed" fracture may not mean a break in the bone. When a skull segment is depressed more than 6 mm below the surrounding bone, surgical evaluation and probably elevation by direct attack is indicated to prevent continuing pressure on underlying cortex.[25]

Bucy[5] said that he had never seen it correct itself spontaneously and thought it should be elevated.

Skull fractures are usually the result of severe trauma, difficult forceps or breech extraction in a contracted pelvis. They may, however, occur in spontaneous and entirely normal delivery, as first recorded by Hirt[15] in 1815. Cerebral hemorrhages and cranial nerve injuries may result from a fracture of the skull or may occur without evidence of fracture after unusually prolonged and difficult delivery, often with application of high forceps. When symptoms of intracranial hemorrhage appear after a spontaneous delivery and normal labor, one must suspect either a hemorrhagic diathesis or a period of anoxia.

Cerebral hemorrhage is the greatest cause of death in newborns. Nesbitt[24] said, in reference to intracranial hemorrhage, that although the improvement of obstetric methods in recent years has cut down greatly the damage from traumatic intracranial hemorrhage, there has been no appreciable reduction of intracranial hemorrhage in infants dying of anoxic injury. Hemorrhage and cranial nerve injuries are discussed in Chapter 87.

Injury to the 7th cranial nerve can result from pressure of the shoulder into the face when the infant's head is kept for long periods, during birth, in sharp lateral flexion. It may also result from pressure of the forceps blade on the course of the facial nerve between the stylomastoid foramen and the parotid gland.[20,24] The incidence of such damage to this nerve has been reported to be as high as 6% in some forceps applications.[20] Treatment in these cases consists chiefly in protection of the cornea from injury until function of the eyelid returns and adequate closing of the eye during sleep can be achieved. The eventual prognosis is good, and function usually returns within

Fig. 7-1.—Paralysis of left leaf of diaphragm accompanying brachial plexus injury in a 1-day-old infant. The diaphragm is high on the left side and shows paradoxical motion on fluoroscopy. Left-sided paralysis is rare; such paralysis is almost always on the right. (Figs. 7-1–7-5, courtesy of Dr. John L. Gwinn.)

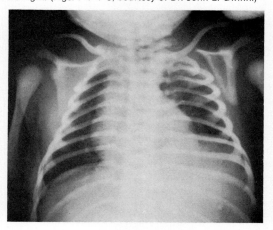

a few days if the paralysis is due to transient pressure from forceps blades. Spontaneous facial paralysis due to pressure from the fetal shoulder is more apt to be prolonged, and the injury may be permanent.[30]

Injury to the phrenic nerve may be present with or without brachial plexus injury. The results of phrenic nerve paralysis are a high leaf of the diaphragm with paradoxical motion of the involved leaf accompanied by varying degrees of respiratory distress (Fig. 7-1). Most patients can be treated medically, but those with severe of recurring respiratory problems should be operated on forthwith[3] (see Chapter 27, Diaphragmatic Hernia). Imbrication of the hemidiaphragm can be accomplished by the transabdominal or thoracic approach. Bilateral eventrations are rare.[19] A 5-day-old infant with this condition was successfully managed in the Childrens Hospital of Los Angeles by a staged transthoracic approach performed by Bertrand W. Meyer.

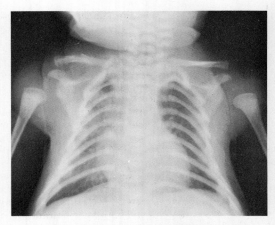

Fig. 7-2.—This 10-day-old infant seemed to have pain with movement of the right arm. The roentgenogram shows fracture of the midportion of the right clavicle. No callus is evident but probably will appear in a few days.

Skeletal Injuries

When the forces exerted during delivery are severe, damage to bones, spinal cord and especially to the brachial plexus should be feared. The association of presumed bleeding into a torn sternocleidomastoid muscle and subsequent shortening are discussed in Chapter 23 (Torticollis).

Large infants may have large shoulders, difficult to deliver. In shoulder presentations or in case of heavy traction on a laterally displaced head or a prolapsed upper extremity, a fracture of the clavicle can result, usually in its lateral or middle third. The clavicle is fractured more often than any other bone in birth injuries (Fig. 7-2). Minimal therapy of this fracture, with a simple restraining bandage, will regularly give a good functional and anatomic result.

Fracture of the humerus or, rarely, of the femur occurs almost always in the middle third of the shaft and often with over-riding of the fragments.

Treatment of humeral fractures consists of simple immobilization in the correct position. Proper alignment without shortening will result. Fractures of the femur may require some traction to overcome the muscle pull and over-riding. Treatment must be instituted quickly, as callus forms with great rapidity. Treatment usually consists of gentle immobilization, since authorities agree that even with inadequate correction of the deformity, callus formation and growth will, in time, give satisfactory alignment and there will be no permanent deformity. Fractures of the leg and forearm have also been reported, although rarely; and when obstetric traction has been sufficient to cause such fractures, there is likely to be damage to the brachial or even to the lumbosacral plexus.

Separation of the epiphysis occurs most often in the femur.[8,22,38] This usually follows breech extraction, and usually in primiparas. Shulman and Terhune[36]

reported four cases and referred to a number in the literature, the largest percentage of which followed breech delivery. Periosteal elevation results, with hemorrhage between the periosteum and the bone. Ordinarily, callus replaces the hemorrhage by the fifth day, and no treatment is needed. Resorption of the callus may take as long as 6 months. However, if there is much displacement, the dislocated epiphysis may be placed in better position and an attempt made to immobilize the limb. These authors warn that during callus formation, supplementary calcium may be needed in the diet to avoid tetany.

Nerve Injuries

Damage to the brachial plexus is responsible for the most common type of birth palsy, the Erb-Duchenne paralysis, which results from damage to the 5th and 6th cervical nerves and their roots. Injury can be so extensive as to paralyze the whole arm. Klumpke paralysis results from damage to the 8th cervical and 1st thoracic nerves. Trauma of the lower cervical roots may give rise to Horner's syndrome.

Treatment of such nerve injuries consists in keeping the part immobilized in a corrective position. For Erb's palsy, the sleeve of the infant's gown may be pinned to the pillow in such a way that the arm remains abducted and the elbow flexed. Radial nerve palsy demands immobilization in a cock-up splint. Recovery usually follows in about 10 days.

Rarely, as in difficult breech deliveries, severe and even fatal injuries may be sustained by the spinal cord and vertebral column. The injury occurs most often at the low cervical or high thoracic level.[21,24] Clinical manifestations of spinal cord injury include paraplegia below the level of injury, paradoxical breathing and loss of sensation.

Internal Injuries

THORACIC INJURIES

Pneumothorax, (Fig. 7-3) sometimes occurs, and about half of the cases are regarded as "spontaneous" without recognizable trauma. The incidence of pneumothorax in newborns has been reported as 0.7% in prematures and 0.1% in full-term infants.[2] The causes differ but are probably, in the main, related to the pressure changes taking place during the adaptation of the infant to extrauterine life.[34] Attempts at resuscitation are responsible in some cases, the use of excessive pressure causing rupture of pulmonary tissues. Rupture of emphysematous tissues near the lung periphery and rupture of lung cysts are also causes of pneumothorax.

Differential diagnosis in cases of respiratory embarrassment must include such causes as subglottic edema or laryngomalacia, chylothorax, lung cysts, pulmonary compression by abdominal viscera herniated through the diaphragm, central nervous system depression and cardiovascular disease.

TREATMENT.—Rarely is pneumothorax of great enough degree to cause symptoms, and treatment should be supportive under careful observation. Aspiration of air is not often necessary, but when the leak is large, with greater than 25% collapse of the lung, or if it persists after initial aspiration, a small plastic indwelling catheter should be inserted promptly through an upper anterior intercostal space and connected to a tube beneath 3 cm of water in a bottle trap. Tension pneumothorax requires continuous aspiration.[16]

Pneumomediastinum may be more serious than simple pneumothorax (Fig. 7-4). Tension pneumomediastinum causes compression of the vena cava and pulmonary veins with consequent shock and death. Rudhe and Ozonoff[34] emphasized that pneumothorax and pneumomediastinum often coexist, and when one is present the other should be looked for. Pneumomediastinum may follow pulmonary interstitial emphysema resulting from rupture of alveoli. The pathway of the escaped air, when there is great enough volume, is by way of the sheaths of the great vessels in the mediastinum.[2] Extension may also occur into the *peritoneal cavity* and be *wrongly interpreted as rupture of a hollow viscus.*

Hemothorax may, very rarely, result from a very traumatic delivery. Chylothorax also occurs and is discussed in Chapter 47.

HOLLOW VISCUS INJURY

Perforations of the gastrointestinal tract (Fig. 7-5) have been the subject of interest for many years.[7] A classic paper is that of Thelander,[40] published in 1939, in which he reviewed 85 cases, of which 16 were of the stomach, 30 of the duodenum and 39 of the remaining intestinal tract. The majority of these are due to obstructive or inflammatory lesions, and trauma is incidental or nonexistent.

Injury to the stomach and upper intestinal tract may result from a number of different factors. The common ones are: the use of air under pressure from mouth-to-mouth breathing or from a respirator, and catheterizations done for investigative purposes or for feeding that result in esophageal and gastric perforations. Spontaneous perforation of the stomach in the newborn is discussed in Chapter 52.

Traumatic perforation of the intestinal tract occurs principally in underdeveloped or premature infants,[28] [32, 33] and it is always an extremely serious condition.

Fig. 7-3—**A,** anteroposterior view of newborn with pneumothorax on the right. **Upper arrows** indicate border of compressed lung; **lower arrows,** bleb within the lower lobe. A nonfunctioning chest tube is visible. **B,** lateral view, showing air compressing the lung and mediastinum posteriorly. **Arrows** indicate position of the bleb in the lower lobe.

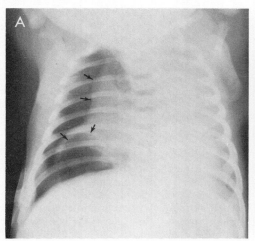 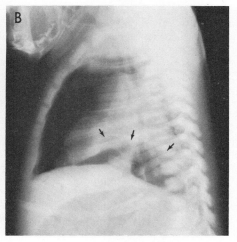

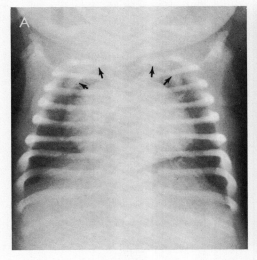

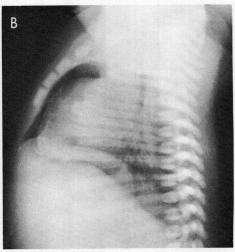

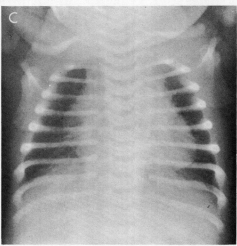

Fig. 7-4 — A, anteroposterior view of 1-day-old infant with air in the mediastinum. **Arrows** indicate position of the thymus, pushed upward, which probably plugs the inlet to the neck and prevents upward displacement of air. **B,** lateral view, showing air filling the anterior mediastinum. **C,** anteroposterior view, taken 3 days later, showing absorption of mediastinal air. No treatment was given.

Perforation may become manifest within a few hours to a week after birth. When the condition is suspected, demonstration of pneumoperitoneum by radiographic studies is diagnostic. Air is not always seen, but the presence of peritoneal fluid and bowel distention are helpful signs. Parker and Mikity[29] state that it is almost impossible to demonstrate the site of the perforation radiographically and advise against the use of contrast medium. The dangers from its use are spillage into the peritoneal cavity, the production of shock and delay in definitive surgical measures. Needle aspiration will often establish the diagnosis and in case of pneumoperitoneum of severe degree will relieve the respiratory embarrassment prior to surgery.

Perforation of the colon is discussed fully in Chapter 57. Treatment of any intestinal perforation must be by prompt surgical intervention. Recognition usu-ally occurs relatively late in the illness, so the mortality is high, varying from 40 to 80% according to some reports.[32,33] The most important step toward improving the survival rate in this condition is diagnosis by radiographic examination.[29]

A recent good explanation of perforations is the diversion of blood from the intestines to more essential areas for survival during intra-uterine stress, "the diving reflex."

INJURY TO SOLID VISCERA

The incidence of injury to solid viscera resulting from birth trauma has been reported as varying from 0.9 to 3.5%.[6] The signs—blood loss accompanied by abdominal distention in the newborn—point to hemoperitoneum. Radiography shows free intraperitoneal fluid without air. Accurate identification of the source

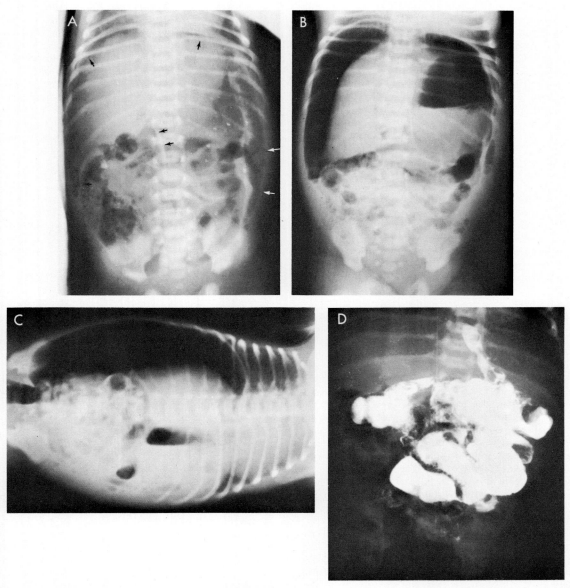

Fig. 7-5—A, flat abdominal roentgenogram of 6-day-old infant with increasing abdominal distention for 2 days (pneumoperitoneum). **Lateral and superior arrows** indicate air accumulation outside the viscera. **Central arrows** indicate falciform ligament outlined by air. This is the so-called football sign. Operation revealed a perforated stomach. **B,** upright abdominal roentgenogram, showing persistence of air between the diaphragm and abdominal viscera. Liver and viscera are compressed medially, giving the so-called saddle sign. Air is also seen in the stomach, even though it was found to be perforated at operation. **C,** lateral decubitus roentgenogram, showing free air compressing the viscera to the left side. **D,** gastrointestinal series taken at 1 month of age shows normal passage of barium.

of the bleeding, whether liver, spleen or adrenals, cannot usually be made except by laparotomy.

Of all solid viscera reported injured during birth, the liver is most frequently affected. In his monograph of 1928, Ehrenfest[9] stated that by far the commonest of intra-abdominal traumatisms were injuries to the liver. He listed these in degree of severity and frequency from small petechial hemorrhages to subcapsular hemorrhages, lacerations of the capsule and actual rupture of the liver.

Potter[31a] found in 2,000 autopsies on newborns that 28 were due to intra-abdominal lacerations with hemorrhage, and of these, 22 were lacerations of the liver. Most authors report similar proportions,[9] though Sieber and Girdany[37] had a different experience in both autopsy and clinical material. They found no rupture of the liver in their institution over a 7-year period, but reported six ruptures of the spleen, three of which were operated on successfully.

Usually the cause appears to be severe trauma in the course of birth. However, prematurity, difficult labor and unusually large size of the infant are all factors. Charif[6] reported on 41 infants, studied at autopsy, who died of subcapsular hemorrhage of the liver; 88% of these infants were immature or premature, and 24% had been delivered by breech extraction. Ehrenfest[9] mentioned several predisposing factors, among them large infants born by breech delivery and high forceps extraction. Gruenwald[13] believed that asphyxia and increased bleeding tendency are factors in producing increased fragility of the liver. Arden,[1] too, mentioned congestion of the liver in asphyxia as predisposing in all probability to hemorrhage of the liver.

Liver lacerations characteristically develop a subcapsular hematoma and then rupture after a delay of several hours to a few days. One such rupture was reported after 5 days, and Parmelee reported on an 11-week-old baby with a large hematoma which ruptured during surgery. The hemorrhage was successfully controlled, and the baby recovered.

Clinically, the condition may be recognized by signs of shock and fluid-filled abdomen. Needle aspiration may disclose blood without evidence of free air. Sometimes the umbilical area may be discolored by leakage of blood into it. One such infant with liver laceration was thought to have torsion of the testicle because of discoloration of the scrotal sac.[10]

Operative treatment is taken up in Chapter 39. Blood replacement through the umbilical or saphenous vein is essential.

Hemangioma of the liver in the newborn presents as an abdominal mass or massive hemoperitoneum. Eight such cases requiring hepatic resection were recorded by Graiver, Votteler and Dorman.[11] There were 7 survivors.

Next in frequency to liver lacerations are injuries to the adrenal glands. The explanation may be that at birth the adrenals are relatively large and have a rich blood supply. Their position, "just below the diaphragm resting on the upper pole of the kidney exposes them to pressure and traction when the thorax is compressed excessively during birth."[30] At any rate, a hematoma forms which may rupture into the retroperitoneal tissues or into the peritoneal cavity. The symptoms are hyperpyrexia, rapid respirations and sometimes petechiae and vomiting and evidence of blood loss.

Adrenal hemorrhage may be unilateral or bilateral. Some cases have been attributed to hypoxia or to infection; some seem to have a spontaneous origin.

Treatment has rarely been effective because of the difficulty of diagnosing the condition in time. Neuroblastoma must be excluded in the diagnosis, and this is sometimes hard to do because hemorrhage may occur as well into the neuroblastoma.[12] Hemorrhage may be massive and in the presence of adrenal insufficiency may be quickly fatal. Occasionally, conservative measures, without operation, have been successful.

Treatment consists of evacuating the hematoma, ligating the bleeding vessels and, if necessary, adrenalectomy. The patient can tolerate this well, since it lowers adrenal function by only about 30%. It is advisable to give antibiotics because there is danger of overwhelming infection and patients with adrenal disease have lowered resistance to infection.

The spleen is much less frequently involved in birth trauma than are the adrenals, according to most statistics.[6,31a] A number of cases have been recognized in newborns and operated on successfully.[10,37,39] When the spleen is torn, hemorrhage is usually not delayed, as in liver lacerations, but is immediate and surgical intervention and splenectomy must be prompt.

The kidney and pancreas are rarely affected by birth trauma. The very rarity of such injury and the vague clinical signs may delay the diagnosis until lethal complications have developed.[18] Eraklis[10] has reported a case of transected kidney with hemorrhage from this organ and from the adrenal which was first thought to be a Wilms tumor. It has been stated that rupture of the kidney or bladder rarely occurs except in the presence of pathologic obstruction of the urinary flow.

REFERENCES

1. Arden, F.: Rupture of liver in newborn, M. J. Australia 1:187, 1946.
2. Bargh, W.: Pneumothorax in the neonate; A presentation of two cases, Brit. J. Anaesth. 36:456, 1964.
3. Bishop, H. C., and Koop, C. E.: Acquired eventration of the diaphragm in infancy, Pediatrics 22:1088, 1958.
4. Brown, J. J. M.: *Surgery of Childhood* (Baltimore: Williams & Wilkins Company, 1963).
5. Bucy, P. C.: in Nelson, W. E. (ed.): *Textbook of Pediatrics* (5th ed.; Philadelphia: W. B. Saunders Company, 1950), p. 313.
6. Charif, P.: Subcapsular hemorrhage of the liver in the newborn: An inquiry into its causes, Clin. Pediat. 3:428, 1964.

7. Cruze, K., and Snyder, W. H., Jr.: Acute perforation of the alimentary tract in infancy and childhood, Ann. Surg. 154:93, 1961.

8. Denes, J., and Weil, S.: Proximal epiphysiolysis of the femur during caesarean section, Lancet 1:906, 1964.

9. Ehrenfest, H.: *Birth Injuries of the Child* (D. Appleton & Co., 1928), p. 196.

10. Eraklis, A. J.: Abdominal injury related to the trauma of birth, Pediatrics 39:421, 1967.

11. Graiver, L.; Votteler, T. P., and Dorman, G. W.: Hepatic hemangiomas in newborn infants, J. Pediat. Surg. 2:209, 1967.

12. Gross, M.; Kottmeier, P. K., and Waterhouse, K.: Diagnosis and treatment of neonatal adrenal hemorrhage, J. Pediat. Surg. 2:308, 1967.

13. Gruenwald, P.: Rupture of liver and spleen in newborn infant, J. Pediat. 33:195, 1948.

14. Hall-Smith, P., and Foulkes, J. F.: Traumatic cicatricial alopecia in an infant girl: Result of the use of a vacuum extractor (ventouse), Arch. Dermat. 89:473, 1964.

15. Hirt: Cited by Ehrenfest.[9]

16. Howie, V. M., and Weed, A. S.: Spontaneous pneumothorax in the first 10 days of life, with review of the literature, J. Pediat. 50:6, 1957.

17. Krebs, W., and Jager, G.: Retinal hemorrhages in newborns: The mode of delivery, Klin. Monatsbl. Augenh. 148:483, 1966.

18. Lorber, J.: Massive bilateral adrenal haemorrhage in the newborn with recovery, Proc. Roy. Soc. Med. 58:125, 1965.

19. Lundstrom, C. H., and Parker, A. R.: Bilateral congenital eventration of the diaphragm, Am. J. Roentgenol. 97:216, 1966.

20. McHugh, H. E.: Facial paralysis in birth injury and skull fracture, Arch. Otolaryng. 78:443, 1963.

21. Melchior, J. C., and Tygstrup, I.: Development of paraplegia after breech presentation. Acta paediat. scandinav. 52:171, 1963.

22. Mortens, J., and Christensen, P.: Traumatic separation of the upper femoral epiphysis as an obstetrical lesion, Acta orthop. scandinav. 34:238, 1964.

23. National Center for Health Statistics: Infant Mortality Trends, United States and Each State, 1930–64 (Washington, D.C.: U.S. Department of Health, Education and Welfare, Public Health Service pub. no. 1000, series 20, no. 1, 1965).

24. Nesbitt, R. E.: *Prenatal Loss in Modern Obstetrics* (Philadelphia: F. A. Davis Company, 1957), p. 203.

25. Nixon, H. H., and O'Donnell, B.: *The Essentials of Pediatric Surgery* (2nd ed.; Philadelphia: J. B. Lippincott Company, 1966), p. 9.

26. O'Neill, E. A.; O'Brian, E. R., and Hyun, B. H.: Rupture of the spleen in the newborn infant: Report of a survival, J.A.M.A. 193:959, 1965.

27. Paine, R. S.: Neurologic conditions in the neonatal period: Diagnosis and management, Pediat. Clin. North America 8:577, 1961.

28. Parker, J. J.; Mikity, V. G., and Jacobson, G.: Traumatic pneumoperitoneum in the newborn, Am. J. Roentgenol. 95:203, 1965.

29. Parker, J. J., and Mikity, V. G.: Radiographic diagnosis of intestinal perforation in early infancy, California Med. 104:35, 1966.

30. Parmelee, A. H.: *Management of the Newborn* (2nd ed.; Chicago: Year Book Medical Publishers, Inc., 1959).

31a. Potter, E. L.: Fetal and neonatal deaths; a statistical analysis of 2,000 autopsies, J.A.M.A. 115:996, 1940.

31b. Potter, E. L.: *Pathology of the Fetus and Infant* (2nd ed.; Chicago: Year Book Medical Publishers, Inc., 1961).

32. Reams, G. B.; Dunaway, J. B., and Walls, W. L.: Neonatal gastric perforation with survival, Pediatrics 31:97, 1963.

33. Rogers, C. S.: Pneumoperitoneum in the newborn, Surgery 56:842, 1964.

34. Rudhe, U., and Ozonoff, M. G.: Pneumomediastinum and pneumothorax in the newborn, Acta radiol. diagn. 4:193, 1966.

35. Schenker, J. G., and Gombos, G. M.: Retinal hemorrhage in the newborn, Obst. & Gynec. 27:521, 1966.

36. Shulman, B. H., and Terhune, C. B.: Epiphyseal injuries during breech extraction, Pediatrics 8:693, 1951.

37. Sieber, W. K., and Girdany, B. R.: Rupture of the spleen in newborn infants: Recovery after splenectomy, New England J. Med. 259:1074, 1958.

38. Siffert, R. S.: Displacement of the distal humeral epiphysis in the newborn infant, J. Bone & Joint Surg. 45A:165, 1963.

39. Spencer, R.: Personal communication.

40. Thelander, H. E.: Perforation of the gastrointestinal tract of newborn infant, Am. J. Dis. Child. 58:371, 1939.

W. H. SNYDER, JR.
N. HASTINGS

8

Physical Abuse During Childhood
(The Battered-Child Syndrome)

INTEMPERATE VIOLENCE directed against the immature has undoubtedly been an element of varying importance in all cultures and has never been foreign to our own. Recognition of the extent and protean manifestations of the malady has come as a shock to the community over the past two decades so that current interest transcends any single profession and involves medicine, the law, sociology and the several behavioral sciences.

The frequency with which wanton injury is visited upon infants and children cannot be estimated with precision since data have accumulated in patterns skewed by the interests and experiences of individuals, e.g., the relation of fractures to subdural hematoma[2] or the incidence of multiple skeletal defects for which no reasonable explanation was readily available.[7] It was to correct this imbalance that Kempe and his colleagues[4] coined the term, battered child, which covers the gamut of physical, as well as emotional and nutritional, abuse recognizable by the alert physician.

This change in orientation has resulted in a veritable deluge of lay and medical literature which gives an impression of a sizable increase in abuse, but such is not documented by rather complete records actively maintained at our hospital for 15 years. A more sensible explanation is a breakdown of former rigid denial that such problems are of major magnitude—a rather common phenomenon with many acts abhorrent to the individual and community conscience.

The Background of Abuse

Man lives in a world of violence, cruelty and disorganized behavior. To much of this, he becomes inured without a deep understanding of motivations. Child abuse is merely a facet of the over-all problem, and it would be strange indeed if universal common denominators were easily elicited. Actually, we are working in an unusually difficult zone of comprehension since we have no clear-cut definition of child abuse, rarely a complainant and frequently no witnesses. Nevertheless, certain patterns are quite clear and others assume sufficient form for definitive discussion.

The vast majority of injuries are inflicted by persons having natural, legal or de facto control of the victim, e.g., parents, other adult relatives and paramours, guardians and baby sitters. Sibs are, in our material, a decidedly poor second and are, when implicated, frequently acting out the pattern of a generally disturbed ménage. When only one person is deemed abusive, it may be either male or female in about equal frequency. However, in many homes, battering seems a conspiracy or, at least, a permissive attitude characterizes the nonviolent partner.

It is very clear that households in which battering occurs are not set apart by the economic status, intellectual or educational level or social heritage of the occupants. Each exerts a quantitative influence, but none is a determinant. The impression that abuse is entirely an urban disease of ignorance and poverty or that it is more common in one racial element than another is largely a figment of present methods for reporting and investigation.

In our current state of incomplete knowledge, we still look upon trauma in infancy and childhood as arising under a spectrum of environmental and interhuman situations. Simplest on the scale can be termed a *generally unprotective environment*. Here active aggression is not as important as a more subtile element: the positive responsibility of parents to provide for their dependents a safe and secure home. Many cannot do this because of low intellectual level, alcoholism or incomplete family units with the excess load thrown on the survivor. These may be compounded by inadequate equipment, slovenly housekeeping and the general defeatism of poverty. The victims of such situations might be regarded as "passively battered."

Dr. Richard Komisaruk,[5] psychiatrist to the Wayne County (Detroit) Juvenile Court, has recently presented conclusions drawn from 100 families in which abuse was reported—largely by urban university centers. Mental deficiency, with its attendant poor judgment and absence of self-control, was most frequently seen and probably would fit a step above

TABLE 8-1.—DATA DERIVED FROM 55 CONSECUTIVE CASES OF PHYSICAL ABUSE SEEN AT THE CHILDREN'S HOSPITAL OF MICHIGAN (DETROIT)

	No.	%
Age		
under 3 mo.	12	21.8
3–6 mo.	13	23.6
6–12 mo.	14	25.5
12–24 mo.	7	12.7
24–36 mo.	5	9.1
over 36 mo.	4	7.3
Race		
Colored	32	58
White	23	42
Sex		
Female	32	58
Male	23	42
Anatomic injury		
Skeletal only	15	27.2
Skull only	2	3.6
Skeletal and skull	8	14.5
Subdural hematoma	4	7.3
Subdural and skeletal	9	16.4
Skeletal and visceral	3	5.5
Soft tissue alone	9	16.4
Skeletal and soft tissue	5	9.1
Results		
Died	6	
Known permanent damage	4	

pure unprotectiveness since active aggression was present.

Homes in which poverty and lack of education or intelligence are not major problems have been studied in relatively small numbers and a variety of characteristics have been stressed. One report from an Armed Service Facility[3] emphasized the young age of marriage, the rapidity of child-bearing and the lack of close or wholesome ties with family and community. Others are impressed by the number of parents who themselves were rigidly and sternly dealt with during childhood or were deprived of a close and dear person while developing, the latter leaving a void or hiatus in some aspect of adult maturity. Every-day terms, such as "angry personality," "easily frustrated," "in a period of unusual stress," "heavy drinker," and the like, appear recurrently in histories taken of families in which injury has occurred. Overt psychoses are rare in the experience of most observers, and in the last 60 families studied here appeared only twice, involving 3 children with 1 death.

The victim himself forms part of the background of abuse. In many instances, a single child is selected from several to bear the brunt of violence while the remainder are carefully protected. We have seen one of twins repetitively battered while the litter mate was adored. Parenthetically, however, we do not believe this whipping-boy situation is as prevalent as we did a few years ago; when abusive families are studied over longer periods of time, we find recurring violence against new children and an unusual number of "crib" and unexplained sudden deaths. In the families of the 55 patients tabulated (Table 8-1), there have been 7 such fatalities. It is self-evident that when ease of frustration is a major part of abuse, some children are more frustrating or abrasive than others. "Irritable," "poor sleeper," "stubborn," "hard to train," are terms frequently used to characterize injured children, while several here had been admitted earlier for eczema, cerebral palsy, vomiting or chronic diarrhea.

Lesions Associated with Physical Abuse

Inflicted injuries provide the same gamut of tissue and organ damage as do those purely accidental. In our experience, most infants survive the first year or two of life without major tissue disruption, and when an accident does occur, all damage can be explained by a single vector of force. With active aggression, on the other hand, (1) injuries tend to be repetitive and cumulative, and (2) the lesions resulting from a single episode frequently do not conform to a uniform vector. To illustrate, an infant is examined after the mother supposedly fell down six steps while carrying the baby. We would not be surprised to find a fractured skull and a midthigh fracture of the femur. However, we would be most alarmed to find a fractured skull plus small metaphyseal disruptions at both knees, since these usually come from torsion, not from a fall. It should also be disturbing to find the fresh skull fracture but to note callus around the break in the femur!

Some idea of the range of injuries can be gathered from Table 8-1 based on the last 55 patients studied at our hospital.

SKELETAL LESIONS.—These can be of any type, but attention is called to the frequency with which metaphyseal injuries are present. These are caused by such torsion as arises from shaking or twisting and are explained anatomically by the firm attachment through Sharpey's fibers of the fibrous periosteum to the cartilage of long bones, in contrast to the loose arrangement along the diaphyses. These fractures vary in appearance from small triangular chips to more linear fragments called "bucket handles" (Figs. 8-1 and 8-2, A). They are frequently accompanied clinically by pain and periarticular swelling, but associated ecchymoses are rare. Calcification along the adjoining shaft where periosteum has been stripped by the related hematoma appears within 7–10 days. New bone forms rapidly, so that the injury within 2–4 months appears as thickening of the cortex and this, in turn, gradually remodels with complete healing. Discovery of one area of metaphyseal damage should automatically suggest a search for other similar lesions. It was this classic pattern which earlier suggested an increased metaphyseal fragility and led to confusion between traumatic changes and scurvy, a condition in which all bones are evenly involved by the underlying deficiency.

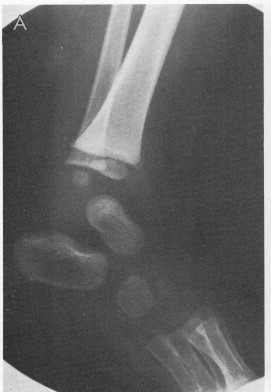

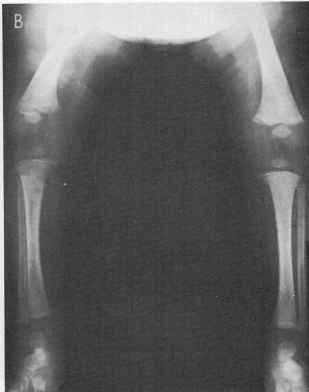

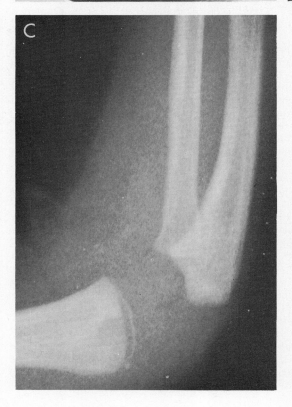

Fig. 8-1.—A, insufficient significance was placed on this single area of metaphyseal injury found at first contact with this 9-month-old girl. She died of a fractured liver 2 weeks later. B, separations at the distal metaphyses of both femurs and left tibia, and healing midshaft fracture of the right femur, in a 4-month-old infant. Bilateral subdural effusion without skull fracture was present. C, recent "bucket-handle" separation of right humerus in a 6-week-old infant. The mother, young, 6 months pregnant when married, was emotionally disturbed.

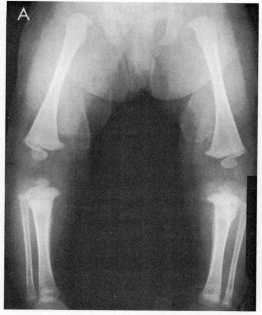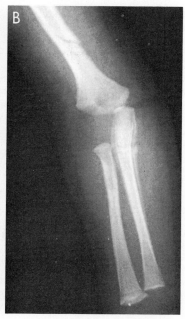

Fig. 8-2.—Injuries in the 7-week-old infant of a mother of 13 years! **A,** fresh metaphyseal fractures of both femurs and older diaphyseal injuries of both tibias. **B,** left arm, with recent oblique fracture of humerus, old greenstick fracture of ulna and recent damage to distal end of radius.

We have been impressed by the rarity with which fractured ribs are encountered after accidents as compared with the relative frequency in battering: 9 of the 55 patients tabulated had one or more such lesions. Probably, distortion by compression leads to this deformity rather than a direct blow or fall such as would commonly occur accidentally (Fig. 8-3). Skull fractures vary in form and extent, but the majority are linear or stellate rather than depressed. Rarely are these accompanied by swelling or contusion, and most likely they result from angulation of cranial bones rather than from direct blows. The usual lack of correlation between roentgenologic evidence of fracture and the presence or extent of underlying damage is illustrated by our material; the calvarium was intact in 6 of 13 patients with subdural hematoma or brain contusion or both.

We carried out, at the time of our initial interest in trauma to the skeleton, an extensive survey of bone pathology seen in infancy and came to the conclusion that rarely must a serious differential diagnosis be entertained. This view, in general, is still current provided good quality films of the entire skeleton are available and the interpreter has had reasonable experience with the younger age groups. Baker and Berdon[1] have studied and illustrated a variety of generalized and local skeletal lesions which predispose to fracture.

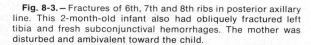

Fig. 8-3.—Fractures of 6th, 7th and 8th ribs in posterior axillary line. This 2-month-old infant also had obliquely fractured left tibia and fresh subconjunctival hemorrhages. The mother was disturbed and ambivalent toward the child.

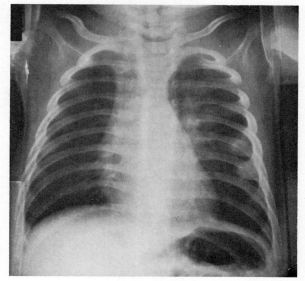

INJURIES TO THE NERVOUS SYSTEM.—These rank next to skeletal lesions in frequency and account for the major part of permanent disability. They occur separately or in conjunction with other evidence of trauma. Acute or chronic subdural hematoma is the form most commonly encountered, but such are frequently the obvious anatomic expressions of brain injury or the remainder of earlier brain contusion. It is self-evident that any infant with skeletal injury should have complete studies to rule out the possibility of brain injury and that the converse is equally important—any infant with brain injury should have a complete roentgenographic survey of the skeleton.

CUTANEOUS AND SOFT TISSUE INJURY.—This is more common in older children than in infants and usually is seen as bruises. Frequently, they occur in interpretable patterns when an object such as a belt or hairbrush has been employed. Four children, in whom skeletal defects were found, had been referred for study of coagulation problems, and in none had trauma received serious consideration. Burns are also encountered, and one of the deaths recorded in Table 8-1 was due to scalding. Small circumscribed burns are frequently attributed to lighted cigarettes.

INJURY TO VISCERA.—In our experience, this type of injury is rather uncommon but extremely serious when present. Two deaths within the past year, 1 from fracture of the liver, the other from rupture of a viscus, have been recorded.

Recognition of Physical Abuse

There is no sine qua non for physical abuse. The thought that adults, especially parents, can exert serious physical brutality on infants is foreign to most physicians and so repulsive that many deny, consciously or unconsciously, the possibility in an individual patient. This is especially evident when there is close parent-physician rapport or if the family is identified as being of the same economic or cultural group as the examiner—a colleague, for instance. Parenthetically, such attitudes explain many of the vagaries in reporting.

The taboo, with wider recognition of the problem, is breaking down. This is a most salutary trend which can only benefit patient, parent and physician through early detection. Rarely are episodes of battering isolated, and repetition is the rule; thus better to be wholesomely suspicious than to run the risk of a truly regrettable incident at a later date.

The following short rules have been helpful to us.

1. Be skeptical when evaluating the volunteered explanation for injury. Recall the formula we learned in high school physics, $F = MA$ (force = mass × acceleration), and decide if the midthigh of a healthy 6-month-old baby (weighing 14 lb) is likely to fracture transversely by being accelerated through the 15 in. separating a couch from a carpeted floor.

2. When one injury is evident, look for others; especially should metaphyseal disruption call for complete surveys.

3. Regard more than one accident resulting in definite tissue injury as rare in a well-regulated household during the first 18 months of life.

4. Remember that battering encompasses more than tissue damage and appraise the over-all growth and nutritional status of the injured infant.

5. Include some medical background in your histories, especially as it relates to the material included earlier on abusive households.

6. Ignore the fact that parents appear to be solicitous and seek your help. This does not eliminate the possibility of a violent rage 2 hours earlier. Do not be misled by the healthy appearance of siblings.

7. Consider the fact that parents have sought your assistance as implied consent to more than immediate care of injury. Utilize the help of colleagues and other health professions (social service, psychologists, etc.) when indicated.

8. Be realistic and don't talk about vague states such as "purpura," "mild osteogenesis imperfecta" or "subclinical scurvy." Each can be proved or disproved scientifically.

Treatment and Prophylaxis of Battering

Therapy for inflicted injuries does not differ from that of similar anatomic deviations acquired accidentally. The primary aim of the physician is to see that no further abuse befalls either the patient or other members of the household, and the best rule we can give in this respect is: *Never relinquish control of a maltreated child until he can be turned over to some other responsible person or agency.* This frequently necessitates appeal to court or to law enforcement departments, but such a certainly justified in view of the repetitive nature of violence and the high mortality among patients released to the same environment in which the initial trouble appeared.

The ultimate disposition of battered children can be made only after careful study of the individual milieu. Rarely is the physician equipped by training, emotional structure or time to undertake such investigations. These are better conducted by individuals with a good background in social work and familiarity with patterns of child abuse. Such are frequently available on the hospital staff, and recently personnel in various courts, the woman's division of the police, and child protective agencies have been trained for these activities. Investigation must be conducted with a purely nonpunitive outlook, since the punishment for offenses is the responsibility of constituted courts and the physician's ends are met when his patient is assured a protective environment.

It is obvious, working with a spectrum of situations, that solutions will cover a broad range of possibilities, and these are currently being evaluated in a number of centers. Sometimes material assistance and moral support for those in whom frustration and immaturity are evident suffices. In others, a close and constant tie to a person skilled in interhuman relations has helped. Some situations benefit from psychiatric approaches at various levels of sophistication; and in a residue, the household is so disturbed that long-term removal of the victim through court action is necessary. Even this is not a cure-all; 3 of the children in our present series were battered in foster homes after having been removed from the natural household because of abuse or neglect.

The increased community interest in abuse has led to a rash of legislative acts and proposals.[6] In general, these are aimed at providing immunity for the physician, who, in good faith, reports to designated agencies or bureaus instances in which he believes mistreatment has taken place. Many take a more active course and make it a misdemeanor for a physician not to report an injury when he has reason to suspect violence. Such acts are constantly undergoing revision, with a trend especially toward broadening the base of reporting individuals or institutions. Thus the onus of reporting in some states can be shifted from the physician, who enjoys a professional or social relationship to the family, to a more impersonal agency, the hospital. It is obvious that no amount of legislation can help unless supported by an enlightened concern on the part of the community, the courts and the medical profession. At present, attitudes vary from an extreme of complete permissiveness or avoidance to one of unconstructive vindictiveness. A mature recognition of the entire problem of child abuse would be much more valuable than any amount of legislation.

Another area of statute with which the physician should be familiar concerns the right or duty of courts responsible for child welfare.[6] Here again there is great variation in interpretation and practice. We have been fortunate in working with two courts whose concept of the law charges parents to provide for their children a safe and wholesome home. The occurrence of physical injury is de facto evidence that this is not being accomplished, and thus it becomes the prerogative of the court to assume jurisdiction. With this philosophy, it is not necessary to name a specific offender or to initiate criminal action to obtain our aim, that is, protective custody of the victim while the home environment is examined and disposition decided.

REFERENCES

1. Baker, D. W., and Berdon, W. E.: Special trauma problems in children, Radiol. Clin. North America 4:289, 1966.
2. Caffey, J.: Multiple fractures in long bones of infants suffering from chronic subdural hematomas, Am. J. Roentgenol. 56:163, 1946.
3. Cohen, M. I., *et al.*: Psychologic aspects of the maltreatment syndrome of childhood, J. Pediat. 69:279, 1966.
4. Kempe, C. H., *et al.*: Battered-child syndrome, J.A.M.A. 181:17, 1961.
5. Komisaruk, R.: Annual Clinic Days Symposium on Trauma, Children's Hospital of Michigan, May, 1967 (unpublished data presented).
6. Paulsen, M. G.: The legal framework for child protection, Columbia Law Rev., 66:678, 1966. (Reprints of this work have been prepared by the Children's Bureau, Department of Health, Education, and Welfare, Washington, D.C.)
7. Woolley, P. V., Jr., and Evans, W. A., Jr.: Significance of skeletal lesions in infants resembling those of traumatic origin, J.A.M.A. 158:539, 1955.

P. V. WOOLLEY, JR.
J. O. REED

9

Burns

Twelve thousand eight hundred individuals died of burns in the United States in 1966, and half of the victims were children under age 14 years.[77] Farmer[37] reported on 3,950 burned children admitted to the Hospital for Sick Children, Toronto. Burns lead the causes of accidental death under the age of 3 and remain in second place to age 14.[2,10,76] About 1 in 4 admissions to the Pediatric Surgical Service at the Boston City Hospital involves injury of some type, and burns are second only to head injuries in this category. *During the period 1954–1967, 1,000 consecutive burned children were treated in this institution with an average stay of 3 weeks.* Most of the burns occurred at home and were preventable: 538 were due to scalding with hot liquids; 358 were caused by open flame, usually associated with the ignition of flammable clothing, and 104 patients sustained burns due to miscellaneous causes, including contact with hot objects, caustics and electricity. In the early years of the series, many fatal burns occurred as the result of exploding, portable, improperly vented, barometric type, single unit space-heaters. This resulted in 19 deaths in 1959. As the result of an intensive local educational campaign and the institution of prohibitive legislation, no children died as a result of spare-heater explosion in 1966. The only hope we see in the further reduction of flame deaths in children lies in massive, urban renewal and recent Federal legislation (P.L. 80–189) making it mandatory to produce children's clothing (i.e., clothing in certain sizes) from nonflammable textiles.[13,24,87,97]

Writing in the 17th Century, Richard Wiseman said: "for however people cry, it's nothing to cure burns: yet, by what I have seen of cures from country or city they are often very ill performed." There is a striking lack of uniformity of burn care at any level. No injury is treated less expertly. Surgeons called upon to treat an occasional burned child commit errors of omission or delay and tragic losses occur. Many of the elements of therapy that seem unimportant have life or death significance.

The burned child usually is cared for in a random way by the accident room attendant, Many die because of improper resuscitation. Patients with full-thickness burns that should be resurfaced in 1 month often spend months, or even years, with infected granulating wounds, dislocations and disabling contractures. Much remains to be accomplished at the postgraduate educational level in providing uniform care for children with burns.

Initial Care

All children with burns involving more than 10% of the body surface and all with burns of the face, hands, feet and genitalia should be admitted to the hospital. No ointments are used. The patient should be bathed or showered, wrapped in a clean sheet and transported immediately to the nearest facility having an experienced, adequately staffed and equipped burn unit. Recently, because of unique funding, "burn hospitals" have been established in key areas under university supervision. Long-overdue research relating to the metabolic, hemodynamic and immune havoc resulting from the burn will be the principal yield of this funding. These burn institutes cannot be expected to assume the burden of burn therapy at the clinical level.

On admission, the height and weight are measured and a surface diagram of the burn is constructed according to the Lund-Berkow method.[11,58] The child is then examined for evidence of respiratory tract injury. The need for tracheostomy comes on exceedingly fast and takes priority over other aspects of initial therapy. A cut-down is established in a vein of an unburned extremity and a polyethylene catheter inserted. Blood is drawn for estimation of hemoglobin, hematocrit, blood urea nitrogen, sodium, chloride, carbon dioxide, potassium and blood type and for direct cross-match with whole blood. In children with burns greater than 40%, a direct central venous pressure line is established. Readings are made hourly on the first day with the aim of staying in the range of 10–15 cm of water.

Intravenous therapy is started with isotonic saline or balanced electrolyte, although, with delay in transportation, colloid as plasma should be used. In burns involving more than 10% of the body surface, we rely entirely on the intravenous route for fluid replacement and have no confidence in the various recommended techniques of oral fluid therapy.

A Foley catheter is inserted into the bladder, and

the color, volume, specific density and sediment of initial bladder urine are recorded. A guaiac test is carried out on the supernatant. Urine sodium and chloride content is estimated at appropriate intervals once urine flow and rate are established. A urine sodium value of less than 40 mEq/liter probably indicates adequate tubular function, while a level of 50 or greater indicates tubular damage unless iatrogenic high levels are produced with lactated Ringer's solution, when levels of 100 mEq/liter or higher may be observed in the first day. Ideally, urine output should be 40 cc/M²/hour. In practical terms, this means 8–20 cc/hour under age 2; 20–30 cc to age 8, and 30–50 cc/hour in older children. The serum sodium level should be kept above 130 mEq, and serum protein content above 5 Gm/100 ml, considering 3.5 Gm/100 ml a critically low level. These measurements can be made on 0.1 cc of serum, using a microrefractometer. The hematocrit should be kept between 40 and 50%; a level of 30, critically low, indicates a need for additional whole blood.

With obvious burns of the respiratory tract, one must monitor arterial Po_2, Pco_2 and serum pH. Patients having an initial Po_2 of less than 75 on admission are placed in 100% oxygen; few will survive.[79] Tracheostomy is mandatory in these patients, with intermittent positive pressure breathing under Demerol sedation (1.0 mg/kg intravenously). Packed cells, Digoxin, Isuprel, prednisolone and ganglionic blocking agents are adjunctive.

Tetanus prophylaxis is given either as toxoid to the already immunized child or as human tetanus immune globulin USP.* Four cc per kilogram is given intravenously, and this is repeated after 4 weeks if open areas remain. Tetanus antitoxin derived from animal sources can now be considered obsolete.

Because of the still present danger of septicemia due to beta hemolytic streptococcus, children hospitalized with burns are given crystalline penicillin, 40,000 units/kg/day intravenously for 3 days. Thereafter, one can shift to procaine penicillin orally or parenterally for 4 more days. A bladder catheter is required for children with major burns and those involving the perineum. We recommend the use of Neosporin bladder irrigant every 6 hours in addition to strict aseptic technique, with a closed disposable gravity collection system changed frequently. In the absence of clinically evident sepsis, no further antibiotic therapy is recommended until grafting begins.

Surface care consists of limited gentle cleansing and removal of char or the remains of broken blisters. The mild surgical soap pHisoHex has satisfactory physical qualities.

All burns are initially exposed regardless of location or circumferential nature. Sedation is not necessary in most children with flame burns but is needed in the child with a superficial dermal burn or scald. The most satisfactory route is by vein (1 mg of morphine for each 5 kg of body weight).

* Hyper-tet, Cutter Laboratories.

A note of caution is valid concerning the use of "behavior modifiers." Substances related to chlorpromazine with a phenothiazine structure should not be given the burned child. They have undesirable autonomic blocking effects which interfere with proper interpretation of the treatment of the shock phase, prolong and intensify the action of narcotics and necessary anesthetic agents and have unpredictable extrapyramidal and cortical effects. Response of the individual child is variable, and bizarre mental patterns have followed the use of these drugs.

Tracheostomy

Twenty-seven children required tracheostomy because of flame burns involving the head and neck area and/or the respiratory tract (Fig. 9-1). The need for tracheostomy usually is evident from the history of the accident and location of the burn. Most of these children were involved in space-heater or other explosions and trapped in an overheated compartment. In addition to obvious burns of the upper thorax, neck and face areas, they have edema and reddening of the pharyngeal mucous membranes, are restless, hoarse and have audible wheezing throughout both lung fields.

It is important that tracheostomy be performed at this stage rather than to try to tide them over with supportive medical measures. No significant morbidity has been attached to the operation, which is usually performed electively under light halothane anesthesia with an endotracheal tube in place. If one is tardy in realizing the need for tracheostomy, it may be done over a bronchoscope at the bedside, where conditions are far from ideal. A short transverse incision is used. A segment of the third tracheal ring is removed. The tracheostomy site must be located low in the neck in children to avoid laryngeal stenosis. The tracheal opening can, however, be located too low, and with return of the hyperextended head to neutral position, pneumomediastinum results. Inadvertent injury to great vessels and unilateral or bilateral pneumothorax have occurred often enough to justify a word of caution about the unrealistic concept of "emergency tracheostomy."

Moistened air and other adjuncts described above provide some hope for a higher salvage rate in children with burns of the respiratory tract. Intermittent suction is necessary in the first 72 hours, observing rigid asepsis. It is usually possible to stopple the tracheostomy tube on the fourth day and to remove it shortly thereafter.

These youngsters do not have ulcerative burns of the tracheobronchial tree. An intensity of heat which produces surface destruction in the moistened depths of the bronchial tree is incompatible with life.[71] We have seen examples of this among the asphyxiation victims of the Cocoanut Grove fire and in autopsy material from incinerated children. We encountered 9 children with fatal pulmonary burns, the leading

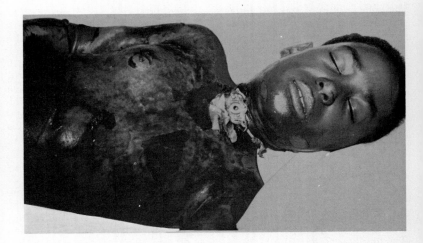

Fig. 9-1.—Tracheostomy was required in 27 children. Edema of pharyngeal mucous membranes progresses rapidly to airway obstruction. This procedure should not be done as an ''emergency'' and is the first consideration in flame burns involving head and neck areas.

cause of death in the first 48 hours. We are indebted to Phillips and Cope,[79] who have done much to elucidate the problem and outline proper care.

The tracheostomy is designed to tide these children over a period of excessive bronchorrhea and obstruction due to edema of pharyngeal membranes.[71] Once through this period, airway continuity can be reestablished. Orotracheal intubation rather than tracheostomy is now under study.[34]

Parenteral Fluid Therapy

The relationship of hemoconcentration to thermal injury was pointed out by Harkins,[44] the significance of surface area involvement by Cope and Moore,[28] and the parameter of body weight was added by Evans[36] in 1952. Out of these various studies came a series of burn "formulas" or "budgets" based to an extent on laboratory and clinical evidence but offered because of their working ability to resuscitate the burn patient adequately in the first days following injury. There is approximate agreement about the total volumes required to accomplish this end but total disagreement about the qualitative aspects. Table 9-1 shows five "formulas" for appropriate amounts of colloid, electrolyte and water to be given for a 50% burn in a 20-

kg (1-M²) child. The formulas of Markley and Moyer have military and civilian disaster considerations but cannot be considered ideal for hospital treatment of the individual burned child.[61,74] Most investigators agree that the static and dynamic extracellular fluid debt and the colloid requirement of the burned child are greater than those of the adult. Consequently, there must be an upward revision of all components of therapy.[31, 45, 91]

Moore[70] suggests therapy calculated at 12% rather than 10% of the initial body weight, and Haynes[45] recommends that the colloid component be revised upward by 30%. There is no question about the clinical value of all of these formulas. More important considerations are time and volume. If a child is brought immediately to the hospital and parenteral fluid therapy is started within the first hour, satisfactory resuscitation can be accomplished with any of these formulas. This is often not the case, and the mere hydraulics of delivering several hundred cubic centimeters of parenteral fluid in an hour to a small child is the chief obstacle to establishment of homeostasis.

For the sake of continuity of burn doctrine, we have relied on a local formula (Table 9-2). In 5 youngsters who had delayed parenteral fluid therapy, we encountered a renal tubular lesion. In each case, it lasted approximately 14 days, with return of normal urine volume, tubular regulation, correction of azotemia and satisfactory burn recovery. The renal lesion in a burned child with previously normal kidneys requires both untreated shock and a heavy load of heme pigments to develop. Dialysis of patients with hyperkalemia (above 8.0) is a useful adjunct. Resins are inefficient because of gastrointestinal difficulties.

In our "formula," the colloid fraction has been increased 50% over the Evans recommendation, giving 1.5 cc of colloid rather than 1 cc for each per cent area of burn. Electrolyte as isotonic saline or commercially

TABLE 9-1.—COMPARISON OF FORMULAS FOR PARENTERAL THERAPY IN A STANDARD BURN PROBLEM*

AUTHOR	COLLOID, IN Cc	ELECTROLYTE, IN Cc	NONELECTROLYTE, IN Cc
Markley	—	2,000	1,500
Moncrief	500	1,500	1,500
Evans	1,000	1,000	1,500
Welch	1,500	1,000	1,500
Cope	2,000	—	2,000

*The greatest variance is in colloid composition, with general agreement about total volume. We are in accord with Haynes, Moore and Cope about the increased colloid requirement in children with thermal burns.

TABLE 9-2.—An Intravenous "Formula"
for the Burned Child*

		A	B	C
"COLLOID"	1.5 cc × % Area × Kg Wt	1/2	1/2	1/2 A & B
"ELECTROLYTE"	1.0 cc × % Area × Kg Wt	0–8 Hr	8–24 Hr	24–48 Hr

"WATER" as 5% D/W = 1,200 to 1,500 cc/M²/24 hr
No burn is calculated in excess of 50% surface area involvement

"Colloid"

I. "PLASMA" IN SCALDS UP TO 30% AND IN FLAME BURNS UP TO 20%

II. WHOLE BLOOD/"PLASMA" IN RATIO OF 1:3 IN FLAME BURNS OVER 20% AND SCALDS OVER 30%

III. WHOLE BLOOD/"PLASMA" IN RATIO OF 1:2 IN FLAME BURNS OVER 40%

Adjust to:

Urine volume	40 cc/M²/hr
Central venous pressure	10–15 cm H₂O
Hematocrit	40–50
Clinical response	

*This formula has served us well as the initial approach to parenteral support in 1,000 consecutive burn admissions. The 5 cases of renal suppression were due to delay in initial therapy. No formula should be rigidly adhered to. (From Welch.[94])

available balanced electrolyte is initially calculated as 1 cc. Water requirement is based on total surface area estimated from kilogram weight.[91] Because burn parameters are not known in the patient with extensive involvement, we do not calculate any burn at more than 50%.

Single unit plasma, Plasmanate or albumin is used in scalds up to 40%, and we give increasing amounts of whole blood in flame burns. Whole blood requirement has been studied by Evans,[35] Quinby,[81] Raker[83] and others.[55] We have made chrome-51 measurements of red cell mass following extensive flame burns in children and have found initial losses to average 300 cc, with a continuing average intrinsic loss of 200 cc of packed cells/M²/week. The validity of such studies has been questioned by Moore, who is uncertain about the ability of heat-damaged cells or cells late in the life cycle to pick up the radioactive tag. This does not include the gram-for-gram replacement that occurs in connection with grafting procedures. The initial red cell losses are due either to immediate destruction from the high local heat in the skin and subcutaneous tissues or to heat damage to blood cells with subsequent dissolution. There is initial capillary sludging, followed by bone marrow suppression, with continued destruction associated with inevitable sepsis after the first week.[25]

The most frequent error in the management of the burned child is failure to appreciate the seriousness of burns of any etiology involving 10–15% of the body surface. The statement is made repeatedly in the literature that burns up to 20% can be treated on an outpatient basis or can be treated entirely by oral liquids taken ad lib. Twenty-five years ago, scalds caused

more deaths in burned children than all other forms of burns combined. Wilson, reporting on 21 burn deaths in children, noted a higher mortality from scalds (36%) than from flame burns (31%). Erb, in 61 autopsies on children, reported 37 deaths from scalds as opposed to 24 deaths from flame burns. Both authors stressed the minor extent of some of the fatal scalds.

Several recent reports include deaths due to scalds involving less than 15% of the body surface in children in the first 2 years of life.[9,37,47] Hitchcock and Horowitz[47] reported on 3 infants less than 1 year of age who died because of inadequate shock therapy, the smallest area of involvement being 5% in a 4-day-old infant. Another died at 1 year with an 8% area and another at 4 months with a 20% area. A similar situation was reported by Barnes,[9] with an adverse mortality grid for the child as compared with that of the young adult. We have treated 538 scalded children without a fatality. Clarkson[23] reported 15 fatal scalds in children 14 years of age or younger in England in 1965. This author has encountered 2 children with immersion scalds involving more than 70% of the body surface; both were infants, both died and are thought to be examples of premeditated homicide or gross parental neglect. Scalds continue to be underread and undertreated, with continuing avoidable deaths in the period of resuscitation.

Estimation of Burn Extent

A common error occurs in the estimation of area involvement. Surface area charts especially adapted to children are necessary. Figure 9-2 is a simplification of our chart and indicates that the head

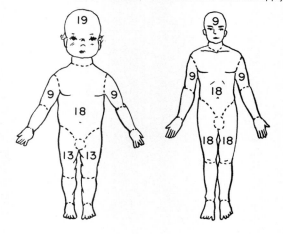

Fig. 9-2.—Simplified diagram taken from more exact working charts used to calculate area of involvement expressed as percentage of total body surface area. **Left,** figure representing a 1-year-old child; **right,** figure representing a 10-year-old child. Because of marked difference in surface area represented by the head and lower extremities, the rule-of-nine does not apply.

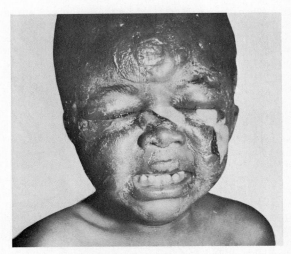

Fig. 9-3.—Toddler scald 18 hours after injury. Because of extensive involvement of the head and neck, this child is a candidate for burn shock unless hospitalized and vigorously treated by the parenteral route.

and neck area of an infant 1 year of age represents 19% of the body surface rather than 9%, as suggested in the overpopular rule-of-nine. With each year of age, the head-neck area decreases by 1% until, at age 10, the child and adult are proportionately identical. The other area of greatest change is in the lower extremities. Here, the 1-year-old child has 13% represented in each lower extremity. This increases at the rate of ½% for each lower extremity a year to age 10. All other areas can be calculated as one would for an adult. It is apparent, then, that scalds involving the head-neck area are shock-producing burns in the range of 15–20% (Fig. 9-3). These children must be hospitalized and vigorously treated with parenteral fluids. Delay results in complications that may be irreversible or fatal. A common one in our experience is central nervous system damage because of diffuse venous thrombosis or the anoxia associated with untreated shock. There are secondary effects on other parenchymatous organs, most obvious in the kidney as a renal tubular lesion and presumably in the liver as well.

Fig. 9-4.—**A,** initial "exposure," used in all children in our series, leads to formation of a comfortable, dry, clean eschar within 48 hours. Discomfort is transient and controlled by intravenous sedation. **B,** in the usual superficial dermal burn due to a hot liquid, spontaneous separation of the eschar occurs in about 2 weeks. This leaves a dry, clean, completely healed wound, with transitory loss of pigment in dark-skinned races.

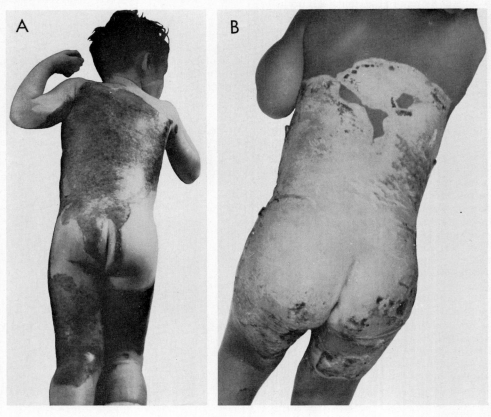

Treatment

CARE OF THE BURN WOUND

EXPOSURE METHOD.—We have initially exposed 1,000 consecutive burned children admitted to the Boston City Hospital. This was done with some misgiving at first because of the strong stand of burn authorities that this method had a limited application. Yet we have had up to 17 in hospital with burns that, by conventional occlusive dressing methods, would require changing at least on alternate days. With limited man-power, we could not keep up this dressing schedule to provide satisfactory occlusive care. We first exposed one-surface burns, then, as the many benefits were observed in terms of clinical improvement, return of temperature to normal, nutritional performance, psychologic attitude and freedom from hours of drudgery, we decided to expose all children admitted, including those with circumferential burns of the trunk, extremities, hands and feet (Fig. 9-4).

Exposure plus daily pHisoHex washes and conservative marginal debridement constitutes the only wound treatment for the majority of patients who have scalds. The eschar is surgically removed or spontaneously discarded in 14–28 days, leaving a completely healed clean surface with loss of pigmentation. Bryant's traction should not be used.[78] In circumferential or very extensive burns involving the trunk and extremities, we use a Stryker burn frame, changing the surface of contact every 2 hours. Other children are allowed to move about freely in a conventional hospital bed, with a change of sheets and perforated plastic film every 8 hours. It is necessary to protect them from bacterial contamination until the burn eschar forms, usually within 72 hours. They are kept on mask, glove and gown, so-called reverse precautions. Once the eschar has formed, we allow those with less extensive burns to be ambulant and mix with other children. This seems to have a beneficial effect on co-operation and attitude toward hospital personnel during the weeks ahead.

We do not take credit for this return to exposure therapy. Copeland reported on this method in 1887, the Sneve[86] described it adequately in 1905, especially in its application to children. Undoubtedly the method goes back to antiquity. Revival of interest can be credited to Wallace,[93] who exposed burns of the face, perineum and buttock in 1947. Eventually others adopted this in their own programs or vigorously attacked it.[5, 80, 85] It is not a competitive form of treatment and constitutes satisfactory closed therapy in the first 2 weeks.

Our experience indicates that it is always successful in children, has not resulted in delay of definitive surgical treatment and has added to the flexibility of our program.

DEBRIDEMENT METHODS

After diuresis has occurred, we are usually in the best position we will be in for the next several weeks. The child is alert, eating well, has a minimal daily temperature variation, a dry wound and no evidence of systemic bacterial invasion. Yet from our experience, this is only the quiet before the storm (Fig. 9-5). Until the latter part of the fourth week, when granulation tissue is firmly established, the patient is vulnerable to invasive sepsis in part thought to be iatrogenic and the cruel dividend of administering multiple "prophylactic" antibiotics.[25, 52] In the 1950's, the offending organism was *Staphylococcus aureus*.[7] From 1960 to 1965, *Pseudomonas aeruginosa* emerged as the killer of children and adults with burns previously thought to be in the salvageable range.[62, 81] Coincident to the awareness of drug-resistant mutant invasive forms of ordinarily saprophytic organisms produced by exposure to broad spectrum antibiotics, there has emerged a return to the use of surface antiseptics. This controversial aspect of burn wound care is discussed later under the heading, New Methods. At this point, it can be said that we are profoundly skeptical about their value and continued use. Whether these agents are used as adjuncts to surface care or not, the goal would seem to be removal of burn tissue only (eschar) and resurfacing as

Fig. 9-5.—Days after burn to initial grafting. The key to burn management after resuscitation and diuresis is rapid debridement and early resurfacing. Early in our series, average time before initial grafting was 26 days; 2 weeks of golden time were lost, and many patients died because of invasive sepsis and an open wound. For the past 8 years, initial grafting has been possible in flame burns by the end of the 2nd week, with every attempt to keep the wound closed with autogenous or donor skin.

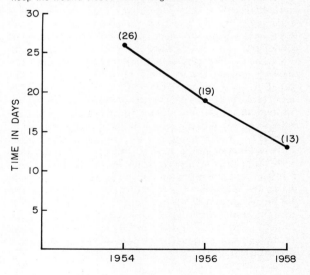

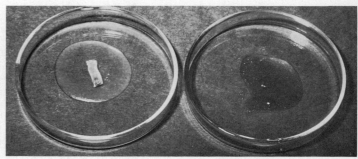

Fig. 9-6. — In vitro study showing effectiveness of ficus protease in dissolving a segment of burn eschar taken down to but not including the adipose layer. **Left**, the biopsy specimen is undisturbed when immersed in the water-soluble vehicle alone. **Right**, 7% enzyme added to the vehicle dissolved the eschar wedge in 72 hours.

rapidly as possible with autologous, allogenic or, rarely, isogenic grafts.

There are several approaches to eschar removal, depending on the area involved and the depth of tissue destruction.

ENZYME DEBRIDEMENT. — Various enzymes and chemicals have been investigated with the hope that they might be useful in hastening the removal of the burn eschar. These include Dakin's solution, pyruvic acid, streptokinase, streptodornase, trypsin, collagenase and various bacterial enzymes, especially those produced by clostridia.[33,42,88] Most of these substances have been discarded because they were ineffective when examined in control series, were toxic in themselves or broke down the sealed routes to bacterial invasion. Objective evaluation is difficult.

The vegetable cathepsins exhibit collagenase or proteolytic activity in an acid medium. Examples are ficus protease, maya protease and the various papain derivatives. We have investigated one of these, ficus protease,† a substance derived from a species of South American fig tree. This material, provided as a powder in 7% concentration, is mixed with a water-soluble base just before application to the eschar. It is most effective in a warm, moist environment, and dressing changes are necessary with reapplication of the enzyme every 12 hours. In vitro and clinical studies indicate that it is selectively proteolytic, does not destroy normal tissue, is not absorbed to any extent or, if it is, does not have toxic manifestations. Its chief drawback in clinical use is that it is locally irritating, although this varies from child to child. Its effectiveness in disposing of burn eschar is shown in Figure 9-6. In this simple study, a biopsy specimen of burn eschar down to normal fat was obtained. One half was placed in a petri dish containing the enzyme vehicle, and the other half was placed in the vehicle with 7% enzyme. The complete dissolution of the eschar fragment in 72 hours in enzyme plus vehicle and the undisturbed appearance in the vehicle alone indicate that the enzyme does have action in excess of moistening achieved by frequent vehicle or saline dressing changes.

---

†Debricin (ficus protease), Johnson & Johnson.

In addition, measurement of the hydroxyprolene content of tissues after enzyme digestion demonstrates that it does have an important collagenase effect. It is not lipolytic and has no effect on burned fat.

Debricin was used by us in more than 150 consecutive flame burns.[20] Split-thickness grafting was necessary in half the patients and was always started by the fourteenth day, using enzymes alone or in combination with surgical debridement.

The most difficult problem in dealing with the flame burn is in estimating its depth. The skin in various areas of the body varies in thickness, and it is important to know whether the basal germinal layer of the skin and epithelial cell groups in accessory skin structures have been destroyed. If not, then as the eschar is removed or is allowed to separate spontaneously, healing can occur from the multiple skin islands that are present in these areas. If there is full-thickness skin destruction, including superficial fat, a very aggressive approach must be taken to remove the culture medium and resurface with homograft or autograft skin.

Only crude clinical methods are available for estimating full-thickness destruction. We speak of the dry, marbleized or cadaver-white, insensitive, painless area as third degree, but this impression is often inaccurate. Ficus protease provided one means for distinguishing between partial and full-thickness destruction in the mixed flame burn. Daily application for 10 days, beginning the second day after the burn, resulted in dissolution of the eschar in areas of partial destruction, providing a halo of pink regenerating skin around the central areas of tough, leathery eschar considered to represent full-thickness destruction. Conway[27] has reported enthusiastically on the use of pyruvic acid paste in estimating the level of destruction in mixed flame burns.

If a patient has sustained a fire burn and we are able to demonstrate the central area of full-thickness destruction, we feel justified in going ahead with early surgical debridement and grafting up to 20% of total body surface. Ficus protease significantly reduced the interval between burn injury and intelligent initial grafting in major flame burns. Satisfactory recipient sites were achieved by the end of the second week in all cases.

Unfortunately, because of high cost and lack of endorsement, ficus protease is no longer produced, nor has any group pushed further into the investigation of the adjunct role of cathepsins in burn management.

SURGICAL DEBRIDEMENT.—Credit for this approach must be given to Wells[95] and the late Harvey Allen,[3] who reported on 1,000 burned children admitted to the Cook County Hospital, Chicago, prior to 1951. Of these, 237 required grafting, and at the time of his report he was carrying out early surgical excision in 30% of his patients. Meeker suggested a series of planing operations with the depth of injury established by the appearance of capillary bleeding.[63] In order to establish a satisfactory recipient site, it is necessary to perform successive dermatome debridements under anesthesia on alternate days after diuresis has occurred. Therefore, starting on the fifth day, it will take 8 days for the planing procedures. A wave of enthusiasm for massive surgical excision followed.[7,60] This is not said in a critical sense because we also were dissatisfied with conventional therapy and reasoned that some radical departure was in order.

Massive debridements were often done in desperation when there was deterioration or a strong clinical suspicion of invasive infection in the absence of positive blood cultures. In our clinic and in most recent reports, the pendulum has swung back to the early surgical excision of areas not in excess of 20%. It is an excellent method in children having noncircumferential flame burns of one extremity or the trunk, excluding burns of the face, hands and feet (Fig. 9-7).

At the Children's Hospital Medical Center, we have had encouragement in a few patients with early excision beyond the 20% level. All were infants with mixed flame burns involving up to 60% of the body surface. We bait the excised area with fresh homograft for 3–5 days before applying the precious autograft material. These infants were in the low survival end of the mortality grid, and the radical departure seemed indicated. Hendren[46] reported similar success and has been combining early massive excision with silver nitrate surface antisepsis. Taylor [92] has investigated the role of staged excision. It may be that infants have a greater and more rapid reparative process and a less vigorous rejection pattern than do older patients, permitting further extension of this method. However,

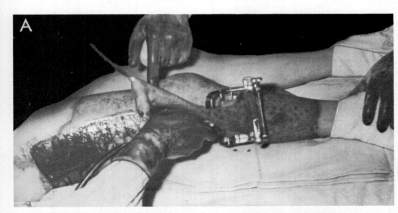

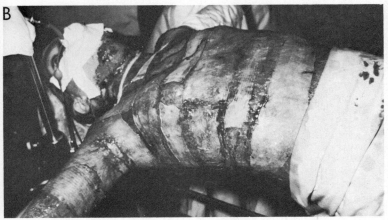

Fig. 9-7.—A, dermatome debridement down to normal-appearing fat or, if necessary, to fascia can be rapidly accomplished, with minimal blood loss at deep levels controlled by electrocoagulation. **B,** more extensive burns involving trunk and extremities require suspension of the patient on a Hawley fracture table, and two teams are used. Superficial knife debridement in the plane of edema below the eschar is tedious, requires massive blood replacement and provides an unsatisfactory base for skin grafting.

we do not have statistical support for this conclusion. Jackson[49] was unable to show increased survival following early excision of burns greater than 35%. Validity or rejection will depend on a prospective study.

HOMOGRAFTS

Brown suggested that cadaver skin be used as a biologic dressing in the burn patient with injury so extensive that he cannot provide sufficient skin for sustained wound closure.[17] This skin can be used fresh or freeze-dried, lyophilized and stored for periods up to 2 years.[18] The latter material has been generously supplied to us by the Tissue Bank of the National Naval Medical Center.

Homografts will provide, as will no other dressing, a dry, clean, burn area free from infection. Combined with autografts, they lead to dramatic improvement of the patient's clinical course. This is a life-saving technique. Zaroff *et al*[96] reported the use of homografts in half of all patients requiring skin grafting. Homografts are applied in several ways: to all debrided, unhealed areas in the presence of suspected infection; to all areas other than the face, neck, hands and flexion creases in burns greater than 40%; in strips alternating with autogenous grafts on a satisfactory

site in a recipient with limited capacity (area or clinical course) to provide autogenous material (Fig. 9-8). In recent years, all areas requiring grafting have been covered initially with homografts to bait the recipient site and to test the ability to adhere before autografts are applied. The postage stamp method is time-consuming and is not effective in closing the wound. The nebulized skin particle technique of Najarian has the same theoretical shortcoming.

In the first grafting procedure in salvageable full-thickness flame burns (30–60%), we attempt to decrease the prepared recipient area by 50%, using the patient's own skin. This requires most of the donor skin available. Areas over bony prominences are infiltrated, plateaus are created, and one can obtain large sheets of extremely thin skin (10 one-thousandths of an inch). We have successfully used the shaved scalp as a donor area. The other half of the burn wound is covered with homografts. We do not expect homografts to last for more than 10 days, and they seldom do. There are reports of fresh material lasting 4–6 weeks, but we have not seen it. Homografts from identical twins last indefinitely.[12, 26] Increased survival has also been reported in patients with total burns, uremia and agammaglobulinemia.

By the fourteenth day, the original donor site can

Fig. 9-8.— A, homografts of either the freeze-dried or fresh variety have been of lifesaving value in our experience. Most patients with flame burns in a salvageable range can provide some autograft skin at the time of the first grafting procedure. **B,** homografts and autografts are laid on in alternate strips and are replaced as necessary to maintain a dry, closed wound throughout the period of resurfacing.

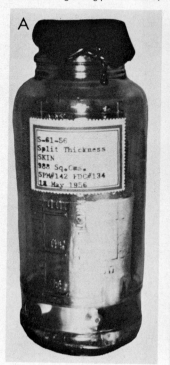
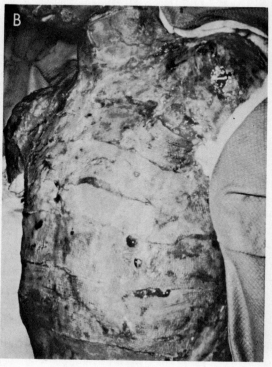

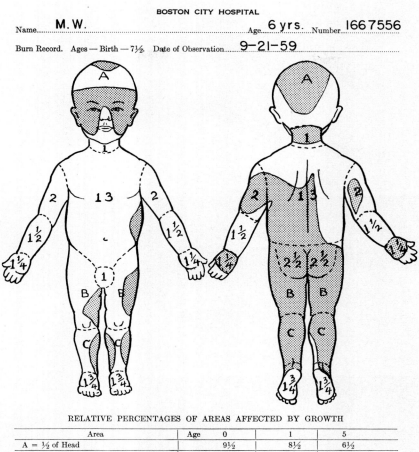

BOSTON CITY HOSPITAL

Name ... M.W. .... Age ... 6 yrs. ... Number ... 1667556

Burn Record.   Ages — Birth — 7½.   Date of Observation ... 9-21-59

RELATIVE PERCENTAGES OF AREAS AFFECTED BY GROWTH

Area	Age	0	1	5
A = ½ of Head		9½	8½	6½
B = ½ of One Thigh		2¾	3¼	4
C = ½ of One Leg		2½	2½	2¾

% BURN BY AREAS

	Head	Neck	Body	Up. Arm	Forearm	Hands
Probable 3rd° Burn	9	1	6	4		1
	Genitals 0	Buttocks 6	Thighs 12	Legs 7	Feet 0	
Total Burn	Head	Neck	Body	Up. Arm	Forearm	Hands
	Genitals	Buttocks	Thighs	Legs	Feet	

Sum of All Areas   Probably 3rd° ... 40 % +   Total Burn ... 46 %

Over for Older Patients

Fig. 9-9. — Surface area chart used at the Boston City Hospital, developed by Lund and Browder, based on Barkow's calculations. This chart can be corrected for exact age and is used for children up to age 5 years. A second chart is used for children aged 5–10. Thereafter, the rule-of-nine is applicable. Only by careful calculation of burn involvement for each of the anatomic parts can a true total be arrived at. Depth as well as extent is important in determining prognosis.

be used to replace the homograft if it has disappeared. If it has not, it is scraped off, all available autograft material is applied, and the remaining areas are filled in with homografts.

An example of the value of homografting is a 6-month-old infant who sustained flame burns of the trunk and lower extremities. He was depleted and ill when transferred and could not stand a definitive grafting procedure. A renal tubular lesion existed with oliguria and azotemia. He had a decerebrate pattern. Exposure of the wound and application of homograft skin brought deterioration to a halt. Autografting was then done, with complete recovery.

Fresh homografts do not have significant advantage over stored material provided a close grafting schedule is adhered to. We have used skin stored in

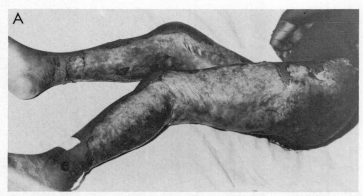

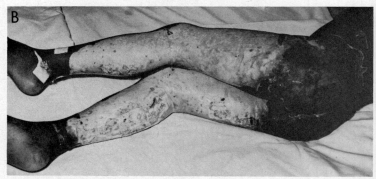

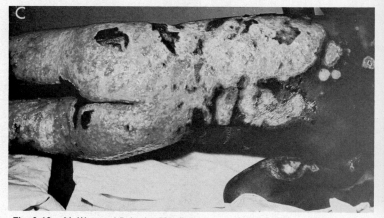

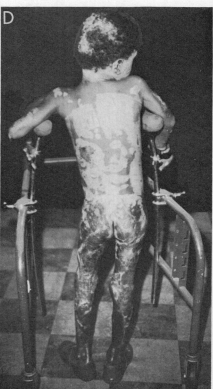

Fig. 9-10. — M. W., aged 5, had a 46% flame burn, of which 40% was third degree. **A,** showing uniform deep involvement of lower extremities. (For total distribution of the burn, see Fig. 9-9.) These areas were marbleized, firm and insensitive. **B,** enzyme debridement was started following diuresis on the 5th day. This photograph shows the contrast of the enzyme-treated area with the untreated area of the back and buttocks. After 72 hours, there is already partial removal of burned tissue. **C,** complete removal of all burn eschar except for two small patches on the buttock and left posterior iliac crest after 8 days of enzyme treatment. The small remaining eschar was removed on the 14th day, at the time of combined grafting. **D,** complete resurfacing of the 40% third-degree area by the 46th hospital day. He was discharged from the hospital 1 week later. We stress early and, whenever possible, continuous ambulation. Because of the rapid debridement and grafting, these youngsters eat ravenously and do not require nasogastric tube feeding; we have not used formula supplements for 10 years.

glycerol and in various nutrient mediums but have found no improvement over the more conveniently stored freeze-dried material.

M. W., a 5-year-old boy, was the only survivor of 5 children in a space-heater explosion, 4 siblings having been incinerated. Forty per cent of the 46% burn area was third degree (Figs. 9-9 and 9-10). Tracheostomy was required because of hoarseness and dyspnea. He was exposed and satisfactorily resuscitated. Diuresis occurred, with return to admission weight.

Enzyme and excision debridement therapy was started and continued until the fourteenth day. He was then equally covered with homograft and autograft skin with a good take. A second combined grafting procedure was undertaken 12 days later. At this time, he could provide the same amount of autograft tissue from healed donor areas and only 10% had to be homografted. The third and final autografting was done on the thirty-eighth hospital day. He was completely healed and ambulant by the forty-sixth day (Fig. 9-10, *D*) and never was a problem in terms of malnutrition or sepsis. He left the hospital 1 week later.

The dramatic effect of closing the wound with skin of any type, or possibly with polyamino acid film as suggested by Walder, is shown in the temperature chart (Fig. 9-11).

This youngster with mixed flame burns and a burn index of 45, treated in 1959 without surface antisep-

tics, remains a model for successful burn treatment. He was resurfaced with his own skin in a period representing 1.3 days for each 1% of full-thickness destruction. The enzyme debridement is of historical interest. Artz established the "burn index" by allowing 1 unit for each per cent of third-degree and 0.5 unit for each per cent of second-degree involvement.[7]

ADJUNCTIVE THERAPY

General management includes the liberal use of whole blood transfusions and intermittent 5-day courses of tetracycline covering each grafting procedure. The daily nutritional goal is 50–100 calories/kg, with 3 Gm of protein/kg plus 1.5 Gm of protein for each per cent of third-degree burn. Donor sites and grafted areas are covered with Adaptic,† followed by rolled mesh gauze soaked in Neosporin solution.[69] Donor sites are exposed after 24 hours. Grafted sites are dressed every second day and are exposed permanently after the fifth day except for areas of contact, which are covered with latticed monofilament mesh.

---

†Johnson & Johnson.

Fig. 9-11.—Chart for M. W. (see also Figs. 9-9 and 9-10) summarizing clinical course and sequence of operations. Closure of the wound at each grafting procedure had a dramatic effect on the temperature course.

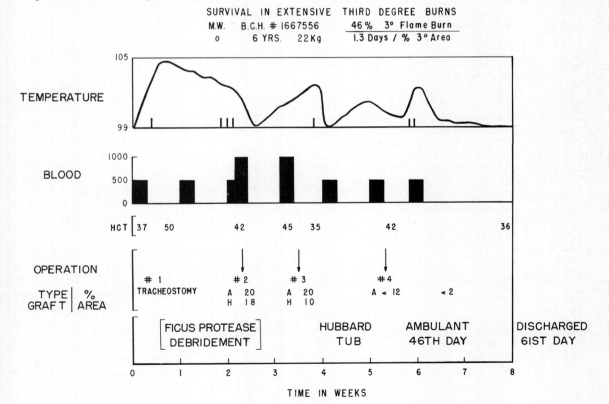

SURVIVAL IN EXTENSIVE THIRD DEGREE BURNS

Complications

The major complications are listed in Table 9-3. Thirty-nine patients had documented septicemia. In 32 patients this was due to *Staph. aureus* and *Ps. aeruginosa* equally divided. Cultures from 3 patients grew *Bacillus proteus*, and from 3 others, Friedländer's bacillus. We have not encountered septicemia due to herellea or other recently reported unusual micro-organisms. The present reprieve from septicemia in burns is, we believe, due to the more intelligent use of antibiotics, although one cannot ignore the possibility that we are enjoying a "bacterial holiday," only to have a new organism mount in virulence to confound new arrivals in the burn field. We have seen a variety of metastatic infections, including ethmoiditis, brain abscess, renal carbuncle and osteomyelitis.

Hemorrhagic bronchopneumonia, or wet lung, occurred in 9 children with respiratory tract burns. Gastrointestinal hemorrhage occurred in 8 patients, with exsanguination in 1. After this experience, we operated on 4 children who lost more than 1 blood volume in 24 hours. Two had vagotomy and pyloroplasty with suture of the ulcer, and 2 had vagotomy and pyloroplasty with Billroth I resection; all died. Thus gastrointestinal bleeding, a 1% complication, usually forecasts disaster. Five renal injuries were due to delay in instituting parenteral fluid therapy. The hepatitis figure is probably low, but jaundice has not been clinically evident or detected in other patients.

Cardiac arrest occurred in 3 patients under anesthesia in connection with dressing changes or grafting. Prompt cardiac massage was effective in 1, and the 40% flame burn was successfully grafted. Two patients could not be resuscitated in spite of thoracotomy and direct cardiac massage with all of the usual pharmacologic aids. Administration of fresh blood, buffering with THAM and use of a warming coil have eliminated this complication in recent years. Cerebral venous thrombosis occurred in 2 children; 1 re-

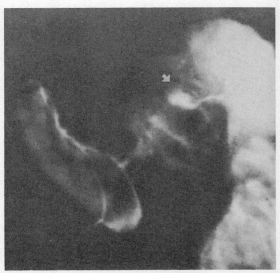

Fig. 9-12.—Curling's ulcer of the stomach observed in 15% of cases with gastrointestinal bleeding and visible as a filling defect. At operation, an actively bleeding branch of the right gastric artery was secured combined with bilateral truncal vagotomy and pyloroplasty. A bleeding Curling's ulcer is the worst prognostic sign in the burn patient; survival is rare.

covered completely, and 1 is an institutional defective. Both had delayed parenteral fluid therapy. Hypertensive encephalopathy was encountered once. This patient was doing extremely well and was 50% grafted within the second week, but 2 days later had a generalized convulsion. The blood pressure was 265/170, and retinopathy was severe. He responded to hypotensive drugs. Because of the convulsive episode, most of his grafts became detached and he then lost the battle with invasive sepsis. He did not have a positive blood culture at the height of the hypertension, but it may be a septic complication we are not familiar with. The patient was not receiving kanamycin, as reported by Lindsay *et al.*[57] The literature on central nervous system complications in burns is sparse and confusing. Autopsy findings in these patients are disappointing. Pneumothorax occurred in 1 youngster who sustained a blast injury as well as thermal burns.

The development of Curling's ulcer is the worst prognostic sign in the burn patient (Fig. 9-12).[1,32,43] We have not encountered an associated perforation, and perhaps youngsters are less vulnerable than are older individuals with a pronounced ulcer diathesis. Extensive flame burns are treated with anticholinergic drugs and antacids after the period of parenteral therapy. Their value is not proved. Bleeding occurred on the fourth day in 1 patient and was evident as massive melena. One patient bled on the eighth day with 6% flame burns of his legs.

At autopsy, children who bleed and those who

TABLE 9-3.—Thermal Burns:
Complications in 1,000 Children

Proved septicemia	39
Tracheostomy	27
Metastatic infection	14
Fatal pulmonary complications	9
Curling's ulcer	8
Tubular necrosis	5
Cardiac arrest	3
Hepatitis (serum)	2
Cerebral venous thrombosis	2
Hypertensive encephalopathy	1
Pneumothorax (blast)	1
Extremity gangrene	1
Bilateral adrenal hemorrhage	1
Total	113

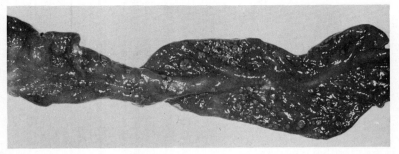

Fig. 9-13.—Gastrointestinal hemorrhage, usually evident as melena, may occur any time after the 4th day and is the worst prognostic sign in thermal burns. In 1 case of exsanguination, several hundred ulcerations were found throughout the gastrointestinal tract. A segment of typically involved small intestine is shown here. Pitressin given intravenously may have some effect in this type of bleeding by lowering splanchnic venous pressure. Perforation at any level is uncommon but is the best indication for successful surgical intervention.

have died with sepsis often have hundreds of ulcerations throughout the gastrointestinal tract (Fig. 9-13). Abramson,[1] reviewing the problem of Curling's ulcer in children, pointed out that 81% of bleeding sites are in the duodenum. Therefore we would not hesitate to explore a child with uncontrolled bleeding, inspecting the stomach and first portion of the duodenum. Direct suture with vagotomy and pyloroplasty would be our choice rather than vagotomy and pyloroplasty with resection in this age group. At this time, only 3 survivors have been reported following surgery for Curling's ulcer in children. Two were operated on for bleeding and 1 for perforation. Of 12 perforations in the literature, 10 occurred in the duodenum. Pitressin administered intravenously has been

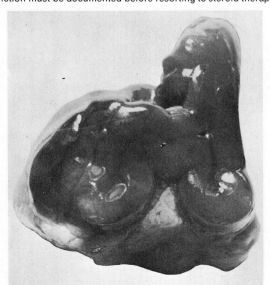

Fig. 9-14.—Hemorrhagic necrosis of adrenal glands in a 5-year-old boy with 45% mixed flame burns. This is the rarest of burn complications (1:1,000). Severely restricted or absent adrenal function must be documented before resorting to steroid therapy.

recommended.[41] Our 1 case of extremity gangrene illustrates a poorly understood entity discussed in Chapter 82. It is usually associated with shock, sepsis, massive transfusions and an inlying vascular tube.

Adrenal substitution therapy has been used in only 2 patients, without success. The need for this medication should be documented with serum and urine sodium levels, eosinophil count and the measurement of steroid output.[44,48,64] Adrenal failure is so much a part of the phase of deterioration in septicemia that it probably is not remediable nor a distinct clinical entity (Fig. 9-14). There is some evidence that adrenal medullary insufficiency can occur and that the hypotension following a grafting procedure or a short period of anesthesia may require epinephrine-like drugs to prevent further injury to parenchymatous organs, notably brain, liver and kidneys. ACTH rather than cortisone may be of help in the postmature or neglected burn.

Fatalities

In our series there were 38 deaths due to septicemia, pulmonary burns, Curling's ulcer and intraoperative cardiac arrest. Twelve children who were dead on arrival (space-heater explosion asphyxia) are not included in the statistics. Table 9-4 shows the predicted

TABLE 9-4.—MORTALITY PREDICTION GRID*

% AREA BURNED	AGE IN YEARS		
	0–4	5–9	10–14
75	1	1	1
70	.9	.9	.9
60	.7	.7	.7
50	.5	.5	.5
40	.3	.3	.3
25	1	1	1
—	0	0	0

*Bull, J. P., and Fisher, A. J., 1954.

TABLE 9-5.—MORTALITY RESULTS: GROUP A
628 CHILDREN, BOSTON CITY HOSPITAL, 1954–1961

% AREA	NO. OF PATIENTS	NO. OF DEATHS	MORTALITY, %
5–15	405	0	0
15–25	158	0	0
25–40	35	4	11.4
40–60	18	9	50.
60–90	12	10	83.4

TABLE 9-6.—MORTALITY RESULTS: GROUP B
368 CHILDREN, BOSTON CITY HOSPITAL, 1961–1967

% AREA	NO. OF PATIENTS	NO. OF DEATHS	MORTALITY, %
5–15	120	0	0
15–25	168	0	0
25–40	62	4	6.4
40–60	13	6	46
60–90	5	5	100

mortality, adapted from the report of Bull and Fisher[19] for children of 14 years and younger. Flame burns with full-thickness destruction are 1.5 times more serious than dermal burns of comparable area produced by hot liquids. No children with burns of any cause involving less than 25% of the body surface died. The 536 patients with scalds survived regardless of extent.

The relationship of surface area of burn to survival is indicated in Tables 9-5 and 9-6. These cover two consecutive periods. The larger number of patients in the first series (Table 9-5) is due to an earlier policy of admitting to the hospital all children with burns greater than 5%. In the second series, children with burns greater than 10% were admitted, as well as children in certain categories (hands, 40; face, 33; feet, 26; infected, 20; genitalia, 13).

Results

Probit analysis is a complex statistical method proposed by Miller and Tainter and applied to the burn problem in a report on 967 patients by Bull and Fisher.[19] It should be adhered to in reporting burn series for the purpose of sound comparison. It throws the proper emphasis on the area of major experience and is a satisfactory method for evaluating progress in burn therapy.[9,39]

There has not been significant improvement in the mortality resulting from burns in children from a review of our experience plus that of the Birmingham Burns Unit, Massachusetts General Hospital, Brooke Army Hospital and the University of Minnesota Hospitals. In combination, there are approximately 6,000 burned patients. When the results are plotted on a logarithmic scale, there is a sigmoid response curve indicating a very low mortality for burns under 30%, then a steep slope pitch in the 30–60% range, with

few survivors above that figure. One can overlay the sigmoid response curve in the various reports. There has been a recent increase in survival time.

Hidden away in the statistical language are pathetically bad results in the management of the burned child. These have been masked by overloading with burns in the intermediate age group from 20 to 35. Two reports have shown a strikingly adverse difference in the performance of the child as compared with that of the young adult. This has led to the erroneous conclusion that burn therapy in the young patient is or needs to be unsatisfactory. A great deal of improvement can be looked for in the care of patients aged 0–14 years, especially in reduction of the period of hospitalization, improved nutrition and morale, elimination of contractures and better cosmetic and functional results. Coming to the hard area of increased survival of the burned child, we have demonstrated that death due to burns involving less than 25% of the total body surface and not involving the respiratory tract should not occur. Occasional patients with respiratory tract burns, bacterial pneumonia and empyema will die with relatively small areas of skin destruction. The greatest improvement has been made in the 30–60% range.

No series yet reported covers enough experience with full-thickness burns involving over 60% of body surface area in children to allow proper appraisal of any method of treatment. If one is an intense student of burns, he will eventually have the satisfaction of treating a burn in the 70–80% range with complete resurfacing and can discharge the patient from the hospital in 6–9 months. We have had 2 such patients and have participated in the care of others in our area.

Individuals in this range who survive seem to have something special. They remain in excellent spirits, eat well and have the immunologic set-up to resist a massive bacterial inoculum. They come back time and time again for grafting procedures. The granulating areas remain flat and clean and continue to accept skin until they are ultimately covered. One youngster with a 70% full-thickness burn was discharged home in 6 months. Her principal complaint now is of excessive sweating of the unburned head and neck because of loss of sudomotor activity in the grafted areas.

New Methods

RESUSCITATION

Markley[62] in 1956 and Metcoff *et al.*[65] in 1961 challenged conventional parenteral support of the burned child. Moyer in published work and Crawford in unpublished investigations have concluded that no blood or other colloid is needed and that equally satisfactory resuscitation is achieved with lactated Ringer's solution. This is buffered to a pH of 8.2 with a ratio 1mEq of potassium to 5mEq of sodium.[74] Enough is given to obtain a urine flow rate of 40 cc/M²/hour and a central venous pressure of 10–15 cm of water. Up to 500% more fluid is given than by conventional formulas. In so doing, body weight increases up to 42% in contrast to the previously accepted increase of 12%. Urine sodium levels may reach 100 mEq/liter in the first day, subsequently dropping to about 40 mEq, thought to be ideal. If the serum protein level falls below 3.5 Gm or the hematocrit below 30, colloid as blood or plasma cannot be given without precipitating pulmonary edema. The work is of theoretical interest and has application in the event of massive civilian or military disaster. It does not represent ideal resuscitation for the individual burned child. We have accomplished adequate resuscitation by conventional methods except in cases of total incineration or rapidly fatal pulmonary burns. A renal tubular lesion was encountered only when institution of intravenous therapy was delayed or given in improper sequence, rate, volume or composition of therapy in the first 24 hours.

Monitoring

In addition to the monitoring of blood gases in patients with pulmonary burns, central venous pressure in all major burns and more concern about serum and urine electrolytes, Gurd and Thal have demonstrated the need for measuring cardiac output, blood pH and lactates in the patient with burn sepsis. Both have demonstrated high-output, low pheripheral resistance shock in this situation. Prompt action must be taken to correct the metabolic (lactic acid) acidosis which precipitates a cycle of anoxia, low perfusion and death.

Surface Antiseptics

No individual whose burn experience extends from the 1940's can fail to recall the less than satisfactory result of application of multiple agents to the burn surface in the hope of preventing surface infection. Aldridge investigated aniline dyes; gentian violet presented a monochrome housekeeping problem, and tannic acid was fatally absorbed. We view the new enthusiasm for topical antiseptics with blunt skepticism. Lindberg and Moncrief and associates[56,69] returned to the method in 1964 when confronted with the uniformly fatal, probably iatrogenic nosocomial septicemia due to *Ps. aeruginosa.* The substance, Lindberg's butter, was synthesized by I. G. Farben Industrie in 1940 and was widely distributed to German combat troops.[50] The American equivalent is closely controlled and is available to a limited number of investigators as Sulfamylon acetate cream.§ The acetate form theoretically presents a 35% smaller acid load than Sulfamylon hydrochloride as it was originally synthesized. However, this expectation has not been realized, and the drug presents a difficult

§Sterling-Winthrop Research Institute, Rensselaer, N. Y.

problem in acid-base control. It is contraindicated in pulmonary burns and is discontinued for 2–3 days when the chloride level rises above 110 mEq/liter, CO_2 falls below 20 mEq/liter, blood pH falls below 7.40 or the respiratory rate exceeds 40/minute. The material must be applied thickly every 3 hours throughout the 24 hours. Patients are exposed throughout the entire process of eschar removal, usually accomplished in 18–21 days. Circumferential burns of the extremity are treated by the closed method.

Although the proposal has considerable merit, as experience has increased there has been growing disenchantment. Small children have a limited pulmonary buffer mechanism and are not entirely cooperative in remaining in any fixed position to keep the material in contact with the burn surface. We were awarded a principal investigator role in studying Sulfamylon and have had experience with approximately 150 children with mixed flame burns. In addition to being unable to demonstrate increased survival in children with flame burns in the range of 30–60%, we noted several other discouraging features. Several children have had convulsions while under Sulfamylon treatment, previously a most rare complication. There is a delay of approximately 1 week in eschar separation compared with the enzyme debridement method. Anaphylactoid deaths have been reported, and skin reactions are common. Bleeding has occurred into the burn bed. A number of patients have had a fatal overgrowth of candida, with visceral moniliasis. The most severe criticism, however, has to do with the rising number of pulmonary deaths. Discontinuation of the treatment does not always change the clinical course. With a steep pitch of serum pH, it is difficult to reverse the pattern even with buffering and assisted ventilation. Inherent in the method is an unacceptably high acid load, in that sulfonamides are excreted as acid salt, have a Diamox effect and are inhibitors of the carbonic anhydrase system. A review of more than 500 patients treated with Sulfamylon at the Brooke Research Center failed to show improved survival with burns of any magnitude.[16] However, patients 14 years and under had an increased survival compared with adults in the standard mortality grid. Brooke childsurvival figures are identical to our experience in group A (1954–1961) when no surface antiseptic was used, and group B (1961–1967) when Sulfamylon was used.

Silver salts have for many years been known to exert an antibacterial effect.[51] Attention was refocused on this problem by Moyer[73] who, in 1965 advocated the treatment of large human burns with 0.5% silver nitrate solution. His arguments were similar to those put forward by Moncrief and associates.[69] In addition, it was thought that debridement could be delayed for periods up to 60 days without adverse effects. Thus spontaneous healing in mixed burns could take place from viable, deep epithelial cell groups. One could, therefore, be certain about areas that would require skin grafting. We have had no experience with silver nitrate but have followed the application of this method to children with interest. Once again, biochemical problems occur and appear to be adverse for young children. Silver nitrate is converted to silver chloride, requiring the excretion of sodium to maintain isotonicity. A closed dressing of thick mesh gauze is saturated every 2–4 hours and completely replaced in 12 hours. In addition to the increased work load imposed by the closed method, there is loss of sodium, chloride, potassium and calcium. These ionic losses must be measured and replaced (sodium chloride to 30 Gm a day, calcium lactate and potassium as contained in Ringer's solution). It is important to monitor bicarbonate every 2–4 hours in any patient under 1 year and with any burn involving over 20% of the body surface. In older children, it is usually sufficient to monitor these levels every 6–12 hours. Once again, reports are filtering in of deaths due to the method because of inability to control pH. Silver storage in parenchymatous organs may be a late problem.[8] There is no reason to expect a differential excess with this method over Sulfamylon, and it is yet to be demonstrated that the method does, in fact, increase survival in burns. Monafo has commented on treatment of 50 patients with burns greater than 30% with a standard MLD of 46%. With the silver nitrate method, the MLD shifted to 64%. However, the series was not broken down into second- and third-degree burns, scalds or flame, and he failed to recognize the burn index. Only by studying silver nitrate application in mixed flame burns with an index of 40 and above can one answer the question of increased burn survival by this method.

Stone and associates[89] recommend gentamicin sulfate as a topical antiseptic in burns. This material has also been given intravenously to patients with documented pseudomonas septicemia. They recognized that examination of the urine with ultraviolet light will disclose a bacterial product of pseudomonas, verdoglobin. Visual identification is allegedly possible 2 days before development of a positive blood culture. Gentamicin is severely ototoxic and nephrotoxic and for this reason will probably not gain wide acceptance. Stone[90] reported on the treatment of 168 children in 1966, but failed to group these as to extent, depth and etiology.

Boles[15] has advocated the surface application of nitrofurazone (Furacin) but has not published a statistical report involving burned children. Mercurochrome has been suggested. Gerow[40] is studying the role of silicone immersion.

A new approach to surface bacterial control is the suggestion of Nagashana[75] that burned patients be exposed to visible multilight. We look forward to the development of this and other physical methods for help in this area.

DEPTH OF BURN

Evans blue and other vital dyes have been used for many years in an attempt to define areas of total skin destruction by demonstrating areas of destroyed circulation.[54] Randolph *et al.*[84] reported experimental and clinical studies utilizing Alphazurine or patent blue V. This material is injected intravenously (0.1 cc/kg of a 10% solution), and one can immediately observe diffusion of dye into skin with an intact circulation. Ten minutes after injection, the area of presumed full-thickness destruction is sketched and recorded by color photography. Later, there is a reverse-coin reading of the same area in that dye diffuses excessively into the area of coagulation necrosis through ruptured capillary membranes. This material is nontoxic and with normal hepatorenal function is completely cleared from the body in about 48 hours. The patient literally turns green. The liver plays an important role in clearance, and the material should not be given to any jaundiced patient or to one with a known history of liver disease.

As a supplement to the injection of patent blue V, we are investigating the value of multiple Hall drill biopsies. The microscopic appearance in an area of partial destruction and in an area of total coagulation necrosis is shown in Figure 9-15. With this added information, one might logically extend the range of early surgical excision.

IMMUNOLOGY

There is a good deal of literature relating to the possible alteration of immune response or its manipulation in the patient with extensive burns. Federoff reported optimistically on the use of convalescent burn serum, but no other investigator has been able to duplicate this experience.[4,29,38,53] Bocenagra *et al.*[14] in a report on the use of convalescent burn serum in 71 children, concluded that it had no value when compared with normal plasma in effect on rate of infection or survival. Antibody titers for pseudomonas in the two groups were identical. At present, convalescent serum seems to have no important role in burn therapy. Kefalides *et al.*[53] suggested from studies carried out at the Children's Hospital of Peru that children especially 3 years old and under, be given supplementary gamma globulin. Once again, the series was random and poorly defined. Stimulated by the report, we have measured 24-hour immunochemical gamma globulin in a number of children with extensive burns and never found a level below 400–600 mg, which is thought to be normal. Therefore a quantitative reduction of gamma globulin would not appear to be involved. On a qualitative basis, there is even less to support the recommendation. The usually available commercial gamma globulin is the S-7 form, which does not contain pseudomonas antibodies. It is possi-

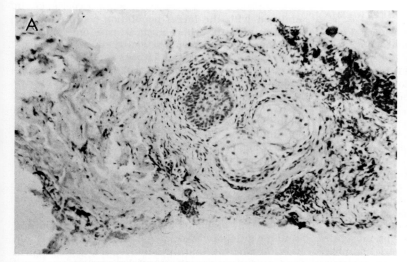

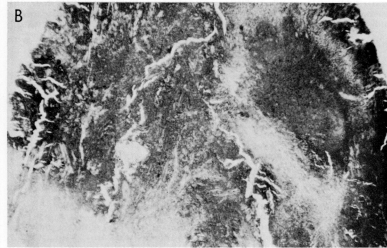

Fig. 9-15. — Photomicrographs of Hall drill biopsy specimen. **A,** an area of partial thickness destruction with viable pilosebaceous structures, intact blood vessels and essentially normal architecture except for edema. **B,** an area of total coagulation necrosis, no skin appendages are identifiable and blood vessels are thrombosed.

ble to fractionate the S-19 form, which has a molecular weight in excess of 1 million and does contain the antibody. Feller and Kamei[38] have investigated the role of pseudomonas vaccine. We tend to discount this as a practical adjunct. Hyperimmune globulin, a fractionated product of convalescent burn serum, would presumably provide the same answer.

One must look for methods to extend the survival of homografts. Murray reported that massive immunosuppression does not prolong the life of the homograft and, adversely, interfered with the ability to control infection. Antilymphocyte serum (ALS) does not prolong survival in small laboratory animals.[67]

Chardak[21,22] was unable to show the value of polyethylene sheeting as a synthetic skin substitute. Recent work by Walder on the use of a polyamino acid film may have some merit.[16]

STEROIDS

Steroids are seldom used or indicated in the management of the burn patient. In our series, 1 child had frank bilateral adrenal hemorrhage, a complication rate of 0.1%. Microscopically, autopsies on many burn patients show adrenal exhaustion. The Addisonian state has not been demonstrated in our series by studies of urine or serum electrolytes, 17-ketosteroid excretion or eosinophil response.[48] In fact, steroid therapy would appear to be contraindicated. Altemeier and associates[4] reported on 380 patients with gram-positive septicemia, the predominant form in burn patients. All patients given steroids died. Of those receiving antibiotics when septicemia developed, 68% died. Only 43% of patients not on either antibiotics or steroids died.

74. Moyer, C. A; Margraf, H. W., and Monafo, W. W., Jr.: Burn shock in association with extravascular sodium deficiency—a report on the treatment with Ringer's solution with lactate, Arch. Surg. 90:799, 1965.

75. Nagashana, T.: Visible multilight treatment of burns, Am. J. Surg. 112:65, 1966.

76. National Fire Protective Association, Boston, Annual Report, 1963.

77. National Fire Protection Association, Boston Annual Report, 1966.

78. Nicholson, J. J., and Foster, R.: Bryant's traction a provocative cause of circulatory complications, J.A.M.A. 157:415, 1955.

79. Phillips, A. W., and Cope, O.: The revelation of respiratory tract damage as a principal killer of the burned patient, Ann Surg., 155:1, 1962.

80. Pulaski, E., *et al.*: Evaluation of the exposure method in the treatment of burns, S. Forum 2:518, 1952.

81. Quinby, W. C., Jr., and Cope, O.: Blood viscosity and the whole blood therapy of burns, Surgery 32:316, 1952.

82. Rabin, E. R., *et al.*: Fatal pseudomonas infection in burned patients, New England J. Med. 265:1227, 1961.

83. Raker, J. W., and Robit, R. L.: The acute red blood cell destruction following severe thermal trauma in dogs: Based on the use of radioactive chromate tagged red blood cells, Surg., Gynec. & Obst. 98:169, 1954.

84. Randolph, J. D.; Leape, L. L., and Gross, R. E.; The early surgical treatment of burns: I. Experimental studies utilizing intravenous vital dye for determining the degree of injury, Surgery 56:193, 1964.

85. Rousselot, L. M.; Connell, J. F., and Whalen, W. P.: The exposure method in the treatment of severe burns, Surgery 33:673, 1953.

86. Sneve, H.: The treatment of burns and skin grafting, J.A.M.A. 45:1, 1905.

87. Southand, S. C., *et al.*: Investigation of fabrics involved in wearing apparel fires, Pediatrics 34:728, 1964.

88. Soutter, R. D.: Chemicals and enzymes in debridement of thermal burns, Arch. Surg. 76:744, 1958.

89. Stone, H. H., *et al.*: Gentamicin sulfate in the treatment of pseudomonas sepsis in burns, Surg., Gynec. & Obst. 120:351, 1965.

90. Stone, H. H.: Pseudomonas sepsis in thermal burns: Verdoglobin determination and gentamycin, Ann. Surg. 163:297, 1966.

91. Talbot, N. B.; Richie, R. H., and Crawford, J. D.: *Metabolic Homeostasis* (Cambridge, Mass.: Harvard University Press, 1959).

92. Taylor, P. H.: The management of extensively burned patients by staged excision, Surg., Gynec. & Obst. 115:347, 1962.

93. Wallace, A. B.: The exposure treatment of burns, Lancet 1:501, 1951.

94. Welch, K. J.: Fluid and electrolyte therapy in the pediatric surgical patient. Internat. Anesth. Clin. 1:237, 1963.

95. Wells, cited by Hendren.

96. Zaroff, L. I., *et al.*: Multiple uses of viable cutaneous homografts in the burned patient, Surgery 59:308, 1966.

97. Zuidema, G. D.: Role of clothing in prevention of thermal injury, Plast. & Reconstruct. Surg. 20:449, 1957.

K. J. WELCH

10

Tetanus and Gas Gangrene
(Clostridial Infections)

GAS GANGRENE and other clostridial infections are among the most dreaded complications of traumatic and surgical wounds. The rapid and fulminating course, profound toxemia, destruction of tissue and high mortality continue to stimulate investigation of new methods of therapy.

The clostridia are widely distributed in nature and may be cultured freely in our environment. They are found in the soil, our homes and clothing and in the intestinal flora of most human beings. They are cultured with high frequency in accidental and military wounds (38%–88% in several studies).[1] In spite of the frequent contamination of surgical and accidental wounds, the incidence of clinical infection is quite low. In a total series of 187,936 major traumatic wounds reviewed by Altemeier and Furste[2] the incidence of gas gangrene was only 1.76%.

The clostridia are saprophytic organisms with minimal invasive capabilities. In man they present as "facultative" pathogens requiring optimal wound conditions for growth and production of their potent exotoxins. Of the 93 species of clostridia identified, less than a dozen cause human disease with any regularity.[4] These include *Cl. perfringens (Cl. welchii)*, *Cl. novyi* and *Cl. septicum*, all capable of producing gas gangrene. In addition, there are *Cl. tetani*, whose exotoxin leads to clinical tetanus, and *Cl. botulinum*, responsible for botulism.

Tetanus

The clinical manifestations of *Cl. tetani* infection are seldom noted in the practice of pediatric surgery. The high rate of induced immunity in the infant population, prophylactic use of tetanus toxoid, meticulous surgical care of wounds and the administration of human tetanus immune globulin when indicated have reduced the incidence of this dreaded infection to the vanishing point. In the World War II experience of the Army, there were only 12 cases of tetanus among 2,734,818 hospital admissions for wounds and injuries, an incidence of 0.00044%. Six of these patients were not previously immunized. This experience must be contrasted with a 3.9% incidence of tetanus in 12,000 injured civilians encountered in Manila (1945) who, as far as is known, had not had tetanus toxoid inoculations before injury.[8]

The prevalence of tetanus in an unimmunized population is emphasized in a report on 226 patients admitted to the Raja Mirasdar Hospital in India in 1 year.[10] Fifty per cent of these patients were children under 12, including 25 infants with tetanus neonatorum.

TETANUS IN THE NEWBORN

Neonatal tetanus, rarely seen in western societies, continues to be a major cause of neonatal death in many parts of the world. In Durban, South Africa, it was the second most common cause of death in the newborn period, accounting for over 14% of all neonatal tetanus mortality.[15] In Japan, the neonatal tetanus mortality was 36.1 in 1945 and, in 1961, 7.1 per 100,000 live births.[8] As tetanus toxoid had been excluded from the Japanese immunization programs, the sharp drop in mortality from tetanus has been attributed to improving obstetric facilities and care of the umbilicus and cord at birth and in the perinatal period.

The cause of tetanus neonatorum has been traced to local infection of the umbilicus resulting from unsterile methods of dividing the cord or delivery in an unclean environment. Certain cultural practices, such as placing camel dung on the amputated cord, are contributory.[9]

The diagnosis of tetanus in the newborn must be made on clinical evidence. The infants commonly are irritable, feed poorly and on examination, in addition to the open umbilical wound, are noted to hold their limbs partly flexed and stiff, with fists clenched. Generalized tonic spasms with some degree of opisthotonos develop on minimal stimulation. The facial expression conforms to the classic risus sardonicus.[15]

Treatment begins with maintenance of adequate ventilation, often requiring insertion of an endotracheal tube and artificial respiration. In advanced cases, the patient is curarized and respirations are controlled. Human tetanus immune globulin* is administered to neutralize the unfixed circulating toxins, and penicillin in high doses is given to kill the toxin-producing bacteria. In a controlled study, corticoids were reported to have produced a significant lowering of mortality.[10]

The mortality for the disease remains high, varying from 56 to 90% despite improved programs of management. Anoxia and exhaustion due to uncontrolled spasms account for deaths within the first 48 hours; thereafter, the causes may include oversedation, pulmonary infections and inanition due to the long convalescent period with a limited caloric intake.

CHILDHOOD TETANUS

Tetanus in the older child follows improper treatment of a contaminated wound in an unimmunized patient. Regardless of immunization status, the wound must be treated meticulously, with removal of all devitalized tissue and foreign bodies and, if necessary, the wound left open. Every patient should receive tetanus toxoid intramuscularly as an initial immunizing dose or as a booster if the patient has not received a booster within the past 12 months. Human tetanus immune globulin for passive immunization may be given if wound conditions warrant and the patient is not or only incompletely immunized; in such cases, penicillin or oxytetracycline therapy must be considered.

Treatment for the established case of tetanus includes prompt care of the offending wound and administration of human tetanus immune globulin, tetanus toxoid, antibiotics and sedatives. Maintenance of adequate ventilation may require a tracheostomy and controlled respirations following curarization. Hyperbaric oxygen has been reported to offer clinical improvement in individual cases; however, the evidence is not adequate to establish it as a useful adjunct to routine treatment.[3]

Gas Gangrene

Clostridial myositis is most often noted in extensive wounds with devitalized muscle due to trauma and arterial insufficiency as a result of injury to a major artery, tourniquet, a tight cast or shock. A common denominator is the lowering of oxidation-reduction potential in tissue that allows the clostridia, obligate anaerobes, to become metabolically active.

In civilian practice, the infection is noted in traumatic wounds which are treated late or incompletely, with devitalized muscle and foreign matter

---

*Hyper-tet, USP, Cutter Laboratories.

left behind. Clostridial infections have been reported following surgery of the biliary tract, large bowel and even gastric surgery for carcinoma. Occasionally, anaerobic myositis develops without evidence of a wound. In such cases, an ulcerating lesion of the colon must be suspected. In the outlining of therapy and recording of results, the degree of infection is carefully documented. Clostridial infections may present as (1) simple contamination of the wound, (2) anaerobic cellulitis and (3) anaerobic myonecrosis. Of these, only anaerobic myonecrosis (gas gangrene) is associated with invasion of muscle, toxemia and shock.

DIAGNOSIS

An early diagnosis of this malignant infection will prevent loss of tissue and lower mortality. There is a variable interval of 12–72 hours between injury and the onset of infection, with an average incubation time of 53 hours. Pain in the affected area is the earliest symptom, followed rapidly by chills, tachycardia out of proportion to the fever, mental confusion and other evidence of toxemia. In the early stages, the skin around the wound is cool, white, edematous and seldom crepitant. Later, the skin develops a bronze discoloration with crepitation in the subcutaneous tissue. The wound exudes a thin, brown fluid with a musty pungent odor. A Gram stain of the fluid will show a uniform population of club-shaped gram-positive rods with spores in a characteristic position (Fig. 10-1). The involved muscle does not bleed when incised and is gray to purple-black and partially liquefied. Thereafter, the area of skin involvement extends rapidly, often several centimeters in an hour, and the patient soon develops a fulminating toxemia, hypotension, oliguria, hemolysis and lapses into coma.

TREATMENT

Since 1960, hyperbaric oxygenation at a pressure of 3.0 atm absolute (30 psi gauge) has been utilized in the treatment of extensive gas gangrene infections. This method of therapy was first implemented and used in 35 patients by Brummelkamp, Boerema and Hogendijk.[7] There were 10 deaths in this series, with 4 directly attributable to the clostridial infections. The causes of the other 6 deaths included renal failure, *Escherichia coli* septicemia, pseudomonas septicemia, massive pulmonary embolism and congestive heart failure.

Observations made during the management of these critically ill patients, in addition to in vitro and in vivo experimental studies, suggest that an elevated tissue oxygen tension has an inhibitory effect on the offending clostridial organism, an obligate anaerobe, which cannot multiply in the presence of a high oxidation-reduction potential.

Another factor responsible for the beneficial effects of high oxygen tension in gas gangrene is suggested by the in vitro studies of van Unnik.[14] Clostridia which were exposed to high oxygen tension for 90 minutes remained viable, but alpha toxin production in broth culture was inhibited.[11] Other investigators have concluded that hyperbaric oxygen does not alter the toxicity of the alpha toxin already formed.[12]

A record of therapeutic achievement similar to that of Brummelkamp was reported by Altemeier.[1] In a series of 42 patients with gas gangrene treated at ambient pressure, early radical surgical debridement, immobilization of the affected part and administration of large doses of penicillin and tetracycline intravenously and of polyvalent gas gangrene antitoxin resulted in the survival of 37.

The treatment of clostridial myositis must begin

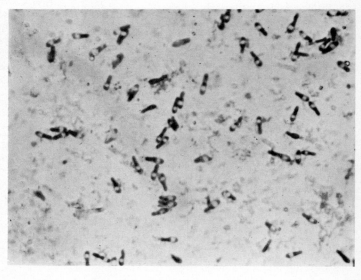

Fig. 10-1.—A Gram stain of wound exudate with uniform population of gram-positive rods.

immediately following the diagnosis based on clinical evidence and a positive Gram stain of the wound exudate. A few hours' delay will cause tissue loss and seriously affect the prognosis. The bacteriologic confirmation of the diagnosis must be made after the fact.

Two intravenous routes are established. Into one are delivered plasma and whole blood to support the intravascular volume lost into the large infected space and by hemolysis. Into the other are given penicillin and chloramphenicol, to which all of our isolates have been sensitive. Tetanus antitoxin is given the previously immunized patient.

The patient is then taken promptly to the hyperbaric chamber for treatment. The patient is first anesthetized with an endotracheal tube in place, the ear drums are incised and the chamber pressure is raised to 3 atm absolute (30 psi gauge).

The patient receives 100% oxygen with halothane for the 90 minute treatment. During the hyperbaric treatment, the operative team explores the wound, estimates the extent of involvement and decompresses involved fascial compartments. Tissue which appeared necrotic at ambient pressure may be obviously viable at 3 atm of oxygen. We limit the debridement of tissue during this initial treatment to avoid resection of possibly viable tissue and to prevent addition of the stress of surgical trauma to the already critically ill patient.

The clinical response to the first hyperbaric and surgical treatment has been most encouraging. The pulse, blood pressure and respiratory and urinary output improve dramatically even though necrotic, bacteria-laden tissue remains in place. The margin of skin necrosis which before treatment would advance several centimeters an hour now remains static. The ability of the clostridia to produce the lethal exotoxins is reduced or completely eliminated by the high concentration of oxygen at the interface of perfused and necrotic tissue.

A second hyperbaric treatment is given within 8 hours of the first, when further debridement of dead tissue is carried out. A third treatment is ordinarily delivered 8 hours after the second. Within the first 24 hours the toxemia is controlled and all necrotic tissue resected. Seldom were more than three treatments needed.

The value of gas gangrene polyvalent antitoxin remains in doubt and carries the dangers of sensitivity reactions. We have not given gangrene antitoxin to our patients.

EXPERIENCE AND RESULTS

The clinical experience at the Children's Hospital Medical Center of Boston consists of a series of 25 patients treated with hyperbaric oxygen. The group includes 4 children 10–17 years of age with advanced clostridial myositis. Three cases followed traumatic wounds involving the extremities and the fourth followed an appendectomy. The last-

mentioned case is reported in detail to bring out important aspects of diagnosis and treatment.

S.O., a 17-year-old girl was admitted to another hospital with a 10-day history of intermittent nausea and lower abdominal pain. Physical examination revealed normal temperature, pulse and blood pressure. Pertinent physical findings were confined to the abdomen and rectum. Palpation of the abdomen revealed severe tenderness in the right lower quadrant and a 7 ×4 cm mass. Rectal examination indicated that the mass extended into the right vault and was not movable.

Several hours after admission, an exploratory laparotomy was carried out through a right, lower paramedian incision. A mass consisting of omentum and terminal ileum was noted, suggesting a diagnosis of regional enteritis. The appendix was seen to enter this mass and was removed along with a portion of adherent omentum. The pathologic diagnoses were: multiple acute microabscesses in the omentum, with subacute and chronic appendicitis.

The course was satisfactory for the initial 48 hours following appendectomy. She was maintained on intravenous fluids during this interval. The second postoperative day the temperature spiked to 103 F, and examination of the abdomen revealed marked tenderness lateral to the incision, a reddish-brownish discoloration of the skin in this area and definite subcutaneous crepitus.

The wound was immediately opened down to the rectus fascial layer, releasing a small amount of thin, foul-smelling brownish exudate. A smear of this discharge disclosed numerous gram-positive, club-shaped rods characteristic of Cl. perfringens. Areas of necrotic muscle were also apparent, so the patient was returned to the operating room, where an extensive debridement of the abdominal wall was carried out. Resection of necrotic muscle included all of the right rectus muscle, half of the left rectus muscle and all of the remaining musculature on the right side (external oblique, internal oblique, transversus abdominis) down to peritoneum. In addition, a large section of necrotic skin and subcutaneous tissue from the right flank area was excised. A 15 × 20 cm section of Vitallium screen was sutured in place over the peritoneum to provide support for the viscera.

Massive doses of aqueous penicillin (12 million units) and tetracyclines (2 Gm) were administered intravenously in addition to 50,000 units of polyvalent gas gangrene antiserum.

Twenty-four hours following wound debridement and initiation of the antibiotic regimen, the patient suddenly became hypotensive and temperature rose to 103 F. She was treated with vasopressors, corticosteroids and a whole blood transfusion, with restoration of normal systemic blood pressure.

On the sixth day following appendectomy (48 hours after wound debridement), the patient complained of severe lumbar back pain and again had spiking temperature to 103 F (per rectum). Inspection of the abdominal wound at this time revealed a small amount of foul-smelling brown exudate and extension of subcutaneous crepitus to the right costovertebral angle. An x-ray of the chest disclosed retroperitoneal air and a right pleural effusion.

At this time she was transferred to the Children's Hospital Medical Center for hyperbaric oxygen therapy (Figs. 10-2 and 10-3).

She was immediately transported to the hyperbaric chamber for the first of six therapeutic compressions (utilizing oxygen ventilation via an endotracheal tube at 30 psi). During each run (60–110 minutes in length), she was lightly anesthetized with halothane accompanied by 100% oxygen to facilitate dressing and culturing of the extensive abdominal wounds. Penicillin (12 million units /24 hours) and chloramphenicol (2 Gm/24 hours) were continued intravenously for an additional period of 5 days, but polyvalent gas gangrene antiserum was not added to the treatment program.

Four cultures of the wound (obtained prior to transfer to the Children's Hospital) grew Cl. perfringens. In addition, spore-bearing, gram-positive rods were identified in the micro-

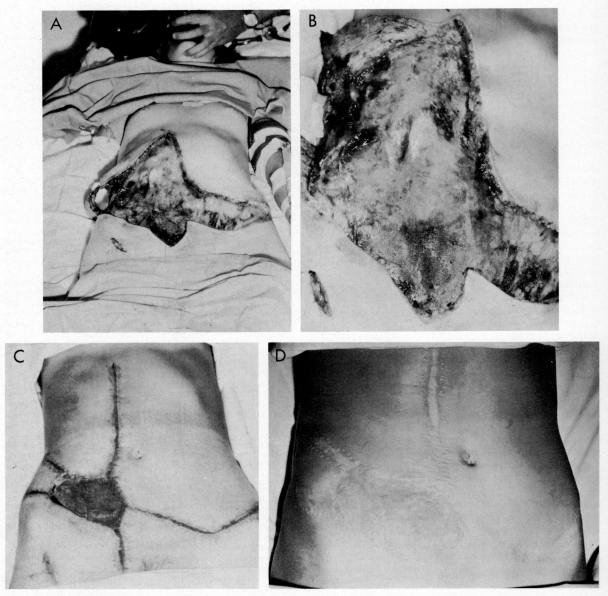

Fig. 10-2.—Patient S.O., with gas gangrene following appendectomy. **A,** wound on admission to the Children's Hospital Medical Center, showing extensive undermined skin flaps and necrotic tissue at margins of resection. **B,** wound 3 days after first hyperbaric treatment; all necrotic tissue has been debrided and edema in viable tissue is reduced. **C,** wound 12 days after hyperbaric treatment. Secondary closure was begun 7 days after admission; final wound closure 5 days later required a split thickness skin graft. **D,** abdomen a year later, showing adequate support and satisfactory contour.

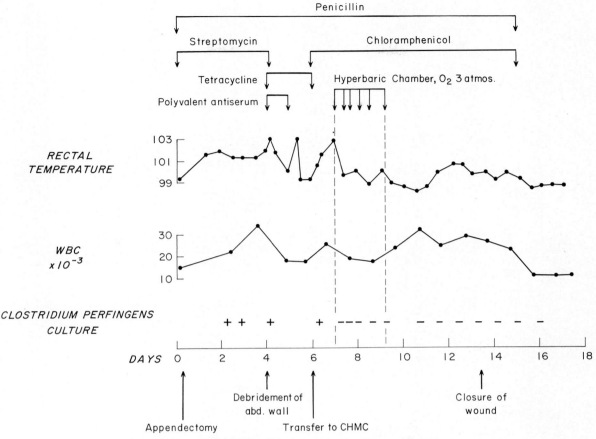

Fig. 10-3.—Patient, S.O.: clinical course and sequence of therapy.

scopic sections of the resected abdominal musculature. It is interesting that cultures obtained after initiation of hyperbaric oxygen therapy failed to grow any pathogenic organisms.

The patient showed prompt and continued improvement after the first period of oxygen breathing in the compression chamber. Although leukocytosis persisted for approximately 10 days, the temperature gradually returned to normal and all evidence of toxicity disappeared.

In our opinion, clostridial infection in this girl had extended beyond control by conventional means despite the adequate surgical excision and antibiotic treatment administered by her original physicians. High pressure oxygen ventilation appeared to be life-saving in this instance.

In the young without underlying systemic diseases, diabetes and arteriosclerosis, gas gangrene is usually a complication of trauma. Three children in our series had gas gangrene in an extremity following a compound fracture which was inadequately treated. The following case is illustrative.

S. R., a 10-year-old boy, fell out of an apple tree and sustained a compound fracture of the left forearm. He was taken to another hospital, where the break in the skin was cleansed,

the fracture reduced and a circular cast applied. Within 48 hours he complained of moderate pain. The next morning, the temperature was 105 F, and 3 days after the accident he was transferred to the Children's Hospital Medical Center.

When the cast was removed, there were discoloration and obvious necrosis of the hand and forearm (Fig. 10-4, *A*). The edema, crepitation and discoloration extended to the axilla and over the deltoid area. A roentgenogram revealed free air diffusely distributed in the tissue compartments of the forearm and complete transverse fractures of the ulna and radius (Fig. 10-4, *B*). Four hyperbaric compressions were given. During the first, the forearm was extensively explored (Fig. 10-4, *C*), and the brachial artery at the elbow was found to be thrombosed, with necrosis in all distal muscular compartments. Amputation was considered, but deferred. During the second hyperbaric treatment, necrotic tissue was excised distal to the elbow. The edema and crepitus in the upper arm diminished progressively, and amputation was done (Fig. 10-4, *D*).

We believe that an amputation carried out at the time of admission as a life-saving procedure would by necessity have been made at the proximal humerus. The apparent ability of hyperbaric oxygen treatment to prevent production of noxious toxins and limit

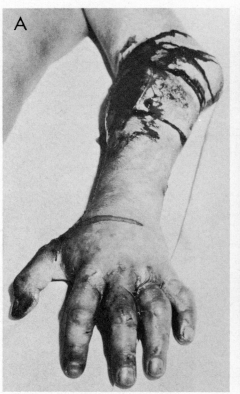

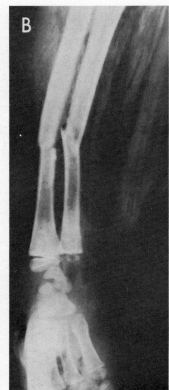

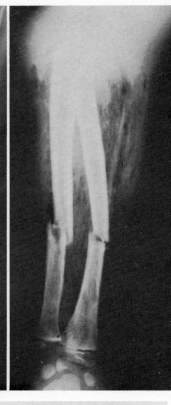

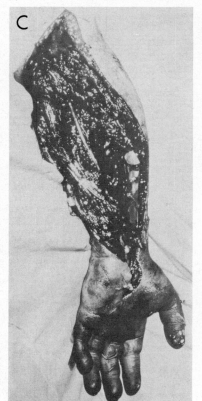

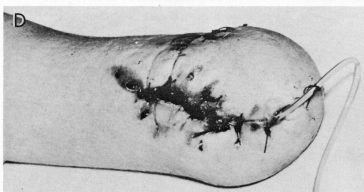

Fig. 10-4.—Patient S.R.: **A,** with discoloration and necrosis of hand and forearm 3 days after fracture. **B,** x-ray, showing diffuse distribution of free arm in tissues of forearm and fractures of radius and ulna. **C,** hand and forearm on extensive exploration during first therapeutic compression. **D,** the amputation stump 10 days after final hyperbaric treatment, with skin closed over the intact humerus. A catheter is left in place for antibiotic irrigations.

organism proliferation permits the preservation of questionably involved tissue without increasing the threat to life.

CONCLUSION

The plan of management of patients with gas gangrene at our institution adheres to the principles of debridement and massive antibiotic therapy, with hyperbaric oxygen utilized as a supplement to conventional therapy. The treatments are administered under light, general anesthesia and repeated at 8–12 hour intervals, until the signs of systemic toxicity have subsided and the infected area is completely free of necrotic muscle. Usually two or three exposures suffice.

Although all obvious necrotic muscle is removed at the initial operation, the use of hyperbaric oxygen allows some latitude in the decision to excise tissue of questionable viability. Occasionally an amputation or sacrifice of a major muscle group can be avoided. In those infections which have extended beyond the boundaries of possible surgical excision, hyperbaric oxygen combined with surgical drainage, antibiotics and supportive therapy may be life-saving.[5, 6, 13]

REFERENCES

1. Altemeier, W. A.: Diagnosis, Classification, and General Management of Gas-Producing Infections, particularly those produced by *Clostridium perfringens*, in Brown, I. W., Jr. (ed.): *Proceedings of the Third International Conference on Hyperbaric Medicine* (Washington, D. C.: National Academy of Science-National Research Council, 1966), Publ. 1404, p. 481-491.
2. Altemeier, W. A., and Furste, W. L.: Gas gangrene, Surg., Gynec. & Obst. 84:507, 1947.
3. Behnke, A. R., and Saltzman, H. A.: Hyperbaric oxygenation, New England J. Med. 276:1479, 1967.
4. *Bergey's Manual of Determinative Bacteriology* (7th ed.; Baltimore: Williams & Wilkins Company, 1957).
5. Bernhard, W. F.: Current status of hyperbaric oxygenation in pediatric surgery, S. Clin. North America 44:1582, 1964.
6. Bernhard, W. F., and Filler, R. M.: Hyperbaric oxygen: Current concepts, Am. J. Surg. 115:661, 1968.
7. Brummelkamp, W. H.: Treatment of Anaerobic Infections with Hyperbaric Oxygen, in Brown, I. W., Jr. (ed.): *Proceedings of the Third International Conference on Hyperbaric Medicine* (Washington, D.C.: National Academy of Science-National Research Council, 1966), Publ. 1404, p. 492-500.
8. Furst, W.; Skudder, P. A., and Hampton, O.P., Jr.: The evolution of prophylaxis against tetanus from the Civil War to the present, Bull. Am. Coll. Surgeons 52:315, 1967.
9. Haggarty, R. J.: Bacterial infections in the newborn, Pediat. Clin. North America 8:481, 1961.
10. Kanakaraj, J. D.: Compression fractures of the spine and tetanus, Indian J. Surg. 27:683, 1965.
11. MacLennan, J. D., and MacFarlane, R. G.: Toxin and antitoxin studies of gas gangrene in man, Lancet 2:301, 1945.
12. MacLennan, J. D.: The histotoxic clostridial infections of man, Bact. Rev. 26:177, 1962.
13. Trippel, O. H., *et al.*: Hyperbaric oxygenation in the management of gas gangrene, S. Clin. North America 43:17, 1967.
14. Van Unnik, A. J. M.: Inhibition of toxin production in *Clostridium perfringens* in vitro by hyperbaric oxygen, Antonie Leeuwenhoek 31:181, 1965.
15. Wright, R.: Tetanus Neonatorum, South Africa M. J. 34:111, 1960-.

ANGELO J. ERAKLIS

Head and Neck

PLATE I

A. Congenital Anophthalmia. This infant was born with extensive craniofacial defects, including bilateral anophthalmia, bilateral complete cleft lip and cleft palate. A central nervous system deficit was suspected.

B. Cleft Lip and Palate. An infant boy with a unilateral cleft lip, cleft palate and typical nasal deformity. The defect was repaired at 1 month of age with the use of an inlay flap; particular attention was paid to the correction of the nasal deformity. The associated cleft palate was repaired when the child was 1 year old.

C. Burn Scald. A toddler sustained this injury of the head and neck areas from hot coffee. Because of the proportionately large surface area represented at this age, such a burn is capable of producing shock. Hospitalization and intensive supportive care are necessary. This photograph was taken 48 hours after the scald, when burn fluid sequestration is maximal.

D. Platelet-Trapping Hemangioma. Infant showed no evidence of hemangioma at birth, but 1 month later an uncomplicated lesion appeared in the perioral region. This spread rapidly and, because of platelet trapping, extravasation and infection occurred, resulting in the loss of important features and ultimately in death.

E. Mixed Hemangioma and Lymphangioma of the Parotid and Cervical Region. Frequently, such lesions are occult, deep to the skin layer and invade the parotid gland by direct extension. In this infant, there was a bulky external component. Excision was carried out in two stages, with preservation of the facial nerve.

F. Thyroglossal Cyst. This 2-year-old boy had a classic thyroglossal cyst with a history of sudden enlargement following an upper respiratory infection. The thyroid lobes were normal in size and location. Complete excision of the cyst was performed, including a central block of the hyoid bone. The proximal stalk extended to the base of the tongue at the foramen cecum.

PLATE I

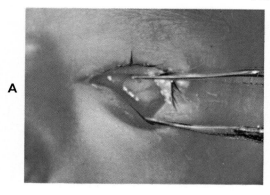

A

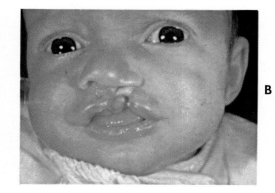

B

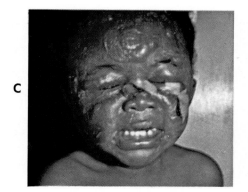

C

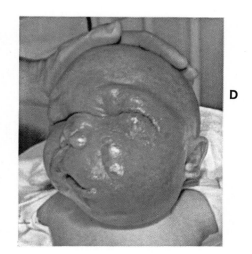

D

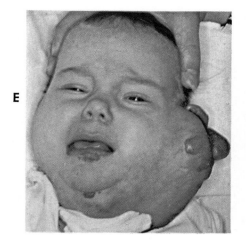

E

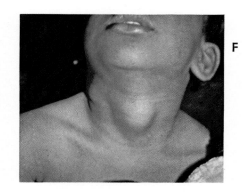

F

11

The Eyes and Lids

Proptosis in Children

MOST DISEASES of and tumors within the orbit are manifested by proptosis of one or both eyes. The term proptosis implies a passive protrusion of the eye by a retrobulbar mass. The term exophthalmos is often used synonymously, but exophthalmos should be used to describe the condition seen in hyperthyroidism. Depending on the size or position of the lesion, the eye may be pushed in one or another direction. There may be limitation of ocular motility, either by nerve involvement or by interference with muscle action. An orbital mass may press on the back of the globe, affecting vision. Pressure around the optic nerve may cause papilledema, and if this persists, optic atrophy may result. If proptosis is severe, the cornea may be endangered by exposure.

INCIDENCE AND ETIOLOGY.—Proptosis in 257 chil-dren seen at the Hospital for Sick Children, Toronto, in 24 years was caused by the following conditions, in order of frequency: acute ethmoiditis, hyperthy-roidism, craniostenosis, neoplasms, Hand-Schüller-Christian disease, hemorrhages of the orbit from trauma. Table 11-1 lists the diagnoses in these cases.

INFLAMMATORY CAUSES: ACUTE ETHMOIDITIS

Proptosis in these cases results from orbital cellulitis secondary to inflammation of the accessory sinuses, usually the ethmoids, following a cold. Infection passes through the thin paper-like medial wall of the orbit from the ethmoid sinuses. These children have an elevation of temperature, periorbital inflammation and proptosis. There is a purulent nasal discharge with pus coming from the sinuses. The ethmoids are likely to appear clouded in the roentgenogram.

Fig. 11-1 (left).—Bilateral proptosis from oxycephaly in a child of 8 months.
Fig. 11-2 (right).—Bilateral exophthalmos from hyperthyroidism in a child of 6 months.

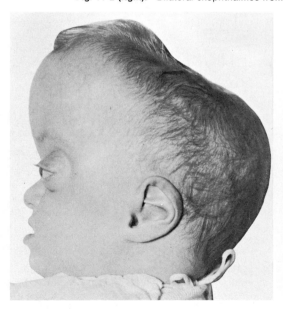 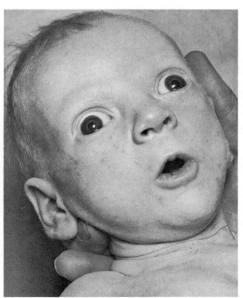

TABLE 11-1.—DIAGNOSIS IN 257 CASES WITH PROPTOSIS

1. Developmental	23
2. Inflammatory	78
3. Metabolic	35
Involvement in general disease	19
4. Neoplastic	41
5. Vascular	50
6. Miscellaneous	1
7. Unknown	10
TOTAL	257

PROPTOSIS

1. Developmental
   a) Dysostosis of Cranial Bones — 3
      1) Meningocoele and encephalocoele
      2) Cleidocranial dysostosis
      3) Hereditary craniofacial dysostosis
         (Crouzon's disease)
   b) Craniostenosis — 17
      1) Turricephaly
      2) Scaphocephaly
      3) Plagiocephaly
   c) Hypertelorism — 3

2. Inflammatory
   Acute ethmoiditis (orbital cellulitis) — 57
   Cavernous sinus thrombosis (orbital cellulitis) — 5
   Orbital cellulitis from injury — 6
   Orbital cellulitis (cause unknown) — 6
   Subperiosteal orbital abscess — 1
   Osteomyelitis of roof of orbit — 1
   Mucocele of ethmoids — 2

3. Orbital Involvement in Metabolic Disorders
   and General Disease
   a) Hyperthyroidism — 35
   b) Histiocytosis-X
      1) Eosinophilic granuloma — 2
      2) Hand-Schüller-Christian disease — 16
      3) Letterer-Siwe disease — 1
   c) Diseases Involving Bone
      1) Rickets — 0
      2) Infantile cortical hyperostosis
         (Caffey's disease) — 0
      3) Osteopetrosis (Albers-Schönberg) — 0
      4) Fibrous dysplasia of bone — 0

4. Neoplastic
   a) Primary Orbital
      1) Benign: Dermoid and epidermoid — 3
         Teratoma — 1
      2) Malignant: Optic nerve glioma — 4
         Sarcoma — 5
         Lymphosarcoma — 1
         Melanoma of orbit — 0
         Lacrimal gland tumor — 0
         Chronic granuloma — 1

PROPTOSIS

   b) Secondary and Metastatic Orbital
      1) Benign: Dermoid of lid — 0
         Recklinghausen's disease — 1
         Osteoma of antrum — 1
         Juvenile angiofibroma of
            nasopharynx — 1
      2) Malignant: Neuroblastoma — 6
         Chloroma — 5
         Nasopharyngeal Ca. or
            sarcoma — 1
         Lymphoma — 2
         Retinoblastoma — 1
         Hodgkin's disease — 3
         Sarcoma of ethmoids — 1
         Sarcoma of antrum — 0
         Ovarian sarcoma — 1
   c) Intracranial Tumors Involving the Orbit
      Temporal lobe tumors — 1
      Craniopharyngioma — 0
      Frontal lobe tumors — 0
      Pituitary tumors — 0
      Middle cranial fossa tumors — 0
      Sphenoid ridge meningiomas — 0
      Dermoid of sphenoid ridge — 2

5. Vascular
   Angiomas: Cavernous hemangioma — 9
      Lymphangioma — 2
   Cavernous carotid fistula — 1
   Sturge-Weber — 3
   Hemorrhage into orbit from:
      scurvy — 3
      leukemia — 10
      hemophilia — 0
      trauma — 22
      hemorrhagic disease of newborn — 0

6. Miscellaneous
   Subdural hematoma — 1
   Subarachnoid cyst — 0
   Osteitis fibrosa cystica — 0
   Paget's disease — 0

7. Unknown — 10

TOTAL 257

For treatment a massive systemic antibiotic therapy is started. Drainage from the ethmoid sinuses is improved by the use of decongestant nose drops. If the maxillary sinuses are involved, they may need irrigation.

CONGENITAL DISORDERS OF THE ORBIT

Certain congenital disorders of the orbit result in proptosis due to shallowness of the orbits. The condition is bilateral but may be worse on one side. An example is craniostenosis, the result of abnormal fusion (synostosis) of the bones of the skull. Early syn- ostosis of the transverse sutures results in oxycephaly (Fig. 11-1). Overgrowth and early ossification of the lesser wing of the sphenoid fixes the orbits in the fetal position and results in hypertelorism.

ORBITAL INVOLVEMENT IN GENERAL DISEASE AND METABOLIC DISORDERS

HYPERTHYROIDISM.—Hyperthyroidism occurs less frequently among children than in adults, but still has a significant incidence in the pediatric age group. The diagnosis is based on the clinical signs of goiter, exo-

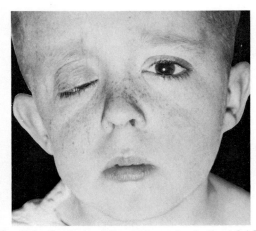

Fig. 11-3.—Proptosis of the right eye due to Hand-Schüller-Christian disease in a boy of 13.

phthalmos (Fig.11-2), tachycardia, tremor and weight loss plus a serum protein-bound iodine level greater than 8 μg/100 ml. In questionable cases, an elevated rate of uptake of radioactive iodine (I^{131}) by the thyroid gland helps to confirm the diagnosis. The only absolute diagnostic test is proof of inability to suppress the I^{131} uptake with triiodothyronine.

HISTIOCYTOSIS-X.—This is a systemic disorder of fat metabolism and storage. The histiocytes of the reticuloendothelial system acquire fat in the form of fine droplets (foam cells). Eosinophilic granuloma of bone, Hand-Schüller-Christian disease and Letterer-Siwe disease are variations of this condition. Masses simulating neoplasms occur in the orbit (Fig. 11-3).

EOSINOPHILIC GRANULOMA OF BONE.—This is essentially a skeletal lesion of weeks' or months' duration, marked by development of cystic areas of bone filled with granulation tissue. This tissue is characterized by a great number of histiocytes having phagocytic properties and by accumulations of eosinophils. The clinical feature is a rapidly developing, painful swelling in the skull, ribs or long bones of a child or young adult. The youngest person in our series was 2 years old. When a lesion involves the orbital bone, proptosis frequently results (Fig. 11-4). When the lesions are in the frontal bone, swelling is in the upper lid and the globe is pushed downward. If the lesions are in the floor of the orbit, the eye may be elevated. Roentgenograms are helpful in diagnosis (Fig. 11-5), but the greatest help comes from biopsy. The lesions heal without treatment and the prognosis is good. At the time of biopsy, the area should be vigorously curetted, followed by irradiation.

HAND-SCHÜLLER-CHRISTIAN DISEASE.—This condition (diabetic exophthalmic dysostosis) is a chronic systemic disease characterized by xanthomatous deposits in the orbit, diabetes insipidus and defects in the membranous bones of the skull (Fig. 11-6), and there may be deposits elsewhere in the skeleton. The disease occurs in children and produces proptosis, which is usually bilateral. Symptoms include polydipsia and polyuria. Some of the children improve, but others die of the disease. Irradiation can be used for symptomatic control of the bony lesions but may not improve the proptosis.

Fig. 11-4 (left).—Eosinophilic granuloma of bone in a girl of 5. Swelling of brow and upper eyelid had been present 1 month. Eye is displaced downward with slight proptosis. An incision was made into the swelling and a biopsy specimen taken; the area was then curetted and irradiated. (Figs. 11-4–11-9, 11-12–11-14, 11-19, 11-27 and 11-40 from Hospital for Sick Children, Toronto:

The Eye in Childhood Chicago: Year Book Medical Publishers, Inc., 1967.)

Fig. 11-5 (right).—Same patient as in Figure 11-4. Roentgenogram shows bony erosion in roof of right orbit; margins show no evidence of reactive sclerosis.

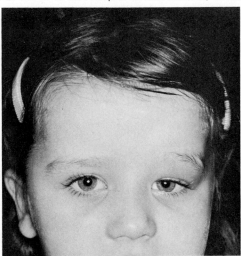

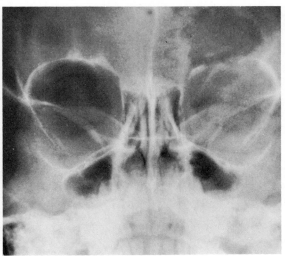

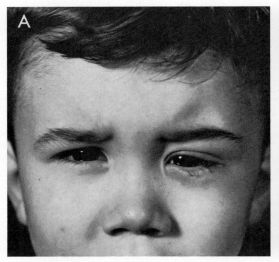

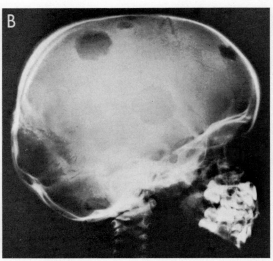

Fig. 11-6.—Left, Hand-Schüller-Christian disease. Five-year-old boy had slight proptosis of left eye due to granulomatous tissue in the orbit. **Right,** roentgenogram shows large deficiencies in the membranous bones of the skull, associated with xanthomatous plaques.

Neoplastic Disease; Tumors; Cysts

Dermoid cysts.—Dermoid cysts are sometimes known as epidermoid cysts. They arise from a con-

Fig. 11-7.—Dermoid cyst in lateral and superior walls of left orbit, causing proptosis. This girl of 11 had had progressive proptosis for 8 months. Changes in bone in upper lateral wall are clearly seen. At operation through a right frontal bone flap, the cyst was removed.

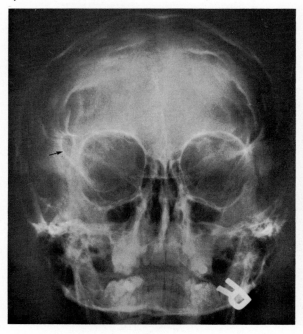

genital rest of primitive ectoderm at the closure of a fetal cleft. The wall is composed of an inner epidermal layer and an outer connective tissue layer. In the connective tissue layer may be sebaceous glands, hair follicles, elastic fibers and smooth muscle. These cysts are often located around the orbital margins and attached to bone. Occasionally, they may be deeper in the orbit, and it may be necessary to take off the lateral wall of the orbit to remove them (Krönlein's operation). An 11-year-old girl had a 6 mm proptosis due to a dermoid cyst in the lateral portion of the roof of the orbit (Fig. 11-7). The tumor was removed by the neurosurgeons through a small left frontal bone flap. Usually, however, dermoid cysts can be removed through a skin incision.

Teratoma.—Teratomas are multipotential tumors that are believed to arise from totipotential or multipotential cells that differentiate into a variety of tissues representing more than one germ layer. They may contain cartilage, connective tissue and fat of mesodermal origin; skin, hair, sebaceous glands of ectodermal origin; and may have typical intestinal epithelium of endodermal origin. The possibility of carcinomatous and sarcomatous change requires that the lesion be excised as early as possible. Teratoma does occur in the orbit (Figs. 11-8 and 11-9); the child is born with the condition. The eye is proptosed by the tumor behind the eye, and the orbital wall is stretched. The eye may be microphthalmic or of normal size.

Neurofibromatosis (Recklinghausen's disease).—In Recklinghausen's disease, tumors arise from the nerves and from the nerve sheaths. Lesions occur in the peripheral nerves and may be noted in the sympathetic and cranial nerves. Neurofibromatosis of

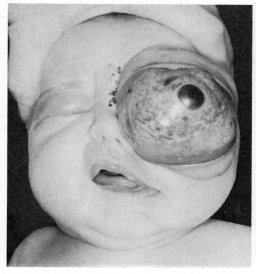 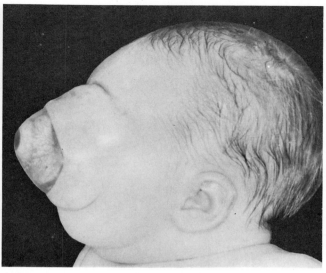

Figs. 11-8 and 11-9. — Teratoma of the orbit. Proptosis is caused by tumor behind the eye. Orbital walls are distended.

the orbit is frequently a solitary neurofibroma. It may arise in association with any nerve and hence may occupy any position in the orbit, displacing the eye in various directions. Slowly progressing proptosis without any other evidence of neurofibromatosis should lead to a search for a solitary neurofibroma (Fig. 11-10).

CAVERNOUS HEMANGIOMA. — This is the most frequent tumor of the orbit causing unilateral proptosis (Fig. 11-11). It is a congenital tumor and may cause proptosis any time after birth. Thrombosis of the vascular spaces may occur, leading to rapid development of proptosis. The proptosis is variable and may be increased by any increase of jugular pressure, as from bending of the head, crying or coughing. A bluish discoloration of the skin of the eyelid may be present;

this is the result of disintegration of a thrombotic portion of the angioma. Angiomas of the orbit may be associated with angiomas in other parts of the body. Most of these tumors reach a certain size and then remain static, generally coinciding with the stopping of body growth.

OPTIC NERVE GLIOMA. — Optic nerve gliomas arise from cells in the glial network separating the nerve fiber bundles composing the optic nerve. Most appear during the first 10 years of life. There is a slowly progressive unilateral proptosis (Fig. 11-12, A), and vision deteriorates owing to optic atrophy. Occasionally, the fundus may show an elevated disc having the appearance of papilledema instead of that of optic atrophy. If the tumor has eroded bone, enlargement of the optic formen may be visible in roentgenograms.

Fig. 11-10 (left). — Child of 18 months with proptosis since birth. Radiographs showed enlargement of superior orbital fissure. Neurosurgeons removed neurofibroma tissue from the middle cranial fossa that had extended there from the orbit.
Fig. 11-11 (right). — Cavernous hemangioma in a 6-year-old

boy. Proptosis had become apparent over the preceding 6 months, and 1 month before this picture was taken, a proptosis suddenly increased as a result of a hemorhage into tumor. Diagnosis was by biopsy. Boy was given 4 roentgen treatments. Tumor gradually disappeared completely

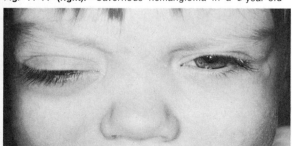 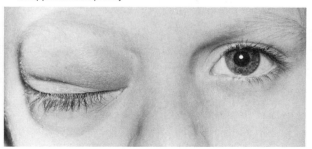

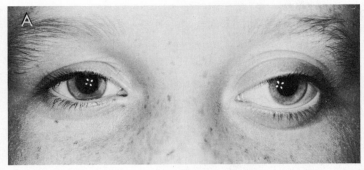

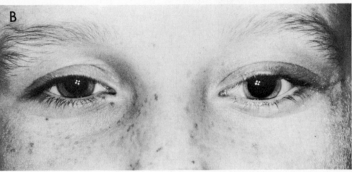

Fig. 11-12.—A, proptosis of the left eye due to glioma of the optic nerve in a girl of 10. Vision in the left eye had become affected about 5 months before this picture was taken. **B,** a neurosurgeon first operated, cutting the optic nerve in front of the chiasm and removing as much as possible of the nerve in the optic chiasm. The part of the nerve including the tumor was then removed from the orbit by removing the lateral wall. The healed scar is seen extending back from the external canthis.

Occasionally, the tumor spreads back in the nerve and involves the optic chiasm. As a point in differential diagnosis from meningioma, vision is affected in glioma, whereas in meningioma vision may not be disturbed.

If the tumor is confined to the optic nerve, it should be removed. It is possible to leave the eyeball in place and remove only the piece of the nerve containing the tumor (Fig. 11-12, *B*). This is done after the lateral wall of the orbit is removed. If the tumor appears in the portion of the nerve inside the optic foramen, a decompression operation may be necessary to preserve vision.

SARCOMA OF THE ORBIT.—Sarcomas of the orbit are malignant and fatal (Fig. 11-13). Rhabdomyosarcomas are the commonest malignant tumors of the orbit among children, 25% of them occurring during the first 10 years of life. Rhabdomyosarcomas have a wide variation in their cytologic characteristics.

The only hope of a cure in these cases is early diagnosis. Exenteration of the orbit should be carried out promptly and followed by irradiation.

MALIGNANT LYMPHOMATOUS TUMORS.—Primary tumors of the lymph nodes are known by the generic term lymphoma. Lymphomas composed only of lymphocytes are known as lymphosarcoma; others, originating in the reticulum cells, are designated reticulum cell sarcomas. Although lymphosarcomas may have widespread metastases, they remain as more or less discrete nodules (Fig. 11-14).

NEUROBLASTOMA OF THE ADRENALS.—This is a malignant tumor of the suprarenal medulla which may metastasize early to the orbit, skull and long bones. Ecchymosis around one or both eyes is one of the commonest signs. Metastases in the bones of the orbit produce proptosis and displacement of the globe. (Fig. 11-15). There is pallor and weight loss, slight elevation of temperature, anemia and a palpable abdominal mass. Confirmation of the diagnosis may be made by biopsy. Roentgenograms of the skull, pelvis and long bones should be taken, as well as pyelograms to learn if the kidney is displaced.

CHLOROMA.—The color of this greenish tumor is due to a pigment chemically related to the porphyrins. It is an atypical form of myelogenous leukemia. Lesions in the subperiosteum of the orbit cause proptosis (Fig. 11-16).

HODGKIN'S DISEASE.—With its liver, spleen and lymph gland enlargement, Hodgkin's disease was seen in 26 cases, in 3 of which there was monocular proptosis (Fig. 11-17).

HEMORRHAGE.—Hemorrhages into the orbit are

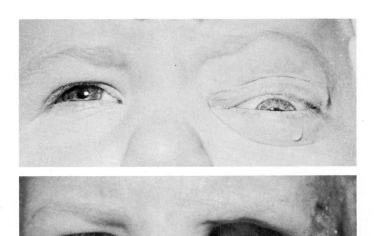

Fig. 11-13.—**Above,** fibrosarcoma of left orbit in a boy of 3 years with rapidly progressing proptosis. **Below,** after exenteration, the tumor recurred, as seen in the floor of the orbit, and the child died.

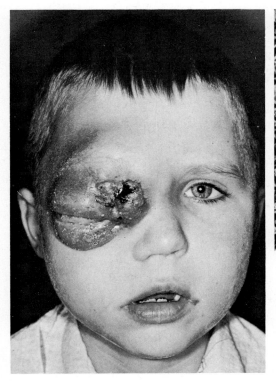

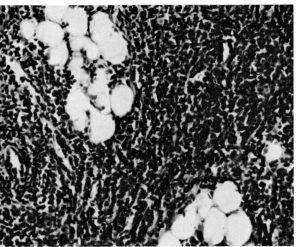

Fig. 11-14.—**Left,** lymphosarcoma, which was inoperable when the patient, a boy of 7, was first seen. He died a month later. **Above,** lymphosarcoma, showing sheets of small lymphocytic cells infiltrating orbital fat and connective tissue. Differentiation from pseudotumors of the orbit may be difficult on microscopy alone.

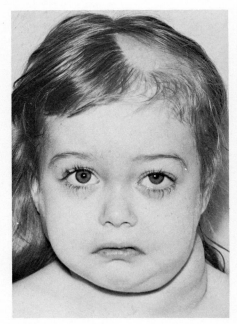

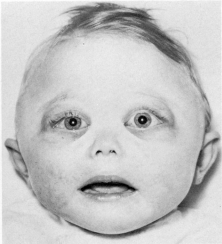

Fig. 11-15 (left).—Proptosis of left eye due to metastasis from neuroblastoma of the adrenal in a child 1 year old. The swelling in the neck is another metastasis.

Fig. 11-16 (above).—Extreme bilateral proptosis from chloroma in a child of 9 months.

Fig. 11-17.—A boy of 7 with proptosis of the right eye and enlargement of liver and spleen due to Hodgkin's disease.

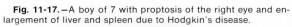

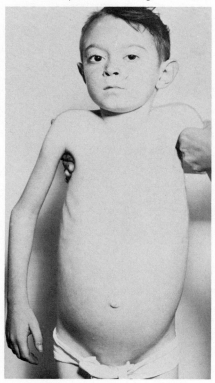

Fig. 11-18.—Retrobulbar hemorrhage with immediate proptosis of 8 mm in a girl of 10, struck on the right eye with a blunt object. Vision was 20/40 but gradually returned to 20/20 as the proptosis disappeared over a 3-month period.

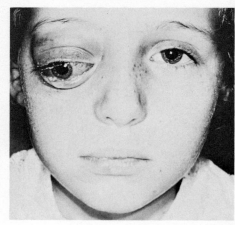

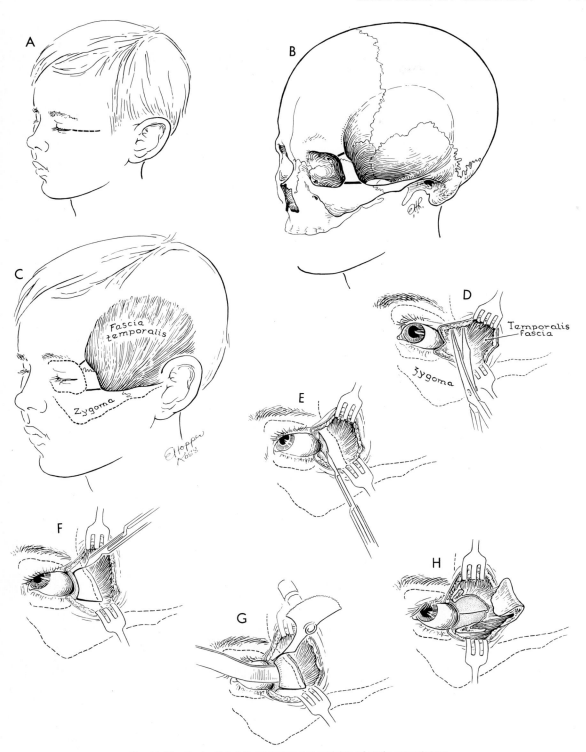

Fig. 11-19.—Berke-Krönlein operation for excision of optic nerve tumor.

most frequently due to trauma (Fig. 11-18) but also occur in leukemia and scurvy.

TUMOR MANAGEMENT.—If a tumor is suspected, a biopsy is desirable but is not always easy to accomplish. The result of biopsy examination indicates the form therapy is to take—irradiation, excision, orbital exenteration—according to the nature of the tumor. Biopsy is usually performed through the fornices to avoid the danger of injuring the levator muscle. Occasionally, the tumor may have to be reached by an incision through the skin of the lids. Tumors behind the globe may require removal of the lateral wall of the orbit (Krönlein operation, see Fig. 11-19). If the exophthalmos is severe enough to cause corneal ulceration, it may be necessary to suture the lid margins together or put in lid adhesions. In the case of hemangiomas, as much of the tumor as possible is removed without damaging the extraocular muscles or nerves; any remnants will usually become smaller.

Krönlein's operation.—Certain tumors deep in the orbit are frequently reached only by removal of the lateral orbital wall: the hemangioma, neurilemmoma, optic nerve glioma and occasionally the meningioma.

Dr. R. N. Berke modified the original Krönlein incision to a horizontal incision (Fig. 11-19, *A*). *B* and *C* show the temporal fossa and muscle and position of the bone cuts.

1. A silk suture (5–0) is placed through the external rectus muscle so that is can be quickly identified. An external canthotomy is done, and the incision in the skin of the face is carried backward and deepened until the fascia covering the temporalis muscle comes into view (Fig. 11-19, *D*).

2. An incision is made in the periosteum along the lateral border of the orbit (Fig. 11-19, *E*) and a periosteal elevator frees the periosteum from the lateral wall of the orbit.

3. Incisions are made through the periosteum (Fig. 11-19, *F*) on the outer wall where the bone is to be cut by the Stryker saw or chisel (Fig. 11-19, *B* and *G*). A metal retractor is placed deep to the bone to protect the orbital structures. The upper cut is directed medially downward; the lower saw cut is medially and slightly upward. This makes the bone slightly wider externally than medially, and when later replaced, it is held in proper position. The lateral wall is then broken with a rongeur and removed. More of the wall posteriorly may be removed with rongeurs.

4. The periosteum lining the orbit (Fig. 11-19, *H*) is cut horizontally to enter the orbit. After the tumor has been removed, the periosteum is resutured, and the bone flap replaced and held by 4–0 chromic catgut; the edges of external periosteum are sutured.

5. The temporal fascia is sutured and the skin wound closed with 5–0 plain catgut.

6. If orbital edema is anticipated, then the lids should be sutured together.

Strabismus

During the first 2 or 3 months of life a baby's eyes do not always remain parallel. After this time, they should work together. Frequently, the eyes appear to be very close together, but this is usually an illusion created by the undeveloped bridge of the baby's nose (Fig. 11-20). More of the white sclera is visible on the outer than on the inner side.

The eyes are examined by having the child look at a light which is directed toward his face from a distance of about 15 in. A spot of light (light reflex) will be seen on the center of both pupils if the eyes are straight. If one eye is turned, the reflex will not be in the center of that pupil. Puppets may be used to attract the child's attention (Fig. 11-21) during the examination.

CONVERGENT STRABISMUS.—The commonest type of strabismus is the convergent (Fig. 11-22); it may be congenital. Many of these children appear to have a paresis of the external rectus muscles. Operation should be done early (10–12 months of age). Experience has shown that lengthening of the medial recti is often enough to straighten the eyes, and in a few

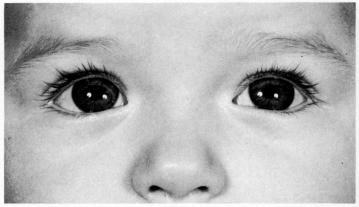

Fig. 11-20.—Pseudostrabismus. The child has a very broad bridge of the nose which covers part of the sclera on the nasal side of both eyes, giving the false impression of strabismus.

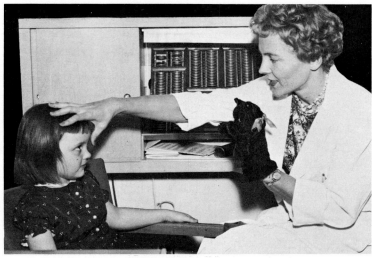

Fig. 11-21.—Method of examination for strabismus with puppets.

months the eyes will abduct freely. Sometimes the medial recti are fibrous bands and the eyes are anchored in the nasal field in the condition known as strabismus fixus. It may be difficult to diagnose the condition until the medial rectus is engaged with a hook and found to be entirely resisting. Occasional cases are seen in which the external recti are replaced by fibrous bands so that when the eye is adducted there is a definite retraction of the eyeball, the so-called Duane retraction syndrome.

Esotropia, which comes on between 18 months and 3 years of age, is often of the accommodational type. It depends on the excessive use of the accommodation which, owing to its synergistic relationship with convergence, excites an excessive amount of convergence. It usually occurs in children with moderate to large degrees of farsightedness (hyperopia). Refraction should be done, using cycloplegic drugs, and if hyperopia is over 2 or 3 diopters, glasses should be prescribed (Fig. 11-23). If the eyes are straight with

glasses, operation usually will not be necessary, but if they are only partially straight, the remaining amount of deviation is to be corrected. If an eye has not been used for some time because of esotropia and the resulting suppression to avoid diplopia, the vision becomes poor in this eye (amblyopia). The vision will be improved (in the poor-vision eye) by patching (occlusion) of the good eye (Fig. 11-24) until the sight is the same in the two eyes.

DIVERGENT STRABISMUS.—This condition is not as common as convergent strabismus, the proportion being about 1 to 4. These children usually have good fusion, and amblyopia is rarer. They hold their eyes straight when looking at near objects, but on looking in the distance, turn one eye outward too far (Fig. 11-25). A lengthening is required for one or both external rectus muscles and should be done early in life. If operation is delayed, a secondary convergence weakness results and one eye gradually assumes a constant divergent position. In this case, a lengthening of

Fig. 11-22 (left).—Convergent strabismus.
Fig. 11-23 (right).—Accommodative esotropia straightened with glasses.

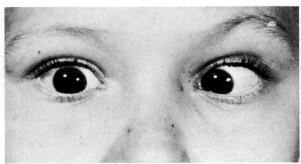
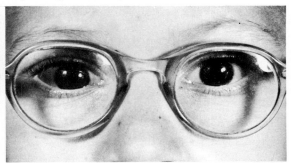

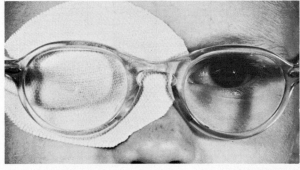

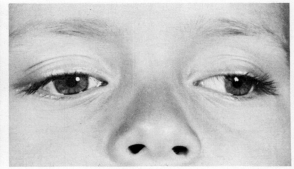

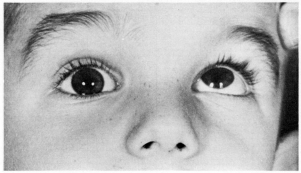

Fig. 11-24 (above left). — Method of occlusion with Elastoplast bandage.

Fig. 11-25 (above right). — Divergent strabismus.

Fig. 11-26 (left). — Left hypertropia.

the external rectus is combined with a shortening operation on the medial rectus.

HYPERTROPIA. — This condition usually is due to an overaction of one or both inferior oblique muscles and can be remedied by lengthening this muscle. Abnormality of any of the other vertical muscles may also result in one eye being higher than the other (Fig. 11-26). The head usually is tilted to compensate for abnormal function of either the inferior or superior oblique muscles.

Eye Injuries in Children

Injuries to the eye cause about 50% of all blindness in one eye and about 20% of blindness in both eyes, hence early proper treatment is extremely important. The various eye injuries and their treatment may be discussed under the following headings: contusions; extraocular and intraocular foreign bodies; lacerations and fractures, and burns.

CONTUSIONS. — Injuries by blunt objects vary in severity from a simple corneal abrasion to rupture of the globe. Any part of the eye may be so injured by contusion as to diminish vision seriously. In some patients, the changes are progressive, so that in all cases a guarded prognosis should be given. Various conditions may follow contusion:

Corneal abrasion is recognized by a roughening of the cornea. When a drop of 1% fluorescein solution is placed inside the lower lid, the abraded area takes up

a greenish-yellow stain. There is much pain and tearing, such as is produced by a foreign body. It is increased on moving the lids, and patients keep their lids forcibly closed. In most cases, the instillation of an antibiotic eye ointment and application of a tight pad to splint the lids suffice.

Hyphema, or blood in the anterior chamber (Fig. 11-27), is frequently seen in children. Most of these cases are caused by flying objects such as BB shot,

Fig. 11-27. — Hyphema.

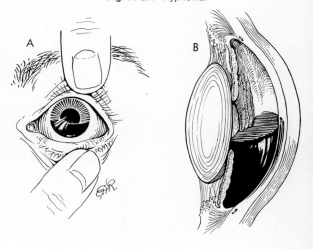

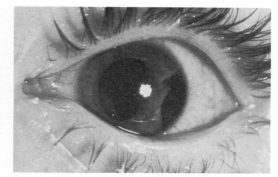

Fig. 11-28.—Iridodialysis. The iris was torn from its root following contusion by a stone.

stones and objects shot by sling-shots. The male to female ratio is about 6 to 1. Secondary hemorrhage is one of the worse complications and in over 75% of our cases occurred on the third or fourth day. It was not noted later than 5 days. When there has been a massive hemorrhage into the anterior chamber, glaucoma may result. In the series studied, glaucoma occurred in 25% of the cases of secondary hemorrhage, and with primary hemorrhage in less than 2%. If the hemorrhage has been massive and glaucoma occurs, blood-staining of the cornea may result. In these cases it may be necessary to evacuate the blood by operation (paracentesis and irrigation of the anterior chamber). When hyphema following injury is noted in a child, he should be put to bed with binocular bandages and kept quiet for several days until the blood absorbs. If glaucoma occurs, an attempt should be made to lower the intraocular tension by use of carbonic anhydrase inhibitors such as Diamox or Daranide. These drugs may lower the tension within the

eye until the blood has absorbed. If the intraocular tension remains high, paracentesis will be necessary. If there is difficulty in washing out the clot, a solution of fibrinolysin will frequently break up the clot and allow its removal from the anterior chamber.

Iris.—Contusions of the eye may cause the pupil to become large and immobile. It may remain moderately dilated for many weeks and sometimes permanently. Iridodialysis (Fig. 11-28) requires no treatment and may not impair vision. Contusions over the ciliary body may cause weakness of accommodation due to paresis of the ciliary muscle. Hypotonia or low intraocular pressure may follow a blow and result in a decrease of aqueous formation.

Lens.—Rupture of the suspensory ligament may cause dislocation of the lens and may be diagnosed by tremor of the iris (iridodonesis) on movement of the eye. Total or partial cataract may result from transmission of the force of the blow through the cornea and aqueous, with or without rupture of the lens capsule. Secondary glaucoma may result either with dislocation of the lens or with traumatic cataract.

Choroid.—Rupture of the choroid may occur as a result of severe contusion. This is seen through an ophthalmoscope as a curved white streak not far from the optic nerve and concentric with it. It usually occurs on the temporal side of the disc. If the macula is involved, loss of central vision results.

Retina.—Hemorrhages into the retina occur and may extend into the vitreous. Detachment of the retina is common after contusion. Commotio retinae, or swelling in the retina at the point of best vision (macula), may result from a blow on the eye. It disappears after several days and vision is usually restored to normal.

Treatment of most of the foregoing conditions is rest. In the case of retinal detachment, operation is required. Cautery burns to the adjacent sclera set up

Fig. 11-29 (left).—Lid laceration involving canaliculus.
Fig. 11-30 (right).—Following repair of lid with Nylon suture (2-0) in lacrimal passages to re-establish patency.

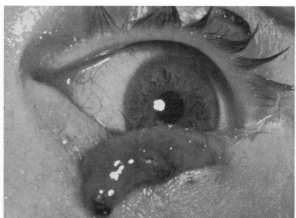

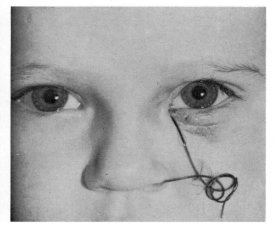

aseptic inflammation to provide adhesions and attachments of the retina. Evacuation of the fluid under the retina may result. Occasionally a piece of silicone rubber is buried under the sclera in order to push the choroid against the detached retina. At present, cryotherapy is much more popular than heat for burning of the sclera to produce adhesions to the retina.

EXTRAOCULAR AND INTRAOCULAR FOREIGN BODIES.— Foreign bodies are frequently seen on the anterior surface of the cornea. Under local anesthesia, the foreign body may be removed with a piece of cotton wrapped on the end of a toothpick or a spud. After removal of the foreign body, a tight pad should be applied to the eye to allow the corneal epithelium to heal over. Particles of steel, stone, glass, and so on, may penetrate the eyeball. Careful examination of the eye with a slit lamp and corneal microscope may reveal the path of the foreign body. X-ray studies are frequently found useful.

Treatment.—Foreign bodies should be removed as soon as possible. If they are magnetic metals, the giant magnet frequently aids in their removal. Occasionally, it may be necessary to leave pieces of glass or nonmagnetic metal in an eye, as too much damage would result from attempts to remove them.

LACERATIONS AND FRACTURES.—During examination of a child with a bad lid laceration (Fig. 11-29), care should be taken to check the eyeball itself for injury. The orbital walls should be examined for possible fracture. A sinking-in of the eye suggests a fracture of the floor of the orbit. Frequently, the inferior rectus and the inferior oblique muscles become caught in the floor fracture and limit the elevation and depression of the eye. The usual x-ray examination often fails to show an orbital floor fracture, so if the signs suggest an orbital floor fracture, tomograms should be taken. Repair of blow-out fractures of the orbital floor is accomplished by making a horizontal incision through the skin just below the bony wall of the orbit inferiorly and then incising the periosteum just below the orbital rim. A periosteal elevator is passed backward under the periosteum until the fracture is located. The contents that are herniating down into the hole should be lifted up and the hole covered with a piece of Teflon or a thin sheet of silicone rubber.

Lacerations in the lids should be repaired as soon as possible after an injury, and if the canaliculi have been cut, the ends may be joined together over a piece of 2-0 Nylon thread (Fig. 11-30). Lacerations in the eyeball require immediate treatment (Fig. 11-31). Care should be taken not to cause herniation of the ocular contents during examination of a child with a bad injury. In such a case, it is best to wait until the child has been anesthetized before carrying out the examination. Tetanus toxoid should be given if the laceration extends into the eyeball. In the management of wounds over the ciliary body, with or without

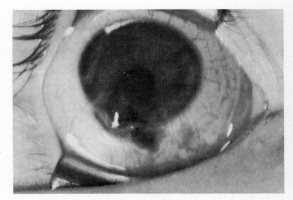

Fig. 11-31.—Perforating injury with prolapsed iris.

incarceration of the structure, good judgment is required. Prognosis must always be guarded, although the outcome can be surprisingly good. The threat of sympathetic ophthalmia (a condition in which the uninjured eye becomes inflamed following the injury to one eye, and the second eye may go on to blindness) is always of concern. The best prognosis is afforded by clean wounds with no incarceration of the ciliary body and little or no vitreous hemorrhage. Sympathetic ophthalmia rarely occurs before 10 days after injury. Injured eyes in which the question of enucleation arises may be observed safely for that length of time.

BURNS AND INJURIES BY CAUSTICS.—Such injuries to the cornea and conjunctiva are detected by the instillation of a drop of 1% fluorescein into the conjunctival sac. A greenish color is taken up by the injured tissues. First-aid treatment consists of copious washing with water. No neutralization of the chemical should be attempted, as valuable time is lost thereby. In hospital, the eye is anesthetized with some non-narcotic local anesthetic agent.

Blepharoptosis

Ptosis of the upper lid indicates a drooping of more than an average amount. The condition may be unilateral or bilateral.

Among ptosis types, only the following are considered here:

1. Congenital ptosis: (*a*) with normal superior rectus action; (*b*) associated with weakness of one or more of the elevator muscles of the eye; (*c*) associated with the jaw-winking phenomenon of Marcus Gunn; (*d*) associated with blepharophimosis.

2. Acquired ptosis: (*a*) local or general disease; (*b*) neurologic causes; (*c*) trauma.

The congenital form is the most common, most cases being unilateral, with fair to good levator action. About 6% of all cases of congenital ptosis demonstrate the jaw-winking phenomenon of Marcus Gunn. These are always unilateral. Here the affected

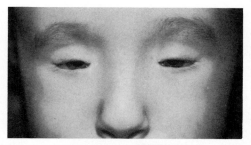

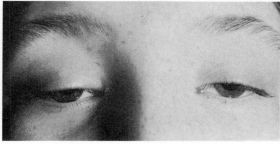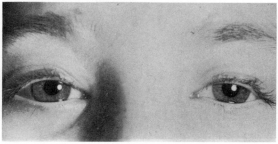

Fig. 11-32 (above).—A child with blepharophimosis and ptosis. The ptosis here is best repaired with fascia lata.
Fig. 11-33 (below left).—A girl aged 9 with bilateral congenital ptosis, with very little levator action.
Fig. 11-34 (below right).—Same girl as in Figure 11-33 after repair with fascia.

lid moves upward when the mandible is either depressed or moved to the opposite side. Ptosis associated with blepharophimosis (Fig. 11-32) is always bilateral and occurs in about 3% of cases of congenital ptosis.

Only a few of the conditions accounting for acquired ptosis will be mentioned, and only those which occur in children. Acquired ptosis may occur with hemangioma, neurofibromatosis and occasionally after enucleation, usually when there has been no implant in Tenon's capsule. Neurologic causes include brain lesions, such as hemorrhage, tumor and trauma. Acquired ptosis may occur with external ophthalmoplegia. Local trauma to the lid may result from injuries or after removal of tumors of the lid.

Preoperative Examination

The corneal reflex and Bell's phenomenon should be investigated. The amount of ptosis is determined by measuring the width of the palpebral apertures, noting how much of each cornea is covered by each upper lid. This may be estimated with the patient looking up, down, but most important in the primary position. Some surgeons record the distance from the rim of the orbit to the lower border of the upper lid.

The range of movement of the lid is estimated by measuring the amount of elevation from looking down to looking up. This is done while preventing frontalis action by holding the muscle with the thumb. The position of the lid fold of the normal lid

should be noted so that at the time of surgery the fold of the ptosed lid will be properly placed.

Operative Procedures

The following procedures are practiced:
1. Procedures utilizing the levator muscle.
2. Frontalis suspension operations (Figs. 11-33 and 11-34).
3. Operation using superior rectus to suspend the lid.

Operations utilizing the levator muscle.—Approach to the levator muscle may be made either through the skin surface[3] or through the conjunctiva (Fig. 11-39).[6] Larger degrees of ptosis are best treated by the external approach through skin (Figs. 11-35 and 11-36). About 2 or 3 mm less correction can be obtained by the conjunctival approach (Figs. 11-37 and 11-38) so that this method is used in cases of small degrees of ptosis (3–4 mm). It is difficult to overcorrect congenital ptosis. Acquired ptosis is more easily overcorrected.

Operations utilizing the frontalis muscle.—Many methods have been used to suspend the lid from the frontalis muscle. The Guyton-Friedenwald suture,[5] which consists of a white silk suture attaching the lid to the frontalis muscle, proved unsatisfactory because a high percentage became infected. Autogenous fascia lata is the best material for the procedure and is much superior to preserved fascia or tantalum wire. This operation[4] gives best results in cases of bi-

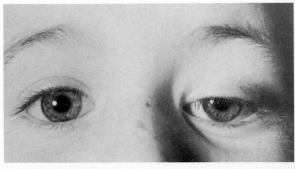
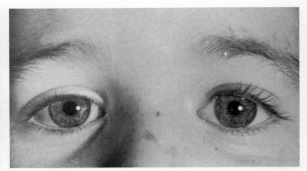
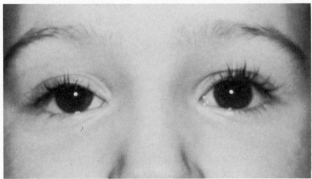
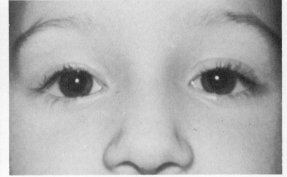

Fig. 11-35 (above left).—A boy aged 4 with ptosis of left upper lid, with good action of levator muscle.

Fig. 11-36 (above right).—Same child as in Figure 11-35 after resection through skin.

Fig. 11-37 (below left).—Slight ptosis of left upper lid of 8-year-old girl.

Fig. 11-38 (below right).—Same patient as in Figure 11-37 after levator resection through posterior surface of lid.

lateral ptosis with little or no levator action (Fig. 11-40). It is a good surgical procedure in blepharophimosis, ptosis occurring after removal of lid tumors where the levator muscle has been damaged, third nerve palsy, and when poor results were obtained from levator resection. In patients with the Marcus Gunn syndrome, a 7 or 8 mm piece of levator muscle is resected by the conjunctival approach, and about 1 month later the lid is suspended to the frontalis muscle with fascia.

Operation utilizing the superior rectus muscle.— The Motais-Parinaud type of operation, in which attachments are made between the superior rectus muscle and the ptosed lid, is frequently complicated by postoperative hypertropia. In view of the good results obtained with the surgical techniques mentioned above, we have stopped using this procedure.

When to operate.—If the lid is completely obscuring vision, early surgery is imperative. Levator resection operations should be carried out after age 3. In frontalis operations in which fascia is used, the thigh must be long enough before good fascia can be obtained, and this again is after 3 years of age. Ptosis due to trauma to the levator should be repaired immediately.

LEVATOR RESECTION THROUGH CONJUNCTIVAL AP-PROACH (Fig. 11-39).—*A*, the position of the desired lid fold is marked to correspond to that on the normal lid. *B*, the lid is everted on a Desmarres retractor. Stab incisions are made lateral to the tarsus edge and a levator clamp is passed across, securing the upper edge of the tarsus. *C*, an incision is made along the distal edge of the clamp which is 3 or 4 mm from the superior tarsal margin. *D*, the dissection is extended backward anterior to the levator tendon and posterior to the septum orbitale. *E*, the conjunctiva is dissected free from the levator. *F*, four double-armed (4-0) plain catgut sutures are placed through all the structures in the clamp 10–14 mm from the cut end of the muscle. Each suture is tied and all tissue is excised distal to the sutures. *G*, the needle is passed into the posterior surface of the tarsus as close as possible to the lid margin. *H*, three double-armed (4–0) plain catgut sutures are used. One arm is passed through the tarsus, levator and skin, and the other arm through the edge of the conjunctiva, levator muscle and skin. These sutures should come through the skin at the line where a skin fold is desired. *I*, two modified Frost sutures close the lids and protect the cornea.

LEVATOR RESECTION THROUGH A SKIN INCISION.— Correction of a greater degree of ptosis is possible through a skin incision. This approach should be used

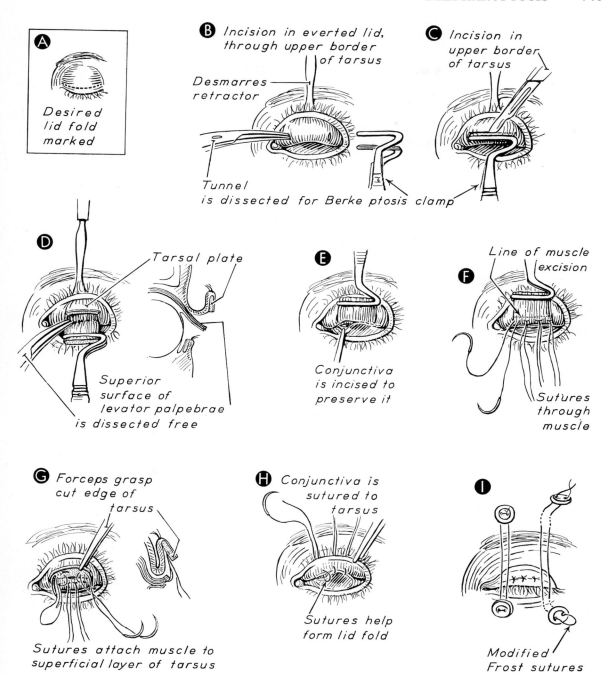

A Desired lid fold marked

B Incision in everted lid, through upper border of tarsus
Desmarres retractor
Tunnel is dissected for Berke ptosis clamp

C Incision in upper border of tarsus

D Tarsal plate
Superior surface of levator palpebrae is dissected free

E Conjunctiva is incised to preserve it

F Line of muscle excision
Sutures through muscle

G Forceps grasp cut edge of tarsus
Sutures attach muscle to superficial layer of tarsus

H Conjunctiva is sutured to tarsus
Sutures help form lid fold

I Modified Frost sutures

Fig. 11-39.—Levator resection through conjunctival approach.

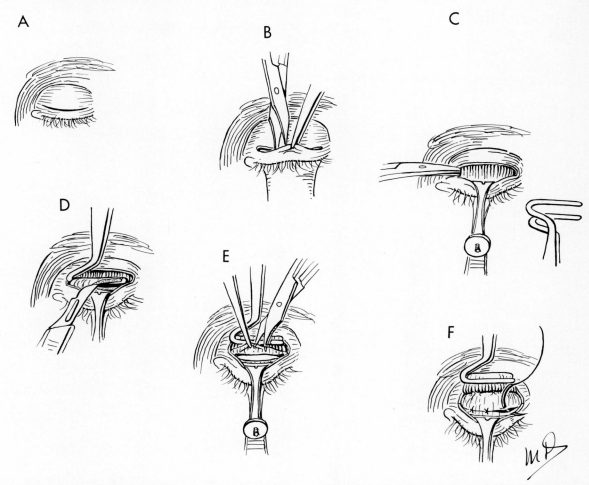

Fig. 11-40.—Repair of ptosis through skin. **A** and **B**, incision through skin and orbicularis oculi; anterior surface of tarsus is exposed. **C**, incisions are made and Berke ptosis clamp is in-serted to secure the whole thickness of lid except skin. **D**, tarsus is incised 4 mm from lid border. **E** and **F**, palpebral conjunctiva is dissected off muscle and sutured to tarsus. *(Continued.)*

when the levator action is poor but not absent. The examiner should place his thumb firmly above the eyebrow to stop the frontalis muscle from raising the lid. A millimeter rule is held vertically over the eye and the patient is instructed to look up as far as possible and then look down also as far as possible. If excursion of the lid is less than 6 mm, the ptosis should be repaired with fascia lata. If there is 6–7 mm of excursion of the lid, the levator muscle should be approached by a skin incision, since more of the muscle can be isolated and excised in this manner.

Technique (Fig. 11-40).—1. Before the levator muscle is resected, one must observe the position of the lid fold on the normal lid. The distance from the lid border should be measured and the skin incision on the ptotic lid made in a similar position. After the site of the incision has been marked on the ptotic lid,

a protective Horn plate is placed under the upper lid and the skin and orbicularis muscles are incised the length of the lid. The orbicularis muscle and the skin are dissected and freed from the tarsus down to the edge of the lid. An Erhardt clamp is placed on the tarsus, the lid pulled down and the skin dissected up from the underlying tissues (*A* and *B*).

2. Two button-hole incisions are then made through the levator and the conjunctiva close to the tarsus, about 25 mm apart. The Berke clamp goes through the incisions to secure the levator muscle. The tarsus is cut across 4 mm from the lid border, and the levator muscle is raised to expose the conjunctival surface (*C* and *D*).

3. An incision is made just below the Berke ptosis clamp (*C*) through the conjunctiva, and the conjunctiva is then dissected free from the muscle (*D*). The

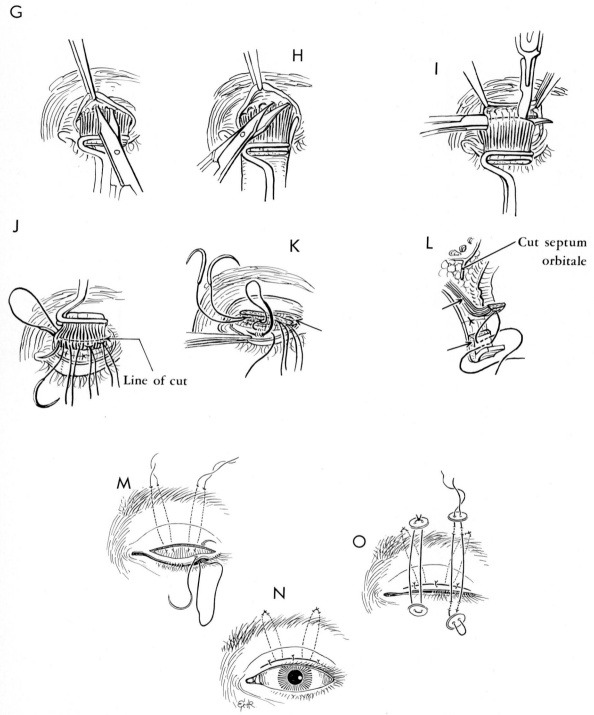

G

H

I

J

Line of cut

K

L

Cut septum
orbitale

M

N

O

Fig. 11-40 *(cont.).* —**G** and **H,** superior surface of levator is dissected free. **I,** septum orbitale is incised. Repair of ptosis through skin. **J,** four 4-0 plain catgut sutures through muscle. **K** and **L,** sutures attach shortened levator to tarsus **(arrows). M,** three 4-0 sutures, through tarsus from conjunctival surface, form skin fold. **N,** three double-armed 4-0 plain catgut sutures through conjunctival surface. **O,** two modified Frost sutures inserted in lower lid and tied.

cut edge of the conjunctiva is resutured to the border of the tarsus with 6–0 plain catgut sutures. This may be done as a continuous suture or as 6 or 7 interrupted sutures (*E* and *F*).

4. The positions of the lateral horn and the check ligament of the levator are now located by palpation through the skin of the upper lid while pulling down on the ptosis clamp. These two structures are cut, freeing the levator muscle.

5. The levator muscle is pulled downward and the septum orbitale is cut free from the levator. This is best done just below the orbital rim where the levator muscle and the orbital septum are separated by a wedge of fat.

6. After that has been done, one may notice the orbital fat to herniate forward. The upper lid is then elevated and the levator muscle pulled down over the lid margin. Four 4–0 double-armed plain catgut sutures are inserted from the deep surface forward through the levator muscle, evenly distributed across the width of the muscle. The sutures are placed in the levator at the level where it crosses the upper border of the tarsus, as a guide to the amount to be resected, which varies between 10 and 15 mm. Two ends of each suture are tied (*J*).

7. The distal end of the levator muscle is excised, and then the sutures are passed horizontally into the tarsus and tied (*G*), thus elevating the lid into its new position. Before the sutures shown in *M* are tied, two 3–0 chromic catgut sutures are placed in the lid as shown in Figure 11-40. These chromic sutures hold the lid up at the desired height until all the reaction in the lid has subsided and usually disintegrate in 2–3 weeks. During the early healing, there is a certain amount of swelling in the lid, and this tends to interfere with the results of the levator shortening that was carried out. Since using these sutures, I have been obtaining better results from my levator shortenings.

8. Three other double-armed 4–0 plain catgut sutures are then placed through the conjunctival surface. One end of the double-armed suture is brought out through the tarsus and the skin below, and the other end through the muscle and skin above, thus closing the skin wound and helping to form a good lid fold.

9. Two modified Frost sutures are inserted in the lower lid and tied (*I*), then a bandage and adhesive strapping are placed over the eye. The bandage should be left in place for 5 days to help minimize the postoperative swelling.

Repair of ptosis with fascia lata.—This operation is used only when there is little or no action of the levator muscle.

Method of placing strips of fascia (Fig. 11-41).— Two pieces of fascia 2 mm wide and 10 cm long are

Fig. 11-41.—Method of placing strips of fascia.

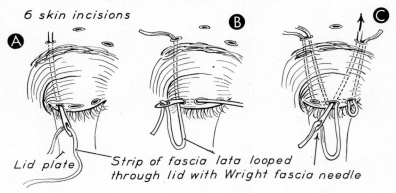

6 skin incisions

Lid plate — Strip of fascia lata looped through lid with Wright fascia needle

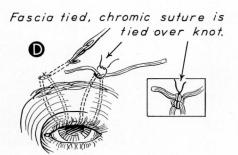

Fascia tied, chromic suture is tied over knot.

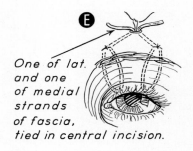

One of lat. and one of medial strands of fascia, tied in central incision.

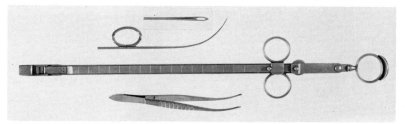

Fig. 11-42. — Wright fascia needle, Crawford fascia stripper and curved forceps for pulling fascia through the end of the stripper.

used for each ptosed lid. Three incisions are made in the lid, 2 mm from the lid margin. The incisions in the forehead are made 7 mm above the brow and parallel to it, the outer being placed 6 mm lateral, and the inner one 6 mm medial to the corresponding incisions near the lid margins. The third incision is made in the brow 6 mm above and parallel to the other incisions, midway between them (A – C). The fascial strips are placed in the lid with the help of the Wright fascia needle as shown in Figure 11-42. When the needle is passed horizontally between the incisions near the lid border (B), the needle is passed through the superficial layer of the tarsus. The purpose of using two pieces of fasica in this method is to have the direction of pull at right angles to the new raised position of the lid border (D). Some authors suggest placing the fascia in the lid in a rhomboid fashion, but in this case a nice curve to the upper lid is not produced. The Wright fascia needle and the Crawford fascia stripper are useful instruments for this operation (Fig. 11-42).

REFERENCES

1. Berke, R. N.: Congenital ptosis: A classification of two hundred cases, Arch. Ophth. 41:186, 1949.
2. Berke, R. N.: Motais-Parinaud type of operation for ptosis: Report on thirty-five cases, Arch. Ophth. 41:324, 1949.
3. Berke, R. N.: Surgical correction of blepharoptosis, Am. J. Ophth. 36:765, 1953.
4. Crawford, J. S.: Repair of ptosis using frontalis muscle and fascia lata, Tr. Am. Acad. Ophth. 60:672, 1956.
5. Friedenwald, J. S., and Guyton, J. S.: A simple ptosis operation: Utilization of the frontalis by means of a single rhomboid-shaped suture, Am. J. Ophth. 31:411, 1948.
6. Iliff, C. E.: A simplified ptosis operation, Am. J. Ophth. 37:529, 1954.
7. Schimek, R. A.: A new ptosis operation utilizing both levator and frontalis, Arch. Ophth. 54:92, 1955.

A. L. MORGAN
J. S. CRAWFORD

Drawings by
MARGUERITE DRUMMOND

12

The Nose

Anatomic Considerations

THE NOSE FORMS the most conspicuous part of the face. It is formed of a bony and cartilaginous vault which rests on the septum. The nasal bones are attached above to the frontal bone. In the midline, they are attached to each other and to the bony and cartilaginous septum. Laterally, they are joined to the frontal processes of the maxillas which arch forward on either side. Below, they attach to the upper lateral or quadrilateral cartilages. These cartilages join each other and the cartilaginous septum in the midline. Below the upper lateral cartilages are the lower lateral or alar cartilages, each of which has a lateral and medial crus. These latter cartilages give form and support to the nostrils. The medial crura are contiguous with each other and the lower border of the cartilaginous septum.

Development

The nose develops in front of the oral fossa, which is anterior to the mandibular processes of the first gill arch. Laterally, the oral fossa is bounded by the maxillary processes and anteriorly by the nasal plate. The latter has a central median portion and two lateral portions separated by deep pits (the nasal pits). A groove separates the nasal process from the maxillary process. Eventually these two fuse. The central part of the nasal plate forms the septum, the philtrum of the upper lip and the premaxilla. The lateral processes form the cheek and the upper lip except for the philtrum. When the maxillary and nasal processes unite, the communication between the nasal pits and the oral fossa is interrupted by the bucconasal membranes. Eventually these membranes disappear and the communication occurs behind the maxillary processes, forming the primitive choanae. Later the palate forms, separating the nasal and oral cavities, and communication is via the pharynx through the posterior choanae.

An understanding of the development of the nose and nasal cavities will help to explain the nasal abnormalities which appear at birth. Some aspects of the development are not, however, completely understood, and for this reason certain anomalies of the nose are difficult to explain.

Congenital Lesions

Absence of the nasal cavities on one (more common) or both sides may occur with bony occlusion. The condition is rare and, if both sides are affected, requires a formidable operative procedure for the construction of an airway. More often, a nostril is obstructed by a membrane of skin within the vestibule. It may be associated with unilateral underdevelopment of the nose and possibly with other defects of the face and ear on the same side (Fig. 12-1). Reconstructive procedures to open the airway should be performed early. Procedures for the modification of the appearance of the nose may be left until later.

CHOANAL ATRESIA.—Occlusion of the posterior nares is called choanal atresia. This is not uncommon, and the subject is dealt with in detail in textbooks on rhinology. It may be unilateral or bilateral (the former being more common) and complete or incomplete. With complete bilateral atresia, the infant must breathe through the mouth and is in danger of suffocation, particularly when suckling. It

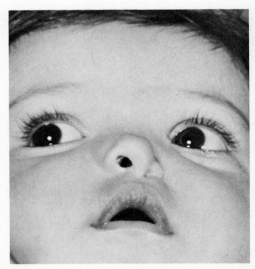

Fig. 12-1.—Unilateral underdevelopment of the nose and face with an incomplete membrane blocking the nares.

should be thought of when an infant has recurrent bouts of asphyxia for which there is no other obvious cause. A fine catheter will not pass through the nose into the pharynx. The need for treatment is urgent. Unilateral atresia may escape detection in infancy but should be considered when there is a constant unilateral nasal discharge. In infancy, difficulty in feeding occurs when the nostril of the unaffected side is closed during feeding by being held against the breast.

ABSENCE OF THE NOSE.—Complete absence of the nose has been reported. It must be an extremely rare anomaly and has never been seen by the author. Absence of half or smaller portions is not uncommon (Fig. 12-1). Various degrees of unilateral absence (or notching of an ala) may also be seen (Fig. 12-2). Plastic reconstruction is indicated for these anomalies.

DOUBLE NOSE.—This rare anomaly may be associated with a midline defect in the lip (Fig. 12-3), the so-called midline harelip, which may also occur without the nasal anomaly. The nasal deformity is associated with an abnormally great distance between the eyes and a broad flat nasal bridge. The latter features may occur alone (ocular hypertelorism). Early operative intervention is indicated to remodel the lip and narrow the nose (Fig. 12-4). Nothing can be done to lessen the width between the eyes.

TUBULAR OR LATERAL NOSE.—Another rare anomaly is one in which a tubular appendage grows from the upper inner portion of the orbital roof (Fig. 12-5). Half of the nose on the same side is missing and the inner canthus is deformed. The free end of the trunk has a dimple in which hair is present, as in the vestibule of the nose. In the case illustrated, there was a cartilaginous bar from the orbital margin into the sausage-shaped mass. Various degrees of the condition may be

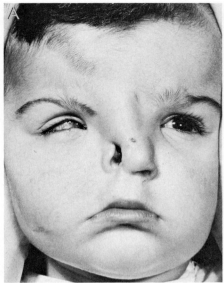

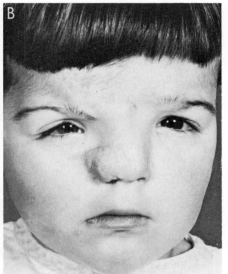

Fig. 12-2. — **A,** notching or coloboma of an ala. This uncommon deformity requires for its correction the addition of tissue trans- ferred from a distance. Small defects can be handled with a composite graft from the ear. **B,** after repair with a forehead flap.

Fig. 12-3 (left). — Double nose with median harelip. Note great distance between the eyes.

Fig. 12-4 (right). — Repair of double nose and midline harelip by excision of central cleft, forceful approximation of parts and addition of a forehead flap.

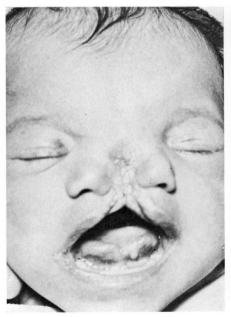

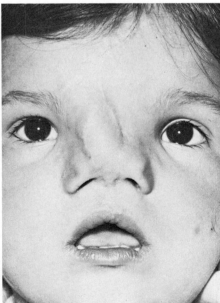

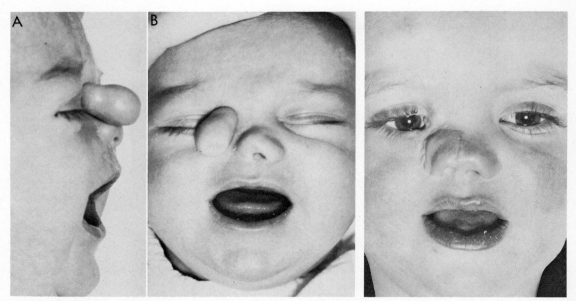

Fig. 12-5 (left).—A, tubular nose, with attachment to region of inner portion of superior orbital ridge. **B,** opposite side of the nose is normally formed.

Fig. 12-6 (right). — Repair of tubular nose by use of the tubular tissue from the orbital region.

seen, so that with hemiabsence of the nose a small amount of tissue may be present at the upper orbital ridge. It is possible to use this tissue in the nasal reconstruction (Fig. 12-6), although some surgeons prefer to discard it and to use a forehead flap.

Form.—The form of the nose is largely dependent on ancestry, so that the nasal types are legion. Whether or not extreme variations in form can be designated as defects worthy of operative reconstruction must be decided for each case individually. These

Fig. 12-7.—A, this boy of 12 has had lack of nasal septum support since infancy. The nose is broad and the tip lacks support. **B,** the central portion of the face appears to be underdeveloped.

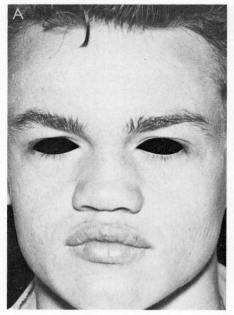
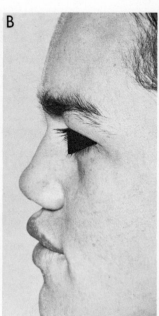

anomalies—hump nose, flared alae and others—are not dealt with in childhood unless they are extreme. One notable exception is *saddle nose* (Fig. 12-7), which may be congenital but is more likely acquired through unrecognized injury of the septum. It is thought that the development of the central portion of the face proceeds more normally when the nose is supported forward. A graft of bone or cartilage is used. From our experience, autogenous bone is perferred. The long limb of the graft becomes the bridge of the nose. It is supported above on the nasal bones and below by a short strut which rests in the region of the anterior nasal spine. Depending on the age at the time of operation, it may be necessary to repeat the procedure with growth.

DEFORMITIES CONCOMITANT WITH CLEFT LIP. — Nasal deformities accompany most single and double cleft lips. With the unilateral defects, the columella and the lower portion of the cartilaginous septum are deflected to the uncleft side with partial obstruction to the airway. The long axis of the nostril is transverse instead of oblique, and the alar cartilage on the cleft side is depressed and flared (Fig. 12-8). With double clefts, the commonest residual deformities are the short columella and flared nostrils.These deformities often require surgical correction later in life. If they are severe, the correction is performed in the preschool period, but if less severe, the correction is delayed until the age of 12 or 14. Many useful procedures have been described for their correction.

Injuries

Injury to the soft tissue only in the form of contusions, abrasions, lacerations, avulsions and burns may occur. The principles of treatment are largely the same in this area as elsewhere. The skin of the nose is molded tightly over the bony-cartilaginous framework with little intervening subcutaneous tissue. That over the upper portion is thin, while that over the tip is thick and well supplied with sebaceous glands. If parts are to be drawn together without deformity there can be no wide debridement of wounds. Cleansing in the usual fashion with minimal trimming is performed, followed by careful approximation of the wound edges with fine suture material. This should be placed intradermally or close to the wound margins. Otherwise, an undesirable ladderlike effect due to necrosis around sutures is produced, particularly in the skin over the lower part of the nose. If the laceration extends into the nasal cavity, additional absorbable sutures are used in the inner layer with knots on the mucous membrane surface. Care must be taken to remove foreign matter which may result in tattooing. If this is neglected, secondary operations of a more difficult nature (abrasion and excision) will be necessary later. Postoperatively the incision should be kept free from blood clot or crusting.

Skin may be raised in flaps (trap-door laceration) which on replacement and healing tend to heap up. Fragmentation of shatterproof glass in automobile

Fig. 12-8.—**A,** previously repaired double cleft of lip, showing the short columella and splayed nostrils. **B,** previously repaired unilateral cleft, showing residual nasal deformity commonly seen —splayed alar cartilage on the cleft side and deviation of the tip of the septum and columella to the uncleft side.

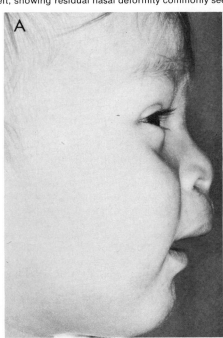
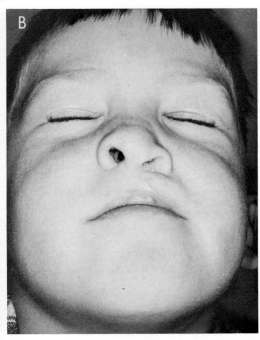

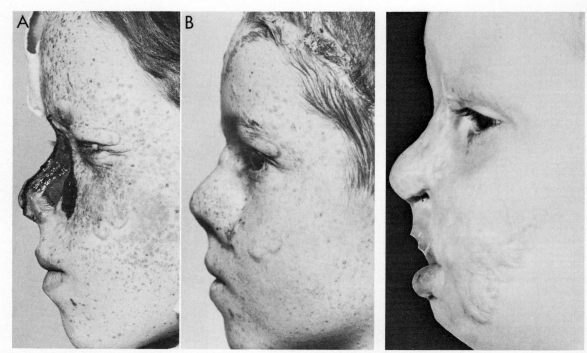

Fig. 12-9 (left). — **A,** loss of a large portion of the nose due to a dog bite. **B,** immediate result after repair by means of a forehead flap.

Fig. 12-10 (right). — Healing after deep second-degree burn. Contracture obliterates the normal contour between nose and surrounding areas — lips, cheeks and forehead.

accidents frequently produces lacerations of this variety. Secondary revisionary procedures often are necessary. For small lesions, excision with direct suture may be satisfactory. For larger lesions, different procedures may be used, including interruption of the line of contracture with various plastic maneuvers (e.g., z-plasty), excision with grafting, or the removal and replacement of the skin after flattening of the base by excision of excess subcutaneous tissue.

Skin may be missing. Replacement by split- or full-thickness skin grafts gives satisfactory coverage. If small portions of the tip or alae are missing, free composite grafts from the ear may be considered as an immediate or secondary procedure. For larger defects (Fig. 12-9), subtotal or total nasal reconstruction is necessary. Such losses in children may be due to the violence of motor vehicle accidents and occasionally to animal bites.

Skin loss due to burning is quite common. A deep partial thickness loss will leave bands of contracture extending from the nose to the forehead, cheeks and lips (Fig. 12-10). If these are not severe, rearrangements of the local tissues by standard plastic procedures may suffice. If they are severe, replacement by extensive split-skin grafting is indicated. The patchy appearance resulting from multiple small grafts is less attractive than when such an area is completely replaced.

Total skin loss due to burning is not uncommon and is dealt with by split-skin grafts as soon as the surface is suitable. Subtotal or total nasal loss from burns with survival is rare in children. This type of injury has been seen in epileptics who fall against a hot stove or into an open fireplace during a seizure.

FRACTURES. — The combination of soft tissue, cartilaginous and bone injury is more common. It may be confined to the nose or may be part of a more extensive lesion involving fractures of the facial bones, such as those that occur in motor vehicle collisions. If the child has a history of nasal injury associated with soft tissue swelling and bleeding from the nose, a fracture is most likely to have occurred. If cartilaginous or bony deformity is left unreduced, it may become more apparent with growth and later in life may require procedures for relief of nasal obstruction and reshaping of the nose. Because of this possibility, such injuries should not be neglected. Initially, the displacement can be easily corrected by simple manipulations, and no complicated splinting is necessary. Elevation of the nasal bones with replacement of the frontal processes of the maxillas and the shifting of the septum to the midline is usually all that is required. On occasion, this may be supplemented by light nasal packing for a short period.

Nasal injuries rarely occur at birth. The cartilaginous septum may be dislocated from the anterior nasal spine. If this is recognized, the deformity should be corrected by manipulation before the healing process leads to consolidation of the tissues in the displaced position.

All patients with such injuries should be referred immediately to those competent to diagnose and treat them.

The nasal damage may be part of a more extensive lesion with smashed facial bones. There may be associated injuries to the brain, the orbit and to the lacrimal apparatus. These require early referral to specialists trained in this type of work. Consolidation of the tissues in the deformed position with the overproduction of bone takes place particularly rapidly in children. Unless contraindicated by the general condition of the patient, the replacement and splinting of the parts in their anatomic position should be planned immediately. Complicated external appliances attached to plaster head caps are of little use for children. They require the use of apparatus which does not interfere with the general activities and which cannot shift or be tampered with by the child. This implies internal fixation of fragments by fine wire or the use of padded lead or aluminum buffers held in position by through-and-through wire sutures. These hold the nasal and lacrimal bones and the frontal processes of the maxillas in their proper positions during healing. Late operations for the correction of any deformity which may result from unreduced displacement of bone, particularly in relation to the medial orbital rim, are difficult to perform and give results which are less than ideal.

Infections

Infections are dealt with in texts on rhinology and do not normally come under the purview of the surgeon. A chronic infective lesion of a nonspecific nature occasionally occurs in infants in the region of the columella and can result in complete loss of the tissues in the area (Fig. 12-11). After the lesion has become quiescent, repair is effected by plastic reconstruction.

Tumors, Nevi and Cysts

Benign tumors of the nose arise chiefly from the soft tissues.

SINUSES AND CYSTS.—Dermoid cysts and sinuses are not infrequently found along developmental fusion lines. The most common of these are in the midline along the dorsum of the nose (Fig. 12-12). If a sinus is present, hairs growing from the wall of the cyst may protrude. A few cysts are superficial, but most of them are situated deeply in a cavity in the septal cartilage and communicate with the surface via a sinus. Occasionally, a mass is present which communicates with the dura through a defect in the skull (encephalocele). These tumors should be removed early in life as they tend to become infected and are then more difficult to handle.

HEMANGIOMAS.—Hemangiomas not uncommonly involve the nose in children. There are many varieties of these blood vessel anomalies. The treatment of these lesions is dealt with elsewhere.

Nevus flammeus or port-wine stain usually affects other portions of the face in addition to the nose. If such an area is small and confined to the nose (which is unlikely), it may be excised and replaced by local flaps or a free graft. Tattooing has been used, but the results are still equivocal. By this method, pigment is placed in the dermis with the hope that it will act as a permanent cover of the birthmark. Other forms of local treatment of the skin (carbon dioxide snow, frostbite) leave scars which are little more attractive than the original lesion, and at the same time the wearing qualities of the skin are materially reduced. Various cosmetics have been developed which in females give a fairly satisfactory disguise.

The so-called *strawberry nevus* has a bright red, slightly raised surface. The natural history for most of these is of increasing size for a few months, followed by cessation of spread and slow involution. Occasionally, such a lesion will increase quickly in size. Ulceration of the central portion will commence and spread rapidly. When this occurs on the nose, the tissue loss may be so serious as to necessitate a total nasal reconstruction (Fig. 12-13). Therefore, if the growth appears to be spreading rapidly, some form of treatment should be instituted to bring it under control. The methods include surgical excision with grafting, electrocoagulation, carbon dioxide snow freezing and radiation. Radiation carries the danger of permanently slowing the rate of growth of the tissues affected. While the initial result may be satisfactory, great distortion can make its appearance with the passage of years. It should be used only by those with experience, the dosage being kept to a minimum.

The *cavernous hemangioma* is a mass of vasoformative tissue in the subcutaneous area often accompanied by some skin involvement (Fig. 12-14). The natural history is of a few weeks or months of growth followed by a slow retrogression which may be complete or may leave some discoloration and redundancy of tissue. A large, fast-growing mass may be excised or treated by electrocoagulation, injection of sclerosing solutions or by radiation. Residual deformities can be dealt with by secondary operative procedures.

The so-called *spider nevi* are a form of hemangioma which are quite common on the nose of children. They may disappear spontaneously. If they re-

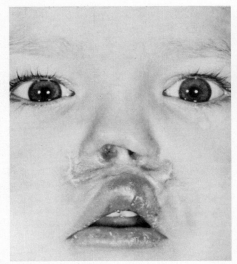
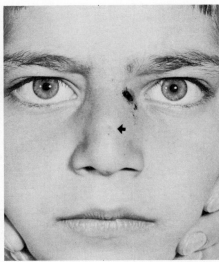

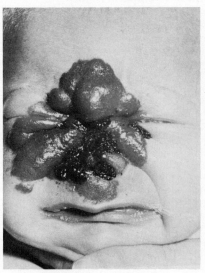
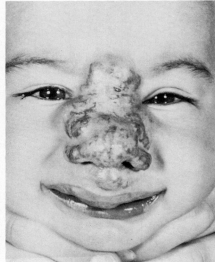
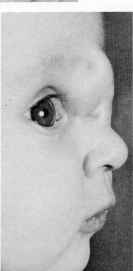

Fig. 12-11 (above left).—Destruction of columella by nonspecific infection.

Fig. 12-12 (above right).—Dermoid cyst of nose. A dimple **(arrow)** is present in the midline. A discharging sinus developed near the medial commissure of the eye which communicated with a cyst high in the nose.

Fig. 12-13 (below left).—Occasionally, rapid lysis occurs in a hemangiomatous area. In this case, there was total destruction of the nose.

Fig. 12-14 (below center).—Hemangioma involving all of the covering of the nose. The tumor is slowly regressing.

Fig. 12-15 (below right).—Fibrosarcoma of the nose commencing in the region of the glabella.

main, however, for many months or years and present a defect to appearance, they may readily be ablated by electrocoagulation of the central area with a fine needle. Such nevi occasionally present a problem in children due to troublesome bleeding when traumatized by scratching.

Pigmented nevi may be present at birth on the nose as elsewhere. When removal is indicated due to change in characteristics of the mole or solely due to

appearance, surgical excision is the method of choice. As there is little loose skin on the nose, direct suture is rarely possible. A full-thickness graft from either the postauricular or the supraclavicular region is employed. Small raised intradermal nevi may be treated by electrocoagulation.

WARTS.—Warts may occur around the nares in children. If they do not respond to medicants employed by the dermatologist, they may be removed by electrocautery under local anaesthesia or nonexplosive general anaesthesia.

TUMORS.—Malignant tumors of the nose are extremely rare in children. We have seen squamous cell carcinoma in a child of 4 years. This was assumed to have arisen from the tissue in the region of the anterior nasal spine or the buccal sulcus above the incisor teeth. It involved the nose and mouth. *Fibrosarcoma* commencing in the region of the glabella (Fig. 12-15) was also seen, in an infant under 1 year of age. These must be regarded as rare occurrences.

Juvenile angiofibroma is a peculiar type of tumor which occurs in the region of the facial bones in children. Most cases come to the attention of the rhinologist first because of epistaxis or nasal obstruction. Occasionally, the first sign is painless swelling in the region of the frontal process of the maxilla. It occurs chiefly in males. While this tumor may infiltrate locally and displace tissues, it does not metastasize. It tends to retrogress after all body growth has ceased. Its removal may present difficulties, but surgery alone with use of electrocoagulation with or without subsequent irradiation can be successfully employed.

REFERENCES

1. Boo-Chai, K.: The bifid nose: With a report of three cases in siblings, Plast. & Reconstruct. Surg. 36:626, 1965.
2. Borsony, S.: Nasal glioma, Arch. Otolaryng. 72:376, 1960.
3. Boyle, T. M., *et al.*: The management of nasopharyngeal chordoma by repeated irradiation, J. Laryng. & Otol. 80:533, 1966.
4. Brauer, R. O., *et al.*: Another method to lengthen the columella in the double cleft patient, Plast. & Reconstruct. Surg. 38:27, 1966.
5. Brown, R. F.: A re-appraisal of the cleft lip nose with the report of a case, Brit. J. Plast. Surg. 17:168, 1964.
6. Canick, M. L.: Major soft tissue injuries to the nose, Plast. & Reconstruct. Surg. 32:549, 1963.
7. Champion, R.: Reconstruction of the columella, Brit. J. Plast. Surg. 12:353, 1960.
8. Coetzee, T.: Proboscis lateralis: A rare facial anomaly, South African J. Lab. & Clin. Med. 10:81, 1964.
9. Crawford, H. R., *et al.*: Congenital choanal atresia, South. M. J. 58:1402, 1965.
10. Crosby, J. F.: Unusual nasal tumors in children: Gliomas and rhabdomyosarcoma, Plast. & Reconstruct. Surg. 19:143, 1957.
11. Deutsch, H. J.: Intranasal glioma, Ann. Otol., Rhin. & Laryng. 74:637, 1965.
12. Esser, E.: Median fissure of the nose, Plast. Chir. 1:40, 1939.
13. Fogh-Andersen, P.: Rare clefts of the face, Acta chir. scandinav. 129:275, 1965.
14. Friedberg, S. A.: Vascular fibroma of nasopharynx (nasopharyngeal fibroma), Arch. Otolaryng. 31:313, 1940.
15. Gibson, T.: Early free grafting: The restitution of parts completely separated from the body, Brit. J. Plast. Surg., 18:1, 1965.
16. Glanz, S.: Hypertelorism and the bifid nose, South. M. J. 59:631, 1966.
17. Jennes, M. L.: Corrective nasal surgery in children: Long term results, Arch. Otolaryng. 79:145, 1964.
18. Kazanjian, V. H.: Treatment of dermoid cysts of the nose, Plast. & Reconstruct. Surg. 21:169, 1958.
19. Klaff, D. D.: Surgical correction of septal deformation in newborn infants and children, South. M. J. 58:1276, 1965.
20. Littlewood, A. H. M.: Congenital nasal dermoid cysts and fistulae, Brit. J. Plast. Surg. 150:1007, 1959.
21. McGillicuddy, O. B.: Encephalomeningoceles in the nasal cavities, Ann. Otol., Rhin. & Laryng. 51:516, 1942.
22. McGovern, F. H., and Fitz-Hugh, G. S.: Surgical management of congenital choanal atresia, Arch. Otolaryng. 73:627, 1961.
23. McLean, G. E.; Broadbent, R. F., and Wolff, R. M.: Dermoid cysts of the nose, Ann. Surg. 30:203, 1964.
24. Marcks, K. M., *et al.*: Nasal defects associated with cleft lip deformity, Plast. & Reconstruct. Surg. 34:176, 1964.
25. Millard, D. R., Jr.: The unilateral cleft lip nose, Plast. & Reconstruct. Surg. 34:176, 1964.
26. Nydell, C. C., Jr., and Masson, J. K.: Dermoid cysts of the nose: A review of 39 cases, Ann. Surg. 150:1007, 1959.
27. Paletta, F. X., and Van Norman, R. T.: Total reconstruction of the columella, Plast. & Reconstruct. Surg. 30:322, 1962.
28. Pratt, L. W.: Midline cysts of the nasal dorsum: Embryologic origin and treatment, Laryngoscope 75:968, 1965.
29. Rees, T. D., *et al.*: Repair of the cleft lip nose: Addendum to the synchronous technique with full thickness skin grafting of the nasal vestibule, Plast. & Reconstruct. Surg. 37:47, 1966.
30. Riggs, R. H.: Pediatric nasal surgery, J. Louisiana M. Soc. 115:329, 1963.
31. Smith, K. R., Jr., *et al.*: Nasal gliomas, J. Neurosurg. 20:968, 1963.
32. Webster, J. P., and Deming, E. G.: The surgical treatment of the bifid nose, Plast. & Reconstruct. Surg. 6:1, 1950.

A. W. FARMER

13

Cleft Lip

HISTORY.—A list of only the names associated with the development of cleft lip repair would be an extensive history of itself. The list then would probably be unfair, as a little-noted or omitted contributor may have designed the basis for the next "new method of repair."

Without personal reference then, cleft lip repair until about 1840 consisted in excision of the cleft as a "V," with maintenance of approximated edges by "hare-lip pins." At the middle of the 19th century the surge of methods, designs and modifications began. The face and nose were mobilized to relieve the tension of the repair. Flaps, triangular and quadrilateral, were designed to give fullness to the vermilion and avoid the straight line scar. Shortly, anesthesia allowed the surgeon to use all of his skills, inventiveness and dreams of duplicating the normal. The possibilities of a superior repair by meticulous closure with fine sutures in layers now were recognized.

This century has been occupied with variations of these methods, refinement of techniques and improvement of individual skills. The goal remains the same: to duplicate the normal. The means to that end is use of the simple design that the surgeon can adapt with his variations to fit the individual deformity. Different methods, old and new, of repair are described in the literature.[1, 8, 11, 12, 15, 17-20] The method presented here is simple, adaptable and proved in long-term follow-up.

Embryology

The varieties of cleft lip are explainable from the embryologic development of the face and mouth (Fig. 13-1). The frontonasal process from above and the maxillary processes on each side surround a cavity which will form the mouth and nose after the second week of embryonic life. A central and two lateral processes develop from the lower end of the frontal process about the fifth week in embryo. The lateral nasal groove separates each lateral process or tubercle from the central. Later, two other tubercles develop on the lower border of the central processes separated from each other by a central groove. The forehead, external nose and central part of the lip will be formed from the frontonasal process and the nasal processes. The orbital fissure, extending into the mouth, separates the maxillary process from the lateral nasal and globular processes derived from the frontal. This fissure is joined in its lower part by the lateral nasal groove and together they make the Y-shaped cleft. The upper median limb of the Y, as described above, separates the lateral and central nasal processes while the single lower limb extends into the mouth and the upper lateral into the eye.

Cleft lip of any variety is produced by failure of closure by any part of the Y-shaped fissures, and this process is completed usually by the second embryonic month. There will be a cleft from the mouth through the lateral part of the upper lip to the eye if the maxillary fails to unite with the frontal process throughout

Fig. 13-1.—**Left,** drawing showing possibilities of facial and lip clefts. **Right,** head of fetus in 7th week. The central nasal processes are separated from the lateral on each side by the lateral nasal grooves, which represent the anterior nares. (Redrawn from Robinson, A. [ed.]: *Cunningham's Textbook of Anatomy*, 6th ed.; courtesy of Oxford University Press.)

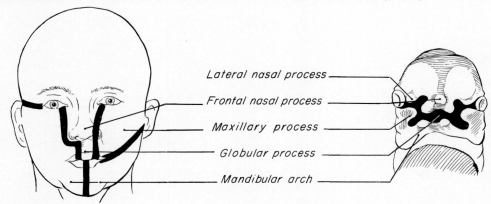

Lateral nasal process

Frontal nasal process

Maxillary process

Globular process

Mandibular arch

the extent of the fissure. The usual cleft lip results if the maxillary fails to unite with the globular process and the cleft extends through the lateral part of the lip to or into the floor of the nose. A midline cleft results if the two globular processes fail to unite. Macrostomia results from failure of closure of the lateral parts of the transverse mouth cleft.

Contributing Causes and Incidence

Heredity has a definite influence on the occurrence of cleft lip. Parents who have one child with a cleft lip are told their chances of having another are definitely greater in any future pregnancies. Often a carefully taken family history reveals some member with a cleft lip; it may be a distant relative. A mixed and changing population, as in the United States, makes prognosis as to cleft lip offspring in any family difficult. Fogh-Andersen[10] investigated cleft lip inheritance in a relatively closed population.

Nutrition of the mother during the first few weeks of pregnancy might be a possible cause. The number of clefts is greatly out of proportion, however, to those mothers who have nausea or vomiting or are in a poor nervous condition. *Vitamin* metabolism is receiving some emphasis and may well have more than a casual relationship.

Mechanical causes are a possibility to be considered. The tongue might fail to recede from its nasal position. Before the palatal ridges develop, the tongue occupies the whole mouth and nasal cavity.

Tumors, amniotic bands and adhesions occasionally are associated with clefts of the lip and other deformities.

Infection and injury are mentioned as possibilities.

Frequency is reported to vary from 1 in 500 to 1 in 1,000 live births. Cleft lip occurs more commonly in boys than in girls and more often on the left side than on the right, but the ratio between the sexes as to laterality is almost the same. Double clefts of the lip are about half as frequent as single clefts.

Preoperative Care and Time for Repair

The parents' acceptance of the infant with a cleft lip is of such importance that repair is done as soon after birth as possible. Repair may be done during the first few hours of life, although this is not the general policy. Postponement of the operation to make it technically easier for the surgeon is unwarranted. It is usually wise to wait until there is a progressive weight gain. Double clefts of the lip usually are repaired at about 1 month or when the infant weighs 10 lb.

Bleeding time, clotting time, hemoglobin, red and white cell counts and urinalysis are included in the general evaluation preoperatively. A normal feeding is given 6 hours before operation. Feeding can be done with a dropper. Gavage rarely is necessary. Infections of the skin and respiratory tract, fever, malnutrition and blood irregularities are contraindications to early operation, as may be the presence of other congenital abnormalities.

Methods of Repair

Simple measurable markings placed on a cleft lip allow the surgeon to plan accurately the details of repair. A small triangular flap just above the vermilion border saves the most lip, yet brings full thickness of lip together from both sides. Mirault[16] in 1845 described the use of a triangular flap, but though it is not clear from which side it came, it provoked thought. Blair and Brown[2] in 1930 published a method of marking, using the triangular flap. The "small triangular flap" with definite measurable marks was developed by Brown and McDowell.[3,4] These authors were the first to mention nasal deformities associated with cleft lip and to describe in detail their primary correction.

Hagedorn[11] in 1884 described another method for the repair of cleft lip (this method was later modified by Le Mesurier[12]). It involves the use of a quadrilateral flap cutting back into the substance of the lip. In recent years there has been a deluge of vague and many times overcomplicated modifications of this method.

A collective review by Davis[7] gives an excellent summary of progress beginning with the writings of Celsus and Galen.

Operation

Cleft lips are primarily repaired by following simple measurable markings on the lip and nose. Though what is available for repair is an important factor, by concentration and accuracy one can convert an acceptable into a superior result. *The method of repair should be fitted to the deformity rather than the reverse.* The aim is a normal lip. The objectives are: the alae of the nose should be symmetrical in curve, level and direction; the floor of the nose should be closed and the columella straight; the upper lip should be full and placed out ahead of the lower lip; the vermilion also should be full and smooth.

Anesthesia is most safely accomplished with ether by the open-drop method. Adequate depth of anesthesia can be maintained throughout the operation by blowing a mixture of ether vapor and oxygen in the region of the infant's nose and mouth. It produces a very light stage of anesthesia supplementing regional nerve block. Infraorbital procaine with epinephrine block makes deep anesthesia unnecessary as well as helping to control the bleeding. The airway is maintained throughout the operation and during the postoperative period by controlling the tongue by means of a suture placed after induction, and suction of the blood and other drainage from the hypopharynx.

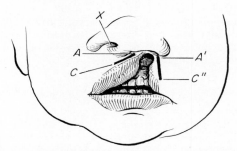

Fig. 13-2.—Cleft lip repair: the V-excision operation.

REPAIR OF UNILATERAL CLEFT LIP

V-EXCISION OPERATION (Fig. 13-2).—While the columella is held over straight, A is marked at the junction of the skin and vermilion at the level of the base of the columella. X is in the same relation to the columella on the sound side. A' bears the same relation to the ala on the cleft side that X bears to the ala on the normal side. C is on the mucocutaneous junction at the point where the vermilion first begins to thin out. C'' is on the mucocutaneous junction, the same distance from A' that C is from A. To perform the V-excision operation, A' is brought over to A and C'' to C, after excision of the edges of the cleft.

THE FLAP OPERATION (Fig. 13-3).—The V-excision operation is marked out first. c' is on the mucocutaneous junction at the most medial point of good full vermilion. b' is on the line $a'-c^2$, equidistant from c' and c^2. The incision is $a'-b'-c'$, saving the amount of lip indicated by the isosceles triangle. b is on the mucocutaneous junction, the same distance from c that b' is from c'.

The lip and nose are mobilized through incisions in the fornix. a, b, c and a', b', c' are incised. a and a' are approximated with a deep stitch of #0000 white silk with the knot tied on the mucosal side and a surface suture of #0000 black silk. b and b' are approximated with a fine deep white stitch and a black one on the surface. Intervening fine surface sutures are placed and an oblique cut is made in the vermilion flap from c'. For the incisions and fine trimming, very sharp scissors are most useful. c and c' are united and the vermilion flaps are interdigitated in a zigzag fashion, fitting them so that they lie naturally together without any pull or stretching. Suturing is then continued on around the vermilion border and up the inside to the fornix. The little flap in the nostril is trimmed to fit with the one from the opposite side, and they are sutured together to form the floor. A few key mattress sutures are placed through the ala to unite the lining and covering (which were separated during the undermining). The mucosal suturing is important and is done with fine interrupted stitches and careful trimming to fit the edges together. The upper corners are rounded somewhat, and the suturing is continued to pull some mucosa into the lip from either cheek. This advances the whole lip and thrusts it forward. If the superior edge of the mucosa is tight, vertical slits are made on either side and allowed to spread open.

REPAIR OF BILATERAL CLEFT LIP

SET-BACK OF PREMAXILLA.—When the premaxilla is too far forward to permit closure of the lip (Fig. 13-4), it may be set back by submucous excision of a block of bone from the vomer. This removal of a block, rather than a wedge, permits the pushing of it directly back like closing a drawer, rather than tilting it back. This factor is of some advantage, as the finished lip should slant forward in the profile view from above downward.

MEASUREMENTS AND MARKING.—With the columella in the midline, a transverse line is imagined across the prolabium at the level of the base of the columella, and the points a are marked on either side where this line crosses the mucocutaneous junction (Fig. 13-5). a' is marked just inside the lower point of the nostril rim on each lateral side of the cleft, being careful to place it in such position that a good nostril will be formed when a' is approximated to a, and marking it

Fig. 13-3.—Cleft lip repair: the flap operation.

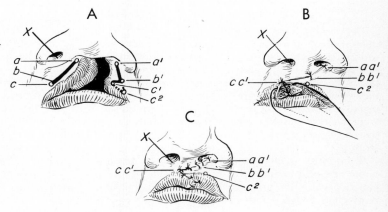

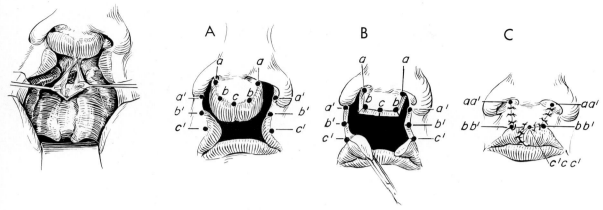

Fig. 13-4 (left).—Operation to set back premaxilla.
Fig. 13-5 (right).—Repair of bilateral cleft lip.

symmetrically on the two sides. The point c is at the bottom of the skin of the prolabium in the midline and equidistant from the two a points. b is one third the distance from c back to a on the curved lower border of the skin of the prolabium on either side. c' is on the mucocutaneous line of the lateral part of the lip and is opposite the most medial point where there is still full thickness of the vermilion. To locate b', the straight line distance ab is measured with small calipers. One point of the calipers is then set on a' and the calipers are rotated until the other point is bc distance from c. The above can be considered a standard marking and can be altered when necessary. For instance, when the cleft is partial on one side, the line $a'b'c'$ is sometimes a straight one, so that b' can be omitted and a straight incision made from a' to c' and a "V" closure done on that side.

The above points are punctured in and the lines scratched in with 5% alcoholic methylene blue, using a fine mechanical drawing pen. The lines are then lightly incised with a knife, with care not to cut the points out. An incision is then made in the buccal fornix on each side and carried upward to separate

the lip from the upper jaw. This undermining is carried upward almost to the orbital border until the cheek is separated from the underlying facial bones, and the space between them is packed temporarily with gauze soaked in 1:5,000 epinephrine solution. The buccal fornix incision is then carried upward inside the lateral wall of the nostril to divide the mucosa between the upper and lower lateral cartilages of the nose until the nostril can be rotated into position and a' can be brought over to a without tension. A small fine scissors is introduced through the buccal fornix and the lower lateral cartilage of the nostril is separated from the skin covering by alternate spreading and dissection up to the midline. The lines $a'b'c'$ (Fig. 13-5, B, C) are then incised through the full thickness of the lip, a stab blade knife being used with a perpendicular sawing motion. The small flap $a'b'c'$ is rotated 180 degrees into the nostril floor. The vermilion of the prolabium is turned backward as a flap to use for lining and $a-a'$ and $b-b'$ are approximated on both sides. $c-c'$ are approximated directly under c and fine interrupted black silk skin sutures are placed all along between $a-b-c$. The vermilion

Fig. 13-6.—**A,** complete cleft of lip, closed in one operation a few hours after birth. **B** and **C,** appearance 10 years later.

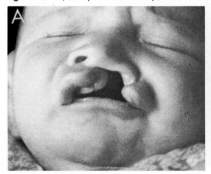 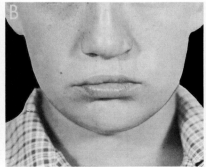 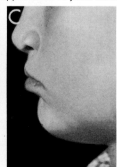

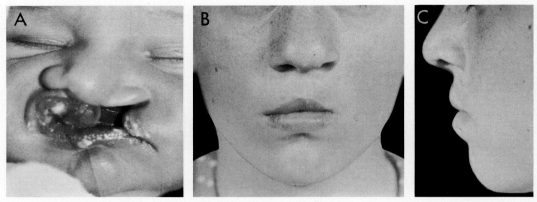

Fig. 13-7.—A, complete cleft of lip with marked deformity of nose, closed shortly after birth. **B** and **C,** appearance 15 years later.

closure is done by interdigitating zigzag flaps from the two sides. The inside mucosa from the two sides is sutured to the prolabium vermilion which was turned back. The nostril floor flaps are trimmed and sutured to the portion of the prolabial skin inside the nostrils. Stay sutures may be put clear across the lip from the inside, encompassing the full thickness of the lip except the skin, to avoid any visible suture marks on the outside.

The lip is marked with a small triangular flap just above the vermilion border to give proper direction and a flexion crease in its normal position. Other essentials are: adequate mobilization of the lip and nose; approximation of squarely cut raw surfaces by fine deep sutures and in the skin close to the edges of the wound, and careful closure of the mucosa. Results of following these simple directions are shown in Figures 13-6 to 13-8.

Mobilization of the lip and nose is done through incisions in the upper fornix, after the markings have

been placed in the lip and lightly incised. The lip must be loose enough to heal with fine approximating sutures. Mobilization of the nose can be done through the fornix and allows the skin to slide on the cartilages and be later rolled into a tube at the proper level and direction without external incisions.

Closure of the lip is done after the incised markings are cut through the full thickness of the lip, including the mucosal lining. Fine silk deep sutures are placed in the floor of the nose approximating a to a' and b to b'. Fine black silk sutures placed close to the edges of the skin are not tied tightly but are meant only to hold in approximation. Small flaps of vermilion are interdigitated after c has been closed to c'. The mucosal lining is closed as carefully as the skin edges. Both sides of the lip, skin, vermilion and mucosa must fit together—pulling or stretching is unnecessary. The mucosal closure everts the lip, gives it natural bulk and, because of the small flap above the vermilion border, produces a natural

Fig. 13-8.—A, complete double cleft of lip, closed in one operation after repositioning of prolabial segment, as shown in Figure 13-5. **B,** appearance 18 years later. Major nasal shaping was done at the original operation.

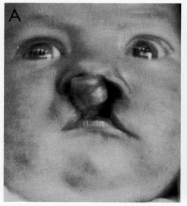

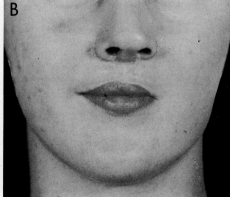

flexion crease. Rotation of the nose into a tube is stabilized by a few mattress sutures placed through the ala and lining.

Double cleft lips are closed in the same manner, uniting previously incised points, after similar mobilization. The varieties of clefts,[5] since they may be asymmetrical, may be more accurately repaired as two single clefts, though both sides are closed at the same time. Complete cleft on one side and incomplete cleft on another may be marked out as a single cleft on the complete side and as a "V" on the incomplete, when a flap above the vermilion border is not available. Whenever possible it is desirable to accomplish the repair of the double cleft lip in one operation for obvious reasons. The general condition of the infant may make this impossible; in this case, of course, it should be done in stages. Too, the particular deformity may require more than one operation to secure the best ultimate result. The trend now seems to be toward a single operative procedure.

Closure of the anterior part of the palate is not done at this time since it may disturb dentition.

POSTOPERATIVE CARE.—Careful observation during the immediate postoperative period is necessary to avoid airway obstruction. Positioning the infant on its side allows proper drainage that may be supplemented by suction if necessary. The hemoglobin and red cell count are checked and fluids and blood replaced as indicated. The suture line should be carefully cleaned at short intervals during this immediate period and regularly after that to promote healing. Feeding, first with sweetened water, is started when the infant can swallow. A dropper is used for the first 7 to 10 days, then a soft nipple is acceptable.

SECONDARY REPAIR OF CLEFT LIPS

Improvements in the lip or nose are made when indicated. Deformities which may increase with growth are surgically corrected as they appear.

Imbalance between the lips usually is correctable by orthodontia, advancement of the lip, or a cross-lip flap. Prosthodontia may be necessary. Figure 13-9 shows balance obtainable by local advancement of the upper lip and avoidance of a cross-lip flap.

Deformities of the nose can be improved at any time, but major surgical alterations are better done after growth of the feature is complete, as shown in Figure 13-10.

Deficiency of the columella is usual in a complete double cleft lip. Occasionally, sufficient height may develop, but usually release of the tip of the nose is necessary when the child is around 3 or 4 years old. A result of this operation is shown in Figure 13-11 with persistence in growth.

Figure 13-12 illustrates, in diagram form, the several steps in the operation to elongate the columella by means of a flap developed from the upper lip.

Marked imbalance between the lips often cannot be improved satisfactorily with tissue available in the upper lip. Advancement of the upper on itself as was done in Figure 13-9 is not possible. The patient in Figure 13-13 was improved by taking excess bulk out of the lower lip and switching it into the upper lip, as

Fig. 13-9.—**A** and **C,** cleft lip repaired primarily elsewhere. **B** and **D,** demonstration of possibilities of secondary repair of lip and nose in one operation. Contour of nose and balance of lips improved without further addition of scars.

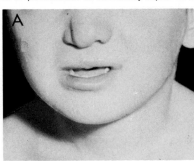
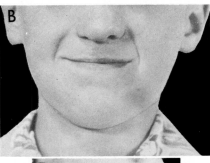
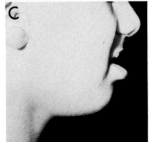
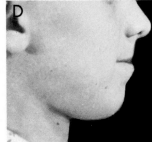

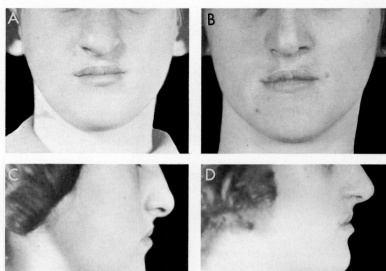

Fig. 13-10.—A and C, acceptable primary repair of cleft lip marred by growth of the nose. B and D, cut-down and shortening of nose relieved "snarling" appearance which annoyed the patient more than the repaired lip.

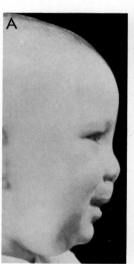
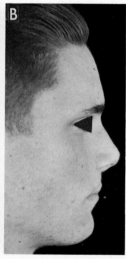

Fig. 13-11.—A, double cleft of lip with acceptable primary repair. Deficiency of columella, present at birth, was exaggerated with growth. Columella elongation (Fig. 13-12) was done when the child was about 4. B, appearance 12 years later.

Fig. 13-12.—Columella elongation out of upper lip. A, flap is outlined in upper lip and elevated. B, tip of nose is mobilized to allow nose to come up out of lip. C, flap is fitted into defect in columella region and sutured. D, E and F, upper lip can be closed or full-thickness skin graft used to cover defect. Transverse incisions in the floor of the nose shorten the lip and add bulk to the elevated tip.

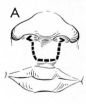 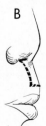 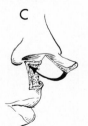 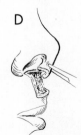 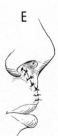 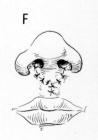

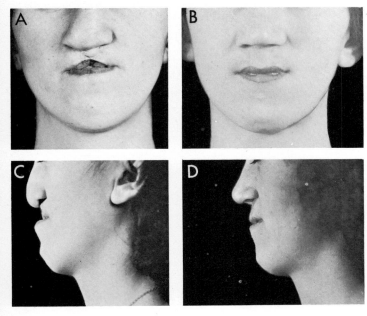

Fig. 13-13.—Deficient double cleft of lip primarily repaired elsewhere. **A** and **C**, marked columella and upper lip deficiency. Columella elongation was done as shown in Figure 13-12. Cross-lip flap, using bulk of protuberant lower lip, was brought into upper lip, as in Figure 13-14. **B** and **D**, balance between lips improved.

a cross-lip flap. In general, this can be accomplished in two operations: the first to open the upper lip and set a designed flap from the lower lip into the defect. After the blood supply has become established, the pedicle can be cut at a second operation, as illustrated in Figure 13-14.

REFERENCES

1. Bell, B.: *System of Surgery* (Edinburgh: Charles Elliott, 1787), Vol. 4, p. 136.
2. Blair, V. P., and Brown, J. B.: Mirault operation for single harelip, Surg., Gynec. & Obst. 51:81, 1930.
3. Brown, J. B., and McDowell, F.: Simplified design for repair of single cleft lips, Surg., Gynec. & Obst. 80:12, 1945.
4. Brown, J. B., and McDowell, F.: Small triangular flaps for the primary repair of single cleft lips, Plast. & Reconstruct. Surg. 5:392, 1950.
5. Brown, J. B.; McDowell, F., and Byars, L. T.: Double clefts of lip, Surg., Gynec. & Obst. 85:20, 1947.
6. Bryant, J. D.: *Operative Surgery* (New York: D. Appleton & Co., 1899).
7. Davis, A. D.: Management of the wide unilateral cleft lip with nostril deformity, Plast. & Reconstruct. Surg. 8:249, 1951.
8. Dieffenbach, J. F.: *Die operative Chirurgie* (Leipzig: F. A. Bockhaus, 1845).
9. Esmarch, F., and Kowalzig, J.: *Surgical Technic* (1st ed. in English; New York: Macmillan Company, 1901).
10. Fogh-Andersen, P.: *Inheritance of Harelip and Cleft Palate* (Copenhagen: Arnold Busck, 1942), p. 39.
11. Hagedorn, A.: A modification of cleft lip operation, Zentralbl. Chir. 11:756, 1884.
12. Le Mesurier, A. B.: Method of cutting and suturing lip in

Fig. 13-14.—Correction of imbalance between lips. **A,** upper lip is opened and desired bulk outlined, taking care to preserve labial artery from one side. **B, C** and **D,** lower lip flap is set into defect in upper lip with blood supply maintained by small artery-carrying pedicle. **E,** 3 weeks later, the pedicle is cut and vermilion closure completed.

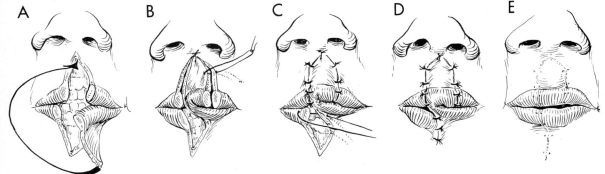

treatment of complete unilateral clefts, Plast. & Reconstruct. Surg. 4:1, 1949.

13. McDowell, F.: Late results in cleft lip repairs, Plast. & Reconstruct. Surg. 38:5, 1966.

14. McDowell, F.; Brown, J. B., and Fryer, M. P.: *Surgery of the Face, Mouth, and Jaws* (St. Louis: C. V. Mosby Company, 1954).

15. Millard, D. R.: Primary Camouflage in Unilateral Harelip, in Skoog, T. (ed.): *Transactions of the First International Congress of Plastic Surgery* (Baltimore: Williams & Wilkins Company, 1957), p. 162.

16. Mirault, G.: Deux lettres sur l'operation du bec-de-lièvre considéré dans ses divers états de simplicité, J. chir. 2:257, 1844; 3:5, 1845.

17. Rose, W.: *On Harelip and Cleft Palate* (London: H. K. Lewis & Co., Ltd., 1891).

18. Schmid, E.: Die Annäherung der Kieferstúmpfe bei Lippen-Kiefer-Gaumenspalten, Fortschr. Kiefer Gesichts. Chir. 1:37, 1955.

19. Tennison, C. W.: Repair of unilateral cleft lip by stencil method, Plast. & Reconstruct. Surg. 9:116, 1952.

M. P. Fryer
J. B. Brown

Drawings by
MURIEL MCLATCHIE MILLER

14

Cleft Palate

HISTORY. — The condition of cleft palate has been recognized for centuries. The history of its treatment is one of continued improvement. As early as the 16th Century these defects were covered or filled with artificial materials, and by the 18th Century the palate had been closed by suture after cauterization. Throughout the 19th Century, even before general anesthesia became available in 1869, efforts were directed toward obtaining adequate lateral relaxation to obtain good midline healing. This culminated in 1861 in the work of Von Langenbeck,[37] who used lateral release incisions and hamular infractions, adding to this elevation of full-thickness and mucoperiosteal flaps and attachment of these flaps to the denuded nasal septum. These techniques improved healing.

During the present century, efforts stimulated originally by Veau[36] have been directed toward making the palate as long as possible, or the velopharyngeal space as small as possible; and improved speech has resulted.

Dental specialists have worked to improve the esthetic and functional end-results of the cleft palate treatment. Speech therapists have developed effective techniques. The care of the cleft palate patient has moved into the realm of rehabilitation medicine, where efforts to integrate the work of the medical and paramedical workers have continued to improve the outlook for these patients. Geneticists and epidemiologists have done more investigation on this than on any other anomaly.

Throughout the years, physical reconstruction has been improved greatly; morbidity and mortality have decreased and become negligible. Speech has improved, but not to the same degree. A significant number of patients with stigmatized speech remain.

Embryology and Development

The development of the whole palate requires a consideration of two areas: the prepalate (primary or labial palate) and the palate proper (secondary or oral palate).

PREPALATE. — The prepalate is related to the development of the face, lips, premaxilla and upper four incisor teeth, that is, the region anterior to the incisive foramen. Development commences during the fourth week of gestation and is completed by the seventh week. There are both classic and modern theories of embryology for this region.

The classic 19th Century treatise of His[17] described the normal development as taking place from masses of ectoderm and mesoderm termed processes, three paired lateral and one central. These processes enlarge, grow together and fuse by ectodermal breakdown. Clefts occur when the mechanism of ectodermal breakdown and fusion is halted. This theory is now considered inadequate because it does not explain some of the variables found in this region such as Simonard's membrane.

The modern 20th Century theory, suggested by Streeter[35] and proved in detail by Stark,[32,33] describes this general region developing between the primitive oral cavity below and the primitive nasal pits above as a series of mesodermal masses underlying ectoderm in such a way as to form furrows. More specifically, the epithelial anlage of the upper lip and premaxilla contains three masses of mesoderm. Each mesoderm mass undergoes a differential surging growth to join the others to form a lip and premaxilla. The process is not one of ectodermal breakdown and classic process fusion. An absence or a decrease in mass volume of either lateral mesodermal mass volume results in some degree of unilateral or bilateral clefting of the lip and the lateral incisor regions of the alveolus. A similar deficiency in the central of the three mesodermal masses results in the rare clefting of the median lip and central alveolar region.

PALATE PROPER.—The palate proper is related to the development of the hard palate, soft palate, uvula and maxillary teeth—the region posterior to the incisive foramen. Development commences during the sixth week of gestation and is completed by 8½ weeks. The newer concepts of mesodermal penetration do not apply. This region develops bilaterally from the palatal processes or plates of the maxillary bones which become prominent during the sixth to seventh weeks, by which time the prepalate has formed. They extend from the prepalate to the tonsillar pillars and hang vertically beside the tongue. Between the eighth and ninth weeks the palatal processes commence positional change from the vertical to the horizontal plane which progresses in a wavelike fashion in a posteroanterior direction under the control of an intrinsic shelf force.[14,38] For a time, the palatal shelves are kept apart by the tongue, but as the tongue lowers in the floor of the mouth and moves forward, the two palatal plates fuse. Alterations of shelf force produce abnormal degrees of palatal arching. Failure of the tongue to lower produces palatal clefts. The best clinical example of this is found in the Pierre Robin syndrome,[10] in which the combined tongue and palate abnormalities are obvious.

Classification

ANATOMIC CLASSIFICATION.—Davis and Ritchie,[7] Veau[36] and others have described anatomic methods of classification. It is common today to refer to: an isolated cleft lip; a cleft lip and cleft palate, unilateral or bilateral, complete or incomplete; and an isolated cleft palate. These methods give little consideration to the alveolus.

EMBRYOLOGIC CLASSIFICATION.—The progress of epidemiologic studies, the need for uniformity of reporting results and the demand for detailed consideration of degree of involvement have led to an embryologic system of classification. The following system of classification is recommended for the future, and the reader should refer to the original papers[2,34] for details.

Clefts of prepalate (primary palate):
   Cleft lip:
      Unilateral; right, left; extent 1/3, 2/3, 3/3.
      Bilateral; right, left; extent 1/3, 2/3, 3/3.
      Median; extent 1/3, 2/3, 3/3.
      Congenital scars.
   Cleft alveolar process:
      Unilateral; right, left; extent 1/3, 2/3, 3/3.
      Bilateral; right, left; extent 1/3, 2/3, 3/3.
      Median; right, left; extent 1/3, 2/3, 3/3.
      Submucous; right, left, median.
   Cleft lip and alveolar process:
      Any combination of foregoing types.
      Premaxilla protrusion; slight, moderate, marked, none.
      Premaxilla rotation; right, left, slight, moderate, marked, none.
      Developmental arrestive prepalate; slight, moderate, marked, total.

Clefts of palate (secondary palate):
   Cleft soft palate; extent, palatal shortness, submucous (occult) cleft.
   Cleft hard palate; extent, vomer attachment, submucous (occult) cleft.
   Cleft soft and hard palate.

Clefts of prepalate and palate (cleft primary and secondary palate):
   Any combination listed under clefts of prepalate and clefts of palate.

Facial clefts other than prepalatal and palatal:
   Mandibular process clefts—including mandibular lip pits.
   Nasal—ocular clefts.
   Oral—ocular clefts.

OTHER CONDITIONS PRODUCING CLEFT PALATE SPEECH.—These include congenital short palate and submucous (occult) cleft palate, both included in the above classification; congenital suprabulbar paresis,[42] acquired palatopharyngeal paresis, diphtheritic and poliomyelitic; congenital absence of tonsillar pillars; changes following tonsillectomy and adenoidectomy; surgical and traumatic loss of palatal and/or pharyngeal tissue; and mimicry of others.

Applied Anatomy

Surgery carried out on a cleft palate patient is concerned primarily with the anatomy of the hard and soft palates, while improvement of speech and total rehabilitation of a patient with cleft palate is concerned, in addition, with the anatomy of the prepalate, the tongue, the nasal pharynx and the oral pharynx.

NORMAL PREPALATE.—The prepalate is covered with mucous membrane which is continuous with that of the palate proper behind, forms the gingiva in front and is densely adherent to the periosteum above. The bone is the premaxilla and composes that portion of the hard palate anterior to the incisive foramen. It thickens in front to form the alveolus, which contains the upper four incisor teeth.

CLEFT PREPALATE.—Prepalatal clefts (Fig. 14-1) are usually associated with vertical lip scars or cleft lips of any degree and may involve alveolar deficiencies varying from a missing lateral incisor tooth in the second dentition to partial or complete clefts of the alveolus unilaterally or bilaterally, to complete absence of the premaxilla (the rare condition of median cleft). The premaxilla, in bilateral complete clefts, will be mobile; and often it is protrusive, since it is attached only by the vomerine or the prevomerine[1] bone.

Fig. **14-1.**—Examples of types of cleft palate: plaster models from dental impressions under 3 months of age. **A,** cleft of prepalate, left, incomplete. **B,** cleft of prepalate, median, complete. **C,** cleft of prepalate, right, complete, and cleft palate, incomplete. **D,** cleft of prepalate and palate, left, complete. **E,** cleft of prepalate, and palate, bilateral, complete; moderate projection of premaxilla and rotation to right. **F,** cleft of palate involving uvula, soft palate and posterior two thirds of hard palate proper.

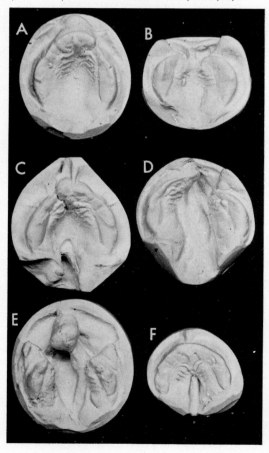

With growth, there will be localized dental disturbance depending on the severity of the prepalatal cleft, manifested by malformation and rotation of the teeth adjacent to the cleft and frequently by the presence of supernumerary teeth in the deciduous dentition and the absence of teeth in the permanent dentition.[20]

NORMAL PALATE.—The palate proper consists of a hard palate, soft palate and uvula. The hard palate is covered with mucous membrane which forms rugae on its surface and meets in the midline as a ridge or raphe and which is continuous with the mucous membrane of the prepalate in front and the soft palate behind. The mucous membrane contains mucus-secreting glands. It is continuous laterally with the gingiva of the maxillary teeth.

Normally, the palatine bones are horizontal with a slight transverse arching. Each is continuous laterally with the maxillary alveolus and superiorly with the vomerine bone in the midline. Posterolaterally, each is separated by a fissure from the pterygoid bone of its side. Each posterior border contains a large and a small foramen for the greater and lesser palatine nerves and vessels.

The soft palate is covered with glandular mucous membrane on both its oral and nasal surfaces, both being continuous with mucous membrane of the oral and nasal cavities. It is firmly fixed to the posterior border of the hard palate and to the maxillary tuberosities by the palatine aponeurosis. It is suspended from the side walls of the posterior oronasal cavities by the tendons of the tensor palatine muscles curving around the hamulus and by the loose areolar attachment of the levator palatine to the medial pterygoid muscle and its fibrous attachments to the eustachian tubes. It has mobile suspension from the lateral and posterior pharyngeal walls and tongue by the palatopharyngeal and palatoglossal muscles. The bulk of the soft palate is made up of mucous membrane and the paired tensor palatine and levator palatine muscles which have their broad origins on the base of the skull on the pterygomandibular ligament and the eustachian tubes and which insert into the midline raphe of the soft palate and the palatine aponeurosis.

All muscles except one are native and are supplied by the same nerve—the accessory nerve via the pharyngeal plexus. The tensor palatine muscles are migrant and are supplied by the mandibular (V3) nerve via the otic ganglion.[15] The blood supply is primarily from the posterior palatine arteries.

The uvula is a midline mass of mucous membrane that contains the small uvulis muscle which appears to have little function and no homologue.

HIGH ARCHED PALATE.—Variation in the transverse arching of the palate is common. Thus the high arched palate is frequently a normal anatomic variation. But it is often associated with submucous cleft palate, craniostenosis and choanal atresia. It is probably due to failure of the complete positional change of the palatine bones from the vertical to the horizontal plane between the sixth and seventh weeks of gestation.

PREPALATAL-PALATAL CLEFTS. — Such clefts always have some involvement of the uvula and soft palate and almost always have some involvement of the hard palate. The hard palate involvement may be a deficiency of one (unilateral) (Fig. 14-2) or both (bilateral) (Fig. 14-3) palatine bones near the midline. The mucous membrane of the septum and the vomerine will be visible on the uncleft side of the cleft. A zone in the region of the incisive foramen extending for varying degrees may be intact (incomplete clefts) (Fig. 14-1, C). Occasionally, this incomplete involvement consists of a midline posterior hard palate deficiency with the vomerine bone lying free in the midline.

Unilateral prepalatal-palatal clefts, after repair of

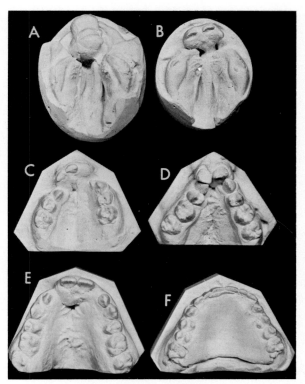

Fig. 14-3. — Appearance of a cleft palate at different ages and after different stages of treatment. **A,** cleft of prepalate and palate, bilateral, complete, with moderate premaxillary projection and mild rotation to right at 3 months of age, immediately before lip surgery. **B,** at 18 months, immediately before palate surgery, to show medial shifting of the lateral maxillary segments that has occurred. **C,** at 5 years, after eruption of deciduous dentition. The model does not show the soft palate repair. **D,** at 8 years, after eruption of permanent dentition, to show the medial displacement of the maxillary segments and lingual tipping of the incisor tooth. The premaxilla has gradually moved posteriorly without surgical section of the vomerine bone. **E,** at 12 years, following orthodontic repositioning of the maxillary segments and tooth realignment. Note that the residual postalveolar palatal defect has enlarged slightly. **F,** an anterior prosthesis to maintain the new premaxillary and dental positions, supply the two missing lateral incisors and cover the residual anterior oronasal fistula.

Fig. 14-2. — Appearance of a cleft palate at different ages and after different stages of treatment. **A,** cleft of prepalate, left, complete, unilateral, at 3 months of age immediately before lip surgery. **B,** at 18 months, immediately before palate surgery, showing narrowing of the cleft palate anteriorly. **C,** at 6 years, with palate healed and primary dentition erupted. The model does not show the soft palate repair. **D,** at 11 years, with secondary dentition erupted, to show the dental deformity due to smallness of the maxillae. **E,** 1 year later, following orthodontic repositioning of the maxillae and minor tooth realignment along with prosthetic replacement of the missing left lateral incisor tooth, which should be removable until 18 years of age and then converted to a fixed bridge.

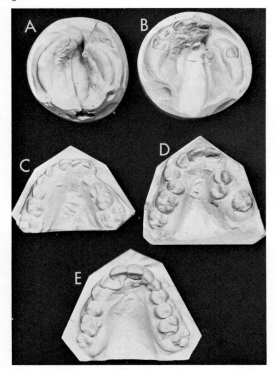

the lip and again after repair of the palate, develop a medial shifting or collapse of the maxillary and premaxillary segments particularly on the cleft side, and the mandible frequently deviates. Associated with this will be dental crowding in the second dentition and decreased vertical growth of the teeth. This complex deformity produces malocclusion and flattening of the upper lip or the whole of the middle third of the face.

Bilateral prepalatal clefts undergo slightly different dental changes.[20] The premaxilla is frequently protruding at birth. Following lip and then palate repair, the premaxilla gradually recedes and its teeth become tipped lingually. Maxillary collapse proceeds somewhat as in the unilateral case but is modified by the final resting place, size and development of the maxillary "wedge." The deformity will be more or less symmetrical.

PALATAL CLEFTS. — Palatal clefts (isolated cleft palate) (Fig. 14-1, *F*) almost always have some involvement of the hard palate in addition to uvular and soft palate involvement. Such involvement may consist of minimal, even submucosal, notching of the posterior border of the hard palate in the midline. Again there may be midline deficiency of the palatine bones extending anywhere up to the incisive foramen.

Palatal clefts may develop dentoalveolar collapse of the posterior maxillary segments with crowding of the teeth. Such developments are particularly likely to occur if the cleft and the surgical repair extended well forward into the hard palate and close to the alveolar margins.

Epidemiology

More information is available on the etiology of the cleft lip and cleft palate than for any other congenital anomaly, perhaps because it is common, obvious and productive of social disability.

INCIDENCE. — Accurate incidence data for any anomaly are difficult to obtain. A continuing study of a segment of Canada,[5] recording only anomalies reported by physicians at birth and therefore probably deficient in isolated cleft palate figures, points out that this anomaly, considering cleft lip and cleft palate together, is the third commonest, being exceeded only by meningomyelocele and clubfoot. The 1959 figures for this study, using cases per 1,000 live births, are: cleft palate 0.25, cleft lip 0.34, cleft lip and cleft palate 0.49, over-all 1.08 (1:930 live births). An earlier study of the same geographic area[18] reported a similar figure. A United States study[31] supplies the following data on the basis of cases per 1,000 live births: cleft palate 0.79, cleft lip 0.29, cleft lip and cleft palate 0.49, over-all 1.57 (1:640 live births). These are comparable to figures from Denmark.[13] Considering these and other variables, it is reasonable to assume a Caucasian incidence of 1:750 live births. It is generally considered that the Negro population incidence is lower than these figures and the mongoloid (Japanese) incidence is higher.

ENVIRONMENTAL FACTORS. — Clefts have been produced by severe alteration of certain environmental experimental factors of small animals from susceptible strains at a suitable period of gestation by means of dietary, vitamin and oxygen deprivation, radiation exposure and cortisone administration.[19, 39, 40] This work cannot be applied directly to humans, although there are reports of decreasing the expected incidence of production of this anomaly in mothers who have a known tendency by avoiding deprivation factors.[6, 10]

A number of clinical environmental factors have been studied in 577 consecutive cases.[4, 24] The mean parental ages were compared with a control obtained from the Report of the Registrar General of Canada. No differences from the control were observed for either maternal or paternal age with or without a family history of cleft. No deviations from the expected were found in the analysis of the birth ranks or in correlating birth rank with maternal age. No significant difference was observed when the mean birth weights of cleft palate infants was compared with the mean birth weights in a large hospital, although the birth weights of the probands were lower than those of their sibs.

With respect to laterality, 43% had left-sided involvement, 24% right-sided involvement and 33% bilateral involvement. The bilateral cases had a greater incidence of both family history and involvement of other members of the family.

The sex distribution is significant. Cleft lip with or without cleft palate is more common in males, whereas the isolated cleft palate is more common in females. No form of sex-linked inheritance satisfies the ratios, and so it must be concluded that for some unknown reason the male factor is more susceptible to cleft lip with or without cleft palate and the female factor is more susceptible to cleft palate alone.

There was a significantly high incidence of severe associated anomalies in both groups, but more so in the isolated cleft palate group. The associated anomalies can be divided into two groups: (1) those occurring in the immediate vicinity: Pierre Robin syndrome (microglossia, micrognathia and cleft palate), Klippel-Feil syndrome (short neck, web neck, cervical spine abnormalities including atlanto-occipital abnormalities),[21] Psaume syndrome[29] or oral-facial-digital syndrome[30] (tongue, floor of mouth, maxillary and mandibular teeth and digital abnormalities); and (2) those occurring elsewhere in the body, particularly congenital heart disease and extremity abnormalities (Ellis-Van Creveld syndrome).[12] This association of a high incidence of congenital abnormalities with cleft palate is suggestive of an over-all disturbance in development.

Studies of the incidence of maternal first trimester disturbances, among which are gestational bleeding, acquired illnesses (rubella, severe nausea, vomiting), operations, accidents and other stresses, have been carried out but have produced no significant data. Similarly, study of social status of the families and previous health of the parents produced insignificant data.

GENETIC FACTORS. — The only established human etiologic factors are genetic. Pioneer work in the field has been reported by Fogh-Andersen.[13]

A study[24] of 750 consecutive cleft cases has shown that approximately 33% of cleft lip patients with or without cleft palate have a history of a similar lesion in the family. Only 25% of isolated cleft palate cases have a similar history.

There is a further evidence to suggest that these two

TABLE 14-1.—GENETIC RISKS OF CLEFT

	CLEFT LIP WITH OR WITHOUT CLEFT PALATE, %	CLEFT PALATE, %
Frequency in general population (ref. 5)	0.08	0.02
Risk of 2nd affected child		
a) if both parents are normal	3.7	2.5
b) if 1 parent has cleft similar to patient's	19.4	14.3
Risk of 3rd affected child (*a* and *b*)	9.0	0.90
Risk of 1st affected child if parent has a cleft	4.04	5.82

groups of lesions are genetically different. A genetic analysis[4] of 413 pedigrees of the above-mentioned series indicates that cleft lip with or without cleft palate is due to at least two pairs of recessive genes if one applies the 40% penetrance observed in cleft twin studies and that isolated cleft palate is due to a simple dominant gene with greatly reduced penetrance.

Chromosome studies.—An abnormal chromosome pattern has been shown for certain severe types of cleft lip and cleft palate usually when associated with other anomalies such as microphthalmia.[28] This work has yet to be confirmed by others.

The epidemiologic data that are available suggest an interplay of genetic, environmental and constitutional factors.[14]

Risk for future siblings.—Reliable estimates for counseling parents of affected individuals and the affected individuals themselves are available[4] (Table 14-1). Such counseling is delimited, however, by the ability to take an accurate pedigree and to consider other variables and should be undertaken in consultation with a geneticist.

Treatment

NEONATAL PERIOD.—In a small proportion of cases, usually those in which the patient has associated anomalies such as the Pierre Robin syndrome, a congenital heart defect, and mental retardation, there will be respiratory and deglutition problems.

If due to local causes, the respiratory distress manifested by cyanosis and sternal indrawing requires manual or elastic traction repositioning of the tongue, and nursing of the baby on the side or face in an assisted environment such as a Croupette. Failure to improve with such careful positioning must be followed by either tracheostomy or surgical forward repositioning of the tongue on the floor of the mouth and the buccal mucosa of the lower lip.[9, 41] Breast feeding is not impossible but usually is contraindicated for both esthetic and mechanical reasons. The majority of the patients do well with a long, large, soft nipple which has a larger than usual hole in it. Assisted feeding by means of a Brecht feeder may be helpful, but the danger of aspiration must be recognized. A small proportion of patients has difficulty in sucking or in swallowing and may require gavage or indwelling plastic tube feedings. The feeding problems do not respond as well to tongue repositioning as do the airway problems. Careful nursing care, requiring great effort and encouragement, is the most important therapeutic factor in the management of this small group of cases. These infants usually learn to suck, swallow and breathe successfully. The mandible becomes acceptable.

Some food will come out of the nose until after the palate is repaired.

PRIMARY SURGERY.—Surgeons agree that it is preferable to have the palate repaired by 2 years of age, before the child has developed many speech abilities and habits. An increasing number of centers operate at 12 months of age. Some dental specialists would like to have the operation postponed until 4–7 years of age to decrease the maxillary and alveolar dental deformity which is allegedly due in part to scar contracture following surgery.

The surgeon has many operations and modifications of operations to choose from. There are two main groups of operations: those producing adequate lateral mobilization to allow midline closure without tension,[37] and those combining these features with complete anterior detachment of the hard and soft palate to allow push-back of the whole palate.[8, 36] The latter type of operation, as described by Le Mesurier,[22] is illustrated in detail (Figs. 14-4 and 14-5) because its results have been reviewed and it has been successful at The Hospital for Sick Children, Toronto. The anterior hard palate is not repaired at the time of the lip operation. Rather, septal flaps are used to close this region at the time of the palate repair, an operation that can be done with an average blood loss of 35 cc, making transfusion unnecessary.

The reader is referred to other worthwhile palate operations, such as closure of the anterior hard palate at the time of lip surgery,[36] and the use of a bone graft to close the bony defect and prevent maxillary and premaxillary collapse.[25, 27]

SECONDARY SURGERY.—Residual oronasal fistulas at, in front of or behind the alveolus may be closed secondarily if they are a cause of foul odors, food impaction or persistent escape of liquids into the nose. This is not recommended routinely because of the possibility of producing dental disabilities, and the region is likely to be reopened if maxillary collapse is to be corrected orthodontically. This region will later have to be covered by a small denture carrying the one or two missing teeth which can be designed to cover the residual prepalatal defect as well. Residual palatal (hard or soft) defects must be closed secondarily.

If the speech result is not acceptable after an adequate trial of speech therapy and after allowing sufficient time for developmental improvement, velo-

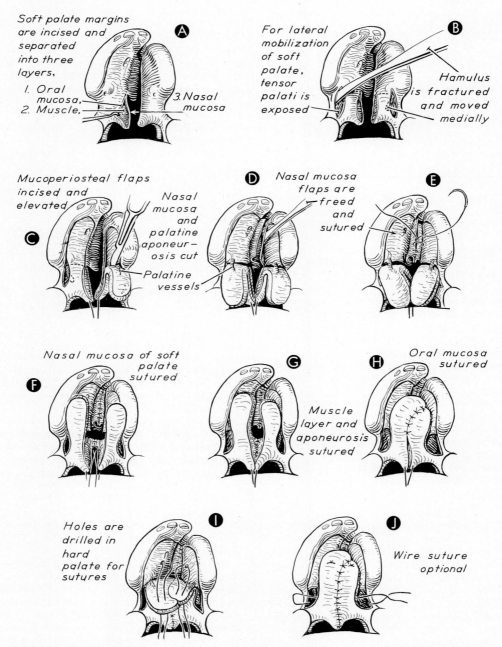

Soft palate margins are incised and separated into three layers.
1. Oral mucosa.
2. Muscle.
3. Nasal mucosa

For lateral mobilization of soft palate, tensor palati is exposed — Hamulus is fractured and moved medially

Mucoperiosteal flaps incised and elevated — Nasal mucosa and palatine aponeurosis cut — Palatine vessels

Nasal mucosa flaps are freed and sutured

Nasal mucosa of soft palate sutured

Muscle layer and aponeurosis sutured

Oral mucosa sutured

Holes are drilled in hard palate for sutures

Wire suture optional

Fig. 14.4.—Repair of a complete unilateral (prepalatal-palatal) cleft palate by a radical one-stage push-back operation combined with a septal-vomerine flap.

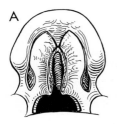 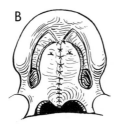 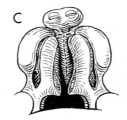 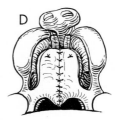

Incomplete cleft palate   *Bilateral, complete cleft palate*

Fig. 14-5. — The operation of Figure 14-4 adapted to an isolated (palatal) cleft of the hard and soft palate (**A** and **B**), and to a bilateral complete (prepalatal-palatal) cleft palate (**C** and **D**).

pharyngeal competence should be reassessed by physical examination and speech cephalometry (Fig. 14-6) or cinefluoroscopy. If the soft palate is short but mobile and the pharynx is of normal size, a secondary pushback procedure may be indicated. If the soft palate is short and immobile and the pharynx is either of normal size or larger than normal, a palatopharyngoplasty (Fig. 14-7) will be indicated. In certain cases, when the palate is both long and mobile but the pharynx is extremely large, pharyngeal augmentation procedures such as the Hynes pharyngoplasty or the insertion of free grafted material beneath the posterior pharyngeal wall[3, 16] may be indicated. Prosthetic speech appliances may be considered when surgery is

contraindicated because of poor anesthetic risk.

REHABILITATION. — Successful treatment involves the consideration of the following factors: the patient's appearance, including both his external facial and dental configuration; the acceptability of his speech; and the success of his rehabilitation, which is a combination of the above as well as his parental and his own mental outlook. The care of other medical and para-medical workers will be required to complete the treatment of many cleft palate patients. Understanding among these people is essential.

Ear, nose and throat. — These children have a higher than usual incidence of otitis media and hearing loss.[4, 11, 26] The early treatment of ear infections is

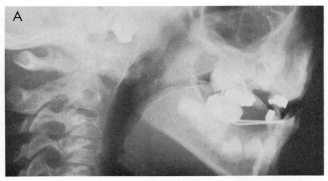

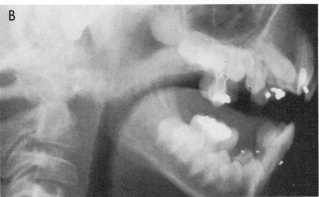

Fig. 14-6. — Speech cephalometric x-ray films. The tongue and pharynx may be coated with radiopaque material such as barium paste. The head is held in fixed position by ear markers. Lateral films are taken in the "rest" position, with the patient "blowing" with closed lips, and saying "ooh" and "ah." **A,** repaired isolated cleft palate in the rest position, showing a short cleft palate which could not make velopharyngeal closure. **B,** 3½ years later, the same patient in rest position after pharyngoplasty, showing the smaller soft tissue mass which unites the posterior pharyngeal wall and the soft palate.

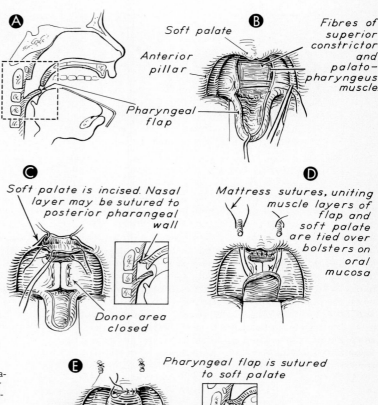

Fig. 14-7.—The palatopharyngeal (pharyngoplasty) operation. The procedure for an anteriorly based pharyngeal flap is outlined, but the pharyngeal flap should be based superiorly for high, very short soft palates.

important. The possibility of hearing loss is watched for and treated by the otolaryngologist. The role of the adenoids and tonsils is given serious consideration. Their thoughtless and traumatic removal is contraindicated because of the possibility of enlarging the velopharyngeal space, but when carefully done will often be of benefit to these children.

Speech therapy.—The function of speech is probably the most important to others although not necessarily to the patient. There is no true objective method to measure speech. Subjective methods should be satisfactory, but they are veiled in the personal interests of the examiner, individual opinions as to what constitutes acceptable speech, the surgeon's tendency to think that his own work is satisfactory and the speech therapist's drive to produce "normal speech."

The outstanding problem in the speech of cleft-palate children is nasality (hypernasality or rhinolalia). Some cannot make the necessary closure between soft palate and pharynx to prevent nasal escape on the production of any of the consonants and

vowels with the exception of the nasal consonants m, n, and ng. Sometimes a muffled tone rather than nasality is produced due to depression of the nasal passages, resulting in lack of resonance.

The sibilant consonants are the most common sound defects in the cleft-palate group. These involve the sounds s, z, sh, zh, ch, and j or soft g. Different types of lisp may develop—the protrusion, the lateral, or the nasal lisp. The explosive consonants p, b, t, d, k, and hard g are frequently affected because there is insufficient breath pressure in the mouth to produce them. The articulation of all consonants may be faulty and then the speech will be unintelligible.[23]

Speech therapy, when indicated, is most valuable between 4 and 8 years of age, although therapists can detect and correct abnormal tendencies in younger children. Advice to parents and demonstration of exercises to build up oral breath pressure are useful in the younger, to be followed by detailed exercises in the older, all followed by tape recordings.

Dental care.—Facial and dental configuration can

TABLE 14-2.—Over-all Subjective* Speech Results of 612 Consecutive Cleft Palate Patients

ACCEPTABLE, 68.5%   UNACCEPTABLE, 31.5%

I, 39.7%   II, 28.8%   III, 21.4%   IV, 10.1%

* I. Normal speech
II. Minor articulation defects not } stigmatizing of cleft palate — Acceptable
III. Intelligible speech, but stigmatized of cleft palate
IV. Unintelligible speech, stigmatized of cleft palate (poor) — Unacceptable

TABLE 14-3.—Factors Related to the Speech Result —612 Consecutive Cases Operated by a One-stage Radical Push-back Palatoplasty, not Subjected to an Intensive Speech Therapy Program and without Dental Reconstruction

VARIABLE	SPEECH ACCEPTABLE, %	SPEECH NOT ACCEPTABLE, %
Type and degree of original involvement		
Palatal clefts		
a) Soft palate alone, or with 1/3 or less of hard palate involved	78	22
b) Soft palate with more than 1/3 of hard palate involved	66	34
c) All palatal only clefts (isolated cleft palate) (a, b)	75	25
Prepalatal-palatal clefts		
a) Cleft lip-cleft palate, incomplete palatal involvement	81	19
b) Cleft lip-cleft palate, complete unilateral palatal involvement	75	25
c) Cleft lip-cleft palate, bilateral mixed involvement, complete on one side, incomplete on other	50	50
d) Cleft lip-cleft palate, bilateral complete involvement	44	56
Intelligence quotient of patient		
120-	82	18
100-119	78	22
80-99	69	31
-80	44	56
Hearing loss		
20 decibels or more bilaterally	56	44
Transient episodes of subjective hard of hearing	62	38
Age of palate operation		
0-36 months	71	29
over 36 months	60	40
Presence of residual defects		
Prepalatal positions	86	14
Palatal positions	35	65
Physical appearance of soft palate (repaired)		
Short	54	46
Scarred	57	43
Decreased mobility	47	53
Visual assessment of velopharyngeal closure		
Decreased closure	47	53
Presence of maxillodental occlusion deformity		
Anteroposterior deformity only	56	44
Lateral deformity only	65	35
Anteroposterior combined with lateral deformity	69	31

frequently be made acceptable.[20] This involves the judicious use of orthodontic repositioning of displaced maxillary segments and malaligned teeth, fixed bridge replacement of missing teeth, removable prosthetic replacement of missing teeth when simultaneous coverage of small anterior residual palatal defects is necessary, sacrifice of hypoplastic teeth, construction of more anterior space by procedures such as the Esser inlay graft techniques, the use of a larger anterior prosthesis in cases with marked maxillary underdevelopment, and the use of a concomitant mandibular resection when this bone is overdeveloped.

RESULTS OF TREATMENT.—Despite all these measures, a certain proportion of patients are left with inadequate speech. Results are fairly constant from main center to main center, variations probably being due to the lack of a standard method of recording results in an unbiased manner.

The speech results of 612 consecutive cleft palate cases have been assessed by the author, who was not one of the operators. Essentially the same operative procedure was used on all cases (Figs. 14-4 and 14-5). The results are summarized in Table 14-2. Avoiding the term "normal," 68.5% of the cases had acceptable speech; 10% of the cases had truly poor speech.

These results have been studied in detail to determine the cause of residual speech defects following palatoplasty. They have been found to be related to many variables not all of which can be controlled, all of which must be taken into consideration when dealing with the rehabilitation of the cleft-palate patient (Table 14-3).

REFERENCES

1. Browne, D.: An orthopedic approach to problems of cleft lip and cleft palate, Tr. Internat. Soc. Plast. Surg., 1955.
2. Bull. Am. A. Cleft Palate Rehabilitation: Report of the nomenclature committee of the American Association for Cleft Palate Rehabilitation, 9:39, 1959.
3. Calnan, J. S.: The surgical treatment of nasal speech disorders, Ann. Roy. Coll. Surgeons England 25:119, 1959.
4. Cleft Lip and Cleft Palate Research and Treatment Center, The Hospital for Sick Children, Toronto, Canada: Five Year Report.
5. Congenital abnormalities reported on Physician's Notice of Birth Form, Prov. of Ontario, Dept. of Health, Courtesy, A. H. Sellers, Director, Division of Medical Statistics.
6. Conway, H.: Effect of supplemental vitamin therapy on the limitation of incidence of cleft lip and the cleft palate in humans, Plast. & Reconstruct. Surg. 22:450, 1958.
7. Davis, J. S., and Ritchie, H. P.: Classification of congenital clefts of the lip and palate, J.A.M.A. 79:1323, 1922.

8. Dorrance, G. N.: The push-back operation in cleft palate surgery, Ann. Surg. 101:445, 1935.

9. Douglas, B.: Treatment of micrognathia associated with obstruction by plastic procedures, Plast. & Reconstruct. Surg. 1:304, 1946.

10. Douglas, B.: The role of environmental factors in the etiology of so-called congenital malformations, Plast. & Reconstruct. Surg. 22:94, 214, 1958.

11. Drettner, R.: The nasal airway and hearing in patients with cleft palate, Acta oto-laryng. 25:131, 1960.

12. Ellis, W. B., and Van Creveld, S.: A syndrome characterized by ectodermal dysplasia, polydactyly, chondrodysplasia and congenital morbus cordis, Arch. Dis. Childhood 15:65, 1940.

13. Fogh-Andersen, P.: *Inheritance of Harelip and Cleft Palate* (Copenhagen: Arnold Busck, 1942).

14. Fraser, F. C., Walker, B. E., and Trasler, D. G.: Experimental production of congenital cleft palate: genetic and environmental factors, Pediatrics 19:782, 1957.

15. Grant, J. C. B.: Vessels and Nerves of Soft Palate, in *A Method of Anatomy* (5th ed.; Baltimore: Williams & Wilkins Company, 1952), p. 748.

16. Hagerty, R. P., and Hill, M. J.: Cartilage pharyngoplasty in cleft palate patients, Surg., Gynec. & Obst. 112:350, 1961.

17. His, W.: Die Entwickelung der menschlichen und thierischer Physiognosen, Arch. f. anat. u. physiol. Anat. part 384, 1892; Beobachtungen zur Geschichte der Nasen und Gaumen-bildung im menschlichen Embryo, Abhandl. d. math. phys. Classe d. kgl. Sachs. Gesellsch. d. Wissensch. 27:347,1901.

18. Hixon, E.: A study of the incidence of cleft lip and cleft palate in Ontario, Canad. J. Public Health 42:508, 1951.

19. Ingalls, T. H.: Causes and prevention of developmental defects, J.A.M.A. 161:1047, 1956.

20. Johnston, M.C.: Orthodontic treatment for the cleft palate patient, Am. J. Orthodontics 44:750, 1958.

21. Klippel, M., and Feil, A.: Un cas d'absence des vertèbres cervicales, Nouvelle Inconographie de la Salpêtrière 25:223, 1912.

22. Le Mesurier, A. B.: The operative repair of cleft palate, Canad. M. A. J. 33:150, 1935.

23. Lewis, R.: Speech and the cleft palate child, Canad. M.A. J. 71:600, 1954.

24. Lindsay, W. K.: The Hospital for Sick Children, Toronto, Canada. Unpublished data.

25. Lynch, J. B.; Lewis, S. R., and Blocker, T. G., Jr.: Maxillary bone grafts in cleft palate patients, Plast. & Reconstruct. Surg. 37:91, 1966.

26. Masters, F. W., Bingham, H. G., and Robinson, D. W.: Pre-vention and treatment of hearing loss in the cleft palate child, Plast. & Reconstruct. Surg. 25:503, 1960.

27. Nordin, K. E.: Bone grafting to alveolar process clefts following treatment of secondary cleft palate deformity, Tr. Internat. Soc. Plast. Surg., 1955.

28. Patau, K., *et al.*: Multiple congenital anomalies caused by an extra autosome, Lancet 1:790, 1960.

29. Psaume, J.: A propos des anomalies fasciales associées à la division palatine, Ann. chir. plast., vol. 2, March, 1957.

30. Ruess, A. L., *et al.*: The oral-facial-digital syndrome: A multiple congenital condition of females with associated chromosomal abnormalities, Pediatrics 29:985, 1962.

31. Shapiro, R. N., *et al.*: The incidence of congenital anomalies discovered in the neonatal period, Am. J. Surg. 96: 396, Sept., 1958.

32. Stark, R. B.: Pathogenesis of harelip and cleft palate, Plast. & Reconstruct. Surg. 13:22, 1954.

33. Stark, R. B., and Ehrmann, N. A.: Development of the center of the face with particular reference to surgical correction of bilateral cleft lip, Plast. & Reconstruct. Surg. 21: 177, 1958.

34. Stark, R. B., and Kernahan, D. A.: A classification of cleft lip and cleft palate based upon newer concepts of embryology, Bull. Am. A. Cleft Palate Rehabilitation 9:45, 1959.

35. Streeter, G. L.: Developmental horizons in human embryos: Age groups XV, XVI, XVII & XVIII, Contr. Embryol. Carnegie Institution 32:133, 1948.

36. Veau, V.: *Divisions Palatine* (Paris: Mason & Cie, 1931).

37. Von Langenbeck, B. von L.: Uranoplastic by detaching the mucous periosteal lining of the hard palate, Arch. klin. Chir. 2:205, 1861.

38. Walker, B. E., and Fraser, F. C.: Closure of the secondary palate in three strains of mice, J. Embryol. Exper. Morphol. 4:176, 1956.

39. Walker, B. E.: Experimental production of cleft palate in animals, Bull. Am. A. Cleft Palate Rehabilitation 7:8, 1957.

40. Warkany, J.: Etiology of Congenital Malformations, in *Advances in Pediatrics* (Chicago: Year Book Publishers, Inc., 1947).

41. Woolf, R. M., Georgiade, N., and Pickrell, K. L.: Micrognathia and associated cleft palate (Pierre Robin Syndrome), Plast. & Reconstruct. Surg. 26:199, 1960.

42. Wynn-Williams, D.: Congenital suprabulbar paresis, Speech Pathol. & Therap., p. 18, April, 1928.

W. K. LINDSAY
Drawings by
MARGUERITE DRUMMOND

15

Auricular Deformities

The external ear consists of three parts, the external auditory meatus, the canal to the drum, and the auricle or pinna. Although all parts of the external ear are involved in major reconstructive undertakings, our discussions will be primarily directed to surgery of the auricle itself and will only incidentally involve other portions of the external ear and surrounding structures.

Congenital anomalies are the most common source of auricular deformities, but traumatic deformities are increasing in frequency. Organized complete discussions of these defects and their correction on an embryologic and anatomic basis are scarce. Excellent discussions of the individual lesions are available, but for a given lesion, there are usually several methods of repair, each advanced as the simplest and best by its proponents.

The following discussion is a summary of the methods we use to correct many of these defects. No claim is made for originality, but we have made a sincere effort to arrive at the least complicated, most practical way of managing each of these problems in our own hands. We realize that with differing conditions, an entirely different procedure might be the method of choice for many of these problems.

Operative procedures on the auricle or external ear are numerous and varied. They range from simple excision of a preauricular tag to a complicated, staged construction of a totally absent auricle. The age of election for these procedures also varies from the newborn period to preschool age, when the growth of the auricle is complete or nearly so. To some extent, most of these procedures are complicated by the fact that the yellow elastic fibrocartilage which forms the scaffolding on which the ear is based is a unique substance in the human body; there is no donor site of comparable tissue with which absent or malformed cartilage can be replaced. As a result of this lack of tissue with similar physical characteristics, most major reconstructive procedures on the auricle are, at best, compromises between the ideal and the attainable. The subsequent discussions summarize the compromises which we have found to be the most satisfactory. Many of these procedures are relatively new and probably will be improved as experience is gained in this area of reconstructive surgery.

Embryology

During the second month of intrauterine life, the first branchial groove loses contact with the first pharyngeal pouch, and as the head of the embryo increases in thickness the groove deepens and narrows to form the funnel-shaped external auditory canal. The entire auricle is formed from the first and second branchial arches which surround the branchial groove, three small hillocks of tissue on each arch. Although embryologists agree that these hillocks are important in formation of the auricle, they do not agree about the role of each of these units in the formation of the final anatomic pattern.

Abnormalities at various stages of this irregular progression from six separate nodules to the irregularly folded thin skin and cartilage structure which is the final form of the auricle cause the different anomalies of the auricle from the simplest malformation or failure of folding of cartilage to the most complicated deformity or microtia. If the disturbance of this area is more extensive, the tissue around the ear and even the entire side of the head may be involved in the deformity, as in the Treacher-Collins syndrome or auriculofacial dysostosis.

In the surrounding tissue changes accompanying ear deformity, the mandible is so frequently involved that when microtia is seen in a newborn, it is important to look carefully for hypoplasia of the mandible, since this is overlooked at times because the auricular deformity is so much more striking.

Anatomy

The most important anatomic features are presented in Figure 15-1 to serve as a reference for the discussions of the various defects.

The auricle is a thin sheet of yellow fibrocartilage folded in an irregular fashion, covered with thin skin which is firmly fixed to the cartilage anteriorly but is quite loose and mobile posteriorly. The most prominent folds in the cartilage can be seen in Figure 15-1. The outer rim of the auricle is known as the helix. This extends from the crus helicus around the anterior, superior and top two thirds to three quarters of the auricle but does not extend down into the lobule,

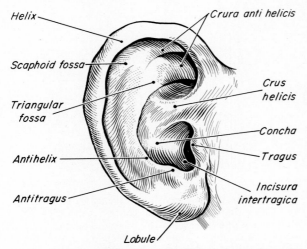

Fig. 15-1.—Anatomy of the auricle. The unusual and complex folds are difficult to attain with reconstructive methods.

which is completely without supporting cartilage. The extension of the antihelix into the superior and anterior crura is important in correction of outstanding ear as well as of lop ear. The tragus is the anterior fold of cartilage which projects posteriorly over the external auditory canal.

Preauricular Tags

Preauricular tags occur relatively frequently. As a rule, they are easily corrected by simple excision and careful closure; but they may be complex and extensive, and their correction consequently more difficult.

Preauricular tags vary from a projection of excess skin, which can frequently be cured by simple ligation in the newborn period (Fig. 15-2, *A*), to larger multiple projections with skin and varying amounts of carti-

lage firmly attached to the supporting cartilage of the ear (Fig. 15-2, *B*).

If the defect is relatively simple, with a small base, it is easily removed under infiltration anesthesia before the newborn baby is discharged from the hospital. As a practical plan of attack, it can most simply be done on the day the baby is to be discharged, since most newborn nurseries will not permit a baby to be transferred to surgery and then brought back to the nursery. Accordingly, the baby goes to surgery from the nursery and, then, after the procedure, is discharged from the hospital with the mother. Three to 4 days later the infant is brought back for removal of all external nonabsorbable skin sutures.

If the tags are broad-based and contain a moderate amount of cartilage which must be removed, or if they are situated so that much care must be used in closure to secure a good cosmetic result, excision is delayed until 3–6 months of age, when a careful excision with plastic closure is performed under general anesthesia. This eliminates the undesirable distortion of tissues which results from the infiltration of large quantities of local anesthetic solution into the operative field.

Preauricular Sinus and Cyst

Preauricular sinuses usually begin in the area between the anterior margin of the helix and the inferior margin of the tragus. Some extend only a few millimeters under the skin surface while others communicate with the middle ear or the external auditory canal or end blindly at the cartilage of the helix or the tragus. Their surgical significance is twofold—cosmetic, and as a blind pouch which too often becomes infected.

Cosmetically, they vary from a barely visible pinpoint opening (Fig. 15-3) on normal skin to a deep depression of the skin with the sinus opening at the bottom of the depression. The larger sinuses, which

Fig. 15-2.—**A,** preauricular ring consisting of skin. This type of anomalous appendage is reasonably well excised under local infiltration anesthesia in the perinatal period. **B,** preauricular tags containing skin and cartilage. The more extensive forms merge with the cartilage framework of the auricle, and operation should be carried out under general anesthesia at the age of 6 months.

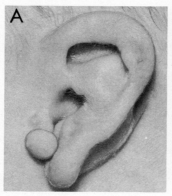
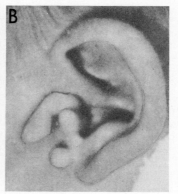

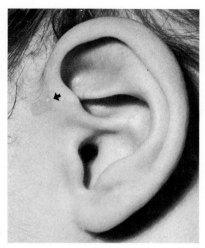

Fig. 15-3.—Preauricular sinus with drainage. These tracts pursue an unpredictable and often complex course. Complete excision of the sinus and tract before development of infection is the key to successful surgical treatment.

Congenital Absence of the Auricle

The most frequently encountered major anomaly of the ear in the newborn period is the so-called absent ear. Almost always, some vestigial structure is present, and usually this contains both soft tissue and cartilage (Fig. 15-5). The cartilage usually is hypoplastic and is always deformed. This anomaly is more common in males, occurring approximately in 5 boys for each 2 girls. Obviously, the cosmetic defect is more of a consideration in boys than in girls, since feminine hair style is such that even a severely deformed ear can be covered quite adequately.

Many forms of therapy have been proposed for this defect, most of which involve bringing tissue from a distant site, usually rib cartilage and cervical skin.[14] Even diced cartilage allowed to assume the contour of a perforated metal mold has been used, since carving of a block of cartilage to resemble the complicated pattern of the normal ear cartilage is difficult to the point of being impracticable.

The numerous stages of such reconstructive attempts and the usual failure to come close to the delicate contours of the normal structure of the auricle have prompted the following compromise program.

The goal in treating this defect is to construct an acceptable replacement for the ear which will withstand the normal trauma of living and remain cosmetically acceptable. For this reason, we have not used homogenous or autogenous cartilage grafts, not only because there is no available cartilage which resembles ear cartilage in its properties but because of the disappointingly frequent occurrence of resorption of grafted cartilage following trauma. This limitation to the use of local tissue as a supporting structure definitely restricts the scope of reconstructive surgery which can be performed.

Our present regimen for these children consists of reconstruction, usually completed in three stages. *The first procedure* is done at 4–6 months of age and consists of operative unfolding of the deformed, furled cartilage to as great an extent as is possible. We try to do this with a minimum of trauma to the thin hypoplastic cartilage and at the same time try to separate the cartilage from its surrounding tissue as little as possible. The unfurled cartilage is then inserted into a subcutaneous pocket under what would normally be the postauricular skin. Usually, the cartilage requires several sutures to secure it in its new unfolded position (Fig. 15-6). The cartilage is then left in this new position for 2–5 years. If growth occurs in this new location, the size of the ear will approximate the normal size even though the contour usually leaves quite a bit to be desired.

The second stage, done at 2–5 years of age, consists of making an incision shaped like a question mark beyond the margin of the cartilage and elevating cartilage along with overlying skin and filling the defect thus created with a thick split-thickness skin

are objectionable because of their appearance, should be excised. The tiny, barely visible openings need no treatment unless they become infected.

If the sinus is infected when first seen, the diagnosis may not be readily obvious unless the sinus opening and its connection to the skin are looked for. Often, the entire area is distorted and inflamed.

Once the diagnosis is suspected, treatment is carried out as for any cellulitis in this area, with massive warm, moist compresses and antibiotics. If an abscess forms in spite of this treatment, it must be surgically drained. It will be easier to obtain an acceptable appearance later if the drainage is performed in the region of the sinus opening so that the incision and drainage scar can be excised at the time of excision of the sinus. Excision then should be delayed for a minimum of 8 weeks, after all signs of inflammation have subsided.

In the presence of a chronically draining sinus, cultures of the drainage will demonstrate the sensitivity of the infecting organisms to antibiotics. If a program of compresses and the appropriate antibiotic therapy does not clear up the infection, excision must then be done in the presence of drainage. The chances of primary healing are improved if the antibiotic to which the organism is most sensitive is given prophylactically, beginning 24 hours preoperatively. Families should be warned that the surgery may be extensive and that recurrences are not uncommon when surgery is performed in the presence of chronic infection.

The Editors wish to present Figure 15-4, illustrating a verified technique for permanent removal of preauricular cysts and sinuses suggested by Rudolf Singer.

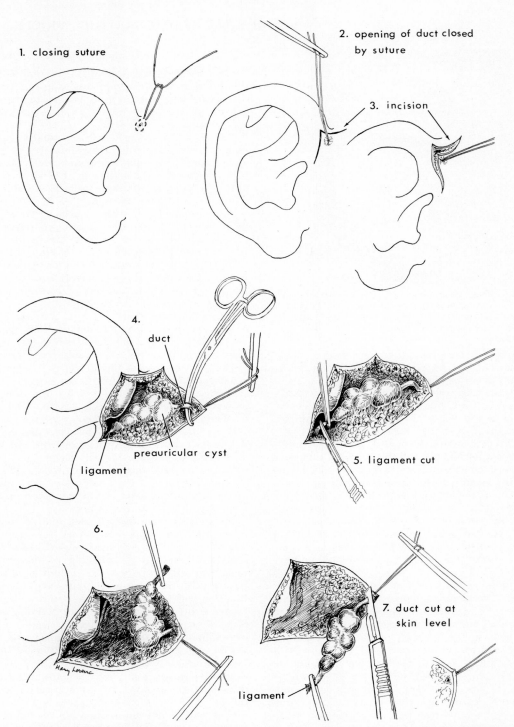

Fig. 15-4.—Total extirpation of a preauricular cyst is effected by first closing the ductal opening with a purse-string or Z suture **(1).** An inverted L-shaped incision is then made **(2 and 3).** The triangular flap formed by the skin incision of cutis and subcutis is elevated and everted, revealing the cyst structure **(4).** Several cysts are arranged around a ligament, which is severed **(5).** This allows the clump of cysts to be easily peeled out of its subcutaneous bed **(6).** The whole complex of duct, ligament and cysts remains connected to skin only by means of the duct, which is cut as closely as possible to the skin **(7).** (Courtesy of Rudolf Singer, M.D., and *American Journal of Surgery* [111:291, 1966].)

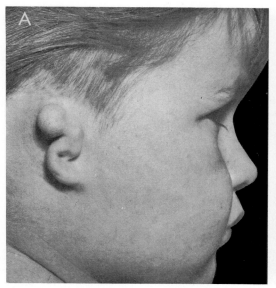
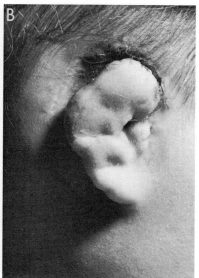

Fig. 15-5. — **A,** congenital hypoplastic ear. Surprising progress in reconstruction can be made by letting out and rearranging the usually abundant skin folds and preserving all available cartilage tissue. **B,** same ear after second stage of reconstruction, usually carried out at age 2–5 years. The "ear" is turned forward and the posterior defect lined with split-thickness skin graft.

graft. This graft then covers the posterior surface of the ear as well as the defect over the mastoid (Fig. 15-5, *B*).

The third stage, done 6–12 months after healing of the second stage, includes construction of an external auditory canal and any minor revisions of contour which seem desirable. The auditory canal is made only for cosmetic reasons and usually is surfaced

Fig. 15-6. — In first stage of reconstruction of missing auricle, the unfolded abnormal cartilage is held in its new position by sutures tied over dental roll bolsters.

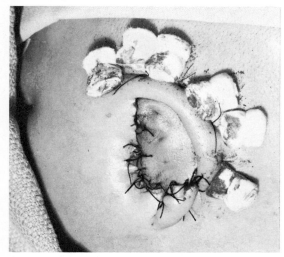

with a small split-thickness graft with a stent for immobilization during healing. At this stage, a fold of skin or, if possible, skin and cartilage should be constructed anterior to the canal to resemble a tragus since either with further surgery or with a prosthesis the tragus and canal are important factors in giving a normal appearance.

We should mention here that malposition is frequently present, and to attain any good cosmetic result by whatever method, the structures which are present should be moved into normal position. This usually requires some displacement of the remnants upward and posteriorly.

X-ray studies are made at this stage to determine whether the middle ear has developed normally, but this is only for information since it does not affect the operative plan. If the structures of the inner and middle ear are normal, and they usually are, bone conduction hearing will be normal and will be superior to air conduction resulting from any attempt to create a functioning external auditory canal and drum if the other ear is normal.

If, as is usually the case, the cosmetic appearance leaves much to be desired, we believe that further attempts at reconstruction by transplanting cartilage and/or skin is probably never worth while unless the ear has been fairly closely approximated to normal by the three preceding operations. In the much more usual situation, when this goal has not been accomplished, we feel that a far more satisfactory answer esthetically, psychologically and financially is the covering of the deformed cartilage and skin with a prosthetic ear which can be quite satisfactory and is

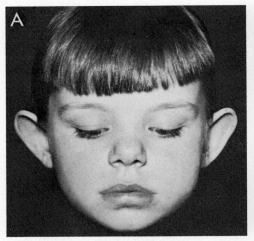
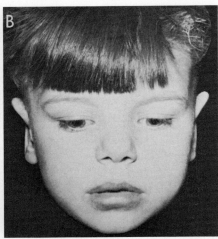

Fig. 15-7.—Protruding auricle. **A,** preoperatively, the auricle stands out at right angles to the head, with failure of reversal of the conchal plate. This defect is usually bilateral and often familial. Age of election for surgery is 4–6 years and should be carried out in both sexes. **B,** an antihelical fold has been created, including the superior crura. Careful external support is required for 3 weeks after operation.

at times hard to distinguish from a normal, natural ear. A plastic prosthesis is used only when it will not be subjected to trauma. Such prostheses are made by a commercial manufacturer from casts of the involved ear and the normal ear.

We realize that this approach to the problem represents a marked deviation from the usual one of autogenous cartilage implants and numerous stages of construction over a long period. Nevertheless we consider this a practical attack on a very perplexing problem and, at least for the present, one that gives the best results to the highest percentage of patients. Furthermore, if additional plastic revision is desired at a later time, nothing has been done to compromise any further procedures; in fact, the most has been made of the available local structures, and they are in the best position to serve as a beginning upon which future construction can be based. If glasses are needed, the reconstructed ear will provide a suitable post for their support.

If therapy were delayed until adult life, the patient could be depended on to keep trauma to a minimum. But this would also leave him with his deformity throughout the portion of his life when the unfavorable reaction to an obvious defect is greatest. When all factors are considered, although there are many disadvantages to this program of reconstruction, it presents the best over-all solution to an exceedingly complex problem.

The problem may be best understood by thinking of the defects of the two methods of final correction. Surgery has the disadvantages of numerous surgical procedures, scars away from the primary defect and appearance which is never a good substitute for normal. Prostheses have the disadvantages of difficulty with retention and the psychologic problem of any "artificial" substitute for a part.

Defects of the Auricle

Outstanding Ear (Protruding Auricle)

The defect of outstanding ear (protruding auricle) is due to a lack of normal folding of the antihelix, which causes the supporting cartilage to hold the ear out at a right angle from the skull or some position between the normal and a right angle (Fig. 15-7, *A*). To some parents this is just another family trait and is not at all objectionable since the child looks just

Fig. 15-8.—Postoperative result of correction of outstanding auricle, showing good antihelix, superior crus and inferior crus.

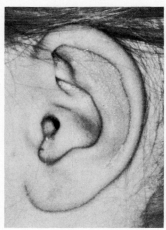

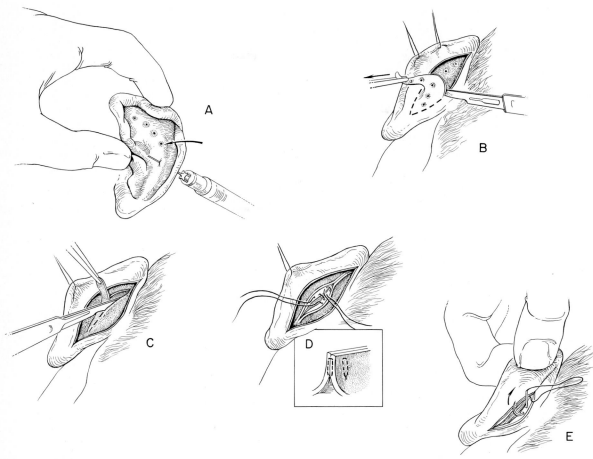

Fig. 15-9.—Correction of outstanding ear. **A,** marking of cartilage and skin after bending to form antihelical fold. **B,** excision of ellipse of postauricular skin. **C,** incision through cartilage.

D, suturing of cartilage to produce permanent antihelical fold. **E,** suturing of postauricular skin with subcuticular continuous suture.

like his father and siblings. But some families, especially when the defect occurs in only one child, are very desirous of cosmetic correction since both they and the child are upset by the defect and the ridicule it evokes in playmates.

Outstanding ear may be unilateral or bilateral. The familial variety usually is bilateral. When the defect is unilateral it is a much more obvious cosmetic defect and almost always should be corrected so that the contour of the two ears is the same.

The cause of outstanding ear is unknown. It certainly has no relation to sleeping with the ear forward, to caps which fold the ear forward or to other external factors. Most often, the defect is evident soon after birth. In fact, the protruding ear usually progresses and is increasingly obvious as ear growth proceeds and its cartilage develops.

Correction of outstanding ear, if it is an isolated

defect, consists of surgical creation of as normal an antihelix as possible (Fig. 15-8). This can be done in the preschool period but frequently is delayed until the self-conscious preadolescent seeks cosmetic correction. A clue to the lack of satisfaction with any one surgical procedure for this defect is evident from the number of operations used for its correction.[3, 4, 13]

Many of these procedures use simple mattress sutures to fold the cartilage and form an antihelical fold.[8, 11] Some others simply score the cartilage to break the spring and hold the fold in place by skin sutures, and some excise portions of cartilage or trim cartilage and use the skin to hold the position in the newly folded contour of cartilage.

Probably the most commonly used procedure, and the one we have found satisfactory for most cases, consists of excision of an ellipse of skin and cartilage marked prior to the skin incision by passing a needle containing methylene blue or brilliant green through the entire thickness of the ear. This is done while the ear is held at its desired position in relation to the head (Fig. 15-9, *A*). Usually the incision in the cartilage must extend from the crus of the antihelix well down on the antitragus. Once this ellipse of cartilage has been excised and skin freed from cartilage, Lembert sutures of 0000 white silk or cotton are placed to fold the cartilage into an antihelix and hold the ear back as far as possible with this one fold in the cartilage (Fig. 15-9, *E*).

The excised ellipse of skin of the same size as, or larger than, the excised cartilage helps to maintain the ear in the proper position while cartilaginous healing occurs. This position is further assured by a protective dressing for 2 weeks, followed by the use of a small circular sleeping cap for 6 weeks to keep the healing cartilage from being broken by forward bending during sleep.

LOP EAR

If the outstanding ear also has a wilted, floppy cartilage in the area of the superior crus, allowing the top of the helix to fall outward, the condition is referred to as lop ear (Fig. 15-10). This is more difficult to correct than outstanding ear, but if, when the antihelix is formed, a new superior crus can be created by extending the incision superiorly and continuing the fold of cartilage in this direction, a very acceptable result is achieved.

DIFFERENCE IN SIZE

In general, differences in size of the two auricles can be corrected best by reducing the size of the larger of the auricles. This results in improvement only if the smaller auricle is not out of proportion to the head size. This reduction in size can be done by a wedge in a superior and posterior direction, as in taking a composite skin and cartilage graft. The incision following reduction in size is less obvious if it is placed in the scaphoid fossa with a small extension across the helix superiorly and down into the concha at the level of the middle segment of the auricle.

DEFORMITY OF THE LOBULE

Deformities of the lobule usually are minor in nature and can be corrected by relatively small plastic procedures.

The most common of these defects is adherent lobule, with the lower pole of the lobule buried within the cheek for varying distances. This is best corrected by generous skin incisions so that local skin may be used to cover the external borders of the lobule and a split-thickness graft used to cover the posterior surface of the lobule and the defect in the cheek under the newly elevated lobule.

Difference in size of the lobules in general is easily corrected by reduction in size of the larger one.

Absence of the lobule occurs as a congenital defect or as a result of trauma. If the local tissue is adequate for use as a flap, this can be elevated from the skin below and posterior to the auricle and a double layer of full-thickness skin and subcutaneous tissue is folded on itself and the postauricular defect closed with a split-thickness graft.

If local tissue is damaged at the time the lobule is lost, it is best replaced by a tubed pedicle of skin from the neck.

Fig. 15-10.—Lop ear. Loss of the superior helical arch plus failure of reversal of the conchal plate adds to difficulty of repair.

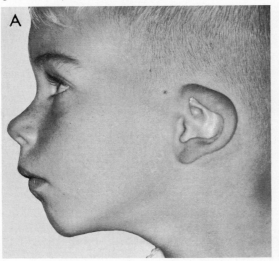
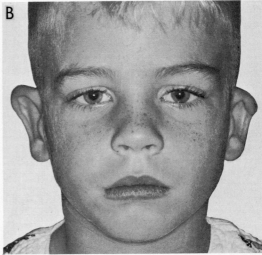

Injuries of the Auricle

TRAUMA

Trauma to the auricle is not as common as might be expected from its extremely exposed position, but it does occur in all degrees of severity.

Lacerations are treated like any other laceration in this region, with careful cleansing and very conservative debridement followed by meticulous approximation of the injured layers. If cartilage needs to be repaired, white silk or cotton is preferable to dark suture material since the dark color may subsequently show through the very thin skin of the auricle. The skin should be approximated accurately with many fine sutures, as in any other exposed area where appearance of the eventual scar is a major consideration. If the sutures are removed within 3–5 days, additional scars from this source are avoided.

Contusion of the auricle occurs rather frequently in some athletic activities. Because of the very loose subcutaneous tissue in the auricle, the resulting hematoma often assumes frightening proportions. This condition is best treated with a contoured compression dressing and is evacuated only if the viability of overlying skin is endangered. Every aspiration has the definite danger of introducing infection into a previously closed injury.

With repeated contusion and eventual organization of hematoma, as well as excess cartilage formation in hematomas between cartilage and perichondrium, the cartilage becomes deformed in the bulky, multi-contoured fashion known as a "cauliflower" ear. This is treated only when at least 12 months have elapsed after the last trauma and no change or inflammation has been present for this length of time; any surgical trauma earlier than this is frequently followed by excessive reaction, and the eventual result is compromised.

The surgical attack is planned to remove all the abnormal scar tissue and cartilage, leaving as much of the normal cartilage as possible. Careful placement of skin incisions will avoid or minimize unsightly scarring. After this excision and closure, carefully contoured pressure dressings are the most important part of the postoperative care. The results from this procedure are usually quite satisfactory, although seldom perfect.

When the entire auricle is torn away by trauma, the avulsed ear is usually a minor portion of the over-all damage to the patient, and its repair is usually less urgent than treatment of the head injury or internal injuries sustained at the same time.

If the auricle is available, the cartilage is removed in the operating room after thorough cleansing and under rigid sterile conditions. When the tissue in the postauricular region is fairly normal, a pocket is created there and the cartilage left in this pocket. If this tissue has been damaged or is likely to become infected, the cartilage is best preserved in an abdominal subcutaneous pocket until a series of reconstructive procedures can be done to replace it in its normal position.

Gilles[6] suggested separation of the skin from the postauricular side of the cartilage and opening of the ear like a book so that it could be placed into a suitable site on a tubed pedicle and later transferred to its original position in stages. Although he had not done this, it seemed too good an idea not to pass on.

If the patient's general condition is critical and it seems advisable to delay even this minor procedure, the cartilage can be preserved at 40 F in serum or saline containing antibiotics for 3-4 days, after which it still has an excellent chance of survival in a subcutaneous pocket.

BURNS

A more frequently encountered traumatic deficiency is absence of all or part of the helix due to third-degree burns. This is best treated by replacement with a cervical pedicle in the form of a narrow roll around the outer rim of normal ear. This will give an acceptable cosmetic result even without replacement of the missing cartilage.

If only local areas of the auricle are lost from burning or trauma, local flaps of postauricular skin or frequently a composite flap of cartilage and skin can be used to replace the defect and the resulting denuded area covered with a split-thickness graft from a distant site.

Exposure to extreme cold may result in loss of auricular tissue comparable to that of thermal burns. Adjacent tissue has subtle vascular injury disproportionate to its healthy appearance and must be used for reconstruction with extreme caution and only if absolutely necessary. In fact, the residual tissue, even though it looks healthy, may have vascular damage so severe that support of pedicles transferred to it is precarious. For this reason, some normal-appearing tissue should be removed back to healthy bleeding tissue if a pedicle is needed. For the same reason, any ear that has been frost-bitten should be protected with great care for 3-4 years after apparent recovery, since a much less severe insult will cause extensive tissue loss during this period of decreased vasculature.

Associated Anomalies

The abnormal shape of the external auricle as a clue to urinary tract malformations was first reported by Potter[12] and has been confirmed by many workers. Probably the most frequent association is that of the so-called pixie ears, including a position slightly lower than normal and a very sharp peak at the top of the pinna. The ears are abnormally soft and flat owing to poor development of the cartilage. They are unusually large and placed low on the head often less upright than normal.

Because this malformation of the auricle is most frequently associated with agenesis of the kidneys, it is always advisable to investigate the urinary tract promptly in a newborn who has "pixie" ears. This should be done by means of an intravenous pyelogram. Recently developed techniques of pyelography are worthy of comment.

The "infusion pyelogram," or injection of the contrast material diluted half and half with 5% glucose in water over a 5–10 minute period, is the best way of obtaining satisfactory films in the newborn in the presence of immature kidneys and their impaired concentrating ability. It is frequently tempting to give an intramuscular injection of the contrast material. From our experience, this should be avoided if at all possible, since the resulting contrast of the x-ray films is frequently equivocal even in the best of circumstances. Of course, this makes evaluation for absence of the kidneys completely worthless, since if no kidneys are demonstrated it is impossible to tell whether the dye was not absorbed rapidly enough or the kidneys are indeed absent.

Other anomalies associated with auricular malformations are local, such as unilateral hypoplasia of the face which includes hypoplasia of the mandible on that side, the Treacher-Collins syndrome, and other local malformations which include deformity of the auricle.

REFERENCES

1. Antia, N. H., and Buch, V. I.: Chondrocutaneous advancement flap for the marginal defect of the ear, Plast. & Reconstruct. Surg. 39:472, 1967.
2. Battle, R.: *Plastic Surgery* (Washington: Butterworths, 1964).
3. Cloutier, A. M.: Correction of outstanding ears; Plast. & Reconstruct. Surg. 28:412, 1961.
4. Converse, J. M., and Wood-Smith, D.: Technical details in the surgical correction of the lop ear deformity, Plast. & Reconstruct. Surg. 31:118, 1963.
5. Cosman, B., and Crikelair, G. F.: The composed tube pedicle in ear helix reconstruction, Plast. & Reconstruct. Surg. 37:517.
6. Gilles, H., and Millard, D. R.: *The Principles and Art of Plastic Surgery* (Boston: Little, Brown and Company, 1957).
7. Gouliam, D., and Conway, H.: Prevention of persistent deformity of the tragus and lobule by modification of the Luckett technique of otoplasty, Plast. & Reconstruct. Surg. 26:399, 1960.
8. Kaye, B. L.: A simplified method for correcting prominent ears, Plast. & Reconstruct. Surg. 40:44, 1967.
9. May, H.: *Reconstructive and Reparative Surgery* (Philadelphia: F. A. Davis Company, 1958).
10. Millard, D. R.: The chondrocutaneous flap in partial auricular repair, Plast. & Reconstruct. Surg. 37:523, 1966.
11. Mustande, J. C.: The treatment of prominent ears by buried mattress sutures: A ten-year survey, Plast. & Reconstruct. Surg. 39:382, 1967.
12. Potter, E. L.: Bilateral renal agenesis. J. Pediat. 29:68, 1946.
13. Straith, R. E.: Correction of the protruding ear, Plast. & Reconstruct. Surg. 24:277, 1959.
14. Tanzer, R. C.: Total reconstruction of the external ear, Plast. & Reconstruct. Surg. 23:1, 1959.
15. Tanzer, R. C.: An analysis of ear reconstruction, Plast. & Reconstruct. Surg. 31:118, 1963.

F. A. McParland
T. C. Chisholm
B. J. Spencer

16

Otolaryngologic Disorders

Surgery of the Tonsils and Adenoids
HISTORY

Excision of the tonsils was mentioned as early as 1000 B.C. in the Hindu literature.[23] Later ancient medical writers, including Hippocrates, Galen and Celsus,[4] described partial tonsillectomy for chronic infection and for symptoms of airway obstruction. Complete faucial tonsillectomy was seldom performed because of the high incidence of severe or even fatal postoperative hemorrhage. Treatment of the tonsils with caustics and live cautery was popular in the

18th Century, but the advent of general anesthesia in the 19th Century was accompanied by a return to the guillotine technique of excision. Surgical removal of the tonsils and adenoids as performed today is a procedure perfected since 1900 and is estimated to be done over 2 million times a year in the United States.[17]

Cryotonsillectomy, using cold for the destruction of tissues, has been described by von Leden and Rand,[20] who advocate its use in patients with blood dyscrasias. The technique has been reported too recently to warrant comment at this time.

EVALUATION FOR SURGERY OF TONSILS AND ADENOIDS

The object of the tonsil and adenoid operation is to remove the diseased adenoid mass and the tonsils with maximum safety in respect to surgical and anesthetic risk, with least discomfort to the patient, with as little tissue damage as possible and with a minimum of postoperative complications. These objectives are interrelated and have a direct bearing on the surgical principles.

Considerable difference of opinion prevails regarding the indications for tonsillectomy and adenoidectomy. Many physicians have seen equivocal or unfavorable results of tonsil and adenoid operations in both local and systemic diseases. Most of the sequelae could have been avoided if adequate preliminary evaluation of the patient and observance of the correct indications for operation had been made.

The anatomic relationships of the tonsils and adenoids have certain peculiar aspects which must be considered in the evaluation of disease of these tissues. Proctor[17] listed four factors of importance: (1) The surface of the tonsils and adenoids is exposed to ingested or inhaled foreign material. (2) The tonsil and adenoid crypts are in close proximity to adjacent blood vessel capillaries. (3) A rich lymphatic connection exists between the tonsils, the adenoids and the regional lymph nodes. (4) The tonsils and adenoids are closely related to the oropharynx, esophagus, nasopharynx, eustachian tubal orifices, nasal passages and paranasal sinuses.

As may be expected from these relationships, the most common childhood diseases of the tonsils and adenoids are acute and chronic infections acquired through inspiration or ingestion of pathogenic organisms, secondary extension of micro-organisms or toxins into the lymphatics or blood stream, enlargement of the tonsils and adenoids with obstruction of the nose, nasopharynx or oropharynx, and direct spread of infection to the nose, paranasal sinuses, eustachian tubes, middle ear or lower respiratory tract.

Evaluation of a complete and careful history may be the major factor in the decision to operate. Attention should be directed to the incidence and severity of upper respiratory infections, tonsillitis, obstructive symptoms (as from nasal obstruction, mouth breath-

ing and eustachian tube obstruction), otalgia, otorrhea, otitis media, cervical adenitis and bronchitis. Pertinent questions in the history should include general health and hygiene, system review, allergies, operations and injuries, drug and food sensitivity, prior infectious disease, developmental and family history.

The physical examination should include a general evaluation of development and health, plus a thorough examination of the neck, cervical glands, ears, nose, nasopharynx, pharynx, hypopharynx, paranasal sinuses and tests of hearing acuity.

INDICATIONS FOR SURGERY

INDICATIONS FOR ADENOIDECTOMY.—Adenoidectomy alone is indicated when symptoms arising from enlarged and/or infected adenoids are present without tonsil infection. Chronic infection of the adenoids is associated with the history of frequent recurrent head colds, especially in the winter, prolonged upper respiratory infections, purulent postnasal discharge with cough and at times bronchitis. The extension of infection may cause fever; symptoms of sinusitis, such as headache, malaise and increased purulent nasal and postnasal drainage; and recurrent otitis media with associated earaches, otorrhea and deafness. Enlargement of the adenoids causes symptoms of obstruction—mouth breathing, snoring, nasal voice quality and accumulation of nasal secretions with subsequent "sniffles" or nasal drip. Blockage of the eustachian tubal orifices may be associated with conductive hearing impairment and/or chronic otitis media.

The child with chronic adenoiditis may present the so-called adenoid facies, with open mouth, high palatal arch and pinched appearance of the middle third of the face. The ears may show signs of middle ear inflammation or infection. The tympanic membranes are often dull, retracted and slightly thickened. The middle ear may be inflamed or contain fluid. Anterior rhinoscopy shows accumulated secretions. The nasopharynx may be examined by mirror, nasopharyngoscope or palpation, it usually will contain a large mass of adenoid tissue covered by mucopurulent discharge. The adenoids may fill the nasopharynx, producing severe signs of obstruction.

In children under 4 years of age, chronic adenoiditis may occur without chronic infection of the tonsils, and adenoidectomy is the operation of choice, even when one or two attacks of acute tonsillitis have occurred. Removal of both tonsils and adenoids in these young children often stimulates hyperplasia of other lymphoid elements in the oropharynx. Recurrent inflammation of such tissue is difficult to treat and may cause persistent sore throat. In children over 4 years, chronic adenoiditis as a rule is accompanied by chronic tonsillitis, and tonsillectomy with adenoidectomy is necessary.

Several conditions must be differentiated from chronic adenoiditis. Thornwaldt's disease, or infected nasopharyngeal bursa, may present a picture of chronic nasopharyngeal infection without adenoid hypertrophy. The diagnosis usually can be made by examination but in some patients only by adenoidectomy.

Retropharyngeal abscess may be confused with a large adenoid mass and should be suspected if a large nasopharyngeal swelling is seen in an acutely ill child who has had a previous adenoidectomy. The abscess is soft and fluctuant in contrast to lymphoid tissue and must be examined with *extreme gentleness* in order to avoid rupture with discharge of the abcess contents into the larynx.

Partial or complete choanal atresia may be confused with obstruction of the posterior nares by adenoids. The clinical examination with trial passage of a nasal catheter will prove or disprove the presence of atresia. The posterior choanae should be checked for patency during every adenoidectomy.

In summary, the conditions for which adenoidectomy is performed are: nasopharyngeal obstruction by enlarged adenoids, recurrent or chronic ear infections[21] or conductive hearing loss secondary to enlarged or infected adenoids, and chronic or recurrent adenoid infection.

Adenoid tissue may undergo regrowth and require secondary removal. Small amounts of lymphoid tissue may recur about the eustachian tubal orifices and produce secondary conductive hearing loss or otitis media. In such instances, the nasopharyngeal radium applicator technique developed by Crowe may be the most effective form of treatment.

INDICATIONS FOR TONSILLECTOMY.—Whereas chronic adenoid infection may occur alone, the experience of most otolaryngologists indicates that chronic tonsillitis is almost always associated with chronic adenoiditis in children. The symptoms of chronic tonsillitis range from frequent recurrent episodes of acute tonsillitis to less clearly recognized complaints, such as swelling of the cervical glands or difficulty in swallowing. The chronically infected tonsil may be enlarged but is generally small, scarred and smooth-surfaced as the result of obliteration of the crypts by infection. The tonsil pillars are partly obliterated by scarring and show capillary injection of their mucosal surfaces. In the course of acute tonsillitis, organisms may break through the tonsil capsule to form a peritonsillar abscess presenting palatal asymmetry, peritonsillar edema and trismus. Most children with chronic tonsillitis or peritonsillar abscess have enlarged cervical lymph nodes, especially those at the angle of the mandible.

The *indications for the combined operation* are:
1. Chronic recurrent tonsillitis—by far the most common indication.
2. Peritonsillar abscess. This situation indicates that the tonsil capsule has been pierced and is no longer a barrier against infection. The authors of several studies[2,11,19] recommend tonsillectomy as immediate treatment for quinsy because of the good drainage and minimal scarring obtained.
3. Nasal airway obstruction from hypertrophic adenoids, in association with chronic tonsillitis. Obstruction of the oropharynx by enlarged tonsils is less commonly seen, but is an indication when severe.
4. Conductive hearing impairment, or recurrent ear infection associated with chronic and/or hypertrophic adenoiditis and tonsillitis. Many adenoidectomies are performed for nerve-type hearing impairment in children who do not have chronic adenoid or tonsil infection. Such needless operations should be condemned.
5. Nephritis, rheumatic fever, iritis and other systemic diseases associated with infections of the tonsils and adenoids. White[21] recommended tonsillectomy and adenoidectomy in patients with chronic rheumatic heart disease who can withstand operation, and in many cases after convalescence from active rheumatic disease.
6. Congenital cardiovascular anomalies, which may predispose to bacterial endocarditis.
7. Diphtheria carriers, who may become bacteria-free following tonsillectomy and adenoidectomy.

Many other indications are invoked to justify tonsil and adenoid surgery, such as recurrent sinusitis, bronchiectasis, asthma, cough, fever, abdominal pain, anorexia, failure to gain weight. In general, those patients who will benefit from tonsillectomy and adenoidectomy will usually have one or more of the indications first listed.

CONTRAINDICATIONS FOR ADENOIDECTOMY AND TONSILLECTOMY

Contraindications of a general nature are:
1. Hemophilia.
2. Blood dyscrasias such as leukemia, anemia, purpura, and disturbances of the bleeding and clotting mechanisms in serum sickness, drug reactions and following multiple transfusions.
3. Active pulmonary tuberculosis.
4. Acute or uncontrolled systemic disease, including diabetes, nephritis and rheumatic fever.
5. General debility.
Contraindications of a transient nature are:
1. History of a concurrent epidemic of poliomyelitis in the local community, especially when the patient has not received full immunization with vaccine.[1,9,18]
2. Acute illness, including upper respiratory infections, pulmonary or cardiac disease, gastrointestinal or renal disease and the acute exanthematous infections.
Functional contraindications are:
1. Peritonsillar or nasopharyngeal vascular anomalies, such as hemangioma.

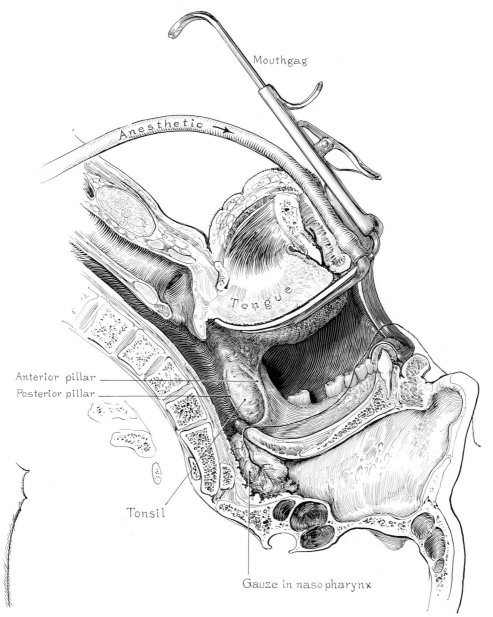

Fig. 16-1.—Tonsillectomy—exposure and packing. The patient is recumbent, the foot of the table slightly elevated. A gauze pack in the nasopharynx prevents saliva, vomitus or blood from entering the nasopharynx. The operator, wearing an electric headlight, stands at the end of the table. By placing the tongue depressor a little to the right or left of the median line of the tongue, an excellent view of the operative field on that side is obtained. (Figs. 1-5, courtesy of the Department of Art as Applied to Medicine, Johns Hopkins University School of Medicine; from original drawings by Max Brödel for the paper by S. J. Crowe.[6])

2. Tumors of the tonsil or nasopharynx which should be treated by more extensive operation or irradiation.

3. Cleft palate. The careful handling of cleft palate patients pre- and postoperatively is often neglected in otolaryngology texts. Exposure of the eustachian tubal orifices via the palatal cleft to pharyngeal food and liquids frequently results in secondary otitis media and hypertrophic adenoiditis. Palatal closure should precede adenoidectomy and tonsillectomy for

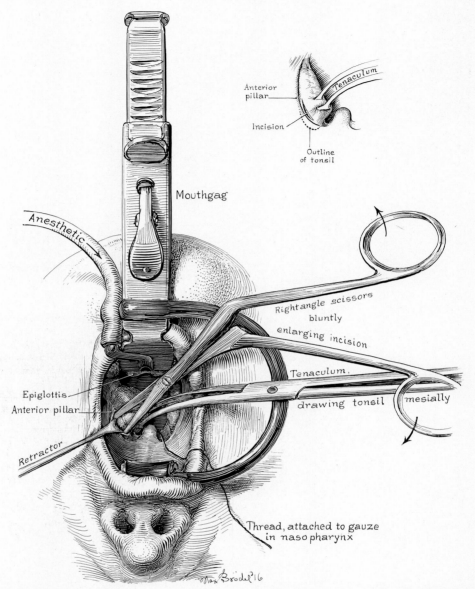

Fig. 16-2.—Tonsillectomy—dissection. The upper pole of the tonsil is gently pulled toward the midline. An incision is then made through the mucous membrane just mesial to the anterior pillar (**inset**). A retractor may be inserted as shown in the large drawing in order to provide better exposure.

several reasons. Closure of the palate may, on the one hand, eliminate the recurrent eustachian salpingitis and otitis media, and on the other, the adenoid tissue may be essential for effective closure of the nasopharynx during deglutition if the postoperative palate happens to be rigid or short. When nasopharyngeal closure is incomplete or barely effective, partial adenoidectomy or irradiation of the nasopharynx, as recommended by Crowe,[5] is the treatment of choice.

Tonsillectomy must be carefully performed to reduce secondary scarring.[3]

PREOPERATIVE CARE

Tonsillectomy and adenoidectomy require the same precautions in preoperative evaluation and preparation as any other operation. Figures of the Baltimore Anesthesia Study Commission indicate an average mortality of 1 in 7,100 patients during or within the first 48 hours after tonsillectomy[17] for the years 1953–1958. This mortality rate is low, but should serve as a reminder that all candidates for tonsillectomy and adenoidectomy deserve a complete history and physical examination as well as adequate laboratory studies.

Preanesthetic medication should include the control of peroral food and fluids in order to avoid the complications of vomiting, and the use of a barbiturate for sedation (such as Nembutal 1 mg./lb. body weight) plus scopolamine or atropine to inhibit respiratory secretions.

ANESTHESIA

The combination of an inexperienced anesthetist, in the absence of a skilled anesthesiologist, plus an inept surgeon often results in unpleasant if not lethal consequences. Tonsillectomy anesthesia is difficult and hazardous; 40% of the deaths studied by the Baltimore Anesthesia Study Commission were associated with difficulties in anesthesia.[17] Student anesthetists, so frequently assigned to tonsillectomy and adenoidectomy procedures, should be adequately supervised.

Inhalation anesthesia is generally preferred for children. The level of anesthesia should be only sufficiently deep to allow for relaxation of the pharyngeal and palatal muscles during adenoidectomy. Thereafter the level may be lightened so that coughing and swallowing occasionally occur and thereby reduce the likelihood of tracheal aspiration.

The decision to use endotracheal intubation should not be an all-or-none rule. The majority of pediatric tonsillectomies can be handled safely without intubation provided both surgeon and anesthesiologist safeguard the airway.[10] Under certain conditions intubation is indicated, but the endotracheal tube does not in itself guarantee adequate pulmonary ventilation or prevent tracheal aspiration.

Davies,[7] summarizing the incidence of mortality following tonsillectomy and adenoidectomy in his series of 21,500 children and 7,200 adults, reported 1 immediate postoperative death. All children were anesthetized by an insufflation technique; nasotracheal tubes were used in all adults. Davies concluded that insufflation without intubation is satisfactory if care and vigilance are observed.

SURGERY

The essentials of tonsil and adenoid surgery are careful adenoid curettage and surgical dissection of the tonsil, adequate hemostasis, gentle handling of tissues and an anesthetic technique which will safeguard the airway and provide minimal risk of aspiration. The use of a properly fitting Davis mouth gag with the patient in the Trendelenburg position will, by elevation of the base of the tongue, maintain an ade-

quate airway and furnish dependent drainage of secretions or blood to the nasopharynx (Figs. 16-1 – 16-5). Efficient suction must be constantly available from the start of anesthesia until the patient leaves the operating room. All manipulations from insertion of the mouth gag to the use of the suction should be performed gently and with a minimum of wasted motion in order to shorten the duration of operation and to reduce postoperative discomfort.

Adenoidectomy is best performed prior to tonsillectomy so that the nasopharynx can be observed for continuing hemorrhage during the remainder of the operation. We have found the curet to be the instrument of choice. Curets must fit between the eustachian tubal orifices and should be positioned by palpation in order to avoid trauma to the tube surface. Following

Fig. 16-3. — Tonsillectomy — dissection. The tonsil is removed by a combination of sharp and blunt dissection, made as close as possible to the capsule of the tonsil and carried down to the lower pole, where the tonsil may be severed by scissors or a snare.

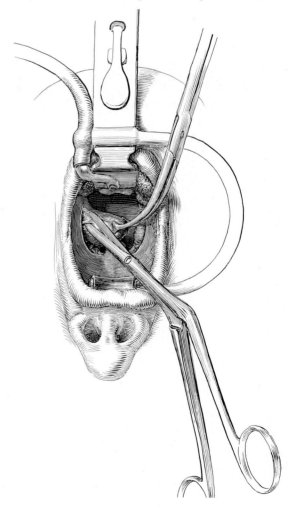

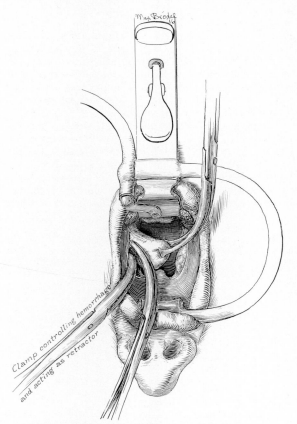

Fig. 16-4.—Tonsillectomy—hemostasis. Every bleeding vessel is clamped as in any surgical operation. This ensures a dry field and lessens the danger of postoperative pulmonary complications.

adenoidectomy, a tagged sponge will usually control bleeding and may remain until the end of the operation.

TECHNIQUE.—The tonsil is grasped with the tenaculum, traction is applied toward the midline, and an incision is made in the mucosa between the anterior pillar and the tonsil, exposing the peritonsillar space. This incision is carried over the upper pole and partly down the posterior pillar. The tonsil is then separated in the fascial plane between the capsule and fossa by meticulous blunt dissection until the attachment with the lingual tonsil is reached. At this point the tonsil may be severed by scissors or with a wire snare. In the presence of scarring, some sharp dissection may be required, but care should be taken to avoid trauma to the fossa musculature. The possibility of large aberrant blood vessels in the fossa should be kept in mind. The throat is kept dry by suction, as necessary. A sponge is gently applied to the fossa for 30 seconds, then all arterial and persistent venous bleeding points are clamped and secured with figure-of-eight sutures

of 00 plain catgut. Only enough tissue to effect hemostasis should be included in the suture. Catgut leads should not be clipped too short because of the tendency of the knot to work loose. Fluothane anesthesia now permits the use of electrocautery to accomplish hemostasis in the tonsil fossae. Magielski[13] used it in 1,054 cases, with an incidence of immediate significant postoperative hemorrhage of 0.4% and no deaths.

When both fossae are dry, the adenoid pack is removed and the nasopharynx is suctioned. In case of persistent nasopharyngeal hemorrhage which cannot be controlled by topical thrombin or clamping of a bleeding point, the insertion of a postnasal pack for 12 hours may be necessary. After all hemorrhage appears to have ceased, the mouth gag is relaxed for

Fig. 16-5.—Tonsillectomy—hemostasis: method of ligating bleeding vessels. Note the small amount of tissue included in the clamp. The sutures are transfixed as superficially as possible and snugly tied. Several operators have found 00 plain catgut to be the best suture material. Because of possibility of slippage, the ends of the catgut suture should be left somewhat longer than shown in the small illustrations.

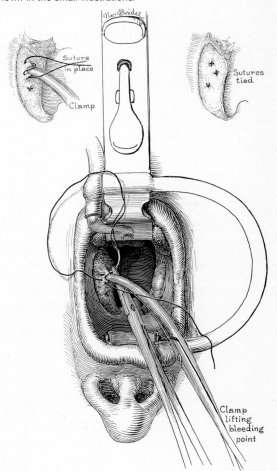

several minutes and, if no further bleeding occurs, the operation is finished. No patient should leave the operating table until all active bleeding is controlled.

POSTOPERATIVE CARE

After operation, the patient is placed in a semi-prone position, with the head turned to the side. (Fig. 16-6). Hemorrhage occurs in about 5% of reported cases.[15] Constant nursing attendance, with a good suction and oxygen nearby, is necessary until the child can handle his own secretions and is in satisfactory condition. The nurse should save all expectorated blood and watch for swallowing of blood, especially in young children. When swallowing movements are observed, when pallor is pronounced or the pulse rate rises, the pharynx should be examined at once.

With this technique Crowe[6] was able to report a 1.2% incidence of postoperative hemorrhage in 1,000 tonsillectomies, and to date we have had no postoperative lung abscess following tonsillectomy at Johns Hopkins Hospital.

Pain may be controlled by codeine or aspirin, or both. It is seldom severe beyond the second postoperative day. An ice collar may provide some comfort. A limited amount of aspirin gum used before meals will ease the discomfort of swallowing. Prolonged pain may be an index of secondary complications and deserves investigation.

No nourishment is given orally until the child is able to swallow without danger of aspiration. Liquids are given first, followed by a soft diet on the second or third day. Parenteral fluids may be necessary,[8] especially in hot weather when body losses are great. Hot, spicy, very acid or rough foods should be avoided for the first 5–7 days. The child's activities should be restricted for the first 2 or 3 days,[12] with a gradual return to normal during the next week. Swimming is not advisable until the tonsil fossae are healed; normally this will take about 2 weeks.

COMPLICATIONS

Most of the complications following tonsillectomy and adenoidectomy occur as phenomena secondary to the healing process. The tonsil fossa and adenoid bed become coated with a yellow-white septic membrane which is gradually replaced by granulation tissue in about 1 week, and then by mucous membrane. Delay in healing may result from diabetes or malnutrition or may follow virulent secondary infection. These factors may be eliminated by control of the diabetes, better than adequate nutrition and chemotherapy, respectively. If the child is taking steroids, these drugs must be continued until healing has occurred.

Severe sore throat may be the result of operative trauma, secondary infection or an impending exanthem. Antibiotics sometimes reduce the soreness by control of the secondary bacterial infection. Earache frequently follows tonsillectomy and adenoidectomy. The ears usually appear normal, in which case the pain is assumed to be of the referred type via Jacobson's nerve to the middle ear. Warm ear drops are sometimes beneficial.

Hemorrhage, the most frequent complication of tonsillectomy, occurs early (in the first 24 hours) or late (from the fifth to tenth day). Most early hemorrhages can be avoided by meticulous hemostasis in the tonsil fossa or by the use of a nasopharyngeal pack if adenoid bleeding persists. Large aberrant vessels in the fossa should be avoided; damage to such vessels may require carotid ligation.

If postoperative bleeding is not controlled by removal of clots from the fossa and the application of gentle pressure with a sponge, the child should be taken to the operating room promptly and anesthetized. The bleeding point is then identified and transfixed. Most patients with postoperative hemorrhage should have blood typing and cross-matching as a precautionary measure.

Fig. 16-6. — Tonsillectomy—postanesthesia position. The patient should remain in semiprone position until fully recovered from the anesthesia. The upper leg and arm may be placed over a pillow to prevent his rolling onto his face. In this position, with head extended, the airway will remain open because the tongue and jaw will fall forward. Secretions and vomitus will tend to run out of the mouth instead of being aspirated. Oxygen, suction and constant nursing care are necessary until the patient is fully awake.

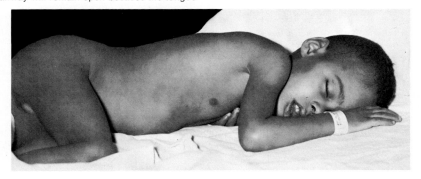

Late postoperative hemorrhage results from sloughing of the granulation membrane or tonsil sutures, and usually occurs 7–10 days after operation. Parents should be advised to watch for bleeding at this time. The treatment is similar to that for immediate hemorrhage. The application of coagulating agents or local tissue infiltration with saline or procaine has been recommended for both types of hemorrhage, but is often ineffectual in late bleeding because the bleeding point is obscured by the septic membrane or granulation tissue in the healing areas. Serious problems may arise from procrastination in the treatment of "tonsil bleeders." Prompt, positive treatment lessens or avoids the possibility of anemia, shock, excessive instrumentation, ingestion of blood and delayed postoperative recovery.

Prolonged acidosis and vomiting are caused by inadequate fluid and food intake. Oral sugar and rectal tranquilizing drugs will often control emesis. Intravenous glucose solutions may be necessary in persistent cases.

Other, but uncommon, complications, such as lung abscess, cervical emphysema[16] and parapharyngeal abscess, are discussed in most otolaryngology textbooks.

Follow-up examinations should be made at 2 weeks, 6 months and 1 year in order to ascertain the condition of the patient and the value of the operation. One of the most frequently performed of operations, the indiscriminate employment of tonsillectomy subjects children to unnecessary risks and unpleasantness, but its performance on good indication frequently transforms children who previously have been repeatedly or chronically ill.[22]

REFERENCES

1. Anderson, G. W.: Tonsillectomy and poliomyelitis, J.A.M.A. 184:80, 1963.
2. Bateman, G. H., and Kodicek, J.: Primary quinsy tonsillectomy, Ann. Otol., Rhin. & Laryng. 68:315, 1959.
3. Berner, R. G.: Hazards of adenotonsillectomy in the child with cleft palate, J.A.M.A. 181:558, 1962.
4. Celsus: *De Medicino*, tr by W. G. Spencer (Cambridge, Mass.: Harvard University Press, 1935), Vol. 3, p. 371.
5. Crowe, S. J., and Burnam, C. F.: Recognition, treatment and prevention of hearing impairment in children, Ann. Otol., Rhin. & Laryng. 50:15, 1941.
6. Crowe, S. J., *et al.*: Relation of tonsillar and nasopharyngeal infections to general systemic disorders, Johns Hopkins Hospital Bull. 28:1, 1917.
7. Davies, D. D.: Anaesthetic mortality in tonsillectomy and adenoidectomy, Brit. J. Anaesth. 36:110, 1964.
8. Faigel, H.: Tonsillectomy—a bloody mess, Clin. Pediat. 5:652, 1966.
9. Fischer, A. E., *et al.*: Poliomyelitic paralysis and tonsillectomy, J.A.M.A. 186:873, 1963.
10. Graff, T. D.: Holzman, R. S., and Benson, D. W.: Acid-base balance during halothane anesthesia for tonsillectomy, Anesth. & Anal. 43:620, 1964.
11. Grahne, B.: Abscess tonsillectomy, Arch. Otolaryng. 68:332, 1958.
12. Heasmon, M. A.: How long in hospital? A study in duration of stay for two common conditions, Lancet 2:539, 1964.
13. Magielski, J. E.: Electrocautery hemostasis in tonsil and adenoid surgery under Fluothane (halothane) anesthesia: 1,054 cases, Laryngoscope 73:595, 1963.
15. Parkinson, R. H.: *Tonsil and Allied Problems* (New York: Macmillan Company, 1951).
16. Pratt, L. W.; Hamberger, H. R., and Moore, V. J.: Mediastinal emphysema complicating tonsillectomy and adenoidectomy, Ann. Otol., Rhin. & Laryng. 71:158, 1962.
17. Proctor, D. F.: *The Tonsils and Adenoids in Childhood* (Springfield, Ill.: Charles C Thomas, Publisher, 1960).
18. Ravenholt, R. T.: Poliomyelitic paralysis and tonsillectomy reconsidered, Am. J. Dis. Child. 103:658, 1962.
19. Volk, B. M., and Brandow, E. C., Jr.: Bilateral tonsillectomy for peritonsillar abscess, Laryngoscope 70:840, 1960.
20. Von Leden, H., and Rand, R. W.: Cryosurgery of the head and neck, Arch. Otolaryng. 85:93, 1967.
21. White, P. D.: *Heart Disease* (3rd ed.; New York: Macmillan Company, 1946).
22. Wilson, I. I.: A review of the indications for tonsillectomy, New Zealand M. J. 61:603, 1962.
23. Wise, T. A.: *Review of the History of Medicine* (London: J. & A. Churchill, Ltd., 1967), Vol. 2, p. 225.

Otitis Media and Mastoiditis

ANATOMIC CONSIDERATIONS

The primary route for extension of infection to the mastoid cells of the temporal bone is by way of the eustachian tube, which connects the nasopharynx to the middle ear cavity. From the middle ear, infection may extend into the mastoid cells through the atticotympanic space. At birth, the mastoid region contains primitive marrow which is gradually replaced in the normal process of development by air-filled cells lined with mucous membrane and which connect with the middle ear. Early infection of the middle ear may prevent the development of the normal air-cell structure and result in a sclerotic or infantile mastoid. The various theories of mastoid development have been discussed by Fowler,[4] who pointed out that some sclerotic mastoids are produced by infection; some, by failure of development following infection; and others, by congenital failure of pneumatization.

Certain factors make the child more susceptible to otitis media than the adult. During infancy, the eustachian tube is straight, horizontal and relatively wide open. Initially, the tubal orifice lies at the level of the palate and assumes a more superior and posterior position in the nasopharynx only as growth of the face proceeds. Thus nasal secretions are more likely to enter the eustachian tube in the younger child. In addition, enlargement of the adenoids and adjacent lymphoid tissue around the eustachian orifice may occlude the tube and prevent proper drainage from the middle ear, or adenoid infection may by direct extension involve the eustachian tube and middle ear space.

OTITIS MEDIA

Otitis media, or inflammation of the middle ear space, occurs as serous otitis media and purulent otitis media. In both types, acute and chronic forms are seen.

SEROUS OTITIS MEDIA.—Acute serous otitis media is a serous effusion into the middle ear space resulting from blockage of the eustachian tube. The condition may arise from an acute head cold, enlarged adenoids, vasomotor or allergic rhinitis or from barometric pressure changes associated with flying. Occasionally, a nasopharyngeal tumor compressing the tubal orifice, or dental malocclusion may be an etiologic factor.[3]

The *signs* and *symptoms* of serous otitis media include decreased hearing, a sense of fullness and pressure in the affected ear and occasionally tinnitus or pain. On examination, the tympanic membrane is usually in normal position or slightly retracted. The membrane may be dull, slightly yellow or straw-colored if fluid is present, and may show air bubbles in the middle ear. When hemorrhage has occurred, the tympanic membrane may be a dusky blue, dark gray or black. The audiogram usually will show a conductive type of hearing impairment. Radiographs of the temporal bone may show diffuse clouding in the affected mastoid cells.

The *treatment* of serous otitis media is primarily directed toward removal of the underlying causative factors, such as enlarged adenoids. In the majority of children, this treatment will effect resolution of the process, but in all cases the child should be followed to ensure that the otitis has cleared. In persistent cases, myringotomy with aspiration of the middle ear fluids may be necessary, and inflations of the middle ear may be helpful.[7] The trans-tympanic drainage tube is occasionally employed to permit prolonged aeration of the middle ear cavity.

PURULENT OTITIS MEDIA.—Acute suppurative otitis media is a purulent infection involving the middle ear space and adjacent cells in the mastoid bone. The most common infecting organisms are *Streptococcus pyogenes*, *Staphylococcus pyogenes aureus* and *albus*, and *alpha hemolytic streptococci*. Purulent otitis media usually results from an acute upper respiratory infection and is often seen in the course of one of the acute contagious diseases, such as measles and influenza.

The *signs* and *symptoms* of acute purulent otitis media are: a sensation of fullness in the ear, decrease of hearing, otalgia, and fever. As the infection progresses, pain becomes more severe and tinnitus may appear. Some children may have tenderness over the mastoid bone. With rupture of the tympanic membrane and escape of pus from the external auditory canal, pain and fever decrease. In the early stages, the tympanic membrane will show dullness, marked erythema and slight retraction of the membrane. As the infection progresses, the tympanic membrane bulges at first in the pars flaccida, and later the entire membrane is pushed outward with loss of all landmarks except the malleus. In late stages, the membrane may become whitish or yellow and a pulsating discharge may be seen if spontaneous perforation has occurred.

The audiogram or tuning fork tests will show a conductive hearing impairment, and, in general, mastoid radiographs will show diffuse clouding of the mastoid air cells. Such clouding can persist for some time and may lead to an erroneous diagnosis of acute mastoiditis.

The *treatment* of acute otitis media depends upon the stage of the infection. When signs of middle ear pressure, such as severe pain, are absent and the tympanic membrane is not bulging, treatment is directed toward control of the infection with antibiotics. Nasal drainage is promoted by the use of nasal decongestants. Anodynes, including glycerin-base ear drops, are used to alleviate discomfort. The patient should be closely followed to make certain that complete resolution of the inflammation occurs. Lumio[9] pointed out that chronic adhesive changes may occur in the middle ear if the inflammatory process does not clear up and that a permanent conductive hearing impairment will result from subsequent scarring and adhesions.

When the middle ear infection has progressed to the stage of severe pain with bulging of the tympanic membrane, myringotomy is performed in addition to the other measures mentioned. Drainage of the middle ear should be done under a short-acting general anesthetic such as vinethene or fluothane. The ear canal is cleansed with alcohol or Zephiran, and an incision made in the posteroinferior part of the tympanic membrane in its midportion and parallel to the external margin. The entire thickness of the membrane should be incised and the opening made large enough to permit good drainage. As a rule, purulent material under considerable pressure will be obtained. Cultures of the discharge are made for identification of organisms and their drug sensitivities. If the middle ear is already discharging, the otologist must make certain that the spontaneous opening is adequate for drainage. Hydrogen peroxide ear drops have been recommended when drainage is present, but our experience suggests that aural medication is rarely needed after myringotomy.

Antibiotic therapy must be sufficient to combat the infection adequately and should be continued until the infection is resolved. Bozer,[1] reporting in 1948 on a series of children with otitis media which had progressed to acute mastoiditis at the Buffalo Children's Hospital, stated that only 3% had received adequate antibiotic therapy. With so many infections by drug-resistant bacteria today, a minimum of adequate therapy is the drug manufacturer's recommended daily therapeutic dosage per pound body weight for at least 5 days and for longer periods of time if resolution is slow. The chemotherapeutic agent chosen should provide prompt and adequate initial blood levels of the drug. Changes in therapy should be made if there is no improvement within 48 hours of treatment, and mastoiditis should be suspected if otorrhea persists more than 2 weeks.

All patients must be followed until complete resolution has occurred, at which time any predisposing conditions are corrected.

MASTOIDITIS

Acute mastoiditis generally is a complication of acute otitis media and less commonly results from chronic otitis media. The most frequent causative organisms are *S. pyogenes, Staph. pyogenes aureus, Diplococcus pneumoniae* and *Klebsiella pneumoniae*.[11] Two pathologic forms are seen: the coalescent type associated with breakdown of the mastoid air-cell walls, and the hemorrhagic or thrombophlebitic type which has been seen more frequently since antibiotics have come into general use.

The frequency of acute mastoiditis has decreased markedly since the introduction of chemotherapeutic agents. Davison[2] noted an incidence of 58.9% of cases with acute otitis media requiring mastoidectomy in 1937 in contrast to an incidence of 3% in 1954. This change is attributed to arrest of the middle ear infection before extension to the mastoid bone has occurred.

The *signs* and *symptoms* of acute mastoiditis include otorrhea, pain and tenderness over the mastoid bone, conductive hearing impairment, fever and roentgenographic evidence of cloudiness and opacity of the mastoid cells, usually with breakdown of the cellular structure, although this is not always present in fulminating infections. In mild infections, the symptoms may be only persistent otorrhea following acute otitis media of 3 weeks' duration, but in more virulent disease, rapid bone destruction with subperiosteal abscess or intracranial complications may appear before otorrhea is present.[1] Bozer[1] and Hoople[6] noted that in many cases of acute mastoiditis, rupture of the tympanic membrane occurred or myringotomy was performed only late in the course of the infection. To quote Rutherford[12]:

> The complacent acceptance of the antibiotic as a cure-all in acute otitis media has led to a state where the younger pediatricians do not know the art of cleansing the ear canal, of observing and recognizing the changes in the tympanic membrane which indicate pathologic conditions in the middle ear, or how to do a myringotomy.

This statement may be applied to mastoiditis, which is now considered by some physicians to be treatable solely by chemotherapy. Mastoiditis is osteomyelitis. The primary and best treatment of acute mastoid infection is adequate drainage supplemented, to be sure, by appropriate antibiotic therapy.

Complications of acute mastoiditis arise from spread of the infection to adjacent areas, directly or by propagating thrombophlebitis. The most common extension is through the mastoid cortex to form a subperiosteal abscess in the postauricular area. Occasionally extension will occur to the zygomatic cells to form a preauricular abscess, or medial to the mastoid tip to present as a Bezold abscess in the upper cervical area. Erosion of the facial nerve canal will produce facial paralysis. Extension to the lateral sinus plate may cause a perisinus abscess or phlebitis and occasionally benign intracranial hypertension. Involvement of the posterior or middle fossa surfaces may produce epidural abscess, meningitis or brain abscess. Extension to the inner ear may produce a serous or suppurative labyrinthitis, and spread to the petrous apex will produce petrositis, often associated with sixth nerve paralysis (Gradenigo's syndrome).[1, 2, 8, 10] In Bozer's series during 1945 and 1946, 94 patients with acute mastoiditis required operation. Two of these had cerebellar abscess, and each had meningismus, meningitis, epidural abscess, Gradenigo's syndrome, and perisinus infection.

The *prognosis* for complications of mastoiditis and acute otitis media has changed considerably with the use of antibiotics. Watson[13] gave a recovery rate for otitic meningitis of 84.6% in 1944 in contrast to 19.6% in 1922. These results were encouraging, but complete safe recovery requires resolution of the infection in the middle ear or mastoid by operative or other means, and measures must be taken to prevent reinfection.

MASTOIDECTOMY. — The technique of simple mastoidectomy consists of a postauricular incision parallel and about 1 – 2 cm posterior to the sulcus behind the auricle. The incision is carried down to the bone but does not extend to the mastoid tip (Fig. 16-7). The cortex is exposed with a periosteal elevator from the posterior border of the bony external auditory meatus to about 1 cm behind the skin incision. A self-retaining retractor is introduced. The mastoid cortex is exenterated with a burr, and the infected mastoid cells underlying the area are removed. The cavity thus created is enlarged to remove all infected cells between the limits of the lateral sinus plate posteriorly, the dural plate superiorly, the facial ridge and bony external auditory canal anteroinferiorly and the osseous labyrinth medially. The antrum is exposed, but the attic space is not entered. A drain is placed in the cavity and brought out through the lower part of the skin incision, which is then closed above. If examination of the tympanic membrane reveals an intact membrane or a perforation which is too small for drainage, a myringotomy is performed. In patients with intracranial complications, exposure of the lateral sinus, middle cranial or posterior cranial fossae may be necessary.

More extensive operations, such as the radical or modified radical procedures, are seldom required for simple acute mastoiditis. As with otitis media, predisposing conditions are to be eliminated. These are in most cases pathologic conditions of the upper respiratory passages and pharynx.

With the development of drug-resistant strains of bacteria, there has been an increase in the incidence of mastoiditis and its complications.[5] Today, the use

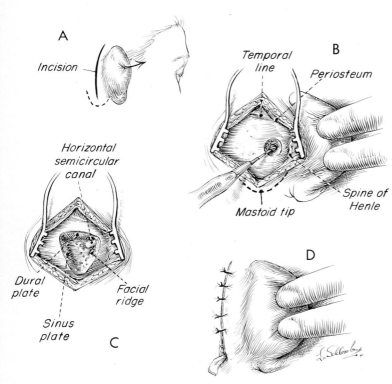

A
Incision

B
Temporal line
Periosteum
Spine of Henle
Mastoid tip

C
Horizontal semicircular canal
Dural plate
Sinus plate
Facial ridge

D

Fig. 16-7.—Simple mastoidectomy. **A,** the usual postauricular incision. **B,** reflection of soft tissue from the mastoid cortex. The spine of Henle on the posterior aspect of the bony external auditory canal represents the approximate level at which excavation of the mastoid bone has begun. **C,** limits of excavation in a simple mastoidectomy: the dural plate of the middle cranial fossa, lateral sinus, facial ridge, and horizontal semicircular canal. **D,** closure of the mastoid. The mastoid cavity has been filled with a drain and a large opening left in the lower part of the incision to provide adequate drainage.

of early and adequate drainage, of sufficient early and continued antibiotic administration and of careful follow-up are essential in the treatment of acute ear infections.

REFERENCES

1. Bozer, H. E.: A study of surgical mastoiditis occurring in children at the Buffalo Children's Hospital during the years 1945 and 1946, New York J. Med. 48:183, 1948.
2. Davison, F. W.: Otitis media—then and now, Laryngoscope 65:142, 1955.
3. Draper, W. L.: Secretory otitis media in children: A study of 540 cases, Tr. Am. Laryng., Rhin. & Otol. Soc., p. 346, 1964.
4. Fowler, E. P., Jr.: *Medicine of the Ear* (2nd ed.; Baltimore: Williams & Wilkins Company, 1948).
5. Goldman, J. L., and Rosenwasser, H.: Current concepts of the management of otitic infections, J.A.M.A. 171:509, 1959.
6. Hoople, G.: In discussion of Bozer.[1]
7. Kapur, Y. P.: Serous otitis media in children, Arch. Otolaryng. 79:38, 1964.
8. Korkis, F. B.: Suppurative mastoid surgery yesterday and today, Lancet 2:833, 1954.
9. Lumio, J. S.: Contributions to the knowledge of chronic adhesive otitis, Acta oto-laryng. 39:196, 1951.
10. Morse, H. R.: Intracranial complications of chronic mastoiditis, Arch. Otolaryng. 63:142, 1956.
11. Palva, T.; Friedman, I., and Palva, A.: Mastoiditis in children, J. Laryng. 78:977, 1964.
12. Watson, D.: Progress in the treatment of mastoid infection and some of its complications, Proc. Roy. Soc. Med. 41:155, 1948.

Choanal Atresia

Congenital atresia of the posterior nares occurs infrequently. Ersner[5] estimated a bilateral incidence of about 1 per 60,000 persons. The low incidence and resultant unfamiliarity with the symptoms of the anomaly have permitted many cases to escape detection and diagnosis. Recent revival of interest in the correction of this anomaly has resulted in uncovering a substantial number of individuals so afflicted and has improved diagnostic techniques.

Unlike harelip and cleft palate, which are known to result from failures of fusion of the maxillary processes and the several parts of the frontal process, the causation of choanal atresia has not been satisfactorily explained. Theories of the mechanisms leading to choanal atresia were reviewed by McKibben.[9]

The obstruction consists of a partition attached superiorly to the body of the sphenoid, laterally to the medial pterygoid process, medially to the posterior edge of the vomer and inferiorly to the horizontal plate of the palatine bone (Fig. 16-8). The obstruction may be little more than a membranous septum or may be a solid mass of bone, or bone and cartilage. Each surface is covered with mucous membrane continuous with that of the nasal and nasopharyngeal surfaces. Minute perforations may be present but are usually nonfunctional. The obstructed side is characteristically associated with narrowing of the nasal and nasopharyngeal cavities due to elevation of the

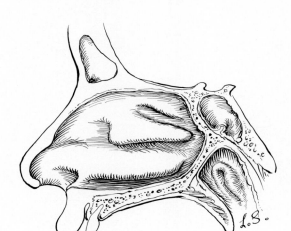

Fig. 16-8.—Sagittal section of the head, made just lateral to the vomer, illustrating an extreme form of choanal atresia with dense bony obstruction between the posterior end of the palate and body of the sphenoid. This is the usual site of choanal atresia, but occlusion by membranes or delicate bony tissue is more common. The obstruction may be unilateral or bilateral.

palatal arch, a more medial position of the medial pterygoid process and an anterior position of the posterior nasopharyngeal wall. Other associated malformations were listed by McKibben.[9]

SYMPTOMATOLOGY.—The infants with bilateral choanal atresia may be divided into four subgroups on the basis of symptomatology.

Cyclic dyspnea.—Newborn infants ordinarily do not acquire the mechanism of mouth-breathing until several days after birth. Dependent upon the nasal airway, they may succumb to asphyxia in the presence of bilateral atresia. The term cyclic dyspnea applies to the recurring phases of asphyxia followed by crying, mouth-breathing, quiet, then asphyxia again. Feeding usually is impossible in these circumstances.

Dyspnea while suckling.—In some cases, symptoms of suffocation occur when suckling is attempted, and oral breathing is necessarily impossible. These infants must learn to suck and breathe alternately. Breathing is heavy, and attacks of suffocation may occur during sleep.

Infants with no dyspnea.—An occasional case in this group has been reported.

Older patients.—The signs and symptoms of complete nasal obstruction are present: mouth-breathing, absence of nasal quality to the voice, poor sense of smell and taste and excessive nasal discharge of mucus or tears. Inability to blow the nose is noted, and dryness of the mouth may be annoying.

As a rule, unilateral atresia is unnoticed until later life unless the patent nostril becomes blocked, as in feeding for example. The symptoms on the obstructed side are similar to those in the bilateral cases.

DIAGNOSIS.—Whenever an infant has difficulty in breathing and cannot nurse, the differential diagnosis should include choanal atresia, tracheoesophageal fistula and tumors or other obstructive lesions in the nose or nasopharynx. Improved breathing after insertion of an oral airway will suggest the presence of an upper respiratory obstruction. Many patients have atrophy and underdevelopment of the turbinates, narrowing of the nasal passages and a high arched palate.

Inability to pass a small catheter through the nostrils into the pharynx is strong evidence that the choanae are obstructed. Posterior obstruction of the nasal cavity may be demonstrated by instillation of iodized oil into the nose followed by roentgenography of the head in the supine position. In older patients, the obstruction may be seen by anterior and/or posterior rhinoscopy when the accumulated nasal mucus has been removed. In small children, it may be necessary to make the examination under anesthesia in order to confirm the nature of the obstruction.

TREATMENT.—The treatment of choanal atresia depends on the seriousness of symptoms in the individual patient.

Infants with bilateral choanal atresia, who are not able to breathe orally, must be provided with an adequate oral airway until mouth-breathing has been established or until operative cure has been effected. Constant nursing attendance is necessary to safeguard the airway. Almost all of these infants require feeding by medicine dropper, spoon or stomach tube until they learn to nurse. Operation on the atresia is performed in most of the severe instances within the first few weeks of life. Bilateral atresia, unnoticed until later in childhood, and not having caused serious symptoms in infancy, is not likely to do so. As in unilateral atresia, the correction of the anomaly may be performed when convenient.

Operative repair.—The technique of the operative procedure to be used varies according to the age of the patient, the type of occluding tissue, and the condition of the nasal structures.

The direct intranasal route for the surgical cure of atresia is the oldest approach, but is chiefly used today for the correction of membranous obstructions. The atretic membrane is curetted away, and a polyethylene stent is inserted between nose and nasopharynx. The stent remains in place until healing has occurred, on the average in 2–3 months.

The submucous intranasal approach has been utilized primarily in adults, but with good results in some children down to 2 years of age. The technique involves incision of the mucosal wall of the inferior nasal septum and floor of the nasal cavity. A tunnel is thus created which is carried posteriorly to the bony atresia plate, and the mucous membrane overlying the plate is elevated in continuity with that of the nasal mucosa. The atresia is then perforated with a chisel and the opening enlarged with rongeurs. The mucosal flap is then returned to its normal position and the mucosa formerly over the bony atresia is incised either in a flap or cruciate incision, in order to cover exposed bony surfaces. A polyethylene stent is inserted through the nose into the nasopharynx and retained in position until healing has occurred.

In most infants and small children with bony atresia, the transpalatal approach, first used in this country by Blair,[2] has been advocated because of the excellent field of view. A palatal flap is created to expose the posterior palatal margin. Owens[10] included the palatal vessels in the flap in order to preserve an adequate blood supply. Removal of part of the hard palate exposes the obstruction, which is removed by rongeurs or burr. Mucosal flaps from the vomer and anterior and posterior surfaces of the obstruction are used to cover the bony surfaces left exposed by removal of the bony wall. The palatal flap is then returned in place.

The chief problem of choanal atresia repair has been postoperative stenosis, which occurs with only slight scar formation because of the congenital narrowness of the nasal passage common to this anomaly. Two main principles of operative repair exist: (1) to open and enlarge the choanae by removal of part of the lateral wall,[12] and (2) to minimize postoperative scarring by the use of mucosal flaps to cover exposed bony areas.[4, 10, 11] The use of stents postoperatively has been subject to debate, but in our experience, a properly fitting stent is essential for good postoperative results.

Few large series of postoperative results have been recorded. Johnson[6] listed two failures and nine cures in patients who were treated by the transpalatine operation. Since few surgeons see this many patients, the need for careful evaluation and handling should be recognized in every instance of choanal atresia that comes to operation regardless of the method of repair elected.

REFERENCES

1. Beinfield, H. H.: Surgical management of complete and incomplete bony atresia of the posterior nares, Tr. Am. Acad. Ophth. 60:778, 1956.
2. Blair, V. P.: Congenital atresia or obstruction of air passages, Ann. Otol., Rhin. & Laryng. 40:1021, 1931.
3. Cherry, J., and Bordley, J. E.: Surgical correction of choanal atresia, Ann. Otol., Rhin. & Laryng. 75:911, 1966.
4. Dolowitz, D. A., and Holley, E. B.: Congenital atresia, Arch. Otolaryng. 49:587, 1949.
5. Ersner, M. S.: In discussion of Beinfield.[1]
6. Johnson, S.: Congenital choanal atresia, Acta otolaryng. 51:533, 1959.
7. Kazanjian, V. H.: The treatment of congenital atresia of the choanae, Ann. Otol., Rhin. & Laryng. 51:704, 1942.
8. Lemere, H. B.: Persistent bucconasal membrane in the newborn, J.A.M.A. 109:347, 1937.
9. McKibben, B. G.: Congenital atresia of the nasal choanae, Laryngoscope 67:731, 1957.
10. Owens, H.: Observations in treating 7 cases of choanal atresia by the transpalatine approach, Laryngoscope 61:304, 1951.

The common signs of laryngeal disease in early childhood are respiratory obstruction, stridor or abnormal quality of the voice and, less often, aspiration of mucous food, or both, into the larynx. Although stridor may result from intrinsic and extrinsic causes, only the intrinsic causes of surgical significance will be considered here. Additional information is available in the chapters on tracheostomy (Chapter 24) and endoscopy (Chapter 30). Before discussing stridor in infancy, we should review differences between the infant and the adult larynx, which explain why stridor is so often the presenting sign of laryngeal disease in children.

EMBRYOLOGY

The earliest indication of the future respiratory tree is observed in the 5-mm embryo (approximately 26 days of gestation) as a groove which runs lengthwise on the floor of the gut, just caudal to the pharyngeal pouches (Fig. 16-9). Externally, the entoderm projects as a ventral laryngotracheal ridge. The boundaries of this primitive sagittal fissure are derived from the six visceral arches or lateral masses. Anterior to the groove, a central mass of condensed tissue (the future epiglottis) lies between the vertical ends of the third and fourth arches. A lateral furrow appears on each side of the laryngotracheal ridge along the line of junction between the ridge and the esophagus. The furrows become progressively deeper and extend craniad; eventually they join, thereby separating a laryngotracheal tube from the esophagus. At the upper end, the laryngeal portion of the tube advances slightly rostrad until it lies between the fourth branchial arches with tissue from the fifth arches as its lateral boundaries. Opening of the cleft does not occur before the second part of the fourth week (Fig. 16-9).

The epiglottis is peculiar to mammals. The 5-mm human embryo shows a rounded prominence which elevates midventrally from the bases of the third and fourth arches. This tissue soon consolidates into the transverse flap that guards the entrance of the larynx during swallowing. The primitive epiglottis becomes concave on its laryngeal surface and, in the middle part of fetal life, differentiates cartilage internally. The slit from the floor of the pharynx into the trachea is the primitive glottis, which becomes bounded on each side by rounded eminences of fourth and fifth arch origin, known as arytenoid swellings. These two swellings grow in a tongue-ward direction. On meeting the primordium of the epiglottis, they turn upward and forward against its caudal surface, as seen in the 12-mm embryo. By the seventh week, the original sagittal slit has added a transverse groove to its upper end, so that the laryngeal aperture becomes T-shaped, as observed in the 16-mm embryo. However,

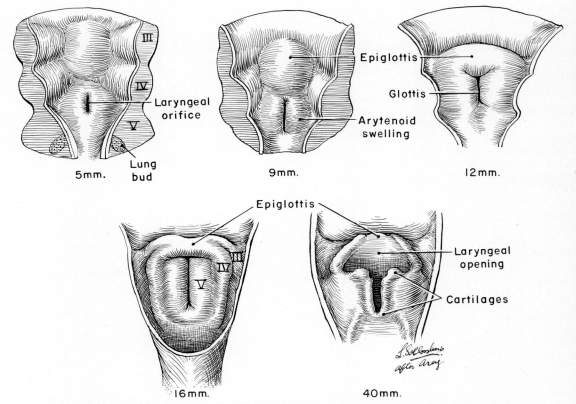

Fig. 16-9.—Development of the larynx in the human embryo at stages from 5 to 40 mm; posterior view.

the entrance to the larynx ends blindly for some time because fusion of the epithelium in the upper larynx has obliterated the lumen there. When the epithelial union is dissolved at 10 weeks of gestation, the entrance becomes more oval in contour (40-mm embryo) and a pair of lateral recesses, or laryngeal ventricles, is evident in the restored cavity. Each of these is bounded cranially and caudally by a projecting lateral shelf. The caudal pair, at the same level as the primitive laryngeal slit, are the vocal folds; these appear at 8 weeks and later differentiate elastic tissue.

The epithelial lining of the larynx is supported by dense mesenchyme derived from the fourth and fifth branchial arches. Early in the sixth week, this mass shows localized condensations that foretell the laryngeal cartilages. By the end of the second or early in the third month, the shapes of the arytenoid cartilages are well defined. During the sixth week, the cricoid cartilage develops from the sixth arches as two separate halves which unite by growth along a vertical lamina. By the end of the second month, the whole ring is chondrified. The arytenoids are separated by a sagittal cleft, but the cricoid anlage is continuous dorsally and ventrally.

The thyroid cartilage originates in the first month as lateral condensations in the fourth arches. At the end of the sixth week, chondrification has progressed considerably. The laryngeal muscles also originate from these branchial arches and are therefore innervated by the vagus nerve.

The trachea and esophagus develop in the cephalic portion of the primitive gut, with separate development of the upper and lower portions of the esophagus. A single tube is formed which eventually divides at 7–8 weeks into two complete hollow tubes—the trachea anteriorly and the esophagus posteriorly.

ANATOMIC DIFFERENCES

1. *Size.*—The principal anatomic difference between the infant and adult larynx is size (Fig. 16-10). The cross-sectional area of the infant larynx and trachea is relatively smaller than that of the adult when related to total body mass. The greatest narrowing occurs in the subglottic region, which predisposes the child to stridor. Before a diagnosis of congenital stenosis can be established, however, it is necessary to correlate the size of the infant to the lumen of his larynx.

2. *Consistency.*—In young children, all laryngeal tissues are softer than in the adult. The cartilages are softer and more pliable; and the mucosa, looser and less fibrous. The relatively narrow lumen and the

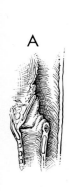
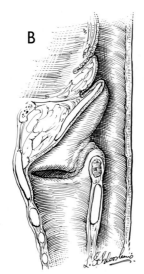

Fig. 16-10.—Growth changes of the larynx. **A,** the 5-week-old infant larynx; **B,** the adult larynx.

TABLE 16-2 – AIRWAY DIAMETERS FROM ANATOMIC SECTIONS AND MOULAGE*

AGE, MO.	GLOTTIS, MM	CRICOID RING, MM	TRACHEA, MM
4	23–26	20	22–25
6	26	20	24
8	24	21	24
10	25	22	26
13	25	22	26

*After Bayeux.[2]

idea of a straighter airway in infants, and the effect of position on the production of stridor is subject to question.

4. *Shape.* — The upper end of the larynx and trachea is funnel-shaped in the infant. This shape disappears in the older child and adult female but reappears in a modified form in the adult male, in whom the backward tilt of the cricoid cartilage is replaced by a forward tilt of the thyroid cartilage. The tracheal lumen, however, no longer diminishes as it descends, as in the infant. Measurements by Tucker indicate that the average newborn subglottic diameter is 6 mm; narrowness is indicated by a 5 mm diameter, and definite stenosis when the diameter is 4 mm or less. There is no uniform agreement as to the relationship of tracheal and laryngeal diameters. Studies by Engel[3] and Bayeux[2] suggest that the cricoid internal diameter is probably the narrowest portion of the airway, although in the newborn, the trachea diameter may not be very much larger (Tables 16-1 and 16-2).

The vocal folds are shorter in the infant than in the adult. The epiglottis overhangs the vestibule less than in the adult and is narrower and generally U-shaped. In addition, the ventricular air sacs of infants are relatively larger in relation to other laryngeal structures than in the adult.

In summary, the infant larynx differs from the adult larynx in its relative size, consistency, position and shape. When infant anatomic characteristics are present to an abnormal degree, the insufficiency of the laryngeal airway, the softness of laryngeal walls and structures, and the weakness of the muscles may result in laryngomalacia with congenital laryngeal stridor. When the normal infant larynx becomes inflamed, as in diphtheria and acute laryngotracheal bronchitis, the relatively small laryngeal lumen is greatly reduced by the edema permitted by the loose areolar tissues of the larynx, especially in the subglottic area. The presenting symptom is stridor.

softness and laxity of the infant's larynx are important causes of stridor when the laryngeal tissues are further narrowed by inflammation and edema.

3. *Position.* — The high larynx of the infant descends continuously during development. In the fetus of 5 or 6 weeks, the larynx is situated opposite the basiocciput, but by the fourth month, the lower border of the cricoid cartilage lies opposite the upper border of the fourth cervical vertebra. At 7 months, the larynx has descended to the middle of the sixth vertebra and is found in this position at term. After birth, further descent occurs until, in adult life, the lower border of the cricoid cartilage lies opposite the lower border of the sixth cervical vertebra, while the tip of the epiglottis, which marks the upper border of the larynx, lies opposite the lower border of the third cervical vertebra.[9]

According to Wilson,[12] as a result of the higher position of the infant's larynx, the line of entry of air current is straighter than in the adult and the epiglottis is less overhanging. In later life, when the larynx has descended to its final position, the axes of the pharynx, larynx and trachea meet at a more acute angle. Wilson noted, however, that not all authors accept the

INDICATIONS FOR LARYNGEAL SURGERY

Respiratory obstruction and hoarseness (or abnormal quality of the voice) are the two principal indications for laryngoscopy in infants, according to Holinger (Chap. 30). Other indications include tracheal aspiration and esophageal (or suspected esophageal)

TABLE 16-1 – TRACHEAL DIAMETERS FROM WOOD'S METAL CASTS*

AGE, MO.	NO. OF CASES	ABT SAGITTAL	ABT CORONAL	ENGEL SAGITTAL	ENGEL CORONAL
0–1	11	3.6	5.0	5.7	6.0
1–3	35	4.6	6.1	6.5	6.8
3–6	37	5.0	5.8	7.6	7.2
6–12	25	5.6	6.2	7.0	7.8

*After Engel.[3]

TABLE 16-3.—INTRINSIC CAUSES OF LARYNGEAL STRIDOR IN INFANCY*

CONGENITAL ANATOMIC ABNORMALITIES	TUMORS AND CYSTS	INFLAMMATORY CONDITIONS	NEUROLOGIC ABNORMALITIES	TRAUMA	FOREIGN BODY
Laryngomalacia	Papilloma of larynx	Acute laryngitis	Tetany	Birth injury	Vegetable
Bifid epiglottis	Laryngeal cysts	Acute Laryngo-tracheo-bronchitis	Neonatal tetany	Post-natal injury	Nonvege-table
Congenital laryngeal stenosis and webs		Diphtheria; postdiph-theritic stenosis	Recurrent nerve paralysis		
Cleft larynx		Exanthema (e.g., measles) and pertussis			
		Tuberculosis			

*After Wilson,[12]

obstruction. The reader is again referred to the sections on endoscopy (Chap. 30) and tracheostomy (Chap. 24) for details regarding the indications and the operative techniques.

CAUSES OF LARYNGEAL STRIDOR IN INFANCY

The lesions which cause stridor in infancy may be divided into intrinsic and extrinsic types. Wilson's classification is shown in Table 16-3 and Table 16-4. The laryngeal causes of stridor in infancy may be classified under the headings of:

Congenital anatomic abnormalities
Tumors and cysts
Inflammatory conditions
Neurologic abnormalities
Trauma
Foreign bodies

Most intrinsic and some extrinsic conditions which require surgical intervention are diagnosed and treated by endoscopic techniques with or without tracheostomy.

Congenital anatomic abnormalities of the larynx that cause stridor include laryngomalacia, bifid epiglottis, congenital stenosis and cleft larynx.

Laryngomalacia is a benign condition which usually disappears by age 2½ and seldom requires surgical intervention. Tracheostomy has been performed in instances of extreme respiratory obstruction, which is unusual. The symptoms appear at birth or soon after and include attacks of inspiratory stridor (often initiated by an external stimulus), cervical soft tissue retraction and a low-pitched sound which ends, at the cessation of the stridor, with the child exhausted and pale. The attack is often precipitated by placing the child in the supine position; cyanosis is infrequent and only temporary when present. The diagnosis is made by direct laryngoscopy: the epiglottis is long and tapering with its lateral folds rolled posteriorly so as to form a long slit. The aryepiglottic folds are found to be closely opposed and to be forced together by any but the slightest inspiratory flow of air. The usual treatment is anticipatory, with gentle handling and positioning of the child plus avoidance of sudden shocks or changes in temperature.

Bifid epiglottis is rare. When laryngeal obstruction is produced by this deformity, tracheostomy and subsequent amputation of the epiglottis have been required.

Congenital *laryngeal webs* are another important

TABLE 16-4.—EXTRINSIC CAUSES OF STRIDOR IN INFANCY*

CONGENITAL ANATOMIC ABNORMALITIES	TUMORS AND CYSTS	INFLAMMATORY CONDITIONS	FOREIGN BODY
Dysphagia lusoria (vascular ring)	Hyperplasia of the thymus	Thymic abscess	In the esophagus
Tracheoesophageal	Cystic hygroma	Retro- and parapharyngeal abscess	
Tracheomalacia	Thyroglossal cysts	Mediastinal adenitis, as in mononucleosis	
Congenital goiter			

*After Wilson.[12]

cause of stridor in infancy. The web may vary in size from complete laryngeal occlusion incompatible with life to a small membranous band across the anterior commissure. Primary symptoms are a poor cry, a weak or aphonic voice and stridor, which may be inspiratory or both inspiratory and expiratory. Feeding problems, dyspnea and cyanosis are also sometimes noted. When the symptoms are mild, the web should probably be left alone. Large webs require division; the chief difficulty encountered is re-formation of the web by scar formation. A variety of operative procedures have been employed to prevent this undesirable complication, including suspension of a plate between the cords, insertion of a laryngeal stent, and tissue grafting to cover the raw surfaces of the cords.[2,7,8]

Cleft larynx, caused by failure of separation of the larynx and trachea from the esophagus by the seventh or eighth week of gestation, may result in a persistent esophagotrachea. This rare condition was first described in 1792, by Richter.[11] The deformity may vary from a minor deepening of the interarytenoid cleft in the body of the cricoid cartilage to a wide cleft extending as far as the bifurcation of the trachea (Fig. 16-11). Successful repair of the latter type of deformity has been reported.[10] Tracheoesophageal fistula has been reported in association with cleft larynx and may obscure identification of the cleft. Symptoms include stridor after birth, aspiration after feeding,

Fig. 16-11.—Newborn larynx with a cleft extending part way through the cricoid cartilage.

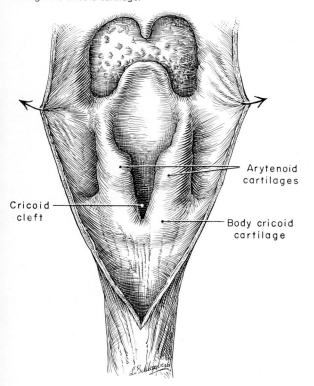

with cyanosis and subsequent pneumonia. Clinically, the picture is similar to that of tracheoesophageal fistula. The larynx is examined, and in the case of small clefts may be mistakenly interpreted as being normal. If tracheotomy is performed, the child may regurgitate through the tracheostoma. The child fails to thrive, has repeated respiratory infections and usually dies in early infancy from aspiration of food material. The diagnosis is best established by direct laryngoscopy when the examiner suspects a possible cleft. Aspiration may be confirmed by cinefluorographic studies of the larynx during the act of swallowing. Small clefts undoubtedly pass unrecognized; the larger defects require closure of the posterior laryngeal or laryngotracheal defect to prevent repeated aspiration pneumonitis.[5]

Tumors and cysts of the larynx may produce infantile stridor. Of these conditions, *papillomas* may be very troublesome. The condition is not usually seen under 2 years of age. The papillomas may be confined to the larynx or may extend above or below the glottic region. Treatment consists of local removal, although a variety of therapeutic regimens have been tried in the past, including local use of escharotics, local hormone applications, radiotherapy, antibiotic and steroid therapy, artificial puberty, to mention a few. Tracheostomy is occasionally required, but the surgeon should remember that papillomas may be implanted into the trachea after this procedure.

The management of *inflammatory lesions* of the larynx is largely nonsurgical except for those instances in which tracheostomy is indicated. Laryngoscopic removal of crusts in diphtheria was advocated by the Jacksons.[6]

Of the neurologic disorders of infancy, *recurrent nerve paralysis* may result from birth injury, infection, maternal disease and surgical injury as well as other causes. When the condition is bilateral, tracheostomy may be required. The prognosis is poor for cases of bilateral paralysis.

Trauma to the infant larynx includes birth and postnatal injury. As with adult fractures of the larynx, restoration of cartilage position and internal stenting is essential to prevent laryngeal stenosis. A temporary tracheostomy is required while the stent is in place.

Stenosis of the larynx has resulted from infection, intubation and following tracheostomy. The majority of such cases are, regrettably, preventable. Management following the development of stenosis includes excision of the stenotic area, skin grafting and the use of an endolaryngeal stent. The prognosis depends on the site and extent of the stenotic area, the age of the patient plus other individual factors, for instance, the duration of the stenosis and tendency to keloid formation.

Foreign bodies in the larynx may produce stridor or respiratory obstruction. Most vegetable foreign bodies do not lodge in the larynx but cause laryngotracheobronchitis or atelectasis after their passage into the tracheobronchial system. Their management, therefore, includes laryngoscopy and bronchoscopic evaluation and treatment.

REFERENCES

1. Baker, D. C., Jr., and Savetsky, L.: Congenital partial atresia of the larynx, Tr. Am. Laryng., Rhin. & Otol. Soc., pp. 14-20, 1966.
2. Bayeux,: Tubage de larynx dans le croup, Presse méd. 20:1, 1897.
3. Engel, S.: *Lung Structure* (Springfield, Ill.: Charles C Thomas, Publisher, 1962).
4. Fearon, B., *et al.*: Airway patterns in children following prolonged endotracheal intubation, Ann. Otol., Rhin. & Laryng. 75:975, 1966.
5. Harrison, H. S.; Fuqua, W. B., and Giffin, R. B., Jr.: Congenital laryngeal cleft: Report of a case, Am. J. Dis. Child. 110:556, 1965.
6. Jackson, C., and Jackson, C. L.: *Bronchoesophagology* (Philadelphia: W. B. Saunders Company, 1951).
7. McHugh, H. E., and Loch, W. E.: Congenital web of the larynx, Laryngoscope 52:43, 1942.
8. McNaught, R. C.: Surgical correction of anterior web of the larynx, Laryngoscope 60:264, 1950.
9. Negus, V. E.: *The Comparative Anatomy and Physiology of the Larynx* (London: William Heinemann Medical Books, Ltd., 1949), p. 175.
10. Pettersson, G.: Inhibited separation of larynx and the upper part of trachea from esophagus in a newborn, Acta chir. Scandinav. 110:250, 1955.
11. Richter, C. F.: Dissertatio medica de infanticidio in artis obstetrica. Thesis for M. D. degree, Leipzig, 1792.
12. Wilson, T. G.: *Diseases of the Ear, Nose and Throat in Children* (2nd ed.; New York: Grune & Stratton, Inc., 1962).

Surgical Treatment of Hearing Impairment

Surgery of the ear is performed for four major purposes: to improve external appearance, to prolong life, to eradicate progressive disease, and to modify hearing function. At the present state of the art, procedures designed to modify hearing impairment are directed to pathology of the external and middle ear. Those designed to improve hearing by modification of cochlear pathology have not proved clinically successful and remain experimental.

Certain types of hearing loss amenable to surgery result from impairment in infancy. Hearing impairment of the infant may be congenital or acquired. In the classification derived from Jay F. Fraser,[1] we find two general types of congenital hearing impairment: (1) endemic (cretinous) *acquired deafness*, and (2) *hereditary degenerative deafness*, of which there are four principal types: (*a*) the Michel type, characterized by complete failure of development of the internal ear, (*b*) the Mondini-Alexander type, with cessation of labyrinthine development after the sixth or seventh month of gestation, (*c*) the Bing-Siebenmann type, in which inner ear development produces a normal bony labyrinth but malformation of the membranous inner ear is found, and (*d*) the Scheibe or cochleosaccular type, in which maldevelopment of the cochlear sensory epithelium exists to varying de-

grees and in which a limited amount of hearing may be found.

In addition to these congenital types of deafness, there are the acquired impairments of infancy, including: *intrauterine hearing impairments* secondary to meningitis, syphilis, virual infections (notably rubella), Rh incompatibility, toxemia of pregnancy, prematurity, and chemical poisons transferred from the mother, and the *postfetal hearing impairments* associated with acute inflammatory diseases causing labyrinthitis, with severe trauma, dystocia and exposure to ototoxic drugs. In the postfetal category, meningitis, particularly meningococcic, is the most common type. Lesser degrees of hearing impairment may be caused by the same diseases which produce the severe forms — otosclerosis, subacute or chronic catarrhal otitis media, chronic otorrhea and drug toxicity.

Surgery of the external ear and middle ear is performed for the modification of hearing impairment in four major etiologic categories: deformity, infection, trauma, and otosclerosis. Abnormalities of the middle ear are frequently associated with meatal atresia, while the inner ear may be normal because of its separate development.

EMBRYOLOGY. — Wilson's review of the embryology may prove helpful.[6] The epithelium of the internal ear is developed from ectoderm and is first seen, in the 2-mm embryo, as a thickened plate lying on the surface of the head just dorsal to the second branchial cleft. This plate invaginates to form the otic vesicle, which differentiates into the cochlea and semicircular canals. At 6 weeks the cochlea consists only of the cochlear duct in the form of a short curved tube. At 7 weeks, a single complete turn of the scala tympani and scala vestibuli have formed out of the surrounding mesenchyme. The cochlea reaches its full two and one-half turns about the ninth or tenth week, and growth continues until the fifth month of gestation. About the eighth week, the epithelium of the cochlear duct begins to differentiate in the basal turn, followed by the apical turn. The organ of Corti and tectorial membrane are recognizable in the basal turn by the twelfth week, when the spiral ganglions and auditory nerve have established connections with the sensory end-organ. At 4 months, the cochlea is almost in its adult form; by 6 months, development is complete.

The auditory tube and tympanic cavity are derived from the tubotympanic recess between the first and third visceral arches. The inner part of the recess is narrowed to form the auditory tube, while the outer part is subsequently differentiated into the tympanic cavity. The tympanum is surrounded by loose connective tissue in which the ossicles develop. Even in adult life, the ossicles are enveloped in mucous membrane. The mastoid antrum appears during the sixth or seventh month, but the mastoid air cells do not develop until the end of fetal life.

The ossicles develop from the condensed mesenchyme of the first and second branchial arches; the malleus and incus develop from the inner ear end of Meckel's cartilage, which is contained in the first arch and separates from the mandible when ossification begins. The stapes is similarly derived from the end of Reichert's cartilage, which is contained in the second branchial arch.

The external auditory meatus develops from the dorsal end of the hyomandibular cleft. The ventral portion of this groove is the primary meatus, a funnel-shaped tube from which the cartilaginous meatus and a small portion of the osseous meatus are formed. From the funnel-shaped tube, a solid core of epidermis extends inward along the floor of the tubotympanic recess. This core hollows out to form the inner portion of the meatus, the secondary meatus, while the blind end forms the outer epidermal layer of the tympanic membrane. The fibrous layer of the membrane is formed by the mesenchyme and the inner layer by the entoderm of the tubotympanic recess.

Congenital abnormalities of the ear include: (1) abnormalities of the auricle, (2) abnormalities of the external auditory meatus and middle ear, (3) abnormalities of the eustachian tube, (4) abnormalities of the tympanic membrane, (5) abnormalities of the middle ear and mastoid process, (6) abnormalities associated with malformations of the skull, (7) dermoids and cholesteatoma of the mastoid, and (8) abnormalities of the internal ear.

ABNORMALITIES OF THE AURICLE

Auricular abnormalities may be associated with other deformities of the ear. One of the simpler deformities is atresia or a collapse of the membranous external auditory meatus, the remaining portions of the external auditory canal, tympanic, middle ear and inner ear being otherwise normal. The resulting conductive hearing impairment is frequently complicated by chronic external otitis because of inadequate aeration of the external auditory canal.

CONGENITAL ABNORMALITIES OF THE EXTERNAL AUDITORY MEATUS AND MIDDLE EAR

Congenital atresia of the external auditory meatus is often associated with microtia. Heredity is not a conspicuous factor in incidence; however, this anomaly appears more often in males than in females. The atresia is usually bony but may be cartilaginous. The meatus may be represented by a blind depression, the bottom of which is occluded by bone covering the deformed middle ear cavity. This condition is often accompanied by normal inner ear function, as demonstrated by bone conduction hearing tests in co-operative children. The pure tone sensitivity by bone conduction will be found to be normal, while a loss of

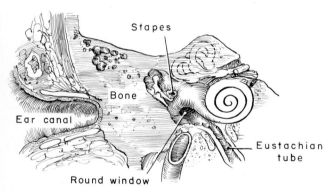

Stapes

Bone

Ear canal

Eustachian tube

Round window

Fig. 16-12.—Above, tympanic bony malformation with mobile ossicles. Below, repair by skin graft to malleus. (Figs. 12–16 redrawn from Goodhill.

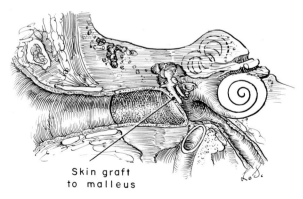

Skin graft to malleus

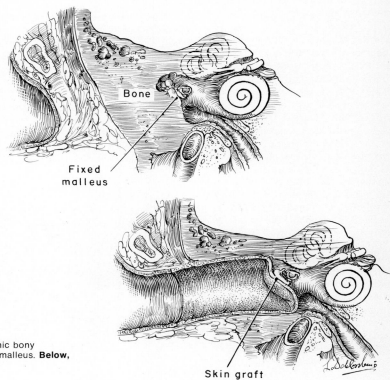

Fig. 16-13.—**Above,** tympanic bony malformation with fixation of malleus. **Below,** repair by skin graft to incus.

50–60 db (ASA) for air conduction is usually present.

In these cases, there is no external meatus and the tympanic membrane is replaced by bone which overlies the entire middle ear. The incus and malleus are almost invariably deformed and are often fused together. The malleus may be fused to the bony plate which replaces the tympanic membrane. The stapes, which is separately derived from the second branchial arch, may be normal and mobile in the oval window. The internal ear, which is developed separately from the auditory plate of neuroectoderm, is also usually normal. The shape of the tubotympanic cavity is abnormal, the tympanum being smaller than usual and the fenestra partially occluded by fibrous tissue. The eustachian tube is sometimes normal but may be malformed. The facial nerve may be normal in size and position or may be small and take a very abnormal course.

Treatment.—Until recently, otologists had little to offer in the way of treatment for bilateral atresia of the auditory conductive mechanisms except in the occasional patient in whom stenosis was caused by narrowing of the external auditory canal at the junction of the cartilaginous and bony portions of the meatus, the middle ear being normal. Here, a plastic reconstruction of the meatus was sufficient to provide a cure.

In the more usual, grossly deformed cases, surgeons have in the past approached the problem with extreme caution, generally advising against an operation even in bilateral cases.

Operative indications and conditions.—The condition must usually be bilateral. The operative hazards, particularly with regard to the facial nerve, are so great that it is seldom justifiable to operate in the unilateral case. Shambaugh, however, believes that unilateral cases could be benefited enough to justify surgery. Inner ear function should be normal, as demonstrated by bone conduction tests. Surgery should usually be deferred in spite of educational problems until the child is old enough to co-operate in audiometry. Recent developments in cortical-evoked-response audiometry may permit an earlier assessment of sensory-neural auditory function. Radiographs must always be taken and should show a normal internal ear shadow. They will also give valuable information as to the degree of pneumatization of the mastoid process.

SURGICAL TREATMENT.—Surgical treatment consists initially in the development of a canal to the inner tympanic wall. Further operative procedures will depend upon the condition of the middle ear as some form of tympanoplasty. The mastoid is explored to demonstrate the mastoid antrum and dorsal plates of the middle and posterior cranial fossae. The tympanic membrane may be absent and replaced by a plate of

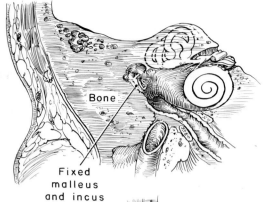

Bone

Fixed
malleus
and incus

Fig. 16-14. — **Above,** tympanic bony malformation with fixed malleus and incus. **Below,** repair by skin graft to capitulum of the stapes.

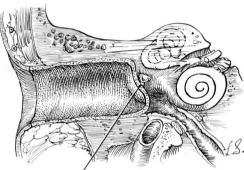

Skin graft to capitulum
of stapes

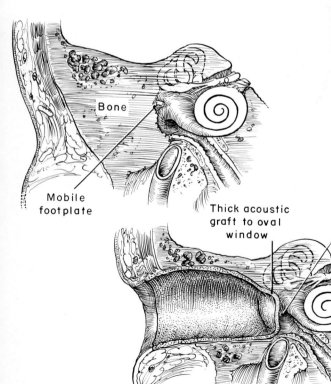

Bone

Mobile
footplate

Fig. 16-15. — **Above,** tympanic bony malformations with deformed fixed malleus, incus and crus but with mobile footplate. **Below,** repair by skin graft to oval window, sealing it from the round-window niche.

Thick acoustic
graft to oval
window

Round
window

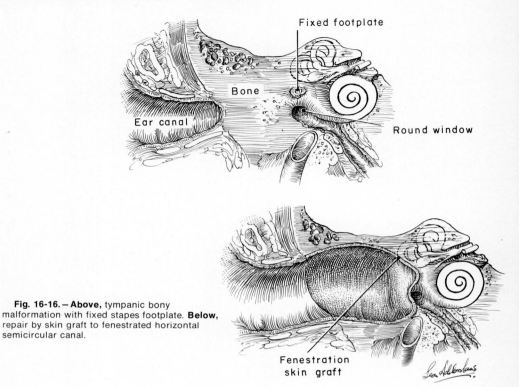

Fig. 16-16.—Above, tympanic bony malformation with fixed stapes footplate. **Below,** repair by skin graft to fenestrated horizontal semicircular canal.

bone. When the bony plate has been removed, several ossicular deformities may be encountered. Upon finding a normal chain with three mobile and connected ossicles, a skin graft is placed deep in the newly formed external auditory meatus to form a new tympanic membrane (Fig. 16-12). The malleus may be fused with the abnormal plate of bone at the site of the tympanic membrane, the incus and stapes being normal; whereupon the malleus is removed and a skin graft is placed in contact with the incus (Fig. 16-13). The incus may be fused with the malleus, both being attached to the bony tympanic plate. In this situation, the fused incus and malleus should be removed and a skin graft placed in contact with the capitulum of the stapes (Fig. 16-14). On occasion, the abnormal tympanic plate may be connected with the crura of the stapes, with a mobile footplate. The round window is isolated by a skin graft extending downward from the promontory, creating a new and lower tympanic membrane (Fig. 16-15). Rarely, the three ossicles are misshapen and fused with a fixed footplate requiring stapedectomy or fenestration (Fig. 16-16).

ABNORMALITIES OF THE EUSTACHIAN TUBE AND TYMPANIC MEMBRANE

Most abnormalities of the eustachian tube are not regarded as surgically operable. Congenital abnor-

malities of the tympanic membrane are usually associated with deformity of the meatus or middle ear, as in microtia; isolated deformities are quite rare. Cysts have been described as small swellings beneath the outer epidermal area of the tympanic membrane. These are not usually true congenital abnormalities.

CONGENITAL ABNORMALITIES OF THE MIDDLE EAR AND MASTOID PROCESS

The auditory ossicles are seldom abnormal in an otherwise normal ear. According to Goodhill,[2] anomalies are more common than hitherto believed. When an abnormality is present, the stapes, which develops separately from the malleus and incus, is usually implicated. It may be abnormally formed or ankylosed or its parts may be defective.

The head of the malleus is occasionally placed abnormally near the tegmen tympani. Malformations and ankylosis of the malleus with the incus and of the stapes with the oval window are not often found except in the microtic ear. Occasionally, the incus is found to be elongated and to end freely without articulating with the stapes. In other cases, the incus and stapes may be hypoplastic, and sometimes no clearly defined intra-tympanic structures are found. These conditions may accompany normal external ears and can only be disclosed by laminagraphy (tomography) or exploration of the middle ear. In some cases these conditions may be helped by tympanic reconstruction.

Abnormalities of the auditory muscles, arteriovascular abnormalities and venous abnormalities are not usual causes of hearing impairment.

CONGENITAL ABNORMALITIES OF THE MIDDLE AND INTERNAL EAR

The internal ear is occasionally involved in the Siebenmann type of middle ear deformity. These cases result from hormone deficiency, usually in cretins. The incidence is three times as common in Switzerland as elsewhere in Europe. There is a myxomatous thickening of the tissues in the middle ear, and various degrees of deformity of the ossicles may be found. The stapes is most often malformed, resembling the columella of the birds' ear, or the footplate may be hypertrophic and ankylosed with the oval window. Nager described a case in which the cochlear duct was collapsed in the basal coil and distended in the apical. Others have described degeneration of the organ of Corti. In the great majority, the vestibule is normal.

DERMOIDS AND CHOLESTEATOMA

Dermoid tumors of the middle ear and mastoid have been mentioned in the *current* literature. Cholesteatoma may be congenital or acquired. Other malformations of the ear are associated with congenital malformation of the skull.

Congenital malformations of the inner ear are not ordinarily amenable to surgery and will not be discussed.

INFECTIOUS DISEASE AND HEARING IMPAIRMENT

Most hearing impairments of childhood and infancy are associated with nasopharyngitis, chronic adenoiditis and otitis media. In this antibiotic era, physicians are likely to regard acute otitis media as a nonsurgical disease. Although antibiotics and chemotherapy prevent complications in many cases of otitis media, these agents may fail to control or cure some infections because of bacterial resistance or delay in therapy. As a result, the symptoms of mastoid disease may be sufficiently masked to permit progress of the pathologic process without appreciable signs or symptoms. The resulting chronic adhesive otitis media can lead to permanent hearing impairment. In many cases the serous exudate in the middle ear is rendered sterile by antibiotics. The exudate fails to resolve and in time becomes organized. This illustrates the need for adequate treatment plus follow-up until resolution of the middle ear effusion. When pain or pressure is evident, a myringotomy can be a hearing-saving procedure and indeed occasionally life-saving. A careful adenoidectomy with or without tonsillectomy may prevent further damage from recurrent middle ear infection.

Chronic serous otitis media is common in children with enlarged tonsils and adenoids and may occur secondary to upper respiratory infection. The eustachian tubal orifices are usually, but not necessarily, obstructed by lymphoid tissue. Allergic factors have been found in some cases. Occasionally, chronic serous otitis media follows adenoidectomy because of scarring in the region of the eustachian tubal orifice. In adults, a possible tumor of the nasopharynx must be considered in the differential diagnosis.

The treatment is important, as persistent middle ear fluids may organize, with development of a progressive and permanent conductive hearing impairment. In time, such a condition may lead to cholesteatosis.

Removal of the adenoids in children is usually curative when hypertrophic adenoiditis is the cause. Occasionally, recurrence of nasopharyngeal adenoid tissue may require a secondary adenoidectomy or irradiation of the nasopharynx. In older children and adults, myringotomy followed by insufflation of the eustachian tube may be necessary to evacuate the fluid. If the process has been long-standing, diagnostic aspiration may be followed by myringotomy and the insertion of a polyethylene drainage tube.

In chronic purulent otitis media, the major goals of therapy have been: to improve hearing, to prevent the spread of infection to the inner ear and to preserve the sound-conducting structures of the middle ear. To achieve these objectives, surgery for chronic otitis media should be based on the following principles: (1) The chronic infection must be eliminated completely and complications prevented. (2) A new closed tympanic cavity properly ventilated through the eustachian tube must be constructed. (3) At the same time, a system for conduction of acoustic stimuli through the middle ear to the cochlea must be created. The surgical procedure must be modified according to the extent of damage to the middle ear structures. This type of surgery, termed by Wullstein[7] *tympanoplasty*, is contraindicated when complications of the middle ear infection are a danger to life or when there is inadequate function of the inner ear and improvement of sound conduction in the middle ear will be without result. Such complications include infection of the meninges or lateral sinus and cholesteatoma of the inner ear.

Several clinical factors affect the indications and prognosis for tympanoplasty. Ranked by audiologic significance, they are: (1) quality of the inner ear; (2) function of the eustachian tube; (3) hydrodynamics of the inner ear, including: (*a*) function of the round window, (*b*) function of the oval window, (*c*) function of the new window; (4) quality of the mucosa; (5) quality of the tympanic membrane, and (6) state of the ossicles.

According to the Wullstein[7] classification (Fig. 16-17), types I, II and III not only furnish protection for the round window but, as far as possible, restore the impedance-matching characteristics of the middle

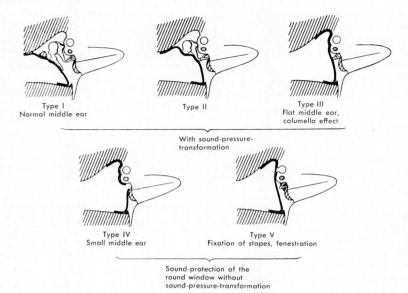

Type I
Normal middle ear

Type II

Type III
Flat middle ear,
columella effect

With sound-pressure-
transformation

Type IV
Small middle ear

Type V
Fixation of stapes, fenestration

Sound-protection of the
round window without
sound-pressure-transformation

Fig. 16-17.—Conditions offering protection of the various inner ear structures. (Courtesy of Wullstein, H.: Ann. Otol., Rhin. & Laryng. 65:1020, 1956.)

ear structures. Types I and II preserve the attic and ossicular chain, and type III produces the so-called columellar effect. Types IV and V only provide protection of the round window.

Successful tympanoplasty with improvement of sensitivity for air-conducted sound is most frequently obtained when the structures of the middle ear are relatively intact, as in type I. In type II and more often in type III, ideal results are fewer and, in type IV and V, become theoretically impossible. Wullstein[7] reported 400 unclassified tympanoplasties with closure of the air-bone gap. The hearing level for speech was 15 db or better in the frequency range of 500–2,000 cycles in one third of the cases. Slightly different results were cited by Proctor. In 1958, Proctor[3] reported an average postoperative hearing level of 50.2 db (ASA) for 50 consecutive radical mastoidectomies. In a review of 122 cases of type IV tympanoplasty, he[4] noted an average postoperative hearing level of 40.2 db (ASA), in contrast to an average preoperative level of 45 db. In a later analysis of type III tympanoplasty, Proctor[5] noted an average postoperative hearing level of 35.4 db compared to an average preoperative hearing level of 40.1 db., a net gain of 4.7 db for the 157 cases. These postoperative results for type III tympanoplasty were short of the theoretical maximal hearing level of 4.5 db for the ideal case. Some of the causes for poor postoperative results cited were: (1) graft perforation (2) frequent presence of sensory-neural loss, (3) impaired window function due to increased stiffness from scars, (4) adherence of the tympanic membrane to the promontory, (5) neural

loss of more than 10 db, (6) inadequate postoperative Eustachian tube function with obliteration of the cavum tympani, (7) graft cholesteatoma, (8) recurrent cholesteatoma, (9) persistence of residual bone infection, (10) nonadherence of the shifted tympanic membrane, (11) progressive necrosis of the stapes, and (12) fracture of the stapes. Proctor concluded: "tympanoplasty is performed to control infection, to prevent recurrent infections and to prevent progression of disease which would result in further hearing loss. In addition, we do what we can to restore some of the hearing loss. The patient should be told that hearing improvement is often minimal and that it may even become worse," a statement with which we concur.

TRAUMA

Certain types of trauma are associated with hearing impairment and require surgical intervention. Removal of a foreign body or cerumen impacting the external auditory canal may immediately improve hearing. Traumatic perforations of the tympanic membrane may follow a blow to the head. If the perforation is a simple slit, healing usually occurs promptly. A large flap-type rupture usually requires careful repositioning for satisfactory healing. In some instances, damage to the ossicles may occur with or without tympanic membrane perforation. If a fracture occurs through the cochlea or if the stapes is driven into the vestibule, vestibular signs may be present: nausea, vomiting and occasionally cerebrospinal fluid drainage through a tympanic membrane perforation or through the Eustachian tube into the nose. Facial paralysis may also occur in temporal bone fractures. In such instances, exploration of the mastoid and repair of the facial nerve are necessary. If a conductive hearing impairment has resulted from trauma and the tympanic membrane is intact, acoustic impedance studies should be undertaken to determine whether or not there is an ossicular disarticulation. Prophylactic antibiotic therapy is indicated in most instances of traumatic injury. In all cases of aural trauma, an otologic examination should be obtained, as well as audiologic and vestibular function studies if indicated.

Otosclerosis

Otosclerosis is not a disease of very young children. In Guild's series of 1,161 routine autopsies, the incidence of otosclerosis in children under 5 was less than 0.6%. In persons over 5 years of age, the incidence was approximately 4%. Occasionally, tympanosclerosis secondary to otitis media is found in children with a conductive hearing impairment which mimics the clinical picture of otosclerosis. After routine otologic, audiologic and radiologic studies, exploratory tympanotomy may be required.

REFERENCES

1. Fraser, J. F.: Studies in the etiology of congenital deafness, Clin. Res. 10:212, 1962 (abst.).
2. Goodhill, V.: *The Modern Educational Treatment of Deafness* (Manchester, England: Manchester University Press, 1960).
3. Proctor, B.: Results in tympanoplasty, Laryngoscope 68:888, 1958.
4. Proctor, B.: Type IV tympanoplasty: A critical review of 122 cases, Arch. Otolaryng. 79:176, 1964.
5. Proctor, B.: What happens in type III tympanoplasty, Tr. Am. Laryng., Rhin. & Otol. Soc., p. 396, 1965.
6. Wilson, T. G.: *Diseases of the Ear, Nose and Throat in Children* (2nd ed.; New York: Grune & Stratton, Inc., 1962).
7. Wullstein, H.: The restoration of the function of the middle ear in chronic otitis media, Ann. Otol., Rhin. & Laryng. 65:1020, 1956.

F. I. Catlin
J. E. Bordley

Drawings by
Max Brodel (Figures 1-5)
Leon Schlossberg (Figures 7 and 8)

17

The Salivary Glands

Surgical lesions of the salivary glands are uncommon in infancy and childhood. One may see recurring or suppurative sialadenitis as well as various types of tumors, benign and malignant. Tumors may arise anywhere one might expect salivary gland tissue to be present, including the floor of the mouth, the palate, the submaxillary and parotid regions. Pathologic processes that involve the parotid are important by virtue of frequency of occurrence and the necessity for skillful surgical management.

From 1937 to 1967, 147 children were encountered with surgical lesions of the major salivary glands at the Children's Hospital Medical Center. Eighty-six patients had neoplasms (Fig. 17-1), 54 had sialadeni-

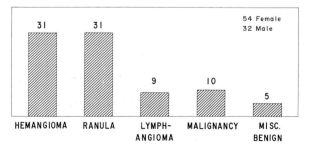
Fig. 17-1.—Neoplasms of the major salivary glands, 86 patients.

TABLE 17-1.—Surgical Lesions of Major Salivary Glands (Children's Hospital Medical Center, 1937–67)

Neoplasms		86
Malignant	10	
Benign	76	
Sialadenitis		54
Acute	20	
Chronic	34	
Miscellaneous		7
Total		147

tis in one of its various forms, and 7 had interesting miscellaneous lesions (Table 17-1). Although most authors have considered neoplasms and sialadenitis separately, it seemed reasonable to combine all surgical lesions of the salivary glands in one chapter because of challenging problems in differential diagnosis and the very important differences in medical and surgical treatment.

Benign Neoplasms

Angioma

From our own survey and other reports, the commonest benign neoplasm affecting the major salivary glands is angioma in one of its several categories.[5,8,13,22,31] We have encountered 31 patients with hemangioma and 9 with lymphangioma, some having mixed angioma. These tumors present most commonly in female infants at birth or within the first months of life. They are usually confined to the intracapsular portion of the gland with only occasional involvement of the overlying subcutaneous tissue and skin (Fig. 17-2). A surface sentinel lesion may provide the clue to diagnosis, thus eliminating the need for biopsy

Fig. 17-2.—A 4-month-old girl with rapidly growing cellular hemangioma of the left parotid gland. Treatment consisted of biopsy and irradiation. There was no residual tumor at age 4 years.

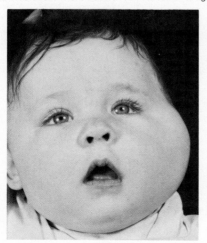

identification. A review of the literature by Wolfe[54] disclosed that of 48 patients operated on for parotid angioma, 2 died intraoperatively because of the prolonged and difficult procedure, and 12–25% sustained permanent 7th nerve palsy. Kaufman and Stout[31] reported on 3 patients with 7th nerve palsy, and Karlin and Snyder[29] stated that 1 patient in 4 sustained anatomic division. It is apparent that surgical removal of a parotid angioma in infancy provides an uncertain result in terms of ablation and recurrence, plus an unacceptably high risk of producing an expressionless face.

Treatment.—Angiomas of the salivary glands may be congenital, but most appear in the first weeks or months of life as a progressive, painless, swelling usually in the region of the parotid gland and only occasionally involving the overlying skin. Provided there is a cutaneous sentinel lesion over the convexity of the swelling, no biopsy identification is necessary. *Group I* lesions are spongy, cavernous, moderately cellular and slowly growing. Open rather than needle biopsy is necessary to provide the correct diagnosis. Following classification from permanent sections, a dose of 200 r is delivered to the area of the swelling with shielding of the thyroid and mediastinal areas. This is repeated in 1 month if growth has not been satisfactorily controlled. Further treatment is unnecessary and, provided there is no lymphangioma component, satisfactory involution occurs with no evidence of the process at age 3–4 years. *Group II* lesions are firm, microscopically cellular, sometimes called hemangioendothelioma (always benign) and characterized by rapid growth. These patients are given 200 r on three successive days. Further therapy is unnecessary. The radiation factors are provided in Table 17-2. *Group III* lesions have large arteriovenous communications and continue to grow in spite of irradiation. For these, we recommend ligation of the external carotid artery, which can be picked up between the branches of the superior thyroid and the lingual arteries. Ligation produces an instant decrease in the size of the tumor, and involution follows at the customary rate.

Recent reports of thyroid malignancy developing many years after therapeutic irradiation of benign

TABLE 17-2.—Treatment of Parotid Hemangiomas

Group I: Spongy, cavernous, slow growth
    BIOPSY ONLY
    200 R; REPEAT IN ONE MONTH
Group II: Firm, cellular, rapid growth
    BIOPSY ONLY
    200 R ON THREE SUCCESSIVE DAYS
Group III: A-V fistulas, rapid, post-irradiation growth
    BIOPSY ONLY
    200 R ON THREE SUCCESSIVE DAYS
    EXTERNAL CAROTID ARTERY LIGATION
    x-ray factors: 250 kvp, 15 ma, 50 cm TSD,
                2.5 mm Cu HVL, filtration Tb-2.

lesions involving the head and neck regions make the foregoing regimens vulnerable to attack. Careful attention to x-ray factors and lead shielding leaves the protocol with some merit. Patient observation may be the best policy after tissue diagnosis for most parotid angiomas in infancy.[25]

Irradiation without biopsy, needle biopsy, injection of sclerosing agents and the introduction of randon seeds are unwarranted because of inability to control the distribution of tissue destruction. The possibility of permanent injury to one or more of the branches of the facial nerve is very real.

LYMPHANGIOMA

We have encountered 9 patients with primary intracapsular lymphangioma or lymphangioma in a juxtaparotid location with histologic invasion of the gland. A review of the literature shows little interest in this angioma subtype, yet in our experience surgical management has been exceedingly difficult. Intracapsular lymphangioma is often a mixed angioma in the perinatal period (Fig. 17-3, *A*). Ultimately the hemangioma component drops out, followed by persistence or vigorous growth of the lymphangioma component some years later (Fig. 17-3, *B*). Juxtaparotid lymphangiomas are a separate entity, not to be confused with the bulky hygroma cysticum coli which involves the major compartments of the neck, infiltrating the floor of the mouth and continuing into the substance of the tongue. Four patients had lymphangioma restricted to and microscopically invading the parotid gland. All were unilateral.

TREATMENT. (Table 17-3).—*Group I*—Neonates

TABLE 17-3.—TREATMENT OF PAROTID LYMPHANGIOMAS

SURGICAL
Group I: Neonate with parotid lymphangioma or mixed angioma
BIOPSY ONLY

Group II: Neonate with juxtaparotid lymphangioma and invasion of gland
SUPERFICIAL EXCISION AND DESTRUCTION OF DEEP CYSTS WITH LIMITED DISSECTION OF 7th NERVE

Group III: Older child with intracapsular tumor
TOTAL PAROTIDECTOMY WITH FULL DISSECTION AND PRESERVATION OF 7th NERVE

IRRADIATION
Mixed angioma, treat as Hemangioma
Pure lymphangioma, NONE

with parotid intracapsular lymphangioma or mixed angioma, as is often the case. Treatment consists of biopsy only for histologic identification and to rule out congenital malignancy of the parotid gland. If permanent sections reveal a mixed angioma, the same x-ray factors and dosage are employed as in the treatment of a pure angioma.

Group II—Neonates with juxtaparotid lymphangioma and histologic invasion of the gland. It is technically impossible to carry out a clean removal of this process without a high risk of 7th nerve palsy. Treatment consists of superficial excision of the lymphangioma in its extraparotid ramifications plus destruction of the deeper intracapsular cysts. This is accomplished by uncapping the cysts and scrubbing the endothelial lining with a mild sclerosing agent under

Fig. 17-3.—Mixed angioma (hemangioendothelioma and lymphangioma). **A,** in this 4-month-old boy, the lesion was identified by open biopsy. Irradiation was withheld because of low cellularity and slow growth. **B,** following near "disappearance" of the tumor at age 2, there was sudden regrowth several weeks after an

upper respiratory infection. Treatment consisted of total parotidectomy with dissection and preservation of the 7th nerve. The histologic diagnosis was pure lymphangioma. No evidence of recurrence 5 years after operation, and no evidence of facial nerve palsy.

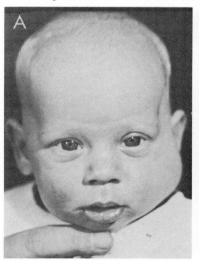 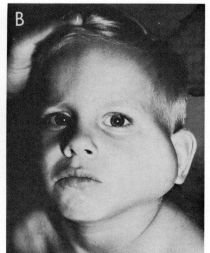

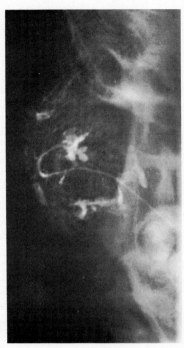

Fig. 17-4.—Sialogram of parotid lymphangioma, showing displacement of ducts, focal sialectasia and filling defects consistent with multiple, spherical, fluid-filled, space-occupying areas of lymphangioma.

careful direct vision. A useful agent is 0.5% iodine applied with a sterile cotton applicator. These tumors form simultaneously with the major neurovascular supply to the head and neck and are found in and around the ramifications of the 7th, 11th and 12th nerves. The 7th nerve trunk measures no more than 0.5 mm in the neonate. While the main trunk of the facial nerve can be identified, the major branches dive into a marsh of multiloculated lymphangioma

tissue. It is technically impossible to free them from the tumor. The limited operation may not be the final answer, and recurrences are common but may not be encountered for months or years after the initial subtotal excision.

In summary, we try to remove the bulk of the tumor without sacrificing any structure of functional or cosmetic importance. Repeated small operations usually suffice. One child went 7 years before a recurrence developed. The second operation was relatively simple, with no difficulty in identifying and preserving essential structures.

Group III—Older children with intracapsular lymphangioma or mixed angioma. Surgical excision is carried out electively at age 4, when most of the hemangioma component has dropped out. This may be a primary definitive operation or reoperation following incomplete removal in infancy. This involves total parotidectomy with dissection and preservation of the 7th nerve. Every attempt should be made to clean out the entire process at the time of full dissection. A preoperative parotid sialogram is mandatory (Fig. 17-4). If elements are left behind, reoperation poses a prohibitive risk of 7th nerve damage since, in addition to residual tumor, there is fibrotic encasement of the nerve and its branches.

No child with pure parotid lymphangioma is irradiated.

RANULA

Thirty-one patients had sublingual cysts (Figs. 17-5 and 17-6). Some of them were of little clinical importance, appearing as pea-sized swellings to the right or left of the midline in the floor of the mouth adjacent to the frenulum. In a number of patients, the ranula achieved heroic proportions. One neonate had a soft blue cystic subglottic swelling that measured 8.0 × 5.0 cm. This produced airway obstruction and required emergency excision.

TREATMENT.—Errors in management have oc-

Fig. 17-5.—Extensive bilateral ranula with suprahyoid projection. The lesion was treated by marsupialization into the oral cavity.

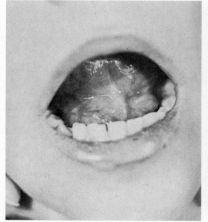
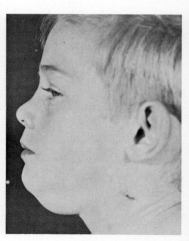

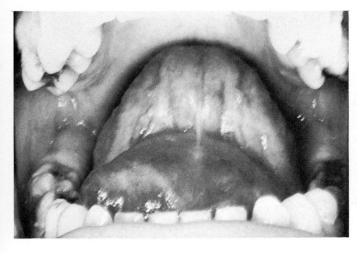

Fig. 17-6.—Large ranula of floor of mouth pushing the tongue dorsally.

curred because of failure to recognize the nature of the process and attempts to excise the cyst completely with a margin of normal tissue. The larger ranulas extend bilaterally or unilaterally from the dental arch to the hypopharynx and under the base of the tongue. Any attempt at total excision results in substantial bleeding and interference with neurogenic apparatus essential to tongue movements and the act of swallowing.

Proper treatment consists of marsupialization of the cyst into the oral cavity.[34] The process may present in a submandibular location (Fig. 17-5) but should always be approached through the oral cavity. This is done under endotracheal general anesthesia with a Dingman double mouth gag and a heavy silk stitch drawing the tongue cephalad after division of the frenulum. The orifice of Wharton's submaxillary duct should be identified with a lacrimal duct probe, and uncapping of the process should be carried out with this probe in place. Upon circumscribing the soft blue dome of the cystic process, a large amount of glairy mucoid material is released, revealing the back wall of the cyst. As the uncapping proceeds, the margin of the cyst is anastomosed to the oral mucous membrane with a running interlocking suture of 4-0 chromic catgut. Most patients leave the hospital the following day, and a ranula cavity of any size is obliterated within 2 weeks. Following this procedure, no patient has required reoperation. The submaxillary duct has not been obstructed in the suturing process in this series.

MISCELLANEOUS BENIGN TUMORS

Two clinical reports account for most of the mixed tumors of the parotid gland in children. Byars *et al*[8] reported 17 patients evenly spread from 7 to 18 years of age. Only 8 were under 14. Howard and associates[27] reported on 6 patients with mixed parotid tumors, but only 1 was operated on before age 14. Mixed tumor is

not uncommon in adolescence. Nine additional cases have been reported.[22,24,40]

There are isolated reports of benign tumors corresponding to all of the organoid structure of the salivary glands deriving from fibrous, neural or acinar tissue (Table 17-4).

Five patients in this series had miscellaneous benign tumors of the major salivary glands. Two had mixed tumors, one involving the parotid and 1 the submaxillary gland. One had a cystadenoma of the parotid and another, a simple cyst. One patient had "benign lymphoepithelial neoplasm" (Mikulicz's disease) but to date has not manifested systemic difficulties.[43] The ophthalmologic features of this disease were identified by Sjögren in 1933. The often associated keratoconjunctivitis results from failure to elaborate tears following obliteration of the acinar structure of the lacrimal glands. The condition may also be encountered with parotid malignancy.[16] Many patients, in addition to keratoconjunctivitis sicca and xeros-

TABLE 17-4.—BENIGN TUMORS OF THE MAJOR SALIVARY GLANDS IN CHILDREN
(94 from the literature to 1967;* 76 from the Children's Hospital Medical Center, 1937–67)

Hemangioma	103
Ranula	33
Mixed tumor	13
Lymphangioma	9
Xanthoma	2
Plexiform neurofibroma	2
Neurofibroma	2
Lymphoepithelial tumor (Mikulicz's disease)	2
Neurilemmoma	1
Cystadenoma	1
Simple cyst	1
Lipoma	1
Total	170

*References: 5, 6, 8, 9, 10, 13, 22, 24, 31, 32, 33, 51, 53.

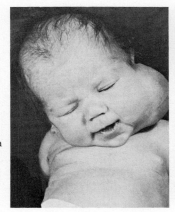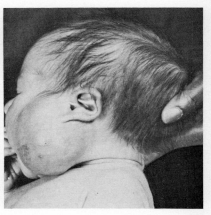

Fig. 17-7.—Congenital duct cell carcinoma in a newborn girl. Treatment consisted of radical parotidectomy with neck dissection. She is well 6 years later.

tomia, are rheumatoid. Grage and Luben[23] reported on 325 patients with salivary gland pathology. Six had Mikulicz's disease with multisystem involvement, but none were children.

Malignant Neoplasms

Ten patients ranging in age from 1 day to 13 years had malignancy of a major salivary gland. There were 7 girls and 3 boys. The congenital variety was encountered in 2 patients; at the time of writing, both were well following radical parotidectomy with neck dissection (Figs. 17-7 and 17-8). One patient, in addition, had excision of the mandible. These cases have been reported by Tefft and Vawter.[49,51] One had adenocarcinoma and the other, duct cell carcinoma. Vawter places these examples of congenital salivary gland malignancy in a special group which he prefers to call embryoma. There were 3 adenocarcinomas, 2 malignant mixed tumors, 2 mesenchymal sarcomas, 1 adenocystic carcinoma and 1 undifferentiated carcinoma. The pathologic classification of 87 malignant neoplasms in children derived from our own experience and a review of the literature is listed in Table 17-5.

The commonest malignant tumor of the major salivary glands in childhood is mucoepidermoid carcinoma, followed in order by undifferentiated carcinoma, undifferentiated sarcoma, adenocarcinoma, adenocystic carcinoma or cylindroma and malignant mixed tumor.[26,46] These tumors present as rapidly growing, often painful swellings in the region of the parotid or submaxillary gland. There is no clinical feature that permits accurate differentation from the more cellular benign tumors or from the fulminant form of chronic sialadenitis. For this reason, all patients with a swelling involving a major salivary gland must have sialography and, if the evidence is not diagnostic of sialadenitis with ectasia, biopsy identification. The biopsy material should be read in permanent sections.

Both in our series and in the literature there have

been many patients without anatomic invasion or interference with the function of the 7th nerve. Normal function of the nerve does not exclude malignancy, but palsy prior to medical or surgical treatment is highly suggestive of a malignant process.

TREATMENT

Treatment of malignant lesions of the salivary glands varies according to the stage of the disease and the histologic nature of the tumor. Some tumors are small and well confined to the superficial lobe of the parotid gland. These require only superficial parotid lobectomy with dissection and preservation of the 7th nerve. The poorest prognosis is encountered in patients having undifferentiated or embryonal carcinomas or sarcomas. In our patients, the disease had in all cases spread beyond the limit of resectability when first seen. Consequently, surgical treatment has been limited to biopsy identification, followed by irradiation and chemotherapy in its various forms. Some

---

TABLE 17-5.—MALIGNANT NEOPLASMS OF THE MAJOR SALIVARY GLANDS IN CHILDREN

(77 from Literature to 1967;* 10 Children's Hospital Medical Center, 1937–67)

Mucoepidermoid carcinoma	36
Undifferentiated carcinoma	11
Undifferentiated sarcoma	9
Adenocarcinoma	7
Adenocystic carcinoma (cylindroma)	6
Malignant mixed tumor	6
Acinar cell carcinoma	4
Squamous cell carcinoma	3
Mesenchymal sarcoma	2
Rhabdomyosarcoma	1
Warthin's tumor	1
Malignant epithelial tumor	1
Total	87

*References: 5, 11, 12, 13, 14, 16, 18, 22, 26, 31, 42, 46, 48.

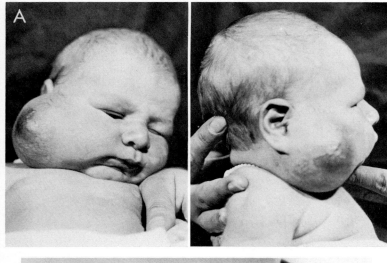

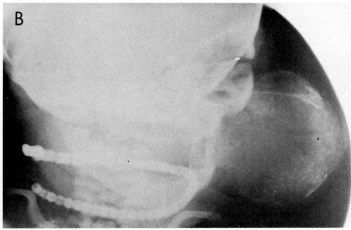

Fig. 17-8.—A, congenital adenocarcinoma of the right parotid gland in a newborn boy. Treatment consisted of mandibulectomy, radical parotidectomy and neck dissection. He is well 16 years later. **B,** roentgenogram of head and neck showing stippled peripheral calcification.

tumors were intermediate in their degree of invasiveness and metastasized late or only to regional nodes. For these patients, one must individualize surgical therapy, which can be offered in a number of combinations. If the 7th nerve is involved functionally or is found to be invaded at the time of operation, it must be sacrificed. Further extension of the operation consists of removing the ramus of the mandible and masseter muscle, thus providing access to the pterygoid fossa and lateral pharyngeal wall. Tumors that have moved in this direction usually have a poor prognosis. Mucoepidermoid carcinoma metastasizes frequently to the lymph nodes of the neck and yet only rarely becomes disseminated. For this reason, wide local excision without neck dissection is recommended. If palpable nodes are subsequently identified in the ipsilateral side of the neck, compartmental nodal dissection can be carried out at a second stage, equaling salvage achieved with neck dissection in continuity.

For all but the highly malignant lesions, we favor compartmental node dissection, sparing the sternocleidomastoid muscle and the internal jugular vein. Decision regarding radical surgery depends on the individual merits of the case and on the interpretation of the tumor tissue by a qualified pathologist. It is possible and, on occasion, desirable to do as extensive a resection as possible to provide the greatest chance for survival. In the extreme form, this consists of radical parotidectomy sacrificing the facial nerve, mandibulectomy, dissection of the contents of the pterygoid fossa, removal of the submaxillary gland and radical neck dissection in continuity on the side of involvement.

RESULTS.—Few details are available about the surgical treatment of the 77 patients with salivary gland malignancy encountered in the literature. It is even more difficult to determine the outcome of any form of therapy. In our series (Table 17-6), at the time of writing, the 2 patients with congenital parotid malignancy were well 3 years and 14 years respectively

TABLE 17-6.—MALIGNANT LESIONS OF THE MAJOR SALIVARY GLANDS

SEX	AGE	LOCATION	TYPE	OPERATION	IRRADIATION	CHEMOTHERAPY	RESULT
M	1 day	Parotid	Adenocarcinoma	Radical parotidectomy, neck dissection	Yes		Well after 14 yr.
F	10 days	Parotid	Duct cell carcinoma	Radical parotidectomy, mandibulectomy	Yes		Well after 3 yr.
F	6 mo.	Submaxillary	Carcinoma	Excision	Yes		Dead in 7 mo.
F	20 mo.	Parotid	Mesenchymal sarcoma	Biopsy	Yes	Yes	Dead in 8 mo.
M	22 mo.	Parotid	Mesenchymal sarcoma	Biopsy	Yes	Yes	Dead in 6 mo.
F	3 yr.	Parotid	Adenocarcinoma	Biopsy	Yes	Yes	Dead in 6 mo.
F	3 9/12 yr.	Parotid	Neurofibro-sarcoma	Biopsy, radical parotidectomy			Dead in 4 mo.
F	9 yr.	Submaxillary	Mixed	Resection			Well after 5 yr.
F	10 yr.	Parotid	Adenocystic carcinoma	Parotidectomy			Well after 6 mo.
M	13 yr.	Parotid	Adenocarcinoma	Radical excision, neck dissection			Dead in 3 yr.

after operation. A 9-year-old girl with a mixed parotid malignancy was well 5 years after wide resection. One girl, age 10, was well 3 years after parotidectomy with preservation of the 7th nerve for a well-localized adenocystic carcinoma. The other 6 patients had highly malignant tumors and were beyond the limit of resectability and cure when first seen. Treatment consisted of biopsy followed by irradiation and chemotherapy with little or no improvement. All died in a matter of months.

MISCELLANEOUS MALIGNANT TUMORS

We have not encountered a child with primary lymphoma involving a major salivary gland.[22]

Fig. 17-9.—Congenital teratoma of cervicoparotid area treated by wide, local resection and closure with rotation flaps. The patient is well and free of disease at age 11.

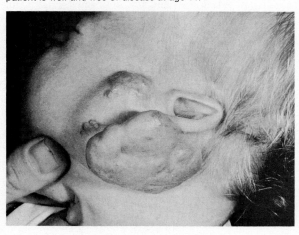

We call attention to a group of malignant tumors that present as swellings in the region of the parotid gland. Some are nasopharyngeal in origin with a mesenchymal ground substance. The epignathi usually contain tissues of all three germ layers.[19,45,53] A third variety is congenital cervicoparotid teratoma[2] (Fig. 17-9).

The diagnosis of juxtaparotid malignancy is aided by sialograpy. In most cases there is external displacement or compression of the gland, but the duct system is normal (Fig. 17-10). Our patient had an undifferentiated sarcoma of nasopharyngeal origin that involved the parotid gland by contiguity. Subsequently, pulmonary and bony metastases developed.

Secondary tumors are found in the region of the parotid gland, notably metastatic neuroblastoma, retinoblastoma and rhabdomyosarcoma. A discussion of these tumors will be found in Chapter 18.

Sialadenitis

Sialadenitis may be encountered as a specific bacterial suppurative infection, a chronic infection without evident etiologic factors or infrequently as granulomatous replacement of the parotid or submaxillary gland.[37,38,41] We have encountered 54 children with sialadenitis (Fig. 17-11). Thirty-seven patients were males and 17, females. Male predilection, especially for chronic parotitis, has been noted in other reports.[28-30]

ACUTE SIALADENITIS

Twenty patients had acute sialadenitis. The parotid gland was involved in 14 and the submaxillary in 6. Parotid abscess requiring incision and drainage was

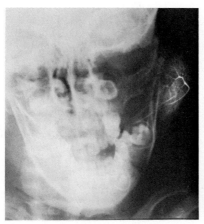 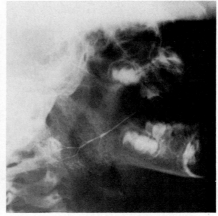

Fig. 17-10.—Sialogram of a patient with a rapidly growing undifferentiated sarcoma of nasopharyngeal origin. Note normal duct structure at all levels and lateral displacement of the parotid gland by the underlying tumor.

encountered in 9. Four patients had incision and drainage of a submaxillary abscess. Acute suppurative parotitis was common in the preantibiotic era and was often the final insult that led to the death of small infants undergoing major surgery for congenital anomalies. Treatment in that era consisted of compresses, incision and drainage, and small amounts of irradiation, usually in the range of 50–75r repeated on several successive days. The low x-ray dosage had little effect on the destructive bacterial infection.

The disease is now most commonly seen in the perinatal period, presenting as a painful, red indurated swelling of the parotid or submaxillary gland. The responsible organism can usually be cultured from the duct orifice. In 12 cases, this was *Staphylococcus aureus,* followed in frequency by streptococcus and d-pneumonococcus. In others, because of the administration of antibiotics before hospitalization, the offending organism was not recovered.

There is often, but not always, a background of dehydration through vomiting or diarrhea and some constitutional impairment related to concurrent disease. One patient had acute glomerulonephritis. Acute parotitis also occurs in the postoperative period in patients who have undergone multiple surgical procedures. Karlan and Snyder[29] encountered 24 patients with acute sialadenitis. In 2, it was a postoperative complication; 1 infant, operated on for pyloric stenosis, died. Two patients had a recent history of mumps. None of their patients required incision and drainage.

Chronic Sialadenitis

Recurring parotitis.—This is a well-documented condition in adults,[7,32,35,50] and a number of authors have described the syndrome as it is seen in childhood, with its variations and considerably better prognosis.[1,21,28,30,37,41] Katzen and DuPlessis[30] reported on 44 children from South Africa with recurrent parotitis. The condition is rare in the Negro. There were 26 males and 18 females. All authors acknowledge that the condition is more common in boys than in girls.

Etiology.—The cause of chronic sialadenitis is unknown. A number of factors have been implicated, but few are applicable in our patients or those in the recent literature.

Allergy, either as a drug sensitivity or food intolerance, has been implicated. There is one report of sialadenitis following periodic treatment of recurring urinary tract infection with sulfisoxazole.[36] Recurring parotitis developed at shorter and shorter intervals after the institution of therapy, and it may be that some drugs are capable of producing distant local tissue sensitization. Opium and other drugs that act on the parotid gland by suppressing secretion may induce parotitis in an indirect way. Many patients had a history of recent pharyngitis and recurring tonsillitis.

Fig. 17-11.—Inflammatory disease of the major salivary glands—sialadenitis.

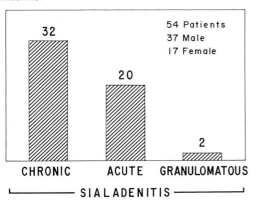

Carious teeth were noted in 5 children. A family history was not noted for any of our patients, and no siblings had the disease.[45]

Parotid gland involvement as a subtype of cystic fibrosis would be a logical entity. The Children's Hospital Cystic Fibrosis Center has under surveillance more than 900 patients; only 2 developed parotitis. Both had sialograms showing minimal ectasia. In both, the parotitis subsided spontaneously and did not recur. Enlarged submaxillary glands are common in patients with cystic fibrosis, and they have increased salivary electrolyte values with abnormally high calcium level. Minute calculi could obstruct the drainage apparatus, producing a stagnation background for sialadenitis.

Culture of material expressed from the parotid duct is of little help in this condition, in contrast to acute sialadenitis. Only nonpathogenic organisms are recovered, and these are not consistent.

Inflammatory or congenital stricture of the salivary duct has been implicated, but only 1 patient in 27 had a stenotic duct orifice.

Mumps presents a problem in differential diagnosis with the first attack, but there are several important differences that make it possible to separate the two conditions. Simultaneous bilateral involvement is rare with chronic parotitis. Mumps was mentioned in the records of only 3 patients. An exudate may be obtained from Stensen's duct during a periodic attack of sialadenitis. None is recovered in mumps. The serum amylase content is elevated with mumps and normal with chronic sialadenitis. With mumps, there is neutropenia; with sialadenitis, there is leukocytosis in the range of 12,000 – 18,000. In addition to mumps, sarcoidosis, tuberculosis and lymphoma must be excluded.

In some patients, chronic parotitis may represent an autoimmune disorder heralding widespread systemic involvement. It may be possible to place some children with sialadenitis in this category. Those showing a marked degree of lymphocytic infiltration and islet formation should be observed for the development of systemic disease. There is striking similarity between this variety of chronic parotitis and lymphoid thyroiditis, or Hashimoto's disease.

SYMPTOMS AND SIGNS. – Recurring, painful attacks lasting 1 – 7 days and aggravated by chewing and swallowing are typical. Physical examination reveals swelling and tenderness limited to the anatomic area of the involved gland without involvement of the overlying skin and subcutaneous tissue. Systemic reactions are variable, but temperature elevation is seldom of more than 1 degree. Examination of the ipsilateral duct orifice at the time of the attack reveals reddening and some pouting. Collected secretions are thick and flocculent, described as snowflake in character. In some cases, the disease is limited to the accessory parotid gland apparatus. This is a small structure centered over Stensen's duct beyond the anterior limits of the true parotid gland. When this alone is involved, it may by local expansion interfere with drainage of the main duct. Between attacks, the gland usually remains somewhat fuller than the uninvolved side and retains local tenderness.

In our series, patients ranged in age from 4 months to 14 years. Fifteen of 27 were 2–6 years old; 12 of the 15 were boys. Eleven children had symptoms from a few weeks to less than 1 year; 9, from 1 to 3 years; 4, from 3 to 6 years; in 3 the duration of symptoms was unknown. Frequency of attacks varied, but they occurred at least every 3-4 months. The side of involvement seemed to be random. Eleven had involvement of the right side, 7 the left, and 5 were bilateral. In 4 cases there was no comment about the side of involvement. Katzen and DuPlessis[30] report on 14 patients with right-sided involvement, 12 left, and 18 bilateral. The higher incidence of bilateral involvement in their series may relate to the older median age. Follow-up of our patients revealed that 5 had gone on to bilateral involvement. Most patients start with unilateral attacks, which become bilateral months or years later. Conversely, they rarely suffer simultaneous attacks on the 2 sides.

DIAGNOSIS. – The diagnosis of chronic sialadenitis rests on the history of the disease, the appearance of a carefully performed sialogram and the histology of the gland determined by open biopsy. At the height of the disease, one sees hyperplasia of duct epithelium and an increased number of mucus-secreting cells. In the periductal tissues there is lymphocytic infiltration, with the formation of some follicles and acinar hypertrophy with fibrosis.

MEDICAL MANAGEMENT. – Treatment of chronic parotitis is in many ways unsatisfactory. Antibiotics are commonly administered at the height of an attack, and the process usually subsides in 3 – 7 days. However, patients not treated with antibiotics do equally well, with no prolongation of swelling or symptoms. Nonspecific supportive therapy includes attention to oral hygiene, massage of the gland and use of acid sweets and chewing gum. Eleven patients had tonsillectomy; 3 improved, and 8 were unimproved. Irradiation for this condition is mentioned only to be condemned. Twenty years ago, 2 patients received 600r in two doses. Steroids were not used by us or in other reported series in childhood.

Katzen followed up 31 of 44 children by recall or questionnaire. Twenty-one had stopped having attacks, usually at age 11 – 13, and all by age 15. Most patients are male; therefore, the hormonal surge at puberty would appear to have significance. Of 10 patients in our series still having attacks, 7 are under 14 years of age. Hopefully, they may go into spontaneous remission at puberty. Karlan and Snyder[29] had good results with nonintervention.

SURGICAL TREATMENT. – The most effective surgical treatment for chronic parotitis is sialolithotomy with removal of one or more opaque calculi identified in a scout film preliminary to sialography. A second procedure of value is the excision of accessory parotid gland apparatus that compresses the midportion of Stensen's duct. If a firm nodule is felt in this location, or if there is evidence of extrinsic compression in the area normally occupied by this tissue, excisional biopsy is indicated, with considerable hope for success. Calibration of Stensen's duct orifice should be routine at the time of sialography, employing graded lacrimal dilators, but we encountered stenosis of the duct orifice in only 1 patient. Meatotomy has been recommended and was carried out in 5 patients in one series without significant improvement. Avulsion of the auriculotemporal nerve was performed in 17 patients by Katzen and DuPlessis.[29] Parotitis recurred in 9; in 3, nerve tissue was not found in the pathologic material, and 3 were lost to follow-up. The improvement that occurred in 2 patients was considered fortuitous; both had bilateral disease, and the disease subsided as rapidly on the unoperated side. Ligation of Stensen's duct is thought to be unwise.[18] This is an attempt to produce autoparotidectomy; however, half the patients have suppuration, and in a considerable number an internal necessitans fistula develops at some point proximal to the site of ligation.

Total parotidectomy with dissection and preservation of the 7th nerve is reserved for advanced disease. Total parotidectomy was carried out in 4 of 28 patients in our series. In 2, the operation was unilateral, and 2 bilateral. In 1 patient, this extensive operation was performed with disease of only a few weeks' duration. The surgeon believed he was dealing with parotid malignancy, yet there was no preoperative sialogram or biopsy examination. Three patients had unremitting disease with advanced sialectasia. Permanent 7th nerve palsy did not occur in any patient.

We believe that parotidectomy for chronic sialadenitis should be reserved for patients with severe, debilitating, recurring attacks, pain, toxicity and total disorganization of the gland.

The surgical procedures carried out in 28 patients with parotid sialadenitis are listed in Table 17-7. The most common procedure was biopsy for identification when sialography was not commonly done or the result was equivocal. The combination of biopsy and irradiation is of historical interest and is mentioned only to be condemned. When calculi were present, sialolithotomy was usually curative. One patient had multiple intraglandular calculi (Fig. 17-12). Local excision of a

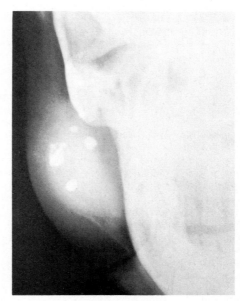

Fig. 17-12.—Sialogram, showing multiple opaque calculi in a boy with recurring parotitis and advanced sialectasia.

small nodule within the substance of the parotid gland without formal parotidectomy was performed in 3 patients. In each case, removal of the process coincided with the abatement of symptoms.

Two patients in the series reported by Katzen and DuPlessis would seem to have been candidates for parotidectomy.[30] One had total disintegration of the gland and a mass compressing the duct suggesting an accessory parotid structure. Another, with disease dating from childhood, and total destruction of the gland, had difficulties in the temporomandibular joint and middle ear, Costen's syndrome. Both appear to be examples of undertreatment.

Of 78 patients reviewed by Maynard[35], 12 had symptoms dating from puberty and 7 were under the age of 14. In 7, Sjögren's disease and xerostomia developed. Therefore nonintervention in childhood would not seem to be appropriate in all cases.

The value of the Currey test for parotid function was recently established by Seward *et al.*,[44] who studied 86 patients with chronic parotitis. In the course of the study they identified a new pathologic condition of the parotid gland consisting of hypersecretion with marked glandular hypertrophy. These patients had a striking increase in the number of zymogen granules, and up to 28 cc of saliva was collected from each side in 5 minutes after pilocarpine stimulation. Treatment of this condition is bilateral superficial parotid lobectomy. There remains enough hyperfunctioning tissue in the deep lobes to provide oral lubrication.

COMPLICATIONS.—Complications of this disorder are largely iatrogenic. The most serious complication,

TABLE 17-7.—TREATMENT OF PAROTID SIALADENITIS

PROCEDURE		No. OF PATIENTS
Biopsy only		10
Sialolithotomy		5
None		5
Parotidectomy		4
Bilateral	2	
Unilateral	2	
Local excision		3
Biopsy and irradiation		2
Irradiation only		5

7th nerve palsy, may result from parotidectomy, the only definitive therapy for advanced sialadenitis with total destruction of the parotid gland. Complications of parotid gland surgery have been minimal in the entire series, whether performed for sialadenitis or neoplasm. Excluding intentional sacrifice of the 7th nerve in patients with malignancy, only 1 patient is left with any degree of nerve impairment limited to the mandibular branch. Two patients developed the auriculotemporal syndrome of Frey. This consists of flushing of the side of the face following mastication. It is painless but may last for several years after parotidectomy.

Complications resulting from the disease itself are not encountered in children. Many adults have decreased to absent salivary output, with distressing dryness, or xerostomia sicca. There is experimental and clinical evidence that absent, defective or deficient parotid gland secretion produces a poor oral hygienic environment leading to a high incidence of dental caries.

Meticulous dental care and the application of fluoride may be helpful.

SUBMAXILLARY SIALADENITIS

Submaxillary sialadenitis occurred in 9 patients. In 3, a calculus was present, and in 2 the gland was replaced by granuloma. One child had a foreign body (timothy grass) blocking Wharton's duct. Karlen and Snyder[29] reported 9 cases of submaxillary involvement; 2 were granulomatous. One had a calculus removed, and 3 required incision and drainage. Treatment of advanced submaxillary sialadenitis is surgical excision; the gland serves no independent function and presents few anatomic hazards in its removal.

Miscellaneous Lesions

Seven patients had unusual salivary gland lesions. One appeared to have a branchiogenic cyst in the lower third of the neck and below this a draining external fistula.[47] This proved to be an ectopic salivary gland with an external duct. Two patients had aberrant parotid gland tissue, and 1 had venous thrombosis of the parotid gland. Branchiogenic cysts were encountered within the parotid gland in 2 patients presenting with sialadenitis (Fig. 17-17).

Sialography

Sialography can be carried out without anesthesia in any child more than 5 years of age. In younger children, a short period of general anesthesia is required.[20] The technique consists of cannulation of Stensen's duct after topical application of Pontocaine and identification of the orifice with a lacrimal duct probe. A blunt lacrimal duct needle attached to a Luer-Lok syringe containing 1 cc of warm Lipiodol is inserted into the duct and 0.5 cc is injected with steady even pressure. At the same time, the duct is drawn into hyperextension by traction on the cheek. There is moderate discomfort at the time of injection, but this lasts only a few moments. When 0.5 cc has been instilled into the normal duct system, there is already some escape of the medium around the hub of the needle. Further injection results in extravasation of Lipiodol into the parenchyma of the gland, not only obscuring the fine network of the duct system but ultimately producing a foreign body reaction and compounding difficulties in the already diseased and fibrotic gland. In one patient, the opaque oil remained in the parotid gland 5 years after sialography. Promi-

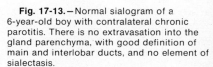

Fig. 17-13.—Normal sialogram of a 6-year-old boy with contralateral chronic parotitis. There is no extravasation into the gland parenchyma, with good definition of main and interlobar ducts, and no element of sialectasis.

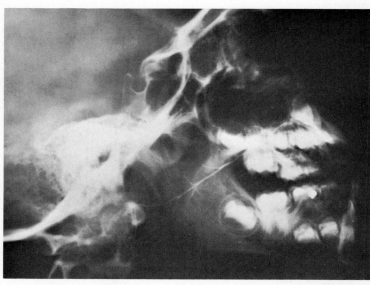

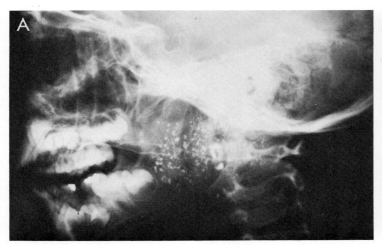

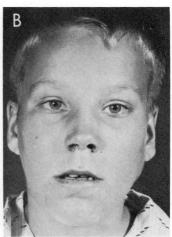

Fig. 17-14.—A, sialogram of a patient with a 6-month history of recurring parotid swelling. Note normal duct system and early but diffuse punctate sialectasia. **B,** photograph, showing notice-able swelling of left parotid region that remains between attacks every 3–4 months.

nent lymphoid follicles associated with long-standing disease may be evident as filling defects.

There have been no complications resulting from sialography in our experience. The children complain of local tenderness and dull discomfort for 1 or 2 days.

Sialography proved to be 96% correct in differentiating chronic inflammatory disease from neoplasm in a recent study of 357 patients by Einstein.[20] A normal sialogram is shown in Figure 17-13 (and see Fig. 17-10), and the various grades of architectural disturbance seen in children with sialadenitis are demonstrated in Figures 17-14–17-17. This condition progresses from punctate sialectasis, to the saccular form, to a widening of the interlobar duct system and, late in the disease, dilation of the major duct system, with progressive disorganization of the gland.

Technique of Parotidectomy

When undertaking parotid exploration, the surgeon should be well rested and unhurried and should have refreshed his knowledge of the anatomy and technical details.[3,4,15] Endotracheal anesthesia is mandatory. The operative field should be draped with sterile transparent plastic sheeting (Steridrape—3M) to expose the entire side of the face, including the corners of the eye and mouth (Fig. 17-18, A) so that facial twitching may be observed when the nerve is stimulated.

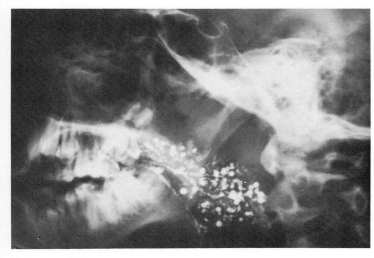

Fig. 17-15.—Sialogram of a patient with advanced saccular sialectasia and widening of interlobar ducts.

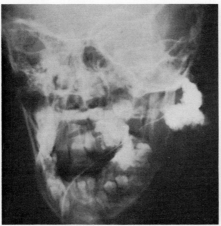
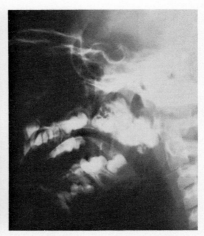

Fig. 17-16.—Sialogram showing total disorganization of the parotid gland. The patient had repeated attacks of sialadenitis over a 4-year period, with fever, toxicity, pain and trismus. The disease is unilateral. Total parotidectomy with dissection and preservation of the 7th nerve was performed.

The Y-shaped incision described nearly 45 years ago provides admirable exposure. When the skin flaps are being elevated, it is important to avoid mobilizing the anterior flap as far forward as the anterior border of the parotid gland, for in so doing one may inadvertently transect small branches of the facial nerve as they emerge from the anterior border of the gland. With upward traction of the ear lobe and anterior traction of the parotid gland, the dissection is carried along the inferior aspect of the external auditory canal, staying very close to this cartilaginous wall. Many small fibrous septae attach the posterior border of the parotid gland to this structure. As these are cautiously transected, the gland may be reflected anteriorly. As the dissection deepens along the ear canal, the main trunk of the facial nerve as it emerges from the stylomastoid foramen is reached (Fig. 17-18, *C*). The main trunk of the facial nerve will be found just a little anterior and a little medial to the tip of the mastoid process, which is less developed in small infants. Furthermore, the facial nerve assumes a more superficial position. One need not injure the facial nerve if one stays close to the auditory canal while reflecting the parotid gland anteriorly.

The styloid process is not a good landmark upon which to rely in identifying the facial nerve. It is absent in approximately 30% of individuals and is extremely small in another 20%. Some authors have recommended identification of the facial nerve by finding its various branches as they emerge from the anterior margin of the parotid gland. This seems less feasible than identification of the nerve as a single trunk, for reasons of both size and variability of peripheral branching.

A nerve stimulator must be available to lend reassurance concerning various septae which at first

Fig. 17-17.—**A,** a boy, aged 10, with recurring sialadenitis caused by an infected intraparotid branchial cleft cyst. He had had attacks for 2 years and grade 3 ectasia. **B,** lateral view, showing the site of biopsy, which provided the unusual diagnosis. Treatment consisted of superficial parotid lobectomy.

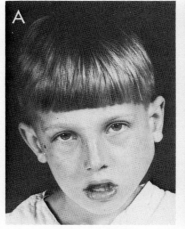
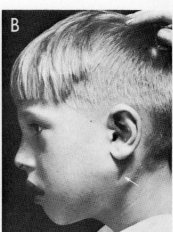

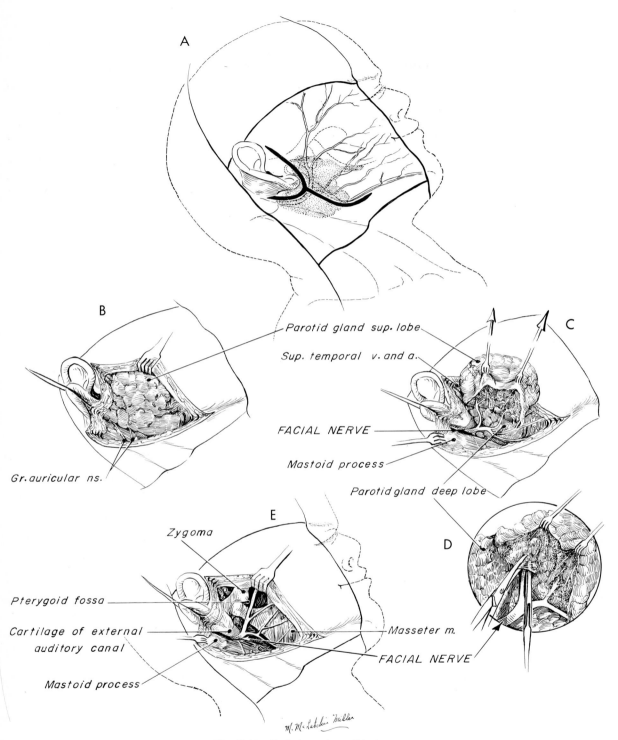

Fig. 17-18.—Technique of parotidectomy.

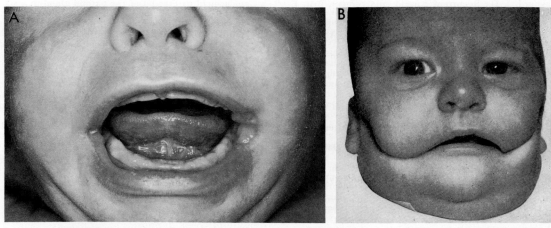

Fig. 18-1.—Lateral facial clefts. **A,** moderate unilateral cleft of the cheek (macrostomia). **B,** extensive bilateral facial clefts extending to temporal areas. (From Blackfield and Wilde.[10])

surgical treatment during the first year of life. They should be operated on between 1 and 3 years of age in order for the postoperative scar to reach its optimal appearance prior to entering school. Usually these clefts are unilateral and the aim surgically is obliteration of the cleft extending from the corner of the mouth into the cheek. It is important to conserve a vermilion flap to line the new, properly located angle of the mouth. The end of this flap is placed as an inlay into the upper surface of the lower lip, thereby avoiding lateral pull on the repaired corner of the mouth as contracture of healing takes place. In other respects the repair requires careful approximation of the deficient orbicularis muscle and the other components of the cheek. A Logan bow is used postoperatively to prevent direct pull on the suture line. Healing generally is complete in a week with a uniformly excellent cosmetic result. If there are associated preauricular tabs or accessory ear structures, they should be excised at the same time. The common type of macrostomia is seen in Figure 18-1, *A,* and a dramatic example of bilateral cleft is seen in Figure 18-1, *B.*

MICROSTOMIA

Microstomia is the rarest of all lip anomalies and represents incomplete development of the primitive blastopore. Surgical treatment consists of unilateral or bilateral extension of the diminutive central opening and construction of a vermilion surface by buccal mucosal advancement.[51] Microstomia may also follow loss of perioral tissue secondary to infection, electrical burns or tumors.

CONGENITAL LIP FISTULAS

This condition, often inherited, may or may not be associated with cleft lip or palate.[60] The consistent location of the fistulas in the central segment of the lower lip suggests a congenital origin; however, the exact embryologic explanation is lacking. Treatment consists of surgical excision with removal of the two mucous tracts and adjacent glandular tissue. Destruction by electrocoagulation is not recommended. Soricelli *et al.*[53] encountered the condition in 6 of 11 members of one family.

Injuries

BURNS OF THE MOUTH

Burns of the mouth by caustics are still common because caustic household cleaning compounds are not always put out of the reach of inquisitive toddlers. If there is no evidence of damage to the esophagus in the usual locations at the level of the aortic arch, midesophagus or the esophagogastric junction, they are given a bland diet. Corroded oropharyngeal surfaces are treated by application of sterile mineral oil and usually heal without scarring. The tissue burn has already taken place by the time these children see a physician, and for that reason attempts at local neutralization usually are ineffective. In addition, one does not always know the nature of the compound that produced the burn.

Burns of the mouth due to flames or hot gases are discussed in Chapter 9. A severe example of such a burn that required early tracheostomy is shown in Figure 18-2.

ELECTRICAL BURNS.—Electrical burns of all types are being seen with increased frequency because of the wide use of electric power. They account for 4–7% of all burns, with the highest incidence in Scandinavian countries, where electricity is widely used. Electrical burns of the mouth have been reported sporadically since Pierre[40] called attention to this entity and reported on 11 children in 1961. Thomson *et al.*[58]

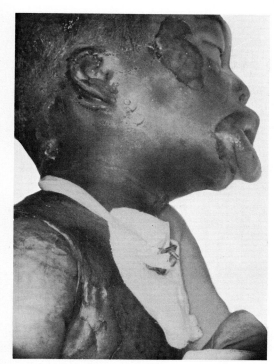

Fig. 18-2.—Flame burn of the airway and oropharyngeal tissues requiring early tracheostomy. Swelling is maximal at 36 hours.

from biting or sucking the free end of a "live" extension cord. Thus electrical burns of the mouth occur most frequently in the creeper or toddler age group, when everything is seen at floor level. The electric cord is a tempting play object, and contact is made at the exposed end or by biting through the insulation. Following completion of the circuit by saliva, there are tetanic contractions of the muscles of mastication, causing the jaws to grip the fixture and maintain contact. Unless the child is exceptionally well grounded, electrocution does not occur. There is destruction of tissue beyond the apparent gross limits of the burn, and eventual loss is always far greater than originally estimated. Children with electrical burns of the mouth should be hospitalized for approximately 2 weeks. During this time, the area of gray coagulation necrosis will slough away, with alarming hemorrhage from the tongue and lips often occurring at this stage (Fig. 18-3). Chewing of the insensitive tissue may be a factor in starting bleeding. Once the danger of hemorrhage has passed, healing occurs rapidly. At this time, the temptation is great to carry out definitive surgical correction, yet deficiency of lip substance is compensated for by cicatricial closure with surprisingly little deformity. Efforts at plastic reconstruction should be deferred approximately 1 year. At that time, usually very little will be required. The tongue will reshape normally and seldom requires surgical treatment. The lip scar can often be improved, and the only long-range problem is damage to permanent tooth buds in the area of burn. Deep destruction with resulting osteomyelitis of the mandible rarely occurs.

A conservative plastic approach should be adopted. Fogh-Anderson[24] found that 12 children required no surgical treatment, whereas 23 had one or more operations. Useful procedures include creation of a sulcus, V-excision of the mature scar, Stein-Estlander-Abbe flap and commissurotomy.

reported that 43 children were encountered in 20 years at the Hospital for Sick Children, Toronto. Fogh-Anderson and Sorenson[24] reported on 35 children treated in Denmark; 20 were aged 1–2 years, 7 were 2–4 years old, and 5 were under 1 year. We have encountered 8 children with this condition, comprising about 1% of burn admissions. Most cases resulted

Fig. 18-3.—A, electrical burn of the mouth in a 5-month-old child. The alveolar ridge and tongue also were involved. Major bleeding occurred on the 7th hospital day. B, 6 months later, showing good cosmetic appearance without surgical intervention.

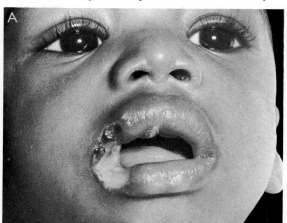
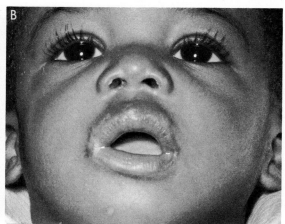

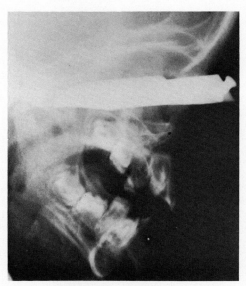

Fig. 18-4.—Knife blade embedded in petrous pyramid of a child of 1 year. Wound entrance was below the right eye.

LACERATIONS

Injuries of the oropharyngeal region are common in childhood, especially in boys. Most are of little consequence, but others may endanger life (Fig. 18-4). Patients with traumatic cleft lip should be hospitalized. Repair must be accurately carried out under endotracheal general anesthesia with careful attention to alignment of the vermilion border of the lip. The children should be hospitalized until the lip is completely healed, and the fresh repair should be supported with a Logan bow to prevent disruption or local injury to the suture line.

Lacerations of the cheek in which Stensen's duct may be severed should be repaired by complete external closure and loose internal closure around a rubber slip drain. If the laceration does communicate with the duct, an internal salivary fistula of no consequence will be established.

Major lacerations of the tongue should be sutured because of the frequent occurrence of delayed hemorrhage.

Lacerations of the palate usually occur in the preschool age group. Children at this age are active, uncoordinated, and usually fall with a spoon or stick in the mouth. The object is driven through the palate, producing a traumatic cleft. The injuries vary from simple perforations to complete detachment of the soft palate, often extending into the tonsillar fossa. If the injury is extensive or perforating, the patient should be admitted to the hospital. Because of the proximity of this area to the central nervous system, tetanus prophylaxis is important. The intraoral tissues are exceptionally resistant to infection, and antibiotics

have little to offer in most instances. The children should be managed like patients undergoing repair of a congenital cleft palate, by suturing the nasal mucous membrane, then approximating the palatal muscle at the base of the uvula, and finally joining the oral mucous membrane. Chromic catgut is used throughout. Only clear liquids are allowed for 5 days following such a repair, and the arms should be restrained with palate cuffs for approximately 4 weeks.

Braudo[12] reported on 4 children who had thrombosis of the internal carotid artery after injury to the soft palate. All patients developed hemiplegia that was transient in 3 and permanent in 1. At postmortem examination, 1 was found to have extensive softening of the corresponding hemisphere.[14] These central nervous system difficulties occurred approximately 3 days after injury.

Hemangioma

Hemangioma may appear as a combined mucous membrane and skin lesion in the region of the oropharynx and is treacherous in this area of rich blood supply. The lesion may be insignificant or absent at birth, first appearing at 1 month of age, and if untreated may progress in several months to massive involvement of the area with secondary infection, ulcerative destruction and loss of important features. Over a long period these combined capillary and cavernous lesions ultimately involute, but en route to that desirable end, loss of important substance of the lips, nose, eyelids and ears may occur. Although difficult to prove statistically, x-ray therapy seems to be of some value in controlling the occasional hemangioma that grows in semimalignant fashion during the first few months of life and cannot be excised because of

Fig. 18-5.—Hemangioma of lower lip and chin, treated with irradiation and conservative surgical excision in stages. Thinning of the lip and reconstruction of the vermilion surface was later accomplished by buccal mucous membrane advancement.

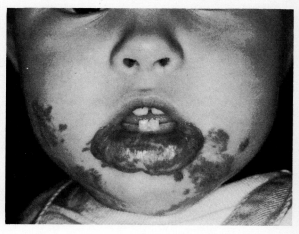

location. During x-ray treatment, there should be careful shielding of tooth buds and eyes. The treatment requires basal anesthesia, using a combination of rectal Pentothal and atropine. The head should be carefully positioned and immobilized by sandbags and the x-ray beam accurately directed. One or two treatments of approximately 200 rads will often impede advance of such tumors.

Surgical treatment of hemangiomas should be conservative unless the lesion is small or pedunculated and can be removed without sacrifice of important structures (Fig. 18-5). The eventual appearance of most facial hemangiomas is much better than one might originally predict, and surgery should be restricted to eventual plastic improvement of stromal elements that remain after regression.[31]

The possible extent of such a lesion is shown in Figure 18-6. No hemangioma was present at birth. At 6 weeks of age there were a few surface blotches, and 3 months later there was massive extension of the lesion. It is now well established that bulky hemangiomas occasionally trap platelets, producing thrombocytopenia and secondary bleeding. In this child, the platelet count fell to 20,000 and the head and neck became monstrously deformed because of continued tumor growth and extravasating hemorrhage. Large doses of cortisone (800 mg daily) were given and the platelet count rose to 50,000. X-ray treatment of the lesion to the limit of skin tolerance (900 r) had no apparent benefit. Splenectomy was performed to raise the platelet count. Following operation, the platelet

Fig. 18-6. — A platelet-trapping hemangioma, not present at birth but evident at 6 weeks. There were transitory, unsustained platelet rises after cortisone therapy, splenectomy and multiple platelet infusions. Death occurred at 3 years due to exsanguination after a minor local injury.

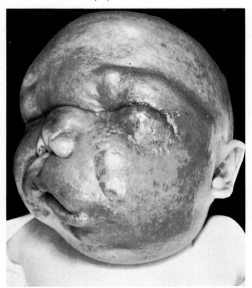

level remained normal for several weeks, then again fell to a pathologic range. Steroid therapy was resumed with little effect. Platelet infusions also failed to achieve a sustained satisfactory level. The child was hospitalized repeatedly over a 3-year period and ultimately died of exsanguinating hemorrhage after inadvertently driving a fork into his cheek.

Today, platelet-trapping hemangiomas can be treated by effective methods of platelet transfusion. Fifteen billion platelets can be given in as little as 15 cc of plasma. Under 1 year of age this results in a normal number of circulating platelets. With this protection, one may wish to excise a hemangioma in which platelet trapping is a threat to life. Diamond has seen 12 such patients, the first recognized some 30 years ago.[18] Good[26] reported on this condition, and there are 72 additional cases in the literature.

NEVUS FLAMMEUS. — Nevus flammeus or port-wine stain, a variant of hemangioma, usually involves the face and may show some tendency to disappear or at least decolorize during the first few years of life, but not as consistently as do capillary hemangiomas. They are usually static by the age of 10 and persist into adult life, developing nodularity with some evidence of continued subcutaneous growth. The relatively pale, blotchy lesion with a smooth surface and uncertain outline is managed best with make-up. The quality and opacity of make-up preparations has improved in recent years. On the other hand, surgical removal may be desirable if the lesion is deep red or purple, has surface nodularity or has been converted into an unsightly lesion by overenthusiastic treatment with sclerosing solutions, dry ice or x-rays. The psychologic reaction to such a lesion is often profound, and any replacement may be considered an improvement. Operation should be deferred until the second decade when the child's face achieves adult proportions.

There are several surgical alternatives. The simplest and often satisfactory solution in the untreated lesion is counter-tattooing of the least objectionable area and excision of the remainder, taking as little subcutaneous tissue as possible to avoid altering the facial contour. The eyelids and angles of the mouth should not be disturbed. The defect may be covered with a thick split-thickness graft which is best obtained with the Reese mechanical dermatome that will cut a graft of perfect uniformity. Lesions involving the eyelids or angle of the mouth may be replaced with full-thickness skin taken from the supraclavicular or postauricular areas. The graft must be carefully stented. The dressing, immobilization and postoperative care have much to do with the final result. Some contracture is inevitable, and appropriate release procedures must be undertaken. Other methods of replacement include pedicle rotation from the cervical area or the forehead. The latter is based on the superficial temporal artery (replacing the forehead defect with a split-thickness graft). A thoracoacromial tubed pedicle graft has been suggested.[25] A full-thickness graft taken from the abdomen has some advantage in the final appearance of the grafted area, but color match is poor. In about 2 years the junction of the graft and adjacent skin smooths out, and except for some increased glossiness and increased pigmentation on exposure to sunlight the result is more acceptable to the patient than the original lesion. No completely satisfactory solution of the problem has been found. Conway[16] reported enthusiastically about counter-tattooing of port-wine stains. MacCollum and Martin[32] did not find this satisfactory, and in our experience the uptake of pigment is irregular and scarring may result.

Lesions of the Jaw

PIERRE ROBIN SYNDROME

The Pierre Robin syndrome consists of hypoplasia of the mandible, posterior displacement of the tongue and often an associated cleft of the soft palate. Inspiratory obstruction with sternal retraction and failure to thrive are common features (Fig. 18-7). The infant hyperextends the neck to breathe more easily. Attacks of alarming cyanosis are frequent and sudden and can be fatal. Glossoptosis diminishes with growth, and in most cases embarrassment of respiration and difficulty with feeding improve in 2 or 3 months. Nevertheless many such infants have died unexpectedly at a time when they seemed to be overcoming their problem.

Tracheostomy should be employed only as a life-saving procedure. If tracheostomy is necessary in the perinatal period, the tube must be left in place for several months; it may result in laryngeal stenosis, especially if the site of tracheostomy is too high and near the cricoid cartilage.

A Stamm gastrostomy should be performed in patients who have marked difficulties with feeding. Repeated attempts at oral feeding in the presence of respiratory distress results in aspiration. In an infant,

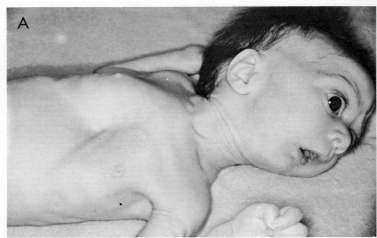

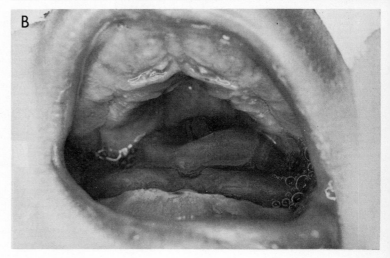

Fig. 18-7.—Pierre Robin syndrome. **A**, 2-month-old infant with micrognathia, glossoptosis and opisthotonic position of the head to improve the airway. **B**, note retrodisplacement of the mandible and tip of the tongue and prominent mouth floor. The associated cleft of the soft palate is thought to be due to abnormal elevation of the tongue during the process of palate closure.

gastrostomy can be accomplished safely under local anesthesia in a few minutes, thereby relieving the nursing staff of many hours of ineffective and dangerous feeding attempts.

Airway obstruction is caused not so much by an oversized tongue as by the hypoplastic mandible and perhaps incomplete development of the intrinsic muscles of the tongue. Micrognathia in itself is an index of immaturity. The jaw steadily lengthens, and at the same time there is marked improvement in the intrinsic operation of the tongue. During this phase of additional local development, surgical procedures have much to offer and indeed may be life-saving. In 1950, Douglas[20] recommended denuding the undersurface of the tongue and the gingivobuccal sulcus, suturing these two structures together. He reported on 6 patients with 1 death. In responses to a questionnaire, he was able to collect 46 additional instances. Twenty-one were not treated surgically; there were 13 deaths in the untreated group. Twenty-five patients were treated surgically by this method, and there were no deaths. Sometimes the Douglas repair does not hold and the tongue falls back into the throat. In 1953, Duhamel[21] added further to the surgical solution of this problem. He described a technique of placing a suture of number 5 silk through the base of the tongue. The ends of the suture are then passed through the alveolar ridge and tied. In order to place this suture, a towel clip may be used to draw the tongue forward. With an index finger below the tongue and a thumb placed on a gauze sponge on the dorsum of the tongue, the suture is placed as far posteriorly as possible in the area where the tongue is thickest. This suture can be combined with the Douglas procedure.[22]

We have utilized this method of surgical treatment in 9 patients and all survived. The Duhamel suture must remain in place for approximately 6 weeks; if properly placed, it does not cut through. The procedure is thought not to interfere with the eruption of permanent teeth.

Moderate cases of Pierre Robin syndrome may be managed by feeding the infant in the upright position and subsequently positioning it prone with the neck extended by applying traction to a skull cap made of moleskin and stockinette to facilitate breathing. Tracheostomy is rarely necessary. A fatality due to this disorder alone is avoidable and tragic.

FRACTURES

Fractures of the maxilla and mandible are uncommon in childhood, in marked contrast to the incidence in adults, who usually incur this injury in automobile accidents. Not only are maxillofacial fractures less common in childhood, but the child's face is inherently more resilient because of the greater cartilage content.

Diagnosis of a fracture of the *mandible* can usually be made by clinical examination. The fracture is ap-

parent as an irregularity in the mandibular arch with loss of proper dental occlusion, and occasionally with a tear of the oral mucous membrane. The commonest site of fracture of the mandible in childhood is the bicuspid area. If there is no significant displacement, no active treatment is necessary. A Barton head dressing is difficult to maintain and involves some degree of danger from aspiration. These children have remarkably little discomfort. A liquid or soft diet should be prescribed for about 4 weeks, following which union usually is sufficiently good to permit a full diet. If displacement is present, and if the child has teeth adjacent to the fracture site, interdental wire fixation can be undertaken. External fixation devices are not recommended. If teeth are absent, stabilization of mandibular fragments can be accomplished by open reduction, placing one or two small steel wires very low in the mandibular ramus. As an alternate method of stabilization, one may pass a wire around the symphysis menti and anchor it to the maxilla through a drill hole in the anterior nasal spine. Central bilateral fractures can be supported by a molded splint held in place by wires circumferentially placed around the mandible and the splint.[41] The splint permits the child to open his mouth and is usually left in place for 4 weeks. These relatively simple techniques avoid the danger of infection and direct injury to tooth buds which may result from more extensive open reduction methods.

The mandible is fractured next most commonly in the subcondylar region, usually with pain and tenderness in the region of the temporomandibular joint, with considerable trismus and displacement of the lower dental arch. Active treatment of such a fracture is seldom necessary. With subsequent growth, a fracture with considerable angulation may be expected to straighten spontaneously without residual deformity. Very rarely there may be complete separation of the fractured surfaces, with rotation of the proximal fragment, which may require open reduction. In an older child, if the proximal fragment consists of merely the head of the condyle, the simplest management may be to remove the head of the condyle, following which pseudarthrosis occurs, with satisfactory function as a result. Occasionally, interosseous wiring is indicated. A fracture in this area in a small child may result eventually in some degree of facial asymmetry by virtue of interference with the growth center in the mandibular head.

Extensive fractures of the *maxilla* are uncommon in childhood, and when seen should be treated much as they are in older individuals. A depressed malar zygomatic arch may be corrected by simple elevation or occasionally by open reduction with placement of wires for external traction within 72 hours. In older children, fixation after reduction by wiring the teeth together is a satisfactory method. The primary objective is establishment of good occlusion without injury to permanent tooth buds. Whenever teeth are wired, the patient must be kept under close observation, with wire cutters at hand to be used in the event of distress from vomiting.[50] Gastrostomy is a useful adjunct in some patients.

If open reduction of a maxillary fracture is considered necessary, and this is rarely the case, one must carefully avoid the site of permanent tooth buds. Good healing can be expected in 3–5 weeks with most fractures regardless of their complexity.

TUMORS OF THE JAWS

Tumors of the jaws are rare in children, and fortunately benign tumors are predominant, especially those related to dental development. The jaws derive from the first branchial arch and are composed of a mesodermal mass covered with ectoderm. Both tissues can produce a variety of neoplasms. In this area of complex development, inclusions of salivary gland or thyroid tissue may occur.

Jaw tumors usually present as asymptomatic swellings. With growth, they cause irregular displacement and ultimate loss of the overlying teeth with complicating sepsis. Radiographic and clinical impressions are notably inaccurate, and all lesions must be identified by surgical biopsy. Jaw tumors in children have been classified as follows:[45]

Tumors of dental origin: follicular cysts; dentigerous cysts; ameloblastoma (adamantinoma).

Benign tumors of nondental origin: giant cell; eosinophilic granuloma; fibroma (fibrous dysplasia).

Primary malignant tumors: carcinoma; sarcoma (endosteal fibrosarcoma, osteogenic sarcoma, unclassified).

Metastatic malignant tumors: neuroblastoma; embryonal carcinoma.

BENIGN TUMORS.—Ordinarily, ameloblastoma is a bulky tissue displacing benign tumor, but it may appear in malignant form and has occurred at the age of 5 months. Giant cell tumors should be carefully cleaned out by curettage and cauterization of the tumor cavity. They have a great tendency to recur; therefore, the first operation should be extensive and definitive. Eosinophilic granuloma is probably part of a general metabolic disturbance related to Hand-Schüller-Christian and Letterer-Siwe disease. It is evident as a swelling of the gums with loosening and bleeding from tooth sockets and ultimate infection. There is no certain method of treatment. Because of the similar histologic and x-ray appearance of jaw fibromas and hyperparathyroidism, calcium, phosphorus and phosphatase blood level determinations are of importance.

Hemangiomas of the mandible and maxilla may present as surgical emergencies. They are usually unsuspected until there is bleeding around a tooth socket either spontaneously or after dental extraction. They are characterized by spurting of arterial blood in large amounts and difficulty with hemostasis by any of the conventional dental techniques. X-ray examination of the jaw reveals the washed-out appearance of bone destruction in the area of the lesion. Ligation of the external carotid artery is of little value. Segmental resection of the maxilla or mandible may be necessary and under some conditions life-saving. Adjunctive hypothermia has been found useful; and, as with nasopharyngeal angioma, freezing of the lesion with a

Fig. 18-8.—A, roentgenogram of infant with exophytic sarcoma of the mandibular region. These congenital tumors present obstetric difficulties but fortunately are not highly malignant and metastasize late. **B**, photomicrograph of mandibular sarcoma, showing mesenchymal ground substance. These have been classified as embryomas. Although locally invasive, they are resectable when exophytic, but seldom are with invasion of the pterygoid fossa. ×100.

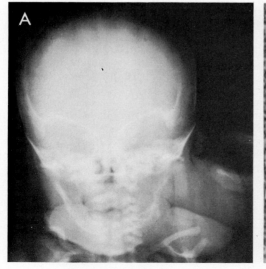

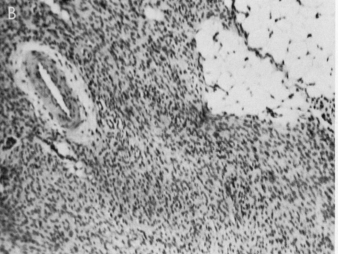

cryoprobe before surgical resection will reduce blood loss substantially.[17,56]

Considerable attention has been devoted to a benign lesion of the jaws considered to be a melanotic neuroectodermal tumor of infancy of neural crest origin. In 1 case this was associated with high urinary excretion of vanilmandelic acid.[11] Historically, these lesions were considered to be odontogenic and closely related to ameloblastoma. Because of their characteristic pigmentation, they appear to represent a separate entity also called melanotic progonoma.[30] In most cases, the tumor has become evident before the age of 1 year, predominantly in the maxilla of female patients.[28] Medenis and associates[35] collected 27 cases from the literature, noting the female preponderance and the fact that all patients were under age 6. Conservative resection with currettage to produce bony bleeding appears to be adequate treatment, with infrequent recurrence.

MALIGNANT TUMORS.—Malignant jaw tumors are rare. Byars reported an endosteal fibrosarcoma in a 3-year-old child, and there are isolated reports of osteogenic sarcoma. Examples of mandibular sarcoma are shown in Figure 18-8.

Burkitt's tumor (the African lymphoma).—In 1958, Burkitt[15] described a primitive and at that time unclassified sarcoma arising in multicentric fashion commonly in the jaws of Negro children in Uganda (Fig. 18-9). He saw 38 patients with the tumor in 7 years, with peak age incidence at age 5. The maxilla is involved more often than the mandible, and loosening of molars is the first clinical sign. These tumors grow to huge size, are locally destructive and do not

Fig. 18-9.—Burkitt's lymphoma involving the jaws of a 3-year-old boy. Death was due to pulmonary metastasis. (From Burkitt.[15])

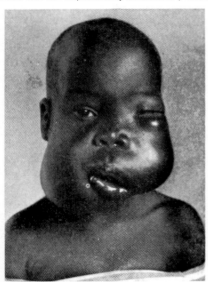

ulcerate. About half metastasize to the abdomen. The regional or distant lymph nodes and spleen are not involved, and there are no changes in peripheral blood. The lesion is essentially osteolytic and is first evident as disappearance of the lamina dura. The obvious relation to neuroblastoma was first considered, but it is a discrete and separate neoplasm. In the relatively small region of Uganda, the tumor attains endemic proportions and is considered the commonest malignant tumor of childhood.

The tendency to jaw involvement has a unique age distribution. Below age 3, the jaw tumor has seldom been observed. In every child 3 years of age, the jaw tumors have been clinically evident; this incidence diminishes with each year of age, the tumors being seen in only 20% of patients at age 12.[14] Few cases have been seen anywhere in the world beyond age 14. Adatia[1] ably reviewed the literature, focusing attention on the multiracial and world-wide distribution.

Burkitt's tumor is very sensitive to relatively small doses of chemotherapeutic agents, placing it in a most favorable category heretofore limited to choriocarcinoma, Wilms' tumor and to some extent pelvic rhabdomyosarcoma.[29,54] Burkitt found a significant response to Methotrexate in two thirds of tumors of moderate size and in four fifths of similar tumors treated with cyclophosphamide (Cytoxan).[13] Of 63 children treated with this agent, 24 had total clinical regression. A relatively small dosage was required, and regression continued after cessation of therapy. A viral etiology has been postulated with a very favorable tumor-host relationship. Irradiation plays a minor role, and surgical excision, except for identification of the process, seems unwarranted.

A word of caution must be inserted because of the current overdiagnosis of the condition in retrospective review of patients with a previous diagnosis of lymphosarcoma or reticulum cell sarcoma.[38] Reclassification has been based on histologic appearance characterized by proliferation of primitive cells of lymphoreticular tissue and by an abundance of actively phagocytosing histiocytes. In addition, a clinical presentation and anatomic tumor distribution similar to that reported in the majority of the African cases has been required. Several patients in our institution have blossomed into full-scale lymphatic leukemia.

Pseudosarcomatous fasciitis.—A perplexing surgical lesion involving the jaws and surrounding mesenchymal tissues initially presenting as a granuloma and later becoming increasingly cellular with a predominance of mesenchymal elements has been called pseudosarcomatous fasciitis.[5] Our patient, a 12-year-old boy, for 5 years had agonizing pain in the distribution of the trigeminal nerve. In addition to stiffening and wasting of tissues, the temporomandibular joint became fixed. Some cases have been thought to be due to aspergillosis and were empirically treated with amphotericin B. Because of the histologic nature of the process, prednisone has been administered to toxic levels. Ultimately, because of the unrelieved pain and nutritional difficulties, surgical treatment must be undertaken. This consists of hemifacial resection including the mandible and appropriate resurfacing. This process is radioresistant.[5]

METASTATIC TUMORS. — These may be found in the jaw region or in the glands of the upper neck. Some are occult in the nasopharynx, or the primary site may never be found. Metastatic spread of neuroblastoma to the skull occurs frequently, but the deposits are most common in the calvarium and the retrobulbar tissues. Rarely, first evidence of the tumor may consist of a swelling of the mandible as a bony metastasis.

SURGICAL TREATMENT. — Accurate diagnosis of jaw tumors is established by surgical biopsy. Most benign tumors can be adequately treated by wide local excision, occasionally taking a horizontal section of the mandibular ramus. Malignant tumors must be treated by wide local excision with hemimandibulectomy. It is important to maintain the symmetry of the face with proper prosthetic support. Iliac bone grafts for older children should not be used until facial growth is complete in the second decade.

Infections

Four types of infection are peculiar to the oropharyngeal region with which all surgeons should be familiar.

LUDWIG'S ANGINA

This infection is aptly named, angina meaning to strangle or suffocate. The causative organism is usually a streptococcus, although there may be a mixed

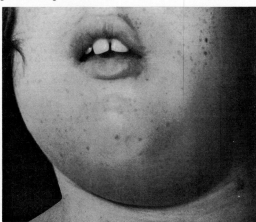

Fig. 18-10.—Ludwig's angina in a girl of 11. Note the brawny edema throughout the submental and submandibular regions. There was elevation of the tongue and mild respiratory embarrassment. The condition responded to antibiotics without need for surgical drainage.

infection. The commonest portal of entry is a carious mandibular molar. Spread through the floor of the mouth is rapid, with involvement of the submaxillary space. In half the patients, Vincent's organisms also are present. A patient with a typical case presents swelling and tenderness of the submaxillary and submandibular regions of the neck, edema of the floor of the mouth and elevation of the tongue (Fig. 18-10). The process may cause complete respiratory obstruction.

Treatment should be started immediately, with large doses of tetracycline and penicillin, to which most patients respond in a gratifying manner. It is seldom necessary to perform tracheostomy or to create large drainage incisions in the submaxillary region, as was formerly done. Pus is rarely encountered early, although at a later stage pus may be found deep between the mylohyoid and geniohyoid muscles or between the geniohyoid and genioglossus muscles.[57] In preantibiotic days, this dread infection occasionally spread along fascial planes of the neck into the mediastinum, with fatal outcome.

NOMA

Noma is a severe necrotizing infection of mucous membranes that may involve the nose, eyelids, auditory canal, vulva, prepuce and anus but is most often encountered in the mouth. It is usually seen in the first decade of life and nearly always in children with a greatly lowered resistance to infection due to a generalized disorder such as malnutrition, blood dyscrasia, parasitic infestation and occasionally following exanthematous disease.[55]

No single organism has been uniformly responsible, and culture usually provides evidence of a mixed infection. Vincent's organisms are nearly always present. The infection starts with ulceration of mucous membranes accompanied by a foul odor and progresses rapidly to necrosis and sloughing of tissues. Destruction of much of the face may result (Fig. 18-11).

Treatment consists of massive broad-spectrum antibiotic therapy and vigorous supportive measures directed toward improving the underlying disease state. Necrotic tissue should be debrided. Before antibiotics were available, most patients with noma died. Today, there are survivors among the group without an ultimately fatal predisposing disease.

PERITONSILLAR ABSCESS

Once a common condition, peritonsillar abscess is seldom seen in this day of early antibiotic treatment of pharyngeal infection. It is extremely rare in small children. Characteristically, there is a history of recent tonsillitis followed by onset of severe pain with unilateral swelling above and medial to the upper

Lesions of the Tongue and Oral Cavity

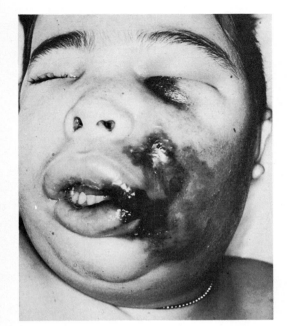

Fig. 18-11.—Noma, or gangrenous stomatitis, destroying a large portion of the left cheek in a 10-year-old child with leukemia.

pole of the tonsil. Trismus or inability to open the mouth widely is common.[44]

Treatment by prompt surgical drainage is mandatory. Drainage should be carried out under full endotracheal general anesthesia, with the patient positioned in a steep Trendelenburg position to prevent aspiration.

RETROPHARYNGEAL ABSCESS

Retropharyngeal abscess is seen in infants and toddlers but rarely in older children. Symptoms may be those of respiratory obstruction, inability to swallow or stiffness of the neck suggesting a cervical orthopedic problem. Once suspected, diagnosis is best made by palpation of the pharyngeal region, gently sweeping the examining finger across the posterior pharyngeal wall.

Treatment consists of surgical drainage. It is best to drain retropharyngeal abscesses without general anesthesia, because induction of anesthesia may be hazardous when respiratory obstruction is imminent. If the patient is in the Trendelenburg position, well wrapped and with the head well extended, the likelihood of aspiration of pus is minimal.

X-ray examination of both soft tissues and vertebrae of the cervical region is indicated to rule out the presence of an opaque foreign body, which may have been ingested, and to exclude cervical osteomyelitis as the underlying cause.

ANKYLOGLOSSIA INFERIOR

This condition, called tonguetie, is common in infancy and often disappears spontaneously or with sucking if the frenum of the tongue is not prominent or is sufficiently thin. In some cases, however, surgery may be necessary to permit normal speech, and operation can be carried out very simply. The handle of a grooved director serves admirably for this purpose. With this instrument, one can elevate the tip of the tongue, permitting the frenum of the tongue to fit between the winglike projections of the handle. The frenum is then cut transversely to release the tip of the tongue. Bleeding is easily controlled by gentle pressure on a gauze sponge for a minute or two. If surgical release of tonguetie is deferred until the child is older, general anesthesia is preferable. Anesthesia of any sort is unnecessary in a small infant.

ANKYLOGLOSSIA SUPERIOR

This condition—attachment of the tongue to the roof of the mouth—is a very rare congenital anomaly. It must be recognized at birth, because severe or total respiratory obstruction is inevitable. There is an associated cleft palate corresponding to the synechial margin. Surgical treatment consists of peripheral freeing and suturing of the raw mucous membrane margins of the palate and tongue. Repair of the cleft palate is deferred until the usual age of 12-14 months.[34,62]

CYSTS

Ranula is a term descriptive of a cyst of the sublingual gland (L., *rana*, frog). It may become very large and interfere with respiration in the newborn. It is fully discussed in Chapter 17.

Cysts of the floor of the mouth are rare except for ranula and lymphangioma in its various forms. Dermoid cysts are uncommon and account for only 2% of head and neck dermoids. These usually are found in the midline deep within the substance of the tongue and, as with dermoids in other locations, are often signaled by the presence of a sinus pore on the surface of the tongue at the junction of the middle and anterior thirds in the midline. Treatment consists of midline longitudinal bivalving of the tongue, tracing the stalk to the dermoid cyst which is embedded deeply in the geniohyoid muscle. These lesions are approached intraorally, although they may present as a midline swelling of the suprahyoid region.[46]

LINGUAL THYROID

Thyroid tissue may be situated in the midline of the tongue posteriorly at the site of the foramen caecum, having failed to descend from its embryonic site of origin. Not only may it cause symptoms of dysphagia or respiratory distress, but it may be subject to the vagaries of normally placed thyroid tissue. Hyperthyroidism, adenoma and even carcinoma may occur. The lingual thyroid should be totally excised, and although this can be performed transorally, it is often preferable to work through a lateral pharyngotomy or transhyoid approach.[61] In the majority of cases, no other functioning thyroid tissue is present lower in the neck (negative scan), and total surgical excision may be expected to produce myxedema. This is not a problem, however, for substitution therapy is both inexpensive and completely satisfactory even in a growing child.

TUMORS

Several tumors of the tongue and floor of mouth are characteristic of infancy and childhood.

CYSTIC HYGROMA.—of the floor of the mouth is often associated with cystic hygroma involving the neck in a collar-like fashion. Although histologically benign, such a tumor may kill by virtue of distribution throughout the vital structures of the neck. These growths do not respect tissue planes or anatomic compartments. A child with cystic hygroma may have involvement of the floor of the mouth, neck and parotid region bilaterally, and in addition the mass may extend caudally into the mediastinum. It is common to see hemangiomatous elements mixed with cystic hygroma, usually recognizable by a bluish discoloration of the overlying skin. Spontaneous hemorrhage into such a mass is not uncommon. Potts[42] emphasized that operation is never simple. If involvement of the floor of the mouth is extensive, tracheostomy and gastrostomy may be necessary in the first few days of life as a life-saving procedure (Fig. 18-12). With an extensive hygroma, it is well to limit one's sights to

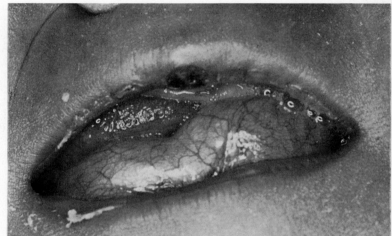

Fig. 18-12.—Cystic hygroma bulging in the floor of the mouth of a 2-day-old infant with a large hygroma encircling the neck. Tracheostomy and feeding gastrostomy were necessary.

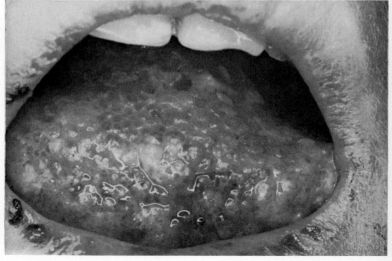

Fig. 18-13.—Diffuse lymphangioma of the tongue of a boy of 10. Note crusting around the lips, indicating poor oral hygiene.

what can be accomplished at a single operation. Thorough cleaning out of a limited area, without injury to such structures as the facial nerve, avoids the necessity for working in that same area subsequently, which is important because reidentification of vital structures may prove difficult. One is never justified in sacrificing important structures which may be surrounded by hygroma, and should be content with removing as much tumor as possible short of injury to important nerves and vessels. Cysts which cannot be safely excised should be opened. Many infants have been needlessly lost by attempts to excise too much hygroma during one procedure. Although it is tempting, it may prove foolhardy. Similarly, an attempt to clean out one entire side of the face and neck in one operation may force the surgeon to hurry unnecessarily, with resultant permanent injury to an important structure.

LYMPHANGIOMA. — is the most common cause of macroglossia in infancy.[4] The tumor may be localized to a small area of the tongue or floor of the mouth, or it may involve these areas diffusely. Characteristically, the gross appearance is that of a raised, firm, mass in the tongue with a warty looking surface composed of many tiny cysts, some of which contain lymph and others blood (Fig. 18-13). Recurring attacks of infection, suppurative glossitis, are common and should be treated with antibiotics. Poor oral hygiene is seen frequently, with gingivitis and dental caries. Bleeding into the oral cavity is not uncommon.

Definitive treatment of diffuse lingual lymphangioma may be very difficult. Radiation may be desirable in cases with diffuse involvement, but in most instances, surgery is the treatment of choice. Radical extirpation is not necessary, since these lesions are never malignant.[36] One should excise sufficient tumor

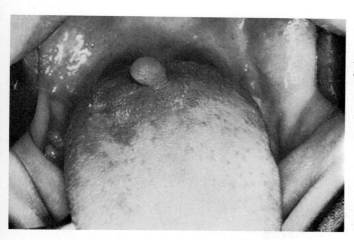

Fig. 18-14. — Benign papilloma of the tongue of a 6-month-old infant, treated by excision.

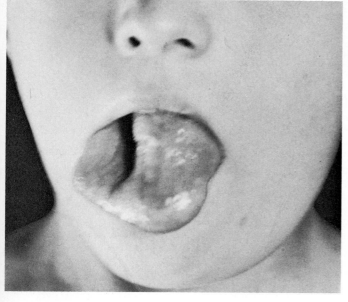

Fig. 18-15. — Plexiform fibroma of the left side of the tongue of a boy of 8. There was no evidence of generalized neurofibromatosis. Treatment was by surgical excision. (Courtesy of Dr. M. M. Ravitch.)

to reduce the bulk of the mass to a reasonable extent, reshaping the tongue to reduce its size and improve speech. This can be done by resection of the tip of the tongue and bilateral marginal V-shaped wedge resection.[47] Surface vesicles are destroyed by electrocoagulation, followed by reepithelization. The size of the tongue may vary from time to time, depending on the degree of lymphatic obstruction and episodes of recurring inflammation. It is often necessary to carry out multiple conservative operative attacks. Several conservative "tailoring procedures" are preferred to widescale definitive excision. Occasionally, one sees a small circumscribed plaque of lymphangioma of the tongue. Surgical excision rids the patient of the annoying mass, intermittent glossitis and considerable worry.

Benign papillomas of the tongue are treated by excision (Fig. 18-14).

Congenital neurofibromatous macroglossia may be seen in childhood, occasionally as a part of generalized neurofibromatosis and in other cases as the only area of involvement.[6] Most cases present with slow-growing hemimacroglossia (Fig. 18-15).

Definitive treatment may be impossible due to the diffuse infiltrative nature of plexiform neurofibroma.[5,43] As in cases of lymphangioma of the tongue, surgical resection is desirable, the goal being to reduce the bulk of the mass and reshape the tongue in such a manner as to improve function. These lesions are not radiosensitive.

Idiopathic macroglossia is occasionally seen with somatic hemihypertrophy. Subtotal glossectomy is required to improve speech. Histologic study shows true hypertrophy of muscle cells and increased stroma. Recurrence has not been observed.

Lesions of the Nasopharynx

A number of surgical conditions arising in the pharynx and nasal cavities are peculiar to childhood. Pharyngeal cutaneous fistula may present with drainage of saliva from a midline cutaneous opening at the level of the hyoid bone. Surgical treatment consists of pursuit of the sinus tract from the level of the skin opening to the pharynx.[59] Schuring[49] reported a spectacular pharyngeal lesion consisting of a completely formed accessory auricle, the lower half presenting just above the epiglottis, with the balance of the ear embedded in the posterior pharyngeal wall. This may have originated from first branchiogenic cleft apparatus between the mandibular and hyoid arches. Elements are usually retained as the Eustachian tube and contribute to the formation of the middle ear. The presence of a completely formed ear in this location more logically relates to the stomadeal plate forming in this bizarre manner.

Nasopharyngeal angiofibroma may be first manifested by a life-threatening bleeding episode both from external loss through the mouth and naries and from flooding of the lungs. Rosen *et al.*[48] have demonstrated the value of bilateral carotid angiography in demonstrating the major source of arterial supply prior to surgery. Treatment consists of peripheral detachment of the palate on one side and elevation of the mucoperiosteal flap, with care to avoid injury to the contralateral palatine vessels. Palatal tissue is adequately nourished from one side. It may be necessary to remove a portion of the hard palate before attacking the extremely vascular tumor. Use of the cryoprobe has been found to have value, freezing the tumor solid and then cutting it away from its bony attachment. This lesion, except for allergic polyps, is the commonest benign tumor of the nasopharynx in childhood but is seldom seen before the age of 7. For this reason, it has been called "juvenile" angiofibroma. Males predominate with sex ratio approximately 4 to 1.[9,33,39] Radiation cannot be given in sufficient dosage to destroy the tumor without damaging ossification centers that are important in adolescence when the nasal feature is determined. Both estrogens and androgens have been shown to have an inhibiting effect on the tumor. Estrogens have been given most often in the postoperative period. With adequate removal of the tumor, palatal healing is usually complete and fistulas are uncommon.

Other solid tumors of the nasopharynx are rare in childhood, although they may arise from the sphenoid bone, maxilla or the soft tissues in this location. A dramatic example encountered in the newborn is nasopharyngeal teratoma. These are often pedunculated and protrude from the mouth as a frightening and often ulcerated, orange-sized mass (epignathi). Sollee[52] reported the successful treatment of one of these tumors in a neonate. Fortunately, they are benign. The simultaneous development of the teratoma and the palate interferes with the proper migration of the lateral halves, so the palate may be moderately cleft or absent. Additional cases in the newborn have been reported by Baugh[8] and Ochsner[37] and their colleagues and by Ehrich,[23] who used the colorful term teratoid parasites of the mouth.

REFERENCES

1. Adatia, A. K.: Burkitt's tumour in the jaws, Brit. D. J., 120:315, 1966.
2. Ahlfeld, F.: Beitrage zur Lehre von den Zwillingen, Arch. Gynäk. 7:210, 1875.
3. Arey, J. B.: Tumors of head and neck, Pediat. Clin. North America 6:2, 1959.
4. Ariel, I. M., and Pack, G. T.: *Cancer and Allied Diseases of Infancy and Childhood* (Boston: Little, Brown & Company, 1960).
5. Arons, M. S., *et al.*: Hemi-facial resection for rare inflammatory diseases of parotid gland: I. Aspergillosis; II. Pseudosarcomatous fasciitis, Am. Surgeon 32:496, 1966.
6. Ayres, W. W.; Delaney, A. J., and Backer, M. H.: Congenital neurofibromatous macroglossia associated in some cases with von Recklinghausen's disease: Case report and review of the literature, Cancer 5:721, 1952.
7. Bardwil, J. M.: Sarcomas of the head and neck, Am. J. Surg. 108:476, 1964.

8. Baugh, C. D., and O'Donoghue, R. F.: Teratoma of tonsil causing respiratory obstruction in newborn, Arch. Dis. Child. 30:396, 1955.
9. Bennett, T. V.: Juvenile angiofibroma of the nasopharynx, Straub Clin. Proc. 32:7, 1966.
10. Blackfield, H. M., and Wilde, N. J.: Lateral facial clefts, Plast. & Reconstruct. Surg. 6:68, 1950.
11. Borello, E. D., and Gorlan, R. J.: Melanotic neuroectodermal tumor of infancy—A neoplasm of neural crest origin, Cancer 19:196, 1966.
12. Braudo, M.: Thrombosis of the internal carotid artery in childhood after injury in region of the soft palate, Brit. M. J. 1:665, 1956.
13. Burkitt, D.: The African lymphoma, J. Roy. Coll. Surgeons Edinburgh 11:170, 1966.
14. Burkitt, D.; Hutt, M. S. R., and Wright, D. H.: The African lymphoma, Cancer 18:399, 1965.
15. Burkitt, D.: Sarcoma involving jaws in African children, Brit. J. Surg. 46:218, 1958.
16. Conway, H., and Docktor, J. P.: Neutralization of color in capillary hemangioma of the face by intradermal injection (tattooing) of permanent pigments, Surg., Gynec. & Obst. 84:866, 1947.
17. Davies, D.: Cavernous hemangioma of the mandible, Plast. & Reconstruct. Surg. 33:5, 1964.
18. Diamond, L. K.: Personal communication.
19. Douglas, B.: Treatment of micrognathia associated with obstruction by plastic procedure, Plast. & Reconstruct. Surg. 1:300, 1946.
20. Douglas, B.: Further report on treatment of micrognathia with obstruction by plastic procedure: Results based on reports from 21 cities, Plast. & Reconstruct. Surg. 5:113, 1950.
21. Duhamel, B.: *Chirurgie de nouveau-né et du nourisson* (Paris: Masson & Cie, 1953), p. 55.
22. Economopoulos, C.: The value of glossopexy in Pierre Robin Syndrome, New England J. Med. 262:1267, 1960.
23. Ehrich, W. E.: Teratoid parasites of mouth, Am. J. Oral Surg. 31:650, 1945.
24. Fogh-Anderson, P., and Sorenson, B.: Electric mouth burns in children, Acta chir. scandinav. 131:214, 1966.
25. Gillies, H., and Millard, R.D.: *The Principles and Art of Plastic Surgery* (Boston: Little, Brown & Company, 1957).
26. Good, T. A.; Carnozzo, S. F., and Good, R. A.: Thrombocytopenia and giant hemangioma in infancy, Arch. Dis. Childhood 90:260, 1955.
27. Gorlin, R. J., and Redman, R. S.: Chromosomal abnormalities and oral anomalies, Am. J. Surg. 108:370, 1964.
28. Kerr, D. A., and Weiss, A. W.: Pigmented ameloblastoma of the mandible, Oral. Surg. 16:1339, 1963.
29. Koop, C. E., and Tewarson, I. P.: Rhabdomyosarcoma of the head and neck in children, Ann. Surg. 160:1, 1963.
30. Körlof, B., and Bergström, R.: Melanotic progonoma of the maxilla, Acta chir. scandinav. 129:292, 1965.
31. Lampe, S., and LaTourette, H. B.: Management of hemangiomas in infants, Pediat. Clin. North America 6:2, 1959.
32. MacCollum, D. W., and Martin, L. W.: Hemangiomas in infancy and childhood, S. Clin. North America, p. 1647, 1956.
33. MacComb, W. S.: Juvenile nasopharyngeal fibroma, Am. J. Surg. 106:754, 1963.
34. Marden, P. M.: The syndrome of ankyloglossia superior, Minnesota Med. 49:1223, 1966.
35. Medenis, R.; Slaughter, D. P., and Barber, T. K.: Melanotic progonoma in childhood, Pediatrics 29:600, 1962.
36. Morfit, H. M.: Lymphangioma of tongue, Arch. Surg. 81:761, 1960.
37. Ochsner, A., and Ayers, W. B.: Case of epignathus, Surgery 30:560, 1951.
38. O'Conor, G. T.; Rappaport, H., and Smith, E.B.: Childhood lymphoma resembling "Burkitt tumor" in the United States, Cancer 18:411, 1965.
39. Osborn, D. A., and Sokolovski, A.: Juvenile nasopharyngeal angiofibroma in a female, Arch. Otolaryng. 82:629, 1965.
40. Pierre, M.: Brulures électriques des lèvres, Ann. chir. plast. 6:21, 1961.
41. Pickett, L. K., and Stark, D. B.: Trauma in and about the mouth in children, Pediat. Clin. North America 3:905, 1956.
42. Potts, W. J.: *The Surgeon and the Child*, (Philadelphia: W. B. Saunders Company, 1959).
43. Rasi, H. B.; Herr, B. S., and Sperer, A. V.: Neurofibromatosis of the tongue, Plast. & Reconstruct. Surg. 35:6, 1965.
44. Richards, L. G.: *Otolaryngology in General Practice* (New York: Macmillan Company, 1939).
45. Richardson, R. J.; Robinson, D. W., and Masters, F. W.: Tumors of the mandible in children, Plast. & Reconstruct. Surg. 23:576, 1959.
46. Rise, E. N.: Dermoid cysts of the tongue and floor of the mouth, Arch. Otolaryng. 80:12, 1964.
47. Robinson, F.: Lymphangioma of the tongue, Brit. J. Plast. Surg. 6:48, 1953.
48. Rosen, L.; Hanafee, W., and Nahum, A.: Nasopharyngeal angiofibroma, an angiographic evaluation, Radiology 86:103, 1966.
49. Schuring, A. G.: Accessory auricle in the nasopharynx, Laryngoscope 74:111, 1964.
50. Sleeper, E. L.: in Cohen, M. (ed.): *Pediatric Dentistry*, (St. Louis: C. V. Mosby Company, 1957).
51. Smith, L. K.: Correction of microstomia, Plast. & Reconstruct. Surg. 14:302, 1954.
52. Sollee, A. N., Jr.: Nasopharyngeal teratoma, Arch. Otolaryng. 82:49, 1965.
53. Soricelli, D. A.; Bell, L., and Alexander, W. A.: Congenital fistulas of the lower lip, Oral Surg. 21:511, 1966.
54. Stobbe, G.D., and Dargeon, H. W.: Embryonal rhabomyosarcoma of the head and neck in children and adolescents, Cancer 3:826, 1950.
55. Stark, S.: Noma or gangrenous stomatitis, Oral. Surg. 9:1076, 1956.
56. Taylor, B. G., and Etheredge, S. N.: Hemangiomas of the mandible and maxilla presenting as surgical emergencies, Am. J. Surg. 108:574, 1964.
57. Thoma, K. H.: *Oral Surgery* (3d ed.; St. Louis: C. V. Mosby Co., 1958).
58. Thomson, H. G.; Juckes, A. W., and Farmer, A. W.: Electric burns of the mouth in children, Plast. & Reconstruct. Surg. 35:466, 1965.
59. Tscheschmedjiev, J., and Chlebarov, S.: Fistula congenita pharyngocutanea, Dermat. Wchnschr. 142:764, 1960.
60. Wang, M. K. H., and Macomber, W. B.: Congenital lip sinuses, Plast. & Reconstruct. Surg. 18:319, 1956.
61. Ward, G. E.; Cantrell, J. R., and Allan, W. B.: Surgical treatment of lingual thyroid, Ann. Surg. 139:536, 1954.
62. Wilson, R. A.; Kliman, M. R., and Haryment, A. F.: Anklyoglossia superior (palato-glossal adhesion in the newborn infant), Pediatrics 31:1051, 1963.

K. J. Welch
W. H. Hendren

resembles lymphosarcoma, yet it most likely is caused by some specific infectious agent. Tumors very like these are now being found in the United States.[14,21] The syndrome includes initial presentation as a jaw or orbital tumor, with a concomitant abdominal tumor.

DIAGNOSIS.—The diagnosis of lymphosarcoma is made on the basis of malignant node involvement with the small lymphocyte series (Fig. 19-7, *B*) together with the exclusion of leukemia by the finding of normal bone marrow, and the exclusion of Hodgkin's disease by the lack of the clinical picture and lack of Sternberg-Reed cells. The lymph nodes may show invasion of the capsule and of blood vessels. The cells seen in the lymph nodes of reticulum cell sarcoma are approximately twice the size of those seen in lymphosarcoma.

CLINICAL PICTURE.—In childhood, this condition may be first manifest in the cervical region in about one third of the cases (Fig. 19-7, *A*). Other involvement will be in the chest, abdomen, bone or other lymph node groups. The disease spreads much more rapidly in childhood than in adult life. If unchecked, a fatal termination may occur within 6 months as opposed to nearly 30 months in the average adult case.

TREATMENT.—A review of the literature reveals a less hopeful attitude toward local treatment of lymphosarcoma in the neck than in the case of Hodgkin's disease. While it is well known that lymphosarcoma occurring in the gastrointestinal tract may at times be excised with a good possibility of cure, the results reported by Slaughter[22] and Rosenberg[19] and their colleagues demonstrate that there is a rare chance of successful surgical excision from the neck. Slaughter reported no success in 11 attempts, although others have reported an occasional 10-year survival.

There are reports of successful palliation of reticulum cell sarcoma with cyclophosamide[9] and with vincristine sulfate.[24]

The surgeon's responsibility lies first in diagnostic biopsy and then in consideration of the disease as a whole. If there appears to be localization in the neck, the patient deserves every attempt at surgical or radiologic eradication of the disease. It is possible that such attempts may be rewarded. Occasionally, it is worth while to attempt to destroy recurrent disease if it is also localized.

METASTASES TO LYMPH NODES FROM CARCINOMA OF THE THYROID

At times, carcinoma of the thyroid is first manifested in children by involvement of cervical lymph nodes. The condition is actually rare in children but increases in frequency until the third decade. Most carcinoma of the thyroid in children is adenocarcinoma. This malignancy is remarkable chiefly for its variation in rate of growth among different patients. In some instances it is rapidly fatal, while in others

(papillary adenomas) there may be extensive metastases to such areas as the lungs or bones and yet the patients may live quite comfortably for as long as 15 years. Treatment of carcinoma of the thyroid is considered in Chapter 20.

REFERENCES

1. Bill, A. H., Jr., *et al.*: Common malignant tumors of infancy and childhood, Pediat. Clin. North America 6:1197, 1959.
2. Burkitt, D., and O'Conor, G. T.: Malignant lymphoma in African children, Cancer 14:258, 1961.
3. Charache, H.: Lymphosarcoma in infancy and childhood, Am. J. Roentgenol. 75:594, 1956.
4. Curry, F. J.: Atypical acid-fast mycobacteria, New England J. Med. 272:415, 1965.
5. Dargeon, H. W.: *Tumors of Childhood* (New York: Paul B. Hoeber, Inc., 1960).
6. Davis, S. D., and Comstock, G. W.: Mycobacterial cervical adenitis in children, J. Pediat. 58:771, 1961.
7. Debré, R., and Job, J. C.: La maladie des griffes de chat, Acta paediat. 43:1, 1954.
8. Gelhorn, A.: Hodgkin's disease: Management with chemotherapeutic agents, J.A.M.A. 191:139, 1965.
9. Hyman, G. A., and Cassileth, P. A.: Efficacy of cyclophosphamide in the management of reticulum cell sarcoma, Cancer 19:1386, 1966.
10. Jones, B., and Klingberg, W. G.: Lymphosarcoma in children, J. Pediat. 63:11, 1963.
11. Kaplan, H. S.: Role of intensive radiotherapy in the management of Hodgkin's disease, Cancer 19:356, 1966.
12. Karnofsky, D. A.: Chemotherapy of Hodgkin's disease, Cancer 19:371, 1966.
13. Lukes, R. J.; Butler, J. J., and Hicks, E. B.: Natural history of Hodgkin's disease as related to its pathologic picture, Cancer 19:317, 1966.
14. O'Conor, G.T.; Rappaport, H., and Smith, E.B.: Childhood lymphoma resembling "Burkitt tumor" in the United States, Cancer 18:411, 1965.
15. Peters, M.V.; Alison, R. E., and Bush, R. S.: Natural history of Hodgkin's disease as related to staging, Cancer 19:308, 1966.
16. Peters, M. V., and Middlemiss, K. C. H.: A study of Hodgkin's disease treated by irradiation, Am. J. Roentgenol. 79:114, 1958.
17. Pitcock, J. A., *et al.*: Hodgkin's disease in children: A clinicopathologic study of 46 cases, Cancer 12:1043, 1959.
18. Pollak, A., and Buhler, V. B.: Fatal atypical acid-fast infection, Am. J. Path. 27:753, 1951.
19. Rosenberg, S. A., *et al.*: Lymphoma in childhood, New England J. Med. 259:505, 1958.
20. Runyon, E. H.: Anonymous mycobacteria in pulmonary disease, M. Clin. North America 43:273, 1959.
21. Sachs, R. L.: Burkitt's tumor (African lymphoma syndrome) in California, Oral Surg. 22:621, 1966.
22. Slaughter, D. P., *et al.*: Surgical management of Hodgkin's disease, Ann. Surg. 148:705, 1958.
23. Smith, D. H., *et al.*: Unclassified mycobacterial infection and disease in children residing in Massachusetts, J. Pediatrics 67:759, 1965.
24. Yount, W. J., and Finkel, H. E.: Treatment of refractory reticulum cell sarcoma with low doses of vincristine sulfate, J.A.M.A. 197:107, 1966.
25. Warwick, W. J., and Good, R. A.: Cat-scratch disease in Minnesota, Am. J. Dis. Child. 100:228, 1960.

A. H. BILL, JR.

20

The Thyroid and The Parathyroids

The Thyroid

HISTORY. — Of all the endocrine glands, the thyroid is the one most commonly affected by pathologic changes in size and function both in children and in adults. Thyroid enlargements are obvious and have long been remarked upon. Incantations against goiter are found in the Hindu *Atharva-Vedu* dating about 2000 B.C. Shakespeare took note of endemic goiter in *The Tempest*: "Who would believe that there were mountaineers dew-lapped like bulls, whose throats had hanging at them wallets of flesh; or that there were such men whose heads stood in their breasts?"

Renaissance artists often portrayed their women with a full smooth goiter at the throat. Cretins appealed to artistic curiosity. Velasquez left a classic depiction of a goitrous cretin, a dwarf of Philip IV, which hangs in the Prado today. A vivid picture of endemic goiter and cretinism was captured by Felix Platter (1536-1614) in his *Praxeus Medicae*, "and in the Carinthia valley called Buntzgerthal, many infants are wont to be afflicted who besides their innate simplemindedness, the head is now and then misformed, the tongue immense and tumid, dumb, a struma often at the throat, they show a deformed appearance and seated in solemn stateliness, staring, and a stick resting between their hands, their bodies twisted variously, their eyes wide apart, they show immoderate laughter and wonder at unknown things."*

The thyroid was described by Galen in his *De Voce* in the 2nd Century A.D., but his descriptions of the gland were vague. No further descriptions of the thyroid appeared until a much fuller and more accurate account was given by Vesalius in 1543 in Book VI of the *Fabrica*.

In *Adenographia*, a treatise dealing with the glands of the human body, published in 1656, Thomas Wharton gave the gland its present name from its fancied resemblance to a shield. Wharton made several guesses as to the function of the gland, but the best remembered, and the most often quoted is, "It contributes much to the rotundity and beauty of the

*Translation by Major, R. H.: *Classic Description of Disease* (3d ed.; Springfield, Ill.: Charles C Thomas, Publisher, 1945).

neck, filling up the vacant spaces round the larynx and making its protruding parts almost to subside and become smooth, particularly in females, to whom for this reason a larger gland has been assigned, which renders their necks more even and beautiful."

1. Goiter

Goiter means simply an enlargement of the thyroid, whether due to neoplasm, inflammation, colloid accumulation or hyperthyroidism. Most commonly the term is used to refer to the compensatory enlargement associated with a relative decrease of thyroxin production and increase of colloid which may arise from a lack of iodine or a number of other defects or deficiencies. The histologic picture in goiters called simple, colloid, endemic, sporadic, congenital, familial, juvenile and pubertal is essentially the same.

PATHOLOGY. — Early in the course of the development of goiter, the gland may show diffuse enlargement and is soft and very vascular. The follicles are small; the colloid often is scanty. The follicular cells are tall and the interfollicular blood vessels prominent. This very early stage of goiter is rarely seen in surgical pathology specimens. At this period, treatment of the deficiency which has resulted in goiter formation will restore the gland to normal. After a time, the changes in the gland become irreversible, and treatment, such as replacement of iodine in a subiodic goiter, results in accumulation of increased amounts of colloid in enlarged follicles, the typical colloid goiter.

If the impairment of thyroxin formation persists, the diffuse enlargement and hyperplasia is replaced by focal areas of hyperfunction scattered through the gland. Microscopically, these areas may be seen as patchy areas of hyperplastic follicles with tall columnar cells, sometimes with the formation of numerous small adenoma-like masses, resulting in a nodular goiter. Often there is considerable fibrosis, and areas of colloid goiter may alternate with areas of hypertrophy and hyperplasia, and minute adenomas which are often poorly defined. Foci of intense activity proceed to hemorrhage followed by central necrosis, fibrosis and sometimes calcification. In some instances, the necrotic nodule may be replaced by a single lake of colloid, or new follicles of varying size may grow in it. The multinodular goiter of the older patient is the end-result of this cycle of hyperplasia and destruction recurring repeatedly, and usually presents a multiphasic pathologic picture, with different stages of the early and late process being represented in sections throughout the gland.[36]

INCIDENCE.—Goiter is more common in females than in males. The incidence among children varies greatly in endemic and in nonendemic goiter areas. In endemic areas, the highest incidence in all age groups is in girls from 12 to 18 and in boys from 9 to 13.[9,10,21] In the endemic areas of the United States, before the use of iodized salt, the thyroid of children commonly became moderately enlarged in early childhood, and by the age of 5, one fourth of the boys and one third or more of the girls presented goiters. In a nonendemic area, advanced goiter in childhood, severe enough to require hospital treatment, is relatively infrequent. Wilkins[39] reported that in a 20-year period at the Pediatric Endocrine Clinic of the Johns Hopkins Hospital, 44 children with goiters were treated. Surveys of children in the general population in nonendemic areas report an incidence of goiter of from 1 to 4%.[9] In 30 years at the Lahey Clinic, 79 children were seen with nontoxic goiters (of whom 22 were proved to have cancer);[1] 58 of the 79 children were girls.

ETIOLOGY.—Compensatory goiter is considered to result from hypertrophy of the thyroid gland in response to a relative lack of thyroxin in the body caused by iodine lack, to goitrogen intake, to stress or to inborn errors of metabolism.[4]

Iodine lack.—The world over, the commonest cause of goiter is iodine lack. The normal requirement for the thyroid is 100–200 μg of iodine per day in the adult, and in childhood and puberty the requirement is probably substantially greater.[24] In a good many parts of the world, the content of soil and water is inadequate to supply the normal needs of the thyroid gland, notoriously in the high mountain regions of the Alps, the Pyrenees, the Himalayas and the Andes. In the United States, before endemic goiter was eradicated by the addition of iodine to table salt as a result of the work of Marine,[20] endemic goiters existed in the Ohio River valley and the Great Lakes region. With the supplementation of iodine intake, the incidence of goiter in children in Ohio fell from 32.3% in 1925 to 4.05% in 1954.[9] When goiter occurs in the presence of adequate iodine intake, other factors must be looked for.

Goitrogens.—A number of naturally occurring substances as well as some drugs are known to block the normal formation of thyroid hormone in the gland, resulting in goiter. Such of these goitrogens as pass through the placenta may cause goiter in the fetus. Iodine excess, curiously, may act to inhibit thyroxin synthesis and thus provoke TSH (thyroid-stimulating hormone) production and thyroid hyperplasia in both children and adults and in the fetus.[6,26] Calcium, fluorine and chloride are other inorganic ions which have been demonstrated to be capable of causing goiter when taken in large amounts. With the exception of calcium, they have not been clinically demonstrated to cause goiter. It is possible that the intake of water with high calcium content in low iodine areas may potentiate iodine lack in the development of goiters.[4,21]

A number of foods are known to contain goitrogens, among them cabbage, rutabaga, rape seed and soybeans.[31,37] Infant feeding formulas derived from soybeans have been reported to cause goiter formation.[31]

An increasing number of drugs and other therapeutic agents are known to cause goiter: thiocyanate, potassium perchlorate, sulfonamides, para-aminosalicylic acid, resorcinol, cobalt,[17] arsenic[30] and BAL (British anti-lewisite),[11] all of which appear to be thyroid blocking agents.[4] With the possible exception of para-aminosalicylic acid, most of them are not likely to be given for a long enough period to produce goiters, except possibly in the fetus. The most commonly known goitrogens are the drugs of the thiourea family in which the thyroid blocking factor is potent and which are therefore used in the treatment of hyperthyroidism. Hyperthyroidism in the mother treated with thiourea drugs may result in goiter in the fetus.

Stress.—Apparently it is possible for the thyroid, while receiving a normal allotment of iodine, to become hyperplastic simply because of excessive demand by the cells for large amounts of thyroxin. This circumstance may occur in children with so-called puberty goiter, a response to the need for extra hormone during this period. Puberty goiter is especially common in girls and may be more frequent and severe where there is a relative deficiency of iodine as well. The increase in size of the thyroid, which occurs repeatedly during the menstrual period in some women, and the stepwise enlargement of goiters in women during repeated pregnancies probably represent a similar response to demand for increased thyroxin formation.

Inborn error of metabolism—This group probably represents the chief cause for the sporadic goiter of nonendemic regions. The etiology of these goiters has been elaborated,[33] and active research continues to unravel the responsible types of deficiency in the formation of thyroxin.

At least five errors of metabolism have been identified, and there are probably many others.[5,13–15] The five specifically identified are: (1) Inability to trap iodide in the thyroid gland[12] (2) Ability to concentrate iodide in the thyroid gland, but inability to oxidize it to iodine[15,33] (3) Normal production of mono- and diiodotyrosine, but inability to convert these substances to thyronines—thought to be due to an impaired coupling enzyme.[15,22] (4) Although all the steps through production of thyroglobulin and its breakdown are believed

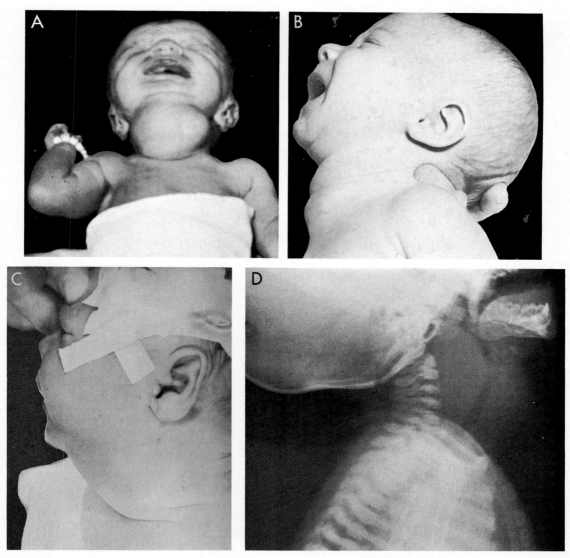

Fig. 20-1.—Congenital goiter: differential diagnosis. **A**, teratoma of thyroid. This infant was born with the huge midline cervical mass causing severe respiratory embarrassment. Diagnosis of congenital goiter was said to have been made and expectant treatment followed. The child died of respiratory obstruction; autopsy revealed teratoma in the position of the thyroid. **B**, hemangioma of neck. A 5-week-old boy, with a swelling present since birth and gradually leading to severe respiratory obstruction. He was admitted in acute distress, with stridor and sternal obstruction. He was intubated without anesthesia, and operation was immediately undertaken for what was thought to be congenital obstructing goiter. An extremely vascular tumor anterior to the thyroid was totally removed; it proved to be a highly cellular hemangioma. Irradiation was given because the tumor seemed to be infiltrating. He was well 12 years later. **C**, congenital obstructing goiter. This infant was referred at 30 hours of age because of increased difficulty in breathing caused by pressure from a large collar-like mass filling the upper neck. He lay on his left side with head in extreme hyperextension. The mother had a history of asthma and took saturated potassium iodide, 24 drops a day. An attempt to treat the child by position and oxygen failed, dyspnea persisted, and cyanosis developed. He was successfully treated by partial excision of the thyroid. (From Packard et al.[25]) **D**, congenital obstructing goiter. Lateral roentgenogram of 2-month-old infant born with a mass in the neck that had recently doubled in size. The mass was large, lobulated, irregular, suggestively cystic, obscured the trachea anteriorly and extended posteriorly to the angle of the mandible. There was marked respiratory difficulty. Subtotal thyroidectomy with removal of the isthmus and portions of the lateral lobes relieved all symptoms. Tumor sections were reported to show a thyroid adenoma of Hürthle cell type. The film shows clearly the large cervical mass and potential airway obstruction from elevation of the base of the tongue and from direct tracheal compression. (Courtesy of Dr. Paul Holinger, Chicago.)

to be normal, iodotyrosine deiodase is deficient: iodine cannot be retrieved from some of the compounds formed in the metabolic chain, and these compounds are excreted from the body with their iodine, thus creating an iodine deficit.[8,34,35] (5) Abnormal release of thyroxin from the thyroid associated with abnormal iodinated polypeptides in the serum.[38]

Clinical features.—Congenital goiter.— The term applies not only to the infant born with goiter but as well to the infant in whom a goiter begins to develop during the first few weeks of life. Congenital goiter (Fig. 20-1), which is very rare in the United States, is common in endemic goiter areas in Europe. According to Aschoff,[3] goiter was present in 50% of all newborn babies in parts of Switzerland as late as 1935, and in Freiberg, Germany, goiter accounted for 10% of the neonatal mortality.

Goiter in the newborn in endemic areas is due mainly to a gross deficiency of maternal iodine intake.[9] In the sporadic goiters of the newborn seen in nonendemic areas, a variety of causes have been observed.[23,24] Iodine intake by the mother, usually as saturated potassium iodide for asthma or as an expectorant, has led to goiter in the infant.[6] Intake of goitrogens by the mother is an increasing cause of neonatal goiter. Cobalt, thiourea drugs and para-aminosalicylic acid given the mother have all led to

goiter in the newborn.[6,18,28] It is likely that prolonged intake of any goitrogen which passes the placental barrier will induce goiter in the fetus.

In most instances, no history of maternal goitrogen intake or iodine lack can be elicited. In normal circumstances, maternal thyroxin crosses the placental barrier in small amounts, and the embryo supplies its own thyroxin from the developing thyroid gland.[7] If a severe error of fetal thyroid metabolism is present, a large goiter may develop in utero. Rarely, a congenital goiter is so large as to cause dystocia at delivery. The head of the fetus cannot flex, and a mental presentation occurs.

Goiter in the newborn due to maternal intake of antithyroid drugs will disappear in 1 or 2 months without treatment. If there is no respiratory obstruction and a valid history of appropriate maternal drug intake is obtained, nothing need be done. Diagnosis of a congenital goiter due to an inborn error of metabolism is based on the negative maternal history and on specialized tests of thyroid function. In these infants, therapy with desiccated thyroid (120–180 mg daily) is important to shrink the goiter and to avoid the complications of hypothyroidism.

Respiratory obstruction with goiter in the neonate, as with any other cervical tumor, is the surgeon's first concern. Stridor, suprasternal, epigastric and

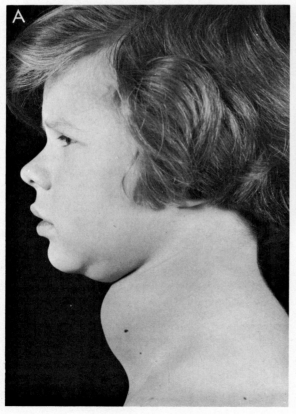

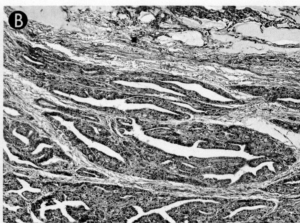

Fig. 20-2.—Sporadic goiter. **A,** this girl of 13 had a history of hypothyroidism diagnosed at age 7 months. Goiter was first noted at age 6. She had taken desiccated thyroid sporadically over this period. Analysis of thyroid function suggested an inborn error of metabolism due to inability to couple iodotyrosines. (From Mosier *et al.*[22]) **B,** the variable microscopic picture is illustrated. Empty follicles lined by cuboidal cells with papillary infoldings are seen in the lower part of the section. Thin-walled follicles lined with flattened cells containing quantities of thin, poorly staining colloid are seen in the upper portion.

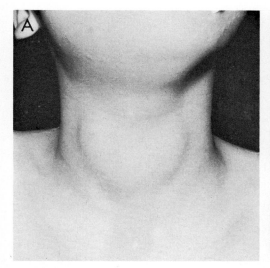
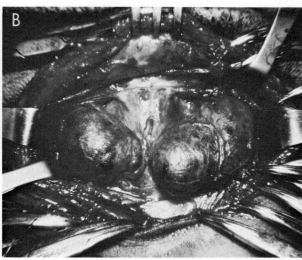

Fig. 20-3. — Colloid goiter. **A**, this 11-year-old girl was euthyroid, but the goiter was nodular and firm, strongly suggesting carcinoma. The mass is clearly visible and symmetrical. There were no palpable lymph nodes. **B**, operative view of bilaterally enlarged gland. Size of the mass and its compression by the strap muscles probably caused the feeling of firmness, because on exposure, the nodules were quite soft. Frozen section revealed colloid goiter, so only a little of the prominent portion was removed from each side. Permanent section confirmed the diagnosis, but areas of normal-appearing thyroid acini were found around a bit of attached ribbon muscle. This was considered to represent a benign phenomenon. After thyroid therapy for a year, the gland was much smaller and firmer but still palpably enlarged, although no longer readily visible.

intercostal retraction and the maintenance of cervical hyperextension characterize the infant with tracheal compression. For some days, an infant with severe respiratory obstruction may appear to compensate for the obstruction, only to grow fatigued and succumb suddenly. Operation should be undertaken if obstruction exists, whether the child "tolerates" it or not. The tracheal intubation is probably the most hazardous moment of the procedure and should be performed without anesthesia. A formal exposure of the thyroid is undertaken and, at a minimum, the isthmus is resected. As Louw[18] has pointed out, the goiter may completely surround the trachea and it may be necessary to perform a bilateral subtotal thyroidectomy. Schifrin and Hurwitt[29] reported an instance of hypothyroidism developing in a child who had had an extensive thyroidectomy for an enormous obstructing goiter. It is worth remembering, however, that goiter may be the presenting symptom in congenital cretins.[19] Tracheostomy for the child with congenital goiter and respiratory obstruction is difficult until the isthmus has been divided and after division, may be unnecessary.

Juvenile goiter. — An enlargement of the thyroid appearing after the neonatal period and before the onset of puberty requires the exercise of substantial clinical discernment. If the gland is nodular, whether the nodule is single or multiple, soft or hard, in addition to the usual tests of thyroid function, an open biopsy should be performed to rule out the possibility of cancer. If the gland is smoothly and diffusely enlarged and not hard, or if biopsy has shown the nodule or nodules to represent colloid goiter (Fig. 20-3), the treatment is with iodine in endemic areas, and with thyroid hormone for children with sporadic goiters presumably due to metabolic thyroid defects. Desiccated thyroid, 120–180 mg daily taken orally, through the familiar suppression of TSH secretion causes suppression of thyroid activity and regression of the goiter. Several months of therapy may be required to bring about a significant decrease in size of the goiter, and occasionally the ultimate size of the goiter may still be such as to justify a thyroidectomy for cosmetic and symptomatic reasons.

Puberty goiter. — Probably the commonest type of goiter encountered in children in endemic areas, it is much more common in girls than in boys and usually regresses spontaneously when the period of adolescence is past. As a rule, the goiter is of small to moderate size, diffuse, soft and asymptomatic. If it becomes quite large, desiccated thyroid, 120–180 mg daily orally, will reduce the size of the gland. Operation should not be required and is likely to result in thyroid insufficiency.

REFERENCES

1. Adams, H. D.: Non-toxic nodular goiter and carcinoma of the thyroid in children 15 years of age and younger, S. Clin. North America 47:601, 1967.
2. Anderson, G. S., and Bird, T.: Congenital iodide goitre in twins, Lancet 2:742, 1961.
3. Aschoff, L.: cited by Clements, *et al.*[9]
4. Berson, S. A.: Pathways of iodine metabolism, Am. J. Med. 20:653, 1956.
5. Blizzard, R. M.: Inherited defects of thyroid hormone syn-

thesis and metabolism, Metabolism 9:232, 1960.

6. Bongiovani, A. M., *et al.*: Sporadic goiter of the newborn, J. Clin. Endocrinol. 16:146, 1956.

7. Carr, E. A., *et al.*: The effect of maternal thyroid function on fetal thyroid function and development, J. Clin. Endocrinol. 19:1, 1959.

8. Chovfoer, J. C.; Kassemaar, A. A. H., and Querido, A.: The syndrome of congenital hypothyroidism with defective dehalogenation of iodotyrosines: Further observations and discussion of the pathophysiology, J. Clin. Endocrinol. 20:983, 1960.

9. Clements, F. W., *et al.: Endemic Goiter* (Geneva: World Health Organization, 1960).

10. Crawford, J. D.: Goiters in childhood, Pediatrics 17:437, 1956.

11. Current, J. V.; Hales, I. B., and Dobyns, B. M.: The effect of 2,3-dimercaptopropanol (BAL) on thyroid function, J. Clin. Endocrinol. 20:13, 1960.

12. Federman, D.; Robbins, J., and Rall, J. E.: Some observations on cretinism and its treatment, New England J. Med. 259:610, 1958.

13. Floyd, J. C., *et al.*: Defective iodination of tyrosine: A cause of nodular goiter? J. Clin. Endocrinol. 20:881, 1960.

14. Fraser, R.: Endocrinology: The thyroid, Ann. Rev. Med. 11:171, 1960.

15. Gardner, J. U., *et al.*: Iodine metabolism in goitrous cretins, J. Clin. Endocrinol. 17:638, 1959.

16. Godwin, I. D.; Newland, C. I., and Folger, J. R.: Congenital goiter, North Carolina M. J. 23:67, 1962.

17. Kriss, J. P.; Carnes, W. H., and Gross, R.T.: Hypothyroidism and thyroid hyperplasia in patients treated with cobalt, J.A.M.A. 157:117, 1955.

18. Louw, J. H.: Congenital goitre, South African M. J. 37:976, 1963.

19. Lowrey, G. H., *et al.*: Early diagnostic criteria of congenital hypothyroidism, Am. J. Dis. Child. 96:131, 1958.

20. Marine, D., and Kimball, O. P.: The prevention of simple goiter in man, J. Lab. & Clin. Med. 3:40, 1917.

21. McGavack, T. H.: *The Thyroid* (St. Louis: C. V. Mosby Company, 1951).

22. Mosier, H. D.; Blizzard, R. M., and Wilkins, L.: Congenital defects in the biosynthesis of thyroid hormone: Report of two cases, Pediatrics 21:248, 1958.

23. Norris, W. J., and Pollock, W. F.: Nodular goiters in children, Am. J. Surg. 90:345, 1955.

24. Oliner, L., *et al.*: Thyroid function studies in children: Normal values of thyroidal I[131] uptake and PBI[131] levels up to age of 18, J. Clin. Endocrinol. 17:61, 1957.

25. Packard, G. B.; Williams, E. T., and Wheelock, S. E.: Congenital obstructing goiter, Surgery 48:422, 1960.

26. Paris, J., *et al.*: Iodide goiter, J. Clin. Endocrinol. 20:57, 1960.

27. Pemberton, J. DeJ., and Black, B. M.: Goiter in children, Surg. 16:5, 756, 1944.

28. Riley, I. D., and Sclare, G.: Thyroid disorders in the newborn, Brit. M. J.: 1:979, 1957.

29. Schifrin, N., and Hurwitt, E.: Hypothyroidism following thyroidectomy for congenital obstructive goiter, J. Pediat. 39:597, 1951.

30. Sharpless, G. R., and Metzger, M.: Arsenic and goiter, J. Nutrition 21:341, 1941.

31. Shepard, T. H., *et al.*: Soybean goiter: Report of 3 cases, New England J. Med. 262:1099, 1960.

32. Southwell, J. and Pollack, W. F.: Recurrent benign nodular goiter in children, Surgery 54:815, 1963.

33. Stanbury, J. B., and Hedge, A. N.: A study of a family of goitrous cretins, J. Clin. Endocrinol. 10:1471, 1950.

34. Stanbury, J. B.; Weijer, J. W. A., and Kassenaar, A. S. H.: The metabolism of iodotyrosines: II. The metabolism of mono- and diiodotyrosines in certain patients with familial goiter, J. Clin. Endocrinol. 16:848, 1956.

35. Stanbury, J. B., *et al.*: The occurrence of mono- and diiodotyrosine in the blood of a patient with congenital goiter, J. Clin. Endocrinol. 15:1216, 1955.

36. Taylor, S.: Physiologic concepts in the genesis and management of nodular goiter, Am. J. Med. 20:698, 1956.

37. Van Wyk, J. J., *et al.*: The effects of soybean products on thyroid function in humans, Pediatrics 24:752, 1960.

38. Whitelow, M. J.; Thomas, S., and Reilly, W. A.: A nongoitrous cretin with a high level of serum PBI and thyroidal I[131] uptake, J. Clin. Endocrinol. 16:983, 1956.

39. Wilkins, L.: *Diagnosis and Treatment of Endocrine Disorders in Childhood and Adolescence* (2d ed.; Springfield, Ill.: Charles C Thomas, Publisher, 1956).

2. Ectopic Thyroid Tissue

LINGUAL AND SUBLINGUAL THYROID GLANDS.—The thyroid derives embryologically from a midline diverticulum in the ventral wall of the pharynx, first noted about the third week of embryonic life, at a point ultimately marked by the foramen caecum at the base of the tongue. This anlage grows downward as a tubular duct descending in the midline and coming to rest in the familiar location, essentially as a paired organ with a midline connecting bar. Two lateral masses of cells which derive from paired out-pouchings of the fourth pharyngeal arch join this midline tissue in its migration but seem not to contribute significantly to the formation of the thyroid gland. If the diverticular character of the tract from the base of the tongue to the region of the thyroid persists, there remains a thyroglossal duct with or without a cyst. Ordinarily in association with such a patent thyroglossal duct sinus, one does not find thyroid tissue (6 of 105 surgical specimens in one series[18]).

Two clinical patterns are associated with maldescent of the thyroid anlage. Lingual thyroid is the result of total failure of migration and presents a solid or cystic mass of varying size at the base of the tongue. If this is large early in childhood or if there is a hemorrhage within it, or cyst formation, respiratory obstruction and death may result. More commonly, the patient complains merely of a lump in the throat and, in most instances, is euthyroid. However, Lucot *et al.*[13] reported on 4 children with clinical hypothyroidism and lingual thyroid tissue demonstrable by scintiscan, in the apparent absence of a palpable mass. In essentially all other reports, the presenting sign has been a mass which was digitally palpable and accessible to inspection through the mouth. In some instances, the mass is large enough and its substance sufficiently characteristic to be identifiable as thyroid tissue through the thinned-out pharyngeal mucosa. Niemann *et al.*[19] report a staggering series of 165 cases of infantile hypothyroidism, of whom 75% were demonstrated to have ectopic thyroid tissue, usually nonpalpable.

SUBHYOID MEDIAN ECTOPIC THYROID.—This presents as a rubbery midline mass at the level of the hyoid or just below it, again in patients who are euthyroid. More often than not, until very recently, these masses have been diagnosed as thyroglossal duct cysts and excised, with belated histologic revelation of their nature and the subsequent development of myxedema in those patients not treated appropriately. The differential diagnosis includes subhyoid median ectopic thyroid, midline cervical dermoid, thyroglossal duct cyst and an occasional enlarged lymph node.

It is of prime importance to realize that in essentially all cases of lingual thyroid and subhyoid median thyroid, there is no other normal thyroid tissue and that removal of the ectopic tissue inevitably results in hypothyroidism. As Ward and his group[17] pointed out, this throws great doubt on the significance of the contribution of the lateral thyroid anlagen to the formation of the thyroid gland. If the diagnosis is suspected, it can be confirmed by scintiscan with I[131], which will both establish the identity of the sublingual or subhyoid mass and indicate the absence of normally placed thyroid tissue.

Treatment.—The indication for treatment in the case of lingual thyroid is the annoying pharyngeal mass, together with the danger of respiratory obstruction from it. There are a number of reports of cancer developing in a lingual thyroid,[1] most in male patients and all in adults.

The only effective treatment for the mass lesion of the lingual thyroid is excision, and since this is generally the patient's only thyroid tissue, excision requires life-long replacement therapy. In at least 1 reported case,[11] a 1.5-cm mass at the base of the tongue in a euthyroid 8-year-old girl with no detectable thyroid tissue in the neck was treated with L-thyroxin and the mass decreased in size. The obvious hazards of a pharyngeal mass of thyroid tissue would argue against this type of therapy. Excision can be done satisfactorily through the mouth for the smaller tumors. Ward's lateral pharyngeal approach would seem to be the most satisfactory for the large tumors.[17]

As with any other lesion of the base of the tongue and epiglottis, postoperative edema may threaten the airway so that a tracheostomy may be required, preferably prophylactically. The mucous membrane over the sublingual thyroid will generally not be separable from it, and direct closure of the pharyngeal wall and floor of the mouth is required. The unpleasant cosmetic appearance of subhyoid median ectopic thyroid is the indication for operative treatment.

Median cervical ectopic thyroid, whether below or above the hyoid, is most satisfactorily treated by splitting the two halves of the thyroid gland, which retain their bilateral arterial supply, so that each half can be placed under its corresponding ribbon muscle, relieving the cosmetic complaint without injuring the gland.[8,9]

PYRAMIDAL LOBE NODULES.—The pyramidal lobe is the last persistence of the thyroid migration, and adenomas and other nodules may form in it as in any other portion of the thyroid. In such instances, however, one will be able to feel the normal thyroid gland at either side, which is not possible with either the lingual or the subhyoid gland.

LATERAL ABERRANT THYROID.—For some 25 years we have been confident that apparently innocent or papillary-looking thyroid tissue and cervical lymph nodes always represented metastases from a carcinoma of the thyroid, occasionally so small as not to be palpable.[3,12] The relatively benign nature and long life history of these tumors led earlier clinicians to mistake these lymph nodes, frequently totally replaced by thyroid tissue, for lateral "rests." In the last few years a number of reports have appeared, discarding the term "lateral aberrant thyroid," abandoned a generation ago, but describing "benign metastasizing thyroid follicles," "thyroid follicle inclusions in cervical lymph nodes," "primary thyroid tumors in cervical lymph nodes," "non-neoplastic thyroid tissue within cervical lymph nodes."[4,14,15] The suggestion, as in the former designation of lateral aberrant thyroid, is that this is non-neoplastic and nonmalignant tissue and has no bearing on prognosis or treatment. A study from the M. D. Anderson Hospital seems extraordinarily apropos and would appear to dispose of this argument.[2] Thyroid carcinoma was found unexpectedly in the thyroid gland or lymph node at autopsy or in the material removed at operation from 22 patients with squamous cell carcinoma of the head or neck or the lung. Twenty of these had mixed papillary and follicular or pure follicular thyroid carcinoma in the thyroid gland or lymph nodes. Carcinoma was demonstrated in the thyroid glands of 15 of the 22 patients, and in the 7 patients in whom no primary carcinoma was demonstrated, only a portion of the thyroid or none of it was removed. Carcinoma was discovered in every case in which the whole thyroid gland was available for study, but this often required serial section. Although the primary tumor might be mixed papillary and follicular, the metastases could be either predominantly papillary or predominantly follicular. The conclusion was: "Any thyroid tissue found in a lymph node represents metastatic cancer." The life history of these tumors is so long that no ordinary follow-up study will resolve the question as to whether or not there may be conditions in which non-neoplastic thyroid is found in the neck outside of the thyroid gland. Block *et al.*[1] found benign thyroid tissue within the carotid sheath in 2 patients in whom total thyroidectomy had failed to disclose any tumor, although serial sections were not made. The occurrence of what appears to be normal thyroid tissue in the strap muscles of children without any apparent relation to tumors of the thyroid[10] has also been reported.

REFERENCES

1. Block, M. A., *et al.*: Does benign thyroid tissue occur in the lateral part of the neck? Am. J. Surg. 112:476, 1966.
2. Butler, J. J., *et al.*: Significance of thyroid tissue in lymph nodes associated with carcinoma of the head, neck or lung, Cancer 20:1, 1967.
3. Clay, R. C., and Blackman, S. S., Jr.: Lateral aberrant thyroid: Metastasis to the lymph nodes from primary carcinoma of the thyroid gland, Arch. Surg. 48:223, 1944.
4. Gerard-Marchant, R.: Thyroid follicle inclusions in cervi-

cal lymph nodes, Arch. Path. 77:633, 1964.

5. Goetsch, E.: Lingual goiter, Ann. Surg. 127:291, 1948.
6. Gricouroff, G.: Primary thyroid tumors in cervical lymph nodes, Acta Unio internat. contra cancrum 20:847, 1964.
7. Grieve, J. A.: A subhyoid median ectopic thyroid, Arch. Dis. Childhood 34:173, 1959.
8. Gross, R. W.: *The Surgery of Infancy and Childhood* (Philadelphia: W. B. Saunders Company, 1953), Chap. 66.
9. Haller, J. A., Jr.; and Williams, G. R.: Isolated midline thyroid in the thyroglossal duct, Surgery 46:437, 1959.
10. Hazard, J. B., and Smith, D. E. (Eds.): *The Thyroid* (Baltimore: Williams & Wilkins Company, 1964) p. 12.
11. Hung, W., *et al.*: Lingual and sublingual thyroid glands in euthyroid children, Pediatrics 38:4, 1966.
12. King, W. L. M., and Pemberton, J. de J.: So-called lateral aberrant thyroid tumors, Surg., Gynec. & Obst. 74:991, 1942.
13. Lucot, H, *et al.*: Quatre cas de thyroides linguales chez l'enfant, décélées à l'occasion d'un retard psycho-motor J. radiol. et électrol. 46:807, 1965.
14. Nicastri, A. D.; Foote, F. W., Jr., and Frazell, E. L.: Benign thyroid inclusions in cervical lymph nodes, J.A.M.A. 194:113, 1965.
15. Roth, L. M.: Inclusions of non-neoplastic thyroid tissue within cervical lymph nodes, Cancer 18:105, 1965.
16. Steffen, H. L.: The ectopic thyroid gland, Am. Surgeon 30:4, 1964.
17. Ward, G. E.; Cantrell, J. R., and Allan, W. B.: The surgical treatment of lingual thyroid, Ann. Surg. 139:536, 1954.
18. Ward, G. E.; Hendricks, J. W., and Chambers, R. G., Thyroglossal tract abnormalities—cysts and fistulas, Surg., Gynec. & Obst. 89:727, 1949.
19. Niemann, N., Pierson, M., Martin, J., and Sapelier, J.: L'ectopie de la thyroïde, cause principale de l'hypothyroïde infantile, Presse méd. 76:659, 1968.

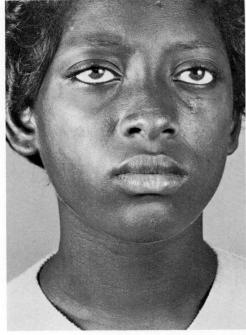

Fig. 20-4.—Hyperthyroidism in a child treated with a thyroid blocking agent. This girl, 14, was first seen with complaint of a mass in the neck, "popping eyes" and sleeplessness for 1 month. The thyroid was symmetrically enlarged. There was mild tremor of the hands. Blood pressure was 125/60, pulse rate 120; PBI was elevated to 13.6 mcg/100 ml and I¹³¹ uptake to 98% in 3 hours. Given perchlorate, 0.5 Gm t.i.d., she became euthyroid in 3 months. Therapy was continued for 24 months, then stopped. She remained euthyroid thereafter. There is still moderate exophthalmos and slight thyroid enlargement. (Courtesy of Dr. R. M. Blizzard, Baltimore.)

3. Hyperthyroidism

INCIDENCE.—Hyperthyroidism is uncommon in childhood. Bram[7] reported that of 1,120 children with goiter, only 7% had hyperthyroidism. He estimated that 2.5% of all cases of hyperthyroidism were found in children. Henoch and Romberg[14] are credited with the first description of hyperthyroidism in a girl of 14, reported in 1851. In 1938, Atkinson[2] was able to collect 208 such cases from the literature. In 1959, Hayles *et al.*[13] reported a total of 253 children treated for hyperthyroidism at the Mayo Clinic between 1908 and 1955, and Saxena, Crawford and Talbot[21] saw 70 cases from 1941 to 1961, accounting for 45% of all goiters seen at the Children's Endocrine and Metabolic Clinic of the Massachusetts General Hospital.

Age and sex.—Hyperthyroidism may occur at any age in childhood but is increasingly common as the preadolescent period approaches (Fig. 20-4). The disease has been described in newborns and in the first few weeks of life in babies born of mothers with one of the several types of thyroid disturbance.[1] About 10% of all reported cases in children occurred between birth and age 5 years, and about two thirds of all cases in childhood are seen between the ages of 10 and 15.[19] There were only 8 male children among Bram's 128 patients. Other series have reported 2 males among 50 patients and 36 males among 253 children.[13,23]

ETIOLOGY.—In adults, hyperthyroidism occurs in two anatomic forms: (1) toxic nodular goiter, the less common of the two, which has not to our knowledge been reported in a child; (2) exophthalmic hyperthyroidism, which presumably is related to pituitary hypersecretion of TSH and takes the same form in children as in adults. The normal depression of pituitary secretion of TSH by increasing levels of thyroxin in the blood is diminished or absent in these patients.

Although it is generally agreed that overstimulation of the thyroid by TSH is a part of the etiology of exophthalmic goiter, it is an oversimplification to assume that the thyroid and pituitary are the only factors in this complex picture. Bioassays of TSH in the blood do not necessarily correlate with the activity of the thyroid gland in hyperthyroidism. Multiple injections of TSH in the experimental animal will not reproduce the whole picture of exophthalmic goiter. In addition, hyperthyroidism has been observed in patients with complete hypophysectomy. It is likely that there are a number of unknown biologic factors operating in this disease.[9,12]

PATHOLOGY.—The acini show increasing height of

the follicle cells with proliferation and hypertrophy of cells leading to an undulating infolding of the epithelium.

In exophthalmic goiter, the follicular colloid, which normally stains deeply, becomes lighter and vacuolated near the periphery or becomes so conspicuously reduced in quantity that it appears frothy. The proliferation and hypertrophy of the follicular cells lead to striking enlargement of the whole gland. A marked increase of vascularity contributes to the gland's increasing size. Lymphocytes are scattered throughout the thyroid parenchyma, and germinal centers may be observed. In some areas of the gland there may be such a dense invasion of lymphocytes that the picture may be confused with struma lymphomatosa. Exophthalmic goiter is an illness which shows cyclic fluctuations, and therefore it is possible to see different degrees of the pathologic picture at different times during the course. Among children, lymphocytic infiltration is found in about 60% of the glands removed.[13]

CLINICAL PICTURE. — No more is known of the etiology of hyperthyroidism in children than of that in adults, but notable is the epidemiologic difference, hyperthyroidism in children being found apparently much more commonly in the United States than in Britain and other European countries. The phenomenon of thyrotoxicosis coming on acutely, shortly after severe stress, is common enough in adults, but possibly more common in children. Saxena and his colleagues[21] reported such a close association in one third of their patients. Six children, for instance, showed evidence of thyrotoxicosis within a few weeks of an automobile accident. Bauer,[5] analyzing 20 instances of hyperthyroidism in children treated at the Children's Hospital, Detroit, found a trigger mechanism in half the cases, varying from acute febrile illness to physical or mental trauma.

The signs and symptoms of hyperthyroidism in children are those seen in adults but with a varying frequency of some of the manifestations. The most common complaint relates to behavioral disturbances. The child is described as nervous, hyperactive, fidgety, fatigable, irritable, emotionally disturbed, doing badly in school. The increase of the size of the thyroid is visible to the parents in at least half of the cases, and increase of appetite is notable. At times, focus on the prominent behavior abnormalities leads to a diagnosis of neurosis or behavioral disorder, and the constant movements have occasionally led to the mistaken diagnosis of chorea. Upwards of three quarters of the children have exophthalmos. A peculiar stare is characteristic, and disappears as the hyperthyroidism is controlled, whereas the exophthalmos takes longer to disappear and may persist. Tachycardia and elevated systolic blood pressure are almost invariable. The gland is soft and diffusely enlarged. Nodular goiter in juvenile hyperthyroidism is rare or nonexistent. A bruit over the thyroid is commonly audible. Sweating, weight loss and tremor are seen in about a third of the patients. Actual cardiac failure is uncommon.

DIAGNOSIS. — Occult hyperthyroidism is not a problem in children, and the diagnosis can be made clinically in almost all instances. Laboratory studies serve as a measure of the effectiveness of therapy. The basal metabolic rate, largely ignored in any case in adults, was never very reliable in children. The chief laboratory tests generally available, and found valuable, are of protein-bound iodine (PBI), butanol-extractable iodine (BEI), the radioactive iodine uptake and the erythrocyte uptake of I[131]-labeled triiodothyronine. Other studies, such as that for LATS (long-acting thyroid stimulator), are still chiefly of investigative interest. In general, these tests are all complementary. The serum PBI level (normal, 3.5–7.5 μg/ml) is significantly elevated in almost every child with thyrotoxicosis and probably serves satisfactorily as a single diagnostic test and measure of response to treatment except in problem cases or in special studies. Both the BEI and PBI tests are invalid in patients who have recently received organic iodine-containing mediums, as for urography. Normal values for both PBI and BEI during the first weeks of infancy are distinctly higher than in adults and remain slightly higher in childhood until adolescence. The thyroid uptake of I[131] (normal, 15–30%) is technically the simplest test and quite satisfactory. In doubtful cases, Werner and Spooner's[25] demonstration that with hyperthyroidism I[131] uptake is not suppressed by exogenous thyroid, offers a useful confirmatory test.

Fig. 20-5. — Hyperthyroidism in a child treated by operation. A boy of 11 had a chief complaint of "nervousness" for 3 years. Enlarged thyroid was noted 9 months before admission. BMR was +43 and cholesterol content 155 mg/100 ml. He was given thiouracil for 6 weeks, then Lugol's solution for 2 weeks, followed by subtotal thyroidectomy. He was discharged the 5th postoperative day. Despite the thiouracil-iodide therapy, the thyroid structure well illustrates the microscopic picture of hyperthyroidism. The follicles are lined with columnar cells, and there is papillary infolding of follicular walls. The colloid shows a lacy lining and vacuolization at the junction with follicular cells.

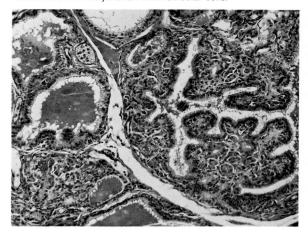

TREATMENT.—Thyroidectomy and the administration of thyroid-blocking agents are at present employed in the treatment of juvenile hyperthyroidism. Radioactive iodine therapy is too hazardous for use in children, apart from the analogy with thyroid cancer developing after external radiation.[8,10,11] Sheline, Lindsay and Bell[22] reported the development of adenomas in 2 of 5 children under age 10 who were treated with radioactive iodine. One of these adenomas was classed as a low-grade carcinoma. Several reports have appeared of carcinoma of the thyroid in patients whose hyperthyroidism had been treated some years earlier with I[131].[17] Nevertheless Saxena and Chapman[20] treated 26 patients under 20 years of age (14 and 15 years) with radio iodine, 100 μg/gm of estimated thyroid tissue: 20 had good control of thyrotoxicosis, 2 poor control, and 4 had recurrence. There were 4 instances of permanent hypothyroidism, and in 1 child, nodules developed in the gland. These workers make a cautious plea for continued use of I[131] therapy. Its chief advantages are simplicity, economy and minimal trauma to the child.

The thyroid-blocking agents such as propylthiouracil and perchlorate can induce a remission but must be taken over a long period of time to establish permanent remission. The Johns Hopkins group[15,26] reported on 33 children treated with thyroid blocking agents. Five failed to respond and ultimately came to operation. Nine were still under therapy at the time of the report. Relapses occurred in 7 (21%) and drug reactions in 4 (17%). Nineteen of the children had achieved what appeared to be a permanent remission of their hyperthyroidism and the drug therapy had been discontinued. The average period required to obtain this remission was 28 months. In Bauer's[5] series of 20 patients treated with propylthiouracil or methimazole, 7 had complete or almost complete remission with treatment durations of 3 years, $3\frac{3}{4}$ years, 6 months, $3\frac{1}{2}$ years, $2\frac{2}{3}$ years and $5\frac{1}{4}$ years. Two were operated on primarily, and 2 because of drug treatment failure, and the others received other drugs with varying effect. The 4 patients operated on had a satisfactory remission and had no relapse after a substantial follow-up; the only complication was mild hypothyroidism in 1. Saxena, Crawford and Talbot,[21] reviewing the reported series of hyperthyroidism in children treated primarily with thiouracils, found a 50% remission rate and a 26% resort to operation. The duration of treatment required was not analyzed, but the individual reports show this to be measured more often in years than in months. In adults, only about half the patients obtain permanent remission from hyperthyroidism under treatment with thyroid-blocking agents, and 2–3% of them will develop skin reactions of significant degree.

Excision of a portion of the gland, bilateral subtotal lobectomy, offers the advantage of prompt solution of the patient's problem. In a substantial number of children it is difficult and at times impossible to maintain constant medical supervision for 2, 3 or more years. There is an ever-present risk of discontinuance of drug therapy with relapse into hyperthyroidism. Proper operative therapy of hyperthyroidism offers a remarkably low incidence of complications. Adequate control of hyperthyroidism in children requires removal of more of the gland than in the adult.

In 95 children with hyperthyroidism treated by subtotal thyroidectomy at the Mayo Clinic between 1934 and 1959, no operative deaths and no laryngeal nerve injuries occurred.[13] Permanent hypoparathyroidism developed in 1 patient. Bacon and Lowrey,[4] from the University of Michigan, reported on 45 children with thyrotoxicosis seen in 20 years. Thirty-three were operated on there, and 2 elsewhere. Only 1 of the 33 was taking thyroid extract. In 1, permanent hypoparathyroidism developed, and 1 developed cord palsy without voice change. Of the 70 patients of Saxena, Crawford and Talbot[21], 52 underwent subtotal thyroidectomy after appropriate preoperative preparation with blocking agents. In 5 patients (10%), hypoparathyroidism did develop. One child with coincident rheumatic heart disease and severe uncontrolled hyperthyroidism operated on in 1947 in an emergency, died 2 days after operation. There were no instances of recurrent laryngeal palsy, thyroid crisis or malignant exophthalmos. Postoperatively in this series, 35% of the 52 children operated on were hypothyroid, although with the increase in length of follow-up, the incidence of hypothyroidism decreased. The reverse is true with I[131]: the longer the follow-up, the higher the incidence of hypothyroidism.

We continue to favor surgical treatment of hyperthyroidism in children after preparation with blocking agents and iodides, although when there are contraindications to operation, the thyroid-blocking agents alone offer an excellent alternative method of therapy. The high incidence of hypoparathyroidism and hypothyroidism after operation in some series is unacceptable and we believe preventable, although possibly at the cost of an occasional recurrence of hyperthyroidism. Ultimately, a nonoperative procedure will prevail, superior to current drugs and operation, but such therapy appears not to be available today.

REFERENCES

1. Adams, D. D.; Lord, J. M., and Stevely, H. A. A.: Congenital thyrotoxicosis, Lancet 2:497, 1964.
2. Atkinson, F. R. B.: Exophthalmic goiter in children, Brit. J. Child. Dis. 35:165, 1938.
3. Arnold, M. B.; Talbot, N. B., and Cope, O.: Concerning the choice of therapy for childhood hyperthyroidism, Pediatrics 21:47, 1958.
4. Bacon, G. E., and Lowrey, G. H.: Experience with surgical treatment of thyrotoxicosis in children, J. Pediat. 67:1, 1965.
5. Bauer, A. R.: Etiology of juvenile hyperthyroidism, Henry Ford Hosp. M. Bull., September, 1961.
6. Beling, U., and Einhorn, J.: Incidence of hypothyroidism and recurrences following I[131], Acta radiol. 56:275, 1961.
7. Bram, I.: Exophthalmic goiter in children: Comments

based on 128 cases in patients 12 and under, Arch. Pediat. 54:419, 1937.

8. Clark, D. E.: Association of irradiation with cancer of the thyroid in children and adolescents, J.A.M.A. 159:1007, 1955.

9. Dobyns, B. M.: Physiologic concepts in the diagnosis and treatment of Graves' disease, Am. J. Med. 20:648, 1956.

10. Doniach, I.: Experimental induction of tumors of the thyroid by radiation, Brit. M. Bull. 14:181, 1958.

11. Duffy, B. J , and Fitzgerald, P. J : Thyroid cancer in childhood and adolescence: Report on 28 cases, Cancer 3:1018, 1950.

12. Gurling, K. J., and Baron, D. N.: Thyroid adenomas and thyrotoxicosis in patients with hypopituitarism following hypophysectomy, J. Clin. Endocrinol. 19:717, 1959.

13. Hayles, A. B., *et al.*: Exophthalmic goiter in children. J. Clin. Endocrinol. 19:138, 1959.

14. Henoch, E., and Romberg, M. H. (1851): Cited by Atkinson.[2]

15. Hung, W.; Wilkins, L., and Blizzard, R.: Medical therapy of thyrotoxicosis in children, Pediatrics 30:17, 1962.

16. Hung, W.: Treatment of hyperthyroidism, Clin. Proc. Child. Hosp., Washington 19:51, 1963.

17. Karlan, M. S.; Pollock, W. F., and Snyder, W. H., Jr.: Carcinoma of the thyroid following treatment of hyperthyroidism with radioactive iodine, California Med. 101:196, 1964.

18. Kunstadter, R. H., and Stein, A. F.: Treatment of hyperthyroidism in children, Am. J. Dis. Child. 76:424, 1948.

19. McClintock, J. C.; Frawley, T. F., and Holden, J. P.: Hyperthyroidism in children: Observations in 50 treated cases including an evaluation of endocrine factors, J. Clin. Endocrinol. 16:62, 1956.

20. Saxena, K. M., and Chapman, E. M.: Proc. 72nd Meet., Am. Pediat. Soc., 1962, abst. 82.

21. Saxena, K. M.; Crawford, J. D., and Talbot, N. B.: Childhood thyrotoxicosis: A long-term perspective, Brit. M. J. 2:1153, 1964.

22. Sheline, G. E.; Lindsay, S., and Bell, H. G.: Occurrence of thyroid nodules in children following I[131] therapy for hyperthyroidism, J. Clin. Endocrinol. 19:127, 1959.

23. Skelton, M. O., and Gans, B.: Congenital thyrotoxicosis, hepatosplenomegaly and jaundice in 2 infants of exophthalmic mothers, Arch. Dis. Childhood 30:460, 1955.

24. Werner, S. C.; Spooner, M., and Hamilton, H.: Further evidence that hyperthyroidism (Graves' disease) is not hyperpituitarism: Effects of triiodothyronine and sodium iodine, J. Clin. Endocrinol. 15:715, 1955.

25. Werner, S. C., and Spooner, M.: A new and simple test for hyperthyroidism employing L-triiodothyronine and the twenty-four hour I[131] uptake method, Bull. New York Acad. Med. 31:137, 1955.

26. Wilkins, L.: *The Diagnosis and Treatment of Endocrine Disorders in Childhood and Adolescence* (3d ed.; Springfield, Ill.: Charles C Thomas, Publisher, 1965).

4. Thyroiditis

Specific thyroiditis is an inflammatory lesion due to an established agent—the organisms of syphilis, tuberculosis or actinomycosis. Until recently, nonspecific thyroiditis has been a wastebasket term applied to inflammatory thyroid lesions without known cause. There is a plethora of synonyms and eponyms—nonsuppurating thyroiditis, granulomatous thyroiditis, Hashimoto's thyroiditis, Riedel's thyroiditis, de Quervain's thyroiditis, giant cell thyroiditis, pseudotuberculous thyroiditis, lymphocytic thyroiditis, struma lymphomatosa. The etiology of some of these conditions is coming to be understood and it is likely that some of these terms will disappear when an etiologic classification can be adopted. For the present, it is useful to continue to use eponyms, and we will discuss the three major forms of nonspecific thyroiditis under the headings of de Quervain's,[7] Hashimoto's[12] and Riedel's[19] thyroiditis.

SPECIFIC THYROIDITIS

Acute bacterial infections of the thyroid gland, uncommon even prior to the days of antibiotics, are today exceedingly rare. Womack[29] pointed out that the thyroid is quite resistant to infection. Injections of pure cultures of staphylococci and streptococci into the superior thyroid artery of dogs rarely induced infection or abscess. When these infections do occur clinically they appear to be chiefly on the basis of hematogenous seeding of the thyroid following acute upper respiratory infections or, accompanying septicemia, from a focus elsewhere in the body. The most common infecting organism is the staphylococcus, but infections due to *Escherichia coli* and the typhoid bacillus (*Salmonella typhosa*) have also been reported.[14]

The clinical picture in acute infective thyroiditis is often dramatic with sudden onset of severe pain in the neck, chills, nausea and headache. The rapid swelling of the gland inside its inelastic capsule tends to induce compression of the trachea with dyspnea and stridor. The gland is extremely tender and stony hard. Pain which radiates to the ear, jaw and face is an early symptom and is almost pathognomonic, occurring in paroxysms and initiated by deglutition. The patient often holds his head acutely flexed. There may be redness of the skin over the area of the gland. The systemic reaction to the infection may be marked to the point of prostration. Necrosis of one or both lobes of the gland, from the increasing pressure within the capsule, has been reported. Suppuration, if undrained, may lead to rupture externally or into the trachea or mediastinum. Symptoms of the milder forms of bacterial thyroiditis and of de Quervain's thyroiditis bear a close resemblance and may only be differentiated by culture and biopsy.

Treatment includes bed rest, hot wet packs to the neck and antibiotics appropriate to the infecting organism. Suppuration is treated by incision.

NONSPECIFIC THYROIDITIS

DE QUERVAIN'S THYROIDITIS.—This form of thyroiditis is known also as subacute nonsuppurative thyroiditis, giant cell thyroiditis, granulomatous thyroiditis, acute nonspecific thyroiditis and pseudotuberculous thyroiditis.

Incidence.—The incidence of de Quervain's thyroiditis is difficult to establish. Of 7,263 patients undergoing thyroidectomy at the University of California Hospital in a 32-year period, 23 patients had this form of thyroiditis.[17] On the other hand, when a clinical rather than pathologic diagnosis is considered, it appears that the disease is thought to be more frequent than the operative figures suggest. The Hitchcock Clinic in New Hampshire reported seeing 2 or 3 patients with de Quervain's thyroiditis each year.[26] The fact is that in the milder forms of this disease symptoms may be mistaken for pharyngitis[10] and may regress spontaneously. Such patients are not usually hospitalized, and in the absence of biopsy, definitive diagnosis has been difficult to establish in the past. The disease appears to be most common in the middle years of life, although instances are noted in children from time to time. Females are much more often afflicted than males.

Etiology.—Despite the microscopic evidence of inflammation and the clinical features of inflammation in patients with de Quervain's thyroiditis, culture of thyroid tissue in these patients has revealed no bacterial organisms. A number of observers have suggested that the disease is of viral etiology, citing the fact that often a number of cases may be recognized within a short span of time in a specific area. Eylan and co-workers[9] suggested that de Quervain's thyroiditis is caused by the mumps virus. They observed a large number of cases of subacute thyroiditis in Israel over a short period in the course of an epidemic of mumps. Ten of 11 patients examined (only 1 child) had positive results of complement fixation tests against mumps virus of substantial degree, compared with only 4 of 52 individuals selected at random from the general population. Culture of biopsies of the thyroid gland of 2 of these patients produced a virus which caused encephalitis in hamsters, and hemagglutination which was prevented by serum from patients who had had mumps.

Pathology.—The thyroid gland usually is not much enlarged but may be adherent to adjacent structures including the trachea and cervical muscles. The muscles and adhering connective tissues are often edematous. Adherence to adjacent structures is often thought of as chiefly characterizing Riedel's thyroiditis but may occur with de Quervain's thyroiditis as well. In the main, the gland is smooth, but occasionally may show bosselations. Varying degrees of fibrous replacement of thyroid parenchyma, often with a fibrous trabeculation, occur interlacing in a red vascular parenchyma. Some segments of parenchyma are circumscribed and appear as small colloid-containing nodules generally measuring less than 1 cm in diameter. Lindsay and Dailey[17] described the evolution of the disease from study of sections taken from patients in varying stages of thyroid involvement. Their view is that the earliest lesion is characterized by loss of epithelium, or single follicles within widely scattered lobules. This is accompanied by localized infiltration of the epithelial layer by many neutrophilic leukocytes. The colloid within the involved follicles gradually disappears and the leukocytes are gradually replaced by monocytes. An invasion of fibroblasts deposits a reticulum of collagen fibers within the follicular spaces. Multinucleated giant cells appear next to the follicular basement membrane and eventually completely occupy the follicular space. Gradually, the giant cells disappear, concomitantly with the appearance of regenerating intrafollicular epithelium. Generally, the inflammatory and proliferative changes within the follicles are accompanied by considerable perifollicular inflammatory reaction characterized by infiltration by lymphocytes and often by numerous eosinophilic leukocytes. Late stages of the disease are characterized by multiple small regenerating follicles embedded in a fibrous stroma.

Clinical features.—In almost every instance the patient complains of a sore throat or occasionally of a painful lump in the throat of several days' to several weeks' duration. As a rule, onset of pain is sudden and may be accompanied by chills and fever. At times restricted to one lobe, the pain may migrate from one side of the gland to the other. Pain on swallowing is often referred to the ears. Examination reveals a swollen, tense and tender thyroid gland. Often the diagnosis may be confused with pharyngitis. Some patients present the symptoms of hyperthyroidism. In the early phases of the disease the PBI level may be considerably elevated, a finding compatible with the symptoms of hyperthyroidism. At the same time, uptake of radioactive iodine by the thyroid will be markedly depressed. This paradox—increased level of thyroid hormone in the serum combined with evidence of depressed function of the thyroid gland—is said to be diagnostic of this form of thyroiditis. Although the PBI level is high, the BEI level has been reported to be low, suggesting that the injured thyroid is producing and spilling into the circulation intermediary products of thyroid hormone metabolism, with depression of thyroxin production.[5,24,25]

Treatment and prognosis.—The disease is self-limiting, and spontaneous resolution ultimately takes place, though symptoms may persist for several weeks or months. Mild forms of the disease may be treated simply with aspirin and restriction of activity. When pain is particularly acute, ACTH and cortisone have consistently led to remission of symptoms. When cortisone is discontinued, the symptoms often recur, so that remission on therapy represents suppression of symptoms. In most instances, the thyroid recovers sufficient function to maintain the patient in a euthyroid state. Most cases of hypothyroidism following de Quervain's thyroiditis have occurred in patients who had subtotal thyroidectomy. Biopsy of the isthmus of the gland may be required to establish the diagnosis. Thyroidectomy is not indicated. In rare instances, the fibrosis and scarring accompanying the disease produce dysphagia, or even dyspnea, which may require subsequent operative therapy.

HASHIMOTO'S THYROIDITIS.—Synonyms of Hashi-

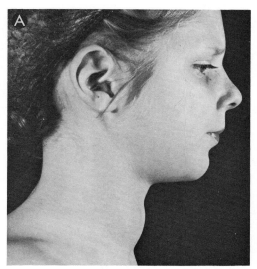

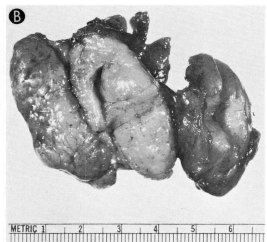

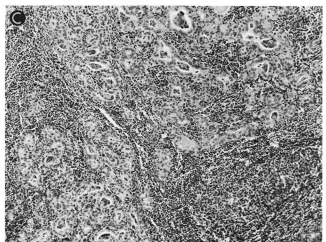

Fig. 20-6. — Hashimoto's thyroiditis. **A,** a girl, 11, with a mass in the neck for a year, was otherwise asymptomatic. The thyroid was enlarged, measuring 11.5×4.5 cm, and soft and fleshy in consistency. The right lobe was somewhat larger than the left. Blood serum was positive for thyroid antibodies on the guinea pig cutaneous sensitivity test. PBI was elevated and BEI depressed. The 24-hour I^{131} uptake was low normal at 17%. An I^{131} scintogram showed equal activity in the two lobes. Clinical diagnosis was Hashimoto's thyroiditis, and operation was elected to confirm the diagnosis. **B,** surgical specimen. Resection of this amount of tissue is unnecessary and only hastens onset of hypothyroidism. The diffuse nature of the glandular involvement is seen, as well as the "fleshy" quality of tissue. Excision of these lesions is temptingly easy because of reduced vascularity and an easily developed plane of dissection. **C,** histologic section, showing marked infiltration by lymphocytes. A germinal center is present in the lower portion of the section. Follicles are small. Follicle epithelium is tall and hyperplastic, a feature characteristic of Hashimoto's disease in young patients.

moto's thyroiditis are struma lymphomatosa, lymphadenoid goiter, and lymphocytic thyroiditis (Fig. 20-6).

Incidence. — This is the most common form of thyroiditis in children.[5,6,11,13] In reported series of patients, mostly adults, undergoing thyroidectomy, from 1 to 7% have been operated on for Hashimoto's disease. Almost exclusively a disease of females, the usual age incidence in adults is in the fourth and fifth decades. There are substantial differences between juvenile lymphocytic thyroiditis and adult Hashimoto's disease. The number of cases discovered in children has increased greatly in recent years; whether they represent an actual increase or greater familiarity in diagnosis is not clear.

Etiology. — The finding of circulatory antibodies

(now at least three) to thyroglobulins by Roitt and Doniach[20] and Witebsky and his colleagues[28] has led to the suggestion that Hashimoto's thyroiditis is due to an autoimmune reaction. Although Witebsky has produced the lesions of Hashimoto's disease in the thyroid of rabbits sensitized to a saline extract of rabbit thyroid, passive transfer to monkeys and dogs of antibody-containing serum has not produced thyroid changes in these animals.[20] It is not established that autoimmunity is the cause of thyroid injury rather than the response to it. Nevertheless the circulating antibodies are so constantly found that the serologic tests for them form an important part of the screening tests for the diagnosis, which ultimately depends on the histologic examination.

Pathology.—Grossly, the gland is symmetrically enlarged, often to a considerable size. The rubbery, firm or hard gland on the cut surface presents a lobular, opaque pale pink appearance. The microscopic appearance of the gland varies somewhat, depending on the stage of the disease. Lymphocytic infiltration, often with the development of intrafollicular germinal centers, is a constant finding.[2,31] Follicles are usually small and colloid is scanty in amount and frequently stains more deeply than usual.[15] Gribetz *et al.*[11] described in 6 patients a variant of this picture which occurs in younger patients, especially preadolescent and adolescent girls. In the glands of these patients, there is hypertrophy of the epithelial cells in addition to the other changes of Hashimoto's thyroiditis. The same changes were observed by Clayton and Johnson[6] in 12 children with Hashimoto's thyroiditis.

Clinical features.—The first symptom noted by the patient is always a swelling of the gland, although occasionally a mild dysphagia calls attention to the condition. There is no history of infection, and the gland is not tender. The gland is diffusely and symmetrically enlarged, firm or, in the later stages, hard enough to suggest the woody feel usually associated with Riedel's thyroiditis.

Laboratory data.—In the early stages of the disease, BMR, I^{131} uptake and PBI level are normal to low normal. As the disease progresses, and with evidence of thyroid failure, the BMR falls, usually associated with a decrease of PBI content and of I^{131} uptake. In the type of lesion that Gribetz described in children, however, there may be an elevated PBI value with a decrease of BEI, suggesting hyperactivity in the gland leading to the production of increased amounts of organic iodides of abnormal form, so that while thyroxin production is falling, the total organic iodine produced is increased. The PBI-BEI discrepancy has come to be recognized as characteristic.[22] These changes in PBI and BEI are also seen in de Quervain's thyroiditis. In children, thyroid I^{131} uptake remains normal or near normal in Hashimoto's thyroiditis, whereas in subacute thyroiditis, I^{131} uptake is depressed. In both conditions, the gland shows little or no response to TSH.[6]

Treatment and prognosis.—The high frequency of thyroid disease in the families of children with chronic lymphocytic thyroiditis, together with the high incidence in these families of apparently well individuals with significant titers of thyroid antibodies, suggests a genetic background. Winter, Eberlein and Bongiovanni,[27] in an interesting study comparing 18 children with acquired hypothyroidism and 33 euthyroid children with chronic lymphocytic thyroiditis (seen in 7 years), found evidence to suggest that both syndromes were variants of the same disease, based largely on the similar PBI-BEI discrepancy. They consider chronic lymphocytic thyroiditis probably the common cause of acquired hypothyroidism in childhood.

The majority of patients with Hashimoto's thyroiditis eventually become hypothyroid. Subtotal thyroidectomy only serves to hasten the appearance of the hypothyroid state.[2] The treatment of choice is administration of desiccated thyroid, continued indefinitely, presumably for life. A number of investigators have reported that under this therapy, the thyroid gland returns to normal or near normal size.[1,18] Operative intervention is designed to obtain thyroid tissue to confirm the diagnosis, to divide the isthmus as prophylaxis against tracheal compression and to perform subtotal thyroidectomy in the occasional patient whose gland is so large and fibrous that its size is not reduced by desiccated thyroid therapy and in whom symptoms or the cosmetic deformity warrants operation. Skillern *et al.*[23] advocated the use of needle biopsy to confirm the diagnosis.

RIEDEL'S THYROIDITIS.—This form of thyroiditis is also known as invasive fibrosing thyroiditis, fibrous thyroiditis and eisenhart struma. Riedel's thyroiditis is rare in children. The general incidence is said to be about 1 for every 2,000 thyroidectomies performed. The disease is commonly encountered in the fourth and fifth decades. Wilkins found only 5 cases described in children. The thyroid is gradually replaced by extensive fibrosis that involves the thyroid and extends to the surrounding structures, the muscles, trachea and carotid sheath. Grossly, the thyroid appears to be white, avascular and woody, and the ribbon muscles may be involved. The parenchyma is replaced by scar tissue in which giant cells are characteristic.

The chief complaint of these patients is of enlargement of the thyroid gland over a period of 3 months to a year without systemic symptoms or pain.

De Quervain's and Hashimoto's strumas are also associated with some fibrosis and firmness but lack the extreme fibrosis of Riedel's struma. Some authors have emphasized the frequency of dysphagia and dyspnea, presumably due to the heavy fibrous envelopment of the trachea and esophagus, but Woolner *et al.*,[30] who reported the largest series on record (20 cases, none in children), found that although these symptoms do occur from time to time, their frequency is perhaps exaggerated. The entire gland may be involved in about a third of the cases, but in many instances, only one lobe or a portion of a lobe is fibrosed.

In patients whose entire gland has been replaced by fibrous tissue, hypothyroidism ensues. But hypothyroidism is not an inevitable sequel of this disease, and many patients may continue to be euthyroid for many years after establishment of the diagnosis. The consistency of the gland in these patients always suggests the possibility of carcinoma. The diagnosis can be made and carcinoma excluded only by biopsy.

The present treatment of choice is resection of the isthmus of the gland, which provides tissue on which to base the diagnosis and releases the trachea from actual or potential encirclement by the fibrotic thyroid.

REFERENCES

1. Astwood, E. B.; Cassidy, C. E., and Aurbach, G. D.: Treatment of goiter and thyroid nodules with thyroid, J. A. M. A. 174:459, 1960.
2. Blake, K. W., and Sturgeon, C. T.: Struma lymphomatosa, Surg., Gynec. & Obst. 97:312, 1953.
3. Blizzard, R. M., and Chandler, R. W.: The history and present concepts of autoimmunization in thyroid disease, J. Pediat. 57:399, 1960.
4. Blizzard, R. M., et al.: Clinical and laboratory response to prolonged cortisone therapy, New England J. Med. 267:1015, 1962.
5. Brown, H., and McGarity, W. C.: Chronic thyroiditis in childhood, J.A.M.A. 171:1182, 1959.
6. Clayton, G. W., and Johnson, C. M.: Struma lymphomatosa in children, J. Pediat. 57:410, 1960.
7. De Quervain, F.: Die akute nichteitrige thyreoiditis, Mitt. Grenzgeb. Med. Chir., supp. 2, p.1, 1904.
8. Doniach, D.; Hudson, R. V., and Roitt, I. M.: Human autoimmune thyroiditis: Clinical study, Brit. M. J. 1:365, 1960.
9. Eylan, E.; Zumcky, R., and Sheba, C.: Mumps virus and subacute thyroiditis, Lancet 1:1063, 1957.
10. Frid, G., and Wijnbladh, H.: Subacute thyroiditis, struma lymphomatosa (Hashimoto's disease) and chronic fibrous invasive goiter (Riedel's disease): A clinical study based on 83 cases, Acta chir. scandinav. 112:170, 1957.
11. Gribetz, D.; Talbot, N. B., and Crawford, J. D.: Goiter due to lymphocytic thyroiditis (Hashimoto's struma): Its occurrence in preadolescent and adolescent girls, New England J. Med. 250:555, 1954.
12. Hashimoto, H.: Zur Kenntniss der Lymphomatosen Veränderung der Schildrüse (Struma Lymphomatosa) Arch. klin. Chir. 97:219, 1912.
13. Hayles, A. B., et al.: Nodular lesions of the thyroid gland in children, J. Clin. Endocrinol. 16:1580, 1957.
14. Hazard, J. B.: Thyroiditis, Am. J. Clin. Path. 25:289 and 399, 1955.
15. Heptinstall, R. H., and Eastcott, H. H. G.: Hashimoto's disease, struma lymphomatosa, Brit. J. Surg. 41:471, 1954.
16. Leboeuf, G. and Ducharme, J. R.: Thyroiditis in children, Pediat. Clin. North America 13:19, 1966.
17. Lindsay, S., and Dailey, M. E.: Granulomatous or giant cell thyroiditis, Surg., Gynec. & Obst. 98:197, 1954.
18. McConahey, W. M., et al.: Effect of desiccated thyroid in lymphocytic (Hashimoto's) thyroiditis, J. Clin. Endocrinol. 19:45, 1959.
19. Riedel, B. M. K. L.: Die chronische zur Bildung eisenharter Tumoren führende Entzündung der Schildrüse, Verhandl. deutsche Gesellsch. Chir. 25:101, 1896.
20. Roitt, I. M., and Doniach, D.: Human autoimmune thyroiditis: Serological studies, Lancet 2:1027, 1958.
21. Roitt, I. M., et al.: Autoantibodies in Hashimoto's disease (lymphadenoid goiter), Lancet 2:820, 1956.
22. Saxena, M., and Crawford, J. D.: Juvenile lymphocytic thyroiditis, Pediatrics 30:917, 1962.
23. Skillern, P. G., et al.: Struma lymphomatosa: Primary thyroid failure with compensatory thyroid enlargement, J. Clin. Endocrinol. 16:35, 1956.
24. Steinberg, F. U. Subacute granulomatous thyroiditis, Ann. Int. Med. 52:1014, 1960.
25. Towerly, B. T.: A study of idiopathic subacute thyroidits, J. Clin. Endocrinol. 16:982, 1956.
26. Vanderlinde, R. J., and Milne, J.: Subacute thyroiditis with special emphasis on the problem of early recognition, J.A.M.A. 173:1799, 1960.
27. Winter, J.; Eberlein, W. R., and Bongiovanni, A. M.: The relationship of juvenile hypothyroidism to chronic lymphocytic thyroiditis, J. Pediat. 69:709, 1966.
28. Witebsky, E., et al.: Chronic thyroiditis and autoimmunization, J.A.M.A. 164:1439, 1957.
29. Womack, N. A.: Thyroiditis, Surgery 16:770, 1944.
30. Woolner, L. B.; McConahey, W., and Beahrs, O. H.: Invasive fibrous thyroiditis (Riedel's struma), J. Clin. Endocrinol. 17:201, 1957.
31. Woolner, L. B.; McConahey, W., and Beahrs, O. H.: Struma lymphomatosa (Hashimoto's thyroiditis) and related thyroidal disorders, J. Clin. Endocrinol. 19:53, 1959.

5. Cancer of the Thyroid

Cancer of the thyroid, once a medical curiosity, has been reported with increasing frequency in recent years. The body over, there are nine sarcomas for every carcinoma reported in surveys of malignancy in childhood, but carcinoma of the thyroid is probably the most common carcinoma found in children. In the area of the head and neck in children, thyroid cancer is challenged in frequency only by cancer of the nasopharynx.

INCIDENCE, AGE AND SEX.—It is estimated that about 4,000 new cases of carcinoma of the thyroid are diagnosed yearly in the United States. About 1 in every 100 of these occurs in a child. Thyroid carcinoma has been reported at every age in childhood but is most common between ages 10 and 14 years. The ratio of females to males is 3 to 1.

PREDISPOSING FACTORS.—Although the etiology of thyroid carcinoma, as of all carcinomas, remains unknown, there appear to be two predisposing factors. The first is goiter, and the evidence for it is chiefly statistical. It is known that the incidence of carcinoma of the thyroid is greater in areas of endemic goiter than in nonendemic areas.[1] Furthermore, since the introduction of iodized salt, the incidence of thyroid carcinoma has tended to decrease from previous levels in endemic areas, whereas it has remained unchanged in nonendemic areas.[3]

The second predisposing factor is especially pertinent to children, and that is exposure of the neck to ionizing radiation during infancy and childhood. This relationship was originally suggested by Duffy and Fitzgerald[5] in 1950. They noted that 10% of 28 children with carcinoma of the thyroid had received prior radiation therapy to the cervical area. Subsequent studies have repeatedly confirmed this observation.[2] Crile[4] found that 11 of 18 children with thyroid carcinoma had received cervical irradiation. Hayles and co-workers[7] observed that of 59 children with thyroid carcinoma, 30 had had such irradiation. In 1951, Horn and Ravdin,[8] reporting from the University of Pennsylvania on 22 patients with thyroid cancer under age 25, found no note in their histories of previous irradiation. Subsequent specific inquiry yielded the information that at least 50% had, in fact, received thymic irradiation in infancy.[12] Hagler *et al.*[6] found that of 19 children operated on for thyroid nodules (15 cancers and 4 adenomas), 18 had received therapeutic irradiation 5–17 years earlier.

Most of these children had been irradiated because of supposed thymic enlargement. Simpson and colleagues[14,15] studied a series of 1,722 children treated with x-rays for thymic enlargement from 1926 to 1951; 1,400 were traced, of whom 67 were dead of all causes. Seven of these children had leukemia, 6 thyroid cancer, and 4 had developed other cancers. In addition, 9 of the traced children had thyroid adenomas. A control group of 1,795 children was also traced. In this group there had been 56 deaths from all causes. None of the children had developed leukemia, none had thyroid cancer, and only 1 thyroid adenoma was found. The radiation exposure of the thyroid in some of the instances was estimated as low as 50 r. It has been concluded that the thyroid in children is peculiarly susceptible to such x-ray exposure. Certainly, unnecessary irradiation of the necks of children should be avoided.

PATHOLOGY.—The major classifications of carcinoma of the thyroid are papillary, follicular, solid and anaplastic (Table 20-1). While true papillary and true follicular tumors are seen, many tumors contain both papillary and follicular elements and are sometimes reported as follicular-papillary or papillary-follicular, depending on the predominating type. In an extensive search for both published and unpublished cases of carcinoma of the thyroid in Europe and America, Winship and Chase[17] collected 285 cases (now 800 cases[9]). Of the lesions observed, 85% were papillary or follicular, or contained both elements; 15% of the lesions seen were undifferentiated carcinoma.

CLINICAL FEATURES.—The classic clinical picture

in a child with thyroid carcinoma is that of a preadolescent girl who presents herself with an asymptomatic nodule in one lobe of the thyroid, the existence of which has been known for months or years. Examination frequently reveals enlarged cervical nodes associated with the lesion, and not infrequently the enlargement of the cervical nodes is the presenting complaint rather than the lesion in the thyroid itself. The incidence of cervical metastases, when these patients are first seen, has been reported to be as high as 70%, this incidence being somewhat higher in children than in adults. Usually the involved cervical nodes are movable, smoothly rounded, nontender and discrete. Matting or fixation is uncommon and is seen only late in the course of the disease. The lesion of the thyroid gland itself is firm to rock-hard, and irregular. Occasionally, the gland is diffusely involved, but a mass in one or the other lobe is more characteristic. A nodule in the thyroid of a child is much more likely to be malignant than a nodule in the thyroid of an adult and calls for immediate operative diagnosis. The histories of these patients are marked by repeated delays because of disbelief that a malignancy is possible. If a nodule in the thyroid is found to be of functioning tissue, on I[131] scintigram, it is less likely to be carcinoma, but the incidence of neoplasms in thyroid nodules in children is so high that operation must still be done. Pulmonary metastases are often present in well-appearing children and do not necessarily contraindicate resection of the primary tumor (Fig. 20-7).

LABORATORY DATA.—These children are almost always euthyroid. Laboratory studies are of little value in the diagnosis.

TREATMENT.—While it is agreed that excision is the most effective treatment available for these lesions, controversy prevails concerning the type of excision to be employed. Operations advised have ranged from thyroid lobectomy alone for lesions without cervical metastases; to total thyroidectomy; to lobectomy plus prophylactic radical neck dissection on the ipsilateral side; to total thyoidectomy plus radical neck dissection. Some have advised the resection of cervical lymph nodes along the jugular chain on a prophylactic basis, while others would avoid all prophylactic operations and would treat cervical nodes when they appear. Even in this instance there is disagreement as to whether a radical neck dissection should be performed or whether only the lymph nodes in the jugular chain and in the bed of the thyroid should be resected. The extremely slow course of this disease makes proper evaluation of the various proposed operative procedures quite difficult.

It is our practice to perform thyroid lobectomy with a modified neck dissection on the side of the lesion. Resection of the sternocleidomastoid is not required, and the jugular vein may often be spared. Biopsy of the lesion at the time of operation, and a frozen section, may allow this procedure to be carried out in one stage. Thyroid carcinoma is often difficult to establish

---

TABLE 20-1.—CLASSIFICATION OF CARCINOMA
OF THE THYROID*

1. Papillary
    a) Predominantly papillary
    b) Mixed papillary and follicular
    c) Predominantly follicular
2. Follicular
    a) Encapsulated
    b) Invasive
3. Solid with amyloid stroma
4. Anaplastic—spindle cell, giant cell, etc.
5. Lymphosarcoma
6. Rare types

*Recommended by the American Goiter Association, 1959.

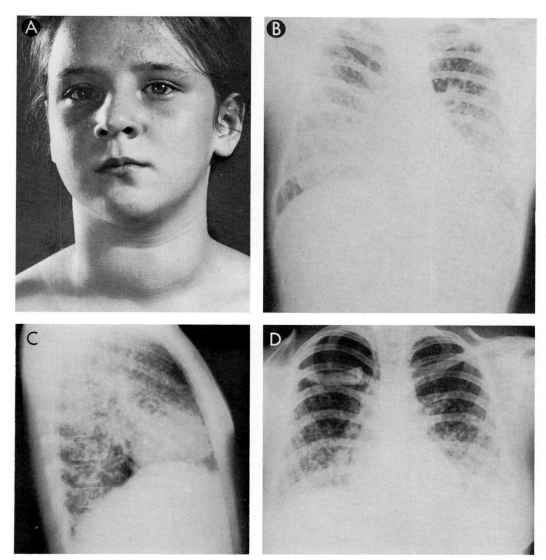

Fig. 20-7.—Juvenile thyroid carcinoma with pulmonary metastases and 16-year survival. **A,** the patient, aged 11, had had a gradually increasing mass in the neck for 4 years and wheezing respiration on exertion and slight dysphagia for 6 months. She had a history of irradiation to the upper anterior chest at 3 weeks of age for an "enlarged thymus." **B** and **C,** chest films on admission showed extensive bilateral infiltration of lung parenchyma by miliary metastases. On Nov. 6, 1947, most of the thyroid was excised. The carotid arteries were encased by tumor and some malignant tissue was left in these areas. She subsequently received large amounts of radioiodine to a total of 1,297 mc between 1948 and 1953. **D,** chest film 2 years later shows the considerable clearing of miliary infiltration of the lungs following I[131] therapy. Apical emphysema is present. The lung lesions picked up I[131] avidly, as demonstrated on scintograms, proving that they were indeed metastatic. The last course of I[131] was in 1953. Later, severe pulmonary fibrosis developed, and she died of respiratory insufficiency in 1963. *(Continued.)*

definitely on frozen section examination, and the dissection may have to be done at a second operation, following confirmation of the diagnosis on examination of the permanent sections. Prophylactic neck dissection is advised since the incidence of positive nodes found in such sections is well over 50% in adults and may be even higher in children.

Sometimes at operation it is found that total excision is not feasible because of the involvement of vital structures. In such instances, a resection of the greater part of the thyroid gland will facilitate the subsequent effective use of radioactive iodine therapy. The remarkably long survival of children with papillary or mixed papillary-follicular carcinoma,

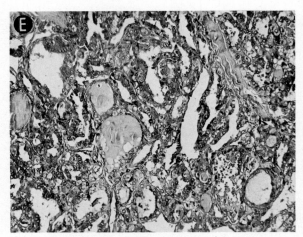

Fig. 20-7 (cont.).—E, microscopic details, showing this to be a moderately undifferentiated follicular carcinoma. The tumor cells are seen to produce considerable amounts of colloid, explaining the effectiveness of I[131] therapy in this patient. Her course was more characteristic of papillary carcinoma than of carcinomas of this type.

even when all cancer could not be removed, suggests caution in applying operative procedures that require tracheal resection and invite laryngeal palsy or hypoparathyroidism. We have 1 patient alive 20 years after incomplete removal of tracheal invasion, and similar cases have been reported.[9,16]

Follicular tumors are the most likely to take up radioactive iodine, and about 3 of every 4 such tumors will do so. Papillary tumors are much less likely to take up iodine, but about 1 out of 4 can be expected to take up some iodine. The very effectiveness of I[131] in the case of pulmonary metastases may be the patient's undoing. If the isotope is taken up by metastases widely dispersed through the lung, destruction of the tumor may be followed by pulmonary fibrosis and progressive pulmonary insufficiency. Since a normal thyroid usually will absorb iodine more rapidly than cancerous tissues, the normal gland must first be eradicated to avoid competition with the carcinoma for the available radioiodine. If the thyroid gland is not excised, its function can be abolished by an initial large dose of I[131]. Residual malignant tissue which does not take up I[131] can sometimes be made to do so by the administration of TSH.[10] In those glands which cannot be resected, and which will not take up radioiodine, external irradiation may offer some palliative aid.[3] In our own experience and that of others, the fate of patients treated 15 and 20 years ago suggests that postoperative irradiation for incompletely removed papillary cancers, recently unpopular, is in fact beneficial and should be employed.

Undifferentiated carcinoma of the thyroid in children, as in adults, is highly malignant. The survival after diagnosis is rarely more than a year. Papillary or follicular carcinoma of the thyroid is an indolent malignancy. Patients may carry metastatic lesions in the neck for many years before metastases appear elsewhere and may continue to live with metastases in lungs or bones for a long time. The lungs are the most common distant site for metastases, and pulmonary involvement occurs at some time in about 20% of the patients. Because of the slowness of growth and development of this tumor, it is probable that at least a 20-year follow-up must be carried out before the results of treatment can be definitely established. Very few such figures are available. Hayles *et al.*[7] reported that among 9 children followed for 20 years, there were 6 survivors, a survival rate of 66.7%. At the end of 30 years, only 1 child was surviving of 4 followed. Available evidence suggests that excess TSH may be a factor in the initiation and growth of thyroid carcinoma. In addition to their primary treatment, all patients with thyroid cancer should receive enough oral thyroid therapy daily to suppress the output of TSH by the pituitary.

REFERENCES

1. Buxton, R. W.: Thyroid disease in childhood, South M. J. 50:1175, 1957.
2. Clark, D. E.: Association of irradiation with cancer of the thyroid in children and adolescents, J.A.M.A. 159:1007, 1955.
3. Clements, F. W., *et al.*: *Endemic Goiter* (Geneva: World Health Organization, 1960).
4. Crile, G., Jr.: Carinoma of the thyroid in children, Ann. Surg. 150:959, 1959.
5. Duffy, B. J., and Fitzgerald, P. J.: Thyroid cancer in childhood and adolescence: Report on 28 cases, Cancer 3:1018, 1950.
6. Hagler, S.; Rosenblum, P., and Rosenblum, A.: Carcinoma of the thyroid in children and young adults: Iatrogenic relation to previous irradiation, Pediatrics 38:1, 1966.
7. Hayles, A. B., *et al.*: Management of the child with thyroidal carcinoma, J.A.M.A. 173:21, 1960.
8. Horn, R. C., Jr., and Ravdin, I. S.: Carcinoma of the thyroid gland in youth, J. Clin. Endocrinol. 11:1166, 1951.
9. Klopp, C. T.; Rosvoll, R. V., and Winship, T.: Is destructive surgery ever necessary for treatment of thyroid cancer in children? Ann. Surg. 165:745, 1967.
10. Maloof, F.; Vickery, A. L., and Rapp, B.: An evaluation of various factors influencing the treatment of metastatic thyroid carcinoma with I[131], J. Clin. Endocrinol. 16:1, 1956.
11. Nishiyama, R. H.; Schmidt, R. W., and Batsakis, J. G.: Carcinoma of the thyroid gland in children and adolescents, J.A.M.A. 181:1034, 1962.
12. Raventos, A.; Horn, R. C., Jr., and Ravdin, I. S.: Carcinoma of the thyroid gland in youth: A second look ten years later, J. Clin. Endocrinol. 22:886, 1962.
13. Rickles, J. A.: Carcinoma of the thyroid gland in childhood, Am. J. Surg. 74:8, 1947.
14. Simpson, C. L., and Hempelmann, L. H.: The association of tumors and roentgen ray treatment of the thorax in infancy, Cancer 10:42, 1957.
15. Simpson, C. L.; Hempelmann, L. H., and Fuller, L. M.: Neoplasm in children treated with x-rays in infancy for thymic enlargement, Radiology 64:840, 1955.
16. Tawes, R. L., and deLorimier, A. A.: Thyroid carcinoma during youth, J. Pediat. Surg. 3:210, 1968.
17. Winship, T., and Chase, W. W.: Thyroid carcinoma in children, Surg., Gynec. & Obst. 101:217, 1956.

M. M. RAVITCH
B. F. RUSH, JR.

The Parathyroids

THE CHIEF CONDITION of surgical concern originating in the parathyroid glands in children is primary hyperparathyroidism. Carcinoma of the parathyroid gland has never been reported in childhood.[10]

The first successful removal of a parathyroid adenoma for hyperparathyroidism in an adult was performed by Mandl[9] in 1926. Four years later, Pemberton and Geddie[11] reported successful removal of a parathyroid adenoma in a 14-year-old girl, the first such procedure reported in a child. Wilkins[19] found 10 children with histologically verified primary hyperparathyroidism in the literature between 1930 and 1954. Nolan *et al.,*[10] in a review of the literature to 1960, discovered 22 children in whom primary hyperparathyroidism had been confirmed histologically and added a case of their own. By 1966, the number of reported cases in children had risen to 30.[4]

The incidence of functioning parathyroid adenomas in children is equal in the sexes, in contrast to adults, in whom 70% of the lesions occur in women.[6,21] The youngest reported patient was 3 years old at the time of diagnosis and had had symptoms for at least a year,[5] but most of the lesions are found in late childhood and early adolescence.

The primary cause of these adenomas is unknown, but some of them have been familial. Multiple adenomas are more common in such instances.[7,14,16] Distinction must be made between familial adenoma and hyperplasia, since the latter is often associated with multiple glandular dysplasia, including pheochromocytoma and medullary carcinoma of the thyroid. This spectacular syndrome can be suspected from the presence of neurogenic tumors at the oral commissure and tip of the tongue.[13]

PATHOLOGY. – The first detailed descriptions of the pathologic changes in primary hyperparathyroidism were reported by Castleman and Mallory in 1935.[3] Woolner and associates[21] expanded these details with an account of the pathologic examination of specimens from 140 patients with hyperparathyroidism in 1952. Two basic pathologic states of the parathyroids lead to hyperparathyroidism. One is the parathyroid adenoma, and the other is primary, *wasserhelle* cell hyperplasia of the parathyroid glands.

In gross appearance, the parathyroid adenoma presents a yellowish brown color somewhat darker than the normal parathyroid. The cut surface is typically homogeneous, but formation of cysts or areas of hemorrhage may occur. The lesions vary greatly in size. An adenoma as small as 120 mg can give rise to serious systemic symptoms.[21] The commonest cell in the parathyroid adenoma is the chief cell, but oxyphilic cells and water-clear cells are also seen.

A striking finding and one that is distinctive of primary hyperplasia is the bulk of parathyroid tissue which is found in the neck. All of the parathyroids are involved, and fusion of the upper and lower parathyroids can produce a single irregular mass on either side. On histologic examination, large, clear cells resembling those of hypernephroma with basally oriented nuclei arranged in an alveolar pattern are seen. Primary hyperplasia is easily distinguished from secondary hyperplasia, for the latter condition usually shows a mixture of all cells with a predominance of chief cells.

PHYSIOLOGY. – Parathyroid hormone appears to have two primary sites of action: the mobilization of calcium from bone, and the promotion of renal clearance of phosphorus. Some evidence exists that these two functions may be performed by two independent hormones which may be present in varying concentrations. In any event, in hyperparathyroidism the osteoporosis of bone, cyst formation, calcinosis, soft-tissue calcium deposits, elevated serum calcium and elevated urinary excretion of calcium are all related to the excessive mobilization of calcium from bone. The decreased serum phosphorus and increased urine phosphorus concentrations are a result of increased renal clearance of phosphorus.

The elevated serum calcium also has its own and poorly understood effect on renal function which results in increased excretion of water, sodium, potassium and chloride, with a lowered urinary specific gravity. Apparently this effect is not a simple osmotic diuresis and cannot be prevented by physiologic amounts of Pituitrin.[17]

CLINICAL FEATURES. – The symptoms of primary hyperparathyroidism are diverse and relatively nonspecific early in disease. Characteristically, the disease has long been present prior to establishment of the diagnosis. In the 23 children reported by Nolan, Hayles and Woolner,[10] the average duration of symptoms prior to diagnosis was 19.4 months. The general symptoms of hypercalcemia are weakness, lassitude, myasthenia, fatigue, anorexia, constipation, abdominal distention, polyuria and polydipsia. Skeletal changes may result in bone pain or loss of stature. Renal calculi and renal colic are seen. Eighteen of the 23 children with hyperparathyroidism showed some evidence of skeletal change roentgenologically, including generalized osteoporosis and bone cysts. Six of the 23 children had renal lithiasis. Alopecia and changes in the fingernails have been noted in a few children.[10] Bone changes have been confused with rickets in some children,[6] and the bone pain has been confused with rheumatic fever.[2]

The most dependable roentgenologic evidence of hyperparathyroidism is subperiosteal reabsorption of bone, which is seen most frequently along the margins of the middle phalanges. The next most frequently observed roentgenologic evidence is the disappearance of the lamina dura of the teeth.

In adults, a varied assortment of associated conditions has been noted accompanying hyperparathyroidism. These include hypomagnesemia,[1,8] pancreatitis[2,7] and peptic ulcer. Of these, peptic ulcer[18] and hypomagnesemia[8] have also been reported in children. Acute parathyroid crisis in children has been reported at least twice. Reinfrank and Edwards[12] reported on a 13-year-old girl with emotional and mental change, drowsiness, generalized weakness, anorexia, abdominal pain and tenderness, BUN of 90 mg and serum calcium of 21.8 mg/ml. At operation, a 6-Gm adenoma was removed, with a dramatic response. Stables, *et al.*[15] observed an acute intensification of hyperparathyroidism and hypercalcemic crisis in a boy with renal osteodystrophy. Removal of three hyperplastic parathyroids and part of a fourth relieved the symptoms.

LABORATORY FINDINGS. — Serum calcium is elevated and serum inorganic phosphorus lowered. In children, normal serum phosphorus levels are a little higher than in adults, being 3.5–4.5 mg/100 ml, compared to 3.0–4.0 mg/100 ml.[17] Thus what would appear to be a low normal value in an adult could be below normal for a child.

The normal serum calcium level is the same in children as in adults, ranging from 9 to 10.5 mg/100 ml. Even slight elevations above this may be significant. Serum calcium and phosphorus levels may fluctuate widely during the course of hyperparathyroidism, and at times may be normal so that serial determinations are of importance. Alkaline phosphatase is elevated when skeletal disease is present. Urinary excretion of calcium and phosphate is high and continues to be high, even when the patient is on a low calcium and/or low phosphorus diet.

DIFFERENTIAL DIAGNOSIS. — The lesions of bone may be confused with congenital bone cyst, polyostotic fibrous dysplasia, giant cell tumors and osteogenesis imperfecta, but the serum calcium is normal in these conditions. Metastatic bone lesions of neuroblastoma or other neoplasms may elevate the serum calcium, but serum phosphorus remains normal. Vitamin D intoxication, and idiopathic hypercalcemia of infancy are accompanied by an elevated serum calcium content, but again the phosphorus level is usually normal and calcium balance studies are normal.

Chronic renal failure, which results in retention of phosphorus and rising serum phosphorus, will stimulate the parathyroid glands to produce secondary hyperparathyroidism and can produce an elevation of serum calcium and many of the clinical features seen in primary hyperparathyroidism. Serum phosphorus content is elevated or sometimes normal, but never low in this situation, and this fact provides a clear differential in the diagnosis of secondary and early primary hyperparathyroidism. In the late course of a functioning adenoma, renal calcification and recurrent renal stones may have so damaged the kidneys that serum phosphorus is not cleared adequately and begins to increase. In this instance, differential diagnosis of primary and secondary hyperfunction of the parathyroids may be difficult or impossible on the basis of clinical findings or laboratory tests. Exploration of the neck and biopsy of the parathyroid tissue is the only recourse in this circumstance.

TREATMENT. — The treatment of hyperparathyroidism is excision of the offending tissues. The neck is entered through a transverse cervical incision exposing the thyroid gland. All four parathyroid areas are explored thoroughly in every instance. The finding of one adenoma does not exclude the coexistent presence of one or more other adenomas. Characteristically, in the presence of an adenoma the remaining parathyroids are atrophic and difficult to identify. If, after a thorough search of the neck, an adenoma has not been found, it is possible that the lesion is in the mediastinum. Mediastinal parathyroid adenomas reported in adults have not been found in children.

If all parathyroid tissue is found to be hypertrophied, one can presume that the diagnosis is primary *wasserhelle* cell hyperplasia. The treatment in this instance is the excision of all of the hyperplastic tissue except for 0.5 cm² or so,[3] an amount adequate to maintain normal calcium and phosphorus metabolism postoperatively. The operation entails little risk, and no deaths in children have been reported from the procedure. Postoperatively, a marked drop of urinary calcium and phosphorus excretion is to be expected. The concentration of serum calcium falls rapidly. Patients with marked bone disease may suffer a transient phase of hypocalcemic tetany.

Following an adequate operation, the prognosis is excellent for long-term survival, provided renal damage from calcium deposits and stone formation has not become severe in the course of the disease. In a few instances in adults, one or more additional adenomas have manifested themselves a number of years after operation. Local recurrence has also been reported when the capsule of the adenoma was opened and bits of the tumor spilled into the wound.

REFERENCES

1. Agna, J. W., and Goldsmith, R. E.: Primary hyperparathyroidism associated with hypomagnesemia, New England J. Med. 258:222, 1958.
2. Bogdonoff, M. D., *et al.*: Hyperparathyroidism, Am. J. Med. 21:583, 1956.
3. Castleman, B., and Mallory, T. B.: The pathology of the parathyroid gland in hyperparathyroidism: A study of 25 cases, Am. J. Path. 11:1, 1935.
4. Chaves-Carballo, E., and Hayles, E.: Parathyroid adenoma in children, Am. J. Dis. Child. 112:553, 1966.
5. Crawford, D.J.M.; Stefanelli, J., and Alvarez, A. F.: Three unusual cases of hyperparathyroidism, Brit. J. Surg. 44:193, 1956.
6. DiGeorge, A. M., and Paschkis, K. E.: Some aspects of tumors of the endocrine glands, Pediat. Clin. North America 6:583, 1959.
7. Jackson, C. E.: Hereditary hyperparathyroidism associated with recurrent pancreatitis, Ann. Int. Med. 49:829, 1957.
8. Harmon, M.: Parathyroid adenoma in a child: Report of a case presenting as central nervous system disease and

complicated by magnesium deficiency, Am. J. Dis. Child. 91:313, 1956.

9. Mandl, F.: Klinisches und experimentelles zur Frage de lokalisierten und generalisierten Ostitis fibrosa, Arch. klin. Chir. 143:1, 1926.

10. Nolan, R. B.; Hayles, A. B., and Woolner, L. B.: Adenoma of the parathyroid glands in children, Am. J. Dis. Child. 99:622, 1960.

11. Pemberton, J. DeJ., and Geddie, K. B.: Hyperparathyroidism, Ann. Surg. 92:202, 1930.

12. Reinfrank, R. F., and Edwards, T. L.: Parathyroid crisis in a child, J.A.M.A. 178:468, 1961.

13. Rush, B. F., et al.: Neuroendocrine dysplasia: Operative experiences with a spectacular syndrome, (in press).

14. Shallow, T. A., and Fry, K. E.: Parathyroid adenoma: Occurrence in father and daughter, Surgery 24:1020, 1948.

15. Stables, D. P., et al.: Parathyroidectomy for hypercalcemic-crisis in renal osteodystrophy, Ann. Int. Med. 61:531, 1964.

16. Stevens, L. E.; Bloomer, A., and Castleton, K. B.: Familial hyperparathyroidism, Arch. Surg. 94:524, 1967.

17. Talbot, N. B., et al.: Functional Endocrinology (Cambridge, Mass.: Harvard University Press, 1952).

18. Tsumori, H., et al.: Juvenile hyperparathyroidism in association with peptic ulcer, J. Clin. Endocrinol. 15:1141, 1955.

19. Wilkins, L.: Diagnosis and Treatment of Endocrine Disorders in Childhood and Adolescence (2nd ed.; Springfield, Ill.: Charles C Thomas, Publisher, 1956).

20. Wood, B.S.B.; George, W. H., and Robinson, A. W.: Parathyroid adenoma in a child presenting as rickets, Arch. Dis. Childhood 33:46, 1958.

21. Woolner, L. B.; Keating, F. R., and Black, B. M.: Tumors and hyperplasia of the parathyroid glands: A review of the pathologic findings in 140 cases of primary hyperparathyroidism, Cancer 5:1069, 1952.

M. M. RAVITCH
B. F. RUSH, JR.

21

Cystic Hygroma

HISTORY. — The word hygroma stems from the Greek, and directly translated means "a moist or watery tumor." *Dorland's Medical Dictionary* defines hygroma as "a sac, cyst, or bursa, distended with fluid." If hygroma is given this definition, then the term cystic hygroma is redundant. Redundant or not, the term has the advantage of priority and long usage to describe a specific tumor of the lymphatic system occurring predominantly in the cervical region of infants and children. On pathologic grounds, cystic lymphangioma would be more correct, but it is unlikely that the term cystic hygroma will be supplanted.

Redenbacker[20] in 1828 described a cystic hygroma which he termed a ranula congenita. Adolph Wernher,[28] of Giessen, in a monograph published in 1843, accurately described the gross pathology of the lesion, noted its common location in the neck and its occasional appearance elsewhere in the body, and distinguished it from branchial cleft cysts, tumors of the thyroid and cervical meningocele. While not certain of its origin, he was sure that it was not due to mechanical factors or to "trespasses of the mother" (Fig. 21-1). He also conferred upon the lesion the name cystic hygroma (which had been suggested a year earlier by von Ammon[27]).

In 1872, Koester[15] suggested for the first time the possible derivation of the lesion from the lymphatic system, but a real appreciation of the relation of these tumors to the lymphatics awaited the detailed and meticulous studies of Sabin,[21,24] which she began to report in 1901. Studying pig embryos in Mall's laboratory, she carefully explored the embryology of the lymphatic system. She emphasized the importance of using fresh embryos and remarked that "we are so near the abattoir that the embryos are often brought with the heart still beating."[21]

In 1913, Dowd[7] published from Roosevelt Hospital in New York an account of 4 patients with cystic hygroma. He incorporated in his paper a collective review which had been prepared by C. E. Farr of all cases reported to that date. In addition, he mentioned exchanging ideas and specimens with McClure[17] of Princeton. From the synthesis of thought of the clinician Dowd and the embryologist McClure, it was proposed that cystic hygromas arose from a sequestration of portions of the "lymph sacs," the growth centers of the primitive lymphatic system.[8] In 1938, Goetsch[11] published a classic account of these tumors. His clinical descriptions and studies of the pathology are still quoted in reviews of the subject.

Embryology of the Lymphatics

According to Sabin,[21,24] the lymphatic system arises from the formation of five primitive lymphatics which she originally called lymph hearts. Sabin stated that these sacs developed from the venous system. Others

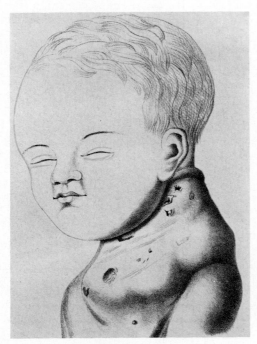

Fig. 21-1.—A neglected, infected and draining cystic hygroma, as illustrated in Wernher's monograph[28] of 1843, the first accurate account of cystic hygroma and its differential diagnosis. The lesion appears to have arisen in the typical location in the posterior triangle of the neck but is so large that most of the neck and a portion of the anterior chest wall are involved. Children with cystic hygroma in Wernher's era usually died when infection occurred, but in some, infection was followed by sloughing of the cyst lining and spontaneous resolution.

have proposed that they develop from the coalescence of clefts in the mesenchyme near the veins. In the human embryo of 2 months, the formation of these sacs is complete; they are the paired jugular sacs lateral to the jugular vein, an unpaired retroperitoneal sac at the root of the mesentery, and paired posterior sacs in relation to the sciatic veins (Fig. 21-2). Outbuddings from these lymph sacs propagate centrifugally to form the peripheral lymphatic system. The head, neck and arms receive a plexus of lymphatics from the jugular sacs. The hip, back and legs are invaded by lymphatics from the posterior sacs, and the mesentery receives its lymphatics from the retroperitoneal sac (Fig. 21-2).

Secondary lymphatic structures developing with or shortly after the development of the primary sacs are the cysterna chyli, the thoracic duct and the subclavian lymph sacs. As is demonstrated by their development, these primitive lymphatic sacs possess a considerable potential for growth. It is believed that cystic hygromas develop from portions of these sacs sequestered from the primary sacs during embryonic life. With a few exceptions, cystic hygromas occur in the area of the primitive sacs. By far the commonest site of formation of cystic hygroma is in the neck, in the area adjacent to the primitive jugular lymphatic sac—the first of these sacs to form and by far the largest. All sacs are formed by the eighth week.

Natural History

Cystic hygromas occur with equal frequency in males and females, and in colored and white chil-

Fig. 21-2.—Lymphatic system in the 30-mm human embryo (about 8 weeks). The major and minor lymphatic sacs are fully developed, and superficial lymphatics are developing from them to spread to the periphery. Prominence of the jugular lymphatic sac in the neck is readily seen. The thoracic duct and cisterna chyli are also present. Sequestration of tissue from any of these structures at this period of development leads to later formation of a cystic hygroma (Sabin[24]).

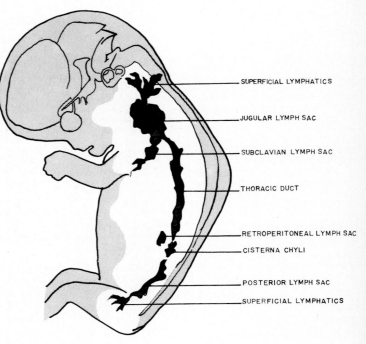

SUPERFICIAL LYMPHATICS

JUGULAR LYMPH SAC

SUBCLAVIAN LYMPH SAC

THORACIC DUCT

RETROPERITONEAL LYMPH SAC

CISTERNA CHYLI

POSTERIOR LYMPH SAC

SUPERFICIAL LYMPHATICS

dren. They are not common tumors. Anderson[1] reported 20 hygromas among 758 benign tumors seen in a children's hospital in a period of 15 years.

The lesion commonly appears quite early, often being observed at birth, and there are reports on record of dystocia at delivery due to the presence of cystic hygromas too large to pass through the birth canal. Fifty to 60% of the lesions reported in the literature appeared before the end of the first year of life, and 80–90% appeared before the end of the second year.[4,12]

Cystic hygromas have been reported in adults, although rarely. We have seen a cystic hygroma in the neck of a woman of 48, and Galofré et al.[10] reported on 8 patients past 50.

Often these lesions become manifest rather suddenly and grow quite rapidly. Growth may then stop for a period, to be followed by another episode of enlargement. Gross[12] remarked that a period of enlargement may be preceded by an upper respiratory infection.

Occasionally, cystic hygromas will partially or completely regress spontaneously, either following infection or at times without apparent cause. This is far too uncommon a happenstance to warrant any delay in treatment in the hope that spontaneous regression will occur. Immediate excision is recommended.

Pathology

There has been much division of opinion as to whether or not lymphangiomas represent true neoplasms. Lymphangiosarcoma itself is very rare, and a sarcoma arising from a previous lymphangioma has, to our knowledge, never been reported.

Nicholson,[18] speaking of angiomas in general, remarked that "angiomata are typical hamartomata, a class of borderline cases between malformations and tumors." Goetsch,[11] in his very careful studies of the pathology of cystic hygroma, pointed out small processes at the fringes of these lesions which he felt represented formation of new tissue by the hygroma. On the other hand, Willis[29] took the view that cystic hygroma represents sequestration of embryonic tissue with no growth potential in the sense that new tissue is formed. He stated: "in my opinion, however, fluid accumulation, the progressive formation of collateral channels and, in some cases, supervening thrombosis and organization, suffice to account for the growth of hygromas. The mingling of lymphatic channels and cysts with the involved tissue is not a proliferative invasive process, but merely a necessary feature of vascular malformation, comparable with that seen in hemangiomas." Landing and Farber[16] classified lymphangiomas as: (1) lymphangioma simplex – made up of many small lymphatic capillaries; (2) cavernous lymphangioma – made up of larger lymphatic channels, and (3) cystic lymphangioma – corresponding to cystic hygroma. They also noted that there is considerable mixing and overlapping since cavernous lymphangiomas may contain many capillary elements, and cystic lymphangiomas may contain both cavernous and capillary elements. They suggest that all these lesions be lumped under the simple term "lymphangioma." The point at which the lesion is too large to be classed as cavernous or too small to be called cystic cannot be defined, and in our opinion the position of the lesion in relation to the original lymphatic centers is as important in distinguishing the cystic hygroma as is its microscopic appearance.

Grossly, these lesions are multilobular, multilocular cystic masses composed of many individual cysts that vary from 1 mm to 5 cm or more in diameter. The locules may or may not communicate. If there has been no infection, the walls are thin and delicate. The cysts are filled with a serous fluid which may be clear to slightly yellow in color and occasionally blood-stained. The mass is often associated with groups of enlarged lymph glands. The lining of the cyst is a thin pearly or gray glistening and almost transparent membrane resembling peritoneum or pleura. In the dissection at operation, it is usually found that the mass is less discrete than anticipated, that sheets and tongues of edematous tissue leaking yellow fluid and at times containing small cysts pass in all directions from the periphery in fascial planes, around and between nerve trunks and vessels. The larger cysts intercommunicate, and trabeculae are often seen with isolated cords traversing the cystic cavities.

Microscopically, the cyst walls consist of a single layer of flattened endothelium. There may be a moderate amount of fibrous reaction in the surrounding tissue. The cords which pass through some of the cystic cavities are actually muscle fibers, thrombosed blood vessels or bits of fascia, presumably from structures entrapped by the enlarging cysts.

Not infrequently, numerous blood-containing capillaries, sometimes few and small, sometimes many and dilated into cavernous spaces, are seen. These suggest that the defect may not be confined to the lymphatic system but may include the vascular system as well. If vascular elements are prominent, the lesion may be termed a lymphohemangioma.

Clinical Course

Most commonly, the presenting complaint of these patients is of a soft mass in the posterior triangle of the neck (Fig. 21-3). The mass can usually be determined to be fluctuant and lobulated, not attached to the skin and not movable on the deep tissue. It is readily transilluminated, unless the accident of hemorrhage into it occurs, which may make it tense and firm, as well as rendering it opaque. Three quarters of the cystic hygromas seen present in the neck and 20% are observed in the axillary region (Fig. 21-4). The remaining 5% are scattered about the body in the

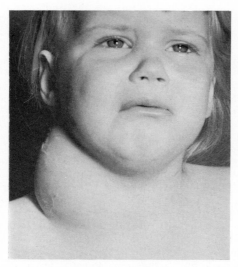

Fig. 21-3.—Cervical cystic hygroma with hemorrhage. A girl, aged 2½, was admitted with a mass in the neck, first noted when she was 15 days old. Originally 2 cm in diameter, the mass gradually increased to 4 cm until 4 days before admission, when she fell and struck the lesion. The mass discolored and rapidly enlarged. The child, previously asymptomatic, developed difficult respirations, especially after exertion, and had to be propped up to sleep. The mass was rather firm but not hard. The clinical impression of cystic hygroma was confirmed at operation, when a large cystic hygroma distended with blood was found. It was adherent to the jugular vein, carotid artery and cutaneous nerves but was fairly well encapsulated, and it could be removed intact and in toto.

mediastinum, retroperitoneal area, pelvis, and groin. The majority of cystic hygromas affecting the neck occur in the posterior triangle, occasionally communicating beneath the clavicle with an axillary hygroma (Fig. 21-5). Some do occur in the anterior triangle and in this location usually appear high in the submandibular region. Often these lesions are associated with intraoral lymphangiomas and are the ones most prone to cause pharyngeal compression and interference with the airway (Fig. 21-6). Cystic hygroma of the parotid region may extend from behind the ear almost to the mouth, and from the jaw line to the eye. These are tumors of the parotid region, not of the gland itself, and are chiefly to be distinguished from large hemangiomas of the same tissues.

Two or 3% of all cervical hygromas are associated with extensions into the mediastinum which in some cases extend to the diaphragm. All patients with cervical cystic hygroma should have a chest film before operation to determine the presence or absence of such mediastinal involvement[6] (Fig. 21-7). Chylothorax and chylopericardium have been complications of cervicomediastinal hygroma.

Except for their visible presence, hygromas usually cause no symptoms. There may be dyspnea and dysphagia and other symptoms indicating compression of the pharynx or structures of the superior thoracic outlet. Rarely, respiratory obstruction had resulted in

death of the child before therapy was instituted. Lymphangiomas of the tongue (Chapter 18) and the floor of the mouth are the most dangerous lesions because of the inherent risk of obstruction to respirations and are the most difficult to treat.

In the preantibiotic era, infection of these cysts was a much-feared complication. Their location adjacent to the drainage areas from the upper respiratory tract presents an easy path for the ingress of infection, and the lymphatic fluid contained in the cavities provides the culture medium. Incision and drainage of the infected cysts usually resulted in a long and debilitating period of lymphatic fluid drainage from the site of incision with maceration of the surrounding skin and continued loss of protein. On the other hand, it sometimes eventuated in destruction of the cyst lining by infection, with ultimate cure.

The location and consistency of the lesion is usually so characteristic that differential diagnosis is not difficult. In addition, this is the lesion of the neck most readily transilluminated. Branchial cleft cysts probably represent the most likely diagnostic alternative. They may usually be differentiated by their preferred location low in the neck along the anterior border of the sternocleidomastoid muscle.

Aspiration of a hygroma yields thin watery fluid that is clear or pale yellow. Aspiration of a branchial cleft cyst yields a thicker fluid. Hamilton Bailey[2] remarked on the constant finding of cholesterol crystals in the aspirate from branchial cleft cysts and believed, as we do, that this is an important distinguishing feature in the diagnosis. Goetsch found that the fluid from cystic hygromas occasionally contained these crystals, though not as frequently.

Fig. 21-4.—Axillary cystic hygroma. A child of 3 months had a 7 × 8 cm mass under the right arm which at birth was about 2 cm in diameter. It was soft and cystic. At operation, the lesion was found to extend under the scapula and clavicle and down the arm for several centimeters. The axillary nerve trunks were involved. All gross tissue was resected. There has been no recurrence.

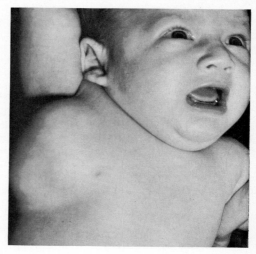

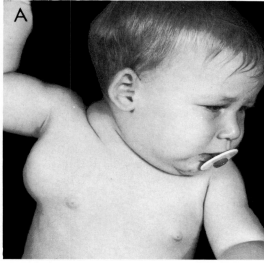

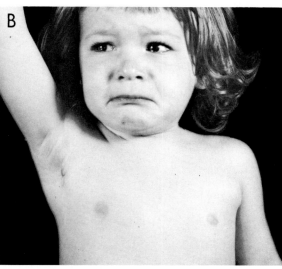

Fig. 21-5.—Cervicoaxillary hygroma recurrent after attempted excision in the neck. **A,** an infant of 9 months immediately before definitive operation, showing the recurrent supraclavicular mass in the posterior cervical triangle and the large communicating axillary hygroma. **B,** 1½ years after operation. Separate incisions were used, transverse in the neck, and in the line of the axillary crease. The pectoral muscle was not divided. There has been no recurrence, and scars are all but imperceptible.

Fig. 21-6.—Cervical cystic hygroma in anterior cervical triangle. Infant at birth had a soft, floppy, cystic mass high in the anterior triangle of the neck, just below the line of the right jaw. In 2½ weeks it had filled rapidly and was now, at age 3 weeks, quite tense. The lesion was excised through a transverse incision; the postoperative course was uneventful.

Fig. 21-7.—Lymphangioma of the neck with mediastinal extension. A boy of 4 years had typical cervical lymphhygroma, with radiologic evidence of a mediastinal mass on the same (left) side. The lesion was completely excised in two operations. There was no recurrence. (Courtesy of the Children's Hospital, Detroit.)

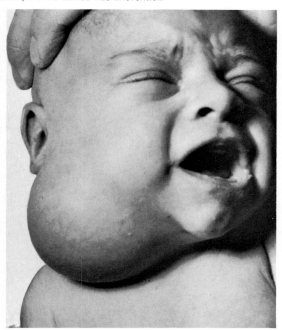

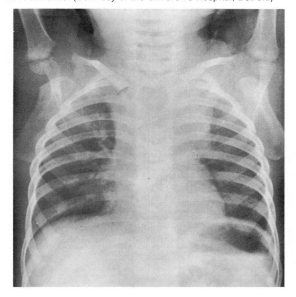

Deep hemangiomas may sometimes present in this location, but they fail to transilluminate, contain blood on aspiration and may be collapsed by constant pressure. Dermoid cysts occur in the neck, may be soft and fluctuant, but are rare in the posterior triangle and are not transilluminated by light. Lipomas occasionally occur in children and may appear to be truly fluctuant, but usually are not transilluminable.

Treatment

Surgical excision is the treatment of choice for these lesions and the only effective treatment available. In an older era, when excision carried great hazards and a mortality of more than 50%,[7,26] many alternative treatments were attempted, including irradiation, incision and drainage, the injection of sclerosing agents and even the injection of boiling water. None of these proved satisfactory.

Because of the hazard of spontaneous infection, of progressive growth leading to substantial disfigurement, with extension into as yet uninvolved areas, and the possibility of dysphagia and suffocation, operative treatment is indicated whenever one of these lesions is encountered. Spontaneous regression is so unlikely as not to be anticipated, whereas increase of size is quite likely, so that operation is certain to have to be performed and delay presents no advantages and some risks. Age is not a contraindication to operation, which should be undertaken just as readily in a newborn as in an older child. The only exception may be the premature infant, in whom operation may await the attainment of normal birth weight.

Cystic hygromas of the neck are best removed through a simple transverse cervical incision under intratracheal anesthesia with a dependable route established for infusion of fluids or blood. Some of the lesions seem fairly well encapsulated and are readily dissected out, but in many instances the lesion is intimately entwined with the structures of the neck, requiring a careful and prolonged dissection to remove the tumor as completely as possible. In some instances, the tumor may closely involve the carotid artery, jugular vein and brachial plexus. Whereas in the removal of other benign cysts it is chiefly the surgeon's pride which suffers if the cyst ruptures, in hygroma, rupture of the cyst may defeat the surgeon. The delicate-walled empty cyst is awkward to handle, the margins difficult to identify.

Axillary hygromas can be approached through incisions in the line of the axillary skin creases. It is not necessary or justifiable to divide the pectoralis major. Adequate exposure in children can almost always be achieved by retraction of the pectoralis.

A special problem occurs if a cervical hygroma extends into the axilla. The infant is draped with that side elevated 15–20 degrees and the arm draped free, the exposed field extending from jaw to nipple and from anterior midline to beyond the posterior axillary line, including the shoulder and upper arm in the field. The cervical portion of the tumor is dissected free above and to either side and dissected off the brachial plexus until the hygroma is seen to pass below the clavicle. The axillary portion is then dissected out through a generous axillary incision and dissection extended up toward the clavicle. By alternate traction and dissection first from above and then from below, the entire specimen is freed and delivered through the passage under the clavicle. A hygroma communicating from the neck into the axilla necessarily has so intimate an attachment to the brachial plexus behind it and to the subclavian vessels in front that a tedious and ticklish dissection is involved.

For a cervical hygroma that extends into the mediastinum, the neck and entire anterior chest are draped out. If the cysts are found in the course of the cervical exploration through a standard transverse incision to extend into the mediastinum beyond reach from above, the incision is carried from its anterior end vertically down the anterior midline and the sternum is split so that the cysts may be removed in continuity. The ipsilateral pleura will almost certainly be simultaneously removed.

Parotid hygromas, so-called, do not involve the gland itself, or no more than its most superficial portion, so that a formal parotidectomy is not required, and there is usually a sharp plane of cleavage between the underside of the hygroma and the superficial surface of the parotid. Incision is made just anterior to the ear as for resection of a parotid tumor (Fig. 21-8 *B*). The facial nerve lies deep to the tumor and should lie bare when the operation is completed (Fig. 21-8 *C* and *D*). The integrity of the nerve must be preserved, but the parents should be warned of the likelihood of temporary paresis after operation.

During dissection of cystic hygromas, particularly those in the neck, any attached structures which suggest lymphatic trunks should be ligated in order to minimize the postoperative accumulation of fluid. If there is any significant accumulation of fluid postoperatively, a small catheter should be inserted into the wound and placed on continuous suction. If the hygroma has been very large, a suction catheter should always be placed at the time of operation, both to handle the fluid which may occur in any large wound and specifically to handle any fluid which may have accumulated from transected lymphatic ducts.

Amputations for extensive lymphangiomas of the arm and shoulder are likely to be in association with an extremely infiltrating lymphangioma which in some cases is surely a mixed hemangioma and lymphangioma.[19]

Cystic hygroma is not a malignant neoplasm and there is no need to sacrifice normal structures in the course of the operation. This is not to be construed as condoning or encouraging a half-hearted attempt at removal. These tumors can and do recur. Neverthe-

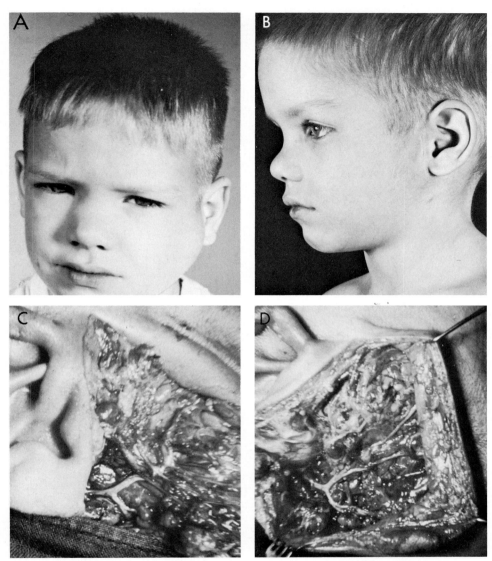

Fig. 21-8.—Parotid lymphangioma. These lesions are usually cystic hygroma, superficial to the parotid gland. **A,** large cystic, transilluminable swelling anterior to and extending beneath the lobe of the left ear, which had recurred rapidly after attempted excision. There is partial paralysis of the lid. **B,** postoperative result, showing the scarcely perceptible scar. The facial nerve branch, divided at the previous operation, was found and re-sutured. **C,** operative photograph of similar lesion being excised from over the right parotid. Traction is being made on the multi-locular cyst downward and forward, and the main trunk and two branches of the facial nerve are exposed. **D,** on completion of the procedure, the facial nerve and its divisions lie cleanly exposed over the surface of the parotid gland. Temporary weakness of the corner of the mouth or of the lids may be expected, but one should confidently anticipate avoiding permanent injury to the nerves.

less it must be recognized that when sheets of edematous tissue enfold nerves and vessels, complete extirpation is technically impossible. Judging from the pathologic studies of Goetsch,[11] it is likely that even when the surgeon believes he has removed all of the lesion, some microscopic bits or pseudopods which are found around the peripheral borders of the tumor do remain. In our experience, if all of the macroscopically identifiable tissue is dissected away, recurrence is rare. This reinforces our belief that the lesion is not a neoplasm in the true sense of the word. If, on the other hand, portions of obvious cystic tumor are left behind, the recurrence rate may be as high as 10 or 15%. If some of the tumor must be left, it is important to leave no intact cysts, and all of the cyst wall should be resected in every instance.

The mortality rate for the excision of hygromas should be nil. When very large lesions involving most of the neck or extending into the mediastinum are included in a series, the postoperative mortality is cited at 2–5%.

REFERENCES

1. Anderson, D.H.: Tumors of infancy and childhood, Cancer 4:890, 1951.
2. Bailey, H.: The clinical aspects of branchial cysts, Brit. J. Surg. 10:565, 1923.
3. Bill, A.H., Jr., and Sumner, D.S.: Unified concept of lymphangioma and cystic hygroma, Surg., Gynec. & Obst. 120:79, 1965.
4. Briggs, J. D., *et al.*: Cystic and cavernous lymphangioma, West. J. Surg. 61:499, 1953.
5. Camishion, R.C., and Templeton, J.Y., III: Cervico-mediastinal cystic hygroma, Pediatrics 29:831, 1962.
6. Childress, M.E.; Baker, C.P., and Samson, P.C.: Lymphangioma of the mediastinum: Report of a case with a review of the literature, J. Thoracic Surg. 31:338, 1956.
7. Dowd, C.N.: Hygroma cysticum colli: Its structure and etiology, Ann. Surg. 58:112, 1913.
8. Farr, C.E.: Personal communication.
9. Freeman, G.C.: Conservative surgical treatment of massive cystic lymphangioma with the report of 8 cases, Ann. Surg. 137:12, 1953.
10. Galofré, M., *et al.*: Results of surgical treatment of cystic hygroma, Surg., Gynec. & Obst. 115:319, 1962.
11. Goetsch, E.: Hygroma colli cysticum and hygroma axillare, Arch. Surg. 36:394, 1938.
12. Gross, R.E.: *The Surgery of Infancy and Childhood* (Philadelphia: W.B. Saunders Company, 1953).
13. Harkins, G.A., and Sabiston, D.C., Jr., Lymphangioma in infancy and childhood, Surgery 47:811, 1960.
14. Kirschner, P. A.: Cervico-mediastinal cystic hygroma: One stage excision in an eight week old infant, Surgery 60:1104, 1966.
15. Koester, K.: Ueber Hygroma cysticum colli congenitum, Verhandl. phys.-med. Gesellsch. Würzb. 3:44, 1872.
16. Landing, B.H., and Farber, S.: Tumors of the Cardiovascular System, *Atlas of Tumor Pathology* (Washington, D.C.: Armed Forces Institute of Pathology, 1956).
17. McClure, C.F.W., and Silvester, C.F.: A comparative study of the lymphaticovenous communications in adult mammals, Anat. Rec. 3:534, 1909.
18. Nicholson, C.W. deP.: *Studies on Tumor Formation* (London: Butterworth & Co., Ltd., 1950).
19. Ravitch, M.M.: Radical treatment of massive mixed angiomas (hemolymphangiomas) in infants and children, Ann. Surg. 134:228, 1951.
20. Redenbacker: Dissertation cited by Wernher.[28]
21. Sabin, F.R.: On the origin of the lymphatic system from the veins and the development of the lymph heart and thoracic duct in the pig, Am. J. Anat. 1:367, 1901.
22. Sabin, F.R.: On the development of the superficial lymphatics in the skin of the pig, Am. J. Anat. 3:183, 1904.
23. Sabin, F.R.: The development of the lymphatic nodes in the pig and their relation to the lymph hearts, Am. J. Anat. 4:355, 1905.
24. Sabin, F.R.: The lymphatic system in human embryos with a consideration of the morphology of the system as a whole, Am. J. Anat. 9:43, 1909.
25. Stratton, V.C., and Grant, R.N., Cervico-mediastinal cystic hygroma associated with chylopericardinum, Arch. Surg. 77:887, 1958.
26. Vaughn, A.M.: Cystic hygroma of the neck: Report of case and review of literature, Am. J. Dis. Child. 48:149, 1934.
27. von Ammon: Cited by Wernher.[28]
28. Wernher, A.: *Die angeborenen Kysten-Hygrome und die ihnen verwandten Geschwülste in anatomischer, diagnostischer und therapeutischer Beziehung* (Geissen: G.F. Heyer, Vater, 1843).
29. Willis, R.A.: *Pathology of Tumors* (2nd ed.; London: Butterworth & Co., Ltd., 1953).

M. M. RAVITCH
B. F. RUSH, JR.

22

Cysts and Sinuses of the Neck

Branchiogenic Cysts and Sinuses

CYSTS, SINUSES AND FISTULAS of the neck which are derived from the branchial clefts are not infrequently seen in childhood. The sinuses and fistulas are encountered more frequently than are the cysts. The branchiogenic cysts seem to make their appearance most often in the age group following childhood, although they have been noted before then.

The first and the second branchial cleft remnants are those most commonly seen. Of these, the abnormalities of the second cleft occur more frequently. For an understanding of these abnormalities, a simple knowledge of their embryology is desirable.

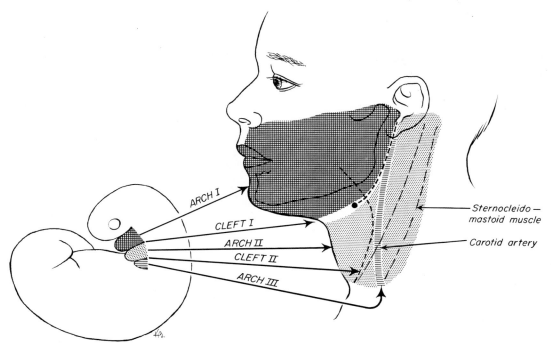

Fig. 22-1.—Derivation of various areas of head and neck from the arches and clefts of the embryo. (Modified and reprinted from *Annals of Surgery* by permission.)

Embryology

The early embryo presents a series of ridges and furrows in the region of the developing neck. These are known as the branchial arches and the branchial clefts respectively. Figure 22-1 shows the parts of the face and neck derived from each of the arches.

As the embryo develops, the arches coalesce and finally give a smooth contour to the cheek and neck. Part of the base of the first branchial cleft remains open as the eustachian tube and the auditory canal. If the first branchial cleft remained entirely open as a cleft, it would leave a defect extending from the auditory canal around beneath the angle of the mandible, ending at a point slightly below the midpoint of the mandible. If the second branchial cleft were not to coalesce, it would leave a cleft exposing the base of the tonsil and, running down parallel to the anterior border of the sternocleidomastoid muscle, would end at a point one quarter of the length of the muscle from its lower insertion.

Evidently the coalescence of these branchial clefts does not always begin from the bottom and extend outward. This seems to be true since the tracts which are found clinically represent a lumen left at the very bottom of what once was the embryologic cleft. Their normal closure can be compared to the gluing together of folds or pleats in a piece of cloth. If the glue did not get all the way down to the base and yet the major part of the surfaces became adherent, a tube or a cyst might be left at the bottom of one of the folds.

From the evidence given us by examining congenital abnormalities of this area, this seems to be a rough analogy to describe the method of their formation. The remnants of the first branchial cleft will appear somewhere along the base of an imaginary fold running from the auditory canal behind and be-

Fig. 22-2.—Areas of the neck in which cysts and sinuses from the first and second cleft are usually found.

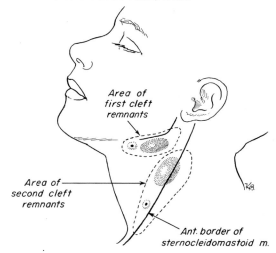

low the angle of the mandible to a point just below its midpoint. The remnants of the second branchial cleft will be found along all or any part of an imaginary line from the tonsillar fossae down to a point on the lower one-third of the anterior border of the sterno-cleidomastoid muscle (Fig. 22-2).

Albers[1] has published a painstaking schematic outline of the branchial clefts and their derivatives, which was published as a color insert to the journal article.

Anomalies of the Second Branchial Cleft

In infancy and childhood, anomalies of the second branchial cleft are seen most commonly in a proportion of about 6 to 1 as compared to anomalies of the first branchial cleft (Fig. 22-3). Most frequently, the abnormality will be evidenced by a tiny pinpoint opening on the anterior edge of the sternocleidomastoid muscle one quarter of its length upward from the sternal end. Attention to the defect will be called by small drops of secretion coming out from this opening (Fig. 22-4). The defect may be either unilateral or bilateral. We have studied 25 such lesions in 24 patients. Of these, 9 were blind sinus tracts, and 16 extended all the way to the tonsillar fossa (Table 22-1).

It should be noted that there are cysts of the lateral neck which are evidently not derived from the branchial clefts. This has been pointed out by Henzel et al.[7] They particularly commented on the cysts which are surrounded by lymphatic tissue, suggesting that these are possibly caused by blockage of the lymphatic outflow of these structures, with subsequent cyst formation. They referred specially to the cyst in the parotid.

Less frequently, one will see a small oval mass presenting anterior to the upper portion of the sterno-cleidomastoid muscle which will represent a cyst derived from this tract. These branchiogenic cysts may

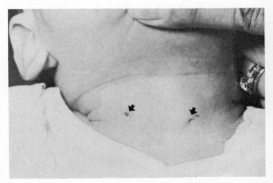

Fig. 22-4. — Child with bilateral branchiogenic fistulas of the second branchial cleft. Each fistula extended up to the upper tonsillar fossa. (Reprinted from *Surgical Clinics of North America* by permission.)

appear at any age. We have studied 6 patients with such lesions.

When a tiny opening is present on the anterior surface of the sternocleidomastoid, it must be recognized that the tract may extend upward all the way into the tonsillar fossa or may extend only a part of the distance. At times such openings may be only 1 cm long.

A cyst represents patency of the central portion of the base of the embryologic cleft. Such a cyst may at times drain into the tonsillar fossa. One of our patients had such a connection.

It has been our experience that in childhood, the tracts which have an external opening rarely become infected. In the older age group, infection has been reported as a problem. The constant drainage of saliva from the neck is undesirable to the patient and his family and is the immediate reason for a visit to the surgeon.

PATHOLOGY. — The lining of a remnant of a second branchial cleft is composed of epithelium which may resemble respiratory epithelium or skin, or some of each, and is surrounded by muscle fibers. Grossly, a fistula of the second branchial cleft may be 5-10 mm in outside diameter, and the wall of the tract is often 2-3 mm thick.

TREATMENT. — The use of sclerosing solutions in such a tract is mentioned here only to be condemned.

Fig. 22-3. — Types of remnants of second branchial cleft. Sinuses and fistulas are seen most often in the young, whereas cysts normally appear at a later age.

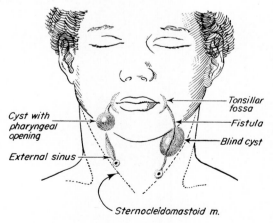

TABLE 22-1. — BRANCHIOGENIC CYSTS, SINUSES AND
FISTULAS (36 PATIENTS)

CLEFTS AND LESIONS	LEFT	RIGHT	TOTAL
First cleft			
Cysts	5	1	6
Second cleft			
Cysts	3	3	6
Sinuses	6	3	9
Fistulas	5	11	16
Total			37
		(One case bilateral)	

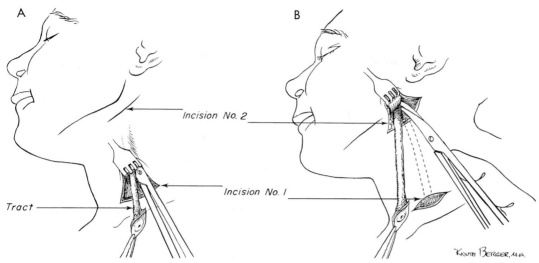

Fig. 22-5.—Operative procedure for removal of fistula of second branchial cleft. **A**, a transverse elliptical incision is made around the mouth of the fistula. Holding this piece of tissue, blunt and sharp dissection is carried directly as far as possible on the fistulous tract. **B**, when the limit of dissection through the lower incision is reached, another transverse incision is made below the angle of the mandible. The platysma muscle is split and the portion of tract already dissected is brought out. The remaining dissection is then completed up to where it can be felt in the mouth by the anesthesiologist's finger. The tract is divided and the upper end closed with one transfixing suture of chromic catgut.

In our experience, surgical excision is the method of choice. The operation may be carried out at any age. On one hand, the larger the patient the easier the procedure since the tract will be stronger and more easily dissected. On the other hand, if the tract extends all the way to the tonsillar fossa, the total distance of the dissection will become greater the greater the size of the child. We have successfully excised fistulous tracts starting from the age of 6 months onward.

Operation.—With the patient in a prone position and with the shoulders elevated on a roll of cloth, the chin is turned away from the side of the branchial cleft sinus. Intratracheal anesthesia is used.

An elliptical incision is made in a transverse direction so that the external opening is removed in the direction of the skin folds (Fig. 22-5). With a probe placed in the fistula, dissection is carried out by means of blunt pointed scissors directly on the tract as high as can be reached through the lower incision. Traction may be applied to the tract in a downward direction, and the incision may be pulled upward so that this dissection can be carried a surprising distance. If the dissection is kept directly on the tract, there is no danger of injuring the vessels which pass close to it.

If the tract is short, the end will be reached through the lower incision. If it extends all the way to the tonsillar fossa, a second and higher incision parallel to the first will be necessary. After reaching the limit of dissection through the lower incision, the second incision is made within the skin folds beneath the poste-rior third of the mandible. Dissection is carried down carefully until the limits of the previous dissection have been reached. The tract is then brought out through the upper incision.

Cox[5] has described the use of a vein stripper as an adjunct in the dissection of these sinuses.

The remainder of the dissection is carried out as previously, directly on the wall of the upper portion of the tonsillar fossa guided by the palpating finger of the anesthesiologist. When this point is reached, a suture ligature of 4-0 chromic catgut on a small round needle is placed through the tract, and the tract is tied off. The short stump of the tract is left intact after the division is made. A rubber band is left as a drain along the plane of dissection. The muscle layers are closed with fine chromic catgut and the skin incisions with silk. The drain is removed the day after surgery.

Anomalies of the First Branchial Cleft

Anomalies of the first branchial cleft are less common than those of the second, yet they comprised 5 of the 18 cases studied by Bill and Vadheim in 1955. They are frequently misdiagnosed and incompletely removed and are followed by repeated infections. We have studied 6 of these lesions in children in addition to 2 in adults included in the study with Vadheim. A study by Lincoln[9] in 1965 described 31 cases of these lesions in a collective survey.

Figure 22-6 shows a photograph of such a case. In this instance there was an abscess which pointed just

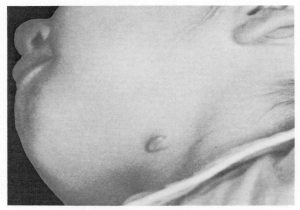

Fig. 22-6.—An infected, draining lesion high in the neck of an 18-month-old child. It proved on surgery to extend upward to the left auditory canal in close relationship to the facial nerve. (Reprinted from *Annals of Surgery* by permission.)

beneath the center of the body of the mandible. The abscess had drained twice previously. Following drainage and subsidence of the infection, a tract was excised around and just behind the angle of the mandible and then upward to end blindly at the lower surface of the cartilage of the external auditory canal. The posterior half of the tract in this case was surrounded by a cartilaginous tube ending blindly at the cartilage of the external auditory canal in the form of a T. The tract just barely passed lateral to the facial nerve (Fig. 22-7).

PATHOLOGY.—Pathologic examination showed the tract to be lined with stratified squamous epithelium. In other cases we have found tissue resembling skin

Fig. 22-7.—Relationships of cyst or sinus of first branchial cleft. Note especially the relationship to the facial nerve and external auditory canal. Others have described passage of the tract *medial* to the facial nerve. (Reprinted from *Annals of Surgery* by permission.)

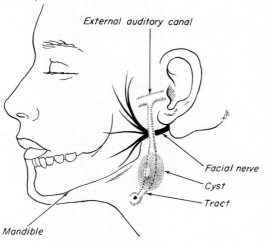

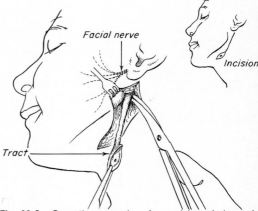

Fig. 22-8.—Operative procedure for excision of sinus of first branchial cleft. A transverse elliptical incision is made around the opening, then posteriorly to a point just beneath the ear. Through this incision the tract is dissected free under direct vision. It is divided at the external auditory canal. The incision is closed with a small drain if necessary.

and containing hair follicles. In every case which we have seen, there has been a surrounding layer of cartilage extending over the posterior portion of the tract and up to the auditory canal.

We have had 2 cases in which there was an actual opening into the auditory canal with infection coming from it. Whether the opening was present at birth or whether it was created by extension of infection is not known. Thus a draining sinus just beneath the middle of the body of the mandible on either side, with or without drainage from the auditory canal, must lead one to suspect a cyst or sinus from the first branchial cleft.

Surgical treatment.—Since the diagnosis of such a cyst or sinus is generally made after repeated infection, adequate drainage and treatment of the infection must be carried out before any excision is attempted. When the infection has subsided, an elliptical incision should be made around the opening of the sinus in the upper neck (Fig. 22-8). This incision should then be extended posteriorly in the skin lines to the angle of the mandible. The anterior portion of the tract can then be excised under direct vision and the posterior portion by retracting the incision upward until the lower portion of the auditory canal is reached. Extreme care should be taken during the dissection in order not to injure the facial nerve or its mandibular branch. The wound is closed in layers, and a small drain should be left in the base of the wound for 24 hours.

REFERENCES

1. Albers, G.D.: Branchial anomalies, J.A.M.A. 183:399, 1963.
2. Bailey, H.: The clinical aspects of branchial fistulae, Brit. J. Surg. 21:173, 1933.

3. Bill, A.H., Jr., and Vadheim, J.L.: Cysts, sinuses, and fistulas of the neck arising from the first and second branchial clefts, Ann. Surg. 142:904, 1955.

4. Byers, L.T., and Anderson, R.: Anomalies of the first branchial cleft, Surg., Gynec. & Obst. 93:775, 1951.

5. Cox, E.F.: Excision of branchial sinus and fistula tracts using arterial intimal strippers, Surg., Gynec. & Obst. 117:767, 1963.

6. DeBord, R.A.: First branchial cleft sinus, Arch. Surg. 81:228, 1960.

7. Henzel, J.H., *et al.*: Etiology of lateral cervical cysts, Surg., Gynec. & Obst. 125:87, 1967.

8. Ladd, W.E., and Gross, R.E.: Congenital branchiogenic anomalies, Am. J. Surg. 39:234, 1938.

9. Lincoln, J.C.R.: Cervico-auricular fistulae, Arch. Dis. Childhood 40:218, 1965.

10. Patten, B.H.: *Human Embryology* (Philadelphia: Blakiston Co., 1947).

11. Small, A.: The surgical removal of branchial sinus, Lancet 2:891, 1960.

A. H. BILL, JR.

Drawings by
KNUTE BERGER, M.D.

Thyroglossal Cysts and Midline Clefts

Thyroglossal Cysts

Cysts and sinuses of the thyroglossal duct are the remnants of the anterior midline structure which formed the origin of the thyroid gland. These remnants are invariably found in or very near the midline of the neck at any level from the tongue down. The relationship of the thyroglossal duct to the midpoint of the hyoid bone is the key to successful treatment of these conditions. The commonest sign is a midline neck mass, but the clinical picture is often obscured by infection. Definitive care requires the total removal of the thyroglossal duct remnants, and this in turn requires removal of the central segment of the hyoid bone. The recurrence rate after incomplete operations is over 20%. Thyroid epithelium in remnants of the thyroglossal duct can reproduce all of the known thyroid disorders, e.g., adenoma, thyroiditis, carcinoma and hyperthyroidism. In general, recurrence or persistence of a thyroglossal duct cyst or sinus is due to incomplete removal. The most common cause of incomplete removal is failure to remove the portions of the tract running through and above the hyoid bone.

ANATOMIC VARIATIONS

There are many anatomic variations of the growth and development of the thyroglossal duct. The abnor-mality known as "lingual" thyroid is discussed in Chapter 20. A lingual thyroid often represents all of the functioning thyroid tissue that the affected individual possesses, and its total removal will inevitably result in myxedema if exogenous thyroid hormone is not supplied.

ORIGIN AND DEVELOPMENT OF THE THYROGLOSSAL DUCT

The entire thyroid gland in the human arises from a single source. It first appears during the fourth week of embryonal development as a midline diverticulum from the pharyngeal floor at the level of the first branchial pouches. As the diverticulum enlarges, it develops a bilobed appearance and descends in the anterior midline of the neck (Fig. 22-9), retaining its attachment to the floor of the pharynx by a narrow stalk called the thyroglossal duct. The second branchial arches meet in the midline anteriorly to form the hyoid bone, which embraces the thyroglossal duct. In the mature individual, the thyroglossal duct is either posterior to the midpoint of the resulting hyoid bone or passes through the middle of it. It is important to recall that the thyroglossal duct arose *above* the hyoid bone The suprahyoid portion of the duct is the part most involved in recurrences.

As the thyroglossal duct elongates, normal cellular proliferation fills the primordial lumen of the stalk, but in some patients a tiny lumen is preserved and can serve as a channel for the transmission of infection or secretions. In the course of normal development, the thyroglossal duct degenerates and disap-

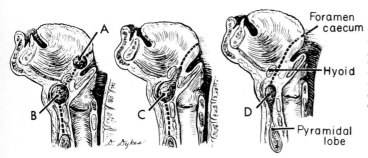

Foramen caecum

Hyoid

Pyramidal lobe

Fig. 22-9.—Representative sites along the thyroglossal duct where functioning tissue may appear. **A**, "lingual" thyroid; **B**, subhyoid median thyroid tissue, may be "ectopic" or a thyroglossal duct cyst; **C**, common location with tract extending above the hyoid; **D**, cyst with continuity to the pyramidal lobe in addition to the extension above the hyoid bone.

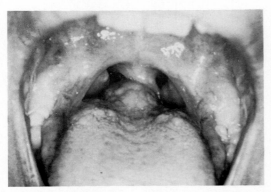

Fig. 22-10.—Lingual thyroid. A large mass is visible at the back of the tongue of this 6-year-old child. Tonsils and uvula nearly block the passageway; however, no symptoms were experienced. A scintogram revealed this to be the only thyroid tissue present.

pears by about the tenth week. The point of origin of the duct remains as the foramen caecum, a small pit on the dorsum of the tongue at the apex of the V-shaped ridge marking the boundary between the vallate and the filiform papillae. Subhyoid median "ectopic" thyroid masses carry many of the same hazards and functional significance as lingual thyroid masses[25] (Fig. 22-10).

A "pyramidal" lobe is a persistent enlargement of the lower end of the thyroglossal duct at its confluence with the thyroid gland. It occurs in one fourth to one third of normal individuals. Either of the lateral thyroid lobes may be partially or completely absent, the isthmus may be absent, and thyroid tissue inclusions may occur within the wall of the larynx or trachea. The complications of hemorrhage and of airway obstruction noted with lingual thyroid masses are also seen with aberrant thyroid tissue in the larynx and trachea. An example may be cited to illustrate these problems. A woman with aberrant thyroid tissue in the wall of her trachea had respiratory obstruc-

tion because of the thyroid tissue hyperplasia during a pregnancy. She survived this pregnancy, but during a subsequent one, further hyperplasia resulted in suffocation and death.[7] Infants who have difficulty in breathing while in the supine position, but can breathe easily in the prone position, have been found to have a thyroglossal duct remnant at the base of the tongue as the cause of the dyspnea[19,24] (Fig. 22-11).

During the second month of embryonal development, follicles and colloid appear in the thyroid gland; after the fifth month, further increase of size of the gland is by proliferation of existing follicles, since no new follicles are formed thereafter. It is generally believed that the lateral growth of the thyroid lobes is limited by the fascial boundaries and great vessels of the neck, and that lateral masses of thyroid tissue are in truth metastatic cancer from a primary cancer in the thyroid gland[30] or originating from midline remnants of thyroid tissue. However, both lateral and midline[16] benign abnormally placed thyroid tissue has been found in the neck without any discoverable primary "carcinoma." This phenomenon has been recently explained on the basis of lymphatic transport or "benign metastasis," the explanation being similar to that used to explain endometriosis in the lungs.[11,18,22]

The epithelium of the thyroglossal duct can develop almost any disease known to occur in the gland itself. Adenoma, carcinoma, thyroiditis, hyperthyroidism and recurrent hyperthyroidism have been reported. It should be noted that many of the thyroid cancers have been located rather low in the thyroglossal duct; some of them may actually have been in a pyramidal lobe that extended a little farther cephalad than usual. The carcinomas that have been reported as arising in remnants of the thyroglossal duct have almost invariably been papillary in pattern.[3,6,10,15,17,28] Occasionally, metastases from thyroid cancers develop a "cystic" appearance, and the discovery of cancer in a "thyroglossal duct remnant" should arouse the suspicion that it might be metastatic rather than primary.

Radioiodine scintigrams have demonstrated functioning thyroid epithelium in midline neck structures

Fig. 22-11.—Effect of child's position on relation of cyst to airway. **A,** supine, the cyst at the back of the tongue drops posteriorly and closes the air passage. **B,** prone, the tongue drops forward, bringing with it the cyst and opening the air passage.

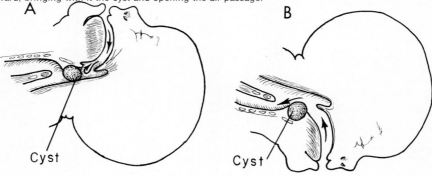

from the thyroglossal duct.[9] Some of these have been very high in the neck, at the level of the hyoid bone. The frequency of the appearance of functioning thyroid epithelium in the thyroglossal duct is variable, the reported incidence varying from 1 to 8% but averaging about 5%. The presence of histologically identifiable epithelium in the thyroglossal duct remnant is not necessarily the same as finding functional tissue. Whether or not the epithelium in the thyroglossal duct is capable of function is determined in part by whether its potential function is overwhelmed by the preponderance of normally placed thyroid tissue. It is easier to demonstrate functioning thyroid epithelium in the thyroglossal duct remnants with the use of radioiodine after most of the normally placed gland has been removed or destroyed and after stimulation with thyrotropic hormone. The rather large size of some thyroglossal duct derivatives was demonstrated in a report of an "elongated banana-shaped thyroid" in a 26-year-old Indian (Bombay) whose entire thyroid gland developed as a greatly enlarged midline mass with no lateral thyroid lobes palpable or identifiable by radioiodine scintigram.[2] This patient was not operated on, but it is probable that all of the functioning thyroid tissue was concentrated in a midline mass of thyroglossal duct origin.

Cysts can occur anywhere along the normal course of the thyroglossal duct from the foramen caecum to the eventual position low in the anterior midline of the neck, but almost all of them occur below the hyoid bone. The presence of the cyst below the hyoid bone does not alter the fact that the original tract came from above the hyoid, and its successful treatment depends on recognition of that anatomic fact. There is no normal connection of the thyroglossal duct to the overlying skin. If infection occurs, some skin fixation may result, and any subsequent incision and drainage will lead to formation of a fistula and a persistent sinus. There is no significant incidence of spontaneous fistulization without preceding infection.

Diagnostic Factors

The outstanding clinical feature of thyroglossal duct remnants is their midline position (Fig. 22-12). A thyroglossal duct remnant may lie far enough off the midline to be mistaken for a *branchiogenic cyst*, but this diagnostic error has been made only once in over 100 cases at the Childrens Hospital of Los Angeles. In the reverse situation, branchiogenic cysts can (rarely) occur so close to the midline that they are mistaken for thyroglossal duct remnants.

Thyroglossal duct cysts may sometimes be seen to rise in the neck when the tongue is protruded. It is most unusual to see a patent foramen caecum or to see any secretions coming from it. A thyroglossal duct sinus usually is too narrow to permit the passage of dyes or radiopaque material, in contrast to the branchiogenic sinuses that will discharge dyes or radiopaque material when suitably placed for such a demonstration.

Cysts of the thyroglossal duct do not usually contain enough fluid to permit aspiration, but if fluid can be obtained, it is usually thick and viscous. There are usually no identifiable epithelial elements or cholesterol crystals. Fluid from a branchiogenic cyst is usually more watery and voluminous; epithelial squames and cholesterol crystals can usually be identified. In the presence of infection, some of these diagnostic differences may be obscured, but the two conditions

Fig. 22-12 (left). — Thyroglossal duct cyst. Swelling overlying the hyoid bone is obvious in this 8-year-old girl. It had been present many months, but there was no infection or symptom — only a concern for her appearance on the part of the patient.

Fig. 22-13 (right). — Thyroglossal duct cyst. Midline swelling at the level of the hyoid bone of a boy of 6. It had been present several years but only recently was recognized as an abnormality by the boy's parents.

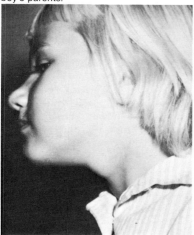
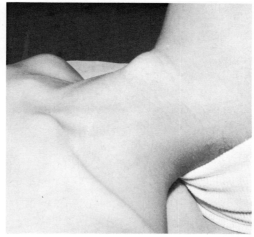

are almost always correctly identified by their location.

The commonest presenting evidence of thyroglossal duct cysts and sinuses is the mass (Fig. 22-13), and this is often heralded by a bout of infection. It is important to emphasize that infection in a thyroglossal duct cyst is not necessarily an indication to drain it. There are some substantial advantages to keeping the cyst intact, because when the time comes for definitive excision, the cure rate for intact cysts is half again as high as it is for sinuses.

Ectopic thyroid, forming a mass overlying the hyoid bone, may be confused with a thyroglossal duct cyst. In some patients, when normal thyroid tissue cannot be palpated, an I[131] uptake study is useful preoperatively. At operation, the differentiation can be made by inspection or on incising the tissue. Removal of all of the patient's thyroid tissue is not advisable.

A potential diagnostic error is that of *dermoid cysts* occurring in the midline of the neck. These cysts are not always attached to the overlying skin; they can occur in the exact midline and have smoothly rounded contour. At operation, one encounters a whitish, cystic structure containing the typical cheesy material but with no demonstrable sinus or tract from the cyst upward toward the hyoid bone. Dermoid cysts are not common, but they can be confusing; they are analogous to the more common dermoid cysts found at the lateral end of the brow. Because of the presence of squamous epithelium in certain thyroglossal ducts, the possibility exists that some of these dermoid cysts may share a common origin with the thyroglossal duct, but no such origin can be considered proved. Dermoid cysts are easily excised intact, but the absence of a duct running up to the hyoid may mislead the unwary surgeon into believing that a thyroglossal duct cyst can also arise without some upward connection. This is anatomically impossible. Rarely a *lipoma,* *hemangioma* or *lymphangioma* may appear as a solitary midline neck structure. Infection of neck nodes in the midline can be confusing, but is also rare. Cellulitis and infection of thyroglossal duct remnants will sometimes obscure the identity of the underlying cyst for several days or weeks. The *midline cervical cleft* has a typical appearance, described later in this chapter, which will rarely be confused with thyroglossal duct remnants.

AGE AND SEX

The average age of the children seen at the Childrens Hospital of Los Angeles with thyroglossal duct remnants has been about 4-1/2 years. Thyroglossal duct cysts have been seen from birth to advanced age, but the majority become clinically evident in the preschool years, often because of infection. Despite statements that thyroglossal duct remnants occur with equal frequency in both sexes, there appears to be a definite preponderance of males in most large series of reported cases, about 60% boys to 40% girls. There does not seem to be any anatomic reason why this should be true, and it may be pure coincidence. It is apparent that the complication rate and the recurrence rate are higher in boys than in girls, and hence the larger centers may receive more boys because they receive more recurrent and complicated cases.

THERAPEUTIC FACTORS

Because the recurrence rate after presumably adequate operations is still at an unsatisfactorily high level (over 20%), it is important to discover if we can why these recurrences develop. Using the term "cyst" for those with intact structures and "sinus" for those with an external opening, the chance of definitive cure with a single operation is 1-1/2 times better for a cyst than for a sinus. We believe that *infected thyroglossal duct cysts* should not be opened unless it is absolutely necessary. Definitive excision should not be undertaken in the presence of active infection. Conservative measures should be used to control infection in order to preserve the anatomic integrity of the cyst and duct.

There is good reason to believe that in some of the children with *open sinuses* seen at the Childrens Hospital, the true nature of the underlying disease was not recognized by the physician who drained the abscess. Some of the children have been referred here because an "abscess" failed to heal and the presence of an underlying thyroglossal duct structure had apparently not been suspected.

The therapeutic ideal is *removal of the entire tract*, and for practical purposes this means removal of the central segment of the hyoid bone in order to get the portion of the tract lying above that level. We recognize the fact that some children with thyroglossal duct cysts have had no recurrence following operations in which the hyoid bone segment was not removed, but these cases are distinctly the exceptions and the practice is mentioned only to be condemned.

Much of the story of recurrence is the story of the retained hyoid segment; this single omission is responsible for more secondary operations than any other cause. There may be some natural reluctance on the part of surgeons to open a bony structure in the presence of infection for fear of osteomyelitis. However, there is only one (possible) example of this complication in the literature, and the risk must be negligible.[4,5] Complete removal of a thyroglossal duct remnant commits the surgeon to removal of the tract by removing that bone segment and then coring the tract out of the musculature of the tongue up to the mucosa of the tongue and the foramen caecum.

After *removal* of the *central portion of the hyoid bone,* there is no need to re-establish continuity of the ends. Some surgeons feel that uniting the hyoid fragments is contraindicated since it unnecessarily distorts the structures of the neck. The lack of the central segment of the hyoid does not produce any disability or interfere with any function.

Suture material. — There does not seem to be any consistent relationship between the recurrence rate and the use of any type of suture material or technique. At the Childrens Hospital of Los Angeles, the surgeons have almost invariably used absorbable sutures if there was any evidence of infection or drainage. In our follow-up studies, we have encountered several cases of transitory difficulty with nonabsorbable suture material, and two patients have come to secondary operations for persistent sinuses which may possibly have been related to nonabsorbable sutures producing a foreign body reaction and persistent drainage.

Drains. — It is our opinion that a soft rubber drain should be used for 24 hours in all cases to prevent a closed space hematoma with compression of the air passages. Such an accident has been reported with a fatal result. While this is a wise precaution, we could not relate the use or nonuse of a drain to the recurrence rate.

Operative Technique (Sistrunk[26])

The choice of anesthetic agents and techniques should rest with the anesthesiologist. At the Childrens Hospital of Los Angeles, endotracheal anesthesia is used without exception in these patients, with a variety of anesthetic agents.

The child is positioned with supports so arranged

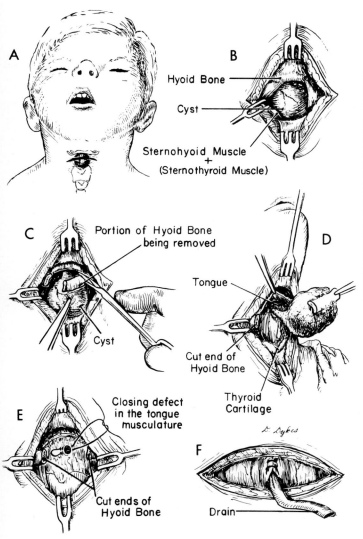

Fig. 22-14. — Operative procedure for removal of thyroglossal duct cyst. **A**, transverse incision directly over an intact cyst, or an elliptical transverse incision around an open sinus. **B**, skin and platysma muscle are cut and the sternohyoid (and sternothyroid) muscles separated and retracted to expose the cyst. Dissection is extended to expose the hyoid bone. **C**, hyoid bone is cut, and the slender tract extending above becomes visible entering the tongue musculature. **D**, example of a cyst lying principally *above* the hyoid with a slender tract extending toward the foramen caecum. The relationship of the duct to the center of the hyoid bone requires complete excision as an integral unit, regardless of whether the bulk of the cyst is above or below the hyoid. Gentle traction on the cyst will help to outline the duct. **E**, thyroglossal duct is removed to the level of the foramen caecum and the defect in the tongue closed with fine catgut sutures. No effort is made to reunite residual hyoid fragments. **F**, a soft drain is left in place for 24–48 hours. Subcutaneous tissues and skin are closed without tension.

that the anterior neck structures are brought anteriorly. With an endotracheal tube in place, it is impossible to compromise the airway in any position, but we have not used extreme hyperextension because it is not necessary and can be hazardous from compression of the spinal cord. A transverse incision directly over the mass (Fig. 22-14) is ideal for intact cysts, and a transverse elliptical excision of the lower opening is best for sinuses. It is better to use a second transverse incision higher up, if necessary, to get all of the tract above the hyoid bone when the initial incision is too low in the neck to permit this. Vertical incisions in the anterior neck are unsatisfactory from a cosmetic standpoint, and a disabling deformity may result if a contracture develops as a result of infection or keloid.

The skin flaps are developed to permit exposure and to permit eventual closure without tension. The thyroglossal duct is identified as it follows its midline course superficial to the ribbon muscles and between them. This dissection is best accomplished by trying to maintain a small cuff of grossly normal tissue adjacent to the duct and trying to maintain the duct intact throughout the operation. Tension on the tract will assist in outlining it, but it is usually not practical or advisable to try to outline the duct with a probe. The injection of methylene blue into the cyst or sinus has, on occasion, been rewarding in outlining the tract, but we do not recommend its routine use.

The central segment of the hyoid bone must be exposed adequately and removed together with the contained or adjacent segment of the thyroglossal duct. (In patients under 3 years, cut with knife, over 3 years with bone cutters.) The dissection of the tract in the musculature of the tongue begins immediately above the hyoid. In dissecting the tract out of the tongue musculature, it is often advantageous to have the anesthesiologist or assistant place a finger on the dorsum of the tongue (Fig. 22-15) at the level of the foramen caecum to serve as a guide as the surgeon approaches the mucosa of the mouth. Any opening into the mouth can be closed with a few fine catgut sutures and similar material used to close the tongue musculature beneath the mucosal closure. It is not necessary to reunite the ends of the hyoid bone. In all cases, a small soft rubber drain should be left in the depths of the incision for a day or two to prevent the accumulation of blood or serum. The subcutaneous tissues can be approximated with catgut and the skin closed with any technique of the surgeon's choice (sutures or clips). In patients with infected sinuses, absorbable sutures should be used in the deeper layers. A standard thyroid dressing is employed and changed as necessary.

RESULTS

Of the 112 patients operated on for thyroglossal duct cysts or sinuses at the Childrens Hospital of Los

Fig. 22-15.—Method for removal of sinus tract extending into the tongue. The anesthesiologist inserts his finger in the mouth and presses anteriorly over the base of the tongue. The tract is coned out of the musculature.

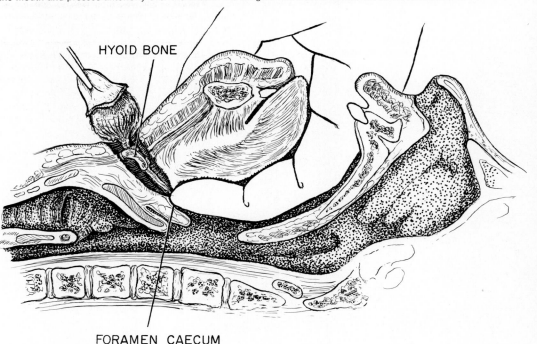

HYOID BONE

FORAMEN CAECUM

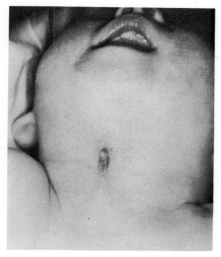

Angeles in the 10-year period, 1957 through 1966,[23] there were 23 who were seen because of recurrent disease requiring further operative treatment. Some of these children had had two and three previous attempts at definitive cure before they were seen here. The central segment of the hyoid bone was still intact in most of these children.

This disease appears to be deceptively easy to treat sometimes, and it is only after critical analysis that we realize that there is a substantial recurrence rate. Most of these recurrences seem to have a clear explanation in the persistent presence of the hyoid bone segment and the portion of the tract that lies in and above it, but some of the recurrences have never been satisfactorily explained. The operation can be undertaken at any age. It should, however, be undertaken as soon after the diagnosis is made as possible, because the delay will increase the risk of infection with its consequent increase in morbidity.

There were no deaths in any of the cases of thyroglossal duct cysts or sinuses seen at this hospital. There were no instances of major bleeding or other major operative complication. The morbidity was brief and uncomplicated in most cases. The best results are obtained by removing intact cysts and tracts

Fig. 22-16.—Midline cervical cleft. This obvious cleft is about 2.5 cm long. At its upper portion there is a tab of skin lying at the level of the hyoid bone. Below this is a longitudinal cleft of denuded skin. With head extended, one can see a continuation of the fibrous cord extending downward nearly to the sternal notch. (Courtesy of Dr. K. J. Welch.)

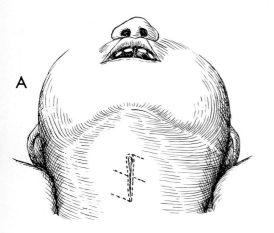
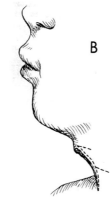

Fig. 22-17.—Technique of Z-plasty for removal and closure of cervical cleft of the neck. **A,** the skin tab at the upper end, the cleft in the skin and the underlying fibrous cord are excised. Lateral incisions are made as indicated. **B,** lateral view of procedure in **A. C,** skin is undermined as indicated by dotted areas and the flaps are elevated. **D,** method of approximating the angles of the Z. **E,** final suturing of the Z-plasty.

Line of incision for cleft removal and double   Z-PLASTY

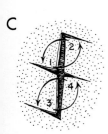
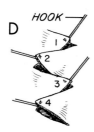
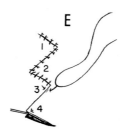

Shaded area
undermined

After rotation
of flaps

Sutured in
reverse position

before infection or incomplete operative intervention complicates the picture.

Midline Cervical Clefts

The usual clinical deformity present in a midline cervical cleft is seen in Figure 22-16. It usually occurs in the female child and consists of a red, raw strip of denuded skin 5–10 mm wide extending from the hyoid bone to just above the suprasternal notch. This superficial defect is accompanied by an underlying thickening and fibrosis of the deeper layers of the skin and subcutaneous tissue forming a fibrous cord which causes some flexion and is made prominent by extending the neck. There is often a skin tab at the upper end of the cleft.

The probable *embryologic* explanation of the defect is a failure of completion of the fusion of the branchial arches in the midline. This concept of origin[13] of the typical lesion also explains some of the unusual variations: a cord without a cleft;[29] a midline mandibular spur or underdeveloped mandible;[1] bony cyst in the central portion of the mandible;[31] cleft of the lower lip and tongue,[21] and absence of the hyoid bone and thyroid cartilage.[8]

Although at one time this defect was considered possibly to be due to an unroofed thyroglossal tract,[14] this explanation is not tenable as the above accompanying defects indicate. Also, no deeply penetrating sinus tract accompanies this condition. There is, however, one report[20] which suggests the probability of the coexistence of the two conditions.

The *surgical treatment* is excision of the defect and all of the underlying fibrotic tissue with a Z-plasty.[12] A double Z-plasty (Fig. 22-17) rather than a single one gives a better plastic result in most hands. The horizontal portions of the scars usually remain thin, but the oblique component of the Z may spread. The *results* are quite satisfactory.

REFERENCES

1. Barsky, A.J.: *Plastic Surgery* (Philadelphia:W.B. Saunders Company, 1938), p. 275.
2. Bhandarkar, S.D., *et al.*: Elongated banana-shaped thyroid, Arch. Surg. 93:654, 1966.
3. Bochetto, J.F.; Montoya, A., and Sunde, E. A.: Papillary carcinoma of the thyroid in thyroglossal duct cysts, Am. J. Surg. 104:773, 1962.
4. Brown, P.M., and Judd, E.S.: Thyroglossal cysts and sinuses: Results of radical (Sistrunk) operation, Am. J. Surg. 102:494, 1961.
5. Brown, P.M., and Judd, E.S.: Thyroglossal cysts and sinuses in children: Results of the Sistrunk operation, Minnesota Med. 44:516, 1961.
6. Clawson, J.: Papillary adenocarcinoma of the thyroglossal duct cyst, Arizona Med. 19:80, 1962.
7. Cooper, T.V.: Case of aberrant thyroid tissue in trachea, J. Clin. Path. 3:48, 1950.
8. Davis, A.D.: Medical cleft of the lower lip and mandible, a case report, Plast. & Reconstruct. Surg. 6:62, 1950.
9. Dische, S., and Berg, P.K.: An investigation of the thyroglossal tract using the radio-isotope scan, Clin. Radiol. 14:298, 1963.
10. Earley, C.M.: Hashimoto's disease (struma lymphomatosa) occurring in a thyroglossal duct cyst, Am. J. Surg. 101:819, 1961.
11. Gerard-Marchant, R.: Thyroid follicle inclusions in cervical lymph nodes, Arch. Path. 77:633, 1964.
12. Gottlieb, E., and Lewin, M.L.: Congenital midline cervical cysts of the neck, New York J. Med. 66:712, 1966.
13. Gross, R.E.: *The Surgery of Infancy and Childhood* (Philadelphia: W.B. Saunders Company, 1953), p. 954.
14. Gross, R.E., and Connerly, M.L.: Thyroglossal cysts and sinuses, New England J. Med. 223:616, 1940.
15. Gurieb, S.R., and Vieta, L.J.: Carcinoma in thyroglossal duct cysts, Arch. Otolaryng. 77:633, 1964.
16. Hathaway, B.M.: Innocuous accessory thyroid nodules, Arch. Surg. 90:222, 1965.
17. Hill, D.P.: Papillary carcinoma arising in thyroglossal tract, Canad. M. A. J. 85:791, 1961.
18. Javert, C.T.: Observations on the pathology and spread of endometriosis based on the theory of benign metastasis, Am. J. Obst. & Gynec. 62:477, 1951.
19. Lewison, M.D., and Lum, D.T.: Apnea in the supine position as an alerting symptom of a tumor at the base of the tongue in small infants, J. Pediat. 66:1092, 1965.
20. Maneshka, R.J.: Congenital midline cervical cleft with a possible thyroglossal duct cyst, Brit. J. Plast. Surg. 14:32, 1961.
21. Morton, C.B., and Jordan, H.E.: Median clefts of lower lip and mandible, cleft sternum and absence of basihyoid, Arch. Surg. 30:647, 1935.
22. Nicastri, A.D.; Foote, F.W., and Frazell, E.L.: Benign thyroid inclusions in cervical lymph nodes, J.A.M.A. 194: 113, 1965.
23. Pollock, W.F., and Stevenson, E.O.: Cysts and sinuses of the thyroglossal duct, Am. J. Surg. 112:225, 1966.
24. Potts, W.J.: *The Surgeon and the Child* (Philadelphia: W.B. Saunders Company, 1959), p. 48.
25. Quigley, W.F.; Williams, L.F., and Hughes, C.W.: Surgical management of subhyoid median atopic thyroid, Ann. Surg. 155:305, 1962.
26. Sistrunk, W.E.: The surgical treatment of cysts of the thyroglossal tract, Ann. Surg. 71:121, 1920.
27. Snedecor, P.A., and Groshong, L.E.: Carcinoma of the thyroglossal duct, Surgery 58:969, 1965.
28. Tanaka, K., and Civia, W.H.: Cancer arising in thyroglossal duct remnant, Arch. Surg. 86:466, 1963.
29. Van Duyn, J.: Congenital midline cervical cord with report of a case and a note on the etiology of congenital torticollis, Plast. & Reconstruct. Surg. 31:576, 1963.
30. Wozencraft, P.; Foote, F.W., and Frazell, E.L.: Occult carcinomas of the thyroid: Their bearing on the concept of lateral aberrant thyroid cancer, Cancer 1:574, 1948.
31. Wyn-Williams, J.D.: Congenital midline cervical cord and web, Brit. J. Plast. Surg. 5:87, 1952.

W. H. SNYDER, JR.
W. F. POLLOCK

Drawings by
DENIS D. DYKES

23

Torticollis

HISTORY. — Torticollis as a deformity was first mentioned by Plutarch in describing Alexander the Great, but the diagnosis is in doubt.[27] Antyllus may have performed tenotomies in about 350 A.D., but the first authentic division of the sternocleidomastoid was done by Isaac Minnius in Amsterdam about 1641.[32] A sternocleidomastoid tumor was first described by Heusinger[12] in 1826, and torticollis was a subject of interest to Dupuytren[8] and many of the German surgeons of the 19th Century.[7,15,18,22,26,28,30,34–36]

There are many causes of torticollis in childhood, for example, cervical hemivertebrae, cervical adenitis, acute fasciitis, abnormal position in utero, and imbalance of the ocular muscles, but the commonest type of torticollis in pediatric practice is the result of fibrosis in the sternocleidomastoid muscle.

Eight theories have been put forward to explain this condition,[1,9,15,18,19,21,24,28,30,33,35] but none is completely satisfactory. All one can say is that the condition is probably an idiopathic intrauterine embryopathy,[16] which merely reveals our ignorance.

Pathology

The basic abnormality is endomysial fibrosis, the deposition of collagen and fibroblasts around individual muscle fibers which undergo atrophy. The sarcoplasmic nuclei are compacted to form "muscle giant cells" which appear to be multinucleated though not necessarily large (Fig. 23-1). Macrophages containing hemosiderin are rarely present.

The severity and distribution of the fibrosis differ widely from patient to patient and from one fascicle to another. In some cases (2–3%) it is obviously bilateral, and in an additional number this is suspected but not easily proved. The fibrosis is always more extensive than the clinical findings indicate, and can be shown to affect the whole length of the muscle even when clinically there is an apparently localized "tumor."[16]

The remarkably mature fibrous tissue in material from neonates strongly suggests that the disease begins well before birth and is probably the cause, not the result, of obstetric difficulties. The reported incidence of breech delivery varies from series to series, but is about 20%, seven times the "normal" incidence, which suggests that the fibrosis may affect the position of the fetus in utero and perhaps prevent normal engagement of the head in the maternal pelvis.

The histologic picture at different ages varies only a little. In those with a tumor, the fibroblasts are more plump, with a mild infiltrate of small round cells; the areas most severely affected are indistinguishable from tendon.

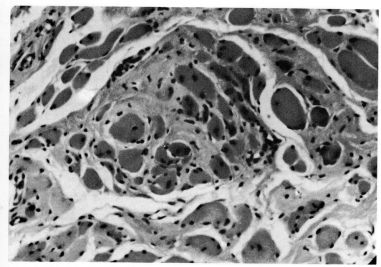

Fig. 23-1. — Specimen from the center of the large persistent tumor in a 9-month-old boy. Note decreased size of muscle fibers undergoing atrophy, some becoming giant cells. The laminae of collagen are thicker than usual.

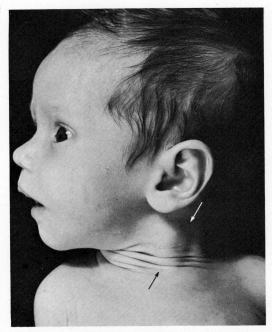

Fig. 23-2.—A tumor affecting both heads of the left sterno-cleidomastoid of a 3-week-old infant. Note the rotation toward the opposite side and absence of angulation. The tumor is more prominent than usual because of loss of subcutaneous fat associated with pyloric stenosis.

In older children, there is some additional interfascicular fibrosis, and little or no infiltration of round cells. Degenerating muscle fibers can be seen at all ages and are probably a form of disuse atrophy produced by limitation of movement by the fibrosis.

The sternal and clavicular portions are affected with almost equal frequency, and although either may be predominantly affected, there is usually more fibrosis in the sternal head.

Clinical Picture

In a prospective series of 100 infants with sternomastoid fibrosis,[16] 66% had a "tumor" in the muscle. In the other 34%, there was fibrosis but no tumor, which would help to explain why only a few of the older children with torticollis have a history of a tumor in the neonatal period (6–20%).

IN INFANTS.—The tumor is a hard, spindle-shaped, painless, discrete swelling 1–3 cm in diameter within the substance of the muscle. It develops some 14–21 days after birth and occurs in about 0.4% of all births, as found in a prospective study.[4] Torticollis is not always present;[16] in the neonate there may be little or no inclination of the head to the side; more often there is pure rotation of the head and face to the side opposite the tumor (Fig. 23-2). The tumor subsequently becomes less discrete and more obviously oc-

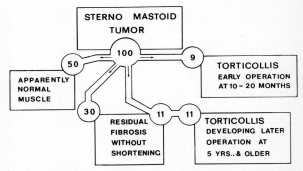

Fig. 23-3.—The outcome in 100 infants with a sternomastoid tumor. These are interim figures, for although the oldest is now 12, the average length of follow-up is 5 years.

cupies the whole length of the muscle which is much thicker than normal.

The natural history of the tumor has been determined by a follow-up of 100 infants[16] (Fig. 23-3). In half of them, the muscle became completely normal clinically by the age of 6 months, without any residual fibrosis detectable by synchronous palpation of both muscles. In another 30%, some fibrosis was still palpable at 12 months of age, but not sufficient to cause torticollis, which may not develop until later, e.g., at 5–10 years of age.

In a few cases (9%), the tumor persisted throughout the first year of life, or even grew steadily larger, to produce torticollis at the age of 9–15 months.

In 2–3% of cases there was a tumor in each sternocleidomastoid, though one of them usually appears earlier, lasts longer and dominates the clinical picture.

In infants with fibrosis but no tumor (34%), torticollis was the presenting symptom. The muscle was uniformly fibrous throughout, part or all of it forming a tight band. The outcome and the clinical categories (Fig. 23-4) are much the same as in those with a tumor, though fewer required early surgery.

Fig. 23-4.—The outcome in 34 infants with fibrotic muscle but no tumor. One infant died of cerebral birth injuries at 3 weeks of age.

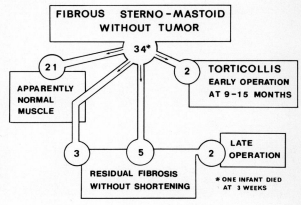

IN OLDER CHILDREN.—Torticollis may develop at any age, and its appearance probably depends on three factors: the severity and the distribution of the fibrosis, and the individual pattern of growth in the particular patient, for example, a sustained spurt in growth at any age may lead to the development of torticollis. In most of the children first seen at 5–10 years of age, fibrous muscular torticollis develops without any known preliminary signs, but in the light of prospective studies it is likely that latent fibrosis was present and that the fibrosis was congenital, regardless of the age at which the torticollis appeared. Because of its slow development and the delay in recognition by parents, secondary effects are usually well established by the time the child is presented for examination, whereas in some infants, these effects develop while under observation, as during follow-up of infants with a sternomastoid tumor.

Secondary Effects

Torticollis in early infancy is manifested by rotation of the head toward the opposite side. If this persists for the first 3 months of life and the infant is permitted to lie in this habitual position, the cranium becomes deformed (Fig. 23-5) by gravitational forces which produce a type of craniofacial asymmetry called plagiocephaly (Fig. 23-6).

PLAGIOCEPHALY.—Plagiocephaly affects all four quadrants of the cranium, and when the flat frontal area is on the same side as the fibrotic muscle, the plagiocephaly is said to be concordant. In children

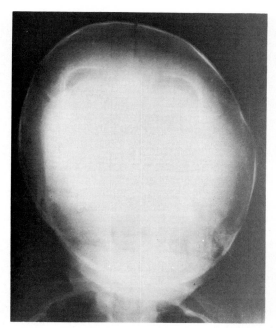

Fig. 23-6.—Radiographic plagiocephaly; a posteroanterior film taken with head fully flexed and beam directed 30 degrees below the horizontal plane.

Fig. 23-5.—The development and nature of one isomer of plagiocephaly. The *interrupted line* indicates the basic symmetrical shape of the cranium as seen from the vertex. *AA*, the normal sagittal axis; *SS*, the surface on which the head rests, with rotation toward the left. The *solid line* depicts the plagiocephaly, and *BB* the new axis of the longest diameter. The right frontal area is flattened; the right ear is situated more posteriorly than the left ear (*line of circles*) which becomes curled forward during rotation. When viewed from in front at *X*, the right half of the face (*R*) appears wider than the left (*L*). The right sternocleidomastoid was fibrotic and the resulting deformity concordant.

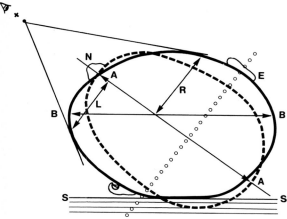

who have plagiocephaly at birth, it may or may not be concordant with the affected muscle.[16]

Plagiocephaly may be accompanied by an apparent increase of width of one half of the face (Fig. 23-5) which may be confused with hemihypoplasia (Fig. 23-7) unless it is appreciated that in plagiocephalic asymmetry of the face, there is no diminution of the orbitomental distance, but rather a wider half on the flattened side (Fig. 23-5). Having been slowly progressive until the infant is 4–5 months old, plagiocephaly is halted when the infant can sit up, and slowly returns toward normal in the next 2 years but may never completely disappear.[5]

FACIAL HEMIHYPOPLASIA.—This form of asymmetry of the face is not confined to individuals with sternocleidomastoid fibrosis, for it also occurs with torticollis due to other causes. In infants with marked sternomastoid fibrosis and angulation of the head, it takes about 8 months to develop and the mechanism is unexplained.

Hemihypoplasia (Fig. 23-7) is progressive as long as the torticollis persists, but is halted as soon as the tension in the sternocleidomastoid muscle is relieved by operation. Immediately after surgery, the parents may think that the hemihypoplasia is more noticeable because the head is now erect, enabling a closer comparison of the two halves of the face. After a few weeks it is apparent that it has halted and is beginning to return toward normal, which probably will

ferior, in 2 other patients, but this subsided slowly in the following 2 years.

REFERENCES

1. André, N.: *Orthopaedia*, 1743 (fascimile edition; Philadelphia: J. B. Lippincott Company, 1961), p. 96.
2. Armstrong, D., *et al.*: Torticollis: An analysis of 271 cases, Plast. & Reconstruct. Surg. 35:14, 1965.
3. Brown, J. B., and McDowell, F.: Wry-neck facial distortion prevented by resection of fibrosed sternomastoid muscle in infancy and childhood, Ann. Surg. 131:721, 1950.
4. Coventry, M.B., and Harris, L.E.: Congenital muscular torticollis in infancy, J. Bone & Joint Surg. 41A:815, 1959.
5. Danby, P.M.: Plagiocephaly in some 10-year old children, Arch. Dis. Childhood 37:500, 1962.
6. Dickson, J.A.: The treatment of torticollis, S. Clin. North America 17:1349, 1937.
7. Dieffenbach, J.F.: *Über die Durchschneidung der Sehnen Muskeln* (Berlin: 1841).
8. Dupuytren: Leçons orales de clinique chirurgicale (Paris: J. B. Bailière et fils, 1839).
9. Golding-Bird, C.H.: Congenital wry-neck (caput obstipum congenitale: torticollis congenitalis), with remarks on facial hemi-atrophy, Guy's Hosp. Rep. 162:253, 1890.
10. Gruhn, J., and Hurwitt, E.S.: Fibrous sternomastoid tumor of infancy, Paediatrics 8:522, 1951.
11. Hellstadius, A.: Torticollis congenita, Acta chir. scandinav. 62:586, 1927.
12. Heusinger, K.P.: Berichte von der königlichen anthropotomischen Anstalt zur Würtzburg, Ber. f. d. Schuljahr 1824/25 (Etlinger, Würtzburg) 4:42, 1826.
13. Holloway, L.W.: Caput obstipum congenitum, South. M. J. 24:597, 1931.
14. Hulbert, K.P.: Congenital torticollis, J. Bone & Joint Surg. 23B:50, 1950.
15. Joachimsthal: Cited by Lidge *et al.*[20]
16. Jones, P.G.: *Torticollis in Infancy and Childhood* (Springfield, Ill.: Charles C Thomas, Publisher, 1967).
17. Kiesewetter, W.B., *et al.*: Neonatal torticollis, J.A.M.A. 157:1281, 1955.
18. Krogius, A.: Zur Pathogenese des muskularen Schiefhalses, Acta chir. scandinav. 56:497, 1924.
19. Lange, C.: Zur Behandlung des Schiefhalses, Wchnschr. orthop. Chir. 27:440, 1910.
20. Lidge, R.T.; Bechtol, R.C., and Lambert, C.N.: Congenital muscular torticollis: Etiology and pathology, J. Bone & Joint Surg. 39A:1165, 1957.
21. Middleton, D.S.: The pathology of congenital torticollis, Brit. J. Surg. 18:188, 1930.
22. Mikulicz, J.: Über die Exstirpation des Kopfnickers beim muskularen Schiefhals neben Bemerkungen zur Pathologic dieses Leidens, Zentralbl. Chir. 1:9, 1895.
23. Moseley, T.M.: Treatment of facial distortion due to wry-neck in infants by complete resection of the sternomastoid muscle, Am. Surgeon 28:698, 1962.
24. Nové-Josserand, and Viannay, C.: Pathogenie du torticollis congenital, Rev. orthop. 7:397, 1906.
25. Oribasius: Cited by Lidge *et al.*[20]
26. Petersen, F.: Zur Frage des Kopfnickerhamatoms bei Neugeborenen, Zentralbel. Gynäk. 10:777, 1886.
27. Plutarch: *Parallel Lives* (Loeb Classical Library) (London: William Heinemann, Ltd., 1958), vol. 7, p. 230.
28. Schubert, A.: Die Ursachen der angeborenen Schiefhalserkrankung, Deutsche Ztschr. Chir. 167:32, 1921.
29. Soeur, R.: Treatment of congenital torticollis, J. Bone & Joint Surg. 38:35, 1940.
30. Stromeyer, G.F.L.: *Beiträge zur operativen Orthopädik oder Erfahrungen über die subcutane Durchschneidung verkürzter Muskeln und deren Sehnen* (Hannover: Helwig, 1838).
31. Tubby, A.H.: *Deformities* (2nd ed.; London: Macmillan Company, 1912), vol. 1, p. 56.
32. Tulp, N.: *Observationes Medicae* (Amsterdam: 1671).
33. Van Roonhuyze, H.: *Encyclopedie Méthodique: Partie Chirurgicale* (1670), vol. II.
34. Völcker, F.: Das Caput obstipum—eine intrauterine Belastungsdeformität, Beitr. klin. Chir. 33:1, 1902.
35. Volkmann, R.: Das Sogenannte angeborene Caput Obstipum und die offene Durchschneidung des M. Sternocleidomastoids, Zentralbl. Chir. 12:233, 1885.
36. Witzel, O.: Beiträge zur Kentniss der secundären Veränderung beim muskularen Schiefhals, Deutsche Ztschr. Chir. 18:534, 1883.

P. G. JONES

24

Tracheostomy

HISTORY.—Tracheostomy, one of the oldest operations known, is primarily a surgical procedure for the establishment of an airway in cases of anoxia due to respiratory obstruction. Secondarily, it provides direct access to the trachea and bronchi for aspiration of retained secretions, or for introduction of a tube to facilitate artificial respiration with a mechanical respirator. Until recently, a tracheostomy was usually considered a last-minute emergency procedure and carried with it a certain aura of desperation. Many factors have combined to change the status of the procedure. Mortality has been lessened by early operation before anoxia has caused irreversible cerebral damage. Chemotherapy and antibiotics play a significant role in eliminating the dangers of fascial plane infections of the neck and anterior mediastinum as well as in healing the illness which necessitated the tracheostomy. Probably it has been the improvement in postoperative care that has been the most significant element contributing to the acceptance of tracheostomy as a clinical therapeutic procedure.

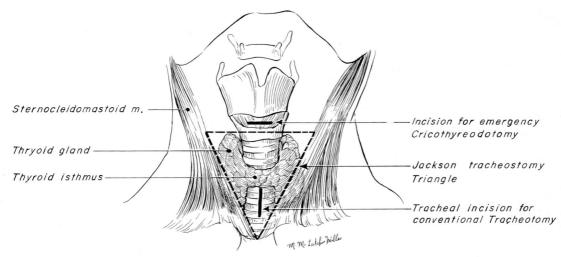

Fig. 24—1.—Anterior view of the neck. Jackson's tracheostomy triangle is outlined, as well as the correct position of the conventional tracheostomy incision and the site of incision for an emergency cricothyroidotomy.

Anatomy

Unless displaced by pathology, the cervical trachea lies in the midline of the neck (Fig. 24-1). Its length is approximately 1½ in. (4 cm) in a 3- to 5-year-old child, 2¼ in. (6 cm) in an 8- to 10-year-old child and 2¾ in. (7 cm) in the adult.[20] These figures vary considerably, particularly in short, heavy individuals in whom occasionally the cricoid cartilage is found to rest almost within the suprasternal notch. In infants, the cartilages of the trachea as well as of the larynx are soft and collapsible, whereas in children

Fig. 24–2.—Lateral view of the neck. Position of the cricothyroid trocar and preferred conventional tracheostomy are shown.

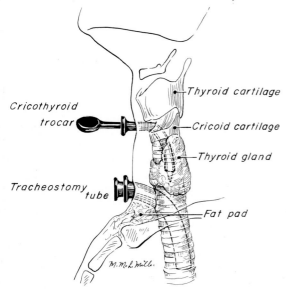

they are more rigid and easily palpated. Covering the trachea are the skin, superficial fascia, linea alba between the pretracheal muscles and the pretracheal fascia. The thyroid isthmus crosses the trachea at varying levels, usually the second to fourth rings. Posterolaterally in the gutter between the trachea and the esophagus, the recurrent laryngeal nerves course upward to enter the larynx. The signet ring-shaped cricoid cartilage, the only complete cartilaginous ring in the airway, is the structure most important in maintaining the patency of the airway. It lies at the level of the third cervical vertebra in infants and gradually descends in the neck, together with the larynx, so that at puberty it lies at the level of the fifth or sixth cervical vertebra.[15] The easily palpated space between the cricoid and thyroid cartilages is the point in the neck of closest approximation between the skin and the airway (Fig. 24-2). Only skin, superficial fascia and cricothyroid membrane cover the airway at this point. In infants, a pretracheal fat pad is generally present, particularly in the suprasternal notch. This is of considerable significance in the performance of a tracheostomy since it may contain blood vessels, particularly inferior to the thyroid isthmus.

Indications for Tracheostomy

GENERAL INDICTIONS.—The primary indication for tracheostomy is progressive respiratory obstruction. Symptoms may be insidious and gradual in their progression, as in the obstruction caused by the slow growth of laryngeal papilloma, or they may be dramatically sudden, as may occur with blockage of the airway on aspiration of a foreign body. A croupy cough, hoarseness, stridor and finally aphonia are the vocal symptoms suggestive of increasing laryngeal obstruction. Restlessness, a rise in the respiratory rate, increasing use of the accessory muscles of respiration and indrawing of the suprasternal notch, intercostal spaces and epigastrium are respiratory signs of obstruction. Anoxia develops when these compensatory efforts fail to provide needed air exchange through the closing airway. The respiratory decompensation that follows is characterized by circumoral pallor and cyanosis, cyanosis of the finger tips and mental hyperirritability progressing to irrational, uncontrollable behavior. Finally, an ashy gray, cyanotic pallor may precede death if the obstruction is unrelieved. Fatigue increases the rapidity of advance of the symptoms and is often the deciding factor in the performance of the operation.[13]

A second indication for tracheostomy is to provide direct access to the airway for frequent aspiration of retained secretions. This has received widest recognition in postpoliomyelitic secretion retention but now is recognized as an important adjunct in the management of such conditions as tetanus, encephalitis, thoracic or brain injury, pharyngeal paralyses, as well as for postoperative bronchial fluid retention, bronchitis and atelectasis.

A third indication for tracheostomy is to permit direct access to the airway to introduce a tube for mechanical respiration. Although such a tube can be inserted through the mouth and through the larynx, prolonged intralaryngeal intubation results in laryngeal trauma and may be followed by chronic laryngeal stenosis. A tracheostomy should be performed if it appears that the indwelling tube must be maintained more than 24 hours; if the intubation is in an infant whose larynx is so small that edema produced by the tube will necessitate a tracheostomy on attempted extubation, the tracheostomy had best be done at once.

SPECIFIC INDICATIONS.—Specific indications for tracheostomy are described according to the respiratory tract lesions themselves.

Congenital malformations.—An increasing number of infants under 1 year of age has been shown to require a tracheostomy because of congenital laryngeal malformations, such as supraglottic fusion, true laryngeal webs, laryngeal cysts, thickening of the glottic and subglottic structures due to deformity of the cricoid cartilage, congenital limitation of vocal cord movements and vocal cord paralysis. Infants with these congenital anomalies may show symptoms of pharyngeal or laryngeal obstruction immediately after birth, and tracheostomy may be required within the first minutes of life. In laryngeal paralysis, the tracheal tube may have to be maintained until such time as the infant develops sufficiently to permit corrective external surgical procedures.

Of increasing importance in modern surgery with its improved techniques is the postoperative tracheostomy required following surgical correction of extensive anomalies not necessarily associated with the respiratory tract. Many of these corrective surgical procedures were not attempted even a relatively few years ago. Operations for esophageal atresia with or without tracheoesophageal fistula, vascular rings, heart disease with abnormalities of the great vessels, enlarged heart with compression of the trachea and prolonged neurosurgical procedures may require a tracheostomy at the completion of the procedure to avoid pulmonary complications during postoperative care.

Inflammatory diseases.—Inflammatory diseases are responsible for most of the obstructing lesions necessitating tracheostomy in older infants and children. Most frequently the disease is acute laryngotracheobronchitis, but laryngeal diphtheria must always be considered, particularly in nonimmunized individuals or populations. Often *Staphylococcus aureus* alone or in combination with other organisms such as *Neisseria catarrhalis, Streptococcus pyogenes* and *Escherichia coli* may be the responsible organisms. The need for tracheostomy in acute laryngotracheobronchitis has definitely decreased with the advent of chemotherapy and antibiotics.[4] The tracheal tube must be in place until the inflammation has subsided, usually 10–30 days, unless some complication makes extubation difficult.

Another indication for tracheostomy in the acute infections is respiratory obstruction in such conditions as poliomyelitis and tetanus.[11] Tracheostomy in bulbar poliomyelitis is of great importance because of hypersecretion of the pharyngeal, tracheal and bronchial mucosa, the weak and ineffective cough, the inability to swallow, the laryngeal obstruction of bilateral vocal cord paralysis and the increase of respiratory embarrassment with general anoxia. Early tracheostomy is indicated in cases of progressive paralysis.

Neoplasms.—The commonest of the benign tumors necessitating tracheostomy in infants and children are laryngeal papillomas. These warty growths are most prolific on the cords themselves. They may cause severe or total obstruction and recur frequently even after the most thorough removal. Other benign tumors within the larynx (fibroangioma, fibroma, hemangioma, lymphangioma, neurofibroma) are occasionally responsible for airway obstruction. External compression of the larynx or trachea by thyroid or mediastinal tumors may necessitate a tracheostomy. Malignant tumors of the larynx and neck of infants and children are very rare. Most of such lesions are sarcomas (fibrosarcoma, rhabdomyosarcoma). Carcinomas of the larynx in infants and children are almost nonexistent.

Miscellaneous indications.—Seldom is tracheostomy necessary in the case of a foreign body in the respiratory tract, although if the object has been present for a long time and has caused remarkable inflammation, or if there has been trauma of the larynx associated with its removal, a tracheostomy may be required. A large foreign body in the esophagus or a retropharyngeal or mediastinal abscess caused by a foreign body may produce severe tracheal pressure necessitating a tracheostomy before the object can be removed esophagoscopically or the abscess drained. Other indications are prolonged coma in skull fractures or barbiturate poisoning, laryngeal edema following burns, particularly flash burns, edema due to an insect bite or an allergy, or external laryngeal trauma.

Technique of Tracheostomy

In *extreme emergency*, the simplest means of opening the airway is to palpate and incise the cricothyroid membrane which lies between the cricoid ring and the inferior border of the thyroid cartilage.[17] In this operation, a knife, scissors or razor blade is used to cut the skin and cricothyroid membrane at right angles to the tracheal axis immediately above the cricoid cartilage. The incising instrument is then twisted to separate the thyroid and cricoid cartilages to open the air passage (Fig. 24-2). Recently, a number of instruments resembling trocars have been described which are designed to facilitate this type of emergency procedure. The immediate danger associated with this technique is the possibility of perforation of the posterior tracheal wall, penetration into the anterior mediastinum or puncture of the pleural cavity with the resultant pneumothorax. Obviously, the smaller the child or infant, the greater is the danger because of the difficulty in locating the trachea owing not only to its small size but also to its flaccidity. These procedures with scalpel or trocar, while life-saving in many cases, should be avoided if possible because of the danger of destroying the all-important cricoid cartilage either at the time of the operation or through infection later. Therefore, whenever this procedure must be used in an emergency, a low tracheostomy should be performed as soon after the cricothyroidotomy as the patient's condition permits.

The conventional tracheostomy is performed under local anesthesia, but if an airway is established with an intratracheal tube or a bronchoscope, general anesthesia may be employed if preferred. The insertion of a bronchoscope or intratracheal tube is also an

TABLE 24-1.—SIZES OF TRACHEOSTOMY TUBES
FOR INFANTS AND CHILDREN

AGE	SIZE OF TUBE FOR ROUTINE TRACHEOSTOMY	SIZE OF TUBE IF RESPIRATOR IS NEEDED
Newborn	00	00-0
6 months	00-0	0-1
12 months	0	1
18 months	0-1	1-2
2 years	1	1-2
3 years	1-2	2
4 years	2	2-3
5-7 years	2-3	3-4
8-12 years	3-4	4-5

invaluable aid in converting an emergency tracheostomy into a tranquil or routine surgical procedure. Although this technique may not be necessary in older children, it is particularly advantageous in infants in whom it is often difficult to locate the collapsible trachea. The standard technique consists of a midline incision in the center of Jackson's tracheostomy triangle[13] (base, the cricoid cartilage; apex, the suprasternal notch; lateral borders, the sternocleidomastoid muscles, as shown in Figure 24-1). A collar incision is an alternative, although there is a little difference between the two in the final scar. The dissection is carried downward in the midline through the fascial planes to the thyroid isthmus. The trachea may be exposed above or below the isthmus or the isthmus may be clamped, ligated and cut and the trachea exposed under it. A tracheal or a thyroid hook is used to grasp the trachea, and the second to fourth rings are incised. The edges of the tracheal incision are then separated with a Trousseau dilator or hemostat and the proper tube inserted (Table 24-1). An infant tracheostomy tube (Fig. 24-3) with a small plate which is rigidly attached to the outer tube at a special 65-degree angle between plate and tube serves best for newborns and small infants.[12] In older infants and children the size, shape and length of tube varies. A correct fit must be obtained (Fig. 24-4). The skin incision is sutured loosely. The edges near

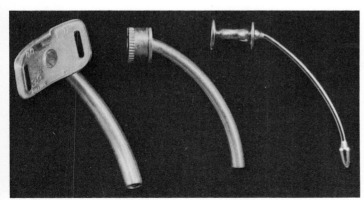

Fig. 24 –3.—Shallow curved infant tracheostomy tubes designed for use in newborn infants and small children.

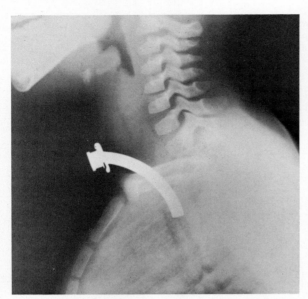

Fig. 24—4.—Lateral roentgen view of the neck, showing correct position of tracheostomy tube in a child with severe obstructing laryngeal edema.

the tube are left open to permit drainage and to eliminate the complications of subcutaneous emphysema which may occur if the skin edges are approximated up to the tube. The tracheal tube is held in place with a twill tape bound around the neck, kept tight enough to prevent the lower end of the tube from coming out of the trachea as the tissues swell or the patient moves.

The plastic tubes[8] developed to replace metal tracheostomy tubes are an effective addition to tracheostomy instrumentarium. The nonadherence of mucus to the surface of some types of tubes makes it possible to eliminate the inner tube. This is desirable in infants because it increases the ventilatory diameter of the tube. However, the disadvantages are that some become soft and easily compressible with use or with resterilization, and occasionally the tube itself does become obstructed with viscid secretions, creating an emergency which can be handled only by complete tube change.

Postoperative Care

The most critical time for infants is after tracheostomy. Constant observation, care and judgment are necessary. Placing the patient in a high-humidity vapor room or humidified tent with temperatures maintained at 70–75 F and humidity above 90% is of the greatest importance. These are the most effective means of combating obstruction due to tenacious bronchial mucopus which has caused many deaths after tracheostomy by plugging the tube and airways.

If necessary, oxygen is added. Special nursing care with an experienced nurse on a 24-hour basis is required in the immediate postoperative period. Repeated catheter aspiration through the tracheostomy tube with an adequate electric suction pump is necessary. The catheter should be provided with a thumb valve to permit intermittent suction. The catheter is passed as far as necessary to reach the secretions and may be directed from side to side into the bronchi by tilting the tube. Three to 5 drops of 0.5 N saline solution are introduced into the tracheostomy tube at half-hour to hourly intervals to liquefy the secretions prior to vigorous catheter suction. Wetting agents to reduce surface tension have been used, but in some cases these appear to cause local irritation and for that reason should be used cautiously. The inner cannula must be removed and cleaned as often as secretions adhere to its walls; the outer surface may be washed with hot water and soap, the inner surface cleaned with a pipe cleaner, rinsed in alcohol and then water before being replaced. After the fourth day, the whole tracheal tube should be changed daily, replacing the tube being worn by a new tube to permit cleaning and sterilization of the outer tube as well. If dyspnea or restlessness persists after tracheostomy, the lower airway may be investigated with a small bronchoscope which may be introduced through the tracheal fistula. Penicillin solution (25,000 units/cc) may be used intratracheally if an infection persists. If the patient's condition necessitates prolonged use of the tracheostomy tube, it is possible to teach the mother of the child to handle the aspirator, clean the inner cannula and the technique of changing the outer tube. After she has had adequate instruction and experience in the hospital under the direction of the nursing personnel, the child may be discharged from the hospital to be controlled as an outpatient.

DECANNULATION.—Extubation is most effectively carried out by using smaller and smaller tubes, finally corking a small tube or using a special decannulating stopper for a test period. Smaller tubes allow a gradual resumption of laryngeal breathing and at the same time reduce the intratracheal obstruction due to the tube itself. Final removal of the tube is done only after a 24-hour test period has been completed with the tube plugged completely. A cosmetic correction of the scar may be carried out later if necessary.

Complications

Complications of tracheostomy per se are uncommon. A serious error in the technique of tracheostomy is making the tracheal incision too high or even cutting the cricoid cartilage. With secondary infection of the cricoid cartilage, laryngeal stenosis and difficult decannulation may follow. On the other hand, if the tracheal incision is made too low, there is danger of ulceration of the anterior wall of the trachea by the tube, erosion of the innominate artery or ulceration of the carina with the formation of granulations on the bifurcation causing an obstruction of the airway below the tracheostomy tube. Pneumothorax also may result from too low a tracheostomy. If the fascial spaces are too widely dissected, air may enter the mediastinum or thorax as the result of severe negative intrathoracic pressure present before the trachea is opened. Similarly, an unusually low incision may be made into the trachea if the head is hyperextended because of the bronchoscope or intratracheal tube inserted to establish the airway. In these circumstances, pneumomediastinum or pneumothorax may occur a few minutes postoperatively as the incised part of the trachea returns below the sternum. This occurs when the bronchoscope or intratracheal tube is removed after the tracheostomy tube is inserted and the head is returned to its normal flexed position.

Gross hemorrhage during the operation or after it may result if anomalies of the great vessels in the neck are present and not recognized during an emergency dissection. Ulceration of the tracheal or carinal mucosa may occur from an improperly fitting tube. Lateral x-rays of the neck and chest with the arms down and back permit the best means of observing the position and fit of a tracheal tube.

Cerebral anoxia may be a complication associated with a tracheostomy if the operation has been delayed too long or if postoperative occlusion of the tube occurs. Hypothermia and the use of agents to reduce cerebral edema are of tremendous advantage in the management of this complication.

Intubation vs. Tracheostomy

The recognized and acceptable use of peroral or nasotracheal intubation to establish an emergency airway is of inestimable value in certain conditions. Laryngoscopes and endotracheal tubes of various sizes and adequate suction facilities have become a permanent part of the instrumentarium of every emergency room, post operative recovery room and intensive care unit. Exposure of the larynx of the unconscious patient requires knowledge and skill to avoid inadvertent intubation or perforation of the hypopharynx or esophagus. This skill can and should be acquired through practice on the cadaver. On the other hand, efforts at intubation of the obstructed larynx of an acutely cyanotic, violently struggling child who is making a desperate, agonal and terminal fight for air, with clenched teeth and maniacal unco-operation, may be contraindicated to avoid loss of time which may better be devoted to a rapid, conventional tracheostomy.

The substitution of nasotracheal or orotracheal intubation as an alternative for tracheostomy for short periods has both enthusiastic advocates[1,5,14,16] and alarmed critics.[2,3,7,9] Advocates stress the relative ease of establishing the airway, the simplicity of introduc-

ing a cuffed endotracheal tube for use with positive pressure respirators, the simplification of extubation and the elimination of such complications as pneumomediastinum, pneumothorax and hemorrhage. Critics point out some of the unfortunate problems associated with or ascribed to intubation: difficulties of maintaining an unobstructed endotracheal tube; the laryngeal complications of hyperemia, edema, ulceration and destruction of the vocal cords, and glottic, subglottic and tracheal stenoses. These admittedly increase in number and severity as recommended or required periods of intubation are increased.

A rational approach with compromise both ways may be considered. Oral intubation and nasal intubation have specific and separate indications and contraindications. Orotracheal intubation is best limited to only temporary 24-hour or less alleviation of obstruction or to provide positive pressure respiratory assistance for the unconscious patient; a large cuff tube may be used which is uncomfortable for the older child but will relieve respiratory deficiency. If, however, the patient is a conscious older child, the ineffective attempts at phonation and the efforts the child makes to remove the tube by oral and lingual manipulation cause sufficient movement of the tube to increase laryngeal trauma. Conversely, nasotracheal intubation to maintain an airway permits use of a smaller diameter (plastic) tube that causes less discomfort and is particularly effective in infants.[21] The airway may be adequately and safely controlled for 5 or 6 days before it is necessary to decide whether tracheostomy is needed or not. The tube is not changed, and every effort is made to eliminate any motion of the tube once it is accurately placed. Thus for temporary alleviation of a noninfectious laryngeal obstruction, for example, following cardiac, neurologic or thoracic surgery, use of a nasotracheal tube may eliminate the need for the additional surgical procedure of tracheostomy. Some even suggest its use for self-limited acute laryngeal obstruction, as occurs in acute epiglottitis; the potential for ulceration in the acute process is, however, great. For the prolonged use of a substitute airway, or if use of positive pressure respiratory apparatus is anticipated, it seems advisable to proceed promptly, or as soon as the patient's condition permits, with the more definitive tracheostomy operation to avoid the laryngeal and tracheal damage which is shown to ensue with long-standing intubation.[6,10] Of interest in this regard is the suggestion that nasotracheal intubation be used to assist in extubating infants who have worn tracheostomies for a period of time and in whom decannulation has apparently been delayed.[18,19]

REFERENCES

1. Allan, T. H., and Steven, I. M.: Prolonged endotracheal intubation in infants and children, Brit. J. Anaesth. 37:566, 1965.
2. Baron, S. H., and Kahlmoos, H. W.: Laryngeal sequelae of

endotracheal anesthesia, Ann. Otol., Rhin. & Laryng. 60:767, 1951.

3. Bergstrom, A., and Orell, S. R.: On the pathogenesis of laryngeal injuries following prolonged intubation, Acta oto-laryng. 55:342, 1962.

4. Bigler, J. A., *et al.*: Tracheotomy in infancy, Pediatrics 13:476, 1954.

5. Conn, A., and Markham, W.: Tracheostomy gets the air, M. World News, p. 105, Oct. 8, 1965.

6. Davenport, H. T.: Management of respiratory obstruction following removal of a tracheostomy tube: A preliminary report of a new technique, Canad. M.A.J. 91:1074, 1964.

7. Fearon, B., *et al.*: Airway problems in children following prolonged endotracheal intubation, Ann. Otol., Rhin. & Laryng. 75:975, 1966.

8. Fischer, N. D., and Hair, G. E.: Tracheostomy tubes of Teflon, Laryngoscope 74:743, 1964.

9. Harrison, G. A., and Tonkin, I. P.: Laryngeal complications of prolonged endotracheal intubation, M. J. Australia 17:709, 1965.

10. Hilding, A. C., and Hilding, J. A.: Tolerance of the respiratory mucous membrane to trauma, Ann. Otol., Rhin. & Laryng. 71:455, 1962.

11. Holinger, P. H., and Johnston, K. C.: Tracheotomy in acute tracheobronchitis and poliomyelitis, Progr. Otol., 1952.

12. Holinger, P. H.: A new infant tracheotomy tube, Ann. Otol., Rhin. & Laryng. 65:239, 1956.

13. Jackson, C., and Jackson, C. L.: *Diseases of the Nose, Throat and Ear* (2nd ed.; Philadelphia: W. B. Saunders Company, 1959).

14. Kuner, J., and Goldman, A.: Prolonged nasotracheal intubation in adults vs. tracheostomy, Dis. Chest 51:270, 1967.

15. Lederer, F. L.: *Diseases of the Ear, Nose and Throat* (6th ed.; Philadelphia: F. A. Davis Company, 1952).

16. McDonald, I. H., and Stocks, J.: Prolonged nasotracheal intubation, Brit. J. Anaesth. 37:161, 1965.

17. Nager, F. R., *et al.*: *Lehrbuch der Hals-Nasen-Ohren-Mundkrankheiten* (Basel: S. Karger AG, 1947).

18. Smith, R. M.: Diagnosis and treatment: Nasotracheal intubation as a substitute for tracheostomy, Pediatrics 38:652, 1966.

19. Smythe, P. M.: The problem of detubating an infant with a tracheostomy, M. Progr. 65:446, 1964.

20. Thomson, St. C.; Negus, V. E., and Batemann, G. H.: *Diseases of the Nose and Throat* (6th ed.; London: Cassell & Co., Ltd., 1955).

21. Way, W. L., and Sooy, F. A.: Histological changes produced by endotracheal intubation, Ann. Otol., Rhin. & Laryng. 74:799, 1965.

P. H. HOLINGER

Drawings by
MURIEL MCLATCHIE MILLER

PART III

The Thorax and Cardiovascular System

PLATE II

A. Congenital Cystic Disease—Left Lower Lobe. Three-and-a-half-year-old child with repeated pulmonary infection. The contrast between the thick-walled scar covering the basal portion of the lobe and the normal upper portion is striking. The diaphragm is at the lower left, just below the lowest of the three white systemic arteries, still undivided, which proceed directly from the aorta to the malformed lobe. These had been demonstrated angiocardiographically. Such systemic arteries may arise from the abdominal aorta and course through the diaphragm. They indicate the congenital nature of cystic disease of the lung and represent a significant operative hazard. There were eight such arteries in all in this patient. Lobectomy was followed by uneventful recovery.

B. Congenital Cystic Disease—Right Lower Lobe. Seven-year-old boy with a lifelong history of repeated severe pulmonary infections, previously diagnosed as bronchiectasis. The entire lobe has been replaced by small and large cysts, lined by a smooth glistening membrane, which histologically showed normal respiratory epithelium. Most of the cysts were filled with a thick glairy mucus, but some also contained air and the roentgenographic films showed multiple fluid levels. Congenital cystic disease causes symptoms usually from repeated infections and occasionally from overdistention of a cyst, particularly in the newborn. Upon diagnosis of the condition, the cyst or lobe should be removed. In this instance, right lower lobectomy was considered curative, for there was no recurrence of symptoms in 14 years.

C. Congenital Deformities of Ribs, Partial Absence of Pectoralis Major, Polythelism. This 12-year-old girl with a complicated defect involving the right portion of the sternum and with deep incurvation of several ribs was successfully treated by multiple osteotomies of the ribs, wedging-out of the incurved segments, and correction of the sternal displacement. The result, 10 years later, was gratifying; the chest wall was smoothly rounded, and on it a small breast has developed. Such bizarre deformities require individually conceived operative procedures. Observation of a number of such patients, over the course of years, who had had no operation, has convinced us that the deformities are progressive and substantial and that they should be anticipated and corrected.

D. Pectus Carinatum, Atypical. Protrusion deformities tend to vary substantially from patient to patient. The depression of the costal cartilages to either side, which is quite conspicuous in this boy, is a fairly constant feature. In him, the sternum is not only prominent, but rotated and there is an extraordinary costochondral prominence on the right. The deformity responded very satisfactorily to staged procedures, involving the resection of the depressed costal cartilages, the excision of chondrosternal prominences and the rotation of the twisted sternum.

E and **F.** Pectus Excavatum, Extreme Form. An 11-year-old girl who has Marfan's disease. Ordinarily we shy away from an operation on the chest deformities of Marfan's disease, but this deformity observed over several years had become progressively more and more embarrassing and disabling. Note the exaggeration of the common asymmetry with the sunken right chest, the rotation of the sternum to the right, and the relative hypoplasia of the right breast. The postoperative view shows the degree of correction which was obtained. The child had an extraordinary increase in vigor and energy and capacity for play and athletics. and a substantial change in personality.

PLATE II

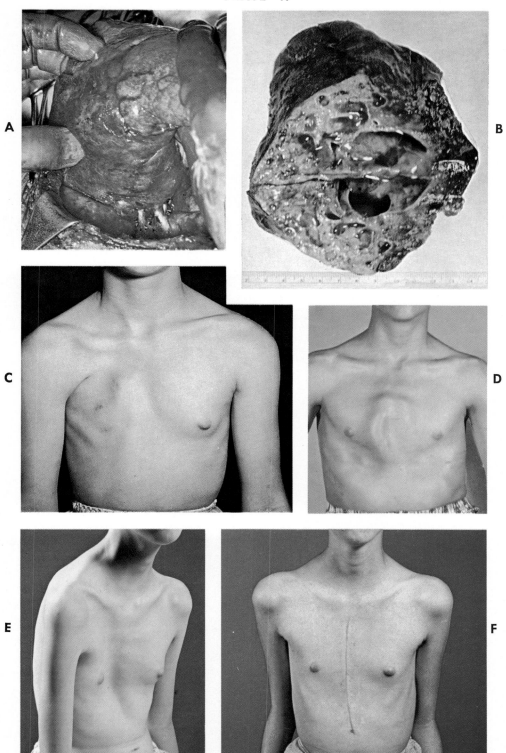

PLATE III

A. Tumor of the Heart. A 5-year-old girl whose heart had been slowly enlarging since infancy demonstrated, on angiocardiography, a filling defect in the left ventricle. A differential diagnosis of tumor of the heart or anomalous origin of the left coronary artery was made. Operation was undertaken, using extracorporeal circulation; and a firm, golf-ball-like tumor was felt in the chamber of the left ventricle, appearing to arise from the anterior surface of the left ventricular wall. At least three quarters of this tumor was excised, and the incision in the left ventricle was carefully sutured. The heart took over well after discontinuance of the extracorporeal circulation. Fatal hemorrhage from the posterior wall of the left ventricle occurred in the recovery room. This photograph, taken in the operating room, shows the tumor being removed; it proved to be an intramural fibroma.

B. Congenital Aortic Stenosis. A boy, aged 12, had limitation of exercise tolerance and a loud aortic systolic murmur, and electrocardiography showed left ventricular strain. With the use of a cardiopulmonary bypass, the aorta was opened, and a markedly stenosed, thickened bicuspid valve was seen. Careful commissurotomies were performed to within 2 mm of the aortic wall on each side, reducing a gradient across the aortic valve of 100 mm to 20 mm One year after operating, the child was asymptomatic, and the electrocardiogram had not reverted to normal.

C. Ventricular Septal Defect. A boy, aged 14, although asymptomatic, had a harsh pansystolic murmur to the left of the sternum, accompanied by a thrill. Cardiac catheter studies revealed a 15% rise in oxygen saturation on passing from the left to the right ventricle and a 35 mm elevation of pressure in the right ventricle. With the use of a cardiopulmonary bypass, the defect, as seen at operation, was closed completely by direct suture; it measured a little over 1 cm in diameter. The patient made an uneventful convalescence and at last examination appeared to be normal, with no evidence of any murmur.

D. Atrial Septal Defect, Secundum Type. A 5-year-old girl who was asymptomatic had a soft-ejection systolic murmur in the pulmonary area, accompanied by a split second sound. A rise in oxygen saturation at atrial level was present on cardiac catheterization, during which no anomalous veins were probed. At operation, hypothermia at a temperature of 30° C was employed, and the atrial septal defect was closed, under direct vision, by a running suture.

E. Transposition of the Great Arteries, Ventricular Septal Defect and Pulmonary Stenosis in a 2 year old. An anastomosis of the superior vena cava to the right pulmonary artery (Glenn procedure) is illustrated. The vena cava is to your left, the end-to-side anastomosis fills the upper and lower branches of the main pulmonary artery; the superior vena cava is ligated at the cavo-atrial junction. The arterial oxygen saturation prior to operation was 53%. Two weeks after operation the arterial oxygen saturation was 77%.

F. Tetralogy of Fallot. A 10-year-old girl, cyanotic since birth, had a catheter-proved diagnosis of tetralogy of Fallot. Open operation for correction was undertaken, employing the artificial heart-lung apparatus. The infundibular area of the right ventricle is seen incised through the pulmonic valve ring to the bifurcation of a small pulmonary artery. The top retractor is at the bifurcation of the pulmonary artery, the retractor on the left exposes the usual large ventricular septal defect with sutures through the inferior margin. The crista supraventricularis is seen to be greatly thickened, as is the wall of the right ventricle. The ventricular septal defect was closed with a teflon patch, and the main pulmonary artery and infundibular of the right ventricle were enlarged with a pericardial prosthesis. The postoperative course, which was uneventful in this case, may be extremely hazardous.

PLATE III

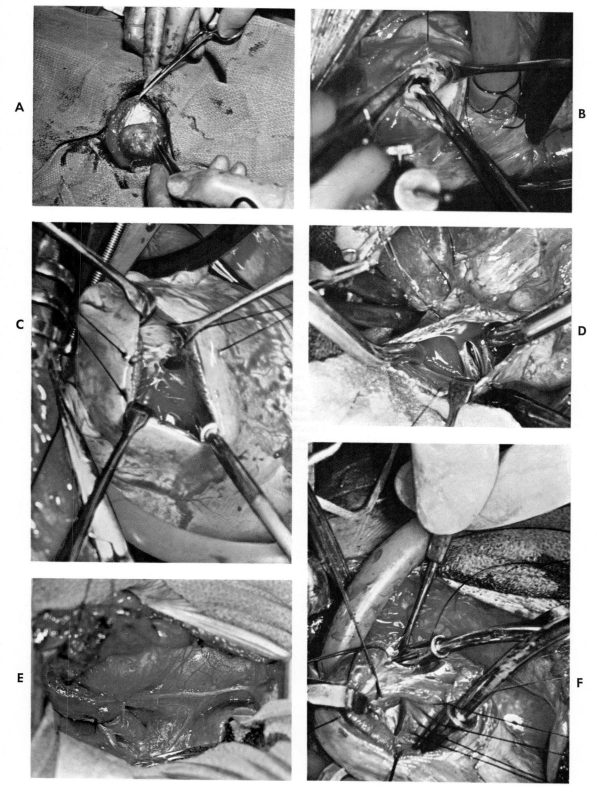

The Breast

Physiologic Considerations

THE BREAST is a modified sweat gland. At birth there is no difference between the sexes. The tiny nipple is surrounded by an inconspicuous areola and usually no breast tissue is palpable underneath. Microscopically, the area beneath the areola, in which there may be palpable an insignificant nodule, contains rudimentary ducts connecting with the nipple, but no acinar development (Fig. 25-1, A). Within a few days of birth, usually at the end of the first week in the majority of infants, a visible swelling of the breast occurs (Fig. 25-4, A), associated with a secretion of milk or colostrum-like fluid, the "witch's milk" of the laity. It may appear from one breast or both and is equally common in infants of either sex. Histologically, this is reflected by hypertrophy and appearance of acini in the duct system (Fig. 25-1, B) and increased vascularity of the stroma. In one way or another, this response is due to the maternal hormones circulating in the infant. It may be due to the mother's estrogen and prolactin still circulating in the infant, or may be due secondarily to the stimulation of hypophyseal activity by the progressive fall of this blood estrogen concentration within the first week of life.

The enlargement of the breasts is frequently accompanied by visible enlargement of the labia and clitoris and, in an occasional instance, by a bloody vaginal discharge.

These changes regress spontaneously as the inciting factors are removed and endocrinologic balance is restored. Breast enlargement and the other manifestations seldom last more than 2 or 3 weeks.

Congenital Anomalies

CONGENITAL ABSENCE OF BREAST OR NIPPLE. — Amastia or athelism occurs occasionally. While it presages a cosmetic problem in females (it is almost invariably unilateral), its chief significance is its frequent association with underlying defects of the chest wall and pectoral musculature. Absence of the pectoralis major, which may also occur independently, is seen with hypoplasia or, more rarely, congenital absence of the breast. Absence of the underlying ribs or costal cartilages is a fairly frequent accompaniment (Fig. 25-2). In such instances there may be total absence of the breast, or merely a decrease in the amount of potential breast tissue so that in females, at puberty, a breast develops on the affected side but is much smaller than the one on the opposite side.

MULTIPLE NIPPLES OR MULTIPLE BREASTS.—Polythelism or polymastia occurs infrequently (Fig. 25-3). Because of the small size of the normal infant breast and even smaller size of the accessory breasts which occur along the embryonic milk line from the axilla to the normal region of the breast, and then down the trunk, in line with the normal breast, the accessory organs are frequently not noticed until puberty or even until pregnancy causes enlargement of the aberrant breast tissue. In childhood, the accessory breast tissue is probably never sufficiently conspicuous to require treatment.

LATERAL DISPLACEMENT OF THE NIPPLES. — Fleisher[2] has seen 7 infants with bilateral renal hypoplasia, in all of whom the nipples were well lateral to the midclavicular line.

MODIFICATIONS OF NORMAL PHYSIOLOGICAL CHANGES

Stimulation of the neonatal secreting breast may cause remarkable hypertrophy which will persist as long as stimulation is continued. The superstition that it is important to remove the witch's milk is responsible for such practice (Fig. 25-4, B).

In girls, the pubertal enlargement of the breasts occurs at a variable period, and at a variable rate, with the onset of puberty, itself variable, anywhere from the age of 9 or 10 to 15 years (Fig. 25-1, D).

In girls at any age before puberty, the breast may respond to the normally present levels of estrogen by

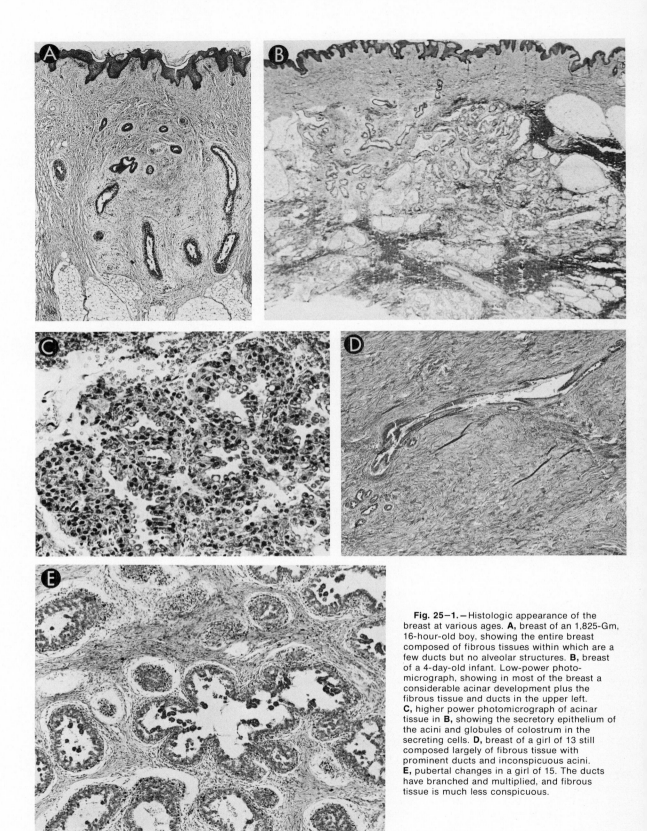

Fig. 25–1.—Histologic appearance of the breast at various ages. **A,** breast of an 1,825-Gm, 16-hour-old boy, showing the entire breast composed of fibrous tissues within which are a few ducts but no alveolar structures. **B,** breast of a 4-day-old infant. Low-power photomicrograph, showing in most of the breast a considerable acinar development plus the fibrous tissue and ducts in the upper left. **C,** higher power photomicrograph of acinar tissue in **B,** showing the secretory epithelium of the acini and globules of colostrum in the secreting cells. **D,** breast of a girl of 13 still composed largely of fibrous tissue with prominent ducts and inconspicuous acini. **E,** pubertal changes in a girl of 15. The ducts have branched and multiplied, and fibrous tissue is much less conspicuous.

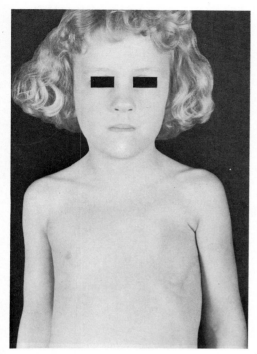

Fig. 25–2.—Congenital absence of the breast (amastia). This child was born without a left breast and nipple, although a faint pigmented area suggests a possible vestige at a point a little lower on the left side than the normal location of a nipple. The conspicuous deformity is due to the frequently associated absence of several ribs and costal cartilages (usually 2nd to 4th) and much of the costal portion of the pectoralis major. The thoracic deformity is susceptible of correction.

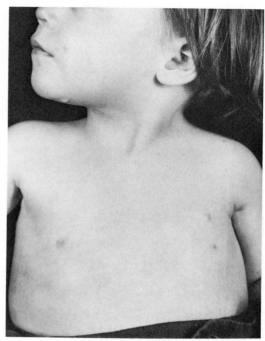

Fig. 25–3.—Polythelism. This child had two well-developed nipples on the left along the course of the embryonic milk line. The supernumerary breast may lactate and, if physically annoying because of proximity to the axilla or cosmetically disfiguring, may be considered for ultimate removal. This patient had a sacral spina bifida and meningocele.

Fig. 25–4.—Neonatal breast hypertrophy. **A,** physiologic hypertrophy in a 12-day-old female with obvious enlargement of the breasts which secreted "witch's milk." The external genitalia were also conspicuously enlarged. This physiologic phenomenon is due to direct stimulation by still-circulating maternal hormones or possibly to temporary stimulation of the pituitary by sudden reduction of the level of these hormones. **B,** exaggerated hypertrophy in a baby of 8 months whose mother constantly milked the breast to express the witch's milk. The more the breasts responded to the mechanical stimulation, the more they were stripped mechanically. The mother could not be persuaded that the condition was self-limited, and manipulation was continued until the child was hospitalized. With application of cold compresses, the breasts soon regressed to normal infantile size.

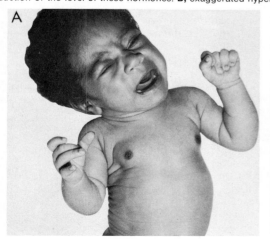

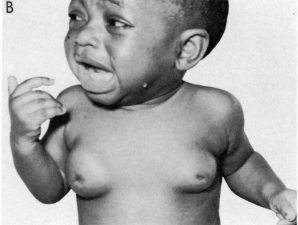

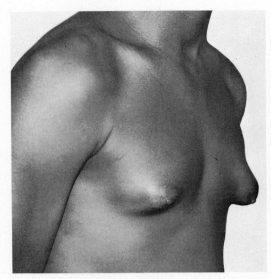

Fig. 25–5.—Pubertal hypertrophy in an adolescent boy. This boy of 11 had normal genital development. Failure of the breasts to diminish in size led to bilateral mastectomy through a subareolar excision. Operation is usually not required.

moderate hypertrophy. A small mass of breast tissue may be felt beneath the nipple on one or both sides without any striking enlargement of the breasts as such. This mass of breast tissue may remain for a period of time or in some instances may persist until it merges with the pubertal hypertrophy of the breast.

The breast of adolescent boys may vary from a firm discoid, perhaps tender, subareolar nodule to a substantial and conspicuous swelling (Fig. 25-5). The peak incidence is at 14 years, with a spread from 10 to 16. In their large study, Nydick *et al.*[6] excluded obese boys. The incidence in Negro boys was lower than in white boys. In the 237 unilateral cases, the right breast was involved twice as often as the left. Probable duration of the mammary enlargement was 2 years. There is a positive correlation between size of testes, penis and thyroid and amount of pubic hair and the mammary hypertrophy of puberty. The breast enlargement is transitory (only 7.7% persist for 3 years) and requires neither hormonal nor surgical treatment. Occasional cases of extreme and persistent enlargement may warrant a subcutaneous excision of the breast.

VIRGINAL HYPERTROPHY OF THE FEMALE BREAST.— This occasionally occurs at puberty and results in the rapid development of enormous mammary glands (Fig. 25-6). These girls present no other evidence of endocrine dysfunction, and the lesion is presumably due to an abnormal local response of the breasts to physiologic stimulation. The enlargement may be unilateral. The breasts may be so huge as to be cosmetically disfiguring and physically disabling. The condition

does not reverse itself and no treatment other than operative removal or a plastic partial excision has been satisfactory.

GYNECOMASTIA.—In occasional adolescent males, one breast or both may hypertrophy to produce a breast which looks and feels remarkably like that of a young woman. This occurs in the absence of any other evidence of endocrine dysfunction, and such hypertrophy usually persists. The social embarrassment that results justifies subcutaneous excision of the abnormal breasts.

KLINEFELTER'S SYNDROME.—The syndrome of dysgenesis of the seminiferous tubules is associated with small atrophic testes deficient in spermatogenesis and showing hyalinization of the seminiferous tubules. Gynecomastia frequently occurs in these patients.

The fat boy with Fröhlich's syndrome has fatty breasts which seem more a part of his general adiposity than actual gynecomastia.

PRECOCIOUS PUBERTY

In girls, various lesions causing physiologic aberrations induce the premature onset of puberty with the usual changes in which the breast takes part, sometimes as the most conspicuous feature.

IDIOPATHIC PRECOCIOUS PUBERTY.—In true idiopathic precocious puberty of unknown etiology, all the physiologic changes of puberty take place. Bilateral breast enlargement is generally the first evidence and is followed by menstruation and the appearance of pubic and axillary hair, and is associated with rapid bone growth and advanced bone age leading to early closure of the epiphyses. Such patients can conceive, as in the famous instance of the 5-year-old Peruvian child reported in the newspapers and commented on by Wilkins.[7]

ALBRIGHT'S SYNDROME (POLYOSTOTIC FIBROUS DYSPLASIA).—In this syndrome, all of the changes associated with puberty may occur in early childhood and are accompanied by the appearance of pathognomonic areas of brownish pigmentation of the skin and diffusely distributed osseous lesions. The basic nature of the endocrine disturbance is unidentified. Ovulation does occur, and apparently these patients may grow to maturity.

PRECOCIOUS PUBERTY ASSOCIATED WITH IDENTIFIABLE NEUROENDOCRINE LESIONS.—*Intracranial lesions.*—Various intracranial lesions may manifest themselves by precocious puberty, of which mammary enlargement is frequently the first sign. Midline brain tumors are most characteristically associated with this syndrome, and precocious puberty has been reported with tumors of the pineal body and of the floor of the third ventricle. Most of these tumors are anatomically or pathologically incurable. Inflammatory lesions of the brain—encephalitis, meningitis—have also been held responsible for the appearance of precocious puberty, possibly because of lesions in the same areas of the brain. Neurologic manifestations, such as signs of increased intracranial pressure or of involvement of the hypothalamus—polydipsia, polyuria—are obvious indications in these patients of the cause of the premature enlargement of the breasts.

Ovarian tumors.—A wide variety of ovarian tumors, the most prominent of which is the granulosa cell tumor, may induce premature onset of puberty with accompanying enlargement of the breasts. Chorioepitheliomas, lutein cell tumors and other ovarian tumors can produce essentially the same sequence of events. In the little patient in whom the entire pelvis can be completely explored in the rectal examination, the enlarged ovary provides a ready clue to the cause of the precocious puberty. Removal of the involved ovary brings a rapid reversal of symptoms. The chorioepitheliomas are usually malignant, and the granulosa cell tumors are occasionally malignant.

Adrenal cortical lesions.—The adrenogenital syndrome, whether induced by cortical hyperplasia or by an adrenal cortical tumor, causes early abnormal development of the breasts and genitalia and hirsutism, with or without other cushingoid changes. A therapeutic trial with cortisone may differentiate hyperplasia of the adrenals from adrenal cortical tumor.

Testicular tumors.—Seminomas, chorioepitheliomas and Leydig cell tumors have all been associated with gynecomastia. Treatment is removal of the involved testis.

Liver factors.—Gynecomastia has occasionally been reported in association with juvenile cirrhosis or with severe chronic malnutrition, presumably due to failure of the liver to destroy estrogen, which occurs also in adult male cirrhotics.

INFLAMMATORY LESIONS

In the neonate, the engorged breast appears to be particularly susceptible to infection, which presumably enters directly through the ducts in the nipple. Staphylococcic abscesses are not uncommon and are one of the lesions which occur with a staphylococcic outbreak in the nursery.

The mild infections in the neonatal breast respond to antibiotics and occasionally compresses. Evidence of suppuration is an indication for incision. In an occasional instance, a neglected breast abscess results in a widespread phlegmon of the chest wall, with devastating consequences.

Pubertal or prepubertal enlargement of the breast, frequently painful, is often improperly given the title of pubertal mastitis.

Fig. 25–6.—Virginal hypertrophy of the breast. This girl of 12 for 4 months had noted rapid enlargement of the breasts, more marked on the right, with some pain and tenderness in both. The breasts were engorged and firm and large veins were seen beneath the skin. **A,** the deformity is obvious. She could not wear normal clothing, and operation was undertaken to transplant the nipples and reduce the size of the breasts. In two stage operations, over 2,500 Gm of tissue was removed. The immediate result was very satisfactory. **B,** in a few months the breasts began to enlarge again and it was evident that a repeat mammoplasty would be necessary. This is unusual, but ordinarily a reduction mammoplasty for virginal hypertrophy is not performed as early as age 12.

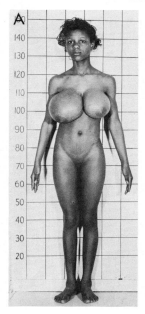

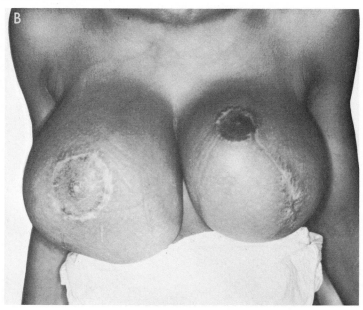

Tumors of the Breast

BENIGN TUMORS.—Tumors of the breast, either benign or malignant, are uncommon in children. There are occasional reports of cysts of the breast. The commonest tumor of the breast in young girls is fibroadenoma, which appears after the onset of puberty. The tumor is benign but in patients of this age group may grow so rapidly and be so large as to suggest, before operation, the possibility that it is malignant. We have seen 2 girls, aged 8 and 10, with bloody nipple discharge due to an intraductal papilloma. Any discrete tumor of the breast should be excised, provided one makes certain that the lesion is not the much more common pubertal mastitis or hypertrophy, which at times produces a firm little mass suggesting a tumor.

MALIGNANT TUMORS.—Carcinoma of the breast has been reported in a small number of children. Herrmann[4] collected 33 cases of breast carcinoma in patients under 20, but only 12 were aged 12 or less, 1 patient was 13 and 1 was 14. Festenstein,[1] reporting a fatal adenocarcinoma of the breast in a Bantu boy of 14, found reports of carcinoma of the breast in 5 boys aged 6, 12, 12, 13 and 14 years 8 months, and in 5 girls, 2 aged 10, 2 aged 11 and 1 aged 12. The number of reported cases has therefore been the same in the two sexes. Although one is inclined to consider cancer of the breast in young women to be more malignant than the same cancer in older women, it is apparent that cancer of the breast in children is less malignant or at least no more malignant than in adults. Of the 12 patients tabulated by Herrmann, 6 at the time of reporting had no evidence of disease, 1 of them 28 years after radical mastectomy at age 4. The patient mentioned by Haagensen[3] had a tumor from the age of 5 which had been under a physician's observation from the time she was 9 until she was 15, with small growth in that period. The tumor was excised locally after this 10-year history and found to be a fairly characteristic carcinoma infiltrating the fat. The patient was well 11 years later. McDivitt and Stewart[5] make a strong case for the relative benignity of breast cancer in children. Their 7 patients, 3–15 years old and all girls, were free from tumor 2–15 years after operation. The tumor recurred in only 1 of 4 treated by local excision; this child had a second local excision and finally a modified radical mastectomy. None of the children had regional or distant metastases. These authors pointed out some of the distinguishing histologic characteristics of cancer of the breast in children.

Sarcoma.—A handful of cases of sarcoma of the breast in young patients has been reported. Herrmann could find only three in patients 12 years of age or under, and all three were reported in the last century. Radical mastectomy is probably advisable.

REFERENCES

1. Festenstein, H.: Adenocarcinoma of the breast in a South African Bantu boy aged 14, South African M.J. 34:517, 1960.
2. Fleisher, D. S., Lateral displacement of the nipples, a sign of bilateral renal hypoplasia, J. Pediat. 69:806, 1966.
3. Haagensen, C. D.: *Diseases of the Breast* (Philadelphia: W. B. Saunders Company, 1956).
4. Herrmann, J. H.: Tumors and other enlargements of the breast, in Ariel, I. M., and Pack, G. T. (ed): *Cancer and Allied Diseases of Infancy and Childhood* (Boston: Little, Brown & Company, 1960), Chap. 7.
5. McDivitt, R. W., and Stewart, F. W.: Breast carcinoma in children, J.A.M.A. 195:388, 1966.
6. Nydick, M., *et al.*: Gynecomastia in adolescent boys, J.A.M.A. 178:449, 1961.
7. Wilkins, L. A.: *The Diagnosis and Treatment of Endocrine Disorders in Childhood and Adolescence* (3d ed.; Springfield, Ill.: Charles C Thomas, Publisher, 1966).

M. M. RAVITCH

26

The Chest Wall

Congenital Deformities of the Chest Wall

DEFORMITIES OF THE thoracic cage are obvious on casual examination and have been known since ancient times. Sporadic attempts to correct some of them in the era of modern elective surgery began in the second decade of this century. The importance to the individual of correction of these defects from the physiologic and orthopedic standpoints as well as the obvious cosmetic and psychologic advantages have only recently been appreciated.

In the past 20 years great interest has been shown in the correction of these deformities, and the surgical principles involved have been well established.

Sternal Clefts

EMBRYOLOGY OF THE STERNUM

In 1919, Hanson[5] published an exhaustive study of the phylogeny and ontogeny of the sternum, and his analysis of the formation of the sternum is generally accepted. The sternum first arises independently of the ribs as two laterally situated sternal bands. These are already present in the 6-week-old embryo. Independent of these, at the cephalad end and in the position of the future manubrium, a single median anterior rudiment develops that is intimately associated with the shoulder girdle. The ventrally growing tips of the ribs gradually approximate the sternal bands, and simultaneously the two sternal bands fuse with each other in the midline. Usually, this fusion is complete by the ninth week of embryonic life. Concurrently, the fused sternal bands unite with the anterior sternal rudiment at their cephalic end. Subsequently, transverse divisions of the cartilaginous sternum result in the differentiation of segmental sternebrae. These lines of division, or sutures, always occur opposite the ends of each pair of ribs, a further indication that the sternum does not grow from the rib elements, as was once thought. Ossification of the sternebrae is an extremely variable process. The centers of ossification regularly appear in the intercostal levels of the sternum, and may either be single and median, or paired. At birth, the sternum is cartilaginous, except for small centers of ossification. Significant sternal marrow spaces are not present until the third year of life, and final ossification of the sternum is usually established by age 14–16 years.

Congenital sternal clefts presumably are the result of a failure of midline fusion of the paired sternal bands. The apparent division of the median anterior sternal rudiment at the cephalic end of the sternum in cases of complete sternal cleft, or of upper sternal cleft, is not explained.

CLINICAL FORMS

COMPLETE FAILURE OF STERNAL FUSION.—This is a rare anomaly. As with the partial defects of sternal fusion, most instances in the past have been reported as cases of ectopia cordis[7,11,16] because of apparent ventral displacement of the heart. Thus instances of failure of fusion of the upper sternum have been reported as cervicothoracic ectopia cordis because of the pulsation in the base of the neck, suggesting cephalad migration of the heart. Clefts of the lower sternum have been reported as thoracoabdominal ectopia cordis because of the apparent caudad migration of the heart. Actually, in these conditions the heart is relatively little displaced except ventrally. The lack of bony covering allows the heart to protrude anterior to the level of the parietes. Cases in which the heart is grotesquely displaced anteriorly, and in which it is not covered by integument, have usually been associated with lethal cardiac malformations, so that no instances of successful correction have been reported. The clefts of the upper sternum suggest ectopia cordis because of the natural association, in the mind of the observer, of the base of the neck with the beginning of the bony sternum so that the area continuous with the neck and not covered by bone appears to be more cervical than thoracic. Actually, when the sternal cleft has been corrected, the heart is completely hidden from view. Essentially the same is true of so-called thoracoabdominal ectopia cordis. The area of chest unprotected by the distal sternum seems to be continuous with the epigastrium and is mistaken for it, and the heart pulsating visibly in this soft area appears to be an abdominal organ.

The deceptiveness of the clinical examination is borne out by observations at operation. For example, in a child with a complete sternal cleft, Maier and Bortone[10] found at operation that what had appeared

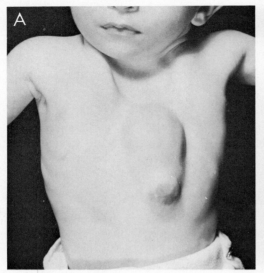
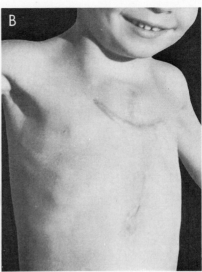

Fig. 26-1.—Complete sternal cleft. **A,** child at age 8 months. There is no bony structure between hyoid and pubis. Rib ends are widely separated, and at this time it was thought, even after operation, that there was no sternum, but some years later, lateral roentgenograms showed sternebrae. Note prominence of the heart and, below it in the pigmented omphalocele-like scar of the umbilicus, the swelling produced by the liver. The heart was encased in the pericardium, but the pericardium was open to the peritoneal cavity and there was a crescentic diaphragmatic defect. **B,** at age 2 years. In the first operation, the ventral ab- dominal portion of the defect was closed by mobilization of local tissues and flaps of the rectus sheath. The edges of the thoracic deformity could not be approximated, so the defect was closed over by a sheet of Teflon felt. A year later, the repair was firm except at the upper end of the Teflon felt, which was lax and, in any case, 2 or 3 cm below the proper upper border of the manu- brium. At the second operation, another sheet of Teflon felt was placed above the first and supported by two rib struts taken from the 4th rib on the right. The result is solid repair.

to be an anterior protrusion of the heart was actually a large outpouching of the pericardium anteriorly with associated increase in the amount of pericardial fluid; and Major,[11] in a patient with a distal sternal cleft, found a pulsating cord in the epigastrium which proved to be a diverticulum of the pericardium with transmitted pulsation.

In the case of complete sternal cleft in which direct suture of the sternal halves satisfactorily repaired the defect, Maier made the important point that whereas 2 weeks after birth, gentle compression of the shoulders toward each other readily approximated the two halves of the sternum, at operation 5 weeks later, at age 7 weeks, it was much more difficult to approximate the sternal halves. The defect had also become much wider, presumably because, with the baby lying on her back, the weight of the shoulder girdle transmitted to the clavicles tended to separate the sternal halves.

Our patient with complete sternal cleft (Fig. 26-1) was not seen until he was 5 months old. The wide defect for the entire length of the sternum was continuous with a large omphalocele-like hernia. Operation disclosed a cleft of the entire sternum, a midline defect of the abdominal wall, a ventral diaphragmatic defect and absence of the diaphragmatic portion of the pericardium. The pericardium and diaphragm were closed and the abdominal defect was repaired

with local fascial flaps. The sternal defect, too wide for closure, was covered with Teflon felt. The Teflon was not brought high enough, so a year later another sheet of Teflon was added above, over split autogenous rib grafts. The result 6 years later was excellent.

Asp and Sulamaa[1] reported an almost identical case in which a good result was ultimately obtained after multiple operations, including transplants of the outer table of the parietal bone. The sternum was said to be completely missing. We had thought this to be the case in our patient, but recent x-ray studies have revealed sternebrae in the lateral view.

Asp and Sulamaa[1] and Larsen and Ibach[8] have reported cases of complete sternal clefts which are little more than narrow fissures.

UPPER STERNAL CLEFTS.—Upper sternal clefts (Fig. 26-2) are rather more common than complete sternal clefts, and a number of patients with this deformity have been operated on successfully. The earlier cases were reported as cervicothoracic ectopia cordis, and particularly when the patients cry or strain the heart seems indeed to be in the neck. No physiologic disability results from the uncovering of the heart by this deformity, but the abnormality is conspicuous and unsightly, and the exposed and unprotected position of the heart is an obvious hazard.

In 1947, Burton[2] reported 2 instances of such ectopia cordis in which the defect was bridged with carti-

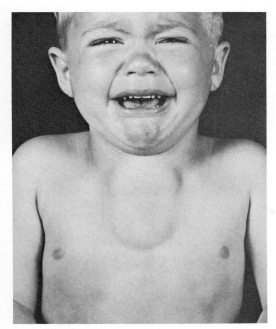

Fig. 26-2.—Upper sternal cleft. Boy of 3 years with a V-shaped cleft in the upper sternum into which the heart bulges, presenting the appearance of cervicothoracic ectopia cordis. Multiple chondrotomies allowed approximation of the sternal edges. Operation in the neonatal period is likely to permit direct closure of such defects without need for chondrotomies or prosthetic materials. (From Sabiston.[15])

lage grafts. The patient of Longino and Jewett[9] (1955) was operated on when 6 days old. The entire sternum except for the xiphoid was found to be split. The fissure was completed and the two sternal halves brought together by direct suture. As in Maier's patient, the lower ends of the sternum tended to override, and this fault was corrected by transverse division of the sternum. Our experience has demonstrated the wisdom of operating early in infancy and the greater difficulty of operating later in life. In the patient reported on by Sabiston,[15] operation was undertaken at 3 years. Direct approximation of the sternal halves was impossible until chondrotomies had been performed in the first, second and third costal cartilages on either side. The ultimate result was excellent. In a 9-year-old patient I operated on in 1958, a broad V-shaped defect was found. Transverse division of the sternal bars at the lower end of the defect, and divisions of several costal cartilages on either side, allowed the sternum to be approximated in the midline with great difficulty and only at the expense of intolerable cardiac compression. The attempt at direct closure was abandoned and the defect was covered with a prosthesis of stainless steel wire mesh with an excellent result, although one would have much preferred direct bony suture. These observations, in conjuction with those of Maier and Longino,

indicate the advisability of operation in the neonatal period because of the progressive increase in difficulty of operation as the children grow older. In a 12-day-old baby, by direct suture Thompson[17] successfully repaired a sternal cleft extending to the xiphoid, and Chang and Davis[4] had similar success in a 4-year-old, although because of the child's age, they had to perform multiple chondrotomies to achieve sternal approximation. Numerous additional cases have been reported in recent years.[6,13,14]

DISTAL STERNAL CLEFTS.—We have seen clefts of the distal sternum only in association with other deformities. The most consistent association, and apparently the commonest, is in a pentalogy of defects (Fig. 26-3) customarily reported as thoracoabdominal ectopia cordis. The five anomalies are: (1) a midline supraumbilical abdominal wall defect; (2) a defect of the lower sternum; (3) a deficiency of the anterior portion of the diaphragm; (4) a defect in the diaphragmatic portion of the pericardium; and (5) an intracardiac defect.

Fig. 26-3.—Distal sternal cleft in pentalogy of defects: sternal cleft, ventral abdominal defect (omphalocele), anterior diaphragmatic defect, pericardial defect, ventricular septal defect (tetralogy of Fallot). The diaphragmatic and midline defects were repaired at once and the cardiac defect left for later repair. (From Cantrell et al.[13])

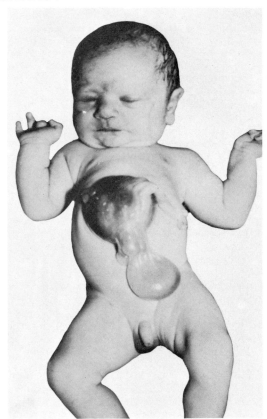

Major[11] collected 13 instances from the literature and reported 2 of his own. Cantrell, Haller and Ravitch[3] reported 4, in addition to the 2 mentioned by Major; and Mulder, Crittenden and Adams,[12] in 1960, presented 3 patients of their own.

From the standpoint of life, the most serious consideration is the intracardiac defect. Usually this is a ventricular septal defect, but there have also been seen tetralogy of Fallot, cor triloculare with a single ventricle, left ventricular diverticulum, tricuspid atresia, and various bizarre anomalies. Interventricular septal defect was present in every recorded instance in which there is an adequate description of the heart. An interatrial septal defect was present in 53% of the cases; valvular or infundibular pulmonary stenosis occurred in 33%. Of the established cardiac snydromes, only the tetralogy of Fallot was seen with any frequency—20% of the patients; and a left ventricular diverticulum was present in another 20%. More or less remote and unrelated congenital anomalies appear to be rare in these patients.

DEVELOPMENT OF THE SPECIFIC DEFECTS.—It has been suggested that the diaphragmatic defect, the pericardial defect and the intracardiac lesions are due to developmental failure of appropriate segments of the mesoderm.

The diaphragmatic defect results from total or partial failure of the transverse septum to develop. When complete, the defect corresponds to that portion of the diaphragm derived from the transverse septum—a ventral defect extending laterally to the region of the pleuroperitoneal folds and dorsally to the point of attachment of the liver and diaphragm. Less extensive defects represent partial rather than total loss of the septum transversum. This anomaly is not related to defects of the foramen of Morgagni.

The pericardial defect involves that portion of the pericardium which normally lies on the diaphragm, and which arises from the somatic mesoderm, immediately adjacent to that region of the same layer from which the transverse septum is derived. Defects of this type, of the diaphragm or of the pericardium, without a corresponding defect in the other, would require a highly specific loss of somatic mesoderm and in consequence are uncommon. It is not surprising, therefore, that coexisting defects of diaphragm and diaphragmatic portion of the pericardium are seen in the great majority of the patients under discussion.

The intracardiac lesions result from faulty development of the epimyocardium, which again is derived from the splanchnic mesoderm corresponding to that portion of the somatic mesoderm from which the pericardium is derived. The reason for the predominant occurrence of ventricular septal defects is not clear.

The sternal defect represents not absence of the sternum but failure of fusion of the distal portion. Similarly, the abdominal wall defect constitutes not an absence of normal elements of the ventral abdominal wall but a failure of complete migration of the myotomes, so that differentiation into the various muscle layers occurs at a point abnormally lateral to the midline. The rectus muscles in these patients arise normally from the pubis but diverge as they run cephalad so that they insert into the costal margin at the midclavicular line.

The basic defect in all of these abnormalities could be an absence or deficiency of ventral midline mesenchymal tissue into which the migrating mesodermal structures would normally grow. The time of origin of this syndrome of concatenated defects would have to be prior to or immediately after the differentiation of the primitive intraembryonic mesoderm into its splanchnic and somatic layers, since derivatives of both of these layers are involved. This would place the time of initiation between the fourteenth and the nineteenth day of embryonic life.

CLINICAL APPROACH.—Apart from the philosophy which has been repeatedly expressed in these pages that congenital anomalies in children are in general most satisfactorily treated as soon as they are seen, provided they are understood and an appropriate operative procedure is available, the children with omphaloceles require immediate operation. At the time of correction of the omphalocele, the ventral abdominal defect can be entirely closed, the fissured sternum repaired and the edge of the diaphragmatic defect sutured to the costal arch. In the present state of cardiac surgery, a direct attack on intracardiac anomalies in the neonatal period is not feasible. A diverticulum of the left ventricle can, however, readily be excised at the time of the repair.

In children not seen until some years after birth, the nature of the defects, the age of the child and its cardiac status will determine whether the parietal defect and the cardiac defect should be operated on simultaneously, or which should take precedence. In a remarkable instance, Mulder[12] operated on a 15-month-old child, completed the sternal cleft in a median sternotomy, excised a diverticulum of the left ventricle, closed a ventricular septal defect, repaired the diaphragmatic and abdominal defects and corrected the sternal fissure at the time of closure of the median sternotomy.

The manner of repair of the ventral defect will vary with its degree. In defects like those of Mulder's patient which represent little more than a diastasis recti, the muscles can be readily approximated in the midline. In others, it may be necessary to make relaxation incisions in the rectus sheath, or even to turn over flaps of rectus sheath, reinforced by fascia lata. In the small patients, it is possible to close the sternal fissure; in older patients, this has not proved possible, and some type of soft tissue or prosthetic repair is required.

REFERENCES

1. Asp, K., and Sulamaa, M.: Ectopia cordis, Acta chir. scandinav., Supp. 283, 1961.

2. Burton, J. F.: Method of correction of ectopia cordis: Two cases, Arch. Surg. 54:79, 1947.

3. Cantrell, J. R.; Haller, J. A., and Ravitch, M. M.: A syndrome of congenital defects involving the abdominal wall, sternum, diaphragm, pericardium and heart, Surg., Gynec. & Obst. 107:602, 1958.

4. Chang, C. H., and Davis, W.: Congenital bifid sternum with partial ectopia cordis, Am. J. Roentgenol. 86:513, 1961.

5. Hanson, F. N.: The ontogeny and phylogeny of the sternum, Am. J. Anat. 26:41, 1919.

6. Herrera, R., and Medina C.: Ectopia cordis toraco-abdominal, Arch. Inst. cardiol. México 32:79, 1962.

7. Kanagasuntheram, R., and Verzin, J. A.: Ectopia cordis in man, Thorax 17:159, 1962.

8. Larsen, L. L., and Ibach, H. F.: Complete congenital fissure of the sternum, Am. J. Roentgenol. 87:1062, 1962.

9. Longino, L. A., and Jewett, T. C.: Congenital bifid sternum, Surgery 38:610, 1955.

10. Maier, H. C., and Bortone, F.: Complete failure of sternal fusion with herniation of pericardium, J. Thoracic Surg. 18:851, 1949.

11. Major, J. W.: Thoracoabdominal ectopia cordis, J. Thoracic Surg. 27:309, 1953.

12. Mulder, D. G.; Crittenden, I. H., and Adams, F. H.: Complete repair of a syndrome of congenital defects involving the abdominal wall, sternum, diaphragm, pericardium, and heart: Excision of left ventricular diverticulum, Ann. Surg. 151:113, 1960.

13. Ongley, P. A., et al.: Partial ectopia cordis simulating tricuspid atresia: Report of a case, Mayo Clin., Proc. Staff Meet. 40:513, 1965.

14. Reese, H. E., and Stracener, C. E.: Congenital defects involving the abdominal wall, sternum, diaphragm and pericardium: Case report and review of embryologic factors, Ann. Surg. 163:3, 1966.

15. Sabiston, D. C.: The surgical management of congenital bifid sternum with partial ectopia cordis, J. Thoracic Surg. 35:118, 1958.

16. Shao-tsu, L.: Ectopia cordis congenita, Thoraxchirurgie 5:197, 1957.

17. Thompson, H. T.: Failure of sternal fusion with herniation of the pericardium, Thorax 16:386, 1961.

Depression Deformities

Depression deformities of the sternum—known under such names as pectus excavatum, funnel chest, trichterbrust, schusterbrust, and thorax en entonnoir—form the group of deformities which are most commonly treated surgically.

Recognition of the deformity goes back to antiquity. Surgical treatment began with Sauerbruch's first patient, operated on in 1913.[31] Lexer's patient was reported by Hoffmeister in 1927,[13] Sauerbruch's second patient was reported in 1931,[32] and in this country Alexander[3] reported 2 in 1931. The classic review of Ochsner and De Bakey[23] appeared in 1938. The analysis of the clinical problem by A. Lincoln Brown[6] the following year, with a simplified description of operative technique, initiated the era of modern surgical management.

Pectus excavatum is a deformity of the thorax marked by a sharp posterior curve of the body of the sternum sweeping down from the manubrium, and deepest just before the junction with the xiphoid. The lower costal cartilages bend dorsally to form a depression, the lateral borders of which are usually angled

more sharply than the superior and inferior portions of the deformity. Asymmetrical deformities are not rare. The concavity is usually somewhat deeper on the right than on the left. Often, the sternum is rotated to the right, in extreme cases by 90 degrees, so that what should be the ventral surface of the sternum forms the left side of the deepest portion of the concavity. The right breast in girls is occasionally somewhat less well developed than the left. The deformity may take the form of a broad, relatively shallow deformity which in an adolescent or a young adult may measure 17 cm in width essentially from nipple to nipple, 14 cm or more in length, and 3–7 cm in depth. Another type presents as a deep narrow central pocket and suggests the easy accommodation of a fist or a large ball. In pectus excavatum in infancy, paradoxical inward motion of the sternum is conspicuous on inspiration, and some degree of deformity persists, even on forced expiration (Fig. 26-4). The deformity is usually present at birth, and progressive.

Infants with this deformity tend to have one of two types of general thoracic configuration. In one, there is a generally well-formed sturdy thorax with a central depression; in the other, the thorax is quite shallow in the anteroposterior diameter even well lateral to the depression. It is quite possible that if left undisturbed, these deformities would develop into the two forms described earlier. Although the patients with the very broad, shallow-seeming deformities almost invariably have a very shallow chest lateral to the deformities, usually a very long thorax and tend to be asthenic, the deep central defects occur in patients of this type as well as in patients with an otherwise well-formed chest. Pot belly is characteristic of children with pectus excavatum, and Harrison's groove is not rare. As the children grow older, a characteristic habitus develops. The chest is sunken, the abdomen protuberant, the shoulders rounded and the neck slouched forward (Fig. 26-5).

OCCURRENCE

Although it appears that the vast majority of instances are sporadic, a definite familial incidence is seen in other cases (Fig. 26-6). We have operated on a father and daughter with the same deformity, and on 3 children with severe deformity in a family with two additional siblings who have had various degrees of somewhat less severe deformity. Sainsbury[30] described a family in which funnel chest was seen in members of 4 successive generations. Occasionally, funnel chest is associated with other skeletal abnormalities. This is particularly true of Marfan's syndrome, the hereditary nature of which is well known. Funnel chest is not rare in association with congenital cardiac malformations. Rickets and scurvy, formerly thought to be causative factors, probably bear no relation to the deformity. Upper airway obstruction early in infancy which persists for a long time with constant inspiratory retraction of the sternum may

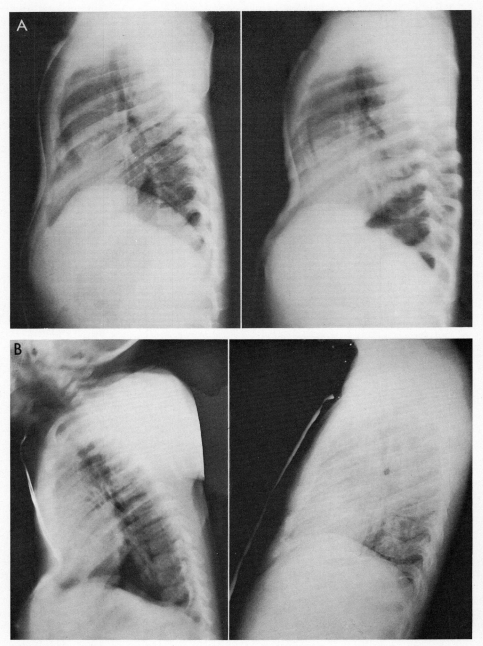

Fig. 26-4.—Pectus excavatum. **A,** C.H., expiration and inspiration showing obvious compression of heart, with the paradoxical inspiratory inward motion of the sternum. **B,** D.P., infant with conspicuous deformity, even in forced expiration during crying. Postoperative roentgenogram shows correction achieved. The lateral views show the depth of the depression but, being essentially sagittal sections, do not indicate the cubic displacement or, of course, the dynamic effects on posture and on heart and lungs.

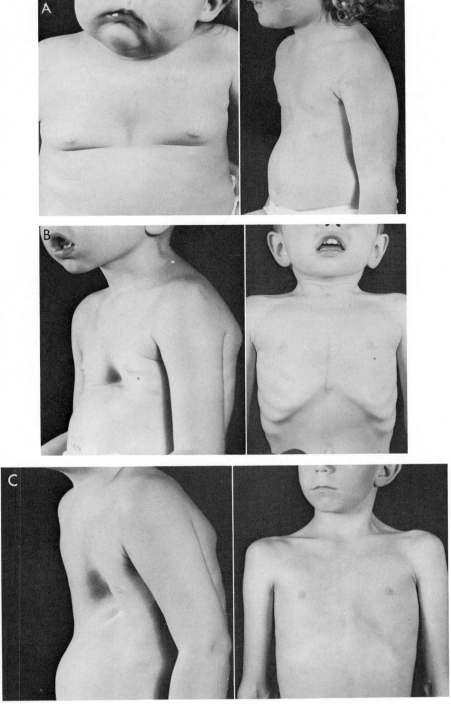

Fig. 26-5.—Pectus excavatum. Types of deformities operated on and results achieved. All left-hand photographs were taken immediately before surgery. **A,** L.P., 3½ years since operation. The deformity had been progressing. **B,** J.A., 5 months since operation, showing disappearance of paradoxical sternal motion on deep inspiration—an optimal result. Posture now assumed was impossible previously. **C,** N.J., 7 years after operation. Note erect posture and inconspicuous scar. A slight subcutaneous prominence of the distal end of the sternum and slight depression of the midline beyond the sternum prevent this from being classified as an optimal result. (*Continued.*)

323

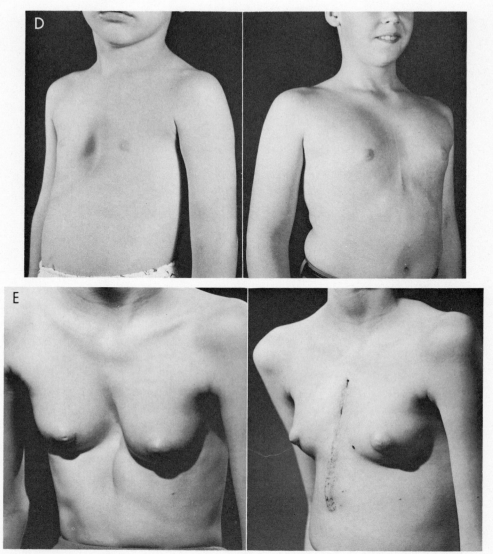

Fig. 26—5 (cont.).—D, G.R., one of two brothers operated on. Before operation, note slumped posture, pot belly and substantial concavity. Satisfactory correction is evident 7 years after operation.` **E,** A.B., age 12, with profound pectus excavatum, agenesis of the left lung and disabling shortness of breath. She had given up bicycle-riding and had difficulty climbing stairs. There was measured restrictive ventilatory defect. Two years after operation, she has striking return of capacity for exercise, riding her bicycle and climbing stairs with ease. There is substantial return of the ventilatory defect toward normal. Because of the pulmonary abnormality, 2 Kirschner wires were placed through the sternal marrow, resting on the chest wall; one was removed in 3 and the other in 6 months, with correction well maintained. This is 1 of the patients whose right breast is smaller than the left.

ultimately result in a fixed deformity. We have seen this in a child with congenital stenosis of the nares.

CLINICAL PICTURE

It is generally stated that pectus excavatum is asymptomatic in infancy and childhood. We have, however, seen 2 infants with severe inspiratory stridor in whom careful study showed no evidence of respiratory obstruction from any of the ordinary mechanisms and in whom the larynx and trachea seemed perfectly normal. Both had marked fixed deformity as well as a severe paradoxical sternal retraction. In both, the stridor disappeared immediately after operation, an event that has been noted by others. In a very small number of infants, a history is volunteered before operation of apparent dysphagia or some impediment to the deglutition of food which is

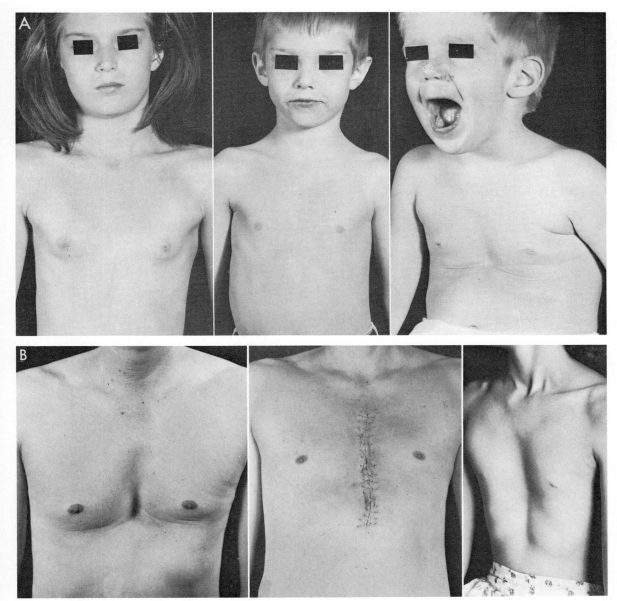

Fig. 26–6.—Pectus excavatum, familial incidence. Most of our cases are not familial, but such incidence is not rare. **A,** B.T. was operated on 9 years earlier at 18 months. Ma.T. was operated on 4 years earlier at 23 months. Mi.T. was operated on shortly after this photograph was taken. Two other siblings had mild deformities, not operated on. **B,** father and daughter. Father was beginning to have some shortness of breath on exertion. Daughter's deformity was still progressing. Both were operated on. Postoperative photograph shows correction of father's deep deformity. Daughter had an equally good result.

relieved by operation. This is perhaps as difficult to explain mechanically as the relief of stridor in our 2 patients. It is almost a regular event for mothers bringing children in for postoperative examinations to state that the children are eating as they never ate before, in terms of avidity and quantity, and that they are more energetic, more vigorous and more outgoing than ever before. This is true in infants and small children as well as in older youngsters. The first evidences of actual physical difficulty appear in childhood. By radiologic study and by electrocardiography with multiple precordial leads and spatial vector cardiography, the heart can usually be found to be displaced to the left and rotated in a clockwise direction.

Presumably as a consequence of the pressure on the heart, and the displacement thus caused, systolic murmurs and cardiac arrhythmias in these children are common. They disappear after operation. Many of the children are thin and asthenic, quiet and do not seem to exercise vigorously. Occasionally, of course, one does see a vigorous, athletic youth with a very deep funnel chest which seems to discommode him not at all, but this is uncommon. More commonly, one is given the story of a child who can hike with his fellows but drops behind on an uphill grade, who can "fool around" a basketball court but not play a game; of a college boy who plays a game or two of tennis but not a set. Exercise tolerance is usually adequate for ordinary activities and moderately reduced for strenuous activities.

The older literature stated, often in the face of obvious published evidence to the contrary (the first surgical patients were all strongly symptomatic and all relieved by operation), that the condition is of no physiologic significance; but gradually mounting evidence attests to the frequency of cardiorespiratory symptoms of varying degrees of severity. We operated on an adult who had twice been in congestive failure with auricular fibrillation and who 10 years after operation was working as a bus driver in the best of health without cardiac symptoms and without medication.[28] In another instance, a young woman of 28 was referred with a history of persistent tachycardia for which a year's treatment with antithyroid drugs had been ineffective. Extensive studies showed no other lesion but a pectus excavatum. Correction of the funnel chest relieved the tachycardia and restored her rapidly diminishing exercise tolerance to normal levels.

The objective evidence of cardiorespiratory abnormality is not as striking as one would wish.[14,33] In our experience,[34] change in the configuration of the QRS complex in VR and V_1 is the commonest electrocardiographic change. Comparison with vector cardiograms in our patients suggests that this is purely a rotational effect. In the milder cases, cardiac catheterization and pulmonary function tests show either normal or low normal values, even in symptomatic patients. Decreased cardiac output has been reported in some of our patients, and a high end-diastolic pressure in the right ventricle in one patient. In the 28-year-old woman mentioned earlier, who was mistakenly treated for hyperthyroidism for a year, cardiac catheterization demonstrated a decrease of cardiac output after 10 minutes of standard exercise on a stationary bicycle, a distinctly abnormal response.

In 1 of our patients, a 12-year-old girl with severe pectus excavatum and agenesis of the left lung (Fig. 26-5, *E*), the combination caused severe symptoms and a serious, measurable restrictive defect in respiratory function. The symptoms were relieved by correction of the deformity, and there was substantial improvement in measured respiratory function.

In a woman of 27 with difficulties suggesting constrictive pericarditis, angiocardiography demonstrated a grotesque compression of the right ventricle, relieved by operation.

Bevegård[4] studied cardiac and respiratory function in 16 adults with funnel chest by cardiac catheterization at rest and during exercise in the sitting and the supine position. He reported a greater reduction of stroke volume during exercise in the sitting position than in normal subjects.

In children, respiratory function tests are difficult to perform and the normal values are not well established. Brown and Cook[7] stated that maximal breathing capacity in adults with pectus excavatum averages less than 50% of normal, but we and others find that the figures tend to be merely in the lower limits of the normal range.

The orthopedic effects of the uncorrected deformity in terms of the slouching, stooped posture are obvious, and the desirability of preventing it is clear, as is the importance of correcting the cardiorespiratory difficulties.

Subject to more argument, perhaps, is the psychologic importance of the cosmetic element of the deformity. It has been a matter of great interest to us that only rarely do parents, or children either, for that matter, present the psychologic effect as reason for operation. In fact, they usually protest that they want the operation only if it is indicated for "reasons of health." But after operation, attention is centered almost entirely on the visible correction of the deformity and the relief this gives, usually to three generations of the family. Many children, both males and females, come for operation in early adolescence, when they become reluctant to undress before their fellows. The father of one patient with a severe deformity allowed me to feel through his shirt his own extremely severe deformity, telling me that because of it he had never undressed before anyone in his adult life and had never gone bathing in a pool or at the beach. The change in personality of a young adult female after correction of a deep deformity is a striking thing. Shy, introverted, almost depressed individuals seem literally to bloom. How much better to prevent this psychologic maladjustment than to wait until adult life to correct it (Fig. 26-7).

INDICATIONS FOR OPERATION

Pectus excavatum causes symptoms in most patients and produces severe symptoms in an occasional one. Operation is recommended (1) to prevent the development of symptoms or to correct those already present; (2) to correct the orthopedic and cosmetic aspects of the deformity, and (3) to prevent or correct the psychologic response to the deformity.

Ample experience has demonstrated to us the ease and safety with which the operation can be performed, even in infants, and has convinced us that

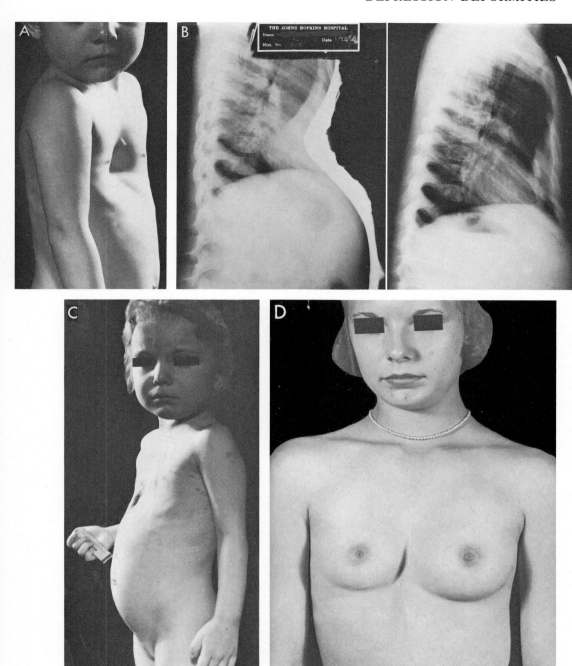

Fig. 26-7.—Pectus excavatum; 12½-year follow-up. **A,** preoperative photograph, showing profound depression and characteristic hunched appearance. **B,** pre- and postoperative roentgenograms, showing extent of the deformity and degree of correction. Contrast is obtained by a midline strip of barium paste squeezed from a tube. **C,** 1 week after operation. **D,** 12½ years after operation. Note the slightly smaller size of the right breast.

the younger the patient, the easier the operation for both patient and surgeon and the more likely a restitution of a normal thoracic contour. For this reason, operation is advised whenever the patient is seen with a severe defect or a defect which is reliably stated to be progressive. In infants, the persistence of the defect during forced expiration in crying is as significant to us as the depth of the defect on quiet inspiration and the degree of paradoxical motion on forced inspiration. A good many children, with relatively minor accentuations of the groove between the pectoral muscles, are merely observed. In most such patients, the defect does not advance, but occasionally a mild pectus excavatum deformity deepens strikingly under observation, and operation is indicated.

The manner of *presentation of operation* to the parents is important. Some parents are incapable of resolving upon an elective operation for their children and will not so resolve, in spite of what may be said; so it is unfair and unwise to present the case for operation so strongly as to leave them feeling guilty when they make the inevitable decision against operation. It is my custom to state that the deformity is usually progressive and that we are unable to predict in which instances it will be progressive; that mild symptoms are extremely common, that real disability is uncommon, and that a serious disability is rare. The parents are informed that the risk of operation in infancy is no different from that in later life, that the operation is easier for the small patient and that early operation affords the best chance of restitution of a normal thoracic contour. They are also told that if operation is not performed, it can be undertaken at any time in the future when symptoms become severe, with the full expectation of relief of all symptoms. But the correction of the sternal deformity will then come after the associated abnormal thoracic configuration has been fixed.

OPERATIVE TECHNIQUE

Operation (Fig. 26-8) is undertaken under endotracheal anesthesia, usually with the patient on a cold water cooling mattress to provide mild degrees of hypothermia and prevent any hyperthermia. In our earlier operations, transfusion was a regular accompaniment, but with development of the operative technique we now transfuse perhaps every third or fourth child. Measured blood loss in a small child may be 20–30 cc, and in a large teenager, 100–200 cc. Transfusion is at times required in the first 24 hours postoperatively to replace blood that oozes into the mediastinum, principally from the sternal osteotomy. Inhalation anesthesia is given with nitrous oxide and halothane so that electrocautery can be used.

A midline incision from just above the upper border of the defect well down to the epigastrium provides the best exposure with the least difficulty. In small girls we employ a transverse submammary incision. This requires more dissection and provides poorer exposure than the midline incision, which is used in all males, in older girls and in younger girls with extensive deformities. Prophylactic postoperative radiotherapy has been recommended, specifically after the operation for pectus excavatum, to prevent the development of keloids.[18] But the incidence of cancer of the thyroid (see Chapter 20) in children treated for enlarged thymus glands with x-ray dosages frequently smaller than would be given to prevent keloid formation, has kept us from adopting this measure.

In the vertical incision, skin, fat and the pectoral muscles are reflected in a single flap; in the transverse incision, the skin flaps are developed and then the pectoral muscles stripped back to either side (Fig. 26-8, *A*). If an alert assistant secures the perforating vessels from the internal mammary as they are brought into view by the stripping of the pectorales, the major source of blood loss is avoided. The pectorales are stripped back to expose the deformed cartilages for the entire extent of their deformity. The lower one or two cartilages covered by the rectus muscle are exposed by splitting the muscle. The involved cartilages are removed subperichondrially for the full extent of their deformity (Fig. 26-8, *B* and *C*), which may be 5 or 6 cm for the lower cartilages and only 2 or 3 cm for the upper cartilages. The fourth, fifth, sixth and seventh cartilages are usually involved, and occasionally the third as well. In the smallest infants, it is sometimes necessary only to resect the fifth, sixth and seventh cartilages to remove all of the deformed cartilages. The xiphoid is now divided from the sternum with scissors (Fig. 26-8, *D*), the small artery on either side secured, and the right index finger inserted into the mediastinum. In common with most authors, we have not been impressed with the frequency with which we can identify a tough midline fibrous structure, corresponding to the substernal ligament, which is thought by some to be a major cause or factor in the deformity.[6] Frequently, the diaphragmatic attachments to the sternum are remarkably light and can almost invariably be separated with the finger. Very occasionally, there is a tough fibrous strand or two which requires cutting. The medial extensions of the pleural envelopes are stripped back with the finger to beyond the sternum on either side, and with the scissors the intercostal bundles are divided from the sternum (Fig. 26-8, *E*). If care is taken to remain close to the sternum, the internal mammary arteries will not be injured and will be exposed on the underside of the intercostal bundles as this dissection continues. Invariably in older children and increasingly often in infants, we then transect the first intact cartilage, usually the third or second, close to the sternum. This permits the transverse osteotomy of the sternum to be performed one interspace higher than otherwise, and allows for a gratifying overcorrection of the deformity. The cartilage is divided by an oblique incision from anteriorly

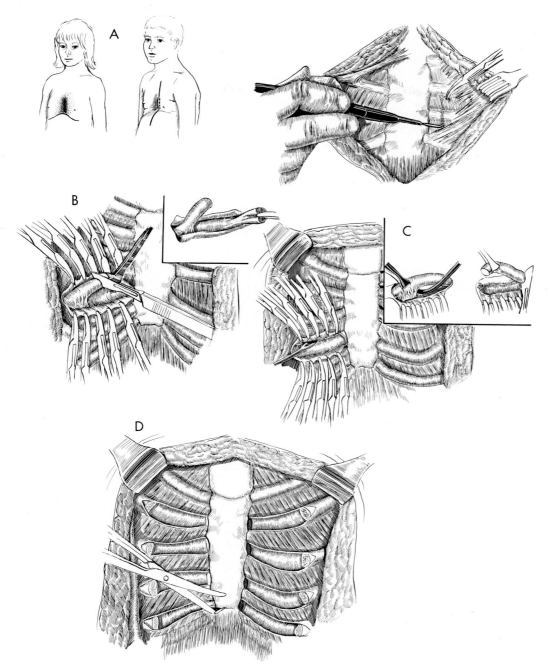

Fig. 26-8.—Operative treatment of pectus excavatum. The slightly bowed, submammary incision is used for little girls; a midline incision for all others. **A,** using the midline incision. After the skin is incised, dissection is carried down to the sternum by electrocautery and the pectoral muscles are dissected back from the sternum and costal cartilages. As the perforating branches of the internal mammary are encountered, they are picked up with a hemostat and coagulated before division. **B** and **C,** the perichondrium is incised longitudinally and a transverse incision made in the perichondrium at either end of the deformed portion of cartilage. If the perichondrial edges are seized with small curved hemostats and dissected away from the cartilage with delicate elevators like a Freer or a slender staphylorrhaphy, the cartilage can be either dissected out in one piece, as in **C,** with the right-angle Brophy elevator slipped under it to complete the dissection, or divided in the midportion, as in **B,** and each half stripped out and divided at its end. **D,** all deformed costal cartilages (in this case, 4) have been excised the full length of their deformity. In infants, this will all be cartilage. In older children and adults, one will go beyond the costochondral junction of 2 or 3 ribs. The xiphoid is shown being divided from the sternum with scissors. A small artery on either side of the xiphoid requires coagulation. (*Continued.*)

329

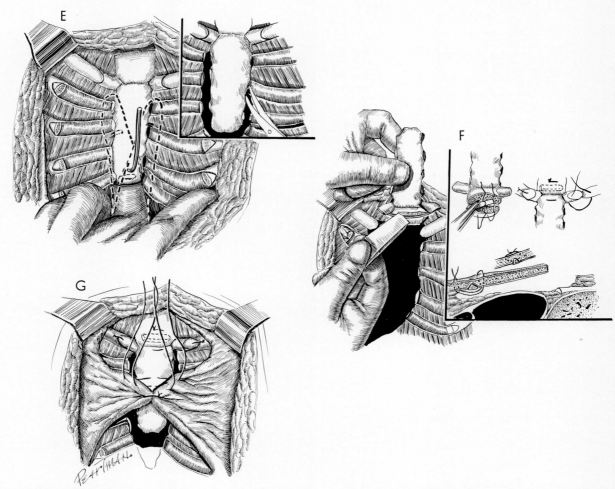

Fig. 26-8 (cont.).—E, the xiphoid having been divided, the sternum is lifted sharply forward with a bone hook, the index finger inserted into the mediastinum, the diaphragmatic attachments, if any, separated and the pleural envelopes displaced back beyond the edge of the sternum on either side. **Insert,** the intercostal bundles are divided from the sternum, with an attempt not to injure the internal mammary vessels. Oblique incisions have been made in the first intact costal cartilage, usually the 2nd or 3rd. The incision is made from medially and in front to laterally and behind. **F,** the sternum is elevated forward and a wire passed around it in the interspace above the obliquely divided cartilage, to serve as guide. Care is taken to be certain that the line of the wire is precisely transverse. The posterior cortical lamella is scored with the corner of a sharp osteotome and the sternum fractured forward. **Insert,** a small piece of bone cut from a rib is inserted in the posterior sternal osteotomy and maintained there by silk sutures passed around the osteotomy and either through the bone fragment or around it. The sternum now sits in good corrected or overcorrected position with the medial ends of the obliquely divided cartilage overlapping the lateral ends to which they are sutured with heavy silk. **G,** the sternum is held in overcorrected position by the chock-block bone graft. The obliquely divided costal cartilages are sutured with medial ends overlapping, and now the pectoral muscles are being sutured to each other and to the sternal periosteum in the midline. Care is taken to close the subcutaneous tissue in at least two layers apart from the skin closure. The xiphoid is not reattached, and no muscle covers the space between xiphoid and sternum. The intercostal bundles are not sutured back to the sternum.

and medially to posteriorly and laterally so that when the sternum is elevated, the medial portion of the cartilage will rest on the lateral (Fig. 26-8, *F* and *G*). The sternum is lifted forward, a wire passed around it in the interspace above the divided cartilage, and the posterior cortical lamella scored with the corner of an osteotome until the sternum fractures forward (Fig. 26-8, *F*). The sternum is now isolated like a peninsula, attached at its upper end only by the anterior cortical lamella and its periosteum. A wedge of bone from an exposed rib is pressed into the osteotomy and retained by a heavy silk suture through or around it, acting as a chock block (Fig. 26-8, *F inset,* and *G*). Wire sutures may necrose the soft bone and cut through or may break. The ends of the obliquely transected second or third cartilage will now be found to have a new relationship to each other, the central ends usually being a little cephalad and resting on the lateral ends. This relationship is maintained by through-and-through sutures of silk, providing additional lateral points of fixation of the sternum to the chest wall.

If the sternum is unusually scaphoid, the result of correction of the first angulation at or near the sterno-manubrial junction is to bring the tip of the sternum well anterior to the level of the chest wall. In such instances, an anterior transverse osteotomy is performed in the distal portion of the sternum at the approximate beginning of the anterior curve. The distal sternum is bent back and held in this position by inserting another wedge of rib bone into the opened linear osteotomy.

We have not used external fixation since our first two operations, the second of which resulted in a fatal infection, the only death in over 250 operations. In adults and large teenagers with extensive rib and cartilage resections, and a long sternum exercising great leverage on the repair, we have experimented with internal fixation. A Teflon sling behind the sternum is difficult to make taut. A rib strut is very effective and has been satisfactory in 2 of our patients. For these cases we have, however, settled upon one or two Kirschner wires[20] passed through the sternal marrow parallel to the anterior chest wall, the ends curled back on themselves so as not to penetrate the skin. The pectoral muscles cover the wires, which are removed in 6 months. We have used these in 2 adults and 2 teenagers. The ingenious Rehbein splints[29] are much more difficult to insert, and the strut bar of steel behind the sternum[2] seems a large foreign body. In any case, such fixation is rarely required or used by us.

Injury to the pleura high on the right is not uncommon. When it occurs, the anesthesiologist is requested to overinflate the lung to expel air from the pleural cavity and the pleural rent is closed. In the deeper deformities, the intercostal bundles which formerly had an extremely indirect course to the sternum, now coming straight across, are found to be redundant and the excess may be trimmed away and one or two sutures placed to tack the intercostal bundles back to the sternum. If there is the slightest appearance of tension, the sutures are released and the intercostal bundles left unattached. The pectoral muscles are sutured to the sternum and to each other in the midline (Fig. 26-8, G) and the skin carefully closed with subcutaneous and cutaneous sutures. As in almost all of pediatric surgery, we avoid dressings. A plastic spray permits daily inspection of the wound and easy examination of the patient. Accumulation of bloody fluid within the mediastinum is not uncommon and requires aspiration, sometimes several times. Although from time to time we employ catheter suction drainage for 48 hours, in general we prefer to keep the wound closed and to aspirate it as necessary.

Breathing is easy after operation and oxygen is not required, but we feel strongly that infants who have been under anesthesia for 1 1/2–2 hours with an intratracheal tube in place should be kept in a moist atmosphere for at least 24 hours. Thus far we have had no instances requiring a tracheotomy or approaching that need, but such a complication has been reported by others. Since the xiphoid is not resutured to the sternum, for fear of re-creating the deformity, there is also an unprotected rhomboidal area just beyond the tip of the sternum and between it and the xiphoid in which paradoxical motion can be observed for perhaps 1 week. This should be explained to the parents to avoid unnecessary concern. We give penicillin and streptomycin routinely for 4 days following operation, although we are well aware of the disputes concerning the use of antibiotics in operations of this kind. The children are allowed feedings and activities as they tolerate them and usually leave the hospital between the seventh and the ninth day. The parents are asked to see to it that older children avoid rough play for 2 weeks after discharge from the hospital. By the end of the third week the chest wall should be fairly firm and activity may be unrestricted. The only complication we have seen after the patient has returned home is the occasional discharge through the incision of a previously unsuspected collection of serosanguineous fluid. The drainage does not persist in such instances and the wound heals over at once.

RESULT

We have operated on 250 patients varying in age from 2 months to 40 years. There has been 1 death in the entire group. Of children 14 years of age or younger, we have operated on 220. Symptoms have always been relieved, and increased vigor and weight and improved eating habits have been commented on frequently. There has been no frank recurrence of the deformity. In a number of patients, the optimal correction obtained after the operation has been lost. In perhaps 6, we have thought that the sternum was sufficiently flattened so that something might be gained by reoperation, but 2 patients and their parents have been too satisfied with the result to agree to reoperation. In the 4 others, reoperation has given gratifying results. In general, we have felt that when less than optimal results were achieved, we had not resected the costal cartilages widely enough, or had not resected enough cartilages, so that the sternal osteotomy was not above the beginning of the downward slope of the sternum.

Our operation as now performed has resulted from progressive modifications without change of the fundamentals of the original procedure, and we have splendid results of 20 years' standing. Mention must nevertheless be made of the evaluation by Moghissi[21] in 1964 of 58 patients operated on at Southampton by the late E. F. Chin, using Chin's[9] modification of the operation we described in 1949.[27] The evaluation was based entirely on cosmetic results. Twenty-seven chests were rated as normal, 18 as fair (70–90% of normal) and 13 as bad (less than 65% of normal). These figures are so far out of line with our results over a much longer period of observation as to raise a question regarding the general applicability of the observations. The wide interest in surgical correction of pectus excavatum in recent years has resulted in numerous suggestions for operative techniques. Some authors[10,16] have insisted on the need for external traction for a longer or shorter time, some have used struts of bone,[35,37] others always secure the chest behind the sternum[24] or through the sternum with a Kirschner wire,[20,26] and some employ a heavy metal strut behind the sternum[15,25] or internal metallic fixation[29] which may be left or removed at a secondary operation. Instead of resecting the cartilages, many authors[1,11,15,19] morcellate the involved cartilages and, on one or another pattern, gridiron the sternum with osteotomies so that when it is pulled into position by external traction, or held by a buried strut, the chest wall appears in normal position without the excision of any of its elements. Actis-Dato's monograph[1] illustrates most of the methods that have been proposed.

We have found external traction to be unnecessary in either the more or the less extensive procedures. Morcellation of cartilages and sternum seems to be an unnecessarily large and possibly bloody procedure. The operation described here, which is a modification of that proposed by Lincoln Brown in 1939, seems the simplest and most effective one.

A word should be said about what has been called the "limited operation," also proposed by Brown. This consists of xiphisternal disarticulation—a freeing of the diaphragmatic attachments to the sternum with the finger, and the resection of parts of one or two of the distalmost cartilages on both sides. It has been suggested that in the smallest infants, this will release the sternum from diaphragmatic traction and allow it to regain its normal position. We have experimented with the limited operation on several occasions and, being dissatisfied with the result achieved in the operating room at the time, have gone on to the formal operation. It has also been our lot to operate on several children on whom the limited operation was said to have been performed and in whom the deformity either persisted or progressed. Our satisfaction with the operation described and its safety, even in infants, is such that we doubt that there is any field for application of the limited operation.

The deformities are sufficiently varied, and atypical instances sufficiently common, that the surgeon should be ready to adapt himself to changing circumstances. The excessively scaphoid sternum is one example. Another is the sternum which is sharply rotated, usually counterclockwise. In minor instances of this kind, the sternum can be rotated at the site of the osteotomy. In others, it is necessary to perform another osteotomy midway in the curve and to rotate the distal portion of the sternum at this level as well, particularly if the rotation is actually spiral.

REFERENCES

1. Actis-Dato, A.; Gentilli, R. X., and Calderini, P.: *Il Pectus Excavatum* (Torino: Minerva Medica, 1962).
2. Adkins, P.C., and Blades, B.: A stainless steel strut for correction of pectus excavatum, Surg., Gynec. & Obst. 113:111, 1961.
3. Alexander, J.: Traumatic pectus excavatum, Ann. Surg. 93:489, 1931.
4. Bevegård, S.: Postural circulatory changes at rest and during exercise in patients with funnel chest with special reference to factors affecting the stroke volume, Acta med. scandinav. 171:695, 1962.
5. Brodkin, H. A.: Congenital chondrosternal prominence (pigeon breast): A new interpretation, Pediatrics 3:286, 1949.
6. Brown, A. L.: Pectus excavatum (funnel chest), J. Thoracic Surg. 9:164, 1939.
7. Brown, A. L., and Cook, O.: Cardiorespiratory studies in pre- and postoperative funnel chest (pectus excavatum), Dis. Chest 20:378, 1951.
8. Brown, A. L., and Cook, O.: Funnel chest (pectus excavatum) in infancy and adult life, California Med. 74:174, 1951.
9. Chin, E. F.: Surgery of funnel chest and congenital sternal prominence, Brit. J. Surg. 44:360, 1957.
10. Effler, D. B.: Pectus excavatum: Surgical treatment, Cleveland Clin. Quart. 20:353, 1953.
11. Gross, R.: *Surgery of Infancy and Childhood* (Philadelphia: W. B. Saunders Company, 1953).
12. Hanson, F. N.: The ontogeny and phylogeny of the sternum, Am. J. Anat. 26:41, 1919.
13. Hoffmeister, W.: Operation der angeborenen Trichterbrust, Beitr. klin. Chir. 141:214, 1927.
14. Howard, R.: Funnel chest: Its effect on cardiac function, Arch. Dis. Childhood 34:5, 1959.
15. Jensen, N. K.; Schmidt, R. W., and Jaramella, J. J.: Funnel chest, a new corrective operation, J. Thoracic & Cardiovas. Surg. 43:731, 1962.
16. Lester, C. W.: The surgical treatment of funnel chest, Ann. Surg. 123:1003, 1946.
17. Lester, C. W.: Pigeon breast (pectus carinatum) and other protrusion deformities of the chest of developmental origin, Ann. Surg. 137:482, 1953.
18. Lindskog, G. E., and Felton, W. L., II: Considerations in the surgical treatment of pectus excavatum, Ann. Surg. 142:654, 1955.
19. Mahoney, E. V., and Emerson, G. L.: Surgical treatment of the congenital funnel chest deformity, Arch. Surg. 67:317, 1953.
20. Mayo, P., and Long, G. A.: Surgical repair of pectus excavatum by pin immobilization, J. Thoracic & Cardiovas. Surg. 44:53, 1962.
21. Moghissi, K.: Long term results of surgical correction of pectus excavatum and sternal prominence, Thorax 19:350, 1964.
22. Morris, J. D.: Surgical correction of pectus excavatum, S. Clin. North America 41:1271, 1961.
23. Ochsner, A., and De Bakey, M.: Chone-chondrosternon, J. Thoracic Surg. 8:469, 1938.
24. Overholt: In discussion of Adkins, P. C., and Gwathmey, O.: Pectus excavatum—an appraisal of surgical treatment, J. Thoracic Surg. 36:714, 1958.
25. Paltia, V.; Parkkulainen, V. J., and Sulamaa, M.: Operative technique in funnel chest, Acta chir. scandinav. 116:990, 1959.

26. Peters, R. P., and Johnson, J.: Stabilization of pectus deformity with wire strut, J. Thoracic & Cardiovas. Surg. 47:814, 1964.

27. Ravitch, M. M.: The operative treatment of pectus excavatum, Ann. Surg. 129:929, 1949.

28. Ravitch, M. M.: Pectus excavatum and heart failure, Surgery 30:178, 1951.

29. Rehbein, F., and Wernicke, H. M.: The operative treatment of the funnel chest, Arch. Dis. Childhood 32:5, 1957.

30. Sainsbury, H. S. K.: Congenital funnel chest, Lancet 2:615, 1947.

31. Sauerbruch, E. F.: *Die Chirurgie der Brustorgane* (3rd ed.; Berlin: Springer Verlag. 1928), p. 735.

32. Sauerbruch, E. F.: Operative Beseitigung der angeborenen Trichterbrust, Deutsche Ztschr. Chir. 234:760, 1931.

33. Therkelsen, F.: Funnel chest, Acta chir. scandinav. 102:36, 1951.

34. Wachtel, F. W.; Ravitch, M. M., and Grishman, S.: The relation of pectus excavatum to heart disease, Am. Heart J. 52:121, 1956.

35. Wahren, H.: The use of a tibial graft as a retrosternal support in funnel chest surgery, Acta chir. scandinav. 99:568, 1950.

36. Welch, K. J.: Satisfactory surgical correction of pectus excavatum deformity in childhood, J. Thoracic Surg. 36:697, 1958.

37. Woods, F. M.; Overholt, R. H., and Bolton, H. E.: Pectus excavatum, Dis. Chest 22:274, 1952.

Protrusion Deformities

Protrusion deformities are much less common than depression deformities of the sternum, and there is apparently less clinical experience in their treatment. There seem to be two types of protrusion deformities quite different in their appearance, probably quite different in etiology and requiring different modes of surgical correction.

CLINICAL FORMS

The first, producing a *pouter pigeon breast*, is undoubtedly congenital. It is marked by prominent forward tilting of the manubrium with what amounts to a manubriogladiolar prominence. Distal to this, the gladiolus inclines posteriorly and actually forms a type of pectus excavatum deformity. It has been pointed out[3] that this deformity is usually marked by abnormal fusion of all of the sternal segments, and the sternum in these patients seems also to be broader than usual.

Treatment of the deformity is directed to correction of the depression component. Elevation of the depressed portion of the sternum produces a normally rounded chest and relieves symptoms when present.[6]

The deformity which is more commonly thought of as pectus carinatum or pigeon breast presents a considerable prominence of the sternum, largely of the corpus sterni, the manubrium being tilted little if at all. This *keeled breast* or *chicken breast* is characterized by a lateral depression of the ribs and costal cartilages to either side of the sternum accentuating the sternal prominence. These lateral depressions or runnels are deep enough to compress the heart and to reduce the thoracic volume substantially (Fig. 26-9). Correction of the lateral depressions restores the volume of the thorax, eliminates any possibility of compression of the heart and lungs and restores the tho-

Fig. 26-9.—Pectus carinatum. D.J., 3 years old. **A,** the keeled sternum is the result of a striking symmetrical depression (the left side is effaced by the lighting). **B,** postoperative result, showing remarkable correction achieved by subperichondrial resection of the deformed cartilages and reefing sutures in the perichondrium. (From Ravitch.[7])

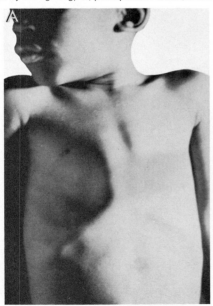
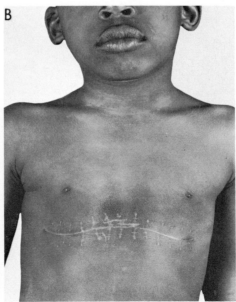

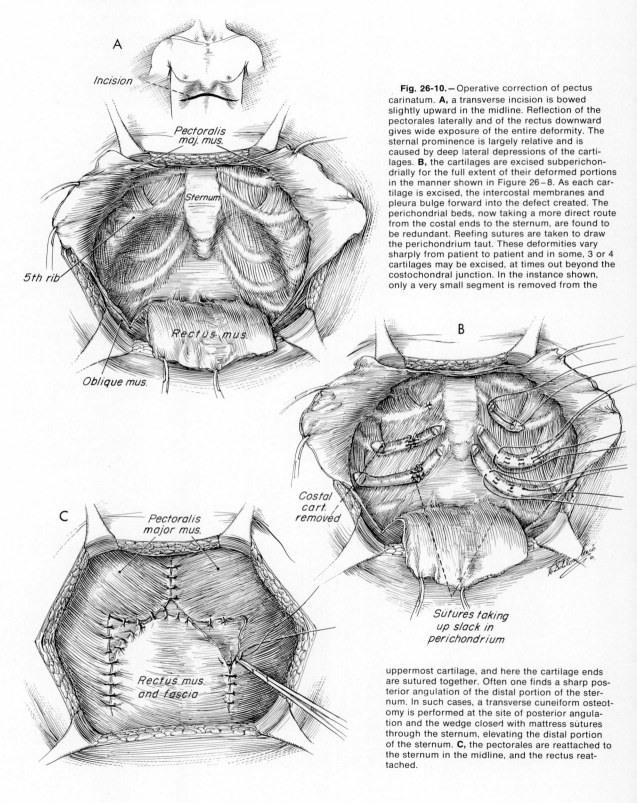

Fig. 26-10.—Operative correction of pectus carinatum. **A,** a transverse incision is bowed slightly upward in the midline. Reflection of the pectorales laterally and of the rectus downward gives wide exposure of the entire deformity. The sternal prominence is largely relative and is caused by deep lateral depressions of the cartilages. **B,** the cartilages are excised subperichondrially for the full extent of their deformed portions in the manner shown in Figure 26–8. As each cartilage is excised, the intercostal membranes and pleura bulge forward into the defect created. The perichondrial beds, now taking a more direct route from the costal ends to the sternum, are found to be redundant. Reefing sutures are taken to draw the perichondrium taut. These deformities vary sharply from patient to patient and in some, 3 or 4 cartilages may be excised, at times out beyond the costochondral junction. In the instance shown, only a very small segment is removed from the uppermost cartilage, and here the cartilage ends are sutured together. Often one finds a sharp posterior angulation of the distal portion of the sternum. In such cases, a transverse cuneiform osteotomy is performed at the site of posterior angulation and the wedge closed with mattress sutures through the sternum, elevating the distal portion of the sternum. **C,** the pectorales are reattached to the sternum in the midline, and the rectus reattached.

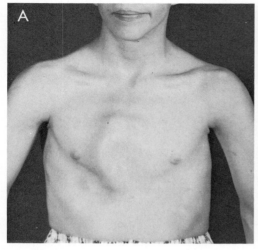
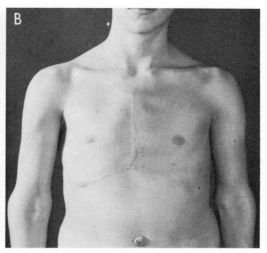
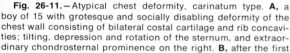

Fig. 26-11.—Atypical chest deformity, carinatum type. **A,** a boy of 15 with grotesque and socially disabling deformity of the chest wall consisting of bilateral costal cartilage and rib concavities; tilting, depression and rotation of the sternum, and extraordinary chondrosternal prominence on the right. **B,** after the first stage. The depressed costal cartilages on the right were excised subperichondrially and the redundant perichondrium reefed and some of the chondrosternal prominence excised. At the second operation, the sternum was rotated and its position corrected; and at the third stage, the left chondral depression was corrected.

racic configuration to one that is essentially normal. The sternum itself need not be disturbed except when, as in 2 of our patients, the distal end of the sternum is turned sharply posteriorly and requires osteotomy for correction.

As in depression deformities, various etiologic mechanisms have been postulated. A number of authors believe that failure of development of muscle in different portions of the diaphragm, these portions then exerting a pull on the attached chest wall as a result of the unopposed action of the muscle on the other side of the central tendon, produces either depression or protrusion deformities. The evidence offered cannot be considered conclusive.[1,2]

SURGICAL CORRECTION

A number of operative procedures have been aimed at the correction of protrusion deformities. Lester[5] excised small portions of the involved cartilages subperichondrially and then excised the entire corpus sterni subperiosteally, allowing redevelopment of the sternum in a depressed position. Chin[2] disengaged the xiphoid and into a slot made for it in the sternum reinserted it at the level of the fourth costal cartilage, a procedure which in small children is said to pull the sternum back into proper position. Our procedure[7] has been the subperichondrial resection of all of the involved cartilages with a reefing suture in the now redundant perichondrium (Fig. 26-10). Howard[4] has combined this with Chin's operation. The variety of protrusion deformities is probably such that, even more than in depression deformities, a certain amount of ingenuity and individuality of approach and operative therapy is required (Fig. 26-11).

REFERENCES

1. Brodkin, H. A.: Congenital chondrosternal prominence (pigeon breast): A new interpretation, Pediatrics 3:286, 1949.
2. Chin, E. F.: Surgery of funnel chest and congenital sternal prominence, Brit. J. Surg. 44:360, 1957.
3. Currarino, G., and Silverman, F. N.: Premature obliteration of the sternal sutures and pigeon-breast deformities, Radiology 70:532, 1958.
4. Howard, R.: Pigeon breast (protrusion deformity of the sternum), M. J. Australia 2:664, 1958.
5. Lester, C. W.: Pigeon breast (pectus carinatum) and other protrusion deformities of developmental origin, Ann. Surg. 137:482, 1953.
6. Ravitch, M. M.: Unusual sternal deformity with cardiac symptoms: Operative correction, J. Thoracic Surg. 23:138, 1952.
7. Ravitch, M. M.: The operative correction of pectus carinatum (pigeon breast), Ann. Surg. 151:705, 1960.

Congenital Absence of Ribs

Numerous anomalies of the ribs are seen, the most common being a supernumerary rib and absence of a rib at one or the other end of the thoracic cage. Except as these are accompanied by spinal malformations (Fig. 26-12), they have no medical importance. Cervical ribs do not cause symptoms in childhood. A deformity which has interested us is the absence of costal cartilages and portions of ribs, usually the second, third and fourth on one side, associated with hypoplasia or absence of nipple and breast, hypoplasia of the subcutaneous tissue and absence of the pectoralis minor muscle and of the costal portion of the pectoralis major (Fig. 26-12). The deformity is made conspicuous by the combination of a soft tissue and an osteocartilaginous defect, and its nature is obvious. If it is large, paradoxical respiration is prominent, but not usually a cause of symptoms. The defect usually extends medially almost to the sternum, the costal cartilages being involved, and laterally to the midaxillary or posterior axillary line. Rickham[6] dignified the paradoxical bulge on inspiration by the designation lung hernia. His patient, a 7-week-old infant with five ribs missing, had fairly severe symptoms. In the first of our patients, seen many years ago in infancy, we delayed operation, not being quite certain of the indications or the procedure. The result has been progressively increasing deformity of the chest wall, so that we have regretted the failure to perform a corrective operation earlier. Since then, we have preferred to operate on these children at whatever age they were seen. In the operation for these deformities, it is important to place the incision be-

yond the area of the defect. A fascia lata graft gave a gratifying immediate result in 1 of our early patients, but the paradoxical motion in the area of the defect recurred in 6–8 months, and we proceeded to the rib-strut operation, which we have preferred ever since.[4] A contralateral rib is removed subperiosteally, either through a separate incision or through a medial continuation of the same incision. With an oscillating saw, the rib of even a small child is easily cut into two strips. Medially, the rib end is inserted into a defect pressed into the edge of the sternum with the point of a hemostat, and laterally the graft over-rides one of the rib ends, to which it is fixed by a through-and-through suture. The medial end is likewise fastened by a suture through rib and sternum. We usually employ two ribs, providing at least three grafts. Over the ribs, to maintain them in position and provide a normal contour by making up for the lack of muscle, we place a sheet of Teflon felt sutured to the rib grafts and to the chest wall on all sides beyond the defect. The results of our last five operations performed

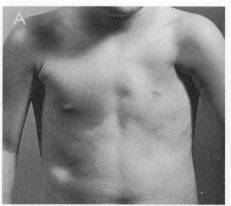

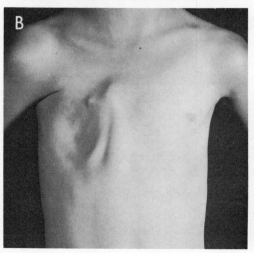

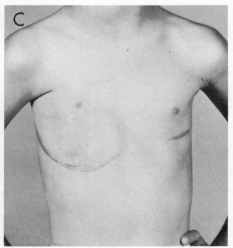

Fig. 26-12.—Syndrome of deficiency of 2nd to 4th costal cartilages, absence of pectoralis minor and costal portion of pectoralis major, upward displacement of hypoplastic nipple and breast, and hypoplasia of subcutaneous tissue. All of our patients have been females, although the condition is reported in males. **A,** A.C., 2 years old. Satisfactory correction was achieved with rib grafts from the same side and a sheet of Teflon felt overlying the defect. **B** and **C,** P.J., 7 years old, with unsightly defect and conspicuous deformity. Paradoxical respiration was obvious, but there were no symptoms. The individual cartilaginous defects were bridged with bone grafts from a rib of the opposite side and the reconstruction reinforced with a sheet of Teflon felt. Absence of the costal portion of the pectoralis major is still obvious, but the chest has normal contour, the chest wall is solid and there is no paradoxical motion on respiration. The breast will probably develop but will be a fraction of the size of the opposite one. Cosmetic augmentation of the breast by prosthetic implant will be postponed until maturity.

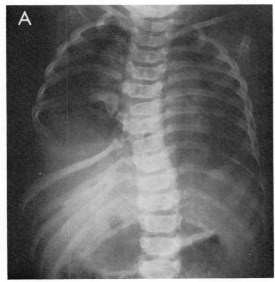

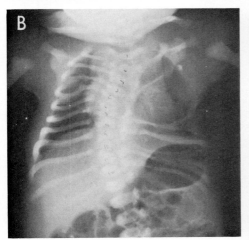

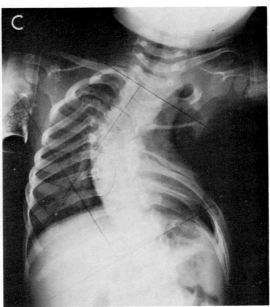

Fig. 26-13.—Absence of ribs. Numerous varieties of real or apparent absence of rib occur, with or without a chest wall bulge that can be interpreted as a lung hernia. **A,** an infant with a wide gap between ribs and a great soft tissue bulge. Actually there are 12 ribs, but some are deformed. These are associated with vertebral deformities. Osteotomies and approximation of the 6th and 7th ribs corrected the herniation and also the scoliosis. **B** and **C,** an infant with multiple absence of bony ribs on the left and abnormalities of bony ribs on the right. There was a large area of symptomatic, paradoxical respiration in the uncovered area. However, the most serious problem was vertebral. Note the large mass of fused bone on the right parallel to the vertebral column and striking progression of scoliosis in 16 months **(C).** Operation was advised, but declined.

in this manner have been particularly satisfying.[5]

A number of these patients have associated anomalies of the vertebrae and the other ribs. In 1 patient, absence of the second to fifth ribs was associated with a sharp depression in the lower ribs, producing a concavity in the chest wall. This was of the kind associated with pectus carinatum.

In a child with numerous hemivertebrae and an enormously wide gap between two ribs, there was an impressive bulge which indeed could have been called a lung hernia. Actually, no ribs were missing. We performed osteotomies of the ribs above and be-

low the defect at their posterior margins and approximated them with heavy pericostal sutures, completing the union by raising and suturing together, periosteal flaps from the two ribs. The hernia was cured; and, what was even more astonishing, the considerable degree of scoliosis which had been present was corrected (Fig. 26-13, *A*). Rickham[6] performed an ingenious procedure in the infant referred to earlier whose sixth to tenth ribs were completely missing. The fifth rib was split as it lay in its bed, and the eleventh rib likewise. The upper half of the eleventh rib, hinged at the anterior end, was swung medially and upward to provide a new costal margin, and the lower half of the fifth rib was approximated to the lower half of the eleventh rib. The mobilized upper half of the eleventh rib was then fixed to the anterior end of the fifth rib and the remaining portion of the eleventh rib.

In many children with grotesque and atypical rib deformities, particularly absence of bony ribs, the associated vertebral anomalies are more significant than the costal deformities because severe scoliosis may result (Fig. 26-13, *B* and *C*).

In some children, the rib deformities are so severe and asymmetrical as to dwarf any sternal deformity, whether protrusion or depression. Some have grotesque local concavities formed by incurvations of the ribs or costal cartilages, sometimes associated with tilting or other deformity of the sternum. These deformities can be corrected by local subperichondrial or subperiosteal excisions of the deformed costal elements or by double osteotomies to wedge out the sunken segments. The associated sternal deformities require special treatment in the individual cases. Some of these bizarre deformities may require special analysis and imaginative operative treatment. Our results with the children operated on and our observations of a number of children over a span of years while withholding treatment have convinced us that the deformities usually become accentuated and that early corrective efforts are well worth while.[5]

REFERENCES

1. Asp, K., and Sulamaa, M.: On rare congenital deformities of the thoracic wall, Acta chir. scandinav. 118:392, 1960.
2. deBenedetti, M., and Chiapuzzo, A.: Malformazione unilaterale dei muscoli pettorali, Arch. ortop. 73:408, 1960.
3. Hecker, W. C., and Daum, R.: Chirurgisches Vorgehen bei kongenitalen Brustwanddefekten, Chirurg 11:482, 1964.
4. Ravitch, M. M.: The operative treatment of congenital deformities of the chest, Am. J. Surg. 101:588, 1961.
5. Ravitch, M. M.: Atypical deformities of the chest wall: Absence and deformities of the ribs and costal cartilages, Surgery 59:438, 1966.
6. Rickham, P. P.: Lung hernia secondary to congenital absence of ribs, Arch. Dis. Childhood 34:14, 1959.

MARK M. RAVITCH

Drawings by
PEARLMAN (Figure 8)
LEON SCHLOSSBERG (Figure 10)

Tumors of the Chest Wall

TUMORS OF THE chest wall proper are moderately uncommon in adults and distinctly more uncommon in children. The paramount observation is this: that malignant chest wall tumors are more common in children than benign chest wall tumors, and that a tumor in the chest wall of a child is more likely to be malignant than a tumor in the chest wall of an adult. Little appears to have been written dealing specifically with chest wall tumors in children. Gleanings from the collected reports of chest wall tumors in patients of all ages indicate that, of the benign tumors, chondromas of the ribs have occasionally been found in children (1 child of 11 years, of 31 collected by Harper[5]). At least one osteoid osteoma has been reported. In 3 children, ribs have been found to be the seat of lesions of the lipoid histiocytoses. Of 10 giant cell tumors of the ribs reported by Buckles and Lawless[2], 3 occurred in children 9, 11 and 14 years of age. Although only 1 of the 10 tumors was frankly malignant, 4 had invaded the soft tissues locally. The numbers in the various series are so small that no suggestion of the frequency of the various malignant chest tumors in children can be given. Ewing's tumor of the bone is in general a tumor of younger patients, and although the rib is one of its less common sites, the proportion of children with Ewing's tumor primary in the ribs appears to be somewhat higher than with this tumor in other bones. Here, as in other bones, the rapidly growing Ewing's tumor produces pain, fever, local heat and erythema, so that the lesion may be mistaken for an inflammatory process. The clinical outlook is bleak. In one series of 8 patients aged 6–59 with Ewing's tumor of the ribs, 4 were less than 30 years of age, 7 were dead and 1 still living with tumor.[11] On the other hand, in a 10-year-old girl with Ewing's tumor, Kinsella *et al.*[9] resected a full thickness of the chest wall, including 3 ribs and portions of the lung. The patient was alive and free from obvious tumor 18 months later. Sarcomas of various kinds comprise the principal group of malignant tumors of the chest wall in infancy and childhood. Most of them are probably chondrosarcomas,[10,12,13] although some of them have been diagnosed as osteogenic sarcomas, and others are undifferentiated anaplastic sarcomas (Fig. 26-14). Hopkins and Freitas[7] described what they considered to be two huge osteochondromas, one on either side, projecting into the thorax of a 3-month-old child, occupying 40% of the hemithorax on the left (8-cm diameter) and 50% on the right and causing dyspnea and cyanosis. The masses were removed in separate operations, taking one rib on the left and three on the right. There was no recurrence after 4 years. The tumor nevertheless was probably a chondrosarcoma. In another 3-month-old child, Hall and Ellison[4] resected an 8 × 10 × 15-cm mass reported to have been growing since birth. The child was well 6 years later. Polk *et al.*[12] reported on a boy of 5 with a tumor involving one rib, previously abandoned as hopeless because

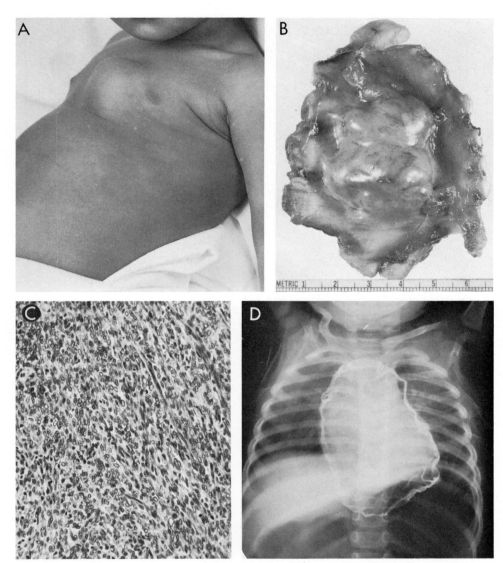

Fig. 26-14.—Undifferentiated sarcoma of ribs or sternum. A pea-sized lump was noted on the chest wall at age 2 or 3 months; at 13 months it was said to be "about as large as 3 almonds, over the ribs, just to the left of the lower end of the sternum." Growth since had been rapid. **A,** at 17 months, the mass, covering the lower chest anteriorly and most of the sternum, was 5.5 cm in diameter, projected outward some 3 cm., was rubbery, firm, fixed to the chest wall, not attached to the skin. Diagnosis was malignancy, probably chondrosarcoma. **B,** the resected specimen. Six cartilages were removed on either side, and bony rib included in 2 of those on the left. The entire gladiolus occupies the center. Note the internal mass, equal to the external mass, and covered by pleura. **C,** photomicrograph, showing highly cellular undifferentiated sarcoma, perhaps of periosteal origin. **D,** postoperative film, showing large tantalum sheet sutured in place. The child had little paradox and was thought to be doing well when she died abruptly 18 hours after operation. This was in 1951. Today we would use a firmer prosthesis, probably perform a tracheostomy and use mechanically assisted respirations for several days until confident the child could aerate effectively, although this baby showed no embarrassment.

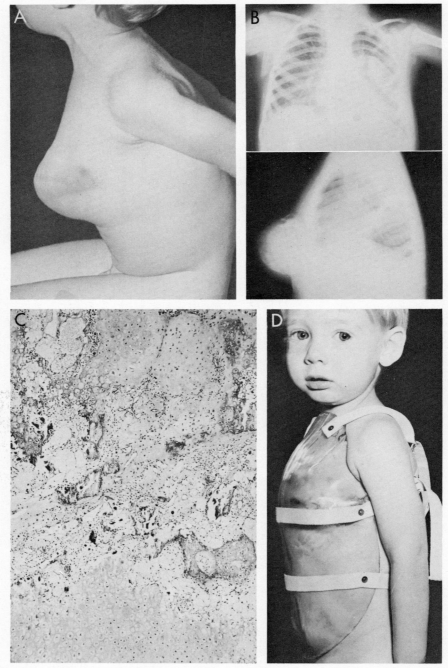

Fig. 26-15.—Chondrosarcoma of ribs and sternum. This boy was born with a cherry-sized mass just left of the sternum. The tumor grew steadily and was removed at age 9 months. Recurrence was obvious in 3 months, and tumor growth continued until hospitalization at age 2 years, when it was 10 × 10 cm and covered most of the anterior chest. **A,** the large tumor and scar of the first operation. The tumor was hard, fixed to chest wall and skin, extended from the 3rd interspace to the costal margin and from the right side of the sternum to the left anterior axillary line.

B, films showing the huge extent of the tumor and calcification within it. **C,** photomicrograph, showing chondrosarcoma. The entire mass was removed with overlying skin and underlying pleura, 5 ribs, distal portion of the sternum and a segment of the opposite costal margin. The free edge of the diaphragm was brought up to the ribs at the upper border of the defect and sutured there, turning the thoracic defect into an abdominal one. The specimen was 11 × 7 × 7 cm. The tumor had destroyed the ribs and cartilage in the area of the mass but was still covered by

of a massive pleural effusion. He was well 15 years after resection of the chest wall and irradiation for the chondrosarcoma. Winter and Tongen[14] reported on a boy who, at age 3-1/2, for an undifferentiated sarcoma of the chest wall, had a wide chest wall resection, including two ribs. He survived an even larger resection for a local recurrence, a right lower lobectomy and a left lower lobe wedge resection for pulmonary metastases, then a third operation on the chest wall and spine for local recurrence. All operations were done in an 11-month period; and, on two occasions in this time, radon seeds were implanted in the chest wall. He was well 15 years later and had had a spinal fusion and Harrington rod correction of the severe scoliosis that had developed. The evidence is good that a number of these tumors were present at birth, that there is an occasional period of delay before rapid growth is manifest, and that a number of patients who died might have been salvaged by an initially decisive and definitive operation instead of a period of observation or a temporizing limited procedure.

Desmoid tumors are rare in children and rarer still in extra-abdominal locations. Keeley et al.[8] operated successfully on a 5-year-old girl with large separate desmoids of the abdominal wall and chest wall. Radically wide excisions appear to have been curative.

TREATMENT.—A chest wall tumor in a child should be assumed to be malignant and should be treated initially by an en bloc full-thickness resection of chest wall. The skin incision should, if possible, be raised as a flap so that after the chest wall has been resected the suture line will fall beyond the defect. If the tumor underlies the muscle belly of the latissimus or the pectoralis, the muscle, if not involved, may be retracted. If the tumor is in the area of muscle attachments, the muscle must be removed with the tumor. An intercostal incision, at least one interspace above or below the apparent extent of the tumor, will allow introduction of the finger to probe the pleural cavity to determine by palpation the apparent extent of the tumor. A block of chest wall is then removed. The only hope of cure in most of these tumors is by obtaining an adequate margin at the first operation; if there is any doubt, one should go an interspace higher or lower or carry the resection farther anteriorly or posteriorly. There is no room for compromise. The sternum must be widely resected, if involved, and the pleura with the chest wall, even if this involves opening both pleural cavities.

With limited resections of the chest wall, particularly if heavy muscles have been preserved, no reconstruction is necessary. If a large segment of chest wall is resected, it is best to repair the defect in part with split rib grafts from the contralateral side with or without an additional fascia lata repair. The prosthetic material that has given us the most satisfaction for this purpose is Teflon felt, although Marlex and other materials are undoubtedly satisfactory. If the rib resection is such as to include the costal margin, we have, on a number of occasions, found it useful to shift the diaphragm to the upper margin of the defect, so that the large defect now becomes abdominal rather than thoracic (Fig. 26-15). This necessarily decreases the volume of the thorax but simplifies the reconstruction and eliminates the likelihood of any significant paradoxical respiration. Figures 26-14 and 26-15 illustrate tumors with which we have had experience, and in Chapter 29, on tumors of the mediastinum, will be found an illustration (Fig. 29-14) of a neuroblastoma perforating the chest wall and presenting as a chest wall tumor.

REFERENCES

1. Bergstrand, H.: Four cases of Ewing sarcoma in ribs, Am. J. Cancer 27:26, 1936.
2. Buckles, M. G., and Lawless, E. C.: Giant cell tumor of ribs, J. Thoracic Surg. 19:438, 1950.
3. Dorner, R. A., and Marcy, D. S.: Primary rib tumors, J. Thoracic Surg. 17:690, 1948.
4. Hall, D. P., and Ellison, R. G.: Osteochondrosarcoma of the chest wall in a newborn infant, Am. Surgeon 30:745, 1964.
5. Harper, F. R.: Benign chondromas of the ribs, J. Thoracic Surg. 9:132, 1939.
6. Herbert, W. P.: Ewing's tumor of the rib: Report of two cases, J. Thoracic Surg. 5:189, 1935.
7. Hopkins, S. M., and Freitas, E. L.: Bilateral osteochondroma of the ribs in an infant; an unusual cause of cyanosis, J. Thoracic & Cardiovas. Surg. 49:247, 1965.
8. Keeley, J. L.; De Rosario, J. L., and Schairer, A. E.: Desmoid tumors of the abdominal and thoracic walls in a child, Arch. Surg. 80:144, 1960.
9. Kinsella, T. J.; White, S. M., and Koucky, R. W.: Two unusual tumors of the sternum, J. Thoracic Surg. 16:640, 1947.
10. O'Neill, L. W., and Ackermann, L. V.: Cartilaginous tumors of ribs and sternum, J. Thoracic Surg. 21:71, 1951.
11. Pascuzzi, C. A.; Dahlin, D. C., and Clagett, O. T.: Primary tumors of the ribs and sternum, Surg., Gynec. & Obst. 104:390, 1957.
12. Polk, J. W., et al.: Malignant lesions of the chest wall, Missouri Med. 58:217, 1961.
13. Watkins, E., Jr., and Gerard, F. P.: Malignant tumors involving the chest wall, J. Thoracic & Cardiovas. Surg. 39:117, 1960.
14. Winter, R. B., and Tongen, L. A.: A malignant chest wall sarcoma with bilateral pulmonary metastases: A fifteen year survival after multiple radical local excision and resection of bilateral pulmonary metastases and a successful treatment of scoliosis secondary to tumor surgery, Surgery 62:374, 1967.

M. M. RAVITCH

pleura on the under surface. **D,** convalescence from this extensive procedure was uneventful. The heart was covered only by skin and fat, and a Plexiglas cuirasse was worn for protection. Two years later, during subcutaneous insertion of rib grafts across the defect, he suffered anoxic cardiac arrest. During only temporarily effective resuscitation by cardiac massage, the left chest was found to be free from tumor.

27

Diaphragmatic Hernia

HISTORY.—The first diaphragmatic hernia was reported by Ambrose Paré in 1579.[6] After that original report, several hundred years elapsed during which the condition remained a pathologic curiosity and was rarely diagnosed during life. In 1761, Morgagni reviewed the pathology of diaphragmatic hernia and described the hernia through the foramen that bears his name.[39] In 1789, an important detailed study of the condition was made by Astley Cooper in his monograph on hernias. He gave an excellent description of the anatomy and symptoms, and his classification of the varieties of this form of hernia is still used today.[45] In 1848, Bochdalek[4] pointed out that some diaphragmatic hernias occur through an opening in the posterior part of the diaphragm. The first case involving herniation of bowel through the diaphragm treated operatively was reported by Naumann in 1888.[32] The patient died. One year later, Walker[44] reported recovery following laparotomy for traumatic diaphragmatic hernia caused by a falling log.

Hedblom[20] reviewed the literature in 1925 and reported a collected series of 378 cases of diaphragmatic hernia. Only 44 of these were classified as "congenital." It is interesting that some of the patients had survived to adulthood, the oldest reported being over 71 years of age. Hedblom pointed out, however, that 75% of children with untreated diaphragmatic hernias failed to live beyond the first month of life and suggested that early operative intervention was the only way to decrease this tremendous loss of life. He reported a surgical mortality of 72.7% in hernias operated on following symptoms of intestinal obstruction, and 38.4% in nonobstructed cases. He urged that obstructed diaphragmatic hernias especially receive prompt operative intervention.

Actually, there were only 22 children in Hedblom's series. They were operated on for diaphragmatic hernias of various types, some congenital and others of traumatic origin. Two children were obstructed preoperatively: 1 died and 1 hernia recurred. Of the remaining 20, 11 were treated by laparotomy with 8 recoveries, 5 were treated by thoracotomy with 3 recoveries, and 4 had combined thoracoabdominal approaches with 1 recovery. These striking salvage rates were used by Hedblom to justify early operative intervention. Hedblom's conclusions are as timely today as they were in 1925. He advised early operation in suspected cases of diaphragmatic hernia before intestinal obstruction or respiratory failure ensued. He encouraged increased use of roentgen examinations to confirm the clinical diagnosis before operation. He felt that operative mortality could be reduced by measures to treat or prevent shock, by differential pressure anesthesia and by postoperative precautions to reduce pneumothorax. He concluded that choice of approach—laparotomy or thoracotomy—depended on the case.

Hedblom's opinions went unheeded at first, but he was supported in his desire for early intervention in children with diaphragmatic hernia by Greenwald and Steiner,[15] who reviewed all cases of diaphragmatic hernia in children, regardless of operative or nonoperative treatment reported from 1912 to 1929. Only 11 of the 82 cases collected were treated operatively and 6 of these recovered. The rest were allowed to follow their natural course. Almost all died. Forty-six were not diagnosed until autopsy. The authors emphasized that most of them might have been saved by early operative intervention. In a similar report during this period, Woolsey[47] drew the same conclusions. Nevertheless operative treatment did not become popular until several successful cases of repair of diaphragmatic hernias in children accumulated.[12,33,43] A decade passed before operative intervention came to be regarded as the treatment of choice. Finally, with increased experience, the operative mortality was gradually reduced. In 1940, Hartzell[19] reviewed the literature and reported an operative mortality of 50%. Ladd and Gross[24] reported 19 cases operated upon with 12 survivors. In 1945, Donovan[13] reported an operative mortality of 24%. Later reports continued to reflect this trend of improvement.[2,17,36,40,49,50] Gross[16] listed 72 patients, with only 8 deaths, 3 of which were due to associated congenital defects.

Embryology

Sometime during the eighth to the tenth week of fetal life the diaphragm is formed and the coelomic cavity is divided into its abdominal and thoracic components. At the same time, the gastrointestinal tract undergoes its major development. The small and large intestines elongate into the umbilical pouch and rotation of the gut takes place. The interrelationship of these two processes—the formation of the diaphragm and the development of the intestine—determines many of the varieties of diaphragmatic hernias encountered in infants and children.

The normal diaphragm results from fusion of several components. At about the eighth week of fetal life the septum transversum forms beneath the heart and grows backward to meet the dorsal mesentery of the foregut, thereby completing the central portion of the diaphragm. Pleuroperitoneal folds then develop on each side and extend laterally and posteriorly, gradually completing division of the thoracic and abdominal cavities. Initially, these folds consist only of membranous pleura and peritoneum. Later, muscle fibers derived from cervical myotomes grow between these membranous layers and reinforce them to form the final diaphragm. As a rule, this process is completed by the end of the ninth week of fetal life. The left side usually closes later than the right. The last portion to be closed on either side is the posterior portion. This triangular area is known as the pleuroperitoneal canal, or foramen of Bochdalek. Although the anterior aspect of the diaphragm usually is completed before the posterior, failure of fusion of the central and lateral portions of the diaphragm may also occur anteriorly. The hiatus in this anterior region is called the foramen of Morgagni. Controversy exists concerning the etiology of diaphragmatic hernias through the foramen of Morgagni. Since most of them have true membranous sacs, it is contended by some that they result not from failure of the diaphragmatic components to fuse, but from failure of muscular elements from the cervical myotomes to reinforce the diaphragm properly. Others contend that these hernias result from trauma, exertion, obesity or other extrinsic causes. Be that as it may, anterolateral diaphragmatic hernias, though rare, do occur in infants and children.[3,5,48]

During formation of the diaphragm, the midgut undergoes rapid elongation into the umbilical cord and develops into its various components. About the tenth week of fetal life the midgut rotates and returns into the abdominal cavity. Premature return of the midgut into the abdominal cavity, or delayed closure of the diaphragm, lays the foundation for many congenital diaphragmatic hernias. Improper muscular reinforcement of the diaphragmatic folds may also be a factor. Furthermore, early in fetal life the esophagus elongates and the stomach enters the abdominal cavity behind the developing septum transversum. Should lengthening of the esophagus be delayed or retarded, it is apparent that the stomach may not enter the abdominal cavity before the lumbar portion of the diaphragm is completed. Lesions such as esophageal hiatus hernia and congenital short esophagus may result. Failure of the pleuroperitoneal folds to be reinforced adequately by invasion of muscle from the cervical myotomes may result in diaphragmatic hernias with true membranous sacs in any portion of the diaphragm. Some observers think that hernias through the foramen of Morgagni, and eventration of the diaphragm, represent this type of embryologic maldevelopment.

Several adventitious diaphragmatic fibromuscular anomalies, including 5 cases of accessory diaphragm reported in the literature since 1951, may represent isolated diaphragmatic remnants resulting from embryonic elements of the diaphragm. Although the ontogeny of these defects is by no means clear, it is felt that the lung bud grows into the septum transversum so as to split off fibromuscular remnants that emerge clinically either as isolated bands in the pleural cavity or as a well-defined accessory diaphragm.[29]

Incidence and Symptoms

It is almost impossible to estimate the incidence of diaphragmatic hernias. They can occur at any age and may be congenital or acquired. Their symptoms vary from vague discomfort to syndromes so severe that life itself is threatened. In children, these hernias are usually congenital, except when associated with severe trauma. Of 116 patients with congenital

TABLE 27-1.—INCIDENCE OF CONGENITAL DIAPHRAGMATIC HERNIA IN INFANTS AND CHILDREN AT CHILDREN'S MEMORIAL HOSPITAL, 1945-66

TYPE	OPERATED ON	NOT OPERATED ON	No.	%
Bochdalek	66	3*	69	59.5
Morgagni	3	–	3	2.6
Hiatus hernia	14	2*	16	13.8
Short esophagus	10	1†	11	9.5
Eventration	13	4†	17	14.6
Totals	106	10	116	100.0

*Died of other congenital defects before operation was considered.
†Asymptomatic.

diaphragmatic hernia observed at the Children's Memorial Hospital of Chicago in 21 years, 106 had symptoms severe enough to warrant operative intervention, 5 were asymptomatic and required no surgical management and 5 died of other multiple congenital defects and diaphragmatic hernia was an incidental finding at autopsy. Distribution of the types of hernia is outlined in Table 27-1.

Symptoms in congenital diaphragmatic hernia vary greatly. They are referable to the respiratory, circulatory or digestive systems. Their severity depends on the size and location of the hernial defect as well as the presence or absence of a hernial sac. These two factors determine the degree of displacement of abdominal viscera into the thoracic cavity and the extent of collapse of the lungs. Indirectly, they determine the age at which intervention becomes necessary. Thus hernias through the pleuroperitoneal hiatus (foramen of Bochdalek), which are usually large and have no hernial sac, cause early and severe symptoms. Most of these patients come to operation within the first week of life, usually in an emergency procedure. Hernias with smaller defects, and with hernial sacs (hiatus hernia and herniation through the foramen of Morgagni), may not manifest themselves until later in life, and their symptoms are usually not as severe. As a result, they rarely come to operation during the newborn period, and the operations can be performed more or less on an elective basis (Table 27-2).

In our experience, the type of surgical approach also depends on the nature of the symptoms and the degree of displacement of the organs into the thoracic cavity. In most of our patients, the approach was through an abdominal incision (Table 27-2) because we believed that this afforded the greatest advantage for returning massively displaced bowel into the abdomen. In a few, the approach was transabdominal because severe or bizarre obstructive symptoms required careful exploration of all the bowel. The remaining patients were explored transthoracically because of the obvious advantages inherent in approaching the hernial defect from above, and because displacement of bowel into the thorax was incomplete. Four patients had a combined thoracoabdomi-

TABLE 27-2.—Diaphragmatic Hernia in Infants and Children at Children's Memorial Hospital, 1945–66: Characteristics of Cases Operated on

| Type | Age at Onset of Symptoms | | Side Involved | | Primary Symptoms | | | Surgical Approach | | |
	Range	Most Frequent	R	L	Cardio-resp.	Obst.	Hemat.	Abd.	Thor.	Comb.
Bochdalek	1 da.–3 yr.	1–3 da.	13	53	57	8	1	50	13	3
Morgagni	1 da.–3 yr.	few mo.	1	2	1	2	0	2	1	0
Hiatus hernia	3 wk.–7 yr.	6 mo.–1 yr.	—	—	3	10	1	3	10	1
Short esophagus	7 da.–2 yr.	Variable, recurrent	—	—	0	6	4	0	3*	0
Eventration	1 mo.–11 yr.	1–3 yr.	4	9	10	3	0	1	12	0
Totals			18	64	71	29	6	56	39	4

*Seven patients with short esophagus were treated with repeated bouginage. Two had operative repair with vagotomy and pyloroplasty.

nal approach. The costal margin was not transected. The combined approach was necessary because the original incision was inadequate for reduction of the hernia or complete repair of the defect. In general, replacement of intestine in a Bochdalek hernia is easier through the abdomen, repair of the hernial defect is easier through the chest.

Management

Management of congenital diaphragmatic hernias can be achieved with low mortality and morbidity only through prompt diagnosis and rapid, effective surgical treatment. Adequate roentgen examination is the foundation of present diagnostic methods. Prompt intervention is the only effective way to save the patient's life in the face of acute cardiorespira-

tory deterioration, or severe obstructive phenomena, which so often occur in these patients. Symptoms vary so much with the site of herniation that management is best discussed on the basis of the type of hernia involved.

Hernias Through the Foramen of Bochdalek

The most common hernia encountered in infants is one through the pleuroperitoneal canal or foramen of Bochdalek. Most of these hernias have no true sac and presumably result from entry of the abdominal organs into the pleural space before the pleuroperitoneal hiatus is completely obliterated. Some, however, result after the pleuroperitoneal membrane has developed but before muscular reinforcement has oc-

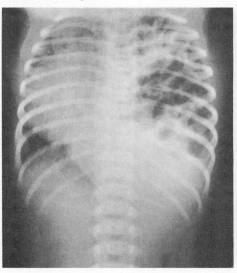

Fig. 27-1 (left).—Bochdalek hernia. This newborn had severe dyspnea and cyanosis, and emergency operation had to be done as a life-saving measure. The intestine obliterates the left pleural space and completely compresses the left lung. The mediastinum and heart are shifted to the right.

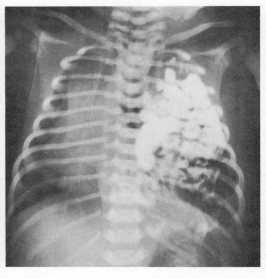

Fig. 27-2 (right).—Bochdalek hernia. Use of radiopaque medium to confirm the diagnosis. In general, this procedure is not necessary and should be avoided. In this patient there was some question of differentiation between diaphragmatic hernia and postpneumonia pneumatoceles.

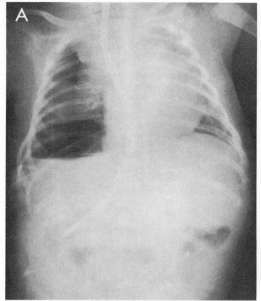 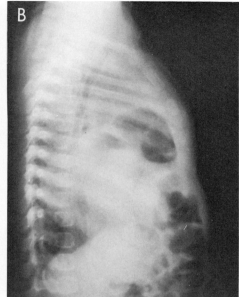

Fig. 27-3.—Right-sided Bochdalek hernia. This 10-day-old patient was admitted with moderately severe dyspnea and cyanosis. Roentgenograms suggested hernia through the right pleuroperitoneal hiatus with a confining sac. The sac was inverted and the defect repaired. **A,** the sharply rounded border of the intestinal gas shadow suggests a confining sac. **B,** lateral view. Note that the right pleural space is not completely obliterated and the right lung is not entirely compressed.

curred, for hernias of Bochdalek occasionally do have membranous sacs. Signs and symptoms vary with the amount of bowel or other intestinal organs displaced into the pleural cavity and the degree of displacement of the mediastinum, or collapse of the lungs. At birth, the infant may seem normal, but as the herniated bowel fills with gas or food, dyspnea and cyanosis develop. Labored respirations pull more and more of the abdominal organs into the open pleural cavity. Cyanosis and respiratory embarrassment become more alarming. Prompt diagnosis and treatment become mandatory if the patient's life is to be saved.

PHYSICAL EXAMINATION.—In addition to the cyanosis, extremely rapid respirations are noted. The abdomen is scaphoid, and instead of the usual diaphragmatic respiration found in infants, a rocking type of respiratory motion occurs with increased intercostal effort. Dullness to percussion is present on the affected side, and there are no respiratory sounds. Heart sounds are displaced in the opposite direction. Peristalsis is not usually heard over the herniated bowel.

DIAGNOSIS.—Roentgenograms (Fig. 27-1) confirm the diagnosis. Gas-filled bowel and often stomach are seen in the pleural space, with collapse of the ipsilateral lung and displacement of the mediastinum toward the opposite side. Ingestion of radiopaque medium is usually not required for diagnosis. In fact, it should be avoided except in unusual circumstances when the diagnosis is not readily apparent. Occasion-

ally it may be used to differentiate between hernia of Bochdalek and congenital lung cysts, postpneumonic air spaces, duplication of the bowel and other anomalies (Fig. 27-2).

TREATMENT.—Operation is the treatment of choice, and more often than not must be performed on an emergency basis. As soon as the diagnosis is made, a catheter is passed into the stomach for constant suction until operation, to attempt decompression and prevent further distention. The patient may also be propped in the semiupright position, lying toward the affected side. This sometimes aids intestinal decompression and improves respiratory capacity. Oxygen, by tent or incubator, also helps relieve dyspnea and cyanosis. Some neonates require intubation immediately after birth and must be maintained with gentle assisted respiration until preparations for immediate operation can be completed. One real key to success is *immediate* surgery, as soon as the diagnosis is made, before progressive respiratory embarrassment or intestinal obstruction leads to deterioration of the patient's condition or to sudden death. Since vomiting is not apt to be serious, dehydration is not a problem unless operation is delayed. An ankle vein is cannulated before operation in order to facilitate blood transfusion and aid parenteral postoperative feedings.

Some controversy prevails as to whether or not these patients should be approached transthoracically or via the abdomen.[23] In our opinion, the matter is determined by the extent of herniation of abdominal organs into the pleural space and the ease with which the surgeon expects to return them into the abdominal cavity. In the unusual instance, with a true membranous sac confining the abdominal organs to less than total obliteration of the pleural space (Figs. 27-3 and 27-4), there is no quarrel with the transthoracic approach. With the usual hernia through the foramen of Bochdalek, however, there is no confining hernial sac, and displacement of the abdominal organs into the pleural space is massive. Since these organs have been in the pleural space for a long time before birth, they have in effect "surrendered the right of domicile" in the abdomen. In order to return them to the abdominal cavity, considerable stretching of the abdominal musculature is necessary. In these circumstances, the abdominal approach is preferable. We used it for most hernias of this type.

A transverse incision is made on the same side as the hernia and the defect in the diaphragm is located. Many operators prefer a vertical paramedian incision. A catheter is inserted through the diaphragmatic hernia into the pleural space.[25] This allows air to enter the pleural space and facilitates delivery of the herniated abdominal organs. These displaced organs are covered with moist laparotomy pads while the hernial defect is repaired (Fig. 27-5).

Fig. 27-4.—Hernia through the left foramen of Bochdalek involving the left kidney in a 3-week-old child. Note demonstration of the left renal pelvis by intravenous pyelography. Symptoms were not referable to the diaphragmatic hernia, which was an incidental finding in a patient with other congenital anomalies.

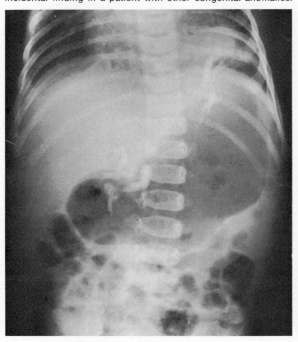

The defect is usually triangular, with base located near the upper pole of the kidney. There may or may not be a posterior shelf. If one is available, closure of the defect is greatly facilitated. Usually, one can find at least a rim of diaphragm rolled against the chest wall. If no posterior shelf is present, the anterior segment of the diaphragm is sutured to the posterolateral chest wall, just above the upper pole of the kidney, with interrupted silk sutures. We strongly recommend that endothoracic tube drainage be introduced before closure of the diaphragmatic hernia is completed. It greatly facilitates postoperative pleural toilet and provides steady gentle suction to help expand the collapsed lung. A small endothoracic catheter is easily introduced through the lower chest wall or through the lateral end of the diaphragmatic hernia repair. It can then be attached to low-level water seal drainage at the termination of the operative procedure. As the last sutures are secured, the anesthesiologist applies very gentle pressure through the endotracheal tube to expand the collapsed lung. It is extremely important that this lung be inflated gently and that vigorous attempts to expand it be scrupulously avoided. In many patients with hernias through the foramen of Bochdalek, development of the lung has been retarded by pressure from the displaced bowel, and both the surgeon and the anesthesiologist may be disappointed to see just a small nubbin of lung which, even after being expanded to its fullest capacity, fails to fill the available pleural space. It has been our experience that pressure on these segments of hypoplastic lung may lead to rupture of the pulmonary alveoli. It is far better to expand the lung only as far as its state of development will permit, then close the diaphragmatic hernia to seal off the pleural space, knowing that some pleural space is left unoccupied. Within a few days postoperatively with continuous intercostal catheter suction, the pleural cavity is completely obliterated (Figs. 27-6 and 27-7) by the fully expanded lung.

Overexpansion of the hypoplastic lung with rupture of the pulmonary alveoli, on the other hand, may lead to tension pneumothorax (Fig. 27-8) not only on the side of the undeveloped lung but occasionally on the opposite normal lung. This is an extremely serious complication and, if undetected, may progress to cause extensive mediastinal displacement. Cyanosis and dyspnea become severe and death threatens.

After closure of the diaphragmatic hernia, the bowel is examined for evidence of abnormal bands, malrotation or other deformities. The displaced bowel may not have had normal rotation, and the duodenum, pancreas or colon may not have developed the usual peritoneal attachments to the posterior abdominal wall. In that case, volvulus is possible and occlusive bands partially or completely obstructing the intestine may be present. Furthermore, it is always an excellent routine to verify the patency of the gastrointestinal tract in the newborn before returning the

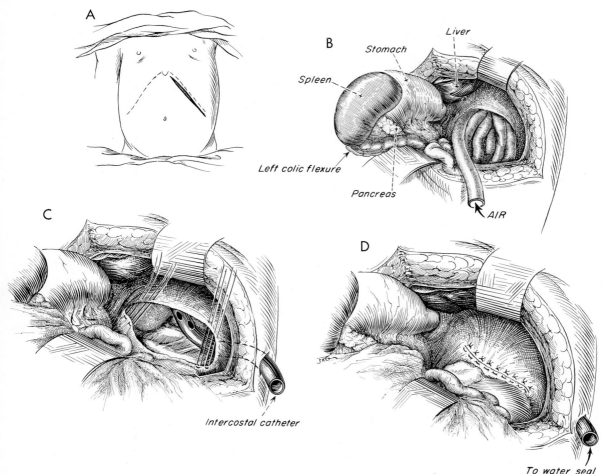

Fig. 27-5.—Bochdalek hernia; operative procedure. **A,** laparotomy incision, paramedian or subcostal, simplifies reduction of the hernia and inspection of the bowel for presence of other anomalies. **B,** intestine being returned to the abdominal cavity by traction. A catheter has been placed into the chest, through the hernial defect, to admit air into the chest and eliminate the nega-

tive pressure which hinders reduction. **C,** the defect exposed. Usually there is a posterior rim, although this may be inconspicuously rolled against the chest wall. **D,** closure of the defect with interrupted sutures. Continuous suction on the intercostal catheter assures evacuation of air and progressive inflation of the often hypoplastic lung.

bowel to the abdominal cavity and closing the operative incision.

Closure of the abdominal incision is sometimes difficult. The abdominal cavity may be too small to accommodate the increased bulk of all the abdominal organs it should ordinarily contain. Manual stretching of both flanks may be helpful, but even with this maneuver the abdominal organs may push up the diaphragm to such an extent that respiratory embarrassment, disruption of the diaphragmatic repair or obstruction of the venous drainage of the lower extremities may occur. If tension of the abdominal wall is so great that the surgeon fears any of these complications, the skin alone may be closed initially, with secondary closure of the peritoneum and fascia 1–2 weeks later.[27] In one instance, an enlarged spleen was

removed prior to closure of the abdominal incision, making it possible to accommodate all the remaining abdominal organs and still achieve primary closure of the incision.

Postoperatively, the patient is placed in an incubator or oxygen tent and receives oxygen with humidified atmosphere. The child's position is changed frequently and pharyngeal aspiration done often. Continuous nasogastric suction and intravenous fluids are continued until efficient abdominal peristalsis begins.

In our series, 66 patients were operated on for herniations through the foramen of Bochdalek (Tables 27-2 and 27-3). Thirteen occurred on the right side; 53 occurred through the left pleuroperitoneal hiatus. Although 1 patient did not have symptoms until 2½

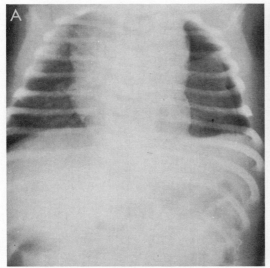

Fig. 27-6.—Bochdalek hernia—hypoplastic lung. This patient, 4 days old, was operated on for a hernia through the left foramen of Bochdalek. **A,** immediately after operation, the hypoplastic lung could fill only a small portion of the left pleural space. It was inflated by gentle suction through the endotracheal tube and the hernial defect closed. Symptoms improved following operation. **B,** 4 days later, air in the pleural sac had absorbed and the pleural cavity was obliterated. The hypoplastic lung was not large enough to replace the absorbed air, and the mediastinum shifted over to help obliterate the pleural space. The patient showed no untoward effects. The lung can be expected to fill the chest in most such cases. Negative pressure intercostal drainage is safe and effective.

Fig. 27-7.—Lung expansion in Bochdalek hernia. The patient, age 4 months, had repair of hernia of Bochdalek on the left side. **A,** roentgenogram of the chest immediately after operation. The left lung was not hypoplastic, but some pneumothorax remained and the lung did not expand fully. **B,** 4 days later the residual pneumothorax had been absorbed and the left lung had expanded to obliterate the pleural cavity. There was no mediastinal shift because the available lung was adequate to replace the absorbed air.

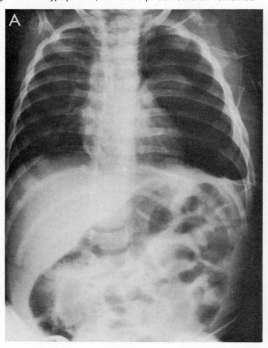

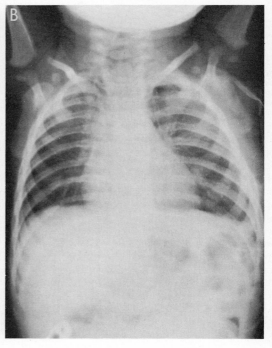

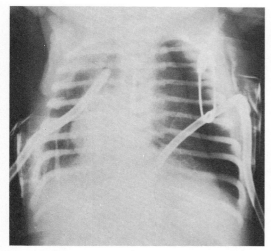

Fig. 27-8.—Bochdalek hernia—postoperative pneumothorax. Roentgenogram of a 2-day-old infant showing pneumothorax from rupture of the contralateral lung following excessive pressure inflation. The diaphragmatic hernia was repaired on the right side. Immediately after operation, dyspnea and cyanosis were not sufficiently improved, and the film demonstrated pneumothorax on the left. This was relieved by insertion of an endothoracic tube and attachment of water-seal drainage. The patient recovered. Forceful inflation is dangerous. Gradual pulmonary expansion by intercostal catheter negative pressure is preferable.

years of age, most of the patients were symptomatic during the first week of life and required emergency operation to save their lives. The majority had symptoms referable to the cardiorespiratory system. Eight also had signs of intestinal obstruction. Fifty were approached through an abdominal incision, 13 transthoracically, and 3 had combined thoracic and abdominal approaches. Thirteen patients died in the immediate postoperative period, although 6 of these deaths resulted directly from other associated congenital anomalies. There was one recurrence following operative repair. This patient died during the second attempt to repair his severe hernial defect.

TABLE 27-3.—DIAPHRAGMATIC HERNIA IN INFANTS AND CHILDREN AT CHILDREN'S MEMORIAL HOSPITAL, 1945–66: MORTALITY RATE AND RECURRENCES

TYPE	No.	RECURRENCES	OPERATIVE DEATHS
Bochdalek	66	1 (1.5%)	13 (19.7%)
Morgagni	3	0	0
Hiatus hernia	14	1 (7.2%)	2 (14.3%)
Short esophagus*	10	0	1 (10.0%)
Eventration†	13	0	2 (15.3%)
Totals‡	106	2 (1.9%)	18 (17.0%)

* Five of these were treated with repeated bouginage.
† One patient who died, expired following a second operation for Bochdalek hernia on the opposite side.
‡ Eight deaths resulted from other associated congenital defects.

Fifty-three patients survived and have done well following operation.

A great deal has been written in recent years concerning the causes of mortality from hernias through the foramen of Bochdalek.[49] A major factor in postoperative mortality has been the presence of aplastic or hypoplastic lung. Short of the observation that agenesis of the lung is frequently associated with multiple congenital anomalies,[14] there is no way to determine preoperatively whether the lung has the capacity to expand sufficiently to contribute to the patient's respiratory welfare in the postoperative period. However, in the absence of multiple congenital anomalies, there should be real potential for postoperative pulmonary expansion and growth.[1] For this reason, postoperative management of the ipsilateral pneumothorax is critical. Attempts at forced insufflation beyond the lung's capacity to stretch, or inadvertent injury to the lung during thoracentesis, can cause disastrous tension pneumothorax.[30] The best method, in our hands, for providing for lung expansion is insertion of an intrapleural transthoracic catheter attached to low-level water seal drainage. It is imperative that the height of the water in the drainage bottle be kept at a minimum (1–2 cm above the lower end of the line attached to the intrathoracic catheter), so that pleural drainage can be effected with minimal effort on the part of the patient. The efficiency of the water seal may be judged by periodic evaluation of the respiratory rate, roentgen study of the chest, the degree of fluctuation of water level in the chest drainage tube and periodic measurement of blood pH and Pco_2.[26]

Estimation of pH and Pco_2 blood levels is a valuable adjunct to postoperative management in diaphragmatic hernia because it quantitates the acidosis resulting from difficulties with pulmonary diffusion. It is not unusual to find a rise of Pco_2 and a fall of pH following repair of diaphragmatic hernia in the first week of life. These patients also become lethargic and require repeated external stimulation to breathe. Assisted respiration with tracheostomy or indwelling endotracheal tube and attempts to correct the acidosis by administration of amine buffers or sodium bicarbonate have been recommended.[10,28]

Meeker and Snyder[26] have also stressed the importance of maintaining adequate intestinal decompression during the immediate postoperative period in infants who have had repair of diaphragmatic hernia. To this end, they strongly recommend gastrostomy because it constantly vents air normally swallowed by the crying infant and helps prevent vomiting and pulmonary aspiration. They are also strong advocates of elective ventral hernia (i.e., delayed closure of the abdominal musculature) in neonates in whom there is difficulty with closure of the abdominal incision.[27]

Our 13 patients who died following operation for hernia of the Bochdalek type illustrate most of the points mentioned above. The deaths were of three types: (1) Six patients had diaphragmatic hernia and other congenital anomalies. Those with the most complicated problems died shortly after operation. Even some who survived the immediate postoperative period, but required numerous other procedures, eventually died. In rare instances, patients with two or more congenital anomalies that were compatible with life managed to achieve enough physiologic recovery to permit useful life. (2) Five patients had hypoplastic lungs and eventually died of inadequate pulmonary diffusion. These very young infants had symptoms at birth, remained in respiratory difficulty throughout the operative and postoperative course and could not be retained in stable acid-base balance despite serial evaluation of Po_2, Pco_2 and pH and use of alkalinizing agents. (3) Two deaths resulted from inadequate space in the abdominal cavity. These patients had intestinal decompression, and 1 had elective ventral hernia, with closure of the skin only over the operative site. Yet the pressure of the confined abdominal organs impeded venous return to the heart via the inferior vena cava and also interfered with respiratory efforts.

There were other patients in this series who survived in spite of similar difficulties. Presumably, they had a lesser degree of pulmonary hypoplasia or reduced abdominal cavity, so that their own compensatory mechanisms and our efforts at postoperative management were able to prevail.

Hernias Through the Foramen of Morgagni

Two of our patients had herniation through the anterior aspect of the leaf of the diaphragm, near the sternocostal junction. These hernias are less common than herniations through the foramen of Bochdalek and have true membranous sacs. The membranous sac confines the herniating bowel and limits the degree of pulmonary compression. In 1 of our patients, however, there were signs of cardiorespiratory embarrassment (Fig. 27-9). In the other, the primary symptoms were those of partial large bowel obstruction (Fig. 27-10). The former occurred in the newborn period. The latter occurred in an older child.

The diagnosis is suspected on routine roentgenograms of the chest and is confirmed by studies with radiopaque material. Surgical treatment is very similar to correction for hernias through the foramen of Bochdalek except that a hernial sac usually has to be excised or inverted and repair of the defect is performed in the anterior, rather than the posterior, portion of the diaphragm. Since the extent of herniation of bowel into the chest is usually small, a transthoracic approach is feasible, although a number of operators prefer an abdominal incision just below the costal margin.[48] Of our 2 patients, in the infant with cardiorespiratory embarrassment, an indefinite diagnosis and a relatively large defect, the approach was transthoracic; in the older child with herniation of colon just deep to the costal margin, the defect was repaired with ease through an abdominal incision.

Eleven instances have been described of associated defects in the diaphragmatic portion of the pericardium so that the intestines herniated into the pericardial sac.[42]

Eventration of the Diaphragm

In some patients, there is no actual hernial orifice in the diaphragm. The leaf of the diaphragm is stretched out, weakened by an apparent diminution of muscular elements, which permits the diaphragmatic leaf to rise high up into the ipsilateral pleural space and obliterate a considerable portion of the lung's breathing capacity. This is known as eventration of the diaphragm (Fig. 27-11).

The etiology of eventration is unknown. It may be the result of failure of muscular migration to reinforce adequately the embryonic pleuroperitoneal fold. Presumably, increased abdominal pressure and possibly increasing negative intrathoracic pressure result in stretching of the relatively weak diaphragm upward into the pleural space. Symptoms vary with the degree of eventration and increase as the extent of pulmonary collapse increases. Often they are minimal or absent; occasionally, moderate or severe. The diagnosis is readily confirmed by roentgenograms of the chest (Fig. 27-11). The elevated leaf of the diaphragm is demonstrated rising into the ipsilateral pleural cavity, while all the abdominal organs lie below a definite arched line which can be made out separating the abdomen from the chest. In case of doubt, pneumoperitoneum has been used to confirm the diagnosis (Fig. 27-13).

Treatment is required only when definite symptoms are referable to the deformity and severe enough to warrant surgical intervention. Operation consists of imbrication of the eventrated leaf of the diaphragm. A transthoracic approach is used. The redundant diaphragm is folded on itself and sutured into place. This gives a strong repair which lowers the diaphragm and restores the lost function of the lung (Fig. 27-12). We have not had occasion to use prostheses to reinforce the leaf of the diaphragm.

This deformity is not akin to injury or absence of function of the phrenic nerve. Newborns have been treated at the Children's Memorial Hospital for paralysis of the diaphragm due to birth injury of the phrenic nerve. Although dyspnea and cyanosis are present and roentgenographic views of the chest are similar to eventration of the diaphragm, fluoroscopy demonstrates a striking difference between the two conditions. Patients with paralysis of the diaphragmatic nerve supply have paradoxical motion of the involved leaf of the diaphragm. Those with eventration of the diaphragm do not.

Partial eventration occurs principally on the right

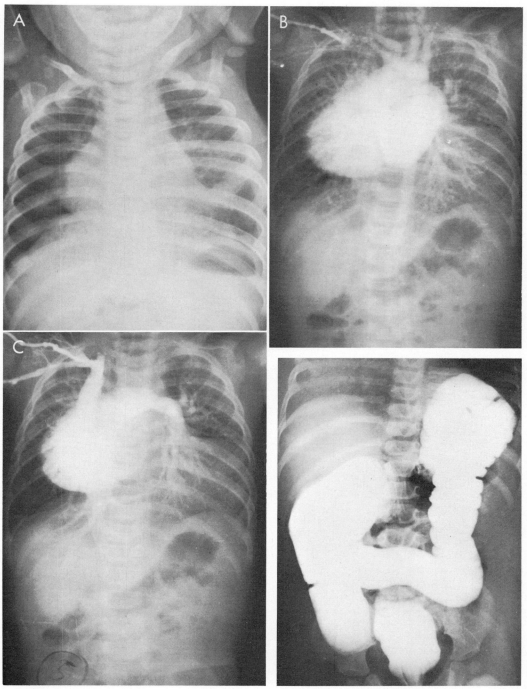

Fig. 27-9.—Foramen of Morgagni hernia. A 1-day-old infant presented symptoms of dyspnea and bouts of cyanosis. **A,** cardiac displacement suggests a tumor in the lower mediastinum. **B** and **C,** angiocardiograms demonstrate that the heart is superimposed on the mass and suggest the possibility of hernia through the foramen of Morgagni. At operation, the large anterior defect was readily repaired through a left thoracotomy.

Fig. 27-10 (lower right).—Hernia of foramen of Morgagni. In this 8-month-old child, the colon protruded through the defect and caused recurrent cramps and abdominal distention. This is the more common picture. There was a confining hernial sac characteristic of these hernias which limited the degree of displacement of bowel into the thorax. A subcostal incision gave excellent exposure.

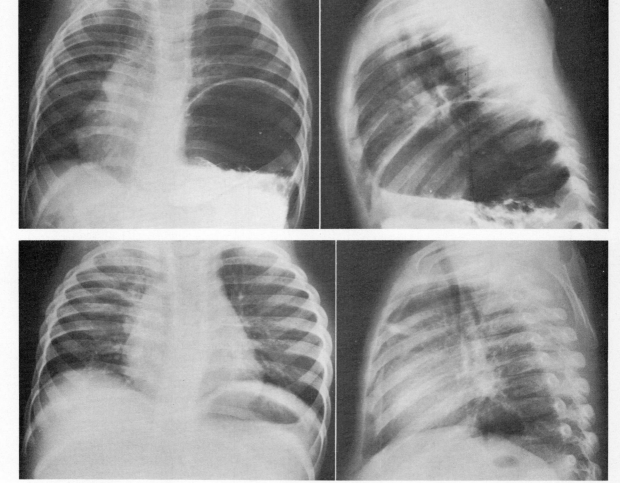

Fig. 27-11 (above).—Eventration of the diaphragm. Roentgenograms of a 5-year-old patient with eventration of the left leaf of the diaphragm. The lung was compressed enough to produce moderately severe dyspnea, especially on exertion. Plication of the diaphragm gave relief.

Fig. 27-12 (below).—Postoperative roentgenograms. The diaphragm is now in normal position.

side.[34] As with complete eventration, the indications for operation are: (1) symptoms, usually respiratory; (2) inability to distinguish eventration from hernia, which is always operated on. Strangulation is possible in such hernias with sacs. If there is time and the baby's condition permits, roentgen examination of the upper gastrointestinal tract may be helpful in establishing the diagnosis preoperatively in questionable cases.[7]

As more thoracic procedures are done in infancy, the danger of inadvertent injury to the phrenic nerve and iatrogenic eventration of the diaphragm in this age group increases. The resulting paradoxical motion of the paralyzed diaphragm during inspiration may seriously impair respiratory function in the postoperative period. Since respiratory function is often marginal in infants, this may be a significant factor in postoperative mortality. When the condition has been detected in time, plication of the paralyzed hemidiaphragm has been done with success.[21]

Congenital Absence of the Diaphragm

Although cases of congenital absence of the diaphragm have been reported, none has been encountered at the Children's Memorial Hospital. With the hernias we have noted which might conceivably fall into this category, sizable portions of the diaphragm have been present anteriorly. They therefore have been considered to be very severe defects in the posterior section of the diaphragm (pleuroperitoneal hiatus). Fortunately, we were able to bring the anterior section of the diaphragm back far enough to complete repair of the diaphragmatic hernia in all but 1 of these patients, although it must be admitted that some of them were extremely difficult to close. In 1 patient in our series, insertion of woven Teflon mesh was required to complete the closure of the diaphragmatic hernia. Nylon,[8] Dacron[38] and also abdominal muscle pedicle flaps[37] have been utilized for the same purpose.

Traumatic Rupture of the Diaphragm

The increased incidence of automobile injuries makes it inevitable that small children will sustain blunt thoracic or abdominal trauma sufficient to rupture the diaphragm. It is important that this possibility be considered in differential diagnosis whenever severe blunt thoracoabdominal trauma occurs. Although traumatic rupture of the diaphragm is rare, it is extremely dangerous and cannot be ignored. The limited experience reported in the literature[22,31] has emphasized the following points: (1) Most reported clinically significant cases of traumatic rupture of the diaphragm have occurred on the left side. (2) The severity of trauma, and particularly other concomitant more urgent injuries, may obscure the fact that the diaphragm has been ruptured; yet symptoms may persist long after the patient has apparently recovered from his initial injuries. (3) Herniation of the stomach or bowel through the ruptured diaphragm is an ever-present danger, either immediately following trauma or long after apparent recovery. When acute herniation occurs, dilatation of the stomach or small bowel may produce intestinal obstruction or respiratory distress sufficient to endanger the patient's life. (4) Prompt diagnosis and treatment can be life-saving. Principles of treatment are no different from those for other types of diaphragmatic hernia.

Esophageal Hiatus Hernia

It is, of course, almost impossible to ascertain exactly how often hiatus hernias occur in children, since most of them are asymptomatic. The suggestion

Fig. 27-13 (left).—Eventration of the right diaphragm in a 3-year-old patient confirmed by pneumoperitoneum. Partial eventration, particularly on the right, may be misdiagnosed as mediastinal, hepatic or diaphragmatic tumor. Pneumothorax provides accurate differentiation.

Fig. 27-14 (right).—Hiatus hernia with esophagus of normal length. The patient had cramps and attacks of nausea. Note small protrusion of esophagogastric junction above diaphragm.

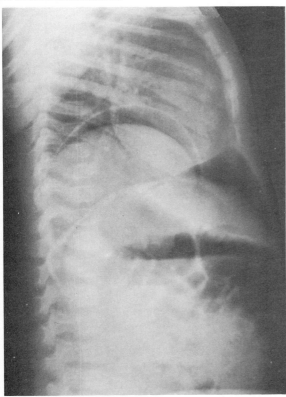

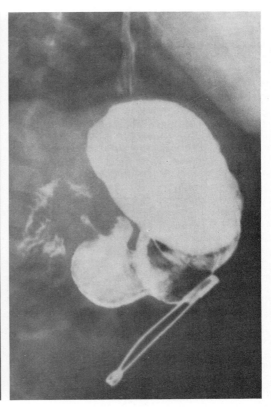

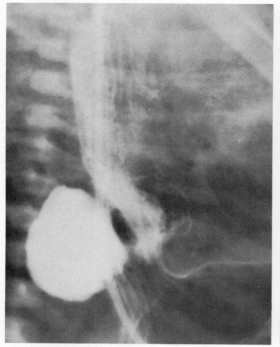 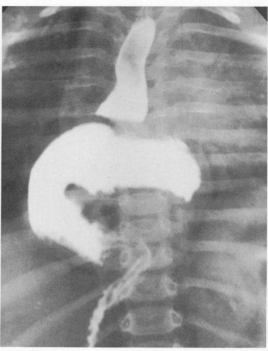

Fig. 27-15 (left).—Hiatus hernia with striking herniations of the upper segment of the stomach through the hiatal defect. Presenting symptoms in this 6-year-old patient were recurrent severe cramps and hematemesis.

Fig. 27-16 (right).—Hiatus hernia. Most of the stomach is in the sac. There is delay of gastric emptying. Although apparently right-sided, such hernias are best reached from the left chest.

by Ritvo,[36] however, that patients suspected of having esophageal hiatus hernia be examined roentgenologically in the Trendelenburg position has greatly facilitated diagnosis of this lesion, and the number of such cases being detected and treated has increased since his suggestion was published. With regard to etiology, in children at least, we may conclude that delay in descent of the stomach into the abdominal cavity may leave the esophageal hiatus abnormally large, even though the length of the esophagus is normal (Fig. 27-14). Symptoms occur, either from regurgitation of acid secretions into the esophagus or because a segment of the adjacent stomach herniates periodically through the hiatal defect (Fig. 27-15). Most patients, therefore, have symptoms referable to the upper gastrointestinal tract—nausea, vomiting, cramps, malnutrition. One patient, however, had sufficient herniation to cause moderate cardiorespiratory distress, and another had hematemesis. Any relationship inferred between enlarged esophageal hiatus defects in children and paraesophageal or esophageal hernias observed in adults would be purely a matter of conjecture. Most observers feel that adult esophageal hernias are acquired rather than congenital.[18,41] We have, however, observed 2 infants with asymptomatic hiatal hernias, discovered on routine roentgenograms of the chest and subsequently studied by

fluoroscopy and barium meal. They differed from the ordinary adult paraesophageal hernia because the esophagus, though normal in length, lay tortuous in the mediastinum, while the esophagogastric junction protruded above the level of the esophageal hiatus (Fig. 27-14). One of these two subsequently developed symptoms and the hernia was repaired. The other is still being observed. A third child with a similar hiatus hernia had associated hypertrophic pyloric stenosis.[35] Presenting symptoms were those of pyloric obstruction associated with congestion and hemorrhage from the upper portion of the stomach. Repair of the diaphragmatic hernia and of the hypertrophic pyloric obstruction relieved the symptoms (Fig. 27-16).

Repair of hiatal hernias in children is adequately accomplished by simple imbrication or excision of the hernial sac and closure of the esophageal hiatus around the distal esophagus (see later in this chapter). We concur with others [18,41] that the transthoracic approach should be used in most patients of this type. In our opinion, asymptomatic patients need not be operated on. In our series, 8 patients had repair of hiatus hernias; 2 died in the postoperative period. These patients were all symptomatic. It is interesting that although 1 had symptoms at the age of 3 weeks, most patients had gone well beyond the newborn period before operation was contemplated. The usual patient was 6 months to 1 year old before symptoms led to diagnosis and surgical treatment of the hiatal hernia. The oldest patient operated on in this series was 15 months old at the time of operation. Five patients were operated on transthoracically, 2 were approached through an abdominal incision, and 1 had a combined approach (Tables 27-2 and 27-3). (See also Hiatus Hernia, p. 392.)

CONGENITAL SHORT ESOPHAGUS

Six of our patients not only had herniation through the esophageal hiatus but also had a congenital short esophagus with the esophagogastric junction located high above the diaphragm in the lower mediastinum (Fig. 27-17). Because of the shortened esophagus, the normal relationship of the cardia and the gastric fundus is lost. Mucosal ulceration and stricture formation occur at the esophagogastric junction. The presenting symptoms consist of regurgitation, poor weight gain and occasionally hematemesis. Symptoms are recurrent, but operative intervention usually is not necessary. All but 1 of our patients with this condition have been successfully managed by repeated dilata-

Fig. 27-17.—Congenital short esophagus. The esophagogastric junction is high above the diaphragm with upper portions of the stomach herniated into the lower mediastinum. A stricture has developed in the esophagus. Although dilations may relieve the obstruction, it will probably be necessary ultimately to resect the distal portion of the esophagus and interpose a segment of colon.

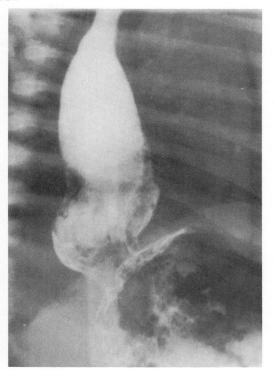

tion by our endoscopy department. Failure of dilatation to relieve the obstruction requires left thoracotomy, with mobilization of the esophagus and elevation of the esophageal hiatus to the level of the gastroesophageal junction.[16] Only 1 of our patients was operated on in this manner. The hiatus was dissected free and brought up to the level of the gastroesophageal junction. It was sutured snugly around the esophagus with interrupted nonabsorbable (silk) sutures. Postoperative roentgen examination demonstrated relief of the obstruction at the esophagogastric junction. Unfortunately, in spite of successful repair, the patient died a month after operation of congenital hydronephrosis and other related anomalies. (See also Hiatus Hernia, p. 392.)

REFERENCES

1. Areechon, W., and Reid, L.: Hypoplasia of the lung with congenital diaphragmatic hernia, Brit. M. J. 1:230, 1963.
2. Baumgartner, C. J., and Scott, R. F.: Surgical emergency of diaphragmatic hernia in infancy, Arch. Surg. 61:170, 1950.
3. Bentley, G., and Lister, J.: Retrosternal hernia, Pediat. Surg. 57:567, 1963.
4. Bochdalek, V. A.: Einige Betrachtungen über die Entstehung des angeborenen Zwerchfellbruches: Als Beitrag zur pathologischen Anatomie der Hernien, Vierteljahrschr. f. d. prak. Heilk. (Prag.) 19:89, 1848.
5. Bonham-Carter, R. E.; Waterston, D. J., and Aberdeen, E.: Hernia and eventration of the diaphragm in childhood, Lancet 1:656, 1962.
6. Bowditch, W.: A treatise on diaphragmatic hernia, Buffalo M. Rev. 9:65, 1853.
7. Canino, C. W., et al.: Congenital right diaphragmatic hernia, Radiology 82:249, 1964.
8. Cerilli, G. J.: Foramen of Bochdalek hernia: A review of the experience at Children's Hospital of Denver, Colo., Ann. Surg. 159:385, 1964.
9. Clay, R. C., and Hanlon, C. R.: Pneumoperitoneum in differential diagnosis of diaphragmatic hernia, J. Thoracic Surg. 21:57, 1951.
10. Creighton, R. E.; Whalen, J. S., and Conn, A. W.: The management of congenital diaphragmatic hernia, Canad. Anaesth. Soc. J. 13:124, 1966.
11. De Nicola, R. R., and Vracin, D. J.: Diaphragmatic hernia through the foramen of Morgagni, J. Pediat. 36:100, 1950.
12. Donovan, E. J.: Congenital diaphragmatic hernia, Ann. Surg. 108:374, 1938.
13. Donovan, E. J.: Congenital diaphragmatic hernia, Ann. Surg. 122:569, 1945.
14. Field, C. E.: Pulmonary agenesis and hypoplasia, Arch. Dis. Childhood 21:61, 1946.
15. Greenwald, H. M., and Steiner, M.: Diaphragmatic hernia in infancy and childhood, Am. J. Dis. Child. 38:361, 1929.
16. Gross, R. E.: The Surgery of Infancy and Childhood (Philadelphia: W. B. Saunders Company, 1953), p. 428.
17. Harrington, S. W.: Diaphragmatic hernia of children, Ann. Surg. 115:705, 1942.
18. Harrington, S. W.: Various types of diaphragmatic hernia treated surgically, Surg., Gynec. & Obst. 86:735, 1948.
19. Hartzell, J. B.: Congenital diaphragmatic hernias in children: Résumé of 68 cases treated by operation, Am. J. Surg. 48:582, 1940.
20. Hedblom, C. A.: Diaphragmatic hernia, J.A.M.A. 85:947, 1925.
21. Jewett, T. C., Jr., and Thompson, N. B.: Iatrogenic eventration of the diaphragm in infancy, J. Thoracic & Cardiovas. Surg. 48:861, 1964.

22. Ker, H.: Closed traumatic rupture of the diaphragm, Brit. J. Surg. 50:891, 1963.
23. Koop, C. E., and Johnson, J.: Transthoracic repair of diaphragmatic hernia in infants, Ann. Surg. 136:1007, 1952.
24. Ladd, W. E., and Gross, R. E.: Congenital diaphragmatic hernia, New England J. Med. 223:917, 1940.
25. Mayo, C. H.: Repair of hernia of the diaphragm, Ann. Surg. 86:481, 1927.
26. Meeker, I. A., and Snyder, W. H.: Surgical management of diaphragmatic defects in the newborn infant, Am. J. Surg. 104:196, 1962.
27. Meeker, I. A., and Kincannon, W. H.: The role of ventral hernia in the correction of diaphragmatic defects in the newborn, Arch. Dis. Childhood 40:146, 1965.
28. Merin, R. G.: Congenital diaphragmatic hernia: From the anesthesiologist's viewpoint, Anesth. & Analg. 45:44, 1966.
29. Minnis, J. F., Jr., and Reingold, M.: Accessory diaphragm: Report of a case, Dis. Chest 44:554, 1963.
30. Morris, J. J.; Black, F. O., and Stephenson, H. E.: The fate of the unexpanded lung in congenital diaphragmatic hernia, Dis. Chest 48:649, 1965.
31. Myers, N. A.: Traumatic rupture of the diaphragm in children, Australian & New Zealand J. Surg. 34:123, 1964.
32. Naumann, G.: Diaphragmatic hernia: Laparotomy; Died, Hygiea 5:524, 1888.
33. Orr, T. G., and Neff, F. C.: Diaphragmatic hernia in infants under 1 year of age treated by operation, J. Thoracic Surg. 5:434, 1935.
34. Ravitch, M. M., and Handelsman, J. C.: Defects in the right diaphragm of infants and children with herniation of the liver, Arch. Surg. 64:794, 1952.
35. Riker, W. L.: Congenital diaphragmatic hernia, Arch. Surg. 62:291, 1954.
36. Ritvo, M.: Hernia of the stomach through the esophageal orifice of the diaphragm, J.A.M.A. 94:15, 1930.
37. Rosenkrantz, J. G.; Cotton, E. K., and Waddell, W. R.: Replacement of left hemidiaphragm by a pedicled abdominal muscular flap, J. Thoracic & Cardiovas. Surg. 48:912, 1965.
38. Schaeffer, J. O.: Prosthesis for agenesis of the diaphragm, J.A.M.A. 188:168, 1964.
39. Sigerist, H. E.: *A History of Medicine* (New York: Oxford University Press, 1951), p. 38.
40. Swenson, O.: *Pediatric Surgery* (New York: Appleton-Century-Crofts, Inc., 1954), p. 196.
41. Sweet, R. H.: The repair of hiatus hernia of the diaphragm by supradiaphragmatic approach: Technique and results, New England J. Med. 238:649, 1948.
42. Thomsen, G.; Vesterdal, J., and Winkel-Smith, C. C.: Diaphragmatic hernia into the pericardium, Acta paediat. 43:485, 1954.
43. Truesdale, P. E.: Diaphragmatic hernia in children with a report of 13 operative cases, New England J, Med. 213:1159, 1935.
44. Walker, E. W.: Diaphragmatic hernia, Internat. J. Surg., September, 1900; abst., J.A.M.A. 35:778, 1900.
45. Watson, L. F.: *Hernia* (St. Louis: C. V. Mosby Company, 1938), p. 390.
46. Weinberg, J.: Diaphragmatic hernia in infants: Surgical treatment with use of renal fascia, Surgery 3:78, 1938.
47. Woolsey, J. H.: Diaphragmatic hernia, J.A.M.A. 88:204, 1927.
48. Baran, E. M.; Houston, H. E., Lynn, H. B., and O'Connell, E. J.: Foramen of Morgagni hernias in children, Surgery 62:1076, 1967.
49. Johnson, D. G.; Deaner, R. M., and Koop, C. E.: Diaphragmatic hernia in infancy: Factors affecting mortality rate, Surgery 62:1082, 1967.
50. Snyder, W. H., Jr., and Greaney, E. M., Jr.: Congenital diaphragmatic hernia: 77 consecutive cases, Surgery 57:576, 1965.

T. G. BAFFES

Drawing by

JANE K. GORDON

28

The Esophagus

Congenital Esophageal Atresia and Tracheoesophageal Fistula

HISTORY.—Congenital atresia of the esophagus without tracheoesophageal fistula was first described in 1670 by William Durston,[8] who observed it in one member of conjoined twins. The usual type of esophageal atresia accompanied by a tracheoesophageal fistula was clearly portrayed by Thomas Gibson[10] in his classic case published in 1697. The variations encountered in anomalies of the esophagus, usually accompanied by a tracheoesophageal fistula, were presented in 1929 by Vogt,[54] whose classification of the anomalies is customarily used. Ligation of the tracheoesophageal fistula, as a step toward eventual correction of the anomaly, was first employed by Richter[45] in 1913. Although Keith[25] in 1910 and Richter envisaged the possibility of correction of the anomaly by an anastomosis of the two portions of the esophagus, a definitive operation of this type was not attempted until the late thirties, when it was employed independently by Lanman[33] and Shaw.[47] During the late thirties, however, a multiple stage plan of treatment consisting of division or ligation of the tracheoesophageal fistula, gastrostomy and cervical esophagostomy was generally employed if operation was done at all. The first two patients to recover were operated on successively by Leven[34] and Ladd[29] in 1939 by the multiple stage plan. An esophagoplasty was done later for both of these patients. The first patient to survive a direct approach to the anomaly by division and closure of the tracheoesophageal fistula and simultaneous primary anastomosis of the two portions of the esophagus was operated upon by the author in 1941 and reported in 1943 by Haight and Towsley.[13] The patient, who is living and well, is married and has a healthy 2-year-old child. The first case of tracheoesophageal fistula unaccompanied by an esophageal atresia was described by Lamb[30] in 1873.

Incidence

The incidence of congenital atresia of the esophagus in reported series of cases varies, but in general has been between 1 in 1,300 and 1 in 4,500 births.[24] Among infants born of residents of Washtenaw County, Michigan, the anomaly has been recognized in 21 during a period of 30 years, the incidence being 1 in 4,425 live births. The anomaly is rarely seen in siblings[18,33,49] but is occasionally seen in one of twins.[5,16,35] Eleven such instances in one twin are known to have occurred among the 288 infants in our series. Woolley et al.[58] reported the anomaly in both members of a pair of twins who appeared to be genetically identical.

Embryology

The embryology of congenital atresia of the esophagus with or without tracheoesophageal fistula is not clearly understood. The anomaly is known to originate in the interval between the end of the third week and the sixth week of fetal life. The presence of vascular anomalies at the level of the atresia has been described by several authors who believe that the localized pressure thereby exerted on the developing esophagus is responsible for the loss of continuity. The tracheoesophageal fistula below the level of the obstruction is attributed to failure of complete closure of the laryngotracheal groove during this stage of development. Langman[31,32] described several cases in which a fibrous cord, believed to be the remnant of an anomalous right subclavian artery, traversed the gap between the two segments of the esophagus. He believed also that an abnormally lengthy persistence of the primitive right descending aorta may be a cause of esophageal atresia. In approximately 5.1% of the cases we have seen, an anomalous vessel, usually an anomalous right subclavian artery, has been encountered at the level of the atresia. A persisting fibrous cord like that described by Langman has been seen only rarely, and in such instances its size has been so small as to make it difficult to identify with certainty.

Types of Anomaly

In 288 cases of esophageal atresia seen since 1935, air was present in the stomach in the preadmission and/or admission roentgenograms in 254 patients

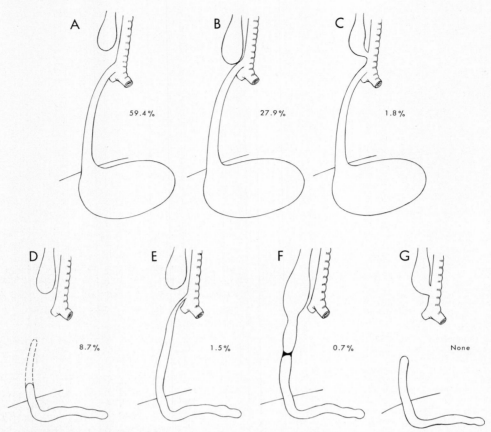

Fig. 28-1.—Esophageal atresia. Types verified in 276 cases. **A,** usual form. Air in stomach; blind upper esophagus; lower esophagus communicates with the trachea or a main bronchus; 2 portions of esophagus separated by variable distance. 164 cases, 59.4%. **B,** same as **A,** but 2 portions of esophagus are in partial muscular continuity; no continuity of esophageal lumen. 77 cases, 27.9%. **C,** fistula between upper esophagus and trachea in addition to fistula between trachea and lower esophagus, the so-called double fistula. Rare. 5 cases, 1.8%. **D,** usual form of esoph-

ageal atresia when air is not present in stomach. Upper end of lower esophagus is a variable but usually short distance above diaphragm; no communication between lower esophagus and trachea. 24 cases, 8.7%. **E,** less common form when air is not present in stomach. Lower esophagus communicates with trachea, but communication is too small to allow passage of air. 4 cases, 1.5%. **F,** complete atresia of esophagus at junction of middle and lower thirds. Rare. 2 cases, 0.7%. **G,** proximal fistula; no distal fistula. No cases in this series.

(88.2%). Four other patients, who did not have air in the stomach, were found to have a fistula between the trachea or bronchus and the lower esophagus. Thus 258 of the 288 patients with esophageal atresia, or 89.6%, had a fistula between the tracheobronchial tree and the distal esophagus. Five of them also had a proximal fistula between the upper esophagus and trachea. Of the remaining 30 patients (10.4%), who did not have air in the stomach, 24 had a lower esophagus that did not extend up to the level of the trachea or a main bronchus, 2 had a complete continuity of the esophageal wall but had a complete atresia at the junction of the middle and lower thirds, and the precise cause of the absence of air in the stomach was not known in the remaining 4 patients.

It was possible to observe, at operation or autopsy, the exact anatomy in 276 of the 288 patients; the

findings are depicted in Figure 28-1. No instance of a proximal fistula but without a distal fistula was seen.

Associated Anomalies

The frequent incidence of other anomalies in infants with atresia of the esophagus coincides with the well-known fact that anomalies are often multiple. Among our 288 patients, 91 (31.6%) had *significant* anomalies in addition to the atresia of the esophagus. The number and the organ system of the significant associated anomalies in the 91 patients are listed in Table 28-1. The total anomalies, significant or not, encountered in all cases are listed in Table 28-2. The number of significant anomalies is greater in Table 28-2 because more than one significant associated anomaly may be present in a single patient.

TABLE 28-1.—PATIENTS WITH SIGNIFICANT ASSOCIATED ANOMALIES IN 288 CASES OF ESOPHAGEAL ATRESIA*

TYPE	TOTAL	PATIENTS LIVING*
Cardiovascular	44	5
Gastrointestinal	31	13
Neurologic	9	0
Genitourinary	4	0
Orthopedic	0	0
Others	3	0
Total	91 (31.6%)	18

*When multiple anomalies have been encountered in a single patient, only the most important anomaly is listed.

For the purposes of classification, the significant anomalies are those responsible for the death of the infant in the immediate postoperative period, or at best they are anomalies that will permit only a limited life expectancy unless correctable by operation. The significant anomalies have included various types of congenital heart disease and lesions of the aortic arch, such as coarctation of the aorta, vascular ring and patent ductus of a size approximating that of the lumen of the aorta. In the gastrointestinal tract, they have included anomalies which have required operative intervention, such as imperforate anus with or without an associated urinary fistula, hypertrophic pyloric stenosis and duodenal atresia due to an annular pancreas. The significant neurologic anomalies have consisted of mongolism, hydrocephalus, craniostenosis, encephalomalacia, cerebellar cyst and spasticity. The urologic anomalies have included polycystic kidneys and stricture of the ureters. The miscellaneous group consisted of 2 patients with adrenal tumors and another patient with Fanconi anemia.

The *nonsignificant* anomalies are those that do not demand immediate surgical treatment and are compatible with a reasonable life expectancy. They have included such conditions as dextroposition of the aorta, dextrocardia, aberrant right subclavian artery, Meckel's diverticulum, anomalies of the vertebrae, ribs or extremities, harelip and cleft palate, horseshoe kidney with or without a single ureter and a number of miscellaneous but less frequently encountered anomalies.

TABLE 28-2.—ASSOCIATED ANOMALIES IN 288 CASES OF ESOPHAGEAL ATRESIA (TOTAL ANOMALIES, 255)

TYPE OF ANOMALY	SIGNIFICANT ANOMALIES	NONSIGNIFICANT ANOMALIES	TOTAL
Cardiovascular	45	21	66
Gastrointestinal	42	22	64
Neurologic	11	2	13
Genitourinary	14	26	40
Orthopedic	0	44	44
Others	2	26	28
Total	114	141	255

Symptomatology

Atresia of the esophagus should be suspected when a newborn infant has unusually profuse oral and pharyngeal secretions which require repeated aspiration. In most patients, the existence of the anomaly is not considered until feedings are first offered. The triad of choking, coughing and cyanosis then becomes apparent. These symptoms are accompanied by the signs of secretions within the tracheobronchial tree. The respiratory rate is often increased and respirations are labored. Aspiration of secretions from the pharynx, together with the clearing of secretions from the trachea by the coughing that frequently accompanies pharyngeal suctioning, will temporarily result in improvement of the infant's breathing and a lessening of the findings on auscultation. The symptoms and findings promptly recur, and with repeated suctioning the sequence continues. In the presence of a fistula between the trachea and lower esophagus, the abdomen is tympanitic; on infrequent occasions the abdomen is tremendously distended so that it greatly interferes with the infant's breathing. When a fistula is not present, the abdomen is scaphoid, and flat on percussion.

Diagnosis

When the possibility of atresia of the esophagus is suspected, the diagnosis can be made promptly or excluded by the passage of a radiopaque catheter into the esophagus. The catheter, of no. 12 F. size, should be new, so that it will not be so soft as to coil up in the proximal segment, thereby deceptively suggesting passage into the stomach. If the catheter passes into the stomach, atresia is obviously not present. If, however, the catheter stops abruptly at a distance of 10 cm, plus or minus 1 cm, from the upper gum margin, the diagnosis is virtually assured. A confirmatory roentgenogram is made to determine the level of the obstruction in relation to the dorsal vertebrae, so that an approximate estimate can be made of the length of the blind upper pouch. For practical purposes, the diagnosis by use of a catheter is sufficient, but the injection of 1 cc of aqueous radiopaque contrast medium (Fig. 28-2) is customary in order to exclude the remote possibility of esophageal obstruction due to a congenital stenosis or web with a lumen too small to permit passage of the catheter. The contrast material may also disclose a fistula between the upper esophagus and trachea in the rare cases in which a fistula is present in this location. The detection of a fistula of this type is facilitated by cinefluoroscopic examination. Provided the contrast material is instilled with adequate caution to prevent overflow into the trachea, the use of contrast material is preferable to the use of a catheter alone, as it permits better estimation of the size of the upper esophagus and on rare occasions reveals unusual abnormalities that might conceivably alter the surgical approach. The contrast ma-

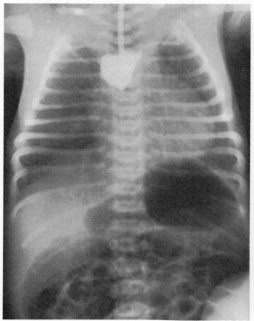

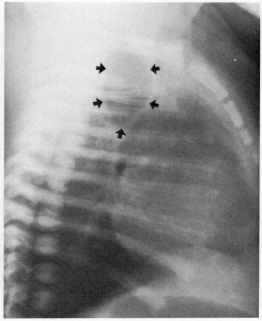

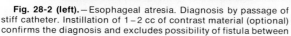

Fig. 28-2 (left).—Esophageal atresia. Diagnosis by passage of stiff catheter. Instillation of 1–2 cc of contrast material (optional) confirms the diagnosis and excludes possibility of fistula between upper esophagus and trachea.

Fig. 28-3 (right).—Esophageal atresia. Distention of upper esophagus by air, indicative of esophageal obstruction.

terial should be aspirated from the upper esophagus before withdrawal of the catheter. If esophageal atresia has not been suspected and a roentgenogram of the chest has been obtained because of the respiratory symptoms, it is not unusual to note a wide dilation of the upper esophagus by air and secretions[22] (Fig. 28-3); this finding alone is indicative of esophageal obstruction and warrants further studies.

The roentgenograms should include the full length of the abdomen, so that the presence or absence of air in the stomach and intestines can be determined. When the upper esophagus is completely obstructed, air in the stomach is pathognomonic of a fistulous communication between the trachea and lower esophagus. Absence of air in the gastrointestinal tract usually signifies that the lower esophagus is only partially developed and does not extend as high as the level of the trachea. In a small percentage of patients who do not have air in the stomach, the lower esophagus communicates with the trachea, but the caliber of the fistula itself, or that portion of the esophagus adjacent to the fistula, is too small to allow the passage of air into the stomach. A roentgenogram of the abdomen is also indicated for the detection of other anomalies, particularly duodenal obstruction.

Preoperative Preparation

The preoperative management occupies a period of 18–24 hours or longer to allow evaluation of the

anomaly by roentgen examination, correction of mild dehydration, cross-matching for blood transfusion and the institution of antibiotic therapy. When hospitalized, the patient is placed in an Isolette into which oxygen is fed through a vaporizer in order to produce a dense fog. The patient's temperature is controlled as required. When air is present in the stomach, the head and chest of the patient are elevated to reduce the tendency to regurgitation of gastric secretions into the trachea. The bleeding and clotting time are estimated on admission, and vitamin K and vitamin C are administered routinely.

If abundant *secretions* are present in the tracheobronchial tree and are not expelled by the coughing induced by pharyngeal suction through the mouth or nose, they should be removed by laryngoscopy and intratracheal aspiration. Intratracheal aspiration is performed with a short metal aspirating tube (Samson-Davis aspirator) (Fig. 28-4) to the end of which a short (3.5 cm) length of a no. 8 F. red rubber whistle-tip catheter is attached by drawing the cut end of the catheter over the open end of the metal tube. During preoperative preparation of the patient, frequent suctioning of the pharynx is necessary to remove accumulating secretions. The aspirating catheter should be advanced well down into the blind upper esophagus to remove secretions that have pooled in it. Continuous aspiration of secretions that gain entrance to the upper esophagus has been advocated by Gross,[12] who has used a nasal catheter, the tip of which is advanced into the upper esophagus and to which continuous suction is applied. A plastic sump catheter has been devised by Replogle[44] for this purpose.

A culture of nasopharyngeal secretions is started on admission so that bacterial sensitivity studies can guide the choice of the antibiotics most effective against the bacteria that have reached the infant's mouth. Routine nasopharyngeal cultures in our patients have revealed the frequent presence of bacteria resistant to penicillin and streptomycin. Because of this finding, an antibiotic management schedule started on admission, before the results of the sensitivity studies will have become available, has been designed to provide as complete antibiotic coverage as is possible. It consists of the use of sodium methicillin, streptomycin, polymyxin B, and one of the broad-spectrum antibiotics, such as erythromycin. In addition, 3 drops of 0.5% neomycin solution are instilled orally every hour. Whereas a positive culture for organisms of one type or another has been obtained in most of the patients admitted more than 12–18 hours after birth, subsequent cultures of the esophagus at operation in the same patients have shown a significant change or decrease of the bacterial flora as a result of the brief period of preoperative antibiotic therapy. This decrease has been particularly striking since the topical use of 0.5% neomycin solution was added to the systemic broad-spectrum antibiotic therapy alone, and as a result of it, the cultures obtained at operation from the proximal pouch during the past several years have usually been negative.

Dehydration, if clinically evident or suspected because of a discrepancy of more than 8 oz between the birth and admission weights, is corrected by the administration of 5% glucose in 0.2% physiologic saline solution given subcutaneously or intravenously. The amount of fluid in such cases should not exceed 15 cc/lb; otherwise no preoperative fluid is given. Physiologic saline solution as such should be avoided, because an excess of salt is provocative of edema in newborn infants. As there is no loss of chlorides from vomiting or diarrhea in infants with congenital atresia of the esophagus, the small insensible loss of sodium chloride is readily replaced by the small amount of 5% glucose in 0.2% physiologic saline solution included with the fluid and blood replacement at the time of operation.

Mild *pneumonitis* or lobular *atelectasis,* particularly in the upper lobe of the right lung, is a common finding. If pneumonitis is present, laryngoscopy and intratracheal aspiration, or occasionally intratracheal intubation for more frequent aspirations, are employed to improve pulmonary aeration before operation. The patient's position is changed at frequent intervals. A fixed position is to be avoided because it will often lead to pneumonitis in the dependent portion of the lung or lungs. The use of alternate lateral decubitus positions is an effective means of preventing atelectasis and of correcting it if already present.

Should pneumonitis be present in the *right* lung on admission, an equal period of time in each lateral position is preferable, but in no instance should the infant be allowed to lie on one side or the other for longer than 30 or 45 minutes. Usually the infant is placed on the right side for 45 minutes, then on the left side for 15 minutes, and the sequence then repeated. The management of the lateral positions should be so designed as to provide for clearing of any pneumonitis which may have been present in the *left* lung on admission and to prevent the development of pneumonitis in the left lung during the brief period of treatment immediately before operation. It has been a common finding that mild pneumonitis or even lobular or lobar atelectasis in the upper lobe of the right lung before operation will often clear completely, at least as demonstrated by roentgen examination shortly after operation, as a result of the positioning of the patient in the left lateral decubitus position during

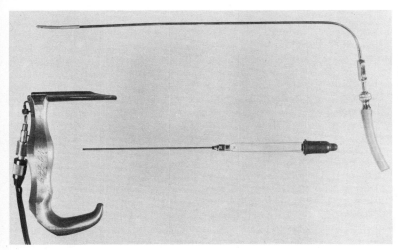

Fig. 28-4.—Esophageal atresia. No. 8 infant laryngoscope and Samson-Davis aspirator for intratracheal aspiration; a Wintrobe pipet for intratracheal instillation of antibiotic solution if indicated by presence of purulent secretions.

the time of the operation. Therefore, on admission or immediately before operation, the finding of pneumonitis in the right lung is not of as much concern as it is in the left lung. If more than 18 hours have elapsed since the admission roentgen examination was made, examination of the chest by portable x-ray apparatus is repeated in order to evaluate the exact status of the lungs immediately before operation.

If *imperforate anus* coexists, its correction is deferred until several days after the repair of the esophageal atresia. Should air not be present in the gastrointestinal tract on admission, a gastrostomy is performed as the initial procedure. Small amounts of air are intentionally introduced into the stomach when hourly feedings of 5% glucose are started 12–18 hours following the gastrostomy. Air will soon reach the rectum, and the length of the anal atresia can then be determined by the customary roentgen measures. A *duodenal* or *pyloric* obstruction, if present, must be relieved promptly, and preferably before operation for the esophageal atresia is undertaken. An elective gastrostomy is done at the time of the abdominal operation.

CHOICE OF OPERATION

AIR PRESENT IN THE STOMACH—When esophageal atresia is accompanied by a tracheoesophageal fistula, the anomaly can be corrected in most cases by *primary anastomosis* of the two portions of the esophagus after the tracheoesophageal fistula has been divided and closed. This is the preferable plan in the robust full-term infant who is in good general condition. It is a matter of personal preference whether the operation is done by the extrapleural[6,38,39,48,52] or the transpleural[12,28,42,53] approach, inasmuch as ample exposure is obtained by either route. The writer, who has favored the extrapleural approach in the past, continues to believe that it is the safer of the two methods. This view has been corroborated by the statistics collected by Holder *et al.*[20] from members of the Surgical Section of the American Academy of Pediatrics. In their analysis, survival with the extrapleural approach (76%) was superior to that with the transpleural approach (66%), although considerably more infants were operated on by the transpleural route than by the extrapleural exposure.

Each of the two methods of exposure of the anomaly has its own advantages. With the *extrapleural approach*, a more stable operative field can be maintained, particularly if any difficulties with the anesthesia are encountered. A quiet operative field is particularly important during the meticulous construction of the anastomosis. After a limited trial with the transpleural approach, it is my opinion and that of others[21] that there has been less trauma to the lung when it is protected by the parietal pleura during the extrapleural exposure than when the transpleural route is used. Furthermore, should leakage of the anastomosis occur after use of the extrapleural exposure, the secretions and inevitable infection remain localized to the extrapleural wound, which can be readily drained by merely removing the sutures in the posterior portion of the incision, whereas with the transpleural approach, a total empyema ensues, with its increased risk and greater difficulties in management. In the collected statistics referred to above, the mortality following anastomotic leaks in patients having the transpleural approach was 63%, whereas it was 40% in those having extrapleural repair. The advantages of the *transpleural* approach are the slightly shorter operating time, the ability to free the lower esophagus to the diaphragm if needed to provide sufficient relaxation in order to obtain a primary anastomosis and the availability of a flap of mediastinal pleura for suturing over the anastomosis. With the extrapleural approach, however, it is readily possible to free the lower segment for a distance of 5 or 6 cm or almost to the diaphragm, and it is debatable whether it should be freed completely to the diaphragm in any case because of the likelihood of producing an iatrogenic hiatus hernia.

An objection to the extrapleural approach is the relative frequency of injury to the parietal pleura. This may occur at the site of the rib resection during the initial establishment of the extrapleural cleavage plane or closer to the mediastinum as the result of the retraction with the ribbon retractor. As a rule, a tear of the parietal pleura, should it occur, is quite small and does not interfere with the anesthesia or the respirations. It usually can be closed securely with one or two sutures of 6-0 silk on vascular needles. At times it is no larger than a pin-prick, and after the edges are grasped with the points of a fine hemostat, it can be closed with a fine silk ligature. The parietal pleura therefore is usually intact at the conclusion of the operation. Pleural tears are more frequent and more difficult to suture in the premature than in full-term infants. Although the extrapleural exposure requires a slightly longer operating time than does the transpleural approach, the difference is of no real significance. A further objection to the extrapleural route is the small amount of paradoxical motion laterally in the early postoperative period, as a result of the resection of a portion of one rib. This objection is believed to be relatively inconsequential. No deformity results from resection of a portion of one rib.

Initial gastrostomy.—On infrequent occasions the gastrointestinal tract of an infant with esophageal atresia and tracheoesophageal fistula is so tremendously distended with air as to interfere seriously with the infant's respirations. In such circumstances, a gastrostomy is performed immediately to decompress the stomach. Repair of the esophageal atresia is deferred until the following day, when the abdominal distention will have largely subsided. Other indications for performance of a gastrostomy in advance of repair of the atresia and fistula are prematurity of less than 4 or 4-1/2 lb, and poor general condition or extensive pneumonitis or both. In the case of mild prematurity or poor general condition, the gastrostomy allows feedings to be started as soon after the repair of the anomaly as is desirable. In instances of extensive pneumonitis, the gastrostomy allows gastric drainage to be employed pending improvement of the infant's condition prior to the repair of the atresia and fistula. Thus, it provides an opportunity for clearing of the pneumonitis by the prevention of further reflux of gastric secretions from the stomach into the trachea. The premise that pneumonitis or atelectasis, so commonly seen in these infants, is largely the result of reflux of gastric secretions into the tracheobronchial tree, rather than aspiration by overflow from the upper esophageal pouch, is based on the observed fact that the incidence of pneumonitis on admission of infants with air in the stomach as a result of a distal fistula is considerably greater (42%) than in infants without a fistula and consequently no air in the stomach (17.4%).[57] Gastrostomy as the initial procedure in all patients with atresia and a tracheoesophageal fistula has been advocated by many surgeons, including Holder and Ashcraft[21] and Martin.[38] In our clinic, initial gastrostomy has been thought to be of particular advantage in the poor-risk and premature infants and is being used in such cases preliminary to repair of the atresia and fistula, although it is not considered necessary in the full-term, good-risk patients in whom repair of the anomaly can be promptly undertaken within a day or so after admission.

Staged operations for the poor-risk patient. — The significant reduction of mortality from esophageal atresia and tracheoesophageal fistula in the past several years has come through the realization that the considerably premature and/or the critically ill infant, from whatever cause, cannot be treated in the same manner as one would treat a full-term, robust infant. from whatever cause, cannot be treated in the same manner as one would a full-term, robust infant. These feeble infants usually do not have the necessary stamina and the respiratory reserve to withstand the rigors of a primary anastomosis and the subsequent recovery period. Instead, the infant must be spared the major operation until his general condition can be materially improved. To accomplish this, Holder, McDonald and Woolley[19] have advocated a *staged approach* as an alternate but preferable plan for the premature or critically ill infant. The plan consists of a gastrostomy for drainage as the initial procedure on the admission of the patient. After an interval of one or several days, the tracheoesophageal fistula is divided and closed under local anesthesia through an extrapleural approach. Gastrostomy feedings can then be started without danger of reflux. During this time and until the patient's condition has improved sufficiently to permit an esophageal anastomosis to be done safely, frequent aspirations of the blind upper pouch are required to prevent overflow of secretions into the trachea, inasmuch as the cervical esophagus is not mobilized to the exterior. The anastomosis is

undertaken through a transpleural approach after the infant has gained 5 or 6 lb, or more, and is in satisfactory condition for the major operative intervention.

The staged plan may also be used when the distance between the two portions of the esophagus is so great that a primary anastomosis cannot be accomplished even after wide mobilization of both portions. In such instance, the tracheoesophageal fistula is divided and closed. An effort is now made to stretch the length of the upper esophagus by intermittent firm pressure exerted with a large, stiff catheter or a Hurst esophageal dilator, as suggested by Howard and Myers.[23] Although our preliminary experiences have not demonstrated any significant and appreciable stretching of the upper esophagus, the inevitable growth of the infant and of the two portions of the esophagus during the interval has resulted in an easier anastomosis, even though the actual measured distance between the two portions of the esophagus has remained the same.

Deferred primary anastomosis. — In the considerably premature or critically ill infant with air in the stomach, an alternate plan is one used by the author and termed a deferred primary anastomosis.[17] In principle, it consists of an initial operation, *gastrostomy*, to allow continuous gastric drainage, and simultaneous *duodenal intubation*, to permit feedings to be given directly into the duodenum or jejunum. Because of the prematurity, it is believed that feedings by the gastrointestinal tract should be started as promptly as

Fig. 28-5. — Esophageal atresia. Prematurity (3½ lb) and poor condition; dextrocardia. Roentgenogram after gastrostomy for drainage and insertion of feeding tube into duodenum and jejunum; contrast material has been injected through the feeding tube (the nonopaque gastrostomy tube is not visible). After gradual improvement, deferred primary anastomosis was done 2 months later; weight was 6 lb and condition excellent.

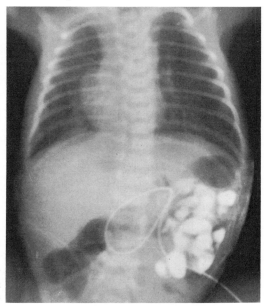

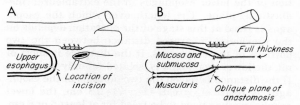

Fig. 28-8.—Esophageal atresia. Telescopic anastomosis. The tracheoesophageal fistula has been divided and the tracheal end closed in 2 layers. **A,** an incision in upper esophagus slightly posterior to its presenting tip allows greater length of anterior wall of upper esophagus to compensate for relatively shorter length of anterior wall of lower esophagus. **B,** inner layer of sutures approximates *full* thickness of wall of lower esophagus to only the *mucosa* and *submucosa* of upper esophagus (knots within lumen). Outer layer of sutures approximates muscularis of upper esophagus to mucularis of lower esophagus 1.5–2.0 mm below level of inner layer of sutures.

will initially have been made at a rather sharp angle if the esophagus has been divided in the plane of the posterior wall of the trachea. When the upper end of the lower esophagus is trimmed, the obliquity is partially preserved in order to increase the diameter of the anastomosis beyond that which would be obtained if the lower esophagus were divided transversely. If the diameter of the lower esophagus is still judged to be too narrow for an anastomosis with adequate lumen, a longitudinal incision downward in the presenting wall of the lower esophagus for a distance of 2 or 3 mm may be made either before the anastomosis is started or during construction of the presenting aspect of the anastomosis.

Telescopic type of anastomosis (Fig. 28-8). — The muscularis of the upper esophagus is incised slightly posterior to its presenting tip to compensate for the relatively shorter length of the anterior wall of the lower esophagus. Excision of a round button of the muscularis exposes the mucosa. The muscularis is then freed circumferentially from the submucosa and mucosa for a minimal distance but enough so that both layers can be readily identified during construction of the anastomosis. The anastomosis is started on that portion of its circumference which is *farthest* from the surgeon. Sutures of 6-0 silk or other nonabsorbable material on fine vascular needles are placed to approximate the outer wall of the muscularis of the lower esophagus to the incised edge of the muscularis of the upper esophagus. These sutures are inserted in the outer wall of the muscularis of the lower esophagus about 2 mm below its uppermost incised edge, and are placed so that the knots will present to the exterior of the suture line. When the sutures are tied, the muscularis of the two portions of the esophagus on the far side of the anastomosis is brought into apposition. The sutures are cut, except for the end sutures, which are left long for identification later, during completion of the outer layer of the anastomosis.

The mucosa of the upper esophagus is now opened and a specimen of secretions is obtained for culture and sensitivity studies. Sutures of material similar to that used for the outer layer are now placed for the inner layer on the far side of the anastomosis, approximating the full thickness of the wall of the lower esophagus to only the mucosa of the upper esophagus and with the knots lying within the lumen so that the sutures will be subsequently discharged. The end sutures are also left long temporarily for identification.

The sutures on the inner layer of the *presenting* aspect of the anastomosis are most readily placed when a catheter is used as a stent. The catheter serves several purposes: it keeps the lumen of the lower esophagus from collapsing during the anastomosis; it prevents the sutures from inadvertently penetrating the inner surface of the opposite side of the anastomosis, and, also, as the mucosa of the presenting aspect of the lower esophagus tends to retract, it allows the sutures to be passed more readily through the full thickness of the wall of the lower esophagus without failing to include the mucosa in the sutures. The flanged end of a no. 8 F., moderately stiff, red rubber Robinson catheter is now excised, and this end is introduced into the lower esophagus and thence into the stomach. The other, or smooth, end is advanced into the upper esophagus until it presents through the nostril or into the mouth to be grasped by the anesthesiologist and withdrawn sufficiently so that it is taut as it passes through the area of the anastomosis. The inner layer of sutures of the presenting aspect of the anastomosis likewise approximates the full thickness of the wall of the lower esophagus to only the mucosa of the upper esophagus and with the knots lying within the lumen.

The outer layer of the anastomosis is now completed by drawing the muscularis of the upper esophagus downward so that it is telescoped over the inner layer, whereupon it is sutured to the outer wall of the muscularis of the lower esophagus 1.5–2 mm below the level of the inner layer of sutures. If the two layers of sutures are situated farther apart, there is a tendency to infolding of the esophageal wall with resultant narrowing of the lumen at the level of the anastomosis. Fewer sutures are used in the outer layer than in the inner layer in order to minimize the tendency to weakening of the wall of the lower esophagus by interference with its blood supply. The anastomosis is now tested by having the anesthesiologist withdraw the catheter until its distal end is just above the anastomosis. The outer end of the catheter is excised and connected to a syringe, and 4–5 cc of physiologic saline solution is now injected, as suggested by Sandblom.[46] This distends the anastomosis and the lower esophagus immediately below the anastomosis and will allow the recognition of any leak that may be present. The maneuver has been valuable in our hands and has at times disclosed a leak that had been completely unsuspected. In such instances, one or two additional sutures in the outer wall ordinarily suffice to prevent further leakage. The catheter is removed on completion of the testing of the anastomosis.

The layer of fascia and areolar tissue that was originally left attached to the azygos vein is now sutured to the upper segment of the esophagus with several interrupted sutures of silk. The presenting aspect of the anastomosis is thereby covered with this layer, which also aids in lessening tension on the anastomosis when the infant cries or swallows. This layer should not be sutured so far around the circumference as to narrow the lumen. The wound is drained with a no. 14 F. whistle-tip catheter which is brought out far posteriorly through the fifth intercostal space and thence through the incision. The catheter tip is held away from the anastomosis by a catgut loop inserted in the parietal wall posteriorly. A dilute solution of sodium methicillin and streptomycin is instilled into the wound, which is then closed in layers. The drainage catheter is connected to a water seal system to which suction of -10 to -15 cm H_2O is applied.

If the ends of the esophagus, even after extensive mobilization, are too far apart to permit an anastomosis to be accomplished satisfactorily, attempt at anastomosis must be abandoned. The less desirable multiple stage plan of gastrostomy, cervical esophagostomy and a later esophageal replacement procedure is resorted to. In this case, the proximal end of the lower esophagus is closed by sutures and a gastrostomy for feeding is done at the same sitting or within the next day or two, if it has not already been provided. A cervical esophagostomy is then performed to allow drainage of pharyngeal secretions to the exterior, and a colon transplant is done later at an optimal time. An alternate plan, when the two portions of the esophagus are too widely separated for a primary anastomosis, is to close the fistula and create a gastrostomy, unless it has already been done. The patient is then managed as mentioned earlier in the staged approach, and an effort is made to elongate the upper pouch by daily stretching with a bougie. If this can be accomplished to an extent that will allow an anastomosis to be obtained satisfactorily at a second attempt several months later, the multiple stage plan can be avoided.

Standard two-layer anastomosis. — When both segments of the esophagus are well developed, a two-layer anastomosis with approximation of the mucosal and muscular layers individually may be used. The collected statistics of Holder et al.[20] showed that this technique resulted in a lesser incidence of stricture than did the telescopic anastomosis (38% vs. 52%), although it was responsible for a greater incidence of leakage (21.4% vs. 10.5%). The ease of performance of the standard type of two-layer anastomosis depends considerably on the thickness of the walls of both portions of the esophagus, particularly the *lower*

esophagus, as well as the ability to differentiate clearly between the muscular layer and the combined mucosal and submucosal layer. When the wall of the lower esophagus is thin, the differentiation may be particularly difficult, especially on the presenting portion of the anastomosis. Also in this latter instance, the holding power of the tissues in each individual layer is less than when the full thickness of the wall of the lower esophagus is included as a combined layer in the other techniques. As a result, the sutures in the standard two-layer technique may cut through the tissues of the lower esophagus when the ends of the two portions of the esophagus are approximated. This is also more apt to happen if there is unavoidable tension when the sutures are being tied.

End-to-side anastomosis. — Interest has been renewed by Ty, Brunet and Beardmore[53] in use of the end-to-side anastomosis originally advocated by Sulamaa et al.[50] In the foreign literature this has been referred to as the "terminolateral" technique. The tracheoesophageal fistula is merely ligated, the upper esophagus is mobilized and a one-layer anastomosis is then constructed between the opened distal end of the upper esophagus and the side of the lower esophagus below the site of ligation. In a modification of this technique used by Berman and Berman,[3] the lower esophagus was divided between double ligatures at the level of the fistula. An advantage of the terminolateral technique over the end-to-end anastomosis is that the lumen at the anastomosis can be made considerably larger than the actual size of the lumen of the lower esophagus. In the literature, the advocates of this technique have not stated the frequency with which it can be used, especially when the two portions of the esophagus are not in close proximity. Nor is the incidence of complications mentioned. I have had no experience with this technique, believing that there would be less chance of effecting a primary anastomosis than with the end-to-end principle which permits the requisite mobilization of *both* portions of the esophagus. Also, the possibility of leakage would seem to be less with the two-layer telescopic technique. In a recent communication, Sulamaa[51] stated that he has not used his technique since 1956–57 because he had seen a recurrent fistula twice at autopsy. He also mentioned that strictures had been rare with this technique and that the indication for its use would be a relatively short gap that would allow an anastomosis without too much tension. In another recent communication, Edward J. Berman[4] said that he and J. K. Berman had abandoned the end-to-side repair, not because of any difficulty with the procedure but because of the difficulty that endoscopists had reported with dilatation of the esophagus postoperatively.

TRANSPLEURAL APPROACH. — In the transpleural approach,[12,42] the pleural cavity is entered through the fourth intercostal space. The incision should not be made so far forward as to allow protrusion of the lung through the anterior portion of the incision. The lung is retracted anteriorly, the mediastinal pleura opened superiorly and the upper segment of the esophagus identified. After double ligation and division of the azygos vein, the incision through the mediastinal pleura is extended inferiorly over the lower esophageal segment, which is mobilized for the required length. The tracheoesophageal fistula is transected and closed, and the esophageal anastomosis is constructed by any of the methods used in the extrapleural approach. The mediastinal pleura is approximated over the anastomosis, leaving an opening superiorly and inferiorly for drainage. If the mediastinal pleura is so thin or frayed that its edges cannot be brought together, a pedicled rectangular flap of the parietal pleura can be fashioned either anteriorly or posteriorly so that it may be sutured over the presenting portion of the anastomosis. An intercostal tube is introduced through a dependent incision and its inner end is advanced close to the anastomosis. It is attached to an air-tight system for continuous negative pressure drainage.

GASTROSTOMY. – In the absence of air in the stomach, the initial operation is a feeding gastrostomy done under a light general anesthesia supplemented by local infiltration of the incision. The anesthesia is readily administered with an infant-size face mask. A transverse incision is made over the left rectus muscle midway between the xiphoid process and the umbilicus. The subcutaneous tissues are reflected from the anterior sheath of the rectus muscle above the level of the incision. The incision is deepened in a transverse direction and the peritoneum is opened. The presenting edge of the left lobe of the liver is retracted upward. In patients without air in the stomach, the stomach will be found to be collapsed and extremely small, usually not larger than one's little finger. A Stamm gastrostomy is employed. After placement of a purse-string suture of 5-0 catgut on an atraumatic needle into the anterior wall of the stomach at as high a level as can be obtained conveniently, the stomach is entered. The length of the lower esophagus is estimated as already described. The mushroom tip of a no. 12–14 F. de Pezzer catheter is trimmed away so that only a narrow flange remains. The catheter is introduced through a short incision in the skin and subcutaneous tissues above the main incision. A track through the rectus fascia, muscle and peritoneum is made by spreading the blades of a small hemostat, and the inner end of the catheter is brought through it into the peritoneal cavity. The catheter is then introduced into the stomach and the purse-string suture is tied. Two sutures of interrupted 5-0 silk on vascular needles are placed in the anterior wall of the stomach on either side of the gastrostomy tube to infold the gastric wall around the tube. The ends of the outermost silk sutures are left long. The omentum is wrapped around the site of entrance

of the catheter into the stomach and the long ends of the sutures are brought through the peritoneum, rectus muscle and anterior rectus sheath. They are tied anterior to the anterior rectus sheath, thereby approximating the anterior wall of the stomach to the peritoneum. After closure of the wound in layers with 5-0 silk, the gastrostomy tube is incorporated within the rolls of an Ace bandage wrapped around the abdomen. The tube is thus held securely by the bandage and cannot be pulled out.

CERVICAL ESOPHAGOSTOMY. – When a primary esophageal anastomosis is not possible, the much less desirable plan of gastrostomy, cervical esophagostomy and esophageal replacement at a later date must be employed. The cervical esophagostomy in this event may be done at the time of the gastrostomy or several days thereafter, or it may be delayed for several or more weeks if the infant is quite premature and the upper esophagus is short, as seen by roentgen examination. The delay allows for further development of the infant and enlargement of the upper esophageal pouch before the cervical esophagostomy is done. Whether or not the delay simplifies the technique of the cervical esophagostomy and allows the esophagus to be brought to the level of the skin more readily is problematical, but this plan has been used in our recent premature infants who have required cervical esophagostomy. Should pneumonitis develop during the waiting period, the operation is performed promptly.

The *anesthesia* for cervical esophagostomy is preferably administered through an intratracheal tube. A small pad is placed beneath the infant's neck. A transverse incision about 3 cm long is made in a skin fold above the left clavicle extending laterally from the midline. The mesial edge of the sternocleidomastoid muscle and the carotid sheath are retracted laterally. The small left lobe of the thyroid gland is retracted mesially. The cervical esophagus is usually located without difficulty. It is freed largely by blunt dissection, except at its distal tip where a fibrous cord extending downward from it may require sharp dissection. After the cervical esophagus has been mobilized, the sternocleidomastoid muscle is split longitudinally in a plane between its sternal and clavicular fibers, and the esophagus is brought out through this opening. The muscularis of the esophagus is sutured to the sternocleidomastoid muscle to prevent retraction of the esophagus. Several sutures are also used for approximation of the esophagus to the platysma. The presenting tip of the esophagus is opened by a transverse incision. The mucosa is everted and meticulously approximated to the edges of the skin. The skin sutures also incorporate the cut edges of the muscularis of the esophagus so that the muscular layer will not retract inward. The ends of the cutaneous incision are closed with one or two sutures. As the suture material throughout the operation consists of 5-0 catgut on atraumatic needles, the sutures in the skin and mucosa will not require removal. A petroleum jelly dressing is applied.

ESOPHAGEAL REPLACEMENT. – The right colon has been used for our patients who have required an esophageal replacement operation. Because of possible pulmonary complications subsequent to this procedure, it is preferred that the patients attain an age of 2 or 2-1/2 years before the operation is undertaken. The technique described by Mahoney and Sherman[37] has been employed. The colon transplant is placed retrosternally, and the proximal anastomosis is made between the cervical esophagus and cecum. It is endeavored to place the cologastric anastomosis high on the anterior wall of the stomach. The lower esophageal segment is resected if this can be readily accomplished, although it has rarely been used for the distal anastomosis. A bilateral vagotomy and pyloroplasty are also performed.

Postoperative Management

The course following esophageal anastomosis for atresia is variable. It can be relatively smooth, as is frequently seen in robust full-term infants without other important anomalies and for whom correction of the anomaly has been undertaken promptly before the development of pneumonitis. More often, the postoperative course may be complicated. This is reflected in two publications, one by Shaw, Paulson and Siebel[48] and the other by Rehbein and Yanagisawa,[43] which are concerned largely with the treatment of the surgical complications. A complication such as overhydration can be prevented. Others such as pneumonitis and atelectasis can be largely prevented, whereas still others, such as leakage, a recurrent tracheoesophageal fistula or a stricture at the site of the anastomosis, must be treated as they arise.

IMMEDIATE POSTOPERATIVE MANAGEMENT. – Following completion of the operative repair of esophageal atresia, the intratracheal tube is maintained in place and oxygen is administered while the infant is being slowly turned on the back. Periods of apnea may occur as a result of the change of position while the patient is beginning to awaken from the anesthesia. The anesthesiologist should ventilate the patient manually until spontaneous normal respirations occur. When breathing is normal and the breath sounds bilaterally have been found to be satisfactory by auscultation, the patient is transferred to a previously heated Isolette which has been brought to the operating room. The oxygen inflow into the Isolette is immediately started at 8 – 10 liters/minute. Because the left lung has been in a dependent position during the operation, secretions may have entered the bronchial tree beyond the point from which they can be removed by aspiration. Also, in some cases, edema may have developed principally in the dependent lung dur-

ing the operation. The infant is therefore positioned on the right side in order to improve the ventilation of the left lung. The intratracheal tube is not removed until the infant has awakened sufficiently to object to its presence. Preferably it is left in place until the patient has been returned to the nursery by the anesthesiologist and surgeon. The anesthesia machine accompanies the patient, to be used en route for ventilating the patient in an emergency, should apnea occur. A chest film made with a portable unit is made in the operating room if there is concern about the presence of pneumothorax on either side, and a roentgenogram is made daily in the nursery for at least the first 4 or 5 days after operation.

Adequate care by nurses who have had particular experience in the postoperative management of infants with this anomaly is one of the most important requirements for the recovery of these patients. It is as important as constant vigilance on the part of surgical and pediatric staffs. Especially within the first few days after operation, these infants require the closest of observation, as their condition, although excellent at the moment, may suddenly deteriorate within the hour, usually as the result of accumulation of secretions within the tracheobronchial tree. It is imperative, therefore, that they be placed in a location, such as an intensive care unit, within the nursery where they can be observed continuously by the nurse in charge, unless they have constant special nursing care.

POSITIONING OF THE PATIENT. – The position of the patient is an influencing factor in the development of atelectasis, and for this reason a constant fixed position should be avoided. Respirations are aided by elevation of the head and chest by inclining the mattress within the Isolette. The alternate lateral positions are used with the infant lying on one side for not longer than 1/2 hour at a time. Frequent auscultation of the chest is important in eliciting rhonchi or a decreased intensity of the breath sounds, either of which suggests the presence of retained bronchial secretions. Even though the secretions can be cleared by tracheobronchial aspiration, the lung in which they arose or were most prevalent is kept uppermost for a longer period than the better aerated lung, in order to favor gravity and ciliary drainage of the secretions into the trachea. Our practice in such instances is to adopt an hourly schedule, with the more involved side uppermost for 40 – 45 minutes and the contralateral side uppermost for 15 – 20 minutes. In so doing, it is particularly important to be certain that atelectasis is not developing in the lung which is in the dependent position for the greater portion of the time. The prone position, which is a natural one for an infant, is used at intervals in conjunction with the alternate lateral positions if bronchial secretions continue to be troublesome. The prone position favors drainage of secretions from the lower lobe and the trachea up to the level of the pharynx, where they can be expelled into the pharynx by the coughing induced by aspiration of the pharynx. This position predisposes to atelectasis of the upper lobes and should therefore not be used for a protracted period in the first few days after operation, when bronchial secretions are usually most troublesome. The prone position has the disadvantage of not allowing dependent drainage from the thoracotomy tube, and accordingly it is customarily not used until the thoracotomy tube has been removed 24–36 hours after operation.

OXYGEN THERAPY.—Oxygen is administered continuously through a vaporizer so that a high humidity is obtained within the Isolette. It is advisable to have the humidity so high that the infant can barely be seen because of the dense fog. If this amount of humidity is not being obtained with a single vaporizer and an oxygen inflow of about 8 liters/minute, oxygen is administered by an ultrasonic nebulizer. The oxygen content in the Isolette is measured at frequent intervals and is preferably maintained at approximately 35%. The concentration of oxygen is gradually reduced until oxygen is no longer necessary. Should a high humidity still be required because of tracheobronchial secretions, a compressed air system is used for vaporization of the inflowing air.

PHARYNGEAL ASPIRATION.—The most frequent complication in the first few days after operation is pneumonitis or atelectasis due to retention of secretions in the tracheobronchial tree. In the robust infant, coughing can be induced by aspiration of the pharynx with a catheter, so that secretions from the trachea are coughed into the pharynx whence they are removed. A narrow band of adhesive tape should be placed as a marker on the catheter 7 or 8 cm from its tip, so that the catheter will not be advanced beyond this distance and thus will not be introduced down to the level of the anastomosis, where it might cause a disruption. Coughing can be stimulated even further by advancing the aspirating catheter through the nares instead of the mouth, as the nasal route often produces sneezing and coughing when the oral route does not do so. It is our custom to use the two routes alternately when employing pharyngeal aspiration.

TRACHEOBRONCHIAL ASPIRATION.—In spite of frequent pharyngeal suctioning, tracheobronchial secretions often continue to be a problem. They are best managed by direct laryngoscopy and removal with a Samson-Davis aspirator introduced into the trachea under direct vision and advanced into both main bronchi. This method is particularly helpful in the prevention of pneumonitis and atelectasis. Tracheobronchial aspiration is started prophylactically 3 or 4 hours after operation and should be used *routinely* at least twice daily in all cases during the first several days following operation, as suggested by Benson.[2] It may be used more frequently if required. The presence of thick mucoid secretions is often surprising

even when there is no more suggestion of them than a faint wet cough during suctioning of the pharynx or an occasional, barely detectable wheeze on auscultation or palpation of the chest. If the aspirated secretions are purulent, 0.5–1.0 cc of a diluted antibiotic solution, such as aqueous penicillin, 100,000 units/cc, is instilled into the trachea under direct vision laryngoscopy and the trachea is again aspirated to remove the excess. The penicillin solution acts not only because of its antibiotic effect but also as an irrigating agent which thins the secretions; the rapid clearing of the amount and purulence of the secretions with this method is often dramatic. Occasionally, when the infant is extremely feeble and the pneumonitis or atelectasis continues or progresses in spite of frequent laryngoscopy and tracheobronchial aspirations, an inlying intratracheal tube is inserted to allow intermittent aspiration through it with a fine-caliber plastic tubing as necessary for several days. Ordinarily this will suffice, but in rare instances recourse must be had to tracheostomy, which may be life-saving. A tracheostomy, however, is avoided as much as possible because of the protracted time that is required before a tracheostomy tube can be removed from an infant.

ANTIBIOTICS.—The systemic preoperative antibiotic schedule is continued postoperatively until the culture and sensitivity reports of the nasopharyngeal secretions obtained on the infant's admission and of the secretions from the upper esophagus at operation are completed. The antibiotic management is then altered as indicated. Because the esophageal anastomosis is performed by an open technique, contamination of the wound is inevitable if bacteria are present within the esophagus. Rarely have the admission nasopharyngeal cultures been negative, and this has been observed only in some infants admitted within 48 hours of birth. More often, the nasopharyngeal secretions of a 1- or 2-day-old infant have contained bacteria. The admission culture studies during the past 5 years have differed from those previously observed, the most frequently encountered organisms being *Streptococcus viridans, Neisseria catarrhalis,* coagulase (−) *Staphylococcus albus, Escherichia coli* and coagulase (+) *Staphylococcus aureus.* The cultures obtained at operation after a short period of systemic and topical antibiotic administration preoperatively are usually negative.

FLUID AND FEEDING MANAGEMENT FOLLOWING PRIMARY ANASTOMOSIS.—The intravenous infusion started in advance of operation is continued postoperatively for 3 or 4 days. For the first day or two, the fluid intake of 5% glucose in 0.2% saline solution is limited to 20–30 cc every 8 hours by means of a Mini-dropper. Between 3 and 5 days after operation, the infant is given a small amount (1–2 cc) of aqueous contrast material to swallow. A roentgenogram is made with a portable unit 1 or 2 minutes thereafter to see if the contrast material has progressed into the stomach and to be certain that there is no leakage at the anastomotic site. If there is no evidence of leakage, oral feedings of 5% glucose are begun at 4 cc/hour. If the feedings are tolerated satisfactorily, equal amounts of boiled skim milk per hour are begun in gradually increasing increments from 4 to 15 cc. The feedings are administered with a medicine dropper and an attached short length of rubber tubing, as advocated by Potts.[41,42] With this method, the feedings are not offered more rapidly than the infant is able to swallow through the small lumen at the level of the anastomosis. The consistency of the feedings is gradually increased until a full caloric intake of 50–60 calories/pound of a 20-calorie/pound formula is usually reached by the tenth to fourteenth postoperative day. At this time, the interval between feedings will have been increased to every 2 hours and shortly thereafter to every 3 hours, the latter interval usually being reached 2–3 weeks after operation. Bottle feedings with a nipple having a small opening are begun when the infant demonstrates that the feedings can be swallowed satisfactorily at a more rapid rate.

GASTROSTOMY.—A gastrostomy, if done as a routine measure in all patients or if used only in selected, poor-risk or premature patients, will ordinarily have been performed on admission, prior to the repair of the esophageal anomaly, as mentioned in the section on Choice of Operation. It has been our practice, however, not to employ a gastrostomy in the good-risk, robust patient preoperatively. Also, in such cases a gastrostomy is not used postoperatively unless specifically indicated as an optional measure if there is concern regarding the security of the anastomosis. In this event the gastrostomy is done 1 or 2 days after repair of the anomaly, rather than immediately on completion of the anastomosis. Should there be leakage of the anastomosis or development of a recurrent tracheoesophageal fistula, a gastrostomy will be mandatory. Ordinarily, a stricture is not an indication for a gastrostomy, as the stricture can be readily managed by antegrade dilatations. If there is doubt in any case regarding the advisability of a gastrostomy, it is better that it be done rather than omitted.

LEAKAGE OF THE ANASTOMOSIS.—An esophageal leak may occur as a result of incomplete approximation of the two segments of the esophagus at operation, disruption of the suture line, or ischemic necrosis of the lower segment of the esophagus immediately below the level of the anastomosis. Factors which favor the development of leakage at the anastomotic site are tension on the two segments of the esophagus as observed at the time of operation, an unusually thin wall of either of the two esophageal segments, particularly the lower segment, undue trauma to either of the segments at the time of construction of the anastomosis, and infection in the wound. Disruption of the lower esophagus immediately below the anastomosis may occur as a result of ischemia due to tension or to the extreme thinness of the esophageal

wall at this level. At times it may result from ischemia secondary to the freeing of the lower esophagus over too great a length. The ability to free the lower esophagus completely is therefore not always without its disadvantages.

Leakage of the esophagus into an *extrapleural* wound (Fig. 28-9) may or may not cause symptoms. It is likely that it will not produce symptoms and that it will not be suspected until a collection of fluid and air is seen in the daily roentgenogram. Because of the silent nature of leakage into the extrapleural wound, the roentgenogram on the third or fourth day after operation is made after 1–2 cc of aqueous contrast material is swallowed in order to see if the contrast material has extravasated into the wound. Leakage of the anastomosis, if it develops, usually does so between the third and fifth postoperative days. If leakage is evident, the sutures are removed from the posterior portion of the wound and the extrapleural wound is readily entered through the incision in the fourth periosteal bed far posteriorly. A small rubber drain is inserted. For a few days there will be profuse drainage of salivary and purulent secretions from the wound. The wound can be irrigated by allowing the infant to swallow small amounts of physiologic saline solution every few hours. The ingested fluid is immediately discharged through the esophageal fistula into the wound. The track through the thoracic wall is kept open until the interior of the extrapleural wound has completely healed. During the process of spontaneous closure of the wound, the esophageal communication with the wound invariably heals, usually within 2 or 3 weeks after its development (Fig. 28-9).

When leakage of the esophagus occurs within a few days after a *transpleural* operation, air and salivary secretions escape into the pleural space which may or may not be partially obliterated by developing adhesions. A tension pneumothorax or pyopneumothorax promptly develops if the drainage tube inserted at operation has been removed or if the air and fluid do not communicate freely with a tube which is still in place. The respiratory distress secondary to a tension pneumothorax becomes alarming, and the patient's condition may suddenly become critical. Drainage of the pleural space is required as an emergency procedure. Management of the inevitable empyema may prove to be difficult if pocketing of the infection occurs.

RECURRENT TRACHEOESOPHAGEAL FISTULA.—A recurrence of a tracheoesophageal fistula results from reopening of the tracheal suture line in the presence of leakage of the anastomosis. Such a recurrence should be suspected in any patient with obvious leakage into the wound. It should also be considered when roentgenograms of the esophagus show an unsuspected small, localized extramural collection of contrast material. The symptoms of a recurrent tracheoesophageal fistula are in some respects similar to those resulting from a tight stricture, in that the infant will

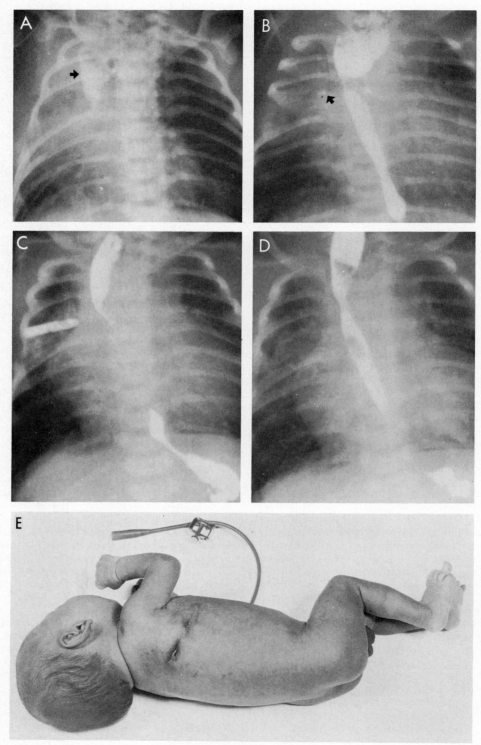

Fig. 28-9. — See legend on facing page.

choke and cough on swallowing, and pneumonitis will develop as a result of aspiration of the feedings. It is important, therefore, to exclude the presence of a stricture by appropriate examinations and to dilate a stricture if present.

The symptoms of a recurrent fistula may vary considerably according to the size of the fistula. With one of very small diameter, the coughing that occurs with feedings is more pronounced when the feedings are thin than when they are thicker. The breath sounds may become quite noisy, particularly during and shortly after feedings as a result of the aspirated material within the tracheobronchial tree. A variable degree of pneumonitis develops. The abdomen becomes distended and tympanitic due to the forceful passage of air from the trachea into the esophagus and stomach when the infant cries, strains or coughs. This occurs because of the increase of intratracheal pressure during forced expiration. The coincident, intermittent partial or complete closure of the glottis forces air from the tracheobronchial tree into the esophagus. It then passes down into the stomach, rather than upward, because of apparent closure of the cricopharyngeus sphincter during the time that the glottis is also closed.

Diagnosis of a recurrent fistula is often difficult, and it may not be established with certainty even when the possibility is suspected. Various maneuvers have been used for detection of a recurrent fistula. With the patient in the prone or slight oblique position, aqueous contrast material is introduced into the upper esophagus through a catheter. As the fistula is on the dependent side of the esophagus, this allows the contrast material to enter the trachea directly from the esophagus by gravitation. The site of the fistula is observed preferably by fluoroscopy with an image intensifier and a permanent recording of the observations. Another method of roentgen examination consists in retrograde filling of the esophagus by means of a Foley bag catheter. The distal end of the catheter is closed with a ligature and a side opening is made in the catheter above the level of the bag. The catheter is introduced into the distal esophagus and the balloon is inflated, thus completely obstructing the esophagus. As the contrast material is being injected into the catheter, it emerges through the new

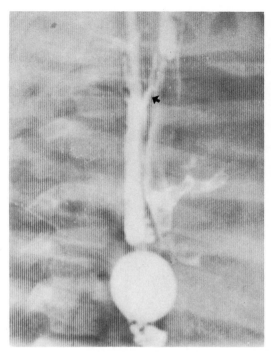

Fig. 28-10.—Recurrent tracheoesophageal fistula **(arrow)**, demonstrated by retrograde filling of esophagus with Foley bag catheter. (Distal end of catheter is obstructed by ligature. Contrast material enters esophagus through new side opening in catheter above level of bag inflated with contrast material.)

side opening above the level of the obstruction and gradually rises to the level of the fistula. It can then be observed to pass directly into the trachea before it has reached the level of the pharynx (Fig. 28-10). The lateral projection is preferred for demonstrating a recurrent fistula roentgenographically. The use of two balloon catheters with one balloon below the level of the suspected fistula and the other balloon above this level has also been suggested.[9] The contrast material is injected so that it emerges between the two balloons.

Tracheoscopy alone may reveal secretions bubbling from the esophagus into the trachea. A more certain method of identifying a recurrent fistula by tracheoscopy consists in the introduction of an opaque catheter such as a no. 5 olive-tipped ureteral catheter down the trachea through the fistula and into the esophagus and stomach, where its presence can be confirmed by roentgenograms. Esophagoscopy has been used for detection of a recurrent fistula, but it has rarely been possible to demonstrate one in this way. During the esophagoscopy, however, an intermittent expiratory blast of air through the fistula can often be heard when the tip of the esophagoscope is positioned immediately above the level of the fistula. The introduction of methylene blue through an intratracheal

◄ **Fig. 28-9.**—Spontaneous closure of esophageal fistula after leakage of anastomosis into extrapleural wound. **A,** wall of *upper* esophagus was extremely thin, and a 1-layer anastomosis was required. Roentgenogram after swallow of aqueous contrast material on 3rd day after operation demonstrates leakage. The extrapleural wound was drained posteriorly and gastrostomy performed. **B,** esophageal fistula almost healed 13 days after its recognition. Faint line **(arrow)** represents residual fistulous track. **C,** roentgenogram 4 weeks after operation shows fistula closed and short tube in drainage track. **D,** roentgenogram 6 weeks after operation and following 4 dilatations shows satisfactory caliber of esophageal lumen. **E,** patient 32 days after operation. Posterior portion of wound at site of drainage of extrapleural space is healed.

tube and simultaneous observation of the region of the suspected fistula by esophagoscopy has been suggested.[1] The methylene blue is seen to enter the esophagus directly at the level of the fistula.

An indirect but useful method for suspecting a fistula is based on the large amount of air that enters the stomach when a fistula is present. If a gastrostomy tube is in place, it is unclamped and its outer end is placed under water. An intermittent and often quite forceful bubbling of air from the gastrostomy tube will be observed during expiration, especially when the infant is crying or struggling. If a gastrostomy has not been done, the same finding can be elicited by means of a catheter introduced into the stomach by way of the esophagus.

Repair of a recurrent tracheoesophageal fistula may prove particularly difficult if less than 2 or 3 months have elapsed since the primary operation. Residual inflammatory reaction in the region of the fistula may still be sufficient to prevent a satisfactory technical closure of the openings into the trachea and esophagus. A gastrostomy should be done as an alternative procedure if one has not already been performed. The feedings are then given via the gastrostomy and the patient's progress is carefully observed. If the patient's condition becomes satisfactory, it may be preferable to delay closure of the recurrent fistula. If symptoms of the fistula continue, there is no recourse other than to attempt closure of it at this time. When the fistula is closed at a considerably later date,

the technical problems of the operation are lessened and satisfactory obliteration of the fistula can be anticipated.

The operation for closure of a recurrent fistula is performed transpleurally. The trachea and esophagus are first separated from each other above and below the level of the fistula; sharp dissection will be required because of the scar tissue that is invariably present. The fistula should be transected as close to the esophagus as possible, thereby preserving a cuff of the fistulous wall to aid in closure of the tracheal end of the fistula. It is preferable that the tracheal and esophageal suture lines not be allowed to remain in apposition. A pedicled flap of mediastinal pleura can usually be fashioned for interposition between the two suture lines. Should this maneuver not be possible, the esophagus can be rotated and approximated to the trachea so that the two suture lines are apart from each other.

STRICTURE AT ANASTOMOSIS.—Roentgenograms of the esophagus taken within the first several weeks after a primary repair of an esophageal atresia will usually show the lumen to be narrow at the level of the anastomosis. The degree of narrowing will depend on the initial size of the lower esophagus, the amount of inversion of the walls of the two segments at operation, and the amount of edema and scarring at the time of the roentgen examination. In the first 7–10 days after operation, the narrowing may be considerable as a result of edema and the original small size

Fig. 28-11.—Enlargement of esophageal lumen following primary anastomosis. **A,** portable roentgenogram of esophagus 4 days after telescopic anastomosis, showing prompt passage of contrast material into stomach, although the lumen is narrow at the anastomosis, which is intact. Three optional dilatations to size 26 F. were performed before discharge 27 days after operation. **B,** the esophagus at 19 months, showing slight indentation at level of anastomosis; no dysphagia.

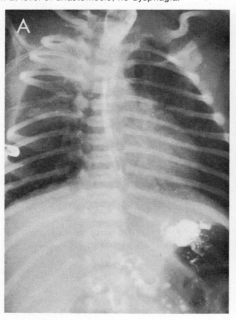
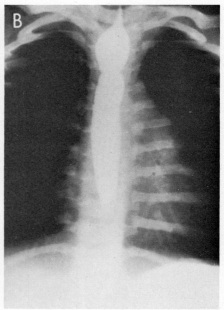

of the lower esophagus. Spontaneous enlargement of the lumen usually occurs (Fig. 28-11) unless the scar formation at the suture line increases. An undesirable degree of fibrous tissue reaction develops particularly when the amount of nonabsorbable suture material that has been used is excessive because of the size or number of sutures. It is advisable, therefore, to use no more sutures at operation than are required to obtain an air-tight and water-tight anastomosis.

If a stricture occurs, it becomes apparent as a rule during the third week after operation. It may first be suspected from the presence of increasing amounts of pharyngeal secretions and mucus. One of the earliest and most common symptoms of a stricture is difficulty in burping the infant. If difficulty in swallowing then develops, the diagnosis is more readily apparent. In such event, the presence or absence of a stricture should be confirmed by roentgen examination. Respiratory stridor may result from tracheal compression secondary to distention of the upper esophagus with secretions and air.

The caliber of the esophagus is tested by passage of progressively larger Robinson urethral catheters, beginning about 2½ weeks after operation. Should a no. 8 F. catheter fail to pass, the presence of a narrow anastomosis or early stricture is evident. Dilatations of the esophagus should then be started by using a Phillips urethral filiform and followers. If the filiform cannot be introduced readily through the stricture, a 4-mm to 20-cm infant esophagoscope is used and the filiform is passed under direct vision. The filiform is left in place and the esophagoscope removed. Followers of increasing size are passed through the stricture until they encounter slight to moderate resistance. The dilatations are repeated at intervals of several days, and it is endeavored to dilate the lumen of the anastomosis one size higher on each occasion, provided too great resistance is not encountered. The dilatation should be done gently to avoid trauma to the esophagus. The interval between dilatations will vary from every 2 or 3 days to once weekly, depending on the ease with which the dilatations are accomplished and the size to which the lumen narrows again prior to each subsequent dilatation.

Although the size of the esophageal lumen in infants without symptoms of a stricture will increase spontaneously in most cases, dilatations have been done almost routinely in our recent patients before they are returned home in order to be certain that the lumen is of an adequate size to prevent the development of subsequent symptoms. In a full-term baby, the lumen at the level of the anastomosis should allow passage of a no. 20–24 F. follower before the infant is discharged from the hospital. In a number of patients, only two or three dilatations are required. If the lumen of the esophagus should not enlarge readily, a longer period of dilatations is necessary. In this event, the dilatations are continued on an out-patient basis and at gradually increasing intervals of 1–3

weeks until the desired no. 26–28 F. size is reached by the time the infant is 2 or 3 months old. The patient is seen at longer intervals thereafter. The size of the lumen may be tested optionally on occasion in order to be certain that it is not decreasing. A roentgenogram of the esophagus is made 3 months after operation and repeated as indicated. This vigorous attitude regarding dilatations has been adopted as a result of the late deaths of 2 patients treated early in our series. The deaths occurred while the patients were at home and presumably resulted from sudden respiratory obstruction as a result of esophageal distention, or aspiration secondary to a stricture.

DEVELOPMENT OF THE PATIENT.— Following repair of an esophageal atresia, an infant shows several significant variations from normal. During the first several months to 2 or 3 years after operation, the patient may have a brassy, barking type of cough. As the parents are necessarily concerned about the cough, they should be reassured that it will disappear spontaneously in time. Solid foods may need to be offered at a later age than with a normal infant, depending on the size of the lumen at the anastomosis. When solid foods such as meat and uncooked fruits and vegetables are given, they may have to be prepared in small pieces. Even though the roentgen examination of the esophagus with barium may show no significant narrowing of the anastomosis, the lumen at the level of the anastomosis lacks the distensibility of the normal esophagus. For this reason, foreign bodies are particularly prone to cause esophageal obstruction. The parents should therefore be cautioned that if the patient suddenly becomes unable to swallow, the presence of foreign material or a foreign body should be suspected and esophagoscopy should be promptly performed.

Roentgen studies of the esophagus in our patients at a late date following repair of esophageal atresia and tracheoesophageal fistula have usually shown good peristalsis of the esophagus except for a short distance of several centimeters below the level of the anastomosis. Although peristalsis does not seem to be present in this area, no interference with swallowing is noted because of the strong propulsive force of the esophagus above this level. Kirkpatrick, Cresson and Pilling[27] have described some degree of inco-ordination of primary peristalsis, particularly below the line of anastomosis. They found that when there was enough contrast material below the anastomosis to distend the esophagus, secondary contractions might occur that were either localized to the point of maximal distention or were more diffuse and involved most of the lower esophagus, thereby resulting in both antegrade and retrograde flow of the contrast material. Similar findings were noted by Desjardins, Stephens and Moes[7] who observed that the primary peristaltic wave faded out at the level of the anastomosis and that segmental contractions were present in the distal segment. The segmental contractions occurred frequently and also caused a reverse flow of the esophageal contents into the upper esophagus. Lind, Blanchard and Guyda,[36] using manometric techniques in an esophageal motility study of 10 children after repair of tracheoesophageal fistula with esophageal atresia, found, in all cases motility patterns indistinguishable from those seen in achalasia. The defective motility in their cases involved the entire esophagus.

Psychometric examinations of selected patients in childhood have revealed some variations from normal, but the late development of patients following repair of an esophageal atresia has been gratifying.

Several of our early patients are now married. There have been three births, and all three infants are reported to be healthy and free from any anomaly.

Results

The results of the management of atresia of the esophagus with or without tracheoesophageal fistula depend largely on the condition of the infant on admission and the proper timing and selection of the operative procedure or procedures (Fig. 28-12). The chances of a successful outcome in the full-term, robust infant without other serious anomalies or pneumonitis should be excellent, whereas the prognosis in the feeble, markedly premature infant, often with serious accompanying anomalies and/or complicating pneumonitis, is correspondingly poor. At present, prematurity and other serious congenital anomalies are the chief obstacles to success. Foremost among the anomalies are those of the cardiovascular

Fig. 28-12.—Infants with esophageal atresia *and* tracheoesophageal fistula being treated concurrently illustrate varying methods of management. **Upper left,** premature with congenital heart disease. Gastrostomy and extrapleural division and closure of fistula because of poor condition (contemplated staged approach). Condition continued to be too poor for anastomosis, so cervical esophagostomy was done 6 months later. Subclavian-pulmonary shunt was then performed. Colon transplant will be required after correction of tetralogy of Fallot. **Upper center,** premature, being treated by gastrostomy for drainage and duodenal tube for feedings **(arrow)** before deferred primary anastomosis. **Upper right and below,** 4 robust patients in good condition, treated by primary anastomosis and without gastrostomy.

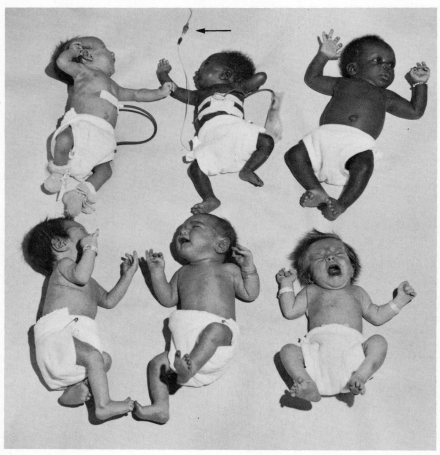

system, since most of the lesions responsible for death are too extensive for correction by open-heart operations in the neonatal period and many of such deaths will occur before the infant has recovered from the esophageal operation. Deaths from postoperative complications, although an important cause of failure in the past, have become progressively less with improved management. Pneumonitis and atelectasis continue to present a problem, but one that can be prevented or overcome in most cases. Leakage of the anastomosis is the most serious of the complications arising at the operative site, especially if it is accompanied by a re-opening of the sutured tracheoesophageal fistula. Although a stricture at the anastomosis was responsible for several of the late deaths in the earlier cases in our series, death from this cause should be preventable by adequate treatment of the stricture.

Collected statistics will show variable recovery rates that depend somewhat on the length of the postoperative evaluation. Of the 284 patients seen at the University of Michigan Hospital since the operation of primary anastomosis was first used in 1939, 148 (52.1%) are living as of the last report. These figures include the deaths of 9 patients who were not operated on, 2 early patients in whom incomplete operations were intentionally performed and 29 who died more than 3 months after operation. Three of the late deaths occurred from congenital heart disease in patients who were still hospitalized; 25 late deaths occurred after the patients had been returned home, and 12 of these resulted from other congenital anomalies.

The results obtained in the last 100 cases, admitted since May, 1956, show a recovery rate of 74% and a late survival rate of 68%. Four of the late deaths in this group were due to other anomalies, 1 to pneumonitis probably secondary to an inadequately treated stricture and 1 to diarrhea and pneumonia. Results during the past 4 years reflect further improvements in management, demonstrated by the fact that 27 (84.4%) of the 32 patients are living. Operation has been undertaken for all of the patients with this anomaly who have been admitted to this hospital during the last 16 years.

Tracheoesophageal Fistula without Esophageal Atresia

TRACHEOESOPHAGEAL fistula of the H type occurs in approximately 3–4% of the anomalies of the upper esophagus. The esophagus is normal except for its fistulous communication with the trachea. The level of the fistula is characteristically higher than that observed with a tracheoesophageal fistula accompanying esophageal atresia.[11] In 9 cases seen at the University of Michigan Hospital, the fistula was situated in the mid-third of the trachea in 2 and at the level of the clavicle or higher in 7 (Fig. 28-13). In an additional infant, a double H-type congenital fistula was situated between the thoracic portions of the trachea and esophagus.

The *symptoms* of choking and coughing with feedings should direct attention to the possibility of a tracheoesophageal fistula of this type, especially when the symptoms are more pronounced with feedings of a thin, rather than a thicker, consistency.[15,55] In the presence of such symptoms, an unusually large amount of air in the stomach and intestines should arouse further suspicions of a tracheoesophageal fistula. The extent of the symptoms and the age at which the patient is referred for treatment depend not only on the size of the fistula but also on its obliquity. If the fistulous communication is of an appreci-able length and not a true esophagotracheal window, the tracheal end of the fistula is usually at a slightly higher level than the esophageal end. Of the 9 patients in this series, 7 were admitted before the end of the third week of life, 4 of them within the first 3 days of life.

The *diagnosis* of a tracheoesophageal fistula alone may be difficult to establish, especially when it is situated in the cervical region. Roentgen examination of

Fig. 28-13.—Tracheoesophageal fistula without esophageal atresia. Location of fistula in 9 cases. **A,** in 7, fistula was at level of clavicle or higher. **B,** in 2, fistula was in mid-third of trachea. In another case, a double H-type fistula without atresia was situated at the latter level.

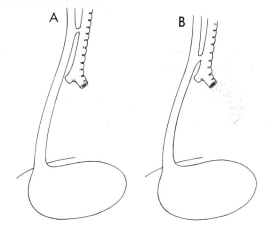

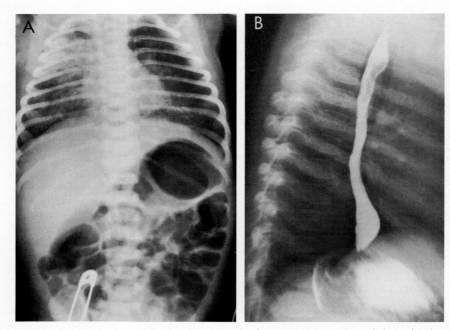

Fig. 28-14.—Tracheoesophageal fistula without atresia. **A,** roentgenogram at age 2 days, showing large amount of air in gastrointestinal tract and right upper lobe pneumonitis. An H-type fistula was recognized on tracheoscopy at age 5 days. Rapid worsening of pneumonitis required operation the following day for transpleural closure of fistula. **B,** roentgenogram 13 months after operation, showing normal esophagus.

the esophagus is the most certain method; this has become more accurate since the image intensifier and a means for the continuous permanent recording of the fluoroscopic observations have become available. It is preferably done with the aid of a Foley bag catheter to allow retrograde filling of the esophagus and fistula (See Fig. 28-10). The fistula may also be detected on a similar roentgen examination following the instillation of contrast material through a catheter with its tip in the cervical esophagus. The examination is made with the patient in the *prone* or slight oblique position. The fistula is accordingly dependent and the contrast material thereby enters the trachea by gravitation.[15] An aqueous contrast solution should be employed, because it is more likely to enter a small fistula than is a thicker, oily type of material. It is particularly important that the level of the fistula be identified, as this information will determine the route for its closure by operation. Tracheoscopy with a 3.5-mm to 16-cm bronchoscope is helpful at times in identifying the fistulous opening into the trachea (Fig. 28-14). Atropine sulfate or scopolamine hydrobromide should be given before tracheoscopy in order to decrease secretions which, when present, interfere greatly with satisfactory observation through an infant-size bronchoscope.

The *operative approach* for correction of a tracheoesophageal fistula will depend on the location of the fistula. If the fistula is at the level of the clavicle or higher, a cervical incision similar to that described for cervical esophagostomy is used. Recent reports[26,40] indicate that most tracheoesophageal fistulas can be closed by a cervical approach. If the fistula is within the thorax, a right transpleural approach is employed. The fistula should be divided flush with its esophageal end, thus preserving an ample amount of tissue for closure of the opening into the trachea. If the fistula is in reality an esophagotracheal window, a small portion of the adjacent esophageal wall should be left attached to its tracheal end to facilitate the tracheal closure. The opening in the esophagus is then closed in a transverse direction without resultant narrowing of the esophagus. A pedicle flap of mediastinal fat or pleura should be interposed between the trachea and the esophagus in order to separate the suture lines.

Six of the 9 patients with a single H-type fistula were operated on and 5 recovered, as did the patient with the double fistula. In the 1 patient who did not recover following operation, the fistula, which was believed to be in the middle third of the trachea, was in reality in the low cervical region and could not be identified through the transpleural approach. The patient died before a cervical operation was done. The diagnosis had not been definitely established in the 3 patients who died without operation. The deaths in these cases occurred 8, 39 and 55 days after birth, 1 of them due to other anomalies. Although a few of the patients with this anomaly may live for months or years with recurring pneumonitis, the life expectancy of most infants with tracheoesophageal fistula without esophageal atresia is quite short. Prompt diagnosis and operative repair are therefore essential if most of these patients are to recover.

REFERENCES

1. Abbott, O. A.: Abnormal esophageal communications: Their types, diagnosis and therapy, J. Thoracic Surg. 14:382, 1945.
2. Benson, C. D.: Personal communication.
3. Berman, J. K., and Berman, E. J.: Congenital atresia of the esophagus with tracheo-esophageal fistula. A simplified method of restoring continuity of the esophagus, Am. J. Surg. 86:436, 1953.
4. Berman, E. J.: Personal communication, Oct. 5, 1967.
5. Brown, R. K., and Brown, E. C.: Congenital esophageal anomalies: Review of 24 cases and report of three, Surg., Gynec. & Obst. 91:545, 1950.
6. Clatworthy, H. W., Jr.: Esophageal atresia: Importance of early diagnosis and adequate treatment illustrated by a series of patients, Pediatrics 16:122, 1955.
7. Desjardins, J. G.; Stephens, C. A., and Moes, C. A. F.: Results of surgical treatment of congenital tracheoesophageal fistula, with a note on cine-fluorographic findings, Ann. Surg. 160:141, 1964.
8. Durston, W.: A Narrative of a Monstrous Birth in Plymouth, Octob. 22, 1670; together with the Anatomical Observations, taken thereupon by William Durston Doctor in Physick, and communicated to Dr. Tim. Clerk, Philosophical Tr., London 5:2096, 1670.
9. Ferguson, C. F.: Congenital tracheoesophageal fistula not associated with atresia of the esophagus, Laryngoscope 61:718, 1951.
10. Gibson, T.: *The Anatomy of Humane Bodies Epitomized.* Wherein all the parts of Man's Body, with their actions and uses, are succinctly described, according to the newest Doctrine of the most Accurate and Learned Modern Anatomists. The Fifth Edition, Corrected and Inlarged both in the Discourse and Figures (London: printed by T. W. for Awnsham and John Churchill, 1697).
11. Giedion, A.: Angeborene hohe Osophagotrachealfistel vom H-Typus, Helvet. paediat. acta 15:155, 1960.
12. Gross, R. E.: *Surgery of Infancy and Childhood* (Philadelphia: W. B. Saunders Company, 1953).
13. Haight, C., and Towsley, H. A.: Congenital atresia of the esophagus with tracheoesophageal fistula: Extrapleural ligation of fistula and end-to-end anastomosis of esophageal segments, Surg., Gynec. & Obst. 76:672, 1943.
14. Haight, C.: Congenital atresia of the esophagus with tracheoesophageal fistula: Reconstruction of esophageal continuity by primary anastomosis, Ann. Surg. 120:623, 1944.
15. Haight, C.: Congenital tracheoesophageal fistula without esophageal atresia, J. Thoracic Surg. 17:600, 1948.
16. Haight, C.: Some observations on esophageal atresias and tracheoesophageal fistulas of congenital origin, J. Thoracic Surg. 34:141, 1957.
17. Haight, C.: In discussion of Holder *et al.*[19]
18. Hausmann, P. F.; Close, A. S., and William, L. P.: Occurrence of tracheoesophageal fistula in three consecutive siblings, Surgery 41:542, 1957.
19. Holder, T. M.; McDonald, V. G., Jr., and Woolley, M. M.: The premature or critically ill infant with esophageal atresia: Increased success with a staged approach, J. Thoracic & Cardiovas. Surg. 44:344, 1962.
20. Holder, T. M., *et al.*: Esophageal atresia and tracheoesophageal fistula: A survey of its members by the Surgical Section of the American Academy of Pediatrics, Pediatrics 34:542, 1964.
21. Holder, T. M., and Ashcraft, K. W.: Esophageal atresia and tracheo-esophageal fistula, Cur. Prob. Surg., pp. 1-68, August, 1966.
22. Holt, J. F.; Haight, C., and Hodges, F. J.: Congenital atresia of the esophagus and tracheoesophageal fistula, Radiology 47:457, 1946.
23. Howard, R., and Myers, N. A.: Esophageal atresia: A technique for elongating the upper pouch, Surgery 58:725, 1965.
24. Humphreys, G. H.; Hogg, B. M., and Ferrer, J.: Congenital atresia of esophagus, J. Thoracic Surg. 32:332, 1956.
25. Keith, A.: A demonstration on constrictions and occlusions of the alimentary tract of congenital or obscure origin, Brit. M. J. 1:301, 1910.
26. Killen, D. A., and Greenlee, H. B.: Transcervical repair of H-type congenital tracheo-esophageal fistula, Ann. Surg. 162:145, 1965.
27. Kirkpatrick, J. A.; Cresson, S. L., and Pilling, G. P., IV: The motor activity of the esophagus in association with esophageal atresia and tracheoesophageal fistula, Am. J. Roentgenol. 86:884, 1961.
28. Koop, C. E., and Verhagen, A. D.: Early management of atresia of the esophagus, Internat. Abst. Surg. 113:103, 1961.
29. Ladd, W. E.: The surgical treatment of esophageal atresia and tracheoesophageal fistulas, New England J. Med. 230:625, 1944.
30. Lamb, D. S.: A fatal case of congenital tracheo-esophageal fistula, Philadelphia M. Times 3:705, 1873.
31. Langman, J.: Esophageal atresia and esophago-tracheal fistula, Acta neerl. morph. 6:308, 1949.
32. Langman, J.: Oesophageal atresia accompanied by a remarkable vessel anomaly, Arch. chir. neerl. 4:39, 1952.
33. Lanman, T. H.: Congenital atresia of the esophagus: A study of 32 cases, Arch. Surg. 41:1060, 1940.
34. Leven, N. L.: Congenital atresia of the esophagus with tracheo-esophageal fistula: Report of successful extrapleural ligation of fistulous communication and cervical esophagostomy, J. Thoracic Surg. 10:648, 1941.
35. Leven, N. L., *et al.*: Surgical management of congenital atresia of the esophagus and tracheo-esophageal fistula, Ann. Surg. 136:701, 1952.
36. Lind, J. F.; Blanchard, R. J., and Guyda, H.: Esophageal motility in tracheoesophageal fistula and esophageal atresia, Surg., Gynec. & Obst. 123:557, 1966.
37. Mahoney, E. B., and Sherman, C. D., Jr.: Total esophagoplasty using intrathoracic right colon, Surgery 35:937, 1954.
38. Martin, L. W.: Management of esophageal anomalies, Pediatrics 36:342, 1965.
39. Minton, J. P., and Clatworthy, H. W., Jr.: Congenital esophageal atresia: A report of improved survival of infants through prompt recognition and surgical correction, Ohio M. J. 58:1262, 1962.
40. Moncrief, J. A., and Randolph, J. C.: Congenital tracheoesophageal fistula without atresia of the esophagus: The diagnosis and surgical correction, J. Thoracic & Cardiovas. Surg. 51:434, 1966.
41. Potts, W. J.: In discussion of Humphreys *et al.*[24]
42. Potts, W. J.: *The Surgeon and the Child* (Philadelphia: W. B. Saunders Company, 1959).
43. Rehbein, F., and Yanagisawa, R.: Complications after operations for oesophageal atresia, Arch. Dis. Childhood 34:24, 1959.
44. Replogle, R. L.: Esophageal atresia: Plastic sump catheter for drainage of the proximal pouch, Surgery 54:296, 1963.
45. Richter, H. M.: Congenital atresia of the oesophagus: An operation designed for its cure, Surg., Gynec. & Obst. 17:397, 1913.
46. Sandblom, P.: Treatment of congenital atresia of the esophagus from a technical point of view, Acta chir. scandinav. 97:25, 1948.
47. Shaw, R.: Surgical correction of congenital atresia of the esophagus with tracheo-esophageal fistula, J. Thoracic

Surg. 9:213, 1939.

48. Shaw, R. R.; Paulson, D. L., and Siebel, E. K.: Congenital atresia of the esophagus with tracheo-esophageal fistula: Treatment of surgical complications, Ann. Surg. 142:204, 1955.

49. Sloan, H., and Haight, C.: Congenital atresia of the esophagus in brothers, J. Thoracic Surg. 32:209, 1956.

50. Sulamaa, M.; Gripenberg, L., and Ahvenainen, E. K.: Prognosis and treatment of congenital atresia of the esophagus, Acta. chir. scandinav. 102:141, 1951.

51. Sulamaa, M.: Personal communication, Aug. 2, 1967.

52. Swenson, O.: *Pediatric Surgery* (2nd ed.; New York: Appleton-Century-Crofts, Inc., 1962).

53. Ty, T. C.; Brunet, C., and Beardmore, H. E.: A variation in the operative technique for the treatment of esophageal atresia with tracheo-esophageal fistula, J. Pediat. Surg. 2:118, 1967.

54. Vogt, E. C.: Congenital esophageal atresia, Am. J. Roentgenol. 22:463, 1929.

55. Ware, G. W., and Cross, L. L.: Congenital tracheo-esophageal fistula without atresia of the esophagus, Pediatrics 14:254, 1954.

56. Waterston, D. J.; Bonham Carter, R. E., and Aberdeen, E.: Oesophageal atresia: Tracheo-oesophageal fistula; A study of survival in 218 infants, Lancet 1:819, 1962.

57. Waterston, D. J.; Bonham-Carter, R. E., and Aberdeen, E.: Congenital tracheo-oesophageal fistula in association with oesophageal atresia, Lancet 2:55, 1963.

58. Woolley, M. M.; Chinnock, R. F., and Paul, R. H.: Premature twins with esophageal atresia and tracheo-esophageal fistula, Acta paediat. 50:423, 1961.

CAMERON HAIGHT

Drawings by
ALFRED TEOLI (Figures 28-1, 28-8 and 28-13)
GERALD P. HODGE (Figure 28-7)

Esophageal Stenosis and Stricture

Congenital Esophageal Stenosis

IT WOULD BE surprising if the esophagus, alone of the cylindrical portions of the gastrointestinal tract, were unaffected by congenital stenoses, whether of muscular, fibrous or membranous type. Most workers in the field believe there is no lack of such instances. It is well to note, however, that with the increasing awareness of the effects of peptic esophagitis associated with hiatus hernia, and the swiftness with which strictures and stenoses can be produced by this mechanism, a number of lesions formerly thought to have been congenital stenoses have been shown to be almost certainly postnatal strictures. Some go so far as to suggest that congenital stenosis does not occur; indeed, that strictures associated with hiatus hernia may be present at birth, presumably due to intrauterine peptic esophagitis (see p. 395).

The problem of differentiating true congenital stenosis of the esophagus from strictures secondary to hiatus hernia and peptic esophagitis was illustrated by Gerbasi[4] in his discussion of 14 cases of congenital stricture seen in 25 years at the University of Michigan. All but 1 were between the middle and lower thirds of the esophagus. Eight patients were seen soon after symptoms developed and were demonstrated not to have a hiatus hernia. Subsequently, 3 of them did have a hiatus hernia. Of 11 patients who were followed, 5 were ultimately proved to have hiatus hernia. Holinger *et. al.*[6] reported 23 cases of congenital esophageal stricture.

The patients we have seen with what we considered to be congenital stricture have followed a uniform pattern. There is no difficulty in swallowing for a variable but relatively short period after birth, when progressive dysphagia and evidence of obstruction appear to progress in a short time to essentially complete obstruction. It is often suggested that symptoms appear with the change to thick feedings, but we have seen these symptoms within 2 or 3 weeks of birth (Fig. 28-15). We think that, with partial obstruction from the first, there has been constant retention of some ingested material proximal to the obstruction, with progressive irritation and edema leading in turn to a complete obstruction.

The roentgenogram (Fig. 28-16) shows smooth, abrupt, complete or nearly complete obstruction to the passage of contrast material, usually in the lower portion of the mid-third of the esophagus. Esophagoscopy may at times show a semilunar or circular valve or web, but in the face of the existing edema, endoscopy is often unrewarding.

TREATMENT. — Early experiences with the impossibility of finding the lumen in the area of the edematous obstruction, whether tubular or due to a diaphragm, and mishaps with esophageal perforation on attempted bouginage, led us to adopt a relatively simple and effective method of treating these patients.

Once the diagnosis has been established by appropriate barium swallows, if a bougie does not fall easily into the stomach, a gastrostomy is performed and nothing is given by mouth for a week or 10 days, while a catheter with constant suction keeps the esophagus empty. At the end of a week, a spool of fine silk thread is suspended above the baby's head and the end of the thread passed into the baby's mouth. As the baby chews and swallows, the thread finds its way through the stenosis and into the stomach, where it is readily fished out, either with a crochet needle or with a suction tip. A heavy silk thread is now drawn

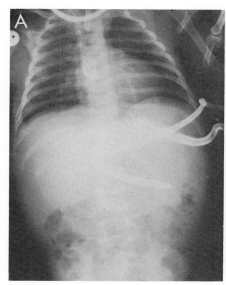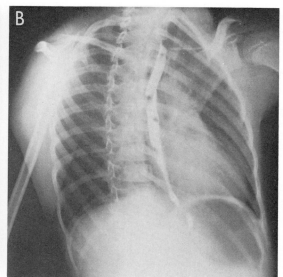

Fig. 28-15.—Congenital esophageal stenosis. A 3-week-old infant with 10-day history of increasing dysphagia culminating in apparent total occlusion. **A,** a catheter passed through the mouth met an obstruction in the midesophagus, and Lipiodol fills the proximal esophagus in a pouch ending at T-7. Esophagoscopy showed what appeared to be a web type of obstruction with a tiny crescentic opening at one portion. Gastrostomy was done, and after 10 days of constant esophageal catheter suction and no oral feedings, the child could swallow a string readily. The esophagus was dilated with graduated plastic beads pulled through on a string, replaced by a Salzer bougie as soon as it could be passed. There was no tendency to recurrence. **B,** barium swallow 3 years later shows no evidence of obstruction or of hiatus hernia. The child has been well.

Fig. 28-16.—Congenital esophageal stenosis. A 3-week-old child with 1-week history of progressive dysphagia culminating in almost complete obstruction. He had regurgitated occasionally since birth. **A,** a small French catheter could not be passed through the obstruction. Esophagoscopy showed extensive edema in which the distal orifice could not be found. Nevertheless some Lipiodol leaks through the incomplete obstruction in the midesophagus. **B,** after gastrostomy, putting the esophagus at rest, followed by ingestion of a thread pulled through the gastrostomy and dilatation by graduated beads, ingested contrast meterial flows readily down the esophagus, although a residual deformity is seen. Dilatations were continued with a Salzer bougie. There is no hiatus hernia. Symptoms have not recurred. Congenital stenoses in general dilate fairly readily and apparently without as much trauma as in dilatation of inflammatory strictures, so dilatation in itself does not produce further scarring and stenosis.

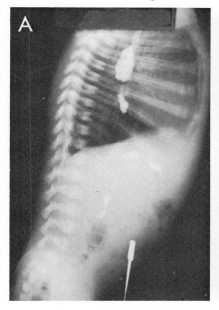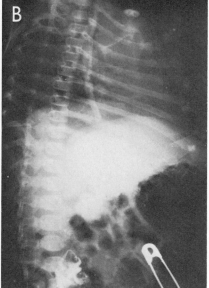

after the fine silk, through the mouth and out the gastrostomy, and tied into an endless loop. Into this loop are spliced sections of thread on which there have been formed olive-shaped beads of cellulose acetate, varying from barely perceptible thickenings of the thread to beads 6 or 8 mm in diameter or larger. These are pulled through the mouth, down the esophagus, through the stricture and out the gastrostomy, or back and forth, in progressively larger sizes. When, after several days, the largest bead passes without difficulty, the daily dilatations are replaced by dilatations every second and every third day, until it is proved that there is no tendency to restricture. As soon as the esophagus will readily accept a Hurst (mercury-filled) or Salzer (shot-filled) bougie, the string is removed and the gastrostomy allowed to close. There has been little tendency to restricture; and after several months of precautionary weekly, followed by bimonthly, calibrations of the esophagus with bougies, treatment may be discontinued. Actually, once the larger sizes of the plastic beads have been pulled through the stricture, one may begin to employ bougies, either the flexible woven, olive-tipped variety or the Salzer, Hurst, shot- or mercury-filled rubber catheters. In most patients with congenital stenosis, as opposed to patients with inflammatory stricture, particularly those which occur after anastomoses, a few dilatations are all that are needed, and there is little or no tendency to restricture. The Tucker soft rubber threaded dilators, essentially tapered tubes of solid rubber with threads incorporated in their centers, serve equally well for dilatation by this method. Angelberger,[1] in a single dramatic case, complemented dilatation with cortisone and penicillin, just as in caustic stricture. We believe this is unnecessary.

In an infant 1 month old with an esophageal web causing obstruction since birth, Lyons *et al.*[9] exposed the esophagus transpleurally, excised the web and closed the esophagus. Seventeen months later the child was well except for some narrowing at the site of esophageal stricture. We and others have successfully treated stenoses of the esophagus by resection, and the specimens have afforded evidence of the congenital and noninflammatory nature of the stenoses. We are impressed, however, by the difference in magnitude between resection and dilatation and are mindful of the fact that stricture following resection is not unknown.[2] Sandblom[11] with success performed a Heineke-Mikulicz esophagoplasty at the site of a localized congenital stenosis.

Congenital esophageal stenoses of a curious kind are due to ectopic tissue. Paulino *et al.*[10] in 2 cases and Kumar[8] in 1 case found congenital esophageal obstruction due to a ring of cartilage with associated respiratory epithelium, treated in 2 cases by segmental resection and in 1 by submucous resection. Schwartz[12] excised a tight stenosis due to a transverse membrane covered by gastric glands.

REFERENCES

1. Angelberger, H.: Angeborene Oesophagusstenose, Ztschr. Kinderchir. 5:56, 1967.
2. Bonilla, K. B., and Bowers, W. F.: Congenital esophageal stenosis, Am. J. Surg. 97:772, 1959.
3. Despons, M. J., and Lasserre, J.: Stenose congenital de l'oesophage: Traitement chirurgical et dilatation postoperative, Ann. oto-laryng. 79:221, 1967.
4. Gerbasi, F. S.: In discussion of Holinger *et al.*[6]
5. Gross, R. E.: Treatment of short stricture of the esophagus by partial esophagectomy and end-to-end esophageal reconstruction, Surgery 23:735, 1948.
6. Holinger, P. H., *et al.*: Conservative and surgical management of benign strictures of the esophagus, J. Thoracic Surg. 28:345, 1954.
7. Huber, P.: Angeborene Esophagusstenose oder Narbenstenose nach Refluxoesophagitis, Wien. klin. Wchnschr. 71:950, 1959.
8. Kumar, R.: A case of congenital esophageal stricture due to a cartilaginous ring. Brit. J. Surg. 49:533, 1962.
9. Lyons, C.; Oschsner, A., and Platou, V.: Segmental resection of the esophagus of infants, South. M. J. 43:585, 1950.
10. Paulino, F.; Roselli, A., and Aprigliano, F., Congenital esophageal stricture due to tracheobronchial remnants, Surgery 53:547, 1963.
11. Sandblom, P.: Plastic repair of congenital esophageal stenosis, Acta chir. scandinav. 97:35, 1948.
12. Schwartz, S. I.: Congenital membranous obstruction of esophagus, Arch. Surg. 85:480, 1962.
13. Wolfrom, I.: Angeborene Oesophagusstenosen, Monatsschr. Kinderh. 107:47, 1959.

Acquired Esophageal Stricture

STRICTURES RESULTING FROM PEPTIC ESOPHAGITIS

Strictures of this type occur chiefly in association with regurgitation of gastric juice in the presence of malfunction of the mechanism at the esophagogastric junction and esophageal hiatus (see p. 395). We saw an interesting variation of this in a child who, during a severe neonatal illness, was fed through an indwelling nasogastric tube for a considerable time. Months later, when the child had apparently recovered from his original illness, he presented the symptoms of esophageal obstruction. He had a very delicate stricture, which was felt to "pop" as an exploratory bougie was passed. It seems almost certain that the indwelling gastric catheter had produced incompetence of the cardia, that he had had esophagitis and this had resulted, quite probably, in kissing ulcers, or areas of esophagitis with adhesion, and that the relatively fresh scar yielded to the bougie. His esophagus has been recalibrated at progressively longer intervals and there has been no tendency to reformation of the stricture, nor has the patient had any symptoms. X-rays have shown no evidence of hiatus hernia.

POSTOPERATIVE STRICTURES

Stricture is common after anastomosis of the esophageal ends in patients with esophageal atresia.

Strictures are particularly prone to occur in patients in whom there has been a fistula, with the inevitable increase in the local inflammatory process. We consider it important for the patient to have a barium swallow within a week or 10 days of operation. If a very marked stricture is found, unless a Salzer bougie can be easily passed, we prefer to pass a silk thread from the mouth through the stricture and out through a gastrostomy for dilatation in the manner described for congenital stenosis. In this manner there is much less danger of injuring the esophagus, a risk which is particularly great because of the frequent angulation of the esophagus at the point of anastomosis. If one delays too long in passing a string or bougie through a postoperative stricture, a dense and impenetrable obstruction may form, requiring the major hazard of formal reoperation. Even less dense postoperative strictures may require relatively long periods of dilatation. If a thread or bougie can be passed through an operative stricture, the ultimate result with persistent dilatation will be excellent, and reoperation need not be considered.

Stricture is not rare after resection of congenital stenoses and constitutes the principal reason for preferring dilatation to operation.

ESCHAROTIC STRICTURES

The widespread use of lye as a cleaning agent, the common practice of storing the solution in old soft-drink bottles, its relative cheapness which makes it most likely to be used in families with numerous children inadequately supervised, all combine to set the stage for the accidental ingestion of this solution of powerful alkali by small children. One of the great difficulties in evaluating the results of various methods of therapy is the uncertainty as to how much solution has been taken, and whether any of it passed beyond the mouth. The mouth may be severely burned in a child who has swallowed none at all.

Children who have swallowed substantial amounts of lye may soon go into collapse, presumably because of the massive necrosis of the esophageal lining, and the large outpouring of fluid into and around the esophagus. Stricture is the inevitable result of the deep burns in a muscular organ whose natural state is collapsed. The strictures which result may take several forms. There may result a twisted, tortuous, narrow passage the entire length of the esophagus, or there may be a single, dense, fairly localized stricture. Total obliteration and the sealing off of the esophagus were not uncommon in former days, and these unfortunate children required cervical pharyngostomies to relieve them of the discharge of the saliva which they could not swallow. The first reconstruction of the esophagus in the Johns Hopkins Hospital[6] was for a child with such a complete escharotic destruction of the esophagus. Acid ingestion differs in its results

from the ingestion of lye, in the frequency with which the esophagus escapes injury while the stomach is severely injured, even to rapid perforation.

The immediate treatment of a child who is said to have swallowed lye begins with careful examination of the lips and mouth for any evidence of burn. There is little enthusiasm for the administration of weak acids as an antidote, although gestures are often made in this direction. Patients who are shocked require appropriate systemic support.

From this point on, treatment is directed to the prevention of esophageal stricture. It was formerly held by many (beginning with von Hacker in 1896), and is still maintained by some, that the esophagus should be allowed to heal without being disturbed, and that then, in the children in whom stricture developed, dilatations could be begun. This approach has the merit of not subjecting every child suspected of having swallowed lye to the uncomfortable indignities of bouginage. On the other hand, it entails acceptance of inevitable stricture formation in most of the children who have actually ingested the lye, and there is the obvious risk that if there is undue delay, or a failure to re-examine such a child, a hopeless stricture may develop before the situation can be dealt with. For many years in the Harriet Lane Home of the Johns Hopkins Hospital a strict routine according to the method of Salzer[17] was observed. Salzer, as far back as 1907, began to use soft rubber catheters filled with fine lead shot before the onset of strictures, and gradually came round to dilatation beginning 2–6 days after the poisoning. In 1920 he reported on 13 children so treated; 12 of whom were entirely well subsequently. One 2-year-old had aspirated some of the lye solution and died of the resultant pneumonia. Gersuny, in 1870, had advocated early bouginage.

All studies of the result of therapy of lye burns of the esophagus are subject to the criticism of the uncertainty whether the esophagus had in fact been exposed to the lye at all, and the uncertainty as to the degree to which it had been burned. Undoubtedly direct esophagoscopy is the most accurate means of evaluating the esophageal burn, but even this procedure is more useful to determine whether the esophagus has been burned or not than it is to determine how deeply it has been burned. Under the plan long employed at the Harriet Lane Home,[9] every child suspected of having swallowed lye was treated as if he had, in fact, swallowed lye, and was admitted to the hospital and dilated with Salzer bougies within 1–3 days of admission. As soon as the child's general condition stabilized and the home had been investigated, the child was discharged home and subsequent dilatation performed in the outpatient department. The interval between dilatations was gradually lengthened so long as there was no evidence of any tendency to stricture formation. The bougies passed were of sizes proportionate to the sizes of the children, up to 36 or 40 in the older children. While some children so treated developed strictures which had to be dilated repeatedly for many months, the majority required only a relatively brief period of treatment. We have not seen the esophagus ruptured by this method, and although it seems perhaps improper to pass instruments through an esophagus whose mucosal surface is healing from severe chemical burns, it is important to keep the esophagus stretched out so that adhesions will not form from wall to wall. It is the prevention of such adhesions which the passage of the Salzer bougies accomplishes in the early weeks, rather than the actual stretching of the strictures.

Bouginage, whether done early or after several weeks, can be done in a variety of ways: (1) per oral blind bouginage; (2) endoscopic bouginage over a thread or a filiform; (3) per oral bouginage over a thread, and (4) retrograde bouginage over a thread passed down the esophagus and through a gastrostomy. Salzer ultimately reported 188 cases with only 4 perforations. The obvious feeling that early dilatations and the swallowing of food irritated the burned tissue, which should be at rest, led to the *methode Bordeaux* of Despons and LeBihan.[7] They performed an immediate gastrostomy to put the esophagus at rest and on day 15 began dilatations over a string.

In 1953, Rosenberg and his associates[16] reported their first experimental studies with cortisone-treated lye burns of the esophagus in rabbits. Their initial results showed that although many of the animals died of invasive infection of the mediastinum, those that survived were almost completely protected against strictures. They repeated the studies 2 years later with the addition of penicillin and eliminated the deaths from infection. Burian and Stockinger,[2] in 1956 reported experiments on lye burns in the esophagus of cats, without treatment, with penicillin alone, and with penicillin and cortisone, and demonstrated a great superiority of the last method. Haller and Bachman,[10] in standard alkali burns in cats, evaluated controls and three treatment groups: steroids only, steroids and antibiotics, and bouginage, steroids and antibiotics. They confirmed Burian's findings and could demonstrate no advantage from the addition of bouginage, which in cats required general anesthesia and resulted in frequent perforation.

Knox and his associates[12] studied severe localized alkali burns of the esophagus in dogs. In addition to antibiotics, the experimental groups were treated by bouginage alone, by prednisone in doses of 0.5 and 0.1 mg/kg/day, and by bouginage plus prednisone 0.1 mg/kg/day. Bouginage was initiated on the seventh day and repeated every 3 or 4 days for 2 months. The best results were obtained in the animals who received bouginage and prednisone in addition to antibiotics. There were no perforations in this group.

Nevertheless 3 of the 15 dogs so treated did develop severe strictures.

A considerable clinical experience has been accumulated with treatment of lye burns of the esophagus with cortisone,[4,8,13,15,18] subject to the ever-present difficulty in analyzing such results because of uncertainty about ingestion in any given instance. We have seen a lye burn of the esophagus which produced a necrotizing slough of the entire esophageal mucosa, as repeatedly viewed through the esophagoscope, which healed under cortisone therapy.

Kohaus and Schurmeyer[13] in 1959 reported 36 cases (27 in children) of esophageal burns, mostly acid. They used cortisone and antibiotics in the more recent cases, usually prednisone in high dosage for 3 days and then decreasing. Daily bouginage began on the twelfth day, antibiotics were continued for 3 or 4 weeks, and steroids for 6 weeks, checked by endoscopy until there was complete mucosal healing.

Schobel[18] in the same year, in a comprehensive review of the subject, indicated his belief that none of the traumatizing dilatation methods could prevent scar tissue formation and recommended early intensive administration of antibiotics and cortisone therapy controlled by weekly endoscopy until there is complete epithelization. He claimed absolute prevention of stricture formation. Ray and Morgan[15] treated 11 children, 10 with cortisone alone, and no stricture occurred. One seemed well but developed a stricture 3 months later and required dilatation. Schobel treated 20 patients in 3 years, and all but 2 healed without stenosis or dilatation. In 1 of the failures, cortisone was begun on the ninth day and discontinued too soon. Cortisone should be continued until healing is complete. One patient with an extremely severe burn had an easily dilated annular stricture. Schobel believed that cortisone dosage should be 50–150 mg a day in adults, and proportionally less in children, and continued for a month or more.

Viscomi and colleagues,[19] in 79 children alleged to have swallowed corrosives, found corrosive burns of lips, tongue, palate or pharynx in 64. Of these, only 16 had esophagoscopic evidence of an esophageal burn; conversely, 1 child without an oropharyngeal burn had a frank burn eschar in the distal esophagus. Similarly, Cleveland and associates[4] obtained esophagoscopic evidence of an esophageal burn in only 37 of 99 children. Again, 1 child with no oropharyngeal burn, not examined with the esophagoscope, developed an esophageal stricture. Viscomi *et al.*, employing a corticosteroid and antibiotic regimen for their 16 esophageal burns, had a stricture develop in only 1, an extremely severe burn. No other complications occurred. In the series of Cleveland *et al.*, five strictures resulted in the 37 esophageal burns treated with a corticosteroid and antibiotics; but three strictures occurred among 6 children not studied by esophagoscopy and not treated, three among 15 children with negative esophagoscopic findings but treated fully, and one among 10 children incompletely treated. Eight of nine strictures responded to dilatation. One perforation occurred on initial esophagoscopy and one in the course of dilating a stricture. One child had a perforated gastric ulcer after 3 weeks of prednisone treatment.

Observations in our clinic have suggested that the barium swallow is a poor guide to the state of the esophagus early after a lye burn; the picture may appear to be relatively normal when esophagoscopy shows a severe mucosal injury.

Holinger and his colleagues[11] reported on 169 patients with caustic burns of the esophagus from the Children's Memorial Hospital, Chicago. Two thirds of the cases were chronic, with original treatment having been given elsewhere. Of the first 96 patients, 27 had complete occlusion of the esophagus at the time of initial hospitalization. These authors pointed out that with care and persistence, it is possible to find a channel and restore an adequate esophageal lumen in almost all of these patients (Fig. 28-17). They reported, as did Gellis and Holt,[9] that with the Salzer method, no stricture forms in patients who have been faithful in their follow-up treatment.

Burford et al.,[1] essentially on a priori grounds, condemned early bouginage, but it seems illogical to allow the esophagus to develop a stricture before any treatment is undertaken.

The immediate necessity is general support of the burned patient, heavy antibiotic therapy and parenteral nourishment. If skilled esophagoscopy is available, it is undertaken as soon as the child's condition has stabilized, within the first 24 hours. Evidence of edema, hemorrhage or ulceration anywhere in the esophagus is an indication for initiation of the intensive therapeutic regimen and prolonged observation. The purpose of esophagoscopy is to discover whether the esophagus has been burned, not how deeply or extensively, so the esophagoscope is withdrawn as soon as a burn is seen. The instrument is not passed through the injured area, thus avoiding perforation. In particularly severe burns, the passage of a thread demonstrates the lumen and allows safe passage of dilating instruments. Controlled animal experiments and clinical reports strongly suggest that intensive antibiotic and heavy corticosteroid therapy will prevent stricture formation. A dose of prednisone of 2 mg/kg/day for 3 weeks, or until esophagoscopy demonstrates mucosal healing, is recommended. The passage of a Salzer or Hurst bougie, as the sole treatment in former days, was found to be free from danger if undertaken before stricture had formed and prevented synechial adhesion of apposed mucosal surfaces and the development of major strictures. It seems reasonable to continue to do this in addition to using cortisone and antibiotics.

Even after cessation of therapy of the child who is known to have ingested lye, his esophagus should be calibrated with bougies at regular intervals for several months and an energetic program of dilations be-

Fig. 28-17.—Lye stricture of the esophagus. A 3-year-old child ingested lye some months previously. **A,** almost complete obstruction. **B,** early result after gastrostomy, passage of a string and retrograde bouginage followed by per oral sounding. Multiple long strictures were successfully dilated and the gastrostomy allowed to close. The child swallows well but remains under ob- servation and has periodic bouginage to make certain that stricture does not recur. She has had one obstruction by a large chunk of unchewed carrot. Slight narrowing persists, but a stricture abandoned elsewhere as hopeless has been successfully dilated and the need for a major reconstruction avoided.

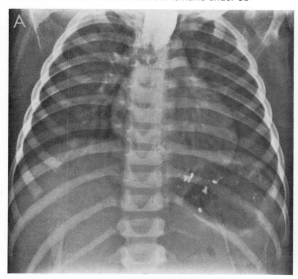
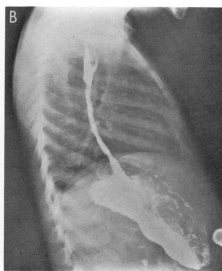

gun at any hint of stricture formation. If expert esophagoscopy is not available, every child with a lye or acid burn of the mouth should be treated as if he had swallowed the material. Each child must then be fully treated.

In patients who are seen late, who have lye strictures which are impenetrable or require continuous dilatations for an indefinite period, esophageal reconstruction is justified. We prefer to replace the esophagus by a loop of right colon. In patients with complete obliteration of the hypopharynx, a cervical pharyngostomy will have previously been performed, and it may be necessary then to perform the reconstruction in stages. The proximal end of the transplanted colon may either be anastomosed directly to the esophageal mucosa or brought next to the pharyngeal stoma and subsequently included with it in a skin tube formed locally. It is not necessary to resect the esophagus, and the sometimes difficult procedure of removing the scarred adherent organ may be omitted. Burford et al.[1] showed that in some cases the stricture is localized and allows of resection and anastomosis.

The situation with respect to the ingestion of bleach is very different from that of the ingestion of lye. Landau and Saunders[14] saw 393 children in 2 years who allegedly swallowed bleach. No strictures and no perforations resulted, although only half of them had any treatment. Two adults who attempted suicide with undiluted liquid bleach had no esophageal sequelae, and no published reports of bleach-produced strictures were found. Dogs had no esophageal strictures when the bleach was run through the esophagus in amounts of 25–100 cc. It seems unlikely that household bleaches will cause esophageal strictures, although it must be pointed out that of 15 dogs whose esophagus was clamped and filled with bleach, 8 "died immediately from perforations into their pleural cavities." The 7 survivors recovered without incident or stricture, untreated.

Our own experiments in cats[20] indicate that bleach can in fact produce severe esophageal injury and stricture, so that we are reassessing our previous casual attitude to bleach ingestion.

REFERENCES

1. Burford, T. H.; Webb, W. R., and Ackerman, L.: Caustic burns of the esophagus and their surgical management: A clinical experimental correlation, Ann. Surg. 138:453, 1953.
2. Burian, K., and Stockinger, L.: Der Einfluss unspezifischer Allgemeinreize auf die Schleimhaut der oberen Luftwege, Monatsschr. Ohrenh. 90:277, 1956.
3. Carver, G. M.; Sealy, W. C., and Dillon, M. L.: Management of alkali burns of the esophagus, J. A. M. A. 160:1447, 1956.
4. Cleveland, W. W.; Chandler, J. R., and Lawson, R. B.: Treatment of caustic burns of the esophagus, J. A. M. A. 186:262, 1963.
5. Daly, J. F.: The early management of corrosive burns of the esophagus, Clin. North America 34:343, 1954.
6. Davis, J. S., and Stafford, E. S.: Successful construction of an extra thoracic esophagus, Bull. Johns Hopkins Hosp. 71:191, 1942.
7. Despons, M. J., and LeBihan, M. J.: Indications de la cortisone dans l'oesophagite corrosive aigue, Rev. laryng. 11/12:1055, 1956.
8. Desports, W., and Ray, E. S.: Lye burns of the esophagus treated with steroid therapy, Arch. Otolaryng. 70:130, 1959.
9. Gellis, S. S., and Holt, L. E., Jr.: The treatment of lye ingestion by the Salzer method, Ann. Otol., Rhin. & Laryng. 51:1086, 1942.
10. Haller, J. A., and Bachman, K.: The comparative effect of current therapy on experimental caustic burns of the esophagus, Pediatrics 34:236, 1964.
11. Holinger, P. H., et al.: The conservative and surgical management of benign strictures of the esophagus, J. Thoracic Surg. 28:345, 1954.
12. Knox, W. G., et al.: Bouginage and steroids used singly or in combination in experimental corrosive esophagitis, Ann. Surg. 166:930, 1967.
13. Kohaus, J., and Schurmeyer, H.: Eigene Erfahrungen mit der Cortison Behandlung bei Speiseröhrenverätzungen, Med. Klin. 54:1018, 1959.
14. Landau, G. D., and Saunders, W. H.: The effect of chlorine bleach on the esophagus, Arch. Otolaryng. 80:174, 1964.
15. Ray, E. S., and Morgan, D. L.: Cortisone therapy of lye burns of the esophagus, J. Pediat. 49:394, 1956.
16. Rosenberg, N., et al.: Prevention of experimental esophageal stricture by cortisone, Arch. Surg. 66:593, 1953.
17. Salzer, H.: Frühbehandlung der Speiseröhrenverätzung, Wien. klin. Wchnschr. 33:307, 1920.
18. Schobel, H.: Zur Therapie der akuten Speiseröhrenverätzungen unter besonderer Berücksichtigung der hormon Behandlung, Ztschr. Hals-, Nasen-, Ohrenh. 7:193, 1959.
19. Viscomi, C. J.; Beekhuis, G. J., and Whitten, C. F.: An evaluation of early esophagoscopy and corticosteroid therapy in the management of corrosive injury of the esophagus, J. Pediat. 59:356, 1961.
20. Weeks, R. S., and Ravitch, M. M.: The pathology of experimental injury to the cat esophagus by liquid chlorine bleach, J. Pediat. (in press), 1969.

M. M. RAVITCH

Esophageal Diverticulum

Pharyngoesophageal Diverticulum

IN ADULTS, the common posterior midline pharyngeal diverticulum, presenting essentially as a mucosa-sub-mucosa-covered hernia in the diamond-shaped area of muscular weakness above the cricopharyngeus fibers, obviously is an acquired lesion. Lahey and Warren[6] carefully described the pathogenesis and development of such pharyngeal diverticula.

In rare instances, congenital diverticula at this level have been reported in children. They are true diverticula with complete muscular walls. The reported instances have manifested themselves in newborn infants by a clinical picture simulating that of atresia of the esophagus. The infants regurgitate mucus and formula, and cough with feedings, but usually without cyanosis. Contrast material fills a pouch high in the thorax and overflows into the trachea, none entering the stomach. There is gas in the stomach. A catheter passed from above enters the diverticulum rather than the esophagus. The two patients of Brintnall and Kridelbaugh[1] were operated on for presumed esophageal atresia, the diverticulum being then discovered and treated definitively. The first died of mediastinitis after excision of the diverticulum, the second died during exploration, with established pneumonia of both lungs. In both instances, the lesion was a true diverticulum, composed of the full thickness of pharyngeal wall, including muscle. Duhamel's[2] first patient was a 3-day-old infant with salivation, strangulation and cyanosis. On endoscopy, an opening was seen behind and to the left of the pharyngoesophageal junction. Lipiodol swallow demonstrated a long sac behind the esophagus, descending in the posterior mediastinum to the third dorsal vertebra. The infant died soon after. Autopsy disclosed a diverticulum opening out of the hypopharynx. A second child had an almost identical lesion, discovered only on endoscopy. The diverticular pouch was longer and narrower, and after endoscopy symptoms disappeared. His third patient had a diverticulum arising from the upper portion of the pyriform sinus and passing anteriorly. This child died of asphyxia after a successful operation for atresia of the right colon. The patient of Rouchy, Crézé and Courtillé[11] was a 24-hour-old full-term infant, presenting difficulty in respiration and salivating abundantly. The diagnosis of esophageal atresia was seemingly confirmed by high obstruction to passage of a catheter and radiologic evidence of a blind esophageal sac. The infant died 24 hours after gastrostomy and proved to have a diverticulum of the hypopharynx behind the esophagus. Review of the films showed a thin stream of contrast material in the esophagus proper.

Rush and Stingily[12] reported on a baby who lived for 20 days with severe respiratory distress. When he cried, a small, soft, fluctuant swelling appeared above the clavicle. This increased day by day until at the time of death it was 7×5 cm. Aspirated through the neck, it yielded air and pus. At autopsy, a large sac was found that led by a narrow isthmus to the esophagus through an opening in the posterolateral portion at the level of the cricoid. The narrow sac filled with air, became infected, and the combination caused obstruction and regurgitation which led to pneumonia and death.

Laurent *et al.*[7] treated a neonate with dysphagia and respiratory distress. A large diverticulum in the usual relationships of a Zenker diverticulum displaced the esophagus and trachea. The diverticulum had a muscular wall. As it was resected, there came into view an esophagotracheal fistula. The infant died.

Diverticulum of the Esophagus Associated with Stenosis

It seems likely that congenital diverticulum of the thoracic esophagus at or above the level of the carina is another variation of those tracheoesophageal anomalies the commonest of which is classic esophageal atresia with tracheoesophageal fistula.

Robb[10] successfully excised a thoracic esophageal diverticulum in a boy of 11. It was associated with what appeared to be a congenital tracheoesophageal fistula. O'Bannon[9] described a diverticular pouch at the level of the third thoracic vertebra in a newborn which was found at autopsy just proximal to a narrow congenital esophageal stenosis. Knox[5] reported an esophageal diverticulum with a tracheoesophageal fistula and without esophageal stenosis in a case somewhat similar to Robb's, and tenKate[13] reported a case similar to O'Bannon's. Grant and Ar-

Fig. 28-18.—True congenital esophageal diverticulum. A 2-year-old girl was subject to respiratory infections from birth, with recurrent febrile episodes, cough and expectoration. Progressive dysphagia appeared at 15 months. The oblique roentgenogram shows the large diverticular sac arising low in the cervical esophagus. At operation the sac was found to arise posteriorly and extend behind the esophagus to a level below the clavicle. The communication with the esophagus was about 2.5 cm in diameter. The excised sac consisted of a full thickness of esophageal wall, thus representing a true diverticulum. True congenital diverticula of the esophagus, of which this is the single example at the Johns Hopkins Hospital, are rare. (Courtesy of Dr. A. R. Nelson.[8])

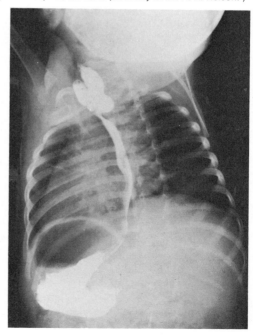

neil's[3] second case was similar to these—in a newborn presenting as an instance of tracheoesophageal fistula with esophageal atresia. The diverticulum at the level of the carina filled with Lipiodol that did not pass into the esophagus. A catheter could be passed into the esophagus to the diverticulum but no farther. A transthoracic resection of the diverticulum, on the day of birth, met with immediate success, and the child was discharged home swallowing well on the 15th day. He died elsewhere at the age of 9 weeks with multiple lung abscesses.

True Congenital Diverticulum of the Esophagus

True diverticula of the esophagus proper, unassociated with any suggestion of tracheoesophageal anomaly, are probably the rarest of all esophageal anomalies. There are several reports of children with signs of recurrent respiratory infection and progressive dysphagia.[3,4,8] Nelson's[8] patient was successfully operated on at the age of 2 by Blalock through a cervical incision, although the diverticulum could not be totally excised through this approach (Fig. 28-18). The 8-year-old patient of Jackson and Shallow[4] died of empyema. Grant and Arneil[3] operated on their patient at age 5. He had had stridor since birth and some dysphagia from the time he began to take solid food. Radiologic studies at age 10 months had shown a large diverticulum rising high in the cervical esophagus. The operation was performed through a left supraclavicular incision, and the large sac was found to communicate widely with the esophagus on its posterior aspect 2 cm below the pharyngoesophageal junction. A one-stage resection was successfully completed.

REFERENCES

1. Brintnall, E. S., and Kridelbaugh, W. W.: Congenital diverticulum of the posterior hypopharynx simulating atresia of the esophagus, Ann. Surg. 131:564, 1950.
2. Duhamel, B.: Deux cas de diverticules congenitaux de l'oesophage cervical: Considerations sur le diagnostic des malformations congenitales de l'oesophage, Arch. franç. pédiat. 6:499, 1949.
3. Grant, J. C., and Arneil, G. C.: Congenital diverticulum of the esophagus, Surgery 46:966, 1959.
4. Jackson, C., and Shallow, T. A.: Diverticula of the esophagus: Pulsion, traction, malignant, and congenital, Ann. Surg. 83:1, 1926.
5. Knox, G.: Congenital tracheoesophageal fistula without esophageal atresia, Surgery 30:1016, 1951.
6. Lahey, F. H., and Warren, K. W.: Esophageal diverticula, Surg., Gynec. & Obst. 98:1, 1954.
7. Laurent, Y.; Schuermans, J., and Brombart, M.: Poche pharyngo-oesophagienne postérieure et fistule oesotracheal chez un nouveau-né, Acta gastro-enterol. belg. 24:618, 1961.
8. Nelson, A. R.: Congenital true esophageal diverticulum: Report of a case unassociated with other esophagotracheal abnormality, Ann. Surg. 145:258, 1957.
9. O'Bannon, R. P.: Congenital partial atresia of esophagus associated with congenital diverticulum of the esophagus: Report of a case, Radiology 47:471, 1946.
10. Robb, D.: Congenital tracheoesophageal fistula without atresia, but with esophageal diverticulum, Australian & New Zealand J. Surg. 22:120, 1952.
11. Rouchy, R.; Crézé, J., and Courtillé, P.: Diverticule congenital de l'oesophage chez un nouveau-né, Bull. Féd. soc. gynéc. et obst. 6:105, 1954.
12. Rush, L. V., and Stingily, C. R.: Congenital diverticulum of the esophagus: Case report, South. M. J. 22:546, 1929.
13. TenKate, J.: Congenital diverticulum of oesophagus, Arch. chir. neerl. 4:277, 1952.

M. M. RAVITCH

Chalasia and Achalasia of the Esophagus

Chalasia of the Esophagus

CHALASIA IS the name given by Neuhauser and Berenberg[5] in 1947 to a condition in newborn infants of apparent relaxation of the cardioesophageal mechanism. On fluoroscopic examination, some infants show a rather free regurgitation of barium from the stomach into the esophagus, up and down for a number of excursions after each bolus of barium is swallowed. This may be unaccompanied by any symptoms. A number of such infants are seen in whom persistent vomiting occurs in the absence of any other discoverable cause, except very free gastroesophageal reflux. Later, Berenberg and Neuhauser[1] discussed 24 such patients seen in 5 years. Regurgitation into the esophagus is noted principally with inspiration, perhaps due to the simultaneous decrease of intrathoracic pressure and increase of abdominal pressure. These children begin to vomit between the third and tenth day of life, the vomiting becoming progressively worse. It appears to be effortless and usually occurs when the child is put down after feeding. The children remain hungry after vomiting and readily accept another feeding. Fluoroscopy is said to show diminished esophageal peristalsis, and the esophageal picture is interpreted as that of a thin-walled, flaccid, large esophagus. The barium column in the esophagus which has filled by reflux during inspiration moves in both directions with expiration, some of the barium passing upward into the mouth, the rest of it down into the stomach. This occurs only when the baby is recumbent. When the baby is in the erect position, there is no regurgitation.

The important differential diagnostic possibility is hiatus hernia. The symptoms are identical and reflux occurs there as well.

Careful fluoroscopy and the use of cinefluorographic techniques are required to demonstrate the presence of a portion of the stomach above the diaphragm in hiatus hernia. In effect, it is reasonable to believe that this relaxation of the hiatus, or of the esophagogastric junction, is in fact the earliest form of hiatus hernia. This is the view taken by Grob,[3] Duhamel,[2] Koncz,[4] Waterston (p. 392) and others. In any case, the symptoms are identical; the hazards in both are malnutrition and starvation, aspiration of vomitus with pulmonary infection, and peptic esophagitis. The treatment is also identical—maintaining the babies in the erect position at all times in an appropriate apparatus (see Fig. 28-26). With the passage of several weeks of such treatment the symptoms are entirely relieved and the radiologically observable phenomena markedly decreased or absent.

REFERENCES

1. Berenberg, W., and Neuhauser, E. B. D.: Cardioesophageal relaxation (chalasia) as a cause of vomiting in infants, Pediatrics 5:414, 1950.
2. Duhamel, B.: Deux cas de diverticules congenitaux de l'oesophage cervical: Considerations sur le diagnostic des malformations congenitales de l'oesophage, Arch. franç. pédiat. 6:499, 1949.
3. Grob, M.: *Lehrbuch der Kinderchirurgie* (Stuttgart: Georg Thieme, 1957).
4. Koncz, J.: in Oberniedermayr, A. (ed.): *Lehrbuch der Chirurgie und Orthopädie des Kindesalters* (Berlin: Springer Verlag, 1959).
5. Neuhauser, E. B. D., and Berenberg, W.: Cardioesophageal relaxation as a cause of vomiting in infants, Radiology 48:480, 1947.

Achalasia of the Esophagus

Achalasia has been known for some 300 years. Von Mikulicz in 1882 named the condition cardiospasm. Hurst in 1915 introduced the term achalasia—absence of relaxation. Langmead in 1920 reported an instance in a 16-month-old child with symptoms from birth, and King in 1955 reported a successful Heller operation in a 9-month-old infant.[8]

SYMPTOMS.—The symptoms of achalasia are those of dysphagia, frequently even for liquids, with regurgitation of food and occasionally aspiration with secondary pulmonary complications.[7] Malnutrition and weight loss result. Initially, there may appear to be periods of remission. The feeding of affected children is slow and tedious, and in fully developed clinical instances, even fluids must be taken in small amounts. Vomiting or regurgitation is without pain or nausea; in advanced cases, the vomitus contains the residue of earlier meals. Radiologic study reveals a substantial or occasionally very great dilatation of the esophagus, with a sharp, smooth tapering at the esophagogastric junction (Fig. 28–19). Passage of a sound easily differentiates this picture from that of esophageal stricture, either congenital or acquired. Despite

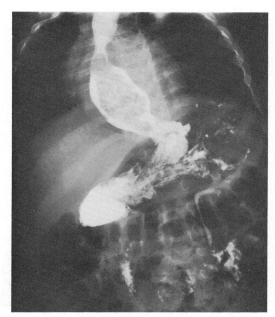

Fig. 28-19.—Achalasia of the esophagus. Roentgenogram after barium swallow by a severely malnourished, 2-year-old child with dysphagia and regurgitation for over a year. Note retained food in the greatly dilated esophagus and the abruptly tapered distal end of the esophagus (superimposed on the shadow of the gastric cardia in this view). The child responded promptly to Heller esophagomyotomy performed through a left subcostal incision supplemented by closure of the esophageal hiatus and attachment of the fundus to the esophagus, recreating the angle of His. Regurgitation ceased and weight gain was prompt.

the severe dysphagia, a sound is readily passed into the stomach of a patient with achalasia. Fluoroscopic examination of the esophagus and study of the peristaltic pattern with balloon pressure tracings show diminished and unco-ordinated peristaltic movements of the esophagus.

In an occasional case in children,[3] as in adults, the onset of symptoms may be abrupt and associated with psychic trauma. This is despite the now well-established fact that in achalasia in adults, the ganglion cells of Auerbach's plexus are deficient or absent and that in the 2 children operated on by Swenson,[9] biopsy of the esophagus showed no ganglion cells. Thibert *et al.*[10] reported two families in each of which well-documented achalasia occurred in two brothers; all 4 patients responded to operation.

TREATMENT.—Dilatation of the esophagogastric junction by distention of a long cylindrical balloon placed partly in the esophagus and partly in the stomach under fluoroscopic control is the preferred initial treatment of achalasia in adults. In children, perhaps because of (justified) timidity in distending the balloon for fear of rupturing the esophagus, dilatation has not been as successful as in adults.[4,6] We and others[4–6,9] resort directly to the Heller cardiomyotomy in infants and children with significant dysphagia and the characteristic roentgen picture.

The approach may be either transthoracic or abdominal (our preference). A long incision is made through the esophageal muscular coat down to the submucosa and carried just barely onto the stomach. Because "recurrences" have been found due to operatively produced hiatus hernia, we routinely place one or two sutures to snug up the hiatus and tack the fundus to the esophagus to recreate the angle of His. Bettex and Stillhart[1] even add a Nissen fundoplasty. The Heller is the simplest and most effective operative procedure and the freest from late complications. Resection of the esophagogastric junction is unnecessarily radical and leads, like all methods of formal cardioplasty and esophagogastric anastomosis, to a high subsequent incidence of peptic esophagitis, commonly with ulceration and stricture or severe hemorrhage. Grob[2] devised a procedure which involves a cylindrical resection of the musculature of the gastroesophageal junction with anastomosis of the divided muscular ends drawn together over the intact mucosa-submucosa tube. This seems interesting, but unnecessary.

The success of treatment, either balloon dilatation or the Heller procedure, is gauged by the relief of symptoms. Dilation of the esophagus may persist but is not an indication for further operation.

REFERENCES

1. Bettex, M., and Stillhart, H., Problemes actuels de chirurgie oesophagienne chez l'enfant, Ann. paediat. 201: 507, 1963.
2. Grob, M.: *Lehrbuch der Kinderchirurgie* (Stuttgart: Georg Thieme Verlag, 1957).
3. Konz, J.: in Oberniedermayr, A. (ed.): *Lehrbuch der Kinderchirurgie und Orthopädie des Kindesalters* (Berlin: Spring Verlag, 1959).
4. Payne, W. S.; Ellis, F. H., Jr., and Olsen, A. M.: Treatment of cardiospasm (achalasia of the esophagus) in children, Surgery 50:731, 1961.
5. Polk, H. C., and Burford, T. H.: Disorders of the distal esophagus in infancy and childhood, Am. J. Dis. Child. 108:243, 1964.
6. Redo, S. F., and Bauer, C. H.: Management of achalasia in infancy and childhood, Surgery 53:263, 1963.
7. Schultz, E. H.: Achalasia in children as a cause of recurrent pulmonary disease, J. Pediat. 59:522, 1961.
8. Steichen, F.; Heller, E., and Ravitch, M. M.: Achalasia of the esophagus, Surgery 47:846, 1960.
9. Swenson, O., and Economopoulos, C. T.: Achalasia of the esophagus in children, J. Thoracic & Cardiovas. Surg. 41:49, 1961.
10. Thibert, F., *et al.*: Forme familiale de l'achalasie de l'oesophage chez l'enfant, Union méd. Canada, 94:1293, 1965.

M. M. RAVITCH

Hiatus Hernia

BY THE TERM hiatus hernia is meant a protrusion of stomach through an abnormally wide esophageal hiatus. The condition has for many years been well described in adults. There are numerous papers describing this condition as one affecting persons in the age group of 60–75 years and suggesting that it is an acquired hernia comparable to a direct hernia in the inguinal region. Such hernias are described as always having a peritoneal sac, and they are of the sliding variety.[1–5,16]

In childhood, the condition appears to be different in many ways. Recent work has tended to simplify descriptively the many lesions at the lower end of the esophagus in children. The term hiatus hernia with or without complications now includes partial thoracic stomach, congenital short esophagus, lax cardia, chalasia, congenital stricture of esophagus, and congenital web in the esophagus.[8–11,14,15,17] There is no doubt that in children this is a congenital disease and the lesion may be demonstrated during the first week of life[18–19] (Fig. 28–20).

The most important abnormality seems to lie in the hiatus itself. At operation, the hiatus in these cases appears to be unduly wide and in many the muscle sling appears to be thin and weak. The stomach protrudes through the diaphragm for a varying degree into the chest, in the majority of cases without a peritoneal sac. The cardia comes to lie at a level above the diaphragm, and in some cases the vagus nerves appear to be unduly lax.

INCIDENCE

The incidence of congenital hiatus hernia in the general population is difficult to assess. Because many infants with small hiatus hernias lose their symptoms in the first few months of life, many hernias undoubtedly are unrecognized in early childhood and may produce symptoms again in adult life. Recognition of the condition in the newborn may therefore depend on how actively these babies are investigated radiographically. The condition, however, seems to have a geographic distribution, being more frequently seen in infancy in some countries than in others.

Since Burke's[8] review of 150 cases seen at the Hospital for Sick Children, Great Ormond Street, up to 1958, 300 more have been seen, bringing the total to

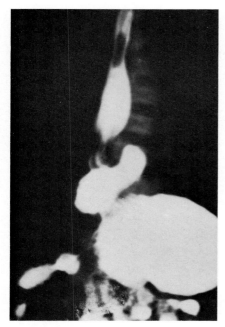

Fig. 28-20.—Typical small hiatus hernia. Lipiodol swallow in a 2-day-old infant who had an excess of mucus in the mouth and was suspected of having atresia of the esophagus. Symptoms disappeared with postural treatment (Fig. 28-26) and operation was not required.

450; operative treatment has been required in less than 50%. Our series shows a male:female ratio of almost 3:1. Most other series in children show not so large a male preponderance. In our series the disease seems to be more severe in the males, half being below the third percentile in weight when first seen, as compared with one quarter in the females.

The mother and sister of one child were found to have hiatus hernias. In another family, identical twin boys were affected. The brother of another child was operated on elsewhere for an esophageal stricture. A history of vomiting in parents and siblings was often obtained.[8]

SYMPTOMS AND SIGNS

VOMITING.—A typical history is one of vomiting from birth. Of the children treated at the Hospital for Sick Children, over 80% vomited during the first week of life and another 15% started to vomit during the first month. In general, the vomiting is forceful, and in the majority of cases the vomit contains altered blood. The mother describes the vomit as being brown or chocolate-colored. A large hematemesis is unusual and the vomit is only rarely bile-stained.[8]

CONSTIPATION.—As a rule, these babies are not constipated, and sometimes this fact is a useful point in the differential diagnosis between hiatus hernia and congenital pyloric stenosis.

TABLE 28-4.—DEGREE OF ANEMIA RELATED TO SEVERITY OF ESOPHAGITIS IN 112 CASES OF HIATUS HERNIA

HG LEVEL, %	ESOPHAGITIS ON ESOPHAGOSCOPY		
	NONE	MILD	SEVERE
<50	1	0	6
50-65	6	5	18
65-80	12	10	14
>80	21	9	10

DYSPHAGIA.—In uncomplicated hiatus hernia, dysphagia is uncommon, and the child will often willingly take another feed after a large vomit. Pain or discomfort on swallowing usually indicates ulceration with stricture formation in the esophagus and a serious prognosis.

WEIGHT.—As a rule, the weight of these children is below average when first seen, the majority falling below the fiftieth percentile.

Severe dehydration is sometimes present during the first few weeks of life. It follows that hiatus hernia is unlikely to be the cause of vomiting in an infant whose weight gain is average or above average.

ANEMIA.—Anemia may be due partly to blood loss and partly to malnutrition. Table 28–4 shows the degree of anemia related to the severity of the esophagitis seen at esophagoscopy in 112 cases at the Hospital for Sick Children, Great Ormond Street.[8]

NATURAL HISTORY OF THE DISEASE.—In uncomplicated cases, the symptoms seem to tend to disappear at about the age of 9 months to 1 year. Vomiting generally tends to diminish when the child starts to sit up and usually has disappeared by the time the child starts to stand and walk. Nevertheless it is common for vomit to be found on the pillow at night for some weeks after vomiting has ceased by day. With stricture formation, the pattern changes and the vomiting becomes more episodic, attacks lasting several days. Dysphagia gradually becomes the predominant symptom, and the child has difficulty in taking solid food.

It is therefore sometimes dangerous to be complacent when the vomiting becomes less manifest at about the sixth to ninth month, since this apparent improvement may mean stricture formation and not spontaneous remission of symptoms.

DIAGNOSIS

A hiatus hernia may be strongly suspected clinically, but the diagnosis can be confirmed only by radiologic examination. Often this examination must be repeated, and the radiologic procedure is not always easy. A certain amount of reflux, especially when the child is crying and when the stomach is full of air, is normal in the first few months of life, but continuous free reflux is not, and its presence is highly suggestive of hiatus hernia. The crucial finding, however, is the pouch of stomach which distends perhaps only momentarily above the phrenic canal (Fig. 28–21).

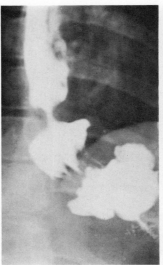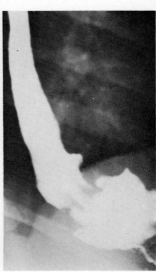

Fig. 28-21. — Hiatus hernia. Roentgenograms taken at about 5-sec intervals during the same barium swallow. That on the left shows well the intrathoracic gastric pouch. On the right, the pouch is not distended and could well be missed. Repeated, careful fluoroscopy and use of cinefluorography or rapid cassette changing techniques, as here, may be required to demonstrate the inconstant hernia.

Some form of rapid cassette changer is therefore essential if radiographs are to show the intrathoracic pouch of stomach. Cineradiography, with image intensification to reduce the amount of radiation, has greatly simplified the radiologic diagnosis.

ESOPHAGOSCOPY. — Esophagoscopy is of no help in confirming the diagnosis. It is essential, however, in assessing the degree of esophagitis, ulceration and stricture formation. Esophagoscopy should be done in all cases prior to operation.

ASSOCIATED CONGENITAL CONDITIONS

CONGENITAL PYLORIC STENOSIS. — Among 150 cases at the Hospital for Sick Children there were 5 of pyloric stenosis with a pyloric tumor demonstrated at operation. In 10 others, laparotomy had been performed previously but without the diagnosis being confirmed. This finding is confirmed in other large series reported in childhood. It may well be that any condition giving rise to vomiting will aggravate the symptoms of an existing hiatus hernia. Olsen and Harrington,[14] reviewing 220 cases of hiatus hernia in adults seen at the Mayo Clinic, noted an apparent etiologic factor in 75%, and in almost one third of these it was some condition giving rise to vomiting. Whooping cough caused an exacerbation of symptoms in several of our cases.

Twelve of our patients have had an unusual type of pyloric stenosis as an additional lesion. This consisted of a "web" of fibromuscular tissue at the pylorus not associated with typical hypertrophy of the pyloric muscle. The deformity was difficult to demonstrate radiologically, the preoperative radiographs showing an appearance similar to that of persistent spasm of the pylorus. This narrowing at the pylorus is not easily seen at laparotomy and can only be demonstrated by opening the stomach and testing the patency of the pylorus with the finger-tip. The obstruction can be relieved by a pyloroplasty, the pyloric canal being incised longitudinally and sewn up with interrupted sutures transversely.

MIGRAINE AND PERIODIC SYNDROME. — Bonham-Carter[7] states that 12 of our patients have developed symptoms of typical migraine with headache and a periodic type of vomiting during the follow-up.

ABNORMALITIES OF THE GLOTTIS OR TRACHEA. — Such abnormalities causing stridor occurred in 5 children in our series, and in 1 child a tight tracheal stenosis necessitated tracheostomy.

MENTAL RETARDATION. — Mental retardation was present in 12 of our first 150 cases. Two of the 12 had phenylketonuria and 4 sucrosuria. Moncrieff and Wilkinson[12] described the association of sucrosuria, mental defect and hiatus hernia, and 3 of our patients presented this syndrome.

Seven of our patients had Down's syndrome (mongolism) as an additional abnormality.

COMPLICATIONS

ESOPHAGITIS. — Without doubt the formation of a stricture in the esophagus above the intrathoracic loculus of stomach is the most important complication of hiatus hernia. Peptic ulceration of the esophageal wall due to the reflux of gastric contents into the squamous cell-lined esophagus is of sinister prognosis. The subsequent fibrosis, which may extend widely through the epithelium and into the muscular coats of the esophagus, makes the outlook for the child very grave. It is therefore vitally important that this serious complication be suspected in all cases and measures taken early to combat the recurrent esophagitis.

ASPIRATION PNEUMONIA. — Pulmonary infections

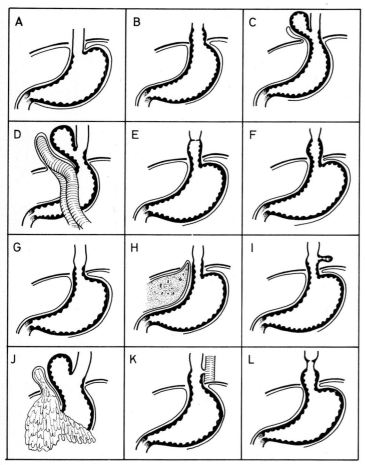

Fig. 28-22. — Varieties of hiatus hernia seen at the Hospital for Sick Children, Great Ormond Street. **A**, normal relationships of esophagus and cardia to diaphragm and peritoneum. **B**, small hiatus hernia, no peritoneal sac (70% of cases). **C**, large hiatus hernia (Fig. 28-23). Cardia is well above the diaphragm; this is not a paraesophageal hernia but a sliding hernia. Half the stomach lies in the peritoneal sac above the diaphragm. Anemia rather than vomiting is the usual presenting symptom.
D, colonic herniation into supradiaphragmatic peritoneal sac. **E**, so-called web in the esophagus. This is invariably a tight, cicatricial stenosis with the causative hiatus hernia below it. **F**, localized ring structure in esophagus above a hiatus hernia. This is always secondary to esophageal ulceration and frequently but incorrectly called a congenital stricture. All in our series have been secondary to a small hiatus hernia.
G, hiatus hernia with fibrous stricture of the esophagus above the hernia due to gastric reflux and recurrent peptic esophagitis (Fig. 28-24). **H**, hiatus hernia with a portion of the left lobe of the liver passing through the hiatus with the stomach. **I**, hiatus hernia with small diverticulum of the thoracic loculus of the stomach.
J, large hiatus hernia with greater omentum prolapsed into the peritoneal sac. **K**, hiatus hernia with a localized deep ulceration in the esophagus which may eventually involve the aortic wall or may perforate and cause suppurative mediastinitis. This type is rare in childhood. **L**, esophageal stricture separated from the hiatus hernia by a segment of normal esophageal mucosa.

due to the reflux and aspiration of gastric contents are not uncommon in small infants. Occasionally, recurrent lung infections may be the presenting symptom in these children.

Types of Hiatus Hernia

In our experience, the hiatus hernia in infants and children is almost invariably a sliding hernia. At the Hospital for Sick Children, we have come to recognize certain characteristic varieties (Fig. 28-22). The most common is the small hiatus hernia without peritoneal sac, which accounts for over 70% of our cases (Fig. 28-22, B). Usually these hernias can be treated posturally (see Fig. 28-26), and operation is not generally required. Very large hernias occur (Figs. 28-23 and 28-22, C). These seem to be commonest in girls. The cardia may remain competent, though it is within the chest, and the hernia is therefore not a paraesophageal hernia. Such patients may present anemia as the chief symptom, as a result of bleeding into the thoracic loculus of the stomach from congestion of

gastric veins at the hiatus. Other abdominal organs may herniate into such large hernias with a peritoneal sac, and we have seen transverse colon (Fig. 28-22, D), the left lobe of the liver (H) and omentum (J) herniating into the sac, alongside the stomach. The thoracic loculus of the stomach may present a small diverticular pouch (I). Stricture of the esophagus in association with regurgitation and peptic ulceration takes a variety of forms. The localized ring stricture (F) is frequently but wrongly called a congenital stricture. Such a stricture is always secondary to ulceration of the esophagus (perhaps in utero), and all of them in our series have been associated with a small hiatus hernia. The stricture may be a very narrow stenosis, the so-called web, but again always with the hiatus hernia below it (Fig. 28-22, E, and 28-25). Long, dense fibrous strictures of the esophagus occur above the hernia as a result of gastric reflux and extensive recurrent peptic esophagitis. This is generally associated with diffuse inflammation of the esophageal wall, mediastinitis and enlarged mediastinal lymph nodes (Fig. 28-24). In some instances, a single

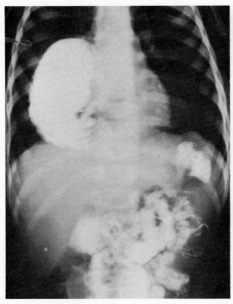 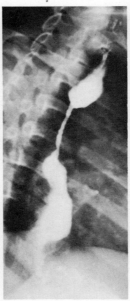 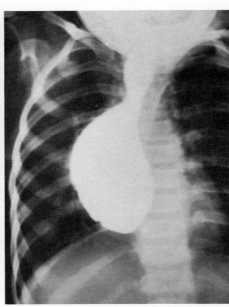

Fig. 28-23 (left).—Large hiatus hernia with most of stomach in the right chest. Such a hernia is easily seen on plain films. This girl of 5 had only mild symptoms of indigestion, without vomiting. Chronic secondary anemia did not respond to iron. Repair of the hernia through the left chest relieved symptoms. The cardia is well above the diaphragm; this is not a paraesophageal hernia.

Fig. 28-24 (center).—Esophageal stricture above a large loculus of stomach in the chest. Barium swallow in a girl of 8 who had had dysphagia since age 1 year. The long narrow stricture was dilated repeatedly from above without permanent relief of symp-

toms. She has since had successful esophagectomy and reconstruction of the esophagus, with relief of symptoms.

Fig. 28-25 (right).—Web stricture. No barium passes the dense stricture. The condition is often thought to be congenital but, as here, a hiatus hernia is present below the obstruction. This baby had had difficulty in swallowing from birth, and through the esophagoscope the esophageal lumen appeared to be completely occluded. At operation, the hiatus hernia was repaired and the stricture dilated by instruments passed upward through a gastrotomy. He was symptom-free thereafter.

discrete deep ulcer of the esophagus is associated with a diaphragmatic hernia. Such ulcers may erode to involve the aortic wall or perforate into the mediastinum with fatal suppuration. This is Barrett's ulcer, more commonly seen in adults (Fig. 28–22, *K*). In a rare group that is difficult to explain, the esophageal stricture is separated from the hiatus hernia by an area of apparently uninvolved esophageal mucosa.

Management

Since the natural course of the disease in infancy is toward spontaneous cessation of symptoms, it is wise to be conservative if the infant is under 1 year and to rely on nonoperative treatment alone. The child should be kept in the upright position and the feeds thickened with corn meal or other cereal. Usually it is impossible to keep a baby or small child propped up safely on pillows, and it is necessary to arrange for the child to be held upright in a small padded seat (Fig. 28–26). This posture may have to be kept until the child is a year old, or until the vomiting ceases.

CHILDREN WITHOUT ASSOCIATED STRICTURE OF THE ESOPHAGUS.—Operation is indicated in any of three circumstances: (1) If the child's symptoms cannot be controlled by medical means, that is, if he continues

to lose weight or if the anemia becomes severe. (2) When the intrathoracic loculus of stomach is large, and certainly when the loculus falls over into the right side of the chest. (3) When the esophagitis as seen on esophagoscopy is very severe or if an actual ulcer of the esophagus can be seen.

CHILDREN WITH ASSOCIATED FIBROUS STRICTURE OF ESOPHAGUS.—All of these patients should be operated on. There is no place for simple dilatation of the stricture which will only tend to make the reflux more severe with further destruction of the esophageal wall.

OPERATIVE TECHNIQUES

SIMPLE GASTROPEXY.—In children with a small hiatus hernia not accompanied by fibrosis and secondary shortening of the esophagus, a simple gastropexy (Fig. 28–27, *A*) is the operation of choice.[6] This procedure reduces the hernia and brings the normal length of esophagus below the diaphragm, thus preventing reflux. Dissection of the cardia is not necessary and the hiatus need not be narrowed.

The abdomen is opened by a vertical left rectus incision, and the anterior wall of the stomach close to the lessor curvature is sutured to the anterior abdominal wall (peritoneum and rectus muscle) by three or

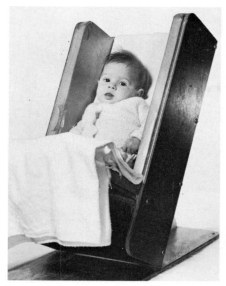
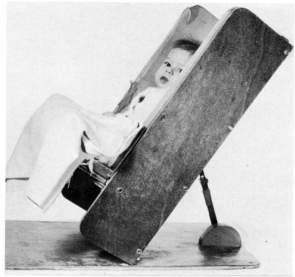

Fig. 28-26.—The esophageal box. A child of 8 months with a small hiatus hernia under nonoperative management. The padded seat is adjusted for tilt. In most infants with hiatus hernia, main-tenance of the erect position in this manner, and careful feeding, will manage the patient until symptoms are permanently relieved.

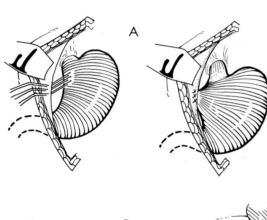

Fig. 28-27.—Operative repair of hiatus hernia. **A,** simple gastropexy. The abdomen is opened by a left vertical incision. The interrupted silk sutures to the peritoneum and rectus sheath pull the stomach and lower esophagus firmly into the abdomen (see Fig. 28-29). **B,** repair of hiatus hernia plus gastropexy. In patients with esophagitis and some shortening of the esophagus, the chest is opened through the 7th interspace and the esophagus freed up to and beyond the aortic arch. The peritoneal cavity is opened all around the hiatus and the stomach freed. The hiatus is then narrowed posteriorly with interrupted silk sutures. The child is then turned on his back and a gastropexy performed, as in **A.**

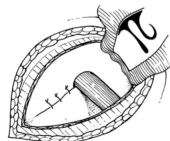
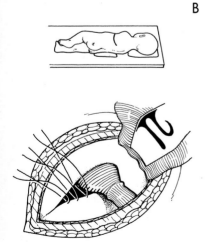

397

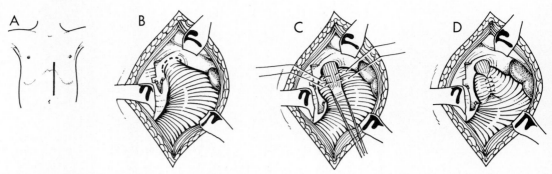

Fig. 28-28.—Fundus plication. **A,** the abdomen is opened through a vertical left rectus incision. **B,** the triangular ligament of the liver is divided and the esophagus freed as it passes through the diaphragm. **C,** a rubber sling is passed around the esophagus to pull it down into the abdomen, and the esophagus is freed up into the chest. **D,** the fundus of the stomach is then folded around the lower esophagus and stitched in front of the esophagus with interrupted silk sutures, which also pick up the esophageal wall.

four sutures of silk. These sutures must be placed so that when they are tied there is very strong tension through the lesser curvature of the stomach, bringing the lower esophagus well into the abdomen.

GASTROPEXY WITH HERNIA REPAIR.—If the hernia is large and/or some shortening or fibrosis in the esophagus is suspected, gastropexy from the abdomen should be preceded by a left thoracotomy through the

seventh space (Fig. 28–27, *B*). The loculus of stomach and the esophagus are dissected free from the mediastinal structures by blunt dissection. The esophageal hiatus is defined and the peritoneal cavity is opened all round the hiatus. A peritoneal sac will be found only in the very large hernias. The esophagus should be completely freed up to and beyond the aortic arch so that the cardia can be brought well below

Fig. 28-29.—Large hiatus hernia treated by gastropexy. This child of 4 had occasional vomiting and became progressively anemic. **A,** roentgenogram demonstrating a large hiatus hernia. **B,** film following gastropexy shows a good length of esophagus below the diaphragm.

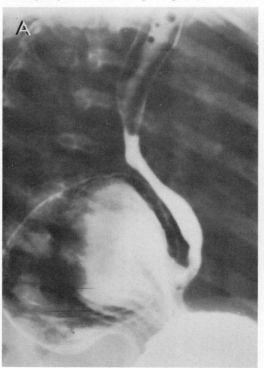

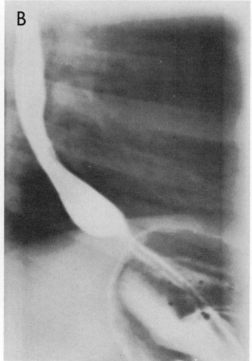

the diaphragm. The right and left edges of the right crus are then approximated posteriorly with thick silk sutures so as to narrow the hiatus, which is too large. These stitches should not be tied so tightly as to devascularize the muscle of the crus, but enough stitches must be inserted to narrow the hiatus firmly against the esophageal wall. The chest wall is then closed with pericostal sutures of catgut, and a pleural drain is inserted to an underwater seal. An abdominal gastropexy as described above is then performed at the same operation.

FUNDUS PLICATION.—After the hiatus hernia is reduced, the cardia may be held securely below the diaphragm by the method of fundus plication (Fig. 28–28), described first by Nissen.[13] This operation can be carried out through either the chest or the abdomen. It consists of folding the stomach around the lower esophagus, where it is stitched with interrupted silk sutures. These stitches are also passed through the esophageal wall to hold it securely in place.

From our experience, it seems that this procedure does not in itself prevent reflux but does so by virtue of the fact that the lower esophagus is held securely below the diaphragm. That is to say, the same result may be obtained (certainly in children) by the more simple gastropexy (Fig. 28–29).

REPAIR OF HERNIA WITH RETROGRADE DILATATION OF STRICTURE.—Before repair of the hernia is carried out metal Hegar dilators are passed in a retrograde manner through a small incision in the stomach wall and through the stricture to dilate it. By this means, a very full dilatation of the fibrous stricture can be undertaken safely with the stricture under direct vision (Fig. 28–30). Any split in the esophageal wall may be repaired at once. The incision in the stomach

Fig. 28-30.—Esophageal stricture; retrograde dilatation. During operation for repair of hiatus hernia when stricture is known to be present, the stomach is opened and dilators are passed retrograde, dilating the stricture as widely as possible. With the stricture under direct observation, rupture of the esophagus is not likely and can be repaired at once if it does occur.

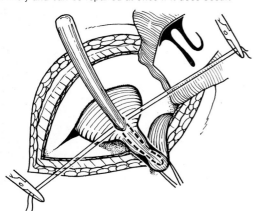

may also be used to examine the lumen of the pyloric canal with a view to pyloroplasty. The hernia is then repaired and gastric fixation carried out as described above.

This type of procedure is suitable for children under age 2. Results in this age group are good. Only a few will require postoperative dilatation of the stricture through an esophagoscope. In older children, however, the results from this procedure are not good. The tendency to reflux esophagitis continues, and the stricture recurs. It is sometimes worth undertaking this operation if the stricture and ulceration of the esophagus are not severe, but the parents must be warned that a further and more radical operation will have to be undertaken.

ESOPHAGOGASTRECTOMY FOR STRICTURE OF THE ESOPHAGUS DUE TO REFLUX ESOPHAGITIS.—Before the development of the safe operation for colonic replacement of the esophagus, we carried out esophagogastrectomy in 15 cases. There was no mortality, and these children are now well with no dysphagia. However, they are all underweight and have to take frequent small meals. We are convinced, therefore, that this operation is unsuitable for children and that replacement of the esophagus with transverse colon is the operation of choice (see the following section, on Reconstruction of the Esophagus). See p. 400.

RESULTS OF OPERATIVE TREATMENT

Of 450 children with hiatus hernia seen at the Hospital for Sick Children up to 1967, 185 have been treated by operation. The rest have received nonoperative treatment. Of the 185 treated surgically, 86 (49%) had a fibrous stricture of the esophagus; this high percentage of stricture may be due to the fact that the more complicated cases are referred to this hospital, and probably does not represent the true proportion in the general population.

HIATUS HERNIA WITHOUT STRICTURE.—Of the 99 children without stricture, 70 had a simple type of repair without gastropexy. Because of recurrence of the hernia, 22 of these required further operative repair, including gastropexy or some other form of fixation of the esophagus below the diaphragm. In 4 of these cases, a stricture developed while the patients were still under treatment. Five other patients have radiologic evidence of recurrence of the hernia but are well, with only minimal symptoms of reflux.

HIATUS HERNIA WITH STRICTURE.—Of 86 patients with esophageal stricture treated up to 1967, 14 had colon replacements (see following section, on Reconstruction of the Esophagus), and 15, esophagogastrectomy. These children cannot eat a large meal and are underweight (see above). The remaining 57 had a hiatus hernia repair with dilatation of the stricture (either retrograde or through an esophagoscope). Of these, 18 still require occasional dilatation because of difficulty with solid food, and 4 of them may eventually require colon reconstruction of the esophagus. The others are well and take a normal diet.

REFERENCES

1. Allison, P. R.: Reflux esophagitis, sliding hiatal hernia and the anatomy of repair, Surg., Gynec. & Obst. 92:419, 1951.
2. Allison, P. R., and Johnston, A. S.: The esophagus lined with gastric mucous membrane, Thorax 8:87, 1953.
3. Barrett, N. R.: Chronic peptic ulcer of the esophagus and esophagitis, Brit. J. Surg. 38:175, 1950.
4. Barrett, N. R.: The lower esophagus lined by columnar epithelium, Surgery 41:881, 1957.
5. Belsey, R.: in Jones, A. (ed.): *Modern Trends in Gastroenterology* (London: Butterworth & Co., Ltd., 1952).
6. Boerema, I., and Germs, R.: Fixation of the lesser curvature of the stomach to the anterior abdominal wall after reposition of the hernia through the esophageal hiatus, Arch. chir. neerl. 7:351, 1955.
7. Bonham-Carter, R. E.: Personal communication.
8. Burke, J. B.: Partial thoracic stomach in childhood, Brit. M. J. 2:787, 1959.
9. Carre, L. J.; Astley, R., and Smellie, J. M.: Minor degrees of partial thoracic stomach in childhood: Review of 112 cases, Lancet 2:1150, 1952.
10. Husfeldt, E.; Thomsen, G., and Wamberg, E.: Hiatal hernia and short esophagus in children, Thorax 6:56, 1951.
11. Kelly, H. D. B.: in discussion on hiatus hernia and esophagitis, Proc. Roy. Soc. Med. 46:941, 1953.
12. Moncrieff, A., and Wilkinson, R. H.: Sucrosuria with mental defect and hiatus hernia, Acta paediat. 43 (supp. 100):495, 1954.
13. Nissen, R., and Rossetti, M.: *Die Behandlung von Hiatushernien und Reflux-Oesophagitis mit Gastropexie und Fundoplicatio* (Stuttgart: Georg Thieme Verlag, 1959).
14. Olsen, A. M., and Harrington, S. W.: Esophageal hiatal hernia of short esophagus type, J. Thoracic Surg. 17:189, 1948.
15. Roviralta, E.: *Hernies hiatales et éctopies partielles de l'estomac chez l'enfant* (Paris: Masson & Cie, 1967).
16. Skinner, D. B., and Belsey, R. H. R.: Surgical management of esophageal reflux and hiatus hernia, J. Thoracic & Cardiovas. Surg. 41:33, 1967.
17. Sawyer, P. R.: Partial thoracic stomach and esophageal hiatus hernia in infancy and childhood, Am. J. Dis. Child. 90:421, 1955.
18. Waterston, D. J.: Hiatus hernia in Gairdner, D., ed.: Recent advances in Paediatrics (London: S. & A. Churchill, Ltd., 1954).
19. Waterston, D. J.: in discussion on hiatus hernia, Proc. Roy. Soc. Med. 47:536, 1954.

DAVID WATERSTON

Drawings by G. LYTH

Reconstruction of the Esophagus

HISTORY. — Esophageal reconstruction was first attempted by Bircher[1] in 1894, using a skin tube. Since then, many methods have been developed, with skin tubes, gastric tubes, jejunal grafts of inert material such as Teflon being employed. Use of the colon, right, left or transverse, is now a well-established procedure. Many positions for the new esophagus have been described, subcutaneous, retrosternal or intrathoracic being the most common. Until 1934, only 20 cases of colon replacement had been recorded,[19] but since then, successful colon replacements have been reported with increasing frequency.[2,3,5,8,13,14,16,18,25] The first successful colon replacement of the esophagus in childhood was reported by Lundblad[12] in 1921. This child had a corrosive stricture of the esophagus, and the colon was placed in a subcutaneous tunnel. The patient lived a normal life until killed in an automobile accident at age 37. At autopsy, the graft was found to be in a satisfactory condition with no evidence of peptic ulceration. Intrapleural colon replacement in a newborn child was first reported by Sandblom[24] in 1948 in a case of esophageal atresia.

Indications for Reconstruction

ATRESIA OF THE ESOPHAGUS. — In cases of atresia of the esophagus without fistula to the trachea, the distance between the upper pouch and the small length of esophagus above the diaphragm is too great for safe primary anastomosis. In a series of cases reported from the Hospital for Sick Children, Great Ormond Street, in 1962,[29] among 19 babies with atresia and no fistula, in only 2 was primary anastomosis possible. Reconstruction of the esophagus is therefore advised in practically every instance of this type of abnormality. In cases of atresia with fistula, the distance between the ends of esophagus is too great for safe primary anastomosis in over 15%. Since the report by Howard and Myers[7] from Melbourne, attempts have been made to carry out a delayed primary anastomosis in such cases, the upper pouch being stretched by intermittent bouginage until a safe anastomosis is possible. In our experience, this delayed procedure carries a high risk due to inhalation of mucus and saliva into the trachea from the upper blind esophagus. Replacement of the esophagus with colon is, in our hands, a safer procedure.

PEPTIC STRICTURE OF THE ESOPHAGUS DUE TO HIATUS HERNIA. — Children who have had recurrent ulceration with fibrosis and shortening of the esophagus may require more radical surgery than repair of the hernia and repeated dilatation of the stricture. If a child has an intractable stricture following an attempt at hiatus hernia repair, the dangers, both mental and physical, of repeated dilatations are great.

ESOPHAGEAL STRICTURE FOLLOWING CORROSIVE BURNS OF THE ESOPHAGUS. — Although repeated dilatations offer a hope of cure in some cases, only the minor degrees of fibrosis affecting a small area of the esophagus can be treated in this manner. Most children who have fibrosis involving the muscular wall of the esophagus due to the swallowing of corrosives require replacement of the esophagus. Certainly all children in whom the strictures are long or multiple require replacement, however high into the pharynx the narrowing extends. It is both dangerous and psychologically harmful to the child to continue with repeated dilatations, either with a gastrostomy and an indwelling thread or through an esophagoscope.

RECURRENT BLEEDING FROM ESOPHAGEAL VARICES DUE TO PORTAL HYPERTENSION. — When portal hypertension cannot be controlled by other means, as a last resort the lower esophagus may have to be replaced.[9,10] We have not had to undertake replacement for this indication, but it may be necessary when all other methods of controlling the hemorrhage have failed.

Methods of Reconstruction in Childhood

COLONIC REPLACEMENT. — This offers many advantages over other methods of reconstruction. The following points briefly summarize these advantages: (1) The cardiac sphincter can be retained in most cases, thus preventing acid reflux into the new esophagus. (2) The whole esophagus (right up to the pharynx if necessary) can be replaced without risk to the blood supply of the transplant.[16,17] (3) The colon can always be used in an isoperistaltic manner. (4) There is evidence that the colon functions well and stands up to the "insults" of feeding better than replacements with other types of tube.[26,15] (5) There is good evidence that the colon grows with the child and continues to function well into adult life.

POSITION OF THE COLON USED FOR RECONSTRUCTION. — The advantages of placing the colon posteriorly in the left thoracic cavity are great: the lower esophagus and cardiac sphincter can be retained, and also it simplifies the anastomosis in the neck with the upper esophagus. When the substernal position is used, the lower anastomosis must be to the stomach

and the upper anastomosis has to be turned posteriorly around the trachea, where it tends to kink; this causes obstruction to swallowing and breakdown with fistula formation.

OTHER METHODS OF RECONSTRUCTION. — *Esophagogastrostomy* should never be used in children (see preceding section, on Hiatus Hernia). This type of reconstruction means that the child can never take a large meal and so remains thin and underweight. It may occasionally be necessary to undertake this kind of operation in children when other methods such as replacement with colon have failed.

Anastomosis of the stomach to the esophagus in the neck[23] should never be done. The stomach fills with swallowed air in the chest, causing collapse of lung and respiratory embarrassment.

Replacement with gastric tube from the greater curvature of the stomach may occasionally be used when colon replacement is impossible, but it has the disadvantages of other methods and is technically difficult in small infants.

Jejunal loops for reconstruction[22,11] offer some advantages in adults, but the dangers in childhood are great. The small intestine has to be anastomosed to the stomach, carrying the risk of subsequent ulceration and stenosis. The marginal arteries are poorly formed in children, making a good pedicle with enough length of graft difficult to achieve.

RIGHT, LEFT OR TRANSVERSE COLON? — The right half of the colon can be used on a pedicle carrying the middle colic artery.[26] This vessel is variable in its anatomy and is often double and very short. The left colon, to have adequate length for total replacement of esophagus, must be used in an antiperistaltic manner, with poor function resulting. The transverse colon on a pedicle consisting of the ascending branch of the left colic artery is the most satisfactory in our hands.[27,29,30] The colon can be approached through the left diaphragm without disturbing the abdominal cav-

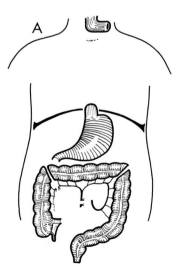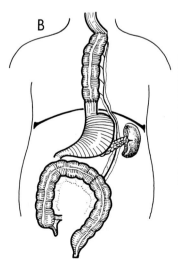

Fig. 28-31. — Reconstruction for esophageal atresia without tracheoesophageal fistula. **A**, the child has had a cervical esophagostomy and gastrostomy (not shown), the middle colic artery has been divided and an appropriate length of transverse colon isolated, the vascular supply coming from an ascending limb of the left colic artery. **B**, the vascular pedicle has been brought behind the pancreas and through an opening in the diaphragm separate from the hiatus. The colon lies in the pleural cavity behind the left lung root and is anastomosed end-to-end to the esophagus above and below. The colon has been reconstructed end-to-end.

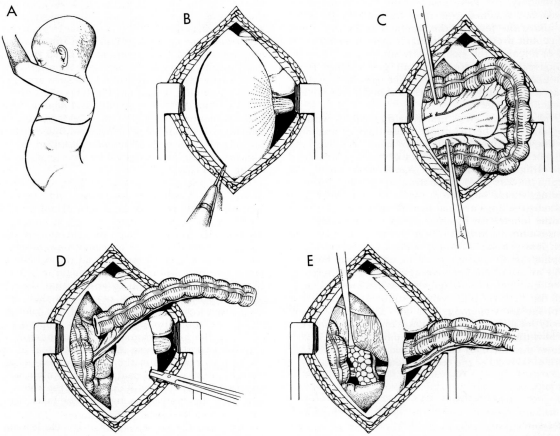

Fig. 28-33.—Esophageal reconstruction; details of technique. **A,** the left chest, neck and arm are draped out and the arm is draped free. A 7th interspace incision in babies of 6 months (the preferred age) allows access both to the abdomen and to the apex of the chest. **B,** the costal margin has been incised (not shown), and the diaphragm is incised around its periphery close to the chest wall. **C,** very satisfactory exposure of the colon has been obtained. The middle colic artery is divided near its origin; however, the transverse colon and splenic flexure now depend on the ascending branch of the left colic artery. The colon is divided at the two flexures. **D,** the colon has been reconstructed. A small opening is made through the diaphragm posteriorly, some 3 cm from the esophageal hiatus. **E,** the colon and its vascular pedicle are brought behind the stomach and pancreas and splenic vessels and through a tunnel made by blunt dissection and drawn into the chest. The distal end of the colonic segment is anastomosed end-to-end to the short stump of residual esophagus. The proximal end of the colonic segment is brought into the neck medial and anterior to the left subclavian artery passing through the pleural cavity behind the hilus of the lung. A one-layer suture line of interrupted silk (like all the other suture lines) between esophagus and colon completes the procedure.

terrupted silk sutures. Before the chest is closed, the position and blood supply of the graft are checked. The ribs are approximated with interrupted pericostal fine catgut, and a tube drain is left in the pleural cavity through a separate stab incision.

POSTOPERATIVE CARE.—The gastrostomy must be kept open and attached to a small funnel about 5 cm above the level of the stomach. These children tend to swallow air postoperatively, and it is important to keep the stomach deflated. The negative pressure in the chest will cause some distention of the colon transplant for a few days, until it regains its normal tone and peristalsis. It is necessary, therefore, to keep a small soft rubber tube through the nostril into the colon in the chest. This tube is attached to an underwater seal beneath the bed; this will give enough negative pressure to prevent any distention of the colon graft. The child is fed intravenously for 48 hours after operation; thereafter, gastrostomy feeds may be started and increased to normal amounts over 48 hours.

The pleural drain may be removed in 48 hours. The tube in the colon may be removed after about 3 days, and oral feeding should be started when this tube is removed. If the child was accustomed to taking food by mouth before operation, the change-over from gastrostomy to oral feeding should present no problem. When a full and adequate intake by mouth has

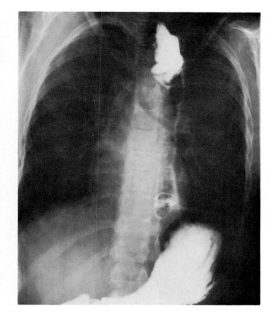

Fig. 28-34.—Esophageal atresia. Roentgenogram after barium swallow following reconstruction of esophagus with transverse colon.

been reached, the gastrostomy feeds may be stopped. Postoperative and long-term results are shown in Figures 28–34 and 28–35.

RECONSTRUCTION FOR PEPTIC OR CORROSIVE STRICTURE

In these cases the principles of the operative treatment are the same as for atresia (Fig. 28–36), but the operation differs in the following details: (1) If the stricture involves the lower part of the esophagus, not so long a segment of transverse colon need be taken (Fig. 28–37, *A*). (2) The pedicle containing the ascending branch of the left colic artery is not taken behind the stomach and pancreas, but in front of the pancreas (*B*). (3) The distal end of the colon is anastomosed to the posterior wall of the stomach, which is turned forward to allow this to be done. This anastomosis is carried out low down on the body of the stomach so that a good length of colon lies below the diaphragm (*C*). This prevents reflux into the new esophagus, the intra-abdominal pressure closing off the lumen of the colon. The anastomosis is carried out with interrupted fine silk sutures. (4) The graft is led through the esophageal hiatus with its pedicle. After the lower esophagus is excised, including the strictured area, the stomach is closed at the cardia, again

Fig. 28-35.—Esophageal atresia. Long-term results of reconstruction with colon in a child now 15. He had esophageal atresia without fistula and also duodenal atresia and underwent duodenoduodenostomy, gastrostomy and cervical esophagostomy at age 1 day. **A,** following colon replacement at age 7 months. **B,** at age 4 years. **C,** at age 13.

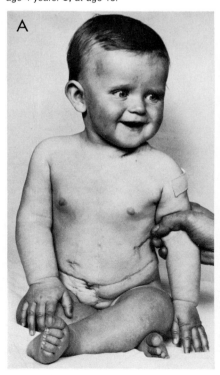
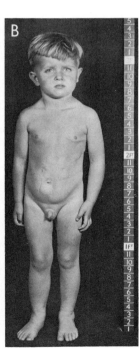
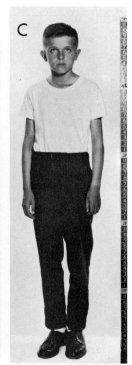

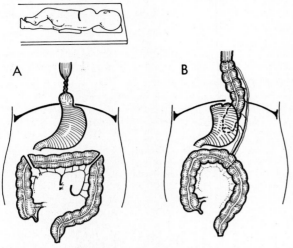

Fig. 28-36. — Esophageal reconstruction for peptic or corrosive stricture. **Inset,** incision and operative approach are as in Figure 28-33. **A,** preparation of the colonic loop is as in Figure 28-33. **B,** only a portion of the esophagus has been resected, but the mechanism of the cardia has been destroyed. The colon is brought anterior to the pancreas and the distal end of the colon is sutured to the posterior wall of the stomach low down on the body of the stomach; the anastomosis between esophagus and proximal end of the colonic segment is in the chest.

with interrupted fine silk sutures in one layer. The upper anastomosis is carried out in the chest, unless the whole esophagus is strictured as in severe peptic esophagitis or corrosive stricture, when it is carried out in the neck as described for esophageal atresia. (5) If gastrostomy has not already been established, it is best to perform one (as described above) at the end of the operation. Postoperative care is then similar to that described for atresia. (6) In patients with corrosive stricture whose whole esophagus is affected, it is sometimes simpler to leave the strictured esophagus in the chest after it has been replaced with colon. The cut ends are closed with interrupted sutures at the replacement operation, and the remains of the esophagus should be removed through a right thoracotomy about 2 weeks after the reconstruction.

Results of Esophageal Reconstruction

Our experience in 60 cases is summarized in Table 28–5.

POSTOPERATIVE COMPLICATIONS. — *Strangulation of the colonic segment* occurred in 3 children, proving fatal in 2. This complication occurred early in the series and has not been met with in later cases. *Intrathoracic leaks* occurred in 4 cases, causing empyema. In 2, the empyema was drained and further progress was uncomplicated. In 1, the leak proved fatal, and in

Fig. 28-37. — Reconstruction of the esophagus for peptic or corrosive esophagitis; details. **A,** the abdomen is approached through the chest, the costal margin incised and the diaphragm opened parallel to the costal margin. **B,** the length of the loop may not need to be as great. The stomach is transected at the cardia and closed over with a single layer of interrupted fine silk sutures. **C,** the diseased esophagus has been resected together with the segment of cardia, and the esophagus and its vascular pedicle have been brought up through the hiatus. The colon is shown reconstructed with a single row of fine interrupted silk sutures. The distal end of the colonic segment is anastomosed to the posterior wall of the stomach well down on the body of the stomach, using a single row of fine silk sutures. This ensures a good length of colon below the diaphragm, which will prevent reflux into the new esophagus. If the vagus nerves have been injured, a pyloroplasty is performed.

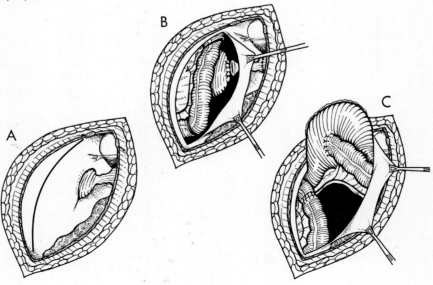

TABLE 28-5.—RESULTS OF ESOPHAGEAL RECONSTRUCTION

CONDITION	ALIVE	DEAD	TOTAL
Esophageal atresia	32	8*	40
Peptic stricture	13	0	13
Congenital stricture	1	0	1
Corrosive stricture	6	0	6
	52	8	60

*This includes 1 patient with mongolism operated on in the newborn period.

another, the colon segment had to be removed and an esophagogastrostomy performed. In 2 cases, the leak occurred not at the anastomotic line but in the colon above the anastomosis. These cases occurred early in the series, before the colon was decompressed by an indwelling tube. *Leakage from the cervical anastomosis* occurred in 17 cases. In the majority, the small fistula closed spontaneously. In 4 cases, surgical closure of the fistula was necessary. *Stricture at the cervical anastomosis* was found in 9 children. In 5, this was treated by esophagoscopy and dilatation; in 4, the cervical anastomosis had to be revised. Symptoms of *pyloric stenosis* were noted in 3 children, and barium examination showed delayed emptying of the stomach. Pyloroplasty relieved the symptoms in all.

Unrecognized cervical tracheoesophageal fistula proved fatal in 1 case. The child had severe tracheobronchitis unrelieved by tracheostomy following colon replacement and he died 2 weeks after operation. Postmortem examination revealed a high cervical congenital tracheoesophageal fistula which had not caused symptoms while he had a cervical esophagostomy.

FUNCTION OF COLON IN THE CHEST.—The use of the transverse colon allows the segment to be isoperistaltic. It has been claimed that, unlike the small bowel, the colon is satisfactory in both isoperistaltic and antiperistaltic fashion.[24] In a large series of colonic reconstructions,[6] however, antiperistaltic operations were followed by a higher incidence of complications in every category. This applied especially to regurgitation in the antiperistaltic cases and was directly related to a high incidence of anastomotic leakage and subsequent stenosis.

Dr. Alan Chrispin has carried out a follow-up radiologic study of our cases of colon replacement at the Hospital for Sick Children, Great Ormond Street. He has shown that the colon empties well into the stomach by a typical "mass movement" type of colonic peristalsis; this occurs with the child in the supine position, and therefore the postulation that the colon acts as a conduit, dependent on its function by the force of gravity,[20] is incorrect. Dr. Chrispin has also shown that when the cardiac sphincter is retained, it prevents completely the reflux into the colon, even with the child supine and with manual pressure being applied to the stomach. He has shown that the

opening of the sphincter is dependent on the act of deglutition. With the colon anastomosed directly to the stomach (i.e., when the lower esophagus has not been preserved), reflux is much less easily elicited when the colon has been anastomosed low down in the stomach and there is a good length of colon beneath the diaphragm.

REFERENCES

1. Bircher, E.: Ein Beitrag zur plastischen Bildung eines neuen Oesophagus, Zentralbl. Chir. 34:1479, 1907.
2. Beck, R. A.; Kreel, I., and Baronofsky, I. D.: Use of left colon to replace esophagus, Ann. Surg. 101:32, 1961.
3. Belsey, R.: Reconstruction of the esophagus with left colon, J. Thoracic & Cardiovas. Surg. 49:33, 1965.
4. Bentley, J. F. R.: Primary colonic substitution for atresia of the esophagus, Surgery 58:731, 1965.
5. Gross, R. E., and Firestone, F. N.: Colonic reconstruction of the esophagus in infants and children, Surgery 61:955, 1967.
6. Hong, P. W.; Seel, D. J., and Dietrick, R. B.: The use of colon in the surgical treatment of benign stricture of the esophagus, Ann. Surg. 160:202, 1964.
7. Howard, R., and Myers, N. A.: Esophageal atresia: A technique for elongating the upper pouch, Surgery 58:725, 1965.
8. Koop, C. E., and Verhagen, A. D.: Early management of atresia of the esophagus, Surg., Gynec. & Obst. 113:103, 1961.
9. Koop, C. E., and Roddy, S. R.: Colonic replacement of distal esophagus and proximal stomach in the management of bleeding varices in children, Ann. Surg. 147:17, 1958.
10. Koop, C. E., and Kavianian, A.: Reappraisal of colonic replacement of distal esophagus and proximal stomach in the management of bleeding varices in children, Surgery 57:454, 1965.
11. Longmire, W. P.: Antethoracic jejunal transplantation for congenital esophageal atresia with hypoplasia of the lower esophageal segment, Surg., Gynec. & Obst. 93:310, 1951.
12. Lundbald, O.: Über antethorakale Oesophagoplastic, Acta chir. scandinav. 53:535, 1921.
13. Mahoney, E. B., and Sherman, C. D., Jr.: Total esophagoplasty using intrathoracic right colon, Surgery 35:937, 1954.
14. Martin, L. W., and Flege, J. B., Jr.: Use of colon as a substitute for the esophagus in children, Am. J. Surg. 108:69, 1964.
15. Nardi, G. L., and Glatzei, D. J.: Anastomotic ulcer of colon following colonic replacement of esophagus, Ann. Surg. 152:10, 1960.
16. Neville, W. E., and Clowes, G. H. A.: Reconstruction of the esophagus with segments of colon, J. Thoracic Surg. 35:2, 1958.
17. Neville, W. E., and Clowes, G. H. A.: Colon replacement of the esophagus in children for congenital and acquired disease, J. Thoracic & Cardiovas. Surg. 40:507, 1960.
18. Neville, W. E.; Smith, A. E., and Storer, J.: Use of transverse colon for reconstruction of the esophagus in tracheoesophageal fistula, Ann. Surg. 144:1045, 1956.
19. Ochsner, A., and Owens, N.: Antethoracic esophagoplasty for impermeable stricture of esophagus, Ann. Surg. 100:1055, 1934.
20. Otherson, H. B., Jr., and Clatworthy, H. W., Jr.: Functional evaluation of esophageal replacement in children, J. Thoracic & Cardiovas. Surg. 53:155, 1967.
21. Petterson, A.: Reconstruction of the oesophagus in infancy and childhood, with a report of primary reconstruction with transverse colon in a premature infant, Acta chir. scandinav. 122:60, 1961.
22. Petrov, B. A.: Retrosternal artificial esophagus from jejunum and colon, Surgery 45:890, 1959.

23. Potts, W. J.: Congenital atresia of the esophagus: Antethoracic placement of the stomach followed by intrathoracic transplantation, J. Thoracic Surg. 20:681, 1950.

24. Sandblom, P.: The treatment of congenital atresia of the esophagus from a technical point of view, Acta chir. scandinav. 97:25, 1948.

25. Scanlon, E. F., and Staley, C. T.: Reconstruction of the cervical esophagus by use of colon transplants, S. Clin. North America 43:2, 1963.

26. Sherman, C. D., Jr., and Waterston, D. J.:Oesophageal reconstruction in children using intrathoracic colon, Arch. Dis. Childhood 32:11, 1957.

27. Sirak, H. D.; Clatworthy, H. W., Jr., and Elliott, D. W.: An evaluation of jejunal and colic transplants in experimental esophagitis, Surgery 36:399, 1954.

28. Waterston, D. J.: In Gairdner, D. (ed.): *Recent Advances in Paediatrics* (London: J. & A. Churchill, Ltd., 1954).

29. Waterston, D. J.; Bonham Carter, R. E., and Aberdeen, E.: Oesophageal atresia: Tracheo-oesophageal fistula: A study in survival in 218 infants, Lancet 1:819, 1962.

30. Waterston, D. J.: Replacement of oesophagus with transverse colon, Thoraxchirurgie 11:73, 1963.

31. Waterston, D. J.: Colonic replacement of esophagus (intrathoracic), S. Clin. North America 44:6, 1964.

DAVID WATERSTON

Drawings by G. LYTH

29

Mediastinal Infections and Tumors

Anatomy

THE MEDIASTINUM is the portion of the thoracic cavity bounded anteriorly by the sternum, posteriorly by the vertebral column, and on either side by the medial surfaces of the right and left pleurae. The thymus, heart, pericardium and the great vessels, trachea, right and left main bronchi, esophagus, vagus nerve, phrenic nerve, sympathetic nerve trunks and the thoracic duct are all in the mediastinum. For anatomic descriptive purposes the mediastinum has been divided more or less arbitrarily into four subdivisions (Fig. 29-1). This is of some clinical significance in view of the observation that the various inflammatory and neoplastic processes have their genesis in specific anatomic divisions and on this account cause differing symptoms.

The *superior mediastinum* is located above the plane connecting the fourth thoracic vertebra with the sternomanubrial junction. Normally, it contains the arch of the aorta, the innominate, carotid and subclavian arteries, the pulmonary arteries and veins, superior vena cava, innominate and subclavian veins, most of the thymus gland, the phrenic nerves and an extensive plexus of lymph nodes and communicating lymphatic vessels.

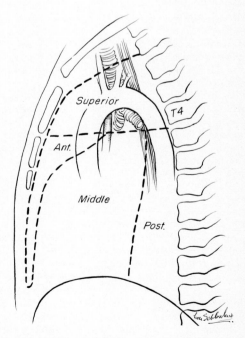

Fig. 29-1.—Diagram of the divisions of the mediastinum.

The *anterior mediastinum* is bounded in front by the sternum and behind by the pericardium. It extends above to the margin of the superior mediastinum, and below to the diaphragm. It contains the remainder of the thymus, numerous lymph nodes and some fatty tissue. The anterior portion of the diaphragm, adjacent to this space, is occasionally the site of a congenital defect (foramen of Morgagni) through which abdominal viscera may herniate.

The *middle mediastinum* is occupied by the heart and pericardium, lymph nodes and lymphatic vessels.

The *posterior mediastinum* is bounded behind by the vertebral column, in front by the posterior aspect of the pericardium, above by the superior mediastinum, with which it is continuous, and below by the diaphragm. Within it are found the trachea, esophagus, thoracic duct, descending aorta, vagus and phrenic nerves, the sympathetic nerve trunks and numerous lymph nodes with their associated lymphatic channels.

Infections of the Mediastinum

ACUTE MEDIASTINITIS. — The mediastinum offers no anatomic barriers to the spread of infection within it, and any kind of suppurative mediastinitis is a grave condition. Bacterial invasion of the mediastinum may follow (1) perforation of the pharynx, esophagus or trachea by disease, ingested foreign bodies, endoscopic injury, penetrating wounds or blunt force in compression injuries of the chest; (2) thoracic and cervical operations complicated by wound infection or suture-line leaks; (3) retropharyngeal or cervical infections breaking through the containing cervical fascia and extending downward, and (4) rupture of suppurative mediastinal lymph nodes.

Mediastinal infection generally evokes a severe systemic response manifested by pain, dyspnea, high fever, striking tachycardia. Infections involving the superior mediastinum, with accompanying edematous compression of the great veins, may result in duskiness and edema of the head and neck. Infections of the posterior mediastinum do not usually cause localizing signs, unless escape of air from esophagus or trachea produces mediastinal emphysema, which appears on the roentgenogram, or dissects upward into the neck, producing crepitation in the supraclavicular fossa. The roentgenogram in acute mediastinitis demonstrates a widened mediastinum and sometimes a pleural thickening or a pleural effusion, which may be a sterile, sympathetic or irritative effusion or may represent actual empyema from direct extension of the suppurative process.

Although the use of antibiotics has sharply decreased the incidence and mortality from mediastinitis, antibiotic therapy alone is not to be relied on except in the less severe infections and those in which treatment has been instituted very early. Incision and drainage is the safest treatment for most suppurative processes, and those in the mediastinum constitute

not an exception but an outstanding indication. An esophageal perforation, for instance, is hazardous chiefly if continued leakage occurs into the undrained mediastinum.

Infection of the anterior mediastinum resulting from an accidental wound, rupture of the lymph nodes or complication of intrasternal therapy or biopsy can be adequately drained through the space left by excision of the third or fourth left costal cartilage.

A supraclavicular incision provides access to the superior mediastinum, the approach being between the esophagus and trachea medially and the carotid sheath laterally. Posterior mediastinal infections may occasionally be drained adequately by this route, but for more dependent drainage the extrapleural and paravertebral resection of an appropriate rib provides direct access to the area of origin of the infection.

TUBERCULOSIS. — Mediastinal tuberculosis is one of the commoner causes of significant hilar lymphadenopathy in childhood. The mediastinal disease represents the result of lymphatic drainage from primary lesions in the pulmonary parenchyma, extending to the nodes along the trachea and bronchi. While the nonspecific systemic effects of tuberculosis may be present, more often than not symptoms may be few or absent in spite of striking radiologic changes. A positive tuberculin skin reaction and evidence of a primary pulmonary lesion in the roentgenogram suggest the tuberculous origin of the mediastinal node enlargement. Not rarely, the parenchymal lesion is inconspicuous or not demonstrable radiographically. Calcification in the parenchymal lesion or the nodes is pathognomonic. The involved nodes usually are in the middle and posterior mediastinum surrounding the main bronchi and trachea and, while usually predominantly on the side of the pulmonary disease, are frequently bilateral.

At times, the mediastinal nodes enlarge so greatly as to compress or erode into the bronchus and produce atelectasis (Fig. 29-2, *A* and *C*). More commonly, the slow scarring of nodes as the process heals leads to a gradual and late bronchial obstruction from the cicatricial process, producing atelectasis and repeated episodes of infection at a time when the tuberculous process is itself inactive.[2] This is the common cause of the middle lobe syndrome, usually seen in middle or late adult years, but occasionally in childhood (Fig. 29-2). Unrelieved atelectasis from this cause, complicated by repeated infections behind the obstruction, with or without the additional radiologic demonstration of bronchiectasis,[6] requires lobectomy. Figure 29-3 illustrates a rare instance of acute, life-threatening compression of the trachea by a tuberculous abscess of the mediastinum. Emergency decompression was required. Except for such rare instances, the treatment of tuberculous mediastinal disease is usually nonoperative, although nontuberculous obstructive sequelae require operation more often than is generally supposed. Joly *et al.*[3] did, however, report on 8

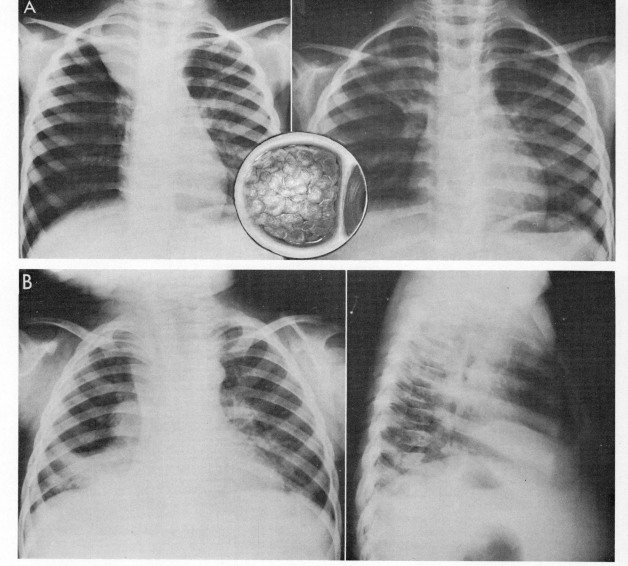

Fig. 29-2.—Mediastinal tuberculosis./**A,** atelectasis of right upper lobe in a 2½-year-old boy. **Left,** the dense shadow looks remarkably like a tumor, particularly since shift of the trachea is prevented by the enlarged paratracheal nodes. **Inset** shows the right main bronchus occluded by granulation tissue, which was removed through the bronchoscope. **Right,** 9 days later, the companion film shows the degree of re-expansion. He made good recovery. Atelectasis in tuberculosis often results from a combination of extrabronchial compression and erosion, with endotracheal obstruction. **B,** rupture into pleural cavity in a 1-year-old boy. Anteroposterior **(left)** and lateral roentgenograms show enlarged mediastinal nodes, generally broadened mediastinal shadow, thickened pleura **(left)** and encapsulated interlobar fluid **(right)**. He was not apparently ill. Tuberculin reaction was positive, and a guinea pig inoculated with pleural aspirate died of tuberculosis. The boy recovered and 7 years later had only a healed and calcified primary focus on the right. *(Continued.)*

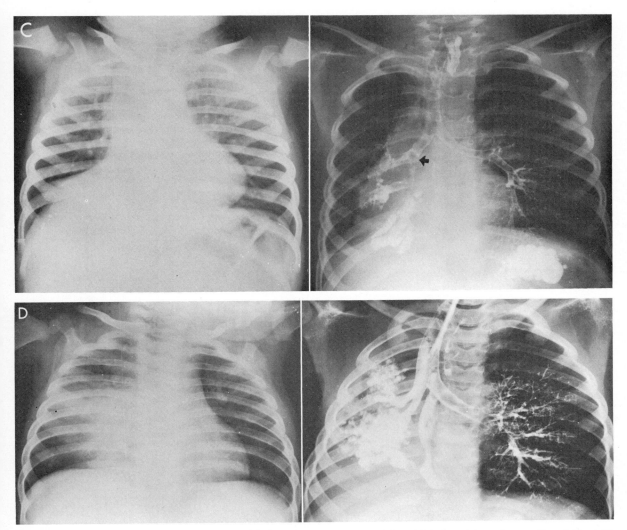

Fig. 29-2 (cont.).—C, bronchial obstruction and atelectasis (RLL, RML). **Left,** at age 21 months this child had a positive reaction to 0.01 mg OT and tubercle bacilli on gastric lavage. The dense triangular shadow at the right base is due to occlusion of the intermediate bronchus by nodes outside it and possibly to bronchial erosion with concomitant endobronchial disease. **Right,** 4 years later. Bronchogram shows narrowing **(arrow)** of intermediate bronchus, atelectasis and bronchiectasis of lower and middle lobes and calcified nodes in right paratracheal region. He did well after right middle and lower lobectomy and a year later was successfully treated for tuberculous meningitis. **D,** bronchial obstruction and atelectasis (RUL, RML, RLL). The child was exposed from birth to a tuberculous mother. **Left,** at 17 months she was tuberculin-positive and had marked enlargement of bronchial lymph nodes on the right and extensive parenchymal shadow. **Right,** 5 years later. This degree of mediastinal shift with entire trachea, esophagus and heart in right hemithorax had been present since age 3. There is severe saccular bronchiectasis throughout the right lung. Most of the bronchial obstruction had long since disappeared, and when the lung was removed to control the secondary infection, no residual tuberculous activity was found. The child did well. (Courtesy of Dr. J. B. Hardy.)

children with large mediastinal tuberculous masses who did not respond to a year's therapy. Thoracotomy, evacuation and resection of the masses were undertaken in the absence of tracheal compression. All of the children did well.

Mediastinal granuloma due to histoplasmosis may simulate mediastinal tuberculosis.[1,7] Woods[8] treated a 4-year-old child with tracheal obstruction by a mediastinal granuloma due to *Histoplasma capsulatum.* A noncalcified mass in the right superior mediastinum displaced and compressed the trachea. Evacuation and partial resection of the granulomatous mass relieved the obstruction, and the child did well. Pate and Haimmon[4] reported on 4 children with mediastinal

fibrosis producing the superior vena cava syndrome and evidence that this was on the basis of histoplasmosis. All 4 were successfully operated on.

SARCOID.—Sarcoidosis is occasionally observed in children.[5] The scarcity of reports makes it difficult to state the relative frequency of the clinical manifestations in children, but both pulmonary and mediastinal lesions appear to be prominent in childhood disease. As in adults, the uveal tract, skin, bones and viscera have been involved. Uveitis, cervical node enlargement or cutaneous nodules on the face of a child with mediastinal lymph nodes suggests the possibility of sarcoid, although the same association of lesions is seen in tuberculosis. The tuberculin and Nickerson-

Fig. 29-3.—Mediastinal tuberculosis; tracheal compression. **A,** chest film of 8-year-old boy shows a lesion in right upper mediastinum. He had been well until 6 days previously, when he had dyspnea, which progressed. Severe tracheal obstruction was obvious. Emergency thoracotomy was required for excision and evacuation of a mass of necrotic nodes and tuberculous pus.

Such a lesion is very unusual. **B,** chest film after 1 year of streptomycin therapy shows clearing of the lesion. **C,** photomicrograph of the mediastinal abscess shows typical appearance of tuberculosis with giant cells, epithelioid reaction and caseation. Acid-fast organisms were demonstrated in the sections.

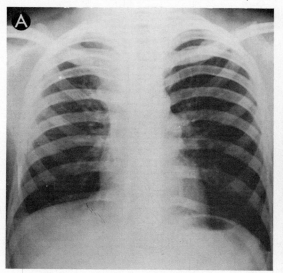
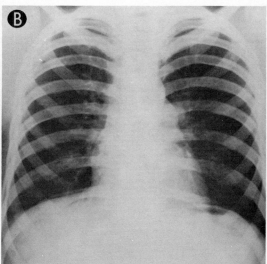
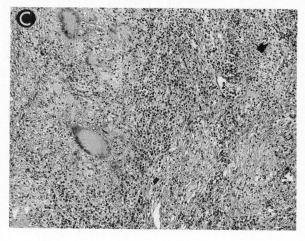

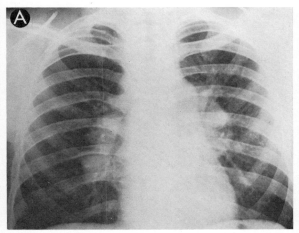

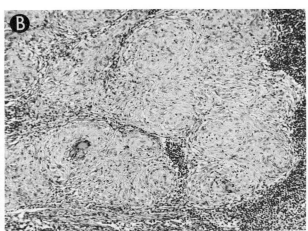

Fig. 29-4.—Sarcoid of mediastinal nodes. Boy of 15 with history of fatigability and blurring of vision. Diagnosis was made by the finding of specific lesions in a small cervical node removed by biopsy, though no cervical nodes were abnormally palpable. **A,** there are bilateral hilar masses. Similar nodes higher in the mediastinum would have been more characteristic of sarcoid. This appearance cannot be distinguished from tuberculosis. **B,** photomicrograph shows hard tubercles and giant cells typical of sarcoid. No Schaumann refractile bodies are seen. Six years later the mediastinal nodes had disappeared and he seemed well.

Kveim tests may differentiate the two diseases. In a boy of 15 with a history of fatigability and blurring of vision, the specific diagnosis was made by biopsy of a cervical lymph node (Fig. 29-4), although no cervical nodes were abnormally palpable.

REFERENCES

1. Gayboski, W. A., *et al.*: Surgical aspects of histoplasmosis, Arch. Surg. 87:590, 1963.
2. Hardy, J. B., and Brailey, M.: *Tuberculosis in White and Negro Children* (Cambridge, Mass.: Harvard University Press, 1958), Vol. I.
3. Joly, H., *et al.*: Traitement chirurgical de certaines adénopathies médiastinales tuberculeuses, Presse méd. 71:2731, 1963.
4. Pate, J. W., and Haimmon, J.: Superior vena cava syndrome due to histoplasmosis in children, Ann. Surg. 161:778-785, 1965.
5. Reeves, R. J.; Baylin, G. J., and Jones, P. A.: Boeck's sarcoid in children, South. M. J. 41:295, 1948.
6. Thomas, D. E., and Winn, D.: Middle lobectomy for tuberculosis in childhood, J. Thoracic & Cardiovas. Surg. 39:175, 1960.
7. Williams, K. R., and Burford, T. H.: Surgical treatment of granulomatous paratracheal lymphadenopathy, J. Thoracic & Cardiovas. Surg. 48:13, 1964.
8. Woods, L. P.: Mediastinal histoplasma granuloma causing tracheal compression in a 4 year old child, Surgery 58:448, 1965.

Thymus

The thymus normally occupies the anterior and superior mediastinum. It is composed chiefly of lymphatic tissue with characteristic Hassall's corpuscles of apparently epithelial origin. The function of the thymus is unknown. The older literature contains numerous accounts of sudden death in infancy due to alleged status thymicolymphaticus. Such deaths are now generally thought to be due to overwhelmingly severe and sudden viral or bacterial infections, to unsuspected suffocation or occasionally to obscure cardiac lesions, such as anomalous or inadequate coronary supply.

In some instances, the thymus has been sufficiently enlarged to present as a cervical tumor.[1,2,7] The roentgenogram of the enlarged thymus characteristically shows a mass with a smooth border projecting on both sides of the anterior mediastinum, although not infrequently chiefly on the right side. With deep inspiration, the thymic shadow decreases in prominence. The thymus diminishes in size with age, but a substantial amount of thymic tissue usually persists.

Formerly, it was common to irradiate an enlarged thymus for real or fancied symptoms or for diagnostic elimination of other lesions producing a similar mediastinal roentgen shadow. The repeated clinical observation of subsequent development of carcinoma of the thyroid in children so irradiated has made this practice totally indefensible. (See Chapter 20.)

Occasionally, thymic enlargement is sufficient to raise the question of tumor of thymic or other origin, and in such instance, operation may be required[3,6] (Fig. 29-5). Tumors of the thymus occur, both malignant and benign (Fig. 29-6). Thymolipoma, a rare benign tumor composed of fat and thymic tissue intermixed, has been reported in a 4-year-old who was without symptoms and was investigated because of a greatly enlarged cardiac shadow.[4] In childhood, the malignant tumors, lymphosarcoma-like or epithelial, outnumber benign thymomas, and the sarcomas outnumber the carcinomas.[5] A thymic tumor originating in the caudal extension of the thymus on the right,

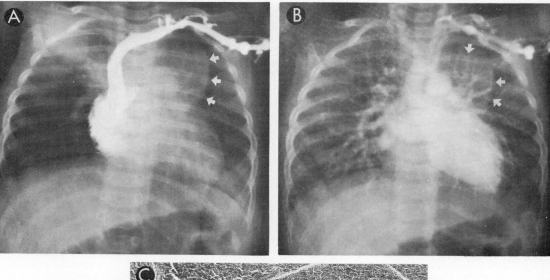

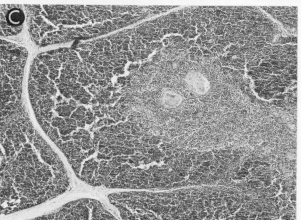

Fig. 29-5.—Enlarged thymus. Thymic enlargement is ordinarily asymptomatic, but the radiologic picture may suggest mediastinal tumor, and operation may be required in doubtful instances. This patient, 6 months old, was being studied because of a cardiac murmur. The plain film showed a large, smoothly rounded mediastinal shadow on the left. **A** and **B**, early and later views in the angiocardiographic series. **Arrows** indicate the mediastinal mass. Angiocardiographic demonstration of both right and left sides of the heart without abnormality clearly indicates that the mass is of nonvascular origin. **C**, the excised mass proved to be an enlarged thymus. The photomicrograph shows normal thymic tissue with characteristic Hassall's corpuscles.

near the diaphragm, may be a source of diagnostic confusion because of its unusual location. In 1 reported case,[8] hemorrhage into a large thymic cyst caused acute distress, presumably due to its sudden enlargement.

REFERENCES

1. Arnheim, E. E., and Gemson, B. L.: Persistent cervical thymus gland: thymectomy, Surgery 27:603, 1950.
2. Behring, C. H., and Bergman, F.: Thymic cyst of the neck, Acta path. et microbiol. scandinav. 59:45, 1963.
3. Fontan, A., *et al.*: La thymectomie chez le nourrisson, Arch. franc. pédiat. 20:1156, 1963.
4. Gunnels, J. C., *et al.*: Thymolipoma simulating cardiomegaly, Am. Heart J. 66:670, 1963.
5. Neale, A. E., and Menten, M. L.: Tumors of the thymus in children, Am. J. Dis. Child. 76:102, 1948.
6. Sealy, W. C.; Weaver, W. L., and Young, W. B.: Severe airway obstruction in infancy due to the thymus gland, Ann. Thoracic Surg. 1:389, 1965.
7. Simons, J.; Robinson, D. W., and Masters, F.: Cervical thymic cyst, Am. J. Surg. 108:578, 1964.
8. Zanca, P., *et al.*: True congenital mediastinal thymic cyst, Pediatrics 36:615, 1965.

Tumors in Mediastinal Lymph Nodes

LYMPHOSARCOMA.—One of the tumors which may originate from lymph nodes in the *anterior* mediastinum is lymphosarcoma. In the majority of instances, this lesion is a *secondary* one in children with primary cervical involvement, but primary mediastinal lesions occur. Characteristically, the anterior mediasti-

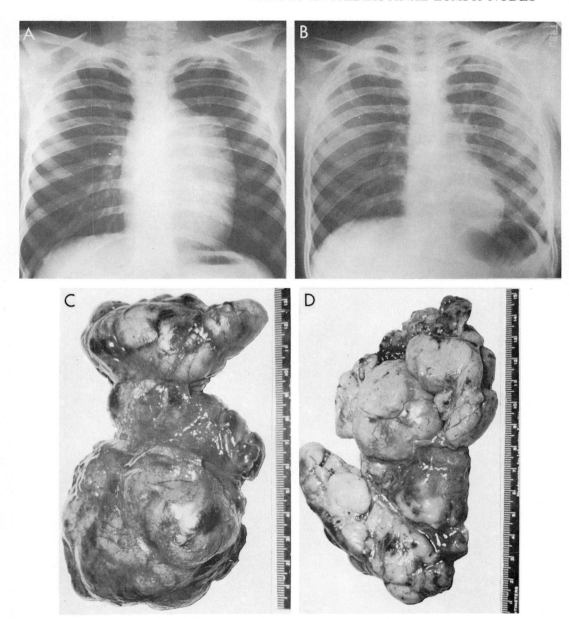

Fig. 29-6.—Benign thymoma. A boy of 11 had x-ray study because of mild cough. **A,** preoperative posteroanterior roentgenogram shows the left border of the heart, superiorly to be continuous with a dense mass, thought on fluoroscopy to be anterior to and separable from the heart, so that angiocardiography was not required. **B,** postoperative posteroanterior roentgenogram shows the cardiac silhouette returned to normal. He was well 3 years later. **C** and **D,** operative specimen. The large, firm, lobulated, anterior mediastinal mass was readily dissected through a left anterior thoracotomy. (Median sternotomy is equally satisfactory for resection of thymic tumors and may be required for thymomas with a large cervical component.) Sections showed characteristic features of benign thymoma. (Courtesy of Dr. J. E. Lewis, Jr.)

num is involved. The chest film of an 11-year-old boy with rather sudden onset of superior vena caval obstruction is shown in Figure 29-7. Bilateral anterior mediastinal lesions were apparent, and at operation, a massive neoplasm infiltrating the surrounding tissues was found. It was not possible to remove it completely. Irradiation produced marked but temporary symptomatic improvement. The lesion diminished considerably in size (Fig. 29-7, *C*), but the child died. The ultimate prognosis in these children is bleak, al-

though considerable symptomatic relief can often be achieved and an occasional cure may follow a combination of operative therapy, irradiation and chemotherapy.

HODGKIN'S DISEASE.—Primary involvement of the mediastinum in Hodgkin's disease is rare in childhood. The lesions in such instances are localized primarily in the anterior mediastinum. The therapy and prognosis of Hodgkin's disease are undergoing hopeful changes with the appreciation of the classification

Fig. 29-7.—Lymphosarcoma. Occasionally, lymphosarcoma begins primarily in the anterior mediastinum and may conceivably justify attempts at operative removal before irradiation and chemotherapy. More often, mediastinal lymphosarcoma is only an episode in a diffuse disease. This boy of 11 developed signs of superior vena cava obstruction. **A,** plain film shows bilateral mediastinal and some pulmonary opacification. **B,** lateral roentgen-ogram shows the bulk of the lesion in the anterior mediastinum. The massive and infiltrating neoplasm could not be extirpated. **C,** irradiation caused marked clinical improvement and obvious clearing of mediastinal enlargement, but the child ultimately died. **D,** photomicrograph of the mediastinal lesion shows closely packed small cells and absence of any germinal centers.

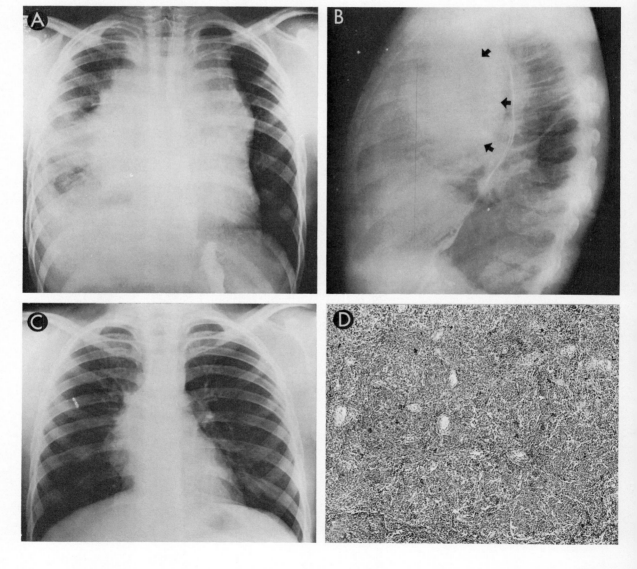

of the forms of Hodgkin's disease, the staging by biopsy, lymphangiography and splenectomy, following the lead of Kaplan[26] and others.

LEUKEMIA.—This may occasionally involve the mediastinum primarily, and lymphadenopathy in this location may appear before characteristic changes in the peripheral blood. Irradiation and systemic administration of antimetabolites may produce remarkable temporary regressions.

Mediastinal Cysts and Tumors

Cysts and tumors of the mediastinum are not rare in infancy and childhood, and extraordinarily large tumors have been successfully removed. The clinical manifestations of these masses are essentially those of expanding, space-occupying lesions and reflect their location. The symptoms most frequently encountered are chest pain, cough, respiratory distress, hemoptysis, dysphagia and weight loss. Remarkably enough, a number of these cysts and tumors, even when large, are asymptomatic and show only incidentally on chest roentgenograms. Table 29-1 shows the various types of mediastinal cysts and neoplasms seen at the Mayo Clinic,[3,4] the Johns Hopkins Hospital[19] and the University of Indiana.[10] The usual

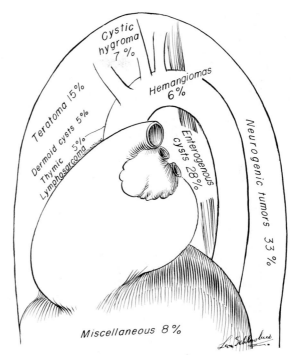

Fig. 29-8.—Mediastinal cysts and tumors. Sites of distribution of lesions in children, from Johns Hopkins,[19] Mayo Clinic[2] and Indiana[10] series. Neurogenic tumors, occurring entirely in the posterior mediastinum, form the largest group, and teratomas and dermoids in the anterior mediastinum, the second largest. The only other large group is composed of the posterior mediastinal cysts of foregut origin (duplications of the esophagus).

TABLE 29-1.—INCIDENCE OF CYSTS AND PRIMARY NEOPLASMS OF THE MEDIASTINUM IN INFANCY AND CHILDHOOD*

TYPE OF TUMOR	No.		%
Neurogenic tumors	39		33
Ganglioneuroma		16	
Ganglioneuroblastoma		2	
Neuroblastoma		10	
Neurofibroma		9	
Neurofibrosarcoma		1	
Ganglioneurosarcoma		1	
Teratomatous tumors	23		19
Teratoma		14	
Dermoid cyst		5	
Teratocarcinoma		4	
Thymic enlargements	6		5
Thymic hyperplasia		6	
Cysts of foregut origin	24		20
Enteric cysts		11	
Bronchogenic cysts		13	
Hemangioma	7		6
Cavernous		3	
Hemangiopericytoma		1	
Hemangioendothelioma		1	
Angiosarcoma		2	
Lymphangioma	7		6
Anaplastic neoplasms (unclassified)	4		3
Miscellaneous	9		8
Lymphosarcoma		3	
Hodgkin's disease		3	
Lipoma		1	
Embryonal rhabdomyosarcoma		2	
Total	119		100%

*Fifty-six cases from the Mayo Clinic,[3] 25 from the Johns Hopkins Hospital[19] and 38 from the University of Indiana.[10]

sites of the more common lesions are diagrammed in Figure 29-8.

Diagnostic studies, important in the preoperative evaluation of these patients, include, in addition to posteroanterior, lateral and oblique roentgenograms, a barium swallow and frequently bronchography. In children with mediastinal lesions, it is not often that esophagoscopy or bronchoscopy will be required. Occasionally, angiocardiography is useful when the question arises of origin of a mass from the heart or great vessels. Precise diagnosis before operation may not be possible. Since some mediastinal tumors have malignant potentialities and most others will sooner or later cause symptoms by virtue of their location, it is our position that all mediastinal tumors and cysts should be removed whenever they are discovered, even though there are no symptoms.

CYSTS OF FOREGUT ORIGIN

A variety of epithelium-lined cysts occurs in the mediastinum.

ENTERIC CYSTS.—Called also enterogenous cysts, gastrogenous cysts and esophageal duplications (see also Chap. 53) these cysts are found in the posterior

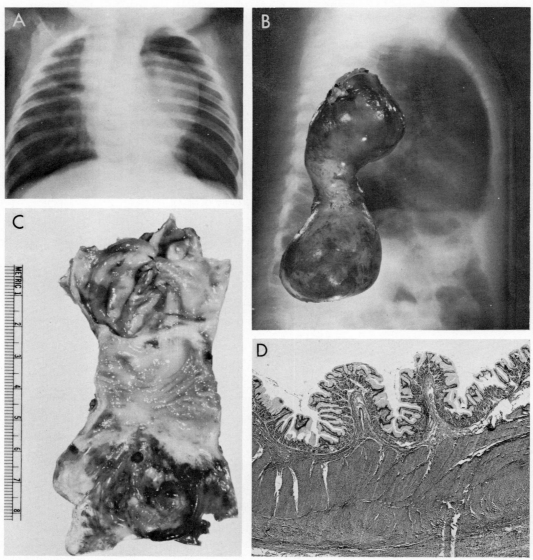

Fig. 29-9. — Mediastinal cyst of foregut origin (enteric cyst). A boy of 4 months had a 3-week history of severe respiratory distress. **A,** the plain film shows a moderately dense, sharply rounded and discrete mass projecting into the left hemithorax. **B,** in the lateral film the mass is seen to be entirely in the posterior mediastinum. The specimen, here superimposed on the roentgen picture, was readily excised. The bulbous caudal portion extended below the diaphragm, which constricted the midportion of the tubular thick-walled structure, whose external appearance was that of bowel. **C,** the interior of the cyst had thick, velvety mucosa with recognizable gastric rugae. The cyst was filled with turbid yellow fluid. **D,** photomicrograph of the lining shows characteristic gastric rugae.

mediastinum. They are muscle-walled, spherical or tubular, have the external appearance of bowel and may be lined by any type of alimentary tract epithelium, or even by ciliated epithelium since portions of the embryonal foregut are lined by ciliated epithelium. The muscle is arranged in layers, complete with myenteric plexuses (Fig. 29-9). Very commonly, cervical or upper thoracic vertebral anomalies are associated,

as hemivertebrae (Figs. 29-10 and 29-11), and not rarely, the same patients have intra-abdominal enterogenous cysts.[1,17,23] Among the most fascinating aspects of the posterior mediastinal enteric cysts is their occasional connection with the alimentary canal.[12] Such apparently purely mediastinal cysts may penetrate through the diaphragm to end blindly in the abdomen[21] or may connect with the jejunum (Fig. 29-10) or duodenum, so that barium and air may enter the long mediastinal diverticulum (Fig. 29-11). As a rule, enteric cysts are closely associated with the esophagus but may be readily dissected away except in rare cases, unlike similar cysts associated with the bowel. Ordinarily, they have no communication with the lumen of the esophagus and therefore, being lined with secretory epithelium, fill with fluid, attain a large size and cause symptoms in infancy or early in childhood. They are more than twice as common on the right as on the left side and, if long enough, show a recognizable constriction due to compression by the azygos vein (Fig. 29-10). Because they are frequently lined by gastric mucosa which secretes an extremely acid solution, peptic ulceration of these cysts occurs, with resultant substernal pain, erosion into lung, bronchus or espohagus, and hemorrhage.[17,25]

Mediastinal cysts of foregut origin of the other two types discussed below are less likely to fill with secretions and expand and cause symptoms from compression or erosion, so that they are not so often discovered in early years.[9,12,13,15]

BRONCHOGENIC CYST. — The second type and perhaps the most common, taking all ages, is composed usually of respiratory epithelium, occasionally with cartilage and a little smooth muscle in its wall, and never with a well-formed muscular wall and myenteric plexus, as seen in the first type.[9,14] Bronchogenic cysts may be located within the lung or, more commonly, along the main bronchi and only occasionally communicate with the bronchial lumen; if they do, the radiographic appearance suggests a pulmonary cyst. They have been reported within the pericardial sac and to have caused death from pressure.[2] Bron-

Fig. 29-10.—Mediastinal foregut cyst communicating with small intestine. A 1-year-old boy with a 1-week history of high fever and frequent vomiting, dyspnea, cyanosis and evidence of pulmonary infection. He had had other such bouts previously. **A,** film taken during a barium meal shows multiple cervical and upper thoracic vertebral anomalies, multiple gas-filled shadows in the right hemithorax, some in the apex of the left chest **(arrow)** and several deposits of barium above the diaphragm. At other stages in the barium study, almost the entire area of opacity and gas in the right chest was filled with barium. **B,** operative specimen. The mass was entirely posterior mediastinal. **Upper arrow** shows the site of constriction by the azygos vein; **lower arrow,** the point where the cystic structure passed through the diaphragm. The caudal end communicated with the lumen of the jejunum in its first loop at the mesenteric border, passing between leaves of the mesentery. The sac contained fluid with an acid reaction. Microscopic sections showed gastric mucosa predominating in the upper half of the specimen and small intestinal mucosa predominating in the lower half, although there were areas of both in each portion. It is well to be aware of such transdiaphragmatic communications. Preoperative confusion with diaphragmatic hernia is obviously possible; approaches to the two lesions are somewhat different, particularly for surgeons who prefer the abdominal approach for hernia. (Courtesy of Dr. J. Snodgrass.)

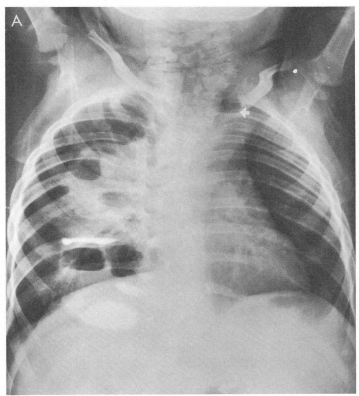
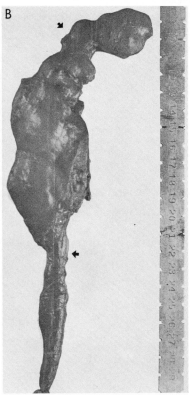

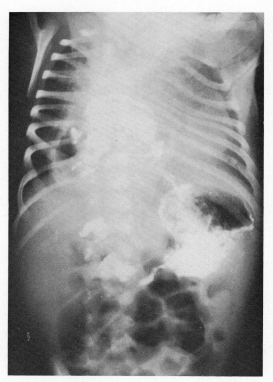

Fig. 29-11.—Mediastinal foregut cyst; neonatal distress, spinal communication. An infant of 1 month had been cyanotic and dyspneic since birth. Roentgen studies showed rachischisis of lower cervical and upper thoracic segments, with marked widening of interpeduncular spacing and abnormal segmentation. The esophagus was displaced anteriorly. In the GI series, the gas- and fluid-filled cystic shadows posterior to the heart are seen to connect with the intestine. At operation, several dilated loops of a bowel-like structure lay in the posterior mediastinum. The caudal end arose from the jejunum, with which it communicated. The mediastinal structure was excised and its infradiaphragmatic attachment to the bowel divided. After 4 uneventful days the baby became acutely ill and *Escherichia coli* was cultured from blood and cerebrospinal fluid. At autopsy, the cephalic end of the cyst was found to communicate with the spinal canal through a bony defect in the T-1 vertebra. The remaining portion of the cyst formed an abscess sac communicating with the spinal canal. There was severe meningitis. This is a clear example of persistence of all the elements of the neuroenteric-canal-residua malformation. (Courtesy of Children's Hospital of Michigan.)

chogenic cysts often are not demonstrable radiologically except for compression of the trachea or bronchus. In a collective review of 31 cases in infants and children, Opsahl and Berman[15] found that 25 patients had symptoms. In 14, the lesion was seen on x-ray films and operation undertaken, successfully in 12. The 11 symptomatic children who were not operated on died.

ESOPHAGEAL TYPE.—The third type of mediastinal cyst of foregut origin is extremely closely associated with the esophagus, and frequently is actually intramural, but contains a ciliated epithelial lining, cartilage in the wall, no intestinal mucosa, no significant amount of muscle in the wall and has no associated vertebral abnormality.

Maier[13] divided the bronchogenic cysts into five groups—paratracheal, carinal, hilar, paraesophageal, and miscellaneous. While the theory of abnormal budding from the respiratory tract readily seems to explain the first groups, it is not as ready an answer to the formation of those cysts which are associated with the esophagus or occur behind it and are attached to the vertebrae. These, like the enterogenous cysts, obviously derive from the primitive foregut, but the precise mode of origin is speculative.

TREATMENT.—The cysts of these three groups cause symptoms by virtue of their size and location and, in the case of the enteric cysts, because of peptic ulceration. Resection is required for all of them, and total extirpation is usually possible. One should be aware of the possibility of transdiaphragmatic extension of the enteric cysts, and of abnormally coursing pulmonary or other vessels, particularly with bronchogenic cysts. Occasionally, dense adherence to esophagus or bronchus or trachea may make total removal of a cyst difficult or impossible. One may then choose to peel the mucosa of the cyst away from the attached structure, leaving the nonepithelial portions of the wall. Chemical cauterization has been employed but is hazardous and uncertainly effective. In an earlier day, Ladd advised marsupialization —establishment of an external fistulous tract. This would rarely be acceptable today. Internal drainage of an enteric cyst into the esophagus has been employed, but if performed in a cyst with gastric mucosal lining would lead to peptic ulceration and the inevitable sequels of hemorrhage and stricture.

CYSTIC HYGROMA (LYMPHOGENOUS CYST)

These multilocular, thin-walled cysts containing lymphatic fluid and dilated lymphatic channels are congenital and characteristically appear in the posterior triangle of the neck (see Chapter 21). Extension of a portion of the process into the mediastinum is not uncommon. Rarely, the lesion arises primarily in the mediastinum; Gross and Hurwitt[7] found 3 instances of this type in 112 patients with cystic hygroma. Total extirpation of the mediastinal portion of a cervical hygroma or of one primarily arising in the mediastinum may not always be possible, but removal of all the grossly recognizable tissue will relieve the symptoms of pressure and prevent the occurrence of infection in the cyst in association with respiratory infections. It would seem that if all of the cyst is removed and no gross tumor is left behind, the remnants may be permanently encased in scar tissue and cause no further symptoms. The results of operation are excellent, and the risks are nonspecific.

Pericardial Cysts (Coelomic Cysts)

In the roentgenogram, these cysts appear usually in the cardiophrenic angle as delicate spherical shadows attached to the pericardium. They are thin-walled, lined by flattened mesothelium, contain clear fluid and may be effortlessly removed. The cysts are asymptomatic and are removed principally to establish their innocent nature. Their occurrence in a child is rare. Such a lesion in a 6-year-old child represents the only childhood example of this type in the records of the Armed Forces Institute of Pathology.

A variety of miscellaneous mediastinal cysts occur. Shidler and Holman[22] described a 4-month-old infant with respiratory distress since birth who had a mesothelium-lined cyst containing clear fluid located between the aorta and vena cava. An unusual transpericardial approach proved successful.

Tumors of Neurogenic Origin

The tumors of neurogenic origin which occur in infancy and childhood are of three histologic and clinical types. All arise in the posterior mediastinum, usually in the more cephalad portion, and present a characteristically dense, sharply circumscribed radiologic appearance. The benign tumors—ganglioneuroma and neurofibroma—may grow to very large size without producing symptoms until Horner's syndrome or marked displacement of the trachea attract attention. The neuroblastoma, the only malignant tumor of the three, may cause pain from involvement of nerve trunks, or may cause symptoms from distant metastases, and occasionally may erode through the chest wall, producing a visible mass (see Fig. 29-14).

Neurinomas, which are not rare in older patients and may occur along the intercostal nerves, even anteriorly, do not seem to develop in children.

There may be clinical and radiologic clues to the nature of these tumors, as indicated below, but in the absence of one or another of these indicative differences it is not possible to make a specific differential diagnosis without operation.[13]

GANGLIONEUROMA.—This is the commonest neurogenic mediastinal tumor of childhood, and most ganglioneuromas reported have occurred in infants or children. It is discovered in infants more commonly than is the neurofibroma. The tumors tend to reach very large size, are discrete, well encapsulated and offer no difficulty in removal, unless they have reached so great a size that this in itself constitutes a problem.[8] The characteristic histologic feature (Fig. 29-12) is the typical ganglion cell, indicative of the origin of these tumors from the ganglions of the sympathetic chain. At least one ganglioneuroma, with an intraspinal extension (dumbbell or hourglass tumor), has been reported. Varying amounts of fibrous tissue are seen within the tumor, and sometimes younger forms of sympathetic cells, so that at times a ganglioneuroma may not be a tumor of a pure cell type, and some of these tumors have malignant potentials, based on a greater admixture of younger sympathetic cells. Tumors with such admixture should be treated by irradiation following operative removal.

NEUROFIBROMA.—The neurofibromas that arise from nerves in the posterior mediastinum—intercostal, phrenic, vagus or sympathetic—may occur as isolated tumors or with the neurofibromatosis of Recklinghausen's disease. In the latter instances, the family history, the presence of the pigmented cutaneous stigmata and the usual multiplicity of lesions all point to this diagnosis (Fig. 29-13). Dumbbell tumors and associated scoliosis are pathognomonic suggestions of the nature of a given tumor in the posterior mediastinum. In such instances, the intervertebral foramina are enlarged and the costovertebral articulations may be displaced. At operation, the tumors are usually sufficiently large, in the area in which intercostal nerves and sympathetic trunks are both located, that it is frequently not possible to be certain of the precise origin of the tumor. Furthermore, in neurofibromatosis, plexiform neurofibromas (rankenneurom) are common, with apparent extensions of the tumor along the sheaths of numerous small nerves, so that total extirpation is impossible. In such cases, one must be content with resection of the principal mass. Although malignant degeneration of neurofibromas is common and to be feared, apparently it takes place mainly in tumors of large size.

NEUROBLASTOMA.—The neuroblastoma is a malignant tumor of sympathetic origin arising from what is conceived to be an immature precursor of the ganglion cell (Fig. 29-14). The majority of neuroblastomas in infancy are found in association with the adrenal gland. When large, such tumors not infrequently extend through or behind the diaphragm into the thorax. Neuroblastomas occurring primarily within the mediastinum and not associated with abdominal tumors are not excessively rare. The presence in the urine of elevated levels of the catecholamines (see Chap. 61) is diagnostic. Although the radiologic appearance frequently suggests a sharply circumscribed lesion, operation usually discloses fairly diffuse infiltration into the soft tissues and involvement of the adjacent ribs and vertebral bodies without evidence of encapsulation. In spite of this, vigorous attempts at operative eradication, with removal of the involved portions of the thoracic wall and electrocauterization of the tumor bed, followed by postoperative irradiation, have resulted in a significant number of apparently indefinite survivals. As with the abdominal neuroblastomas, the period-of-risk formula seems to hold. The best results are in the youngest infants, and the probability of cure is soonest established in them.

TREATMENT.—It is estimated that some 20% of neurogenic tumors of the mediastinum are malignant. The neuroblastomas are malignant from the

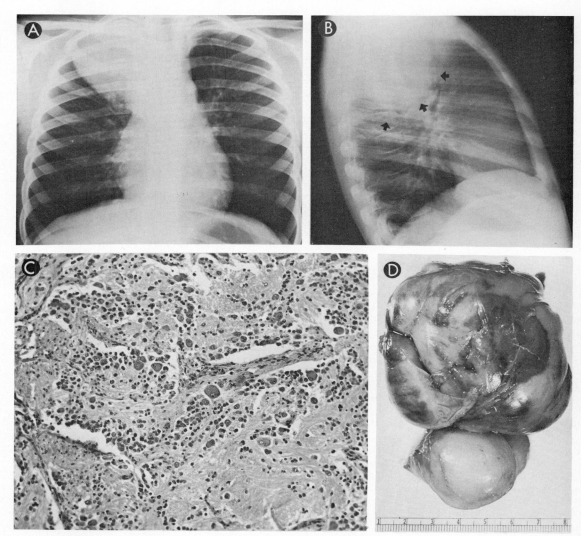

Fig. 29-12.—Ganglioneuroma of mediastinum. A boy of 6 had severe chronic cough. **A** and **B**, roentgenograms show a discrete, dense, rounded tumor filling the posterior mediastinum. Tumors of neurogenic orgin are invariably in the posterior mediastinum, usually in the cephalad portion. **C**, photomicrograph shows characteristic ganglion cells, almost in pure culture, although the few small, round, hyperchromatic cells may represent younger forms in the sympathetic series. A varying amount of neurofibrillary structure is found in these tumors. **D**, operative specimen. The lobulated tumor was readily removed. The attachments were few, loose and not vascular.

start, and the neurofibromas have a potentiality for malignant degeneration which has been claimed to be as high as 40%.[11] All of these tumors can grow to enormous size, in mass alone constituting a threat to life, and at this point create technical difficulties for the surgeon. The tumors should be removed when first recognized. A formal posterolateral thoracotomy affords the best exposure, although occasionally with small tumors a rib resection over the tumor provides direct and satisfactory access. The neurofibromas and ganglioneuromas, which usually are sharply encapsulated, may be removed without much difficulty unless

great size has led to extensive vascular connections. If dumbbell intraspinal extensions are recognized before operation, laminectomy for removal of the intraspinal portion is usually performed first. The neuroblastomas require en bloc chest wall resection, and a vigorous effort at removal or destruction of the tumor, followed by irradiation and chemotherapy (see Fig. 29-14).

TERATOMAS AND DERMOID CYSTS

Second in frequency only to the mediastinal tumors of neurogenic origin, these embryologic malforma-

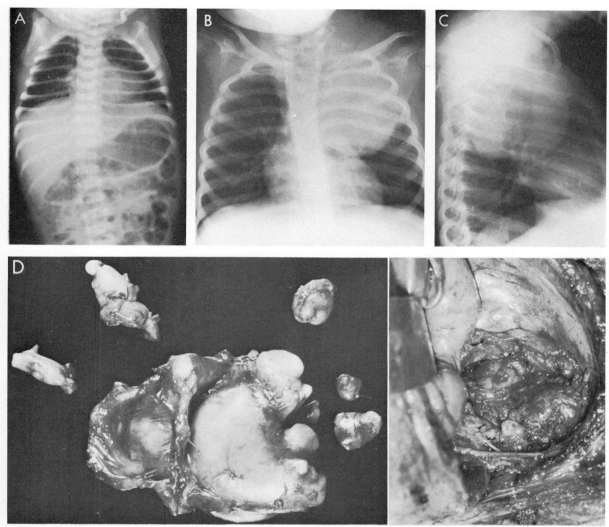

Fig. 29-13.—Mediastinal neurofibroma; Recklinghausen's disease. This 2½-year-old child was one of 8 siblings. The father and one of his brothers have frank Recklinghausen's disease. The mother has no stigmata. Seven of the 8 children have obvious neurofibromatosis. All have multiple areas of cutaneous pigmentation and at least subcutaneous nodules. Four have had large tumors operated on. **A,** roentgenogram in neonatal period shows no obvious tumor. **B,** at age 2½, during routine study of all the siblings, the chest film shows an enormous asymptomatic left supraclavicular tumor, uniformly dense and sharply circumscribed. **C,** the intrathoracic tumor is so large that it would be difficult to say that it arose in the posterior mediastinum, although obviously it is closely applied to the paravertebral gutter. This growth in the short life of the child is remarkably rapid and cause for concern. At operation, the firm spherical mass was found to have numerous pseudopod-like projections posteromedially and posterosuperiorly, extending into the mediastinum and neck. There was no hourglass spinal tumor and no direct invasion by the mass, extension being by innumerable nervelike connections from 1 to 15 mm in diameter ramifying in all directions. These were amputated as far from the tumor as possible. Postoperatively, the child had Horner's syndrome. Microscopic sections showed plexiform neurofibroma. **D: left,** gross specimen, view of the flattened posterior aspect with its pleural covering peeled back, showing a number of the processes which extended into the neck and mediastinum. These were amputated close to the tumor; then additional portions were removed from the tumor bed after delivery of the tumor. **Right,** the tumor bed, showing the upper half of the thorax now empty and the stubs of tumor processes extending into the neck and mediastinum before they were excised.

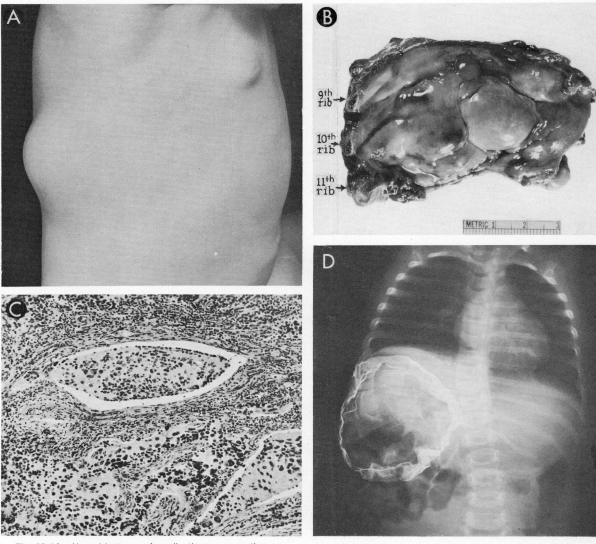

Fig. 29-14.—Neuroblastoma of mediastinum, presenting as a chest wall tumor in a baby of 8 months. **A,** the tumor caused a visible bulge in the posterior axillary line. It was fixed to the deep tissues. **B,** operative specimen, pleural aspect. The diffusely spreading, not localized character of the tumor is obvious. A full-thickness block of all tissues of the chest wall, except skin and fat, was removed. Almost certainly, the tumor infiltrated between the vertebrae. The tumor bed was coagulated with electrocautery. **C,** the tumor is composed largely of very young cells of the sympathetic series and therefore qualifies as a sympathicoblastoma, but here and there occasional ganglion cells were found.

Official diagnosis was ganglioneuroblastoma. Presence of a solid plug of tumor in a vein, plainly visible here, led to an incorrectly gloomy prognosis. **D,** the diaphragm was moved to the 8th rib, the upper border of the operative defect, and the resultant large ventral hernia repaired with tantalum mesh. This film, made some months later, shows the tantalum to be largely fragmented. We no longer use metallic mesh, preferring Teflon felt. The child was free from tumor 10 years later, but resection and heavy irradiation resulted in severe scoliosis.

tions contribute some of the largest and most unusual mediastinal tumors. The term dermoid cyst usually is applied to tumors composed entirely of ectodermal derivatives. The typical dermoid is a thick-walled fibrous sac lined by squamous epithelium in which are seen the various skin appendages, the sac being filled with hair and occasionally teeth—the typical caseous detritus.

Teratomas, which may be solid or cystic, contain derivatives of all three embryonic germ layers. In addition to cartilage and bone, glial tissue is a characteristic component, together with all manner of epithelial structures and many bizarre types of glandular tissue. In fact, it has become apparent that if careful search is made in the wall of most dermoid tu-

mors, whether of the mediastinum or of the ovary, at least a small portion of the wall may be found to contain a solid tumor in which there are derivatives of the other two germ layers. The tumors are almost invariably found in the anterior mediastinum (Figs. 29-15 and 29-16), occasionally within the pericardium. They may reach enormous size, bulging out into one hemithorax or the other, and when the great size and long duration of the tumor have caused a bulging of one side of the chest wall, the clinical diagnosis of teratoma or dermoid may be made with some assurance on inspection of the patient. Only an occasional tumor is recognized to be malignant at birth, but perhaps 20–25% of the reported instances have been called malignant. The criteria of malignancy,

Fig. 29-15.—Teratoma of mediastinum. An 11-year-old girl had no symptoms but repeated episodes of dizziness, possibly attributable to superior vena caval obstruction, although she had no symptoms of the superior vena cava syndrome. In general, this syndrome appears only with malignant tumors and occasional chronic sclerosing mediastinal infections. **A** and **B**, preoperative roentgenograms show the fairly dense, somewhat irregularly nodular mass in the anterior mediastinum projecting into the left hemithorax. **C**, posteroperative film, after uneventful removal of the benign cyst, shows an essentially normal chest.

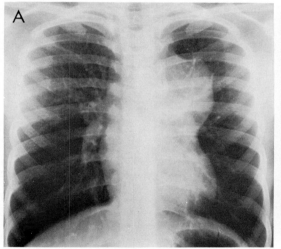
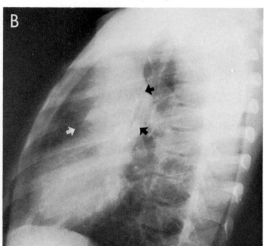
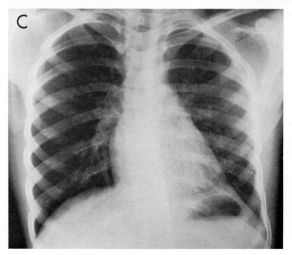

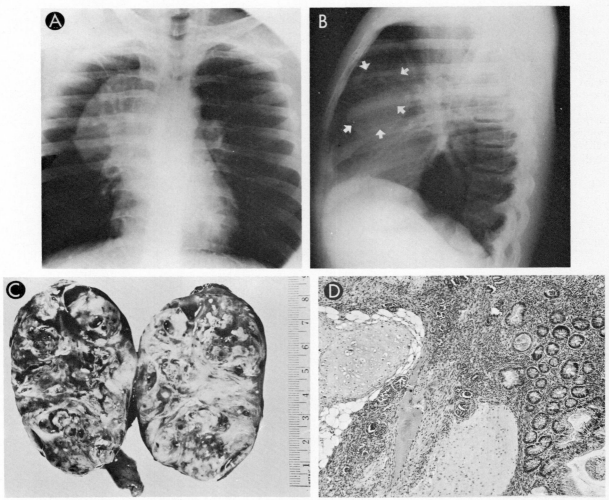

Fig. 29-16.—Mediastinal teratoma. A boy of 12 had a 6-month history of occasional pains in the right chest. Teratomas may reach great size without causing symptoms except those due to displacement or compression of mediastinal structures, and occasionally are so large and have been present for so long in the growing chest wall that the chest bulges asymmetrically on the side of the tumor. **A** and **B**, plain films show the large mass of somewhat varying density in the anterior mediastinum extending into the right hemithorax. **C,** Gross specimen shows areas of varied consistency, but aside from a few frank cysts, this is a solid tumor. **D,** photomicrograph shows the melange of histologic structures characteristic of teratomas—cartilage on the left, glial tissue bottom center, various types of fibrous tissue, glandular structures and fat. But when malignancy occurs (20–25%) it is almost invariably epithelial and usually adenocarcinoma.

based in a few cases solely on histologic evidence within the primary tumor, are somewhat uncertain in view of the bizarre admixture of various elements, so that the actual incidence of malignancy proved by the ultimate clinical behavior of the tumors is a little lower than the figures given. When malignancy occurs, it is almost invariably in the form of carcinoma rather than sarcoma, and usually of an adeno- or papillary type of carcinoma. Death comes from direct extension and pulmonary and other metastases. Symptoms of the benign tumors are caused by dis-

placement of the trachea, esophagus or heart and great vessels or by infection within the cyst and erosion into the pleural cavity or trachea. The coughing up of hair in such instances is a pathognomonic sign. Until either infection or malignant degeneration has occurred, the tumors are quite readily removable.[11,14,18] As in other mediastinal tumors, removal of all of them is required because malignancy may be present or may develop and because continued growth of the tumor leads to serious symptoms from pressure and displacement of mediastinal structures. In addi-

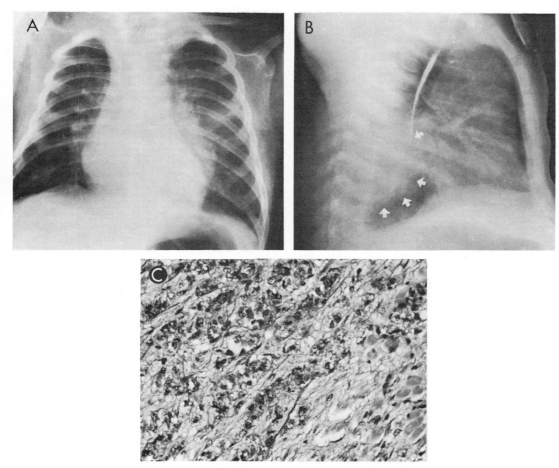

Fig. 29-17.—Embryonal rhabdomyosarcoma. A 2-month-old boy had intermittent fever and rapidly progressive paralysis of the lower extremities. **A,** plain film shows the shadow of a mediastinal mass on the left. **B,** lateral film shows the lesion to be located posteriorly. **C,** photomicrograph of specimen removed at operation for biopsy study only. A few muscle fibers are identifiable in the lower right corner. The extremely anaplastic and embryonal tumor was thought to be probably rhabdomyosarcoma. (Courtesy of Dr. J. E. Lewis, Jr.)

tion, infection of these tumors or erosion into other structures may produce dangerous symptoms and greatly complicate the problem of operative removal.

MISCELLANEOUS NEOPLASMS

A wide variety of additional neoplasms and cysts of all kinds have been described in the mediastinum, usually in isolated case reports.[20,25] These include hemangiomas, lipomas, embryonal rhabdomyosarcomas (Fig. 29-17), osteochondromas and a group of anaplastic carcinomas and sarcomas.

In addition to the lesions discussed in this chapter, it must be remembered that a number of other conditions which occur in the mediastinum require consideration in the differential diagnosis. These include

intrathoracic goiter, aneurysms of the pulmonary artery and other congenital anomalies of the great vessels, and diaphragmatic hernia of any of the several types. Although differentiation may often be made on clinical and roentgenologic grounds, frequently only operation discloses the final diagnosis.

REFERENCES

1. Beardmore, H. E., and Wigglesworth, F. W.: Vertebral anomalies and alimentary duplication, Pediat. Clin. North America, p. 457, May, 1958.
2. Dabbs, C. H.; Berg, R., and Peirce, E. C. II: Intrapericardial bronchogenic cysts, J. Thoracic Surg. 34:718, 1957.
3. Ellis, F. H., Jr., and DuShane, J. W.: Primary mediastinal cysts and neoplasms in infants and children, Am. Rev. Tuberc. 74:940, 1956.
4. Ellis, F. H., Jr., *et al.*: Surgical implications of the me-

diastinal shadow in thoracic roentgenograms of infants and children, Surg., Gynec. & Obst. 100:532, 1955.

5. Elwood, J. S.: Mediastinal duplication of the gut, Arch. Dis. Childhood 34:474, 1959.

6. Fallon, M.; Gordon, A. R. G., and Lendrum, A. C.: Mediastinal cysts of foregut origin associated with vertebral abnormalities, Brit. J. Surg. 41:520, 1954.

7. Gross, R. E., and Hurwitt, E. S.: Cervicomediastinal and mediastinal cystic hygromas, Surg., Gynec. & Obst. 87:599, 1948.

8. Hamilton, J. P., and Koop, C. E.: Ganglioneuromas in children, Surg., Gynec. & Obst. 121:803, 1965.

9. Hardy, L. M.: Bronchogenic cysts of the mediastinum, Pediatrics 4:108, 1949.

10. Heimburger, I. L., and Battersby, J. S.: Primary mediastinal tumors of childhood, J. Thoracic & Cardiovas. Surg. 50:92, 1965.

11. Kent, E. M., *et al.*: Intrathoracic neurogenic tumors, J. Thoracic Surg. 13:116, 1944.

12. Leider, H. J.; Snodgrass, J. J., and Mishrick, A. S.: Intrathoracic alimentary duplications communicating with small intestine, Arch. Surg. 71:203, 1955.

13. Maier, H. C.: Bronchogenic cyst of the mediastinum, Ann. Surg. 127:476, 1948.

14. Morrison, I. M.: Tumors and cysts of the mediastinum, Thorax 13:294, 1958.

15. Opsahl, T., and Berman, E. J.: Bronchogenic mediastinal cysts in infants, Pediatrics 30:376, 1962.

16. Page, U. S., and Bigelow, J. C.: A mediastinal gastric duplication leading to pneumonectomy, J. Thoracic & Cardiovas. Surg. 54:291, 1967.

17. Rhaney, K., and Barclay, G. P. T.: Enterogenous cysts and congenital diverticula of the alimentary canal with abnormalities of the vertebral column and spinal cord, J. Path. & Bact. 77:457, 1959.

18. Rusby, N. L.: Dermoid cysts and teratomata of the mediastinum, J. Thoracic Surg. 13:169, 1944.

19. Sabiston, D. C., Jr., and Scott, H. W., Jr.: Primary neoplasms and cysts of the mediastinum, Ann. Surg. 136:777, 1952.

20. Saini, V. K., and Wahi, P. L.: Hourglass transmural type of intrathoracic lipoma, J. Thoracic & Cardiovas. Surg. 47:600, 1964.

21. Shepherd, M. P.: Thoracic, thoraco-abdominal and abdominal duplication, Thorax 20:82, 1965.

22. Shidler, F. P., and Holman, E. F.: Mediastinal tumors, Stanford M. Bull. 10:217, 1952.

23. Veeneklaas, G. M. H.: Pathogenesis of intrathoracic gastrogenic cysts, Am. J. Dis. Child. 83:500, 1952.

24. Willich, E.:Thorako-abdominale magenduplikatur, Kinderchirurgie 5:115, 1967.

25. Wilson, J. R., and Bartley, T. D.: Liposarcoma of the mediastinum, J. Thoracic & Cardiovas. Surg. 48:486, 1967.

26. Symposium on clinical aspects of Hodgkin's disease, Cancer 19:297, 1966.

M. M. RAVITCH
D. C. SABISTON, JR.

Drawings by
LEON SCHLOSSBERG

Endoscopy

IN THE STUDY and management of conditions involving the larynx, respiratory tract and esophagus of patients of any age, endoscopic procedures are indispensable. The indications for the procedures in infants are usually associated with critical obstruction to respiration or swallowing. Experience, teamwork and an adequate instrumentarium reduce any potential hazard to a minimum, permitting routine examination of even the smallest infants without complications. This concept, long stressed by Chevalier Jackson, has now been accepted universally and an endoscopic team is recognized as an essential part of pediatric surgery.

Pediatric Laryngology

ANATOMIC CONSIDERATIONS. — The larynx in the newborn child lies at about the level of the fourth cervical vertebra, descending in the adult to lie between the level of the fifth and sixth cervical vertebrae. The glottic dimensions in the infant are approximately 7 mm anteroposteriorly by 4 mm across the posterior commissure. Thus the glottic airway during inspiration is a triangle of approximately 14 sq mm; it is important to note that an edema of 1 mm of the

mucosal surfaces will reduce this to 5 sq mm, or only 35% of the original lumen. Mucosa is rigidly adherent to the posterior surface of the epiglottis and loosely attached anteriorly and along the aryepiglottic folds. Therefore supraglottic edema such as is seen in *Hemophilus influenzae* infections results in laryngeal obstruction by extravasation of fluid anterior and lateral to the epiglottic cartilage. This forces the lateral edges of the epiglottis to curl inward and pushes the tip backward to occlude the larynx in a trap-door fashion. A similar soft areolar tissue makes up the subglottic structures immediately below the level of the vocal cords. This tissue is encircled by the rigid cartilaginous ring of the cricoid, the only complete cartilaginous ring in the airway. Inflammatory edema or the trauma of intubation is quickly affected by this factor of rigid encirclement, which is extremely important in laryngeal obstruction. Similar edema occurring in the aryepiglottic fold or the epiglottis has an opportunity to extend laterally into the soft pharyngeal tissues so that supraglottic edema may become much more extensive than subglottic edema before it produces actual respiratory obstruction.

CONGENITAL ANOMALIES. — Commonest of all con-

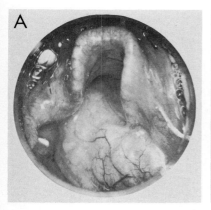 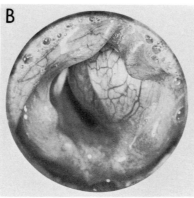

Fig. 30-1. — Laryngocele. **A,** laryngocele dissecting posteriorly and appearing as a cyst in the right aryepiglottic fold. **B,** laryngocele protruding from the right laryngeal ventricle to account for severe dyspnea in a newborn infant.

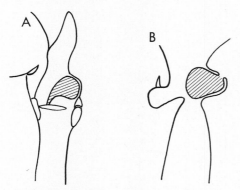

Fig. 30-2.—Laryngocele. **A,** sagittal section. **B,** coronal section through the glottis.

genital anomalies of the larynx is *laryngomalacia.* This is characterized by gradually increasing stridor during the first year of life which spontaneously decreases in intensity and disappears 6 months to a year later. It is important because stridor is the principal symptom of all obstructions of the airway, congenital or acquired, and therefore must be accurately identified to differentiate laryngomalacia from other conditions causing stridor such as laryngeal cysts, paralyses, subglottic stenoses and vascular rings. Other cartilaginous anomalies are absence of the epiglottis and deformities of the cricoid, such as a stenotic cricoid ring, and a laryngoesophageal cleft. Endoscopic resection of the stenotic ring may adequately enlarge the lumen of a deformed cricoid, although it may be necessary to resort to external reconstruction and a skin graft lining after normal growth has taken place. An external pharyngotomy or a thyrotomy approach will be necessary to repair a severe laryngoesophageal cleft.

Cysts and *laryngoceles* (Figs. 30-1 and 30-2) are encountered originating in the anterior aspect of the ventricle of the larynx.[2] Internal laryngoceles protruding from between the true and false cords and those bulging into the aryepiglottic fold generally have some connection with the interior of the larynx. Glot-

tic cysts and internal thyroglossal duct cysts do not have actual or potential communication with the interior of the larynx. Laryngeal cysts may be aspirated endoscopically with a large-bore needle or may be partially marsupialized. External resection through a pharyngotomy is rarely necessary. The external thyroglossal duct cyst presenting in the anterior aspect of the neck at about the level of the hyoid bone is an enlargement of the embryonic thyroglossal duct extending from the isthmus of the thyroid gland to the foramen cecum at the base of the tongue. It lies anterior and inferiorly to the hyoid bone, and the duct may pass through, in front of or behind the hyoid. Infection causes marked swelling of the anterior aspect of the neck and floor of the mouth. It is excised during a period of quiescence through a collar incision over the superficial swelling. Dissection should include removal of the stalks leading to the thyroid isthmus and the stalk extending upward through the hyoid bone. The body of the hyoid bone should be removed routinely to prevent recurrence and the tract followed to the base of the tongue (see p. 285).

Webs are seen as a supraglottic fusion of the false cords, glottic membranes between the true cords (Fig. 30-3,*A*), fusion of the anterior portion of the true cords, or subglottic webs, which are distinct from cartilaginous cricoid obstruction. Congenital glottic atresia is rarely seen in the living because the infant can survive only if the atresia is immediately recognized at birth and relieved at once by tracheostomy. Subglottic stenosis, a thickening of the subglottic structures, is common and accounts for many cases of recurring "croup" or prolonged extubation in infants tracheostomized because of respiratory obstruction early in life. Tracheostomy is necessary often within the first 24 hours in infants with the more severe webs and subglottic stenoses. Slitting of the web and repeated, rapid dilatation without anesthesia, or the use of an internally fixed polyethylene splint are effective.

The *paralysis* of one or both vocal cords in newborn infants is usually a serious manifestation of a gross anomaly of another organ system. Bilateral laryngeal paralysis is associated with cerebral retardation, a meningomyelocele or extensive birth trauma.

Fig. 30-3.—Laryngeal lesions in infancy. **A,** congenital laryngeal web seen through the direct laryngoscope. **B,** papilloma of the larynx of an 18-month-old infant.

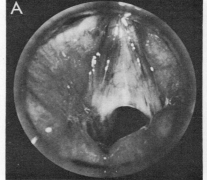
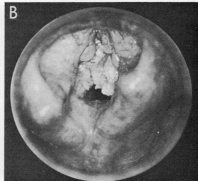

Unilateral left cord paralysis may often be traced to anomalies of the heart or great vessels, the esophagus or the tracheobronchial tree. Unilateral right cord paralysis may be seen in an otherwise normal infant. It should be noted that the voice (cry) of an infant with bilateral recurrent laryngeal nerve paralysis is more normal than that of an infant with unilateral paralysis; but inspiration is stridorous and a large percentage require a tracheostomy.

The prognosis of laryngeal paralysis in infants depends on the etiology. Bilateral vocal cord paralysis is most frequently a part of a generalized central nervous system disorder, and the prognosis is relatively poor. Infants with right cord paralysis may have no other neurologic lesion and the ultimate prognosis for voice function is relatively good. In most infants with left cord paralysis, the prognosis depends on the associated cardiovascular or other intrathoracic pathology. The voice may improve in time through compensatory action of the remaining actively functioning laryngeal and pharyngeal muscles, but when the paralysis is present prior to cardiac or esophageal surgery, or if additional operation is contemplated, the paralysis must be taken into consideration in order to reduce postoperative complications.

Vascular anomalies consist of hemangiomas and lymphangiomas, the former as capillary and cavernous, the great majority associated with other hemangiomas about the head and neck, the latter as laryngeal extensions of a cystic hygroma. They are found in a predominance of females to males in a ratio of more than 5:1 and are recognized soon after birth when infants with obvious skin lesions become hoarse and dyspneic. Tracheostomy is required in most cases, usually before the age of 6 months. Spontaneous involution occurs, and therefore active surgical or irradiation therapy should be avoided or postponed. Improvement of the larynx in cases of lymphangiomas follows only after control of the neck mass.

ACUTE INFLAMMATORY DISEASES.—These include such processes as acute laryngitis, laryngotracheobronchitis and diphtheria which are characterized by edema, exudate and membranous obstruction.[9] Primary management is antibiotic and antitoxin therapy with the patient placed in an atmosphere of high humidity. Steroids have been advocated in the management of acute obstructive laryngitis, but their value is questionable. Tracheostomy is often necessary as an emergency procedure. However, a rapidly introduced intratracheal, oro- or nasotracheal airway may temporarily relieve obstruction sufficiently to permit a tranquil tracheostomy to be performed with routine surgical preparation and adequate instrumentarium.

TRAUMA.—External trauma to the larynx occurs in automobile, sled or bicycle accidents and in sports such as baseball, wrestling and boxing. Massive hematomas may rapidly obstruct respiration, and simple or compound fractures of the laryngeal cartilages occur to cause complete destruction and obliteration of the laryngeal lumen. Open or closed reduction following a tracheostomy can be achieved through an external surgical approach or through peroral laryngeal dilatation. Cartilages must be splinted by an internal laryngeal splint which may be attached to the tracheostomy tube and maintained in place for several months until the lumen is adequately re-formed.

Internal trauma results from vocal abuse. Vocal nodules, singers' nodes and screamers' nodes are synonymous terms for the epithelial thickening of the vocal cords at the junction of the anterior one third and posterior two thirds of the cords. In small children, direct laryngoscopy is necessary to confirm the diagnosis, whereas in older children it is done by simple mirror laryngoscopy. Therapy consists of voice correction and rehabilitation unless the nodules are quite large, when forceps removal through the laryngoscope under general anesthesia is indicated. Removal without adequate voice therapy is often followed by recurrence. The nodules usually disappear as the growth of the larynx during puberty changes the points of stress in phonation.

Commonest of the *foreign bodies* causing mechanical laryngeal obstruction are egg shells, safety pins, fragments of glass, plastic toys and other flat objects that become lodged in the larynx in an anteroposterior plane.[6] Sudden choking, loss of voice and dyspnea indicate their presence, although a large foreign body in the cervical esophagus will cause the same symptoms because of the laryngeal or tracheal compression. Hypopharyngeal and laryngeal foreign bodies constitute 7% of foreign bodies that require endoscopic removal from the air and food passages.

NEOPLASMS.—Commonest of the neoplasms are the laryngeal papillomas[12] (Fig. 30-3, *B*). These verrucous growths slowly fill the larynx, causing hoarseness, dyspnea, then aphonia and finally total respiratory obstruction.[8] They must be removed by direct laryngoscopy with laryngeal cup forceps, although papillomatous obstruction often requires tracheostomy. Radiation should be strictly avoided because of the frequency of subsequent chronic laryngeal stenosis and even malignant degeneration following its use.[1] Malignant lesions, generally sarcomas, rarely are found to be the cause of laryngeal obstruction in infants. Direct laryngoscopic biopsy is necessary to establish the diagnosis.

Direct Laryngoscopy

INDICATIONS.—Respiratory obstruction and hoarseness or an abnormal quality of the voice are the two principal indications for laryngoscopy in infants and children. Since the larynx of patients in the lower age groups cannot be examined with a laryngeal mirror, direct examination with a laryngoscope is necessary.

The examination should be preceded by neck and chest x-ray study. If the obstruction is severe and the diagnosis remains in question, the direct laryngoscopic examination is mandatory. In cases of respiratory obstruction, direct laryngoscopy should not be attempted without adequate preparation for a tracheostomy, not because of the procedure but because of the lesion that might be disclosed by the examination.

TECHNIQUE.—Anesthesia is unnecessary for most direct laryngoscopic procedures in infants, but for prolonged procedures, general anesthesia is most satisfactory. The infant is securely wrapped and the head firmly held with the neck flexed on the chest and the head extended on the neck. In this position the laryngoscope is introduced from slightly to the right of the midline, the blade pointed toward the suprasternal notch. The base of the tongue should be followed until the tip of the epiglottis is seen; the laryngoscope then dips under the epiglottis and the instrument is lifted anteriorly to expose the larynx. The most common error is the advancement of the laryngoscope into the laryngopharynx, compressing rather than exposing the larynx. Introduction of the laryngoscope into the pyriform sinus or too deeply into the vallecula shuts off the airway by closing it with the epiglottis, trap-door fashion. This is best avoided by accurate midline direction of the laryngoscope blade, careful identification of the tip of the epiglottis and a firm advance of the laryngoscope once the epiglottis has been lifted. These steps prevent the rolling of the curled, slippery epiglottis from under the laryngoscope blade.

Bronchoscopy

The lobar, segmental and subsegmental anatomy of the bronchi is already established in the second month of fetal life. A bronchogram of the newborn will identify a lobar and segmental bronchial pattern comparable to the adult configuration (Fig. 30-4). The use of infant laryngoscopes and bronchoscopes makes possible the bronchoscopic examination of an infant of any age. Small instruments are essential and the duration of the examination should be rigidly limited. In infants who merely require removal of tracheal or bronchial secretions, aspiration may be done with a semirigid catheter or a small rubber-tipped metal aspirator passed through the larynx as it is exposed with a laryngoscope. Anesthesia is neither necessary nor desirable for bronchoscopy in the newborn. Oxygen may be administered during the procedure, the oxygen tube with a flow of 2-3 liters/minute being attached directly to the oxygen arm of the bronchoscope.

INDICATIONS.—The principal indication for bronchoscopic examination of infants or children is evidence of *bronchial obstruction:*[10] persistent wheezing, obstructive emphysema or atelectasis. Obstructive emphysema may indicate the presence of a foreign body, an intraluminal congenital web or partial

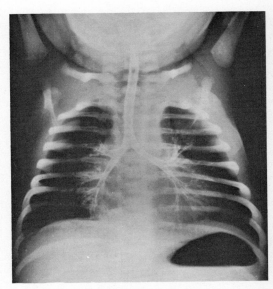

Fig. 30-4.—Bronchogram showing normal tracheobronchial configuration of a newborn infant. (Courtesy of Dr. Harvey White.)

extrabronchial compression by a tumor or a vascular anomaly. The frequency with which the vascular anomalies occur has only recently been recognized, and it is through the pattern of their tracheal, bronchial and esophageal pressure that the preoperative diagnosis of the type of cardiovascular anomaly is made.[3]

Atelectasis in newborn infants has many implications. Normally, it takes from 2 days to 2 weeks for complete aeration of the lung, so that patchy atelectasis is not in itself an indication for bronchoscopy in the newborn. If, in addition to atelectasis, excessive secretions are present on physical examination, or if a segment, lobe or entire lung is atelectatic, bronchoscopic examination is indicated to determine the cause of obstruction and to remove it if possible. Unrelieved obstruction may result in bronchiectasis. Apparent unilateral atelectasis in our series of bronchial anomalies has been due to agenesis of a lung in 11 cases (Fig. 30-5). Duplication of bronchi or lobes may be associated with pulmonary cysts. *Excessive secretions* in the tracheobronchial tree of a newborn infant requiring bronchoscopic aspiration should lead to search for a possible pharyngeal paralysis or a congenital tracheoesophageal fistula. *Spontaneous pneumothorax,* an occasional finding responsible for dyspnea and cyanosis in a newborn infant, is, of course, a contraindication to bronchoscopy. In infants aged 6 months to a year, severe bronchopulmonary suppuration is most probably due to fibrocystic disease of the pancreas. Cystic changes in the bronchial epithelium and the easy entry of infecting organisms into the respiratory tract cause the extensive suppurative bronchitis, atelectasis, bronchiectasis and bron-

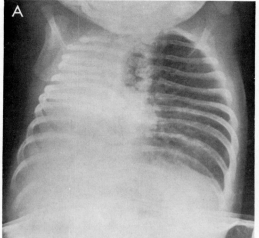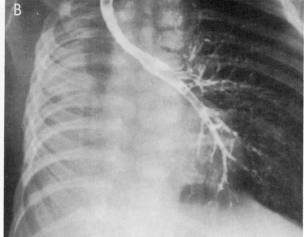

Fig. 30-5.—Agenesis of the right lung. **A,** routine anteroposterior film taken because of suspected atelectasis. The heart is entirely in the right chest, and the left lung has herniated across the midline. **B,** bronchogram of the same infant, showing total absence of the right bronchus.

chopneumonia which characterize the pulmonary findings. Mechanical removal of viscid secretions from the airway is essential, and repeated bronchoscopic aspiration of the main bronchi and of the lobar bronchi assists in reducing the frequency of episodes of bronchopneumonia. Occasional exposure of the larynx with a laryngoscope and aspiration of the trachea with a catheter or small tracheal aspirator is of further value.

Foreign bodies in the pharynx, larynx or tracheobronchial tree are a major cause of sudden death in infants and young children. Twenty-two deaths in children between age 2 months and 7 years, of whom all but 2 were less than 4 years old, were found to be due to objects lodged in the respiratory tract.[14]

Tracheal and bronchial foreign bodies constitute approximately 35% of foreign bodies of the air and food passages requiring endoscopic removal. Commonest of the aspirated foreign bodies are peanuts and other nut meats. These are most frequently seen in the bronchi of infants 1–3 years of age. In our own cases involving 640 bronchial foreign bodies, 244 obstructions were due to peanuts in infants or children under age 4. Small pieces of raw carrot and crisp bacon, on the diet lists of many pediatricians, rank next in frequency as food foreign bodies in the bronchi of younger infants, together with fragments broken from a chicken bone given the infant for "teething." Hardware, tacks, nails, screws and other objects such as BB shot, teeth and beans from a bean blower are generally seen in somewhat older children. There were 280 of these miscellaneous objects in the series of 640 bronchial foreign bodies, most of them in children 3–7 years old. Symptoms almost invariably begin with severe coughing, gagging, choking and wheezing. This stage of the symptomatology is often followed by a symptomless interval as the object becomes fixed in a bronchus, giving a false sense of security and suggesting that the object has been coughed out or swallowed. The third stage of the symptomatology is that of complications: atelectasis, pneumonitis, lung abscess, pulmonary hemorrhage or bronchiectasis. A persistent wheeze, obstructive emphysema or atelectasis, or the visualization of a radiopaque foreign body itself, establishes the diagnosis in most cases. If there is any question of diagnosis, bronchoscopic investigation is indicated.[4]

TECHNIQUE.—A bronchoscopic examination may be made of patients of any age. In newborn infants and in most children, anesthesia is unnecessary, although sedation with the appropriate dosage of morphine is recommended for children, provided there is no contraindication such as respiratory obstruction or general debility. Local anesthesia may be used in children over 10 years and in adults. Atropine or scopolamine may be added to the preoperative medication unless one wishes to evaluate the amount of secretion normally present in the tracheobronchial tree. General anesthesia for a routine bronchoscopic examination is usually not necessary, and often the condition for which the patient is being examined contraindicates its use. General anesthesia may be employed provided the anesthesiologist and the bronchoscopist agree on who is to assume the responsibility of maintaining the airway, because with the bronchoscope in place, the anesthesiologist no longer has access to the airway or control of respiration without the use of a respirator.

In infants and children, it is essential to use small-caliber bronchoscopes to keep possible laryngeal edema at a minimum and to permit inspection of the tiny basilar branch bronchi. With the patient securely restrained, the larynx should first be exposed with the laryngoscope (Fig. 30-6), as described above. Under direct vision, the bronchoscope is then introduced cautiously, using the lip of the bronchoscope to separate the cords. As the bronchoscope enters the trachea, the head is rotated posteriorly and the advancing instrument enters either bronchus upon shifting of the head from side to side. Inspection of the branch bronchi in an orderly progression is essential. Recognition of the mechanical problem involved in a foreign body removal as well as the specific forceps techniques (Fig. 30-7) should be learned through practice on anesthetized laboratory animals. Although many of the complications and failures of attempted foreign body removal arise because of a lack of adequate instrumentarium, fully a half of these difficulties are due to inadequate familiarity with known safe techniques.

COMPLICATIONS.—The commonest complication of bronchoscopy in infants and children is laryngeal edema. The causes are trauma with the laryngoscope on exposure of the larynx, trauma to the cords on insertion of the bronchoscope through the glottis, the use of too large a bronchoscope and prolonged or early repetition of the bronchoscopic examination. Acute laryngeal edema, often the result of a previous unsuccessful examination, is a contraindication to bronchoscopy unless a tracheostomy is to be done before the bronchoscope is withdrawn. Peanuts and other vegetable foreign bodies cause more bronchial and laryngeal edema than do metallic foreign bodies. Pneumothorax or subcutaneous emphysema may follow a traumatic bronchoscopy because of tracheal or bronchial fracture, although subcutaneous emphysema may be associated with the aspiration of a foreign body prior to any instrumentation. Management of the pneumothorax is by closed drainage, although if a tracheal or bronchial tear is present, immediate surgical closure is mandatory. In spontaneous subcutaneous emphysema, removal of the obstructing foreign body and then placing the child in a tent with high oxygen concentration usually suffices, although a tracheostomy and mediastinotomy may be necessary if there is a progression of the emphysema.

Esophagoscopy

Esophagoscopy is an indispensable diagnostic and therapeutic procedure available for the study of infants and children with dysphagia. Its development parallels advances in other fields. While it had its origin with candlelight reflected into a tube, routine esophagoscopic examination has been dependent on electrically lighted instruments, careful preoperative roentgen studies and mechanically safe bougies, forceps and surgical techniques.

INDICATIONS.—Dysphagia, complete inability to swallow, inco-ordination or pain on swallowing, regurgitation of undigested food or fluids, "feeding problems" and hematemesis are indications for esophagoscopy. Frequently, dysphagia first appears at 4-6 months of age when the infant begins taking semisolid food. The feeding time is prolonged and food may even be rejected. The increasing inability to swallow often results in an altered behavior pattern, but before attempting to treat the condition on a psychogenic basis, the possible presence of an organic lesion in the esophagus should be considered.[7]

Conditions affecting the esophagus in the newborn are mechanical and neurogenic. The mechanical lesions are congenital atresia, fistula, stenosis and webs. The neurogenic disorders are the occasionally

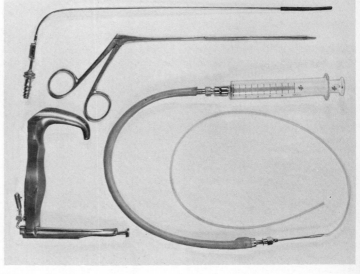

Fig. 30-6.—Equipment for bronchoscopy in infants. The larynx is exposed with the laryngoscope, and the polyethylene tube is guided through the glottis with the laryngeal alligator forceps. Opaque medium is instilled under cinefluoroscopic control. The rubber-tipped metal Samson aspirator is used to clear the tracheobronchial tree of secretions and oil on completion of the procedure.

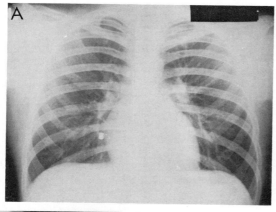

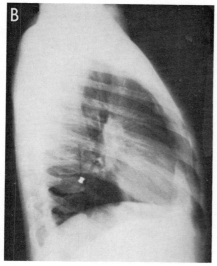

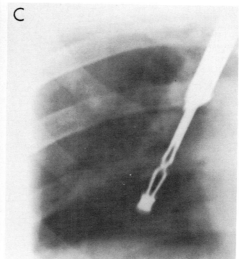

Fig. 30-7.—Bronchial foreign body. **A,** anteroposterior, and **B,** right lateral chest films demonstrate an air-rifle pellet in the posterior basilar division of the right lower lobe bronchus. **C,** film taken during bronchoscopic removal of the foreign body with cross-action forceps. The procedure was done with biplane fluoroscopic guidance.

encountered cardiospasm[13] and the more common failure of the swallowing mechanism due to a congenital lesion of the central nervous system. Chemical burns, foreign bodies and strictures associated with the repair of atresias are the commonest of the acquired lesions.

A fluoroscopic study of esophageal function should precede an original esophagoscopic examination. Other studies include a routine anteroposterior chest film and a lateral neck and chest x-ray taken with the infant's arms down and back to reveal the pharynx, larynx and the retropharyngeal and retroesophageal spaces. Cinefluorography has many advantages over routine fluoroscopy, particularly in infants whose swallowing function cannot be controlled. Prior feedings should be withheld so that the contrast medium is taken eagerly. Esophagoscopy permits direct inspection and confirmation of the lesion seen radiographically, but diagnostic esophagoscopy is also indicated in infants with esophageal symptoms whose x-ray findings are negative, since some mucosal lesions, foreign bodies, varices or other nonobstructing conditions may not be immediately apparent on the contrast study.

TECHNIQUE.—Inspection of the esophagus with an esophagoscope presents problems that are minimized by the availability of an adequate instrumentarium. Anesthesia is unnecessary in infants but, if preferred, the airway must be assured by an intratracheal tube to avoid asphyxia due to compression of the trachea by the esophagoscope. General anesthesia may be desirable for initial esophagoscopy in older children, although most esophagoscopic examinations, particularly repeat procedures necessary for the dilatation of strictures, may be done without anesthesia.[5] The infant or child is firmly wrapped and placed in a recum-

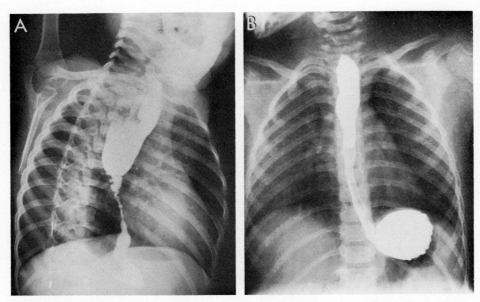

Fig. 30-8.—Congenital esophageal stricture. **A,** long, narrow stricture of lower half of the esophagus. **B,** esophagram following a series of endoscopic dilatations. There is no hiatus hernia.

bent position. The shoulders are held on the table, the neck flexed on the chest and the head extended on the neck. In this position there is a direct, straight line from the mouth, through the pharynx, retrolaryngeal space and the upper thoracic esophagus. The scope, held like a billiard cue, is inserted into the right side of the mouth and directed to the right pyriform sinus. A small bougie may be gently inserted into the cervical esophagus at this point to act as a lumen finder and the scope advanced over it as the cricopharyngeus muscle relaxes. Inspection continues, keeping the lumen in view as the head is rotated posteriorly. The advance through the cardia is also facilitated by first inserting a small bougie into the stomach and passing the scope over it.

Dilatation of strictures.—Congenital strictures of the esophagus may consist of single or multiple webs, or segments of stenosis from 1 to 10 cm long. Congenital webs respond immediately and usually permanently to a single dilatation or a short series of dilatations. The dilatation may be done with an esophagoscope guided through the web over a thread or an esophageal bougie, or with graduated, mercury-filled rubber Hurst bougies that may be increased in size as the web responds to dilatation.[7] Most strictures of whole segments of the esophagus respond to dilatation with mercury-filled bougies, but some are fibrous and require dilatation with the rigid esophagoscope or antegrade or retrograde olive-shaped Plummer bougies, advanced over a previously swallowed thread (Fig. 30-8). In severe cases requiring gastrostomy, the thread is recovered from the gastrostomy opening for more satisfactory control. In these circumstances,

Tucker retrograde bougies may be used. The choice of bougie will depend on a careful consideration of the roentgenologic appearance of the stricture and the age of the patient. For esophagoscopic dilatation, the infant esophagoscope should be used in infants under 1 year of age. A larger tube provides better visualization and would permit passage of dilating esophageal bougies through it, but it is likely to obstruct the airway. If passage of the instruments meets with little resistance and no other lesion is seen, subsequent dilatations may be accomplished with the Hurst type of mercury-filled bougies at intervals of a few days to several weeks as dictated by the response to treatment. Occasionally, the esophagoscope will have to be used several times before a stricture will permit passage of a flexible dilator. When a satisfactory lumen has been obtained, the dilatations are repeated as often as necessary to keep the patient symptom-free or to retain adequate patency.

In rare instances, a very firm stricture that does not respond to peroral dilatation is encountered in early infancy. In such cases, gastrostomy is indicated to maintain nutrition and permit dilatation over a string. If it still fails to respond, direct operation may be necessary. Experience has shown that surgical resection and end-to-end anastomosis often result in a postsurgical stricture, but if dilatation is begun early, the response is better than that of the original lesion. If at all possible, resection of the esophagogastric junction should be avoided.

Stricture formation following the repair of an esophageal atresia and tracheoesophageal fistula presents special problems in endoscopic management.[11]

Half of the surviving patients require some type of dilatation procedure, a percentage steadily declining as techniques of suture of the anastomosis site improve. Maintenance of the lumen is accomplished much more easily than re-establishment once a stenosis at the site of anastomosis has become firm. An esophagogram 10 days postoperatively will indicate the adequacy of the lumen through the anastomosis. If it is tight, dilatations with mercury-filled Hurst bougies are begun biweekly or with longer intervals between dilatations depending on the response to therapy. Failure to follow this regimen often results in stenosis, sometimes first apparent at 4 months of age when semisolids then added to the diet lodge in the stricture. Patients operated on elsewhere, who are referred for dilatation of the anastomosis, are generally in this age group. By this time the anastomosis site is rigid and response to dilatation procedures is much slower. An additional endoscopic problem in some cases consists of severe tracheal stenosis at the point from which the lower esophageal segment was resected from the trachea and the opening into the trachea repaired. Respirations in such cases are loud, labored and rasping and there is a constant, brassy cough. Examination of the trachea with the infant bronchoscope demonstrates an area of stenosis near the bifurcation, with granulation tissue on the posterior wall of the trachea. This area requires gentle dilatation before dilatations of the esophagus can be begun. Upper respiratory infections in such infants cause an alarming respiratory obstruction, and occasional dilatations of the trachea are necessary during the intervals between upper respiratory infections.

Caustic burns of the esophagus.—In cases of acute, early, caustic burns, active dilatation is begun 24–48 hours after ingestion of the caustic, using soft rubber, smooth-tipped, catheter-like bougies filled with mercury. Graduated sizes from 16 to 36 F. are well lubricated before being inserted into the mouth and are allowed to advance to the stomach by their own weight. Two or three bougies are used daily, gradually increasing the size during the first 2 weeks. Dilatations are then spaced twice a week for a month, then once a week for another month. Subsequent dilatations are continued at monthly intervals for a year, and then the period between dilatations is increased. Treatment must be continuous in spite of an absence of symptoms if stricture formation is to be avoided. Strictures will form if for one reason or another treatment is discontinued by the patient or the family, or if initial treatment has been delayed because the patient was seen late.

The use of steroids has been strongly advocated by some for the management of acute caustic burns of the esophagus. The relief of pain, the general improvement of swallowing function and the apparent reduction of scar tissue formation have indicated that this therapy is an important adjunct to the management of these patients. Although the immediate effects with this regimen are dramatic, concomitants are an increase in the incidence of gastric hemorrhage, gastric perforation and gastric and particularly pyloric stenosis.

Retrograde, antegrade and endoscopic dilatations generally have been successful in opening and maintaining the esophageal lumen in patients with chronic strictures resulting from caustics. The most rapid and successful technique for this group, particularly in the presence of a gastrostomy, is the dilatation with a Plummer bougie over a string held taut in the gastrostomy opening.

In the small percentage of patients with congenital or acquired esophageal stenoses in whom it becomes apparent that a functioning esophagus cannot be obtained by conservative measures, reconstruction or replacement becomes necessary.[11] Nevertheless, in view of the frequency with which dilatation procedures are necessary after operative correction, it appears that even an only fairly good esophagus is preferable to food passages which are made by various types of surgical procedures. The techniques of these procedures are described elsewhere (see pp. 377 and 382). It should be mentioned, however, that postoperative endoscopic dilatation is most often necessary following resection of a stricture and simple anastomosis of the adjacent ends, particularly when the stricture involves the cardia. A more difficult though less common problem exists at the cervical anastomosis site of a colon transplant. In either case, early recognition of a beginning stenosis followed by active dilatation procedures may succeed in maintaining the lumen whereas delay, with the resulting firm, tortuous stricture formation, may necessitate reoperation to prevent starvation.

Ingested foreign bodies.—Of foreign bodies requiring endoscopic removal, 57% are esophageal.[4] Almost any object that an infant or child can insert into its mouth may become lodged in the food passage. The initial symptoms of coughing, choking, gagging and excessive salivation suggest a foreign body, but once it has become fixed in the esophagus the symptoms may disappear to give a false sense of security that results in a failure to complete the diagnostic studies. There may be no immediate sequelae and the usual tendency is to pass off the incident lightly, thinking it has no significance. Several hours, weeks or even months later, dysphagia or dyspnea or both may develop when esophageal and paraesophageal swelling have occurred, and a roentgenogram reveals a foreign body in the esophagus.

Roentgenographic study in the case of a suspected foreign body should consist of anteroposterior and lateral views of the neck, chest and abdomen. For the lateral roentgenogram, the chin should be thrust forward and the arms held firmly down and back to present the cervical position of the esophagus in a clear silhouette. If there is no evidence of a foreign body, an esophagogram may be necessary, but if immediate

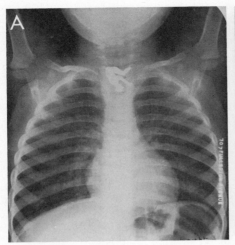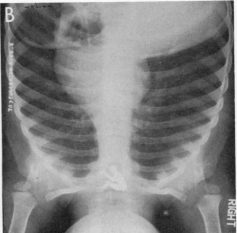

Fig. 30-9.—Esophageal foreign body. **A,** foreign body (toy machine gunner) in cervical esophagus. **B,** study of inverted film clarifies the endoscopic problem, since this will be the approach of the esophagoscopist.

esophagoscopy is anticipated, iodized oil should be used to avoid coating the mucosa and foreign body with white barium paste that makes direct visualization so difficult; otherwise, barium is preferable.

Successful esophagoscopic removal of foreign bodies in infants and children depends to a large extent on the proper choice of instruments and a thorough knowledge of the mechanical problems involved (Fig. 30-9). The use of a large esophagoscope will allow good visualization, but in an infant or a small child a large tube may seriously obstruct respiration or even rupture the esophagus. The forceps must be adaptable to the necessary grasping and manipulation of the particular foreign body and should be of proportionate diameter and length to allow adequate visualization through the esophagoscope employed. A team of experienced assistants will expedite the procedure. In most instances, no anesthesia will be necessary. If the child is more than 2 years old, premedication with morphine sulfate will allow sufficient depression to permit a reasonably quiet procedure. Overdosage may cause severe depression and result in a sudden cessation of respiration during the esophagoscopic procedure. Inhalation anesthesia may be necessary in some instances to obtain increased relaxation, particularly when adequate assistance is not available. Ether is preferred in most cases, administered with an endotracheal tube to ensure adequate ventilation while the esophagoscope is in place.

The esophageal foreign bodies most often found in children are disks, including coins, buttons, washers. Our series comprised 1,209 esophageal foreign bodies in patients of all ages, and in 291 or approximately 50% of the children usually 1–3 years old, the objects were coins. The disk generally lodges in the cervical esophagus, the x-ray showing the circular density at the clavicular level or just above it, while the lateral x-ray shows the edge of the disk. Not uncommonly, two or more coins are seen lying side by side. If the object lodges in any other site in the esophagus, a postoperative esophagram should be made to see if a stricture was responsible.[4]

COMPLICATIONS.—The most serious complication of esophagoscopy is perforation either of the left pyriform sinus or at the level of the cardia. Proper positioning of the patient, careful visual recognition of landmarks as the examination progresses and the use of the "lumen finder" bougie reduce this possibility to a minimum. Perforation during dilatation of strictures is made less likely by use of a previously swallowed thread which serves as a guide. The avoidance of too active a dilatation at any one session reduces the possibility of rupture due to tears between strictures. A perforation will be recognized by rising temperature and pulse and respiratory rates, shock, evidence of subcutaneous emphysema and, in low perforations, mediastinal emphysema, pneumothorax or hydrothorax. Drainage and, if seen early, suture of the tear are indicated. A more conservative approach may be followed in paraesophageal inflammation due to a foreign body or instrumentation. Antibiotics and the temporary withholding of oral feedings usually control this type of infection, although careful x-ray observation of the neck and chest is the only sure means of evaluating the progress or regression of the condition.

As previously mentioned, respiratory obstruction may occur during esophagoscopy in infants because of the easy compressibility of the tracheal cartilages. Constant observation of the respiratory rate and the use of techniques that will permit immediate withdrawal of the esophagoscope should obstruction occur are essential to avoid this complication.

REFERENCES

1. Galloway, T. C.; Soper, G. R., and Elfen, J.: Carcinoma of the larynx after irradiation for papilloma, Arch. Otolaryng. 72:289, 1960.
2. Holinger, P. H.: Clinical aspects of congenital anomalies of the larynx, trachea, bronchi and esophagus, J. Laryng. & Otol. 75:1, 1961.
3. Holinger, P. H.; Johnston, K. C., and Zoss, A. H.: Tracheal and bronchial obstruction due to congenital cardiovascular anomalies, Ann. Otol., Rhin. & Laryng. 57:808, 1948.
4. Holinger, P. H.: Foreign bodies in the air and food passages, Tr. Am. Acad. Ophth. 66:193, 1962.
5. Holinger, P. H., et al.: The conservative and surgical management of benign strictures of the esophagus, J. Thoracic Surg. 28:345, 1954.
6. Jackson, C., and Jackson, C. L.: Diseases of the Air and Food Passages of Foreign Body Origin (Philadelphia: W. B. Saunders Company, 1936).
7. Johnston, K. C., and Holinger, P. H.: Esophageal diseases in infants and children. Postgrad. Med. 25:2, 1959.
8. Majoros, M.; Parkhill, E. M., and Devine, K. D.: Papilloma of the larynx in children—a clinicopathologic study, Am. J. Surg. 108:470, 1964.
9. Meade, R. H., III: Laryngeal obstruction in children, Pediat. Clin. North America 9:233, 1962.
10. Norris, C. M.: Laryngeal and bronchial obstruction in children, New York J. Med. 65:3049, 1965.
11. Potts, W. J., and Idriss, F.: Review of our experience with atresia of the esophagus with and without complicating fistulae, Maryland M. J. 9:528, 1960.
12. Shipkowitz, N. L., et al.: Evaluation of an autogenous laryngeal papilloma vaccine, Laryngoscope 77:993, 1967.
13. Swenson, O., and Oeconomopoulos, C. T.: Achalasia of the esophagus in children, J. Thoracic & Cardiovas. Surg. 41:49, 1961.
14. Weston, J. T.: Airway foreign body fatalities in children, Ann. Otol., Rhin. & Laryng. 74:1144, 1965.

P. H. HOLINGER

Drawing by
ELEANOR KALWEIT

31

Congenital Malformations and Neonatal Problems of the Respiratory Tract

Neonatal Respiratory Distress

THE APPEARANCE of cyanosis or dyspnea in the newborn infant is a justifiable cause for alarm and calls for prompt diagnosis. Excluding pneumonia and congenital heart disease, there are many interesting and urgent conditions that cause respiratory distress in the newborn and some require immediate surgical therapy. Causes for respiratory distress due to decreased pulmonary ventilation may be divided into three general groups: obstruction of the airway, pulmonary displacement, and pulmonary deficiency.

If the cyanosis and rapid, labored respiration are due to an obstruction of the airway, the infant will also have stridor and marked suprasternal and intercostal inspiratory retractions. Examination of the nose, mouth and throat and laryngoscopy may disclose the underlying pathology. The need for x-ray examination of the chest and lateral films of the head and neck is obvious. Bronchoscopy may be indicated if the obstruction appears low in the respiratory tract.

The dyspnea due to pulmonary deficiency or displacement is not accompanied by stridor or severe inspiratory retractions. The infant will have rapid and labored respirations with varying degrees of cyanosis, depending on the amount of pulmonary tissue that is nonfunctioning. Physical examination of the infant and x-ray study of the chest will usually indicate the cause of the respiratory distress.

Obstruction of the Airway

The airway may be obstructed anywhere along the respiratory system from the nasal choanae to the smaller bronchi. The obstruction may be complete or partial, intrinsic or extrinsic.

Choanal atresia, if bilateral, produces alarming respiratory difficulties in the newborn until the infant learns to breathe by mouth. Cyanosis at rest, relieved by crying, is the clue to this condition. Insertion of a plastic anesthesia airway will relieve the symptoms immediately.

The Pierre Robin syndrome with hypoplasia of the mandible may cause obstruction of the upper airway by posterior displacement of the tongue (Fig. 31-1). Macroglossia in itself may lead to respiratory difficulties. A suture in the tongue to hold it forward or positioning of the infant face down on a frame establishes a patent airway.

Tumors of the neck and floor of the mouth often obstruct the airway, either by external pressure, such as results from congenital goiter or large thyroglossal duct cysts, or by actual invasion of the epiglottis, larynx or trachea by tumors, notably hemangiomas and lymphangiomas (Fig. 31-2). (See also Figs. 20-1 and 21-7.) Cysts or abscesses may be aspirated as an emergency treatment.

Intrinsic obstruction of the larynx may be caused by deformity of the epiglottis by stenosis, or by actual atresia. Tracheal and bronchial obstruction can occur from mucous plugs or aspirated vomitus or may be due to stenosis or collapse from deficiency of the cartilaginous support. External pressure exerted by vascular rings or bronchial cysts may produce partial tracheal or bronchial obstruction. Tracheostomy usually after trans oral intubation, may be life-saving in some instances of obstructive lesions involving the pharynx or larynx.

Pulmonary Displacement

Space-occupying lesions in the pleural cavities produce respiratory distress by compressing the normal lung and reducing respiratory reserve.

Paralysis of the diaphragm, usually due to birth injury, results in striking elevation of the diaphragm, compression of the ipsilateral lung and mediastinal shift (Fig. 31-3). Conservative measures usually will tide the patient over until the condition can be toler-

Fig. 31-1 (left).—Pierre Robin syndrome. This newborn had respiratory difficulty, especially during feedings. Gavage through a small plastic feeding tube and positioning to extend the neck with the child in lateral position tided the patient over for several weeks until the condition was better tolerated. At times, it is necessary to advance the tongue, preferably by a plastic procedure on the mucous membrane.

Fig. 31-2 (right).—Lymphangioma infiltrating the neck and tongue, causing respiratory obstruction (preoperative view). Removal was attempted at age 1 week, but widespread extension into trachea, larynx, esophagus, floor of the mouth and mediastinum made complete removal impossible. Tracheostomy was necessary postoperatively, and radiotherapy was given. Three years later, most of the neck deformity was gone. but the tongue was still enlarged and covered by cysts.

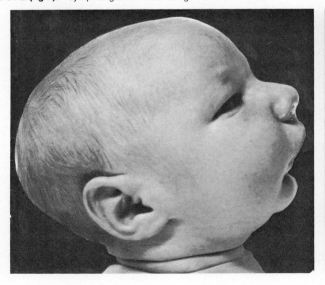
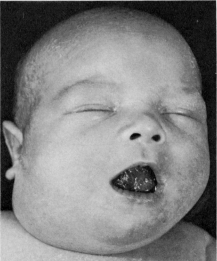

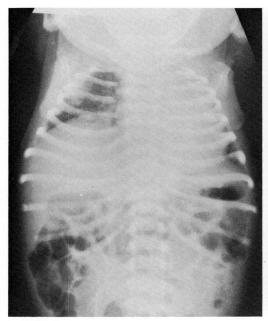

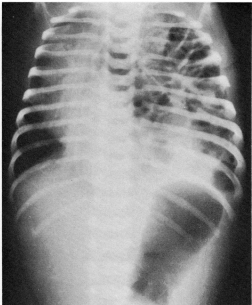

Fig. 31-3 (left).—Right diaphragmatic paralysis due to phrenic nerve injury during a difficult delivery. Dyspnea and cyanosis were present from birth. Elevation of the diaphragm with mediastinal shift and cardiac displacement leaves little aerated lung. Oxygen therapy and semiupright positioning relieved symptoms, and in several weeks the child could leave the hospital. Ultimate outlook should be good, though regeneration of the nerve is unlikely.

Fig. 31-4 (right).—Diaphragmatic hernia on the left, causing progressively severe cyanosis and dyspnea in this 2-day-old child. Loops of bowel collapsed the left lung, herniating across the mediastinum to the opposite side. Only the gas-filled stomach remains in the small abdominal cavity. Immediate laparotomy with reduction of bowel and repair of the defect in the foramen of Bochdalek was done. Recovery was uneventful. (See also pp. 342 ff.)

Fig. 31-5 (left).—Spontaneous pneumothorax in this 3-day-old child caused sudden, very severe respiratory distress. The collapsed lung is seen at the right hilus. The tension pneumothorax has herniated the anterior mediastinum, compressing the opposite lung. Immediate insertion of an intercostal catheter through a trocar, with closed drainage, relieved symptoms, and sealing of the leak with re-expansion of the lung was complete in 24 hours.

Fig. 31-6 (right).—Congenital tension cysts in the right upper lobe caused severe, rapidly increasing respiratory distress in this 4-day-old infant. Septa are seen in the radiolucent area, but no true lung markings. Mediastinal shift has caused compression of the right lower and middle lobes and the opposite lung. Lobectomy at age 5 days gave dramatic relief, and the child was asymptomatic thereafter.

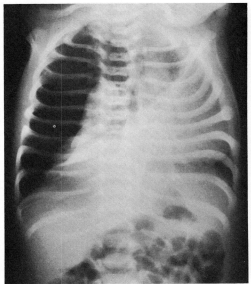

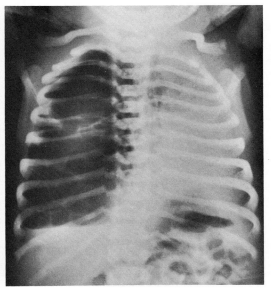

ated. Only once in our experience has imbrication of the diaphragm been considered necessary to save the patient. Eventration of the diaphragm, with thinning of the dome and reduction of peripheral musculature, produces pulmonary compression in a similar manner. Diaphragmatic hernia in the newborn frequently causes severe distress. Diagnosis can be made from an upright roentgenogram of the chest that shows multiple spaces with air-fluid levels (Fig. 31-4). Distress occurs as much from pulmonary inadequacy as from displacement (see p. 349). During the wait for emergency surgical correction, continuous aspiration of the stomach may prevent increasing distress due to swallowed air entering the bowel in the chest. If the respiratory problem is severe, it may be necessary to insert an endotracheal tube and breathe for the infant to make optimal use of all lung tissue that can be aerated.

Pneumothorax[1,9] is usually easy to differentiate since a nubbin of collapsed lung remains at the hilus (Fig. 31-5). The pneumothorax may be due to spontaneous rupture of a surface bleb during vigorous crying; or it is more likely due to the forcing of air into the tracheobronchial tree under excessive pressure during resuscitative efforts in the newborn period (see Fig. 31-9). If the pneumothorax is sufficient to cause respiratory distress from compression of the lung and mediastinal displacement, closed drainage with an intercostal catheter is necessary. Congenital lung cysts may balloon up rapidly; they are characterized by large air-containing cavities with well-defined margins (Fig. 31-6). Treatment of tension cysts in the newborn is immediate resection of the cyst or the involved lobe. Temporary catheter decompression may be necessary as an emergency measure. Lobar emphysema and interstitial emphysema are dealt with in more detail below.

Pulmonary Deficiency

A third cause of neonatal respiratory distress is deficiency in the lungs themselves, as in neonatal atelectasis, pulmonary aplasia and hyaline membrane disease. It is a prime cause of death of infants with diaphragmatic hernia in which the lung is underdeveloped.

ATELECTASIS OF THE NEWBORN.[6,11]—One of the briefest and most precarious periods in an individual's existence is on his entry into extrauterine life. At birth, the lungs suddenly must assume function by inflation of the alveoli. This is accomplished by the positive pressure of crying and by the negative pressure exerted by the contracting diaphragm. The latter pressure, sometimes as high as -50 cm of water, helps to pull apart the moist alveolar walls held together by powerful cohesive forces. This expansion has been shown to be gradual, taking from 24 hours to 3 days for completion.

It should be stressed that the condition being considered is not a resorption atelectasis secondary to

obstruction but a primary lack of expansion. In the lungs of a premature infant there is the additional factor of anatomic immaturity of the lung.

Cyanosis and dyspnea usually appear immediately after birth or within a few hours. These symptoms are relieved by oxygen administration but recur promptly when this treatment is discontinued. Usually there are striking lower sternal retraction ("diaphragmatic tug") and decreased breath sounds. Roentgenograms of the chest may show poorly aerated lungs.

The first step in therapy is a thorough clearing of the airways, using the laryngoscope or even the bronchoscope if necessary and feasible. The tiny lumen of a 3-mm bronchoscope, the size accommodated by a newborn infant's larynx and trachea, in itself offers great resistance to ventilation. Thus insertion should be deft and rapid, suctioning done quickly and the instrument withdrawn immediately. After this, some form of limited pressure ventilation (not over 30 cm of water) may be helpful, and oxygen administration may compensate for the temporary decrease of aeration.

In some newborn infants, especially prematures, the cartilaginous portions of the rib cage may be extremely mobile, and with each piston-like stroke of the diaphragm, the sternum draws inward, preventing an effective build-up of the vital negative pressure, much as in a steering-wheel injury in the adult. In such cases, partial sternal fixation may be helpful,[11,12,14] obtained by fastening a towel clip percutaneously into the fibrous tissue on the anterior surface of the lower end of the sternum. Gentle traction is then exerted upward to the roof of the incubator by means of a rubber band. A second point of traction in the upper portion of the sternum may be necessary occasionally. Traction must be maintained for several days, until pulmonary expansion is complete.

Another factor, thought at times to prevent alveolar expansion, is the rigidity of a small thoracic cage which confines the lungs in spite of positive pressure exerted by vigorous crying or mechanical means. Some surgeons advocate unilateral thoracotomy in the fifth intercostal space to release the lung and allow its expansion under direct vision with positive pressure of 15–30 cm of water.[2] Although this might be applicable in rare and selected cases, I doubt the necessity or advisability of such drastic therapy. At the Children's Memorial Hospital we have never had occasion to employ this type of treatment. It is contraindicated in the premature infant, and bilateral thoracotomy for this purpose is unjustified.

HYALINE MEMBRANE DISEASE.—Characteristically, hyaline membrane disease, or neonatal respiratory distress syndrome, produces tachypnea within 2 hours of birth (Fig. 31-7). As dyspnea increases, cyanosis becomes evident. The lungs are dull on percussion, breath sounds gradually decrease in intensity, and rales become progressively widespread. Diffuse em-

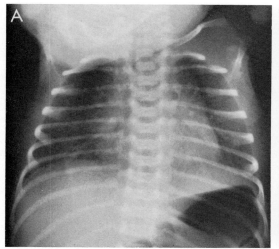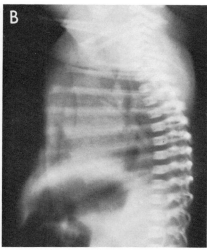

Fig. 31-7.—Hyaline membrane disease (neonatal respiratory distress syndrome). This child, the second of twins delivered by breech, weighed 1,745 Gm. A few hours after birth, there were cyanosis, severe tachypnea, with marked subcostal and sternal retractions. Retraction persisted for 36 hours and tachypnea for 48, followed by gradual improvement. The baby ultimately did well. The only treatment was keeping him in an atmosphere of high humidity for 72 hours. In fatal instances, respiratory difficulty progresses to death in 48–72 hours, often with bloody froth in the air passages. Autopsy in such cases shows atelectasis, with hyaline membrane covering the surfaces of the dilated alveolar ducts. Scattered hemorrhages throughout, with leukocytic proliferation are common. **A,** posteroanterior view, showing diffuse, fine granularity in the lung fields. **B,** lateral view, showing sharp sternal retraction.

physema may be seen with an unexpanded chest and flattened diaphragm. Excessive pulmonary secretions are common. Half the afflicted infants die, usually in 24–48 hours after birth.[14] The condition is of unknown etiology and commonest in premature infants, infants born by cesarean section and infants born of diabetic mothers. Treatment includes use of antibiotics, a moist atmosphere and oxygen. Traction on the sternum has been reported to aid respirations,[12] and tracheostomy with positive pressure respiration has been used successfully.[4]

LOBAR EMPHYSEMA.—Lobar emphysema may cause respiratory distress in infancy.[5,7,8,10,13,15,16] The most interesting and urgent type is the rapidly ballooning emphysema seen in very young infants and almost always confined to a single lobe.[16] It results from incomplete bronchial obstruction that allows ingress of air during inspiration but prevents egress of air during expiration. The obstruction may be intraluminal, due to an intrinsic web or vessel; mural, due to a deficiency of cartilaginous support, or extrinsic, due to pressure from anomalous vessels or a ligamentum arteriosum. The apparent absence of a discernible mechanism in certain instances may be due to the fact that division and suture of the bronchus during lobectomy are at the site of the lesion producing the obstruction, which is thus destroyed, or left behind in the sutured bronchial stump. A localized deficiency of bronchial cartilage is the most likely cause,[11,15] and the occasional patient with symptoms persisting after lobectomy may have similar areas in other bronchi.

Dyspnea, diminished excursion of the affected side with decreased breath sounds and hyperresonance and increasing cyanosis should prompt immediate roentgen study of the chest (Fig. 31-8). A radiolucent

Fig. 31-8.—Lobar emphysema involving left upper lobe, causing increasing dyspnea and cyanosis at age 14 days. Diminished breath sounds were noted over the left chest, with mediastinal shift to the right. This film shows herniation of the mobile anterior mediastinum. A filmy web of lung markings in the radiolucent area suggests emphysema rather than lung cyst. Immediate lobectomy led to uneventful recovery. No specific cause of obstruction was found in the resected specimen.

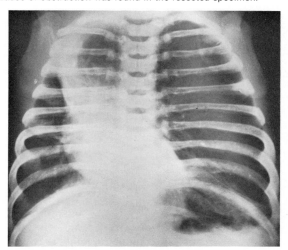

area in the lung fields, with a shift of the mediastinum, is suggestive of lobar emphysema or congenital lung cyst. The appearance of scattered lung markings in the area of radiolucency usually differentiates lobar emphysema from lung cyst and pneumothorax.

The emphysema due to foreign bodies, or inflammatory swelling of the bronchial lining, is usually less severe and more often occurs in the older infant and child. Bronchoscopy should be resorted to in order to establish the causative factor. Visualization of the offending bronchus in lobar emphysema may be impossible, however, since it is the upper lobe which is most often involved.

Many very young infants with rapidly ballooning lobar emphysema present such emergencies that delay of operation is dangerous and unjustified. Lobectomy is the treatment of choice, and since the upper lobe is almost always the lobe involved, the incision is made in the fifth intercostal space. During induction of anesthesia, positive pressure may further overinflate the lobe and reduce respiratory exchange to such an extent that rapid thoracotomy must be done to free the lobe and save the infant. The pulmonary hilar structures usually are well-defined in an infant and unencumbered by inflammatory residua, so that lobectomy is usually easier than in older patients, and the principal burden of technical proficiency rests on the anesthesiologist.

Needle aspiration of the emphysematous lobe has been suggested as definitive treatment,[10] but in the 2 reported instances, pneumothorax occurred, requiring further aspiration. Both patients survived without resection.

When treated by immediate lobectomy, this condition has an excellent prognosis. The only place needle aspiration may have is as an emergency measure while one prepares for operation. All 11 children treated by resection at the Children's Memorial Hospital have survived and are perfectly normal. No discernible effect on growth or activity has been noted. There was one death in 33 reported resections.[8] About 14% are thought to have some respiratory symptoms in succeeding years, perhaps due to other anatomically defective bronchi.

INTERSTITIAL EMPHYSEMA.—In the infant, overinflation of the lungs due to vigorous artificial respiration, the strain of severe coughing or crying, or overenthusiastic positive pressure anesthesia may result in alveolar rupture and leaking of air into the perivascular connective tissues. This interstitial emphysema may rupture into the pleural cavity, producing pneumothorax or dissect into the mediastinal structures, eventually reaching the subcutaneous spaces[3,9] (Fig. 31-9).

If this process continues, increasing dyspnea and cyanosis occur, the cardiac sounds become muffled, and finally the blood pressure falls. This distress is thought to be due to several factors: splinting of the lung by the trapped interstitial air, reduction of the

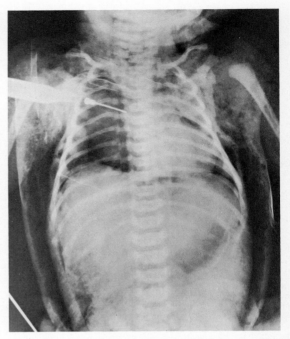

Fig. 31-9.—Pneumomediastinum and subcutaneous emphysema in a newborn who required resuscitation, which was given by mouth-to-mouth insufflation. It was noted that "each time the doctor blew into the child's mouth, the child got bigger." Tubes were put into the anterior mediastinum and both pleural cavities. The air absorbed, and the child left the hospital well.

respiratory volume by the pneumomediastinum or pneumothorax, and compression of veins, especially the pulmonary return, by the air in the mediastinum and pulmonary roots. Pneumopericardium causes the typical picture of cardiac tamponade, necessitating pericardial aspiration. Roentgenograms of the chest show the presence of air in the mediastinum, pleural cavity or pericardium.

Mild degrees of this condition occur and require only oxygen administration. In more urgent cases, aspiration of the larger collections of air in the pleural cavity or mediastinum may suffice, or insertion of a catheter through a trocar may become necessary for tension pneumothorax. Thoracotomy for evacuation of loculated air in the mediastinum, with establishment of adequate drainage, has been described.[3] In our experience, this has never been necessary.

REFERENCES

1. Abramson, H., and Rook, G. D.: Pneumothorax in infancy and childhood, J. Pediat. 36:744, 1950.
2. Berglund, E., and Eder, W. P.: A surgical approach to atelectasis of the newborn infant, Surgery 29:127, 1951.
3. Berman, E. J., and Kahn, A. J.: Pulmonary interstitial emphysema with air block syndrome, J. Pediat. 51:457, 1957.
4. Colgan, F. J.; Eldrup-Jorgensen, S., and Lawrence, R. M.: Maintenance of respiration in the neonatal respiratory

distress syndrome, J. A. M. A. 173:1557, 1960.

5. Ehrenhaft, J. L., and Taber, R. E.: Progressive infantile emphysema in infancy: Surgical emergency, J. Thoracic Surg. 26:1, 1953.
6. Farber, S., and Wilson, J. L.: Atelectasis of the newborn, Am. J. Dis. Child. 46:572, 1933.
7. Fischer, H. E.; Lucido, J. L., and Lynxwiller, C. P.: Lobar emphysema, J.A.M.A. 166:340, 1958.
8. Fischer, W.; Potts, W. J., and Holinger, P. H.: Lobar emphysema in infants and children, J. Pediat. 41:4, 1952.
9. Hurwitz, S., and Greenwood, H.: Pneumothorax and pneumomediastinum in the newborn infant, J. Pediat. 45:437, 1954.
10. Korngold, H. W., and Baker, J. M.: Nonsurgical treatment of unilobar obstructive emphysema of the newborn, Pedi-

atrics 14:296, 1954.
11. Love, W. G., and Tillery, B.: New treatment for atelectasis of the newborn, Am. J. Dis. Child. 86:423, 1953.
12. Michaelson, R. P.: Treatment of atelectasis of the newborn by sternal traction, Laryngoscope 63:379, 1953.
13. Nelson, T. Y.: Tension emphysema in infants, Arch. Dis. Childhood 32:38, 1957.
14. Schaffer, A. J.: *Diseases of the Newborn* (2d ed.; Philadelphia: W. B. Saunders Company, 1965), p. 111.
15. Sloan, H.: Lobar obstructive emphysema in infancy treated by lobectomy, J. Thoracic Surg. 26:1, 1953.
16. Thomson, J., and Forfar, J. O.: Regional obstructive emphysema in infants, Arch. Dis. Childhood 33:97, 1958.

W. L. RIKER

Chylothorax

SUDDEN ACCUMULATIONS OF chyle in the thorax or abdomen occur at three periods of life: (1) in the neonatal period; (2) in later childhood when it is usually due to trauma, either accidental as in compression injuries to the chest or by direct operative injury to the thoracic duct, and (3) later in life when, in addition to trauma, neoplastic and inflammatory obstructions of the thoracic duct lead to extravasation.

SPONTANEOUS CHYLOTHORAX.—A newborn infant or one in the first month of life presenting with dyspnea, mediastinal displacement and a collection of fluid filling one hemithorax, usually the right, may, in the absence of any evidence of infection, be assumed to have a chylothorax. It has been shown[1] that ligation of the vena cava in dogs and cats will cause a chylous pleural effusion in 50% of the animals, and it seems reasonable to suppose that abrupt rises of venous pressure in the course of delivery or during resuscitative attempts immediately after delivery should result in thoracic duct rupture. The extravasated chyle presently ruptures from the mediastinum into the pleural cavity. In a number of instances, operation has disclosed one or several fistulas between the thoracic duct and the pleural cavity. It is probable that some of such openings represent congenital fistulas. Generally, one must assume that a traumatic rupture of the thoracic duct occurred during the birth process.

The very small number of reported cases—5 from the Mayo Clinic,[6] 16 in Boles and Izant's[2] review and 38 in Tischer's[8] review (which failed to find the 2 cases reported here in the first edition)—merely indicates that most clinics see only 1 or 2 of such cases and that most of the individual instances are not reported. Eleven of the 16 patients reviewed by Boles and Izant had effusion and respiratory distress within the first 5 days of life, and 5 of the 11 were in respiratory distress within hours of birth.

Given the observed rate of reaccumulation of chyle, this suggests that in some of these infants the chyle might have been present in the pleural cavity before birth, having leaked through such a fistulous orifice as has been described. We have seen a child with a chylous effusion in the peritoneal cavity— chylous ascites—which caused troublesome distention and respiratory distress from the elevated diaphragm immediately after delivery—obviously an antenatal ascites. It is of more than passing interest that the effusion occurred on the right side in 11 of Boles' 16 patients and was bilateral in 1.

In the chylothorax of the neonatal period, repeated aspiration seems to be all the treatment required (Fig. 31-10). Some patients respond to two or three thoracenteses yielding a total of only several ounces of fluid. The greatest total amount of fluid aspirated from a child who recovered was the 1,955 cc aspirated in 27 thoracenteses over 30 days by Boles and Izant.[2] Both patients of Randolph and Gross[5] were operated on, the only 2 successfully so treated, but in only 1 was it thought that the chylous leaks were closed and the proximal thoracic duct ligated successfully. The 2 patients we saw at the Harriet Lane Home, both with right-sided effusions, responded to aspiration in a few days and presented no therapeutic problem. Among Tischer's[8] 38 collected cases in the first 3 months of life, there were 6 deaths in the 10 cases seen in 1944 or earlier, none of them in patients treated operatively. In the 28 subsequent cases there were 2 deaths, both in infants with bilateral effusions in the immediate postnatal period, 1 treated with bilateral tube drainage, 1 not treated. Of the 26 survivors seen since 1944, only 4 were operated on. Nutrition may become a serious problem in children requiring repeated thoracentesis, because of the loss of both protein and fat.[3] Reinfusion of the aspirated chyle is feasible, and has been done, but at times with catastrophic reactions.

TRAUMATIC CHYLOTHORAX.—The principal experience with traumatic chylothorax has been afforded after thoracic operations and in particular the Blalock

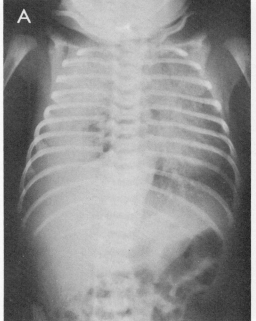 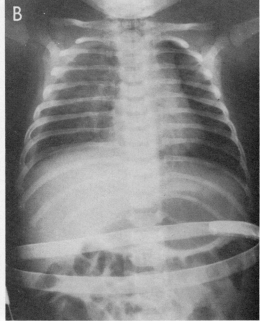

Fig. 31-10.—Spontaneous chylothorax in the neonate. This 22-day-old baby had had respiratory distress for 10 days. Three aspirations on successive days totaling 61 cc of characteristic creamy white chyle relieved her symptoms and there was no reaccumulation. She remained well. **A,** initial film before aspiration. The entire right hemithorax is filled with opaque fluid. The heart is displaced against the left chest wall; the right lung is the small nubbin compressed against the mediastinum. **B,** after aspiration, the lung is almost fully expanded but for a little evidence of fluid or thickened pleura at the periphery.

operation for tetralogy of Fallot performed on the left side. Although Shumacker and Moore[6] assumed an aggressive attitude toward these lesions and operated promptly to ligate the thoracic duct proximal to the fistula, Maloney and Spencer,[4] with an experience of 13 cases of traumatic chylothorax seen on the cardiac surgery service of the Johns Hopkins Hospital, found that 11 of the 13 patients responded readily to repeated aspiration. Only 2 required operative ligation of the duct, both of whom survived.

There seems to be general agreement that underwater-seal catheter drainage to keep the lung expanded and promote its adherence to the chest wall is the soundest therapy. If drainage persists in quantities beyond the tolerance of the child and shows no sign of diminishing, or is persisting after 2 or 3 weeks, one is justified, whether for neonatal or surgically produced chylothorax, in ligating the thoracic duct just above the diaphragm through a right thoracotomy. This is, however, rarely necessary.

REFERENCES

1. Blalock, A.; Cunningham, R. S., and Robinson, C. S.: Experimental production of chylothorax by occlusion of superior vena cava, Ann. Surg. 104:359, 1936.
2. Boles, E. T., and Izant, R. J., Jr.: Spontaneous chylothorax in the neonatal period, Am. J. Surg. 99:870, 1960.
3. Burdette, W. J.: Management of chylous extravasation, Arch. Surg. 78:815, 1959.
4. Maloney, J. V., Jr., and Spencer, F. C.: The nonoperative treatment of traumatic chylothorax, Surgery 40:121, 1956.
5. Randolph, J. G., and Gross, R. E.: Congenital chylothorax, Arch. Surg. 74:405, 1957.
6. Roy, P. H.; Carr, D. J., and Payne, W. S.: The problem of chylothorax, Mayo Clin. Proc. 42:457, 1967.
7. Shumacker, H. B, Jr., and Moore, T. C.: Surgical management of traumatic chylothorax, Surg., Gynec. & Obst. 93:46, 1951.
8. Tischer, W.: Der Chylothorax im ersten Trimenon, Ztschr. Kinderchir. 5:43, 1967.

M. M. RAVITCH

Pulmonary Agenesis

THERE MAY BE complete agenesis of both lungs, one lung, a lobe, or lobes. Minetto *et al.*,[3] in their exhaustive review of the subject, divided the lesions into bilateral pulmonary agenesis, unilateral pulmonary agenesis, pulmonary aplasia, pulmonary hypoplasia and lobar aplasia. Agenesis has been known to exist for several hundred years; Morgagni described it in 1762. In 1907, Von Eiken first made the clinical diagnosis correctly. Boenninger in 1928 first made the diagnosis on the basis of bronchography, and Stokes

and Brown in 1940 first confirmed the diagnosis bronchoscopically.

Bilateral pulmonary agenesis is the rarest malformation, of which some half-dozen cases have been reported. Curiously, the children are not necessarily stillborn and may make respiratory efforts. The trachea may be entirely wanting, or a portion of it may be preserved with or without an associated esophageal anomaly. Cardiac anomalies are usually associated.

Thirty instances of *unilateral pulmonary agenesis* were collected by Minetto and his colleagues, 17 on the left and 13 on the right. Although about half the infants with pulmonary agenesis as their principal

Fig. 31-11.—Agenesis of the left lung. A 12-year-old girl had profound pectus excavatum (see Fig. 26-5, *E*) ectromelia of the hand and disabling dyspnea rapidly progressive for the past 2 years. **A,** posteroanterior film, showing the heart in the left chest, mediastinal hernia into the left chest and opacity of unknown nature in the left upper chest. **B,** bronchogram, showing only a stump of the left main bronchus. This was also observed bronchoscopically, when the right main bronchus showed a yielding external compression, as if by a vessel. **C,** angiocardiogram; catheter in right pulmonary artery. There is no evidence of a left pulmonary artery. **D,** angiocardiogram; left heart phase. The left ventricle and ascending and descending aorta are clearly visible. Some of the opacity remains unaccounted for—possibly thymus. (From Ravitch and Matzen.[4])

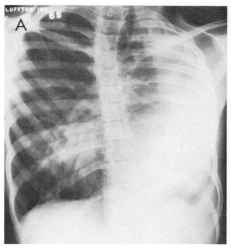
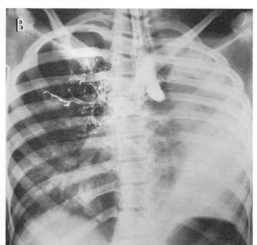
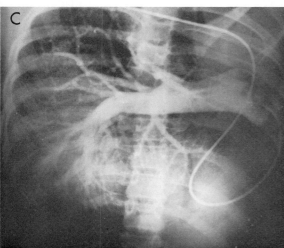
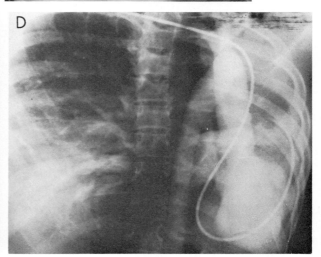

lesion die in infancy or early childhood, the reported cases have included patients aged 60 and 70 dying of other causes. Skeletal, cardiac and other visceral anomalies are commonly associated. Respiratory symptoms—dyspnea, cyanosis, harsh breathing—are common, and even the children who survive frequently show retarded development. Although in some instances the chest on the affected side may be less well developed, it is striking that more often the outward appearance of the thorax does not suggest absence of a lung. The flattening of the chest and narrowing of the interspaces which occur after pneumonectomy are not usually found in pulmonary agenesis. Presumably this is due to the fact that from early intrauterine life the heart has been completely displaced into the hemithorax left empty by pulmonary agenesis, and the thorax is, in a sense, filled. The mediastinum is markedly shifted and the percussion note over the affected side is flat. Roentgenograms show a dense homogeneous shadow on the affected side, with the heart entirely in that hemithorax. The clinical story of respiratory difficulty, with the roentgenogram showing a massive mediastinal shift, is often interpreted as massive atelectasis. Bronchoscopy shows absence of one major bronchus, and bronchography confirms this observation (Fig. 31-11). Collected series suggest a predilection for the left side and for males. As might be expected, absence of the right lung is associated with more symptoms and a shorter life expectancy than absence of the left lung.

The cause of death has been a source of considerable discussion, particularly when other significant anomalies are not found and in view of the fact that in perhaps half the reported cases pulmonary agenesis has been compatible with normal life. The patients who died usually had a history of severe dyspnea, frequently with wheezing and cough. A few had obvious pulmonary infections in the sole lung. Maier and Gould[1] operated on a 10-week-old infant who had been born prematurely and had been subject to frequent and severe bouts of respiratory distress for the previous 4 weeks. The diagnosis of agenesis of the right lung was made correctly, and operation was undertaken in an attempt to relieve the respiratory distress, thought to be due to pressure on the trachea. The child had often held her head in an extended position and tended to tire while feeding. At operation, the trachea was found compressed and deviated by an abnormally coursing aorta lying unusually far toward the right. It was not possible to relieve the compression and displacement, and the infant died. Maier suggested that such kinking of trachea or bronchus, plain at the operating table, obscure at autopsy, may account for some deaths. Anomalies of lobation

and of the bronchovascular patterns of the remaining lung have been reported[4] but the remaining lung is not decreased in size and should be adequate to sustain life.

Minetto counted 93 reports of patients with *pulmonary aplasia*, a condition in which, once more, the lung is absent but there is a rudimentary bronchial stump. The carina is normal, seen bronchoscopically. The main bronchus on the affected side may end blindly or may show a tentative division into several branch bronchi. The symptoms, prognosis and state of the contralateral lung are essentially the same as in total agenesis.

Pulmonary hypoplasia, as analyzed by Minetto, composes a heterogeneous group of conditions, including an underdeveloped lung in association with a diaphragmatic hernia, hypoplastic lung with absence of a pulmonary artery, and a globular malformation in which a mass of poorly differentiated pulmonary tissue is attached to a malformed and underdeveloped bronchus.

Lobar aplasia has been reported some 30-odd times. It may be unilobar or bilobar. A combination of absence of the right upper lobe and right middle lobe is the commonest single type. The heart is markedly displaced to the side of the agenesis, and repeated pulmonary infections seem to be common in patients in this group. If the bronchial connections to the remaining lobe, or lobes, on the affected side are adequate and if angiocardiography shows normal pulmonary vasculature, there is no treatment to be offered. If the bronchi are inadequate, or if no pulmonary artery or an extremely small one is found to the remaining lobe, a resection may relieve the symptoms.

REFERENCES

1. Maier, H. C., and Gould, W. J.: Agenesis of the lung with vascular compression of the tracheobronchial tree, J. Pediat. 143:38, 1953.
2. Marioni, P.: Agenesis of the lung, Dis. Chest 41:232, 1962.
3. Minetto, E.; Galli, E., and Boglione, G.: Agenesia, aplasia, ipoplasia polmonare, Minerva med. 49:4635, 1958.
4. Ravitch, M. M., and Matzen, R. N.: Pulmonary insufficiency in pectus excavatum associated with left pulmonary agenesis, congenital clubbed feet and ectromelia: Improvement following operation, Dis. Chest. 54:58, 1968.
5. Thomas, L. B., and Boyden, E. A.: Agenesis of the right lung, Surgery 31:429, 1952.
6. Valle, A. R., and Graham, E. A.: Agenesis of the lung, J. Thoracic Surg. 13:345, 1944.
7. VanLoon, E. L., and Diamond, S.: Congenital absence of the right lung: Its occurrence in a healthy child, Am. J. Dis. Child. 62:584, 1941.
8. Wexels, P.: Agenesis of the lung, Thorax 6:171, 1951.

M. M. RAVITCH

Abnormal Tracheobronchial Communications and Variations in Lobation

ABNORMAL TRACHEAL COMMUNICATION.—The commonest of this type of abnormality is certainly that associated with esophageal atresia (see Chap. 28).

The single commonest anomalous bronchial origin associated with symptoms is so-called ectopic tracheal bronchus (trifurcation of the trachea), which usually arises on the right side. It is thought sometimes to represent an apical segmental bronchus arising separately proximal to the carina and at other times to be truly supernumerary. The eparterial bronchus of a number of animal species arises from the trachea separately, and the situation then appears to be not unlike that seen in these patients. The abnormally arising pulmonary segments are frequently the site of repeated pulmonary infection which requires resection for relief.[1] Roshe[2] described an unusual variant in which there were one tracheal bronchus and two additional separate bronchi of the upper lobe, one arising essentially from the trachea at the origin of the right main bronchus and the other just below it. Each of the three segments had an anomalous pulmonary vein draining into the superior vena cava. Resection of the three segments cured the repeated attacks of pulmonary infection. The abnormal pulmonary venous drainage had not been anticipated.

A fascinating anomaly of tracheobronchial communication is that in which there is a congenital bronchobiliary fistula. Stigol, Traversaro and Trigo[3] from Buenos Aires reported on a 14-month-old infant with repeated pulmonary infections and yellow sputum. Bronchography demonstrated an anomalous passage downward from the right side of the tracheal bifurcation to the region of the diaphragm. The bronchoscope could be passed into this channel, which was seen to contain bile. At operation, the tubular tract was divided from its origin in the right main bronchus, close to the carina, and the tract followed down through the diaphragm for at least 2 cm. The tract contained bile. Histologically, it was like bronchus proximally and like esophagus distally. Three previously published cases and one unpublished were also mentioned. Weitzman et al.[5] have described an identical case in a child 2 years and 9 months old.

VARIATIONS IN LOBATION.—The lingular segment of the left upper lobe occasionally is entirely separated, as if it were a left middle lobe, and other segments may be so demarcated. The azygos lobe on the right side is not an abnormality of lobation but a radiographic phenomenon created by the passage of the azygos vein in a sulcus in the posterior aspect of the left upper lobe and can be diagnosed from the characteristic, almost vertical shadow of the vein in the plain x-ray film. The condition causes no symptoms and requires no treatment.

Thomson and Aguino[4] treated a newborn infant with severe respiratory distress. The baby died after ligation of a large patent ductus and of the vessels to what appeared to be an unaerated right lung. No right main bronchus arose from the trachea. There was a fistula between the lower third of the esophagus and a bronchus leading to the right lung. The right lung was unilobar, and the vasculature and the bronchial distribution were those of a normal right lower lobe.

REFERENCES

1. Marks, C.: The ectopic tracheal bronchus: Management of a child by excision and segmental pulmonary resection, Dis. Chest 50:652, 1966.
2. Roshe, J.: Bronchovascular anomalies of the right upper lobe, J. Thoracic & Cardiovas. Surg. 50:86, 1965.
3. Stigol, L. C.; Traversaro, J., and Trigo, E. R.: Carinal trifurcation with congenital tracheobiliary fistula, Pediatrics 37:89, 1966.
4. Thomson, N. B., Jr., and Aguino, T.: Anomalous origin of the right main stem bronchus, Surgery 51:668, 1962.
5. Weitzman, J. J.; Cohen, S. E., Woods, L. O., Jr., and Chadwick, D. L.: Congenital bronchobiliary fistula, J. Pediat. 73:329, 1968.

M. M. RAVITCH

Anomalies of the Pulmonary Vessels

A VARIETY OF ANOMALIES of the pulmonary vasculature are of significance particularly in respect to their relation to the lungs and quite apart from the considerations related to cardiovascular surgery.[2]

ANOMALOUS SYSTEMIC ARTERIES SUPPLYING THE LUNG

In the discussion later in this chapter of congenital cystic disease of the lung and of lower accessory lung, instances are mentioned in which these conditions are associated with one or several large arteries from the descending thoracic aorta or the abdominal aorta entering the periphery of the lung. In some of these cases, there is no pulmonary artery; in others, both types of arterial circulation exist.

HYPOPLASTIC LUNG WITH ANOMALOUS SYSTEMIC ARTERIES

Maier[5] reported on a 12-year-old girl with moderate dyspnea and diminished volume of the right lung. Angiocardiography showed a small right pulmonary artery. At operation, two large systemic arteries were found perforating the diaphragm and supplying the right lung. The vessels were divided, and the patient was relieved of symptoms. A 14-year-old boy with frequent respiratory infections, cough, sputum and dyspnea had an anomalous bronchial architecture.[5] At operation, no pulmonary arteries or veins supplying the right lung were found. A number of arteries entered the lung from the diaphragm, and venous drainage was into the superior vena cava. The lung was removed.

ABSENCE OF THE PULMONARY ARTERY TO ONE LUNG

Patients with this anomaly show some reduction in the volume of the abnormal lung and absence of the normal hilar vascular shadows. The mediastinum is displaced toward the anomalous lung, and the contralateral lung is overdistended and emphysematous. Maier reported such an instance in a boy of 9 with recurrent pulmonary infection. There was no pulmonary artery. The pulmonary veins were normal. The arterial supply was from a systemic vessel descending along the trachea and entering the right upper lobe. Absence of the pulmonary artery is more common on the right than on the left. A number of such patients have been seen, some with symptoms of pulmonary infection sufficient to warrant resection. Ferencz[1] in her excellent review reported 25 collected cases of absence of one pulmonary artery in patients with otherwise normal hearts. At least 4 had definite abnormalities of the bronchopulmonary pattern, and only 1 was known to have anomalous pulmonary venous return. Hemoptysis was the most serious symptom and was at times severe, presumably caused by excessive inflow of blood into the lung from systemic channels.

Three of the 25 had bronchiectasis, none had lung cysts or sequestrations.

ABERRANT LEFT PULMONARY ARTERY

Respiratory obstruction caused by compression of the trachea by a vascular ring due to a double aortic arch or other anomaly of the great vessels is well known (see p. 530). Less well known is compression of the trachea by an aberrant left pulmonary artery passing behind the trachea from the right side. Among the 15 cases reviewed by Jackson *et al.*[4] there were only 3 survivals, 2 after division, relocation and suture of the vessel, and 1 without operation.

CONGENITAL PULMONARY ARTERIOVENOUS FISTULA

This condition is uncommon but because of its clinical interest a substantial number of instances have been reported.[7,10] It consists of a direct communication within the lung between a pulmonary artery and vein. The connection usually is in the form of an aneurysmal sac, sometimes quite small but at other times several centimeters in diameter. Of great importance is the fact that the lesions may be multiple, may occur in more than one lobe and in both lungs. They may be associated with obvious telangiectases of the lung (Fig. 31-12). The cases occur sporadically, but Glenn *et al.*[3] reported instances in siblings, and the father of our patient, reported by Sloan and Cooley,[8] had an almost identical lesion. Pulmonary arteriovenous fistulas occur with particular frequency in patients with hereditary hemorrhagic telangiectasia (Rendu-Osler-Weber disease), and perhaps a sixth of the reported cases of pulmonary arteriovenous aneurysms have been associated with this syndrome. Somewhat less than a quarter of the cases have been discovered in childhood; almost all of the others have been diagnosed early in adult life, the symptoms in most cases going back to childhood. Some of the arteriovenous aneurysms suggest cavernous hemangiomas, but others are relatively simple sacs with direct and obvious arterial and venous connections. The walls are extremely thin. The arterial and venous branches supplying and draining the aneurysm may be quite large, and conspicuous enough to show on a plain roentgenogram. In some instances, the arterial supply has been from an aberrant systemic artery.[9]

SYMPTOMS. — The physiologic disturbances produced by pulmonary arteriovenous fistulas depend on the shunt of unoxygenated blood into the peripheral circulation. The shunts may be of very great volume and commonly are sufficiently large to cause clinical cyanosis and to result in unsaturation and anoxemia of a degree to stimulate the bone marrow to produce striking polycythemia. The case illustrated in Figure 31-12 was first correctly diagnosed by a hematologist to whom the patient had been sent with a diagnosis of polycythemia vera. Cardiac enlargement occurs in some patients but as a rule is not severe. Dyspnea is the most common symptom. Epistaxis probably reflects the presence of similar telangiectases in the nasal mucosa. Cerebral symptoms, presumably due to anoxemia or to thrombosis in association with the polycythemia, are common. Brain abscesses occur as in other lesions with pulmonary vascular shunting. Hemoptyses are frequent and severe and occasionally exsanguinating. Fatal hemorrhage has occurred from rupture of an aneurysm into the pleural cavity, the aneurysms being almost always at the surface of the lung.

PHYSICAL EXAMINATION. — Abnormal murmurs are

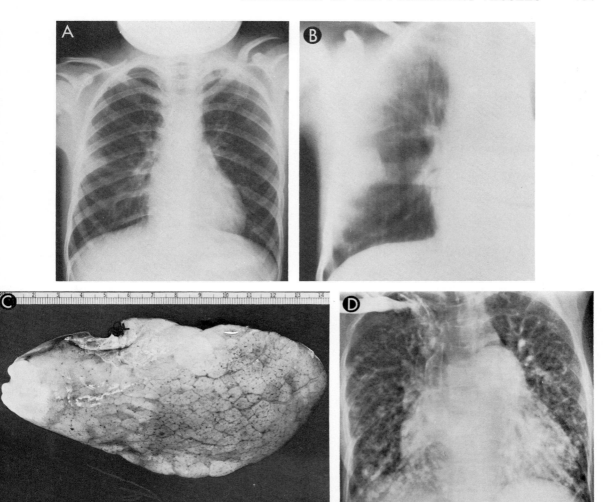

Fig. 31-12.—Pulmonary arteriovenous aneurysm. Child seen at 8 years with polycythemia, cyanosis and dyspnea, temporarily relieved by right middle lobectomy but ultimately developing high-output cardiac failure. **A,** plain film shows a peripheral opacity on the right at the level of the third anterior interspace. **B,** laminagram shows clearly the spherical body of the arteriovenous sac and distinctly outlines the feeding and draining pulmonary vessels. **C,** operative specimen, right middle lobe (1949). At operation, the entire right lung was found to be dotted with numerous telangiectatic and hemangioma-like lesions from 2–3 mm to 1–1.5 cm in size. Some of the larger ones were slightly raised and palpable. The large aneurysmal arteriovenous communication was in the right middle lobe. The specimen was photographed after injection of radiopaque material into the pulmonary artery. The lobulated white area at the posterior tip of the middle lobe is the aneurysmal sac. A pneumonectomy was not performed because of the possibility that similar lesions existed on the other side. **D,** angiocardiogram 8 years after middle lobe resection. (See text.)

commonly heard over the site of the aneurysms, and occasionally a thrill has been palpated. Cyanosis and clubbing are almost invariable, and associated telangiectases or hemangiomas of the skin and mucous membranes have been seen in almost half the patients.

RADIOLOGIC FINDINGS.—The aneurysms are themselves usually visible on the plain film as rounded or lobulated discrete densities connected to the hilus by the cordlike vessels (Fig. 31-12, *A*). Pulsation of the mass can frequently be noted under the fluoroscope. Laminagraphy sharply outlines the sac and its vessels (Fig. 31-12, *B*). Angiocardiography is the most definitive roentgenologic procedure and almost invariably shows the arterial and venous supply and the aneurysmal sac.

TREATMENT.—The lesions are sufficiently dangerous in themselves to warrant operation on diagnosis.

The symptomatic patients, those with severe polycythemia, with cyanosis and dyspnea or history of hemoptyses, obviously require operation. The operation is simple enough and sufficiently free from specific hazard to be equally advisable on a prophylactic basis for patients with diagnosed arteriovenous fistula who have few or no symptoms.

Because of the frequent multiplicity of the lesions, the propensity of previously insignificant lesions to increase in size with the passage of time and the possibility that small lesions, radiologically invisible, exist in the other lung, as little pulmonary tissue as possible should be removed. It is feasible to excise the aneurysmal sac and its vessels without excising any lung tissue at all,[6] and in other instances it may be possible to perform segmental resections. When telangiectases are found, the probability that they exist in the contralateral lung is sufficiently good so that these should be ignored and only the principal aneurysm excised. The immediate result of excision is excellent in terms of mortality, relief from symptoms and physiologic restoration to a normal condition. The resection involves no specific hazard. The ultimate prognosis depends on the existence or development of other systemic shunts in the lung or of other manifestations of hereditary telangiectasia. In this respect, the case shown in Figure 31-12 is of interest.

The child was first seen at age 8 with a 16-month history of fatigability, progressive cyanosis and dyspnea and development of clubbing of the fingers. The hemoglobin was 17.5 Gm., red blood cells 6.1 million and hematocrit 53.2. Eight years after middle lobe resection, she seemed essentially well except for cyanosis on exertion beginning 4 years following operation. Dyspnea on exertion then began to return and increased progressively, with cyanosis and fatigability. In 1955 she was hospitalized with headache and stiff neck. Two brain abscesses were drained, one right frontal, one right parietal. She returned in 1957 because of attacks of paroxysmal nocturnal dyspnea and severe cyanosis. She now had pulsating vascular swellings over the right external malleolus and the mandible. Because of occasional hematemeses, a barium study was undertaken which showed a gastric ulcer.

The progressive high-output failure made it imperative to learn whether her pulmonary arteriovenous fistulas were limited to the right lung, in which case a completion of the pneumonectomy might be considered, or whether they involved the left lung as well, in which case she would be beyond operative assistance.

The angiogram (Fig. 31-12, *D*) shows numerous arteriovenous fistulas in both lungs. Those in the right lung are somewhat larger and more impressive than those on the left, but the involvement on the left side is sufficiently great to make completion of the right pneumonectomy useless. Note the great enlargement of the right side of the heart and the huge pulmonary arteries. The left side of the heart is large also.

The diffuseness of this lesion puts the patient beyond the hope of rescue by operative intervention, and she is doomed to die of cardiac failure if one of the other hazards of her condition does not prove fatal before that occurs.

REFERENCES

1. Ferencz, C.: Congenital abnormalities of pulmonary vessels and their relation to malformations of the lung, Pediatrics 28:993, 1961.
2. Findlay, C. W., Jr., and Maier, H. C.: Anomalies of the pulmonary vessels and their surgical significance, Surgery 29:604, 1951.
3. Glenn, F.; Harrison, C. S., and Steinberg, I.: Pulmonary arteriovenous fistula occurring in siblings: Report of two cases, Ann. Surg. 138:886, 1953.
4. Jacobson, J. H., II; Morgan, B. C., and Humphreys, G. H., II: Aberrant left pulmonary artery, J. Thoracic & Cardiovas. Surg. 39:602, 1960.
5. Maier, H. C. : Absence or hypoplasia of a pulmonary artery with anomalous systemic arteries to the lung, J. Thoracic Surg. 28:145, 1954.
6. Parker, E. F., and Stallworth, J. M.: Arteriovenous fistula of the lung treated by dissection and excision without pulmonary excision, Surgery 32:31, 1952.
7. Shumacker, H. B, Jr., and Waldhausen, J. A.: Pulmonary arteriovenous fistulas in children, Ann. Surg. 158:713, 1963.
8. Sloan, R. D., and Cooley, R. N.: Congenital pulmonary arteriovenous aneurysm, Am. J. Roentgenol. 70:183, 1953.
9. Watson, W. L.: Pulmonary arteriovenous aneurysm, Surgery 22:919, 1947.
10. Yater, W. M.; Finnegan, J., and Giffin, H. M.: Pulmonary arteriovenous fistula (varix): Review of the literature and report of two cases, J. A. M. A. 141:581, 1949.

M. M. Ravitch

Congenital Cystic Disease of the Lung

Discussions of cystic disease of the lung are handicapped by a number of factors. The older authors, particularly, often confused undoubtedly acquired cystic formations, such as bronchiectasis and the pneumatocele of staphylococcic pneumonia, with congenital conditions. Among the undoubted congenital cystic conditions of the lung there are a number of varieties, and simultaneous discussion of these without clear differentiation of the types, particularly in a consideration of embryologic mechanisms, still further confuses the issue.

We will consider bronchogenic cysts, "true" congenital lung cysts, congenital cystic adenomatoid malformation of the lung, miscellaneous congenital cystic malformations and lower accessory lobe.

BRONCHOGENIC CYSTS

These are unilocular, round, thick-walled cysts lined by ciliated respiratory epithelium and are located in the mediastinum or close to the major bronchi but not communicating with them. They probably represent early malformations dating to the time of closure of the primitive foregut, and are dealt with in Chapter 29, in the discussion of mediastinal cysts and tumors. Biancalana[4] has described an intrapulmonary unilocular cyst, without a bronchial communication, which he considers to be an intrapulmonary bronchogenic cyst.

True Congenital Lung Cysts

ETIOLOGY.—The congenital nature of lung cysts is evident from the facts that they have been seen in infants only a few hours old, that cysts in babies only a few hours or weeks old have been found to be lined by tall ciliated columnar epithelium (Fig. 31-13, *B*), that they are associated with other abnormalities such as trilobed left lungs and aberrant systemic arteries arising from the aorta and inserting into the periphery of the involved lobe (Plate II, *A*, p. 217, and Fig. 31-14, *B*) and that, in some of them, abnormal epithelial formations have been found, suggesting hamartomatous structures (see Fig. 31-17). At this point in the experience with lung cysts in children there is no longer discussion as to whether they are congenital or acquired and debate instead centers on the embryogeny of these malformations. Nevertheless it is important to note that most students agree that very few significant lung cysts are found in autopsies on stillborn babies. This can probably be explained by the assumption that the epithelial clefts

which exist are neither large nor conspicuous until dilated in vivo by air or by accumulations of the mucus they secrete. The cysts of which we speak invariably communicate with the bronchus, as demonstrated by air in their cavities, anthracotic pigment in their walls or the admission of contrast medium during bronchographic study. From the standpoint of the thoracic surgeon interested in pediatric problems, the condition is not rare, and our own experience exceeds 20 cases.

CLINICAL PICTURE.—Because the cysts communicate with the bronchial air passages, they almost inevitably become infected. Infection may occur within the first weeks of life (Fig. 31-13) and may be severe, or it may develop quite suddenly years later. A number of our patients with multilocular cysts were treated for years for bronchiectasis (Fig. 31-14). It is not at all uncommon for a large unilocular cyst to become infected and to be diagnosed as a lung abscess or empyema. Three of our patients were sent to us when their "empyema" cavities failed to collapse under long-continued intercostal tube drainage (Fig. 31-15), and we operated on one of our own patients with the thought that he had a lung abscess. In him, the presence of a systemic artery from the aorta to the left lower lobe, and the well-preserved respiratory epithelium lining the cavity, made the diagnosis. The failure of a lung cyst to collapse under tube drainage is characteristic. Not rarely, large thin-walled cysts distend with air which is trapped by a flap-valve mechanism, so that tension cysts develop and necessitate attention because of the resultant respiratory

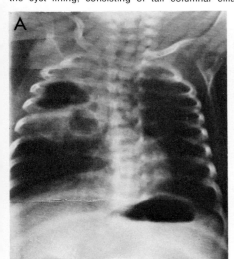
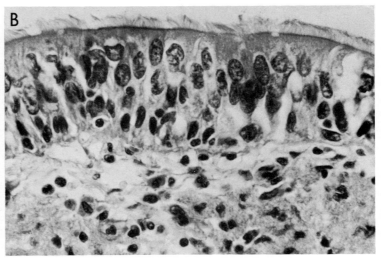

Fig. 31-13.—Congenital cystic disease of the lung. Infection in a 13-week-old infant with 3-week history of cough. At operation, cysts were found to involve the upper lobe, to which the middle lobe was fused; both were removed. The upper lobe was occupied by a pus-filled multilocular cyst 5.5 cm in greatest diameter. **A,** preoperative roentgenogram, showing a number of separate air sacs in the opacified right upper lobe. **B,** photomicrograph of the cyst lining, consisting of tall columnar ciliated bronchial epithelium. There were a few mucous glands in the cyst wall and a thin layer of smooth muscle between the basement membrane and fibrous wall of the cyst. In some areas there was acute inflammation. The child was well and grew normally after operation. It is inconceivable that ciliated epithelium of this kind could have come to line an acquired lesion in this infant's short preoperative life.

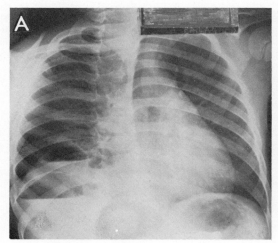

Fig. 31-14.—Congenital cystic disease of the lung simulating bronchiectasis. A 6 1/2-year-old boy with repeated attacks of pulmonary infection variously diagnosed as pneumonia and bronchitis since age 9 months. Nocturnal cough and morning sputum had been constant. He had intermittent bouts of dyspnea and noisy repirations. Bronchiectasis had been diagnosed. Repeated aspirations gave no relief and he was referred for consideration of operation. **A,** roentgenogram showing several large fluid levels at the right base. **B,** at operation, the right lower lobe was found to be firm and covered by old inflammatory tissue. A large systemic vessel, apparently arising from the distal aorta and about the size of a lead pencil, entered the convexity of the posterolateral surface of the lower lobe. In normal position was the usual pulmonary arterial branch to the lower lobe. The lobe is almost entirely replaced by numerous large cysts, many intercommunicating and all filled with glairy mucopus. In addition to the large cysts seen on the roentgenograms, there are numerous smaller ones.

Fig. 31-15.—Congenital cystic disease of the lung misdiagnosed as empyema. A 3-year-old boy with history of severe respiratory infection at age 14 months and repeated subsequent infections, always in the right lung. At age 2, rib resection and drainage were performed for suspected empyema after pus was aspirated from the cavity. There had never been any sputum. The wound had drained constantly since. A second rib resection and catheter drainage had failed to affect the size of the cavity. At operation, a smooth-walled cyst was found in the right lung, which was dissected from the remainder of the upper lobe and removed. Despite the 11 months of drainage, the cyst was lined by well-preserved epithelium varying from tall ciliated, evenly columnar cells to pseudostratified columnar epithelium.

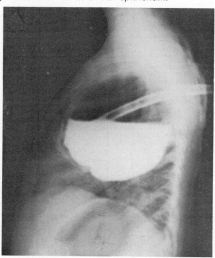

embarrassment (Fig. 31-16). Cysts of the kind under discussion may be unilobar or multilobar and occur somewhat more often in the lower lobes than in the upper lobes and as frequently on one side as on the other. An entire lung may be occupied by cysts. We have not had a patient with proved bilateral congenital cystic disease, and, faced with a picture suggesting bilateral cystic disease, we would be inclined to search carefully for evidence of cystic fibrosis of the pancreas with resultant bronchiectasis.

Clubbing of the fingers is rarely if ever associated with congenital lung cysts. Metastatic infections apparently have not been described. Rupture of the cyst into the pleural cavity with empyema, or tension pneumothorax, also seems not to occur, except as the result of diagnostic aspiration. Hemoptysis is seen, but infrequently. Womack and Graham[39] in 1942 suggested the possibility of carcinoma arising in such a cyst. Bauer[2] reported an unequivocal instance, and several others are on record. Cysts in every way resembling those under discussion have at times become symptomatic only in adult life or have been incidental findings at autopsy on patients who had been entirely asymptomatic. Nevertheless the rule is for the cysts to cause symptoms early in life, either from distention and pulmonary insufficiency or from infection and resultant cough, sputum production, fever and malnutrition. In general, congenital lung cysts are not associated with anomalies elsewhere in the body, cystic or otherwise.

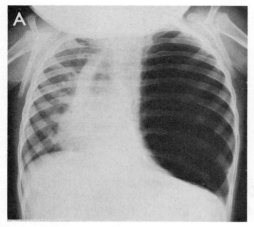
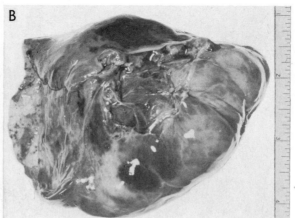

Fig. 31-16.—Congenital cystic disease of the lung—tension cyst in a year-old infant who had repeated attacks of respiratory infection and dyspnea from age 5 months and 2 1/2 months of continuous hospitalization. **A,** roentgenogram shows marked displacement of heart and mediastinum to the right by the air-filled cyst. The cyst edge can be seen in the costophrenic sulcus and medially in the cardiophrenic angle on the left. **B,** operative specimen. The left hemithorax was filled by a large, round, smooth, bluish thick-walled air-containing cyst. Pleural surfaces were smooth and shiny. The cyst was evacuated but refilled rapidly with air, necessitating during operation its deflation by needle and demonstrating a flap-valve mechanism. The cyst occupies the entire lower lobe except for a small fringe of diaphragmatic portion anteriorly. The upper lobe, a tiny compressed nubbin displaced into the mediastinum, expanded nicely and filled the hemithorax. The cyst wall was lined by low cuboidal epithelium. The child had no further difficulty.

DIFFERENTIAL DIAGNOSIS.—Congenital diaphragmatic hernia, also seen chiefly on the left side, may suggest congenital cystic disease of the lung with multiple fluid levels and areas of opacity. Displacement of the mediastinum, intestinal obstruction and severe dysnea are not usual with cystic disease. Postpneumonic pneumatoceles, after staphylococcic or other pneumonia, may be indistinguishable from the cavities of lung cysts, particularly if the history is undependable and a series of films is not available. If a pneumatocele is suspected one should delay operation for several weeks, looking for gradual disappearance of the lesion. A cyst under tension may be indistinguishable from lobar emphysema, but in either case treatment is urgent and surgical. On the right side, a mediastinal foregut remnant (esophageal duplication) communicating through the diaphragm to the bowel, hence containing air, may be confusing, although its shadow should be separable from that of the lung.

PATHOLOGY AND EMBRYOGENESIS.—The cysts usually are lined by respiratory epithelium whose tall columnar character and delicate cilia may be well preserved, even after repeated infection and drainage. On the other hand, some cysts, even in small infants, show signs of erosion and granulation tissue as the result of infection, and these cysts may be lined by pseudostratified squamous epithelium. It is uncommon for lung abscesses to become lined by ciliated epithelium, the epithelium lining an abscess, which evacuates without collapsing, usually being squamous. It has been reported, however, that such cavities can be lined by ciliated epithelium, and this has been alleged to be the source of the epithelium in cysts called congenital. Since this is a process which requires many months for development, it cannot be regarded as the mechanism of the appearance of ciliated epithelium in the cysts of children days or weeks old.

The cyst walls may contain odd bits of bronchial cartilage and smooth muscle but rarely mimic bronchial architecture in any systematic way. Abnormal proliferations of mucus-secreting glands, or of respiratory epithelium, may suggest adenomas or hamartomas (Fig. 31-17). In our report[34] of such an instance in 1949, we suggested that this was merely a variation of the pathologic picture and further evidence that congenital cystic disease of the lung is indeed congenital. The condition has been christened *congenital cystic adenomatoid malformation* of the lung.[3,8,20,21] The reviews of Holder and Christy[20] and Belanger *et al.*,[3] both appearing in 1964, listed 32 and 34 published reports. Craig, Kirkpatrick and Neuhauser[9] thought, as do we, that there is a spectrum of congenital cystic disease varying from cysts with no adenomatosis, through cysts with incidental adenomatosis, to adenomatosis with incidental cysts. The excised left lower lobe of Holder's 7-day-old infant successfully operated on contained no cysts and appears to be unique. The case of Ch'ln and Tang[8] was associated with general anasarca, which has been seen in perhaps half the reported cases. Thus the histologic picture, the frequent location in upper lobes and the absence in these cases of anomalous systemic ar-

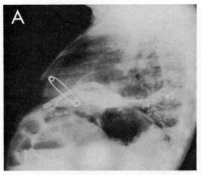

Fig. 31-17.—Cystic adenomatoid malformation of the lung. An 11-year-old boy, known to have had a cystic area in the lung since he was a year old. A tube thoracotomy was performed at age 5, during an attack of "pneumonia" and high fever. The tube had been worn continuously for 6 years, with constant discharge of glairy fluid and an obvious bronchial fistula. **A,** roentgenogram after Lipiodol was injected into the cyst through the catheter shows free communication with the bronchial tree. When the cyst was dissected away from the chest wall and the external opening clamped off, a flap-valve mechanism was demonstrated. The entire left lower lobe was removed and found to be occupied by a large unilocular, fibrous-walled cyst with smooth lining. **B,** the cyst is lined by bronchial epithelium with tall ciliated columnar cells and mucous glands beneath the lining. Masses of malformed cells and frondlike processes of mucous glands project into the lumen. **C,** hamartomatous malformation of mucous glands in the lung are seen at a distance from the cyst wall. (From Ravitch and Hardy.[34])

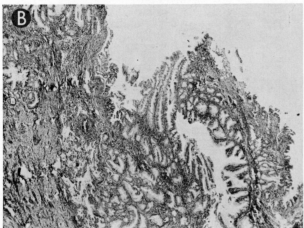

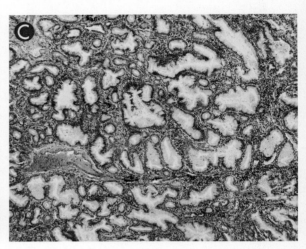

teries supplying the affected lobe all argue for the establishment of congenital cystic adenomatoid malformation of the lungs as at least a special subgroup of cases within the category of congenital cystic disease.

Most interesting, and important from the standpoint of the surgeon, are the anomalous systemic vessels arising from the descending aorta or the abdominal aorta and entering the lung away from the hilus[16,32-35] in the usual congenital cystic disease of the lung. These served Pryce[32,33] as the basis for his theory of pulmonary sequestration, the assumption being that these abnormal arteries have exerted traction on a portion of the lower lobe, divorcing it in varying degrees from its anatomic association with the remainder of the lower lobe. The theory fails to explain the development of the forms of cystic disease which occur without any vascular abnormality. Instances are on record of fatal hemorrhage resulting from avulsion of one of these abnormal aortic branches in the course of delivery of a cystic lobe by an unsuspecting operator. The arteries may be single or multiple and in our experience have been up to 6–8 mm in diameter (see Plate II, *A*). The systemic arteries are usually associated with diminution or abnormality of pulmonary arterial supply to the affected lobe, and

there may be a systemic venous outflow (through the azygos system) as well as pulmonary venous outflow. Boyden[5] thinks the arterial anomaly is essentially a coincidence, and others[14] fail to be attracted to Pryce's theory of primacy of the arterial malformation. Nevertheless the term sequestration is firmly fixed, and congenital cystic disease of the lungs is equated by most with intralobar sequestration (for extralobar sequestration, see later).

Abbey Smith's[37] logical analysis suggests that in the fetus the development of cystic disease, particularly in the posterior section of the basal segment of the left lower lobe, is associated with insufficient or inadequate pulmonary arterial inflow. In these circumstances, he has proposed that there persist and enlarge vessels from the aorta, still present at this early embryonic stage. He has pointed out that such an aberrant systemic artery is rarely if ever seen in the absence of the pulmonary changes of sequestration.

TREATMENT.—The treatment of congenital lung cysts is removal of the cyst or the involved segment, lobe or lobes. The large unilocular cysts which distend with air may, in some instances, be peeled away from the lobes in which they arise without sacrifice of any significant amount of pulmonary tissue. Lobes that are the seat of multilocular communicating cysts of varying sizes which contain much mucus as well as air usually require lobectomy. Operation is specifically advised, even in the absence of symptoms, in the knowledge that symptoms will invariably develop and that operation on a healthy child with an uninfected cyst or system of cysts is safer than operation on a child who is chronically ill and has a grossly infected lung. The only death in a child with cystic disease in the Johns Hopkins series was in 1939 when a child of 8 months was sent home to be "built up" and to return in 2 years but died of "pneumonia" a month after discharge. There are numerous reports of lobectomies in the first weeks of life, and Minnis[27] successfully removed a lower lobe of an infant on the first day of life for cystic disease of the left lower lobe. Preoperative sputum cultures will help to guide antibiotic therapy. The aortogram, demonstrating anomalous systemic arterial supply to the involved lobe, both confirms the diagnosis and forewarns the surgeon (Fig. 31-18).

We do not think there is any place for preliminary drainage of infected cysts, although in the presence of a dangerously overexpanded cyst, venting it with a needle may be necessary while preparations for operation are being made. Ordinarily, the accumulation of air within a congenital cyst is gradual, and the respiratory embarrassment does not suddenly become extreme except in the presence of superimposed contralateral pulmonary infection. Localized congenital emphysema in the newborn, on the other hand, may lead to rapid development of respiratory distress. Pneumatoceles after staphylococcic pneumonia may, at times, distend with great rapidity to produce alarming symptoms. The treatment of lobar emphysema is lobectomy and, of tension pneumatoceles, catheter drainage.

PROGNOSIS AFTER PULMONARY RESECTION IN CHILDHOOD. — It is a truism of thoracic surgery that, technically, pulmonary resection in infants is infinitely easier than pulmonary resection in adults because of the elasticity of the hilar structures and the absence of scar and matted lymph nodes.[7,10,27] Although the issue is perhaps not yet completely resolved, it is thought that the infant can respond to pulmonary resection with an actual increase in the number of his respiratory units and so perhaps suffer less in terms of loss of functioning respiratory tissue than the older child or adult. Engel[13] suggested that in children under the age of 5, new acini and alveoli are formed after pulmonary resection, but that beyond that age lung growth is achieved principally by enlargement of existing alveoli. There is now ample experience with lobectomy and pneumonectomy in infants and children who have gone on to an asymptomatic early adult life.

The function of the residual lung after pulmonary resection early in life has been investigated.[25] In puppies, it has been shown that functional pulmonary diffusing surface is restored from 9 to 12 months after pulmonary resection. This is thought to be both by hyperplasia and by "regeneration" of alveoli in the growing animal. Pneumonectomy in the adult animal leads to an increase of the air space without a corresponding increase of the functional alveolar capillary diffusing surface. Some evidence of emphysema in pneumonectomized puppies developed after a number of years.[15] The early studies of Lester, Cournand

Fig. 31-18.—Congenital cystic disease of the lung. A child of 6 months with repeated history of pulmonary infection. **A,** roentgenogram shows a peculiar triangular opacity in the left lung in the supradiaphragmatic area behind the heart. It was suggested that this might be a "sequestered" lobe. **B,** a catheter aortogram demonstrates a very large branch of the lower thoracic aorta, not much smaller than the aorta itself, feeding directly into the lung. At operation, several systemic arteries were found going into the lower lobe, which was carneous and contracted, with normal-appearing bronchus, pulmonary artery and vein. Resection was followed by uneventful recovery.

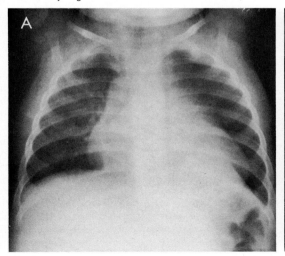
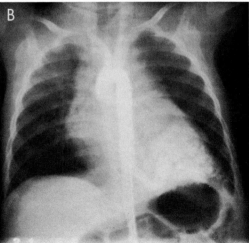

and Riley,[24] and of Peters *et al.*[30] of children who had had pneumonectomies and a healthy remaining lung showed that residual air was increased in some, ventilatory capacity was adequate for extreme physical demands and that maximal breathing capacities were at least as great as the expected normal for one lung. More recent studies by Peters *et al.*,[31] Filler[15] and Giammona *et al.*[17] support the earlier observations. Filler studied 15 adolescents who had had bisegmentectomy, lobectomy or bilobectomy for posttuberculous bronchiectasis. Subjects with bisegmentectomy showed no impairment of pulmonary function even when measured by bronchospirometry; the remaining patients had slight decreases of lung volume and physiologic evidence of hyperdistention of the remaining lung parenchyma without evidence of bronchial obstruction and without effect on maximal breathing capacity. The respiratory function of the lung was unimpaired. Bronchospirometry showed decrease of lung volume and pulmonary perfusion on the operated side, quantitatively proportional to the extent of resection. Distention of the remaining lobe or lobes was proportionately greater in the upper than in the lower lobectomies. Peters and his colleagues compared their studies of 11 patients under 16 at the time of pulmonary resection with those of patients operated on between the ages of 16 and 21. The results in the younger group were excellent, except for 4 with residual disease. These 4 were rated as having good results, with slight exertional dyspnea. Of the 12 older patients, 6 had excellent results, 5 good and 1 fair. And of these, 3 had persistent bronchiectasis. The children operated on at a younger age had lower residual volume-lung capacity ratios and higher maximal breathing capacities, suggesting to Peters that hyper- rather than overdistention occurred in the remaining lung of the younger group. Most of the resections were done for bronchiectasis, only two for lung cysts in the young group and one in the older group, so the possibility of disease in the remaining lung affects these studies. In children with certainly normal residual lung, even slighter defects might be found. Giammona *et al.* studied 8 children who had had pneumonectomy at age 1–15 years and at intervals of 2–15 years after operation. Most of the patients had been operated on for bronchiectasis, only 2 for lung cyst. Their observations demonstrated moderate overinflation of the lung with minimal restriction of respiratory function. The carbon monoxide diffusion capacity was affected. The ratio of pulmonary capillary blood volume to pulmonary arterial blood volume was increased, suggesting overdistention of the pulmonary capillary bed after pneumonectomy. Pulmonary arterial pressure was high normal at rest and elevated with exercise. Pulmonary arterial resistance was normal at rest and with exercise. In sum, pulmonary resection is well tolerated by children and in the absence of disease in the remaining pulmonary parenchyma is associated with minimal physiologic and clinical changes, at least into early adult life.

OTHER TYPES OF LUNG CYSTS

Other and rare types of cystic formations are the inconsequential pleural, thin-walled cysts which communicate with lymphatic vessels and are thought to be congenital cystic dilatations of the pulmonary lymphatics.[28] Occasionally, small cysts of the pleural mesothelium occur. Laurence[22] and Giedion, Muller and Molz[18] reported identical cases of infants who died after a few hours of desperate respiratory distress. The roentgenogram in Giedion's case showed a striking appearance, as of a chest full of soap bubbles. In both infants, there was diffuse pulmonary lymphangiectasis.

A variety of pathologic processes occasionally cause cystic degeneration of the lung. Lung abscess and bronchiectasis have been mentioned. Cysts have been reported also in several of the lipoid histiocytoses.[28] We have seen a child with papillomatosis of the larynx and trachea in whom the papillomatosis extended down into her smaller bronchi, with resultant destruction of the lungs by the formation of cysts lined with these papillomas.[29,36]

LOWER ACCESSORY LOBE (EXTRALOBAR PULMONARY SEQUESTRATION)

The lower accessory lobe is a rare and characteristic anomaly, probably embryologically significant in connection with the possible development of the forms of lung cysts. Characteristically, the accessory lobe is a rounded, smooth, soft mass lying between the dome of the diaphragm and the inferior surface of the lung, almost always on the left. It is covered by what appears to be smooth, glistening visceral pleura. The accessory lobe is not attached to the lung, is not air-containing and is nourished by an artery directly from the aorta. Histologically, the accessory lobe displays a variety of epithelial structures suggesting alveoli and bronchi with occasional areas of cartilage. The lung itself usually is normal in its anatomic conformation and division into lobes.

These anomalies are usually noted as asymptomatic radiographic shadows or may cause symptoms by compression of the lower lobe. Occasionally, such a sequestered accessory lobe has been found within the pericardium[1] or beneath the diaphragm. They have been removed as mediastinal tumors of unknown nature. Operation presents no technical problems.[12,23] In most instances, the pedicle of such a lobe reaches into the mediastinum in close relation to the esophagus. In the cases of Louw and Cywes[26] and Rubin *et al.*,[35] there was an epithelium-lined communication between the esophagus and the sequestered lobe. Boyden[6] had previously suggested, on the basis of a patient operated on by Bill in whom a similar but solid pedicle was found, that extralobar pulmonary sequestrations are probably the result of an abnormal embryonic diverticular out-pouching of the esophagus. Louw and others have pointed out the frequent association of diaphragmatic hernia with this lesion. A lung whose sole bronchus arises from the esophagus[19] is occasionally reported as a sequestration. Such lesions, discussed under abnormal tracheobronchial connections (p. 449), are more probably related to the mechanisms producing esophageal atresia and tracheoesophageal fistula than to those producing sequestration of the lung.

REFERENCES

1. d'Abreu, A. L.: *A Practice of Thoracic Surgery* (London: Edward Arnold, Ltd., 1958), p. 24.
2. Bauer, S.: Carcinoma arising in a congenital lung cyst, Dis. Chest 40:552, 1961.
3. Belanger, R.; La Fleche, L. R., and Picard, J. L.: Congenital cystic adenomatoid malformation of the lung, Thorax 19:1, 1964.
4. Biancalana, L.: Die lungenzysten, Thoraxchir. u. vask. Chir. 11:511, 1964.
5. Boyden, E. A.: Bronchogenic cysts and the theory of intralobar sequestration: New embryologic data. J. Thoracic Surg. 35:604, 1959.
6. Boyden, E. A.; Bill, H. A., and Creighton, S. A.: Presumptive origin of a left lower accessory lung from an esophageal diverticulum, Surgery 52:323, 1962.
7. Burnett, W. E., and Caswell, H. D.: Lobectomy for pulmonary cysts in a 15-day-old infant, with recovery, Surgery 23:84, 1948.
8. Ch'ln, K. Y., and Tang, M. Y.: Congenital adenomatoid malformation of one lobe of a lung with general anasarca, Arch. Path. 98:221, 1949.
9. Craig, J. M.; Kirkpatrick, J., and Neuhauser, E. B.: Congenital cystic adenomatoid malformation of the lung in infants, Am. J. Roentgenol. 76:516, 1956.
10. Crossett, E. S., and Shaw, R. R.: Pulmonary resection in the first year of life, Surg., Gynec. & Obst. 97:417, 1953.
11. Cournand, A., *et al.*: A follow-up study of cardiopulmonary function in four young individuals after pneumonectomy, J. Thoracic Surg. 16:30, 1947.
12. DeBakey, M.; Arey, J. B., and Brunazzi, R.: Successful removal of lower accessory lung, J. Thoracic Surg. 19:304, 1950.
13. Engle, S.: *Lung Structure* (Springfield, Ill.:, Charles C Thomas, 1962.).
14. Ferencz, C.: Congenital abnormalities of pulmonary vessels and their relation to malformation of the lung, Pediatrics 28:993, 1961.
15. Filler, J.: Effects on pulmonary function of lobectomy performed during childhood, Am. Rev. Resp. Dis. 80:801, 1964.
16. Findlay, C. W., Jr., and Maier, H. C.: Anomalies of the pulmonary vessels and their surgical significance, Surgery 29:604, 1951.
17. Giammona, S. T., *et al.*: The later cardiopulmonary effects of childhood pneumonectomy. Pediatrics 37:79, 1966.
18. Giedion, A.; Muller, W. A., and Molz, G.: Angeborene Lymphangiectase der Lungen; Helvet. paediat. acta 22:170, 1967.
19. Hanna, E. F.: Bronchoesophageal fistula with total sequestration of the right lung, Ann. Surg. 159:599, 1964.
20. Holder, T. M., and Christy, M. G.: Cystic adenomatoid malformations of the lung, J. Thoracic & Cardiovas. Surg. 47:590, 1964.
21. Kwittken, J., and Reiner, L.: Congenital cystic adenomatoid malformation of the lung, Pediatrics 30:759, 1962.
22. Laurence, K. M.: Congenital pulmonary cystic lymphangiectasis, J. Path. & Bact. 70:325, 1955.
23. Leahy, L. J., and MacCallum, J. D.: Cystic accessory lobe, J. Thoracic Surg. 20:72, 1950.
24. Lester, C. W.; Cournand, A., and Riley, R. L.: Pulmonary function after pneumonectomy in children, J. Thoracic Surg. 11:529, 1942.
25. Longacre, J. J.; Carter, B. N., and Quill, L. M.: An experimental study of some of the physiological changes following total pneumonectomy, J. Thoracic Surg. 6:237, 1937.
26. Louw, J. H., and Cywes, S.: Extralobar pulmonary sequestration communicating with the esophagus and associated with a strangulated congenital diaphragmatic hernia, Brit. J. Surg. 50:102, 1962.
27. Minnis, J. F., Jr.,: Congenital cystic disease of the lung in infancy, J. Thoracic & Cardiovas. Surg., 43:262, 1962.
28. Moffat, A. D.: Congenital cystic disease of the lungs and its classification, J. Path. & Bact. 79:361, 1960.
29. Moore, R. L., and Lattes, R.: Papillomatosis of the larynx and bronchi, Cancer 12:117, 1959.
30. Peters, R. M., *et al.*: Respiratory and circulatory studies after pneumonectomy in childhood, J. Thoracic Surg. 20:484, 1950.
31. Peters, R. M.; Wilcox, B. R., and Schultz, E. H., Jr.: Pulmonary resection in children: Long-term effect on the function and lung growth, Ann. Surg. 154:652, 1964.
32. Pryce, D. M.: Lower accessory pulmonary artery with intralobar sequestration of lung: A report of seven cases, J. Path. & Bact. 58:457, 1946.
33. Pryce, D. M.; Sellors, T. H., and Blair, L. G.: Intralobar sequestration of lung associated with an abnormal pulmonary artery, Brit. J. Surg. 35:18, 1947.
34. Ravitch, M. M., and Hardy, J. B.: Congenital cystic disease of the lung in infants and children, Arch. Surg. 59:1, 1949.
35. Rubin, E. H., et al.: Intralobar pulmonary sequestration – aortographic demonstration, Dis. Chest 50:561, 1966.
36. Singer, D. B.; Greenberg, S. D., and Harrison, G. M.: Papillomatosis of the lung, Am. Rev. Resp. Dis. 94:777, 1966.
37. Smith, R. A.: Some controversial aspects of the intralobar sequestration of the lung, Surg., Gynec. & Obst. 114:57, 1962.
38. Weisel, W.; Docksey, J. W., and Glicklich, M.: Vascular anomalies associated with intrapulmonary bronchial cysts, Am. Rev. Tuberc. 71:573, 1955.
39. Womack, N. A., and Graham, E. A.: Developmental abnormalities of the lung and bronchogenic carcinoma, Arch. Path. 39:301, 1946.

M. M. Ravitch

32

Infectious Diseases of the Lungs

Pneumonia and Empyema

HISTORY.—The fact that pulmonary infections were followed by empyema and that this required external drainage for cure was known to the ancients. Hippocrates, Paul of Aegina, Fabricius and other ancient authorities were concerned with the optimal time and manner of drainage of the empyema. Lanfranc used the cautery to perforate the chest and to drain the empyema. One of Vesalius' celebrated cases was a cure of empyema. The first formal thoracotomy for empyema in modern time is ascribed to Küster, in 1889. Graham conclusively demonstrated the dangers of early open thoracotomy for empyema in the resultant pneumothorax and collapse; and thereafter, until the antibiotic era, discussion as to therapy largely centered on the relative advantages of open drainage and the various types of closed drainage and the optimal time for employment of these measures.

PATHOGENESIS

Empyema thoracis, or accumulation of pus within the pleural cavity, occurs from (1) hematogenous spread in children with septicemia, (2) direct or lymphatic extension from inflammatory or suppurative processes within the lung, or (3) contamination of the pleural cavity by external trauma, operation or operative sequelae. In addition to the systemic signs of infection, the children show varying degrees of tachypnea and cyanosis. If the collection of fluid is large,

the intercostal spaces may bulge and there may be a striking mediastinal shift. Neglected empyemas may rupture outward through the chest wall (empyema necessitatus), through the lung and the bronchial tree, or through the diaphragm. In ancient times, external drainage of empyema was recognized as no more than an anticipation of this process.

INCIDENCE AND MORTALITY

Fifteen years ago, it appeared that postpneumonic empyema in infants and children was a vanishing disease of historical interest only. Writing in 1961 for the first edition, we stated: ". . . if it were not for the children with staphylococcal empyema, medical students and interns might rarely see a case of empyema, except perhaps on a traumatic or a postoperative basis." We did not realize it then, but the story told by Figure 32-1, reproduced from the first edition, represented the end of a trend and not the remorseless effects of antibacterial chemotherapy and antibiotic therapy. That the use of these agents did, in fact, affect the clinical picture, occurrence and relative incidence of the forms of bacterial pneumonia is clear enough from Figure 32-1 and Table 32-1. The effect of the various antibacterial agents over the period of the study can be summarized somewhat as follows. With the advent of sulfonamides, the need for

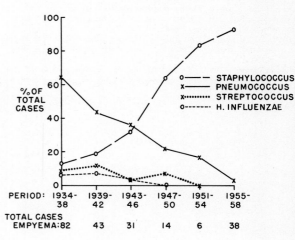

Fig. 32-1.—Empyema: incidence of causative agents. Analysis of 214 cases of empyema among 10,632 diagnosed cases of pneumonia at the Harriet Lane Home of the Johns Hopkins Hospital, Jan. 1, 1934, to Dec. 31, 1958 (see Table 32-1 for time periods according to drug therapy). Empyema had almost disappeared in the 4-year period 1951–54, when 6 cases were seen, 5 staphylococcic, 1 pneumococcic. In the final period there are almost as many cases as in the initial period, 1939–42, but due entirely to an upsurge in occurrence of staphylococcic pneumonia and empyema among infants. Empyema from streptococcus and *H. influenzae* is no longer seen.

TABLE 32-1.—MORTALITY AMONG HOSPITALIZED PATIENTS WITH PNEUMONIA AND EMPYEMA

PERIOD	CASES HOSPITALIZED	NO. OF CASES	DEATHS	MORTALITY, %
I: 1934-38 (presulfonamide)	Pneumonia	864	77	9
	Empyema	82	24	29
II: 1939-42 (sulfonamides)	Pneumonia	958	58	6
	Empyema	43	5	12
III: 1943-46 (penicillin)	Pneumonia	506	54	10
	Empyema	31	5	16
IV: 1947-50 (penicillin and streptomycin)	Pneumonia	205	26	13
	Empyema	14	2	14
V: 1951-54 (penicillin, streptomycin, and chlortetracycline)	Pneumonia	276	36	13
	Empyema	6	0	0
VI: 1955-58 (polyantibiotic)	Pneumonia	266	41	15
	Empyema	38	4	11

hospitalization was not affected, but the total mortality from both pneumonia and empyema dropped somewhat. The introduction of penicillin sharply decreased the need for hospitalization of children with pneumonia, but the mortality from empyema and pneumonia among those who were admitted to the hospital did not change, and essentially the only change in mortality occurred during period V, when there were no deaths from empyema although the mortality rate for pneumonia was still 13% (Table 32-1). The percentages of the empyema patients under 2 years of age underwent a steady increase from the beginning of the study, when the figure was 55%, through the final period, when 89% of the children were 2 years of age. This reflects the predominant affinity of staphylococcic pneumonia and empyema for infants. In period V, during which chlortetracycline was introduced, there were only 6 cases of empyema, 1 due to pneumococcus and 5 to staphylococcus. In the final period, 1955 through 1958, despite no change in the total number of pneumonia patients seen or hospitalized or in the incidence of pneumonia in children under 2, there were 38 cases of empyema, an increase of incidence to 14% of the hospitalized cases. Thirty-five cases were due to staphylococcus, and of the 38 cases, 34 (89%) occurred in patients under age 2. There were no deaths due to pneumococcus after 1947, no deaths due to streptococcus after 1939 and no case of streptococcic empyema after 1948. Infection due to *Hemophilus influenzae* was not seen after 1944.

In the 1934–38 period, the death rate from staphylococcic empyema was 55%. It must be admitted that here, as in other cases of empyema of various kinds, multiple manifestations of the infectious process were often seen and contributed to the deaths that occurred. The death rates from staphylococcic empyema in the successive periods of study were 25%, 0%, 11%, 0% and, in period VI (1955-58), with a sudden upsurge of staphylococcic empyemas, 15%.

The effect of widespread antibacterial therapy appears to have been to decrease the need for hospitalization of children with pneumonia and to eliminate almost entirely the incidence of empyema due to pneumococcus, streptococcus and *H. influenzae*. This was accompanied by a sharp increase of empyemas due to the staphylococcus, almost all in infants (see Table 32-2). Although the increase of staphylococcic pneumonia and empyema may have been the inevitable effect of the proper widespread therapeutic use of antibacterial agents, a general feeling prevailed that indiscriminate use of antibiotics far beyond the specific indication for serious infections may have aggravated the preferential overgrowth of staphylococcus in a large section of the population, thereby accounting for the changes in incidence noted. This rather pat explanation was rudely upset when, almost as soon as it was written, the incidence of staphylococcic pneumonia very sharply decreased. This has been a world-wide phenomenon, and once more the total number of postpneumonic empyemas seen in our hospitals is very small.

TREATMENT OF EMPYEMA

The violent arguments of former years with respect to the preferred method of treatment of empyema have disappeared. The widespread general understanding of the importance of full pulmonary expansion in the treatment of suppurative collections in the chest has been a contributing factor. Further elements contributing to peace came as the result of the work of Graham, with agreement as to the respiratory dynamics involved and with the general decrease of the frequency with which postpneumonic empyema was seen.

It has always been possible to treat an occasional patient with empyema successfully by means of repeated aspiration, with or without instillation of antibiotics. This method is substantially less certain to cure than drainage, likely to require considerably more time and probably causes more discomfort to the patient. In any case, a substantial number of patients so treated will ultimately require a drainage procedure, and there is the risk that in the meantime the pleural exudate will have thickened sufficiently so that it may not be possible to expand the lung. The degree of success in the treatment of empyema should be gauged by the rapidity with which the patient is cured of his suppurative disease and the rapidity with which the hemithorax begins to function normally. Treatment, therefore, combines appropriate systemic antibiotics and effective drainage.

In the face of a frank empyema, or a large and probably infected effusion in association with pneumonia, it is our practice at once to institute intercostal tube drainage running to an underwater seal, usually with additional negative pressure. This may be done as soon as the collection of fluid is found. Since open pneumothorax is not produced, no risk is involved. The largest catheter which the intercostal space can accommodate should be used. If too large a catheter is employed, the pressure of the ribs will occlude it. In older children, the familiar trocar thoracotomy set is used. Since we customarily employ negative pressure drainage, we are not as concerned as formerly about techniques to avoid admission of air. In infants, after a skin incision has been made, the catheter, grasped in a hemostat, may be pressed through the chest wall into the pleura. In patients of all ages, trocar thoracotomy and rib resection and open drainage are performed under infiltration anesthesia. The catheter is inserted posterolaterally in the lowest interspace through which pus has been aspirated, preferably not so far posteriorly as to cause discomfort in the supine position. Formation of empyema in unusual locations requires insertion of the catheter accordingly. From this point on, so long as the patient continues to improve, as measured by subsidence of fever, tachycardia and dyspnea and decrease in the size of the cavity on repeated measurement and roentgen study, no more need be done. The tube is removed when the cavity is reduced to a sheath around the tube. If at any time the patient's condition reaches a plateau short of disappearance of the empyema cavity and complete restoration of the clinical condition to normal, a rib resection and open drainage should be performed at once.

Chronic empyema, in which the lung cannot be made to expand, may occasionally require decortication—the removal of the fibrinous rind over the parietal and visceral pleura. The deforming collapse procedures of the Schede and other types should never be required in children.

STAPHYLOCOCCIC PNEUMONIA AND EMPYEMA

The special nature of staphylococcic pneumonia and its complications, and the likelihood that with another cyclic swing it will become common again, justify specific consideration of its clinical course and management. Staphylococcic pneumonia primarily attacks infants; approximately one quarter of the cases are seen in the first year of life, and there is a direct relationship between age and mortality (Table

TABLE 32-2.—PRIMARY STAPHYLOCOCCIC PNEUMONIA AT HARRIET LANE HOME OF THE JOHNS HOPKINS HOSPITAL, 1955–58: MORTALITY BY AGE GROUPS

AGE RANGE	CASES	MORTALITY, %
0–3 months	25	17
4–12 months	21	5
1–6 years	14	0
Over 6 years	0	0
Totals	60	8

32-2). The history usually is of sudden onset of a respiratory infection with extremely rapid progression. At times, within a few hours of onset the child may manifest tachypnea, fever, dyspnea, cough and cyanosis, and the violent respiratory efforts may lead also to abdominal distention elevating the diaphragm and increasing dyspnea. The physical signs are those associated with any pneumonic infection. Usually, staphylococcus can be obtained from cultures of material from nasopharynx or of pleural fluid obtained by thoracentesis before antibiotic therapy is begun, even when only a little thin fluid is present, and obviously will be cultured in the presence of a frank empyema.

RADIOGRAPHIC CHARACTERISTICS.—A pulmonary infiltrate is present in all these patients, and in our experience is bilateral in approximately 10%. In 67 patients observed at the Harriet Lane Home of the Johns Hopkins Hospital[12] pleural effusion or empyema occurred in 72%. Radiographic visualization of air within the lung parenchyma as excavations or pneumatoceles or within the pleural cavity as pneumothorax (Figs. 32-2 and 32-3) and evidence of a bronchial fistula in the latter are said to be pathognomonic of staphylococcic pneumonia. It is frequently assumed that this is a new phenomenon and peculiar to staphylococcic pneumonia and staphylococcic empyema. Actually, in our experience there have been observed various radiolucent shadows presumed to be parenchymal in occasional pneumococcic and other empyemas. Pyopneumothorax was seen in the Harriet Lane Home in the study period 1934-1958 in at least 23 instances of pneumonia and empyema due to organisms other than staphylococcus, principally pneumococcus.[9] In the same period, there were 24 instances of pyopneumothorax with staphylococcic empyema. The presence, therefore, of a pneumatocele and particularly of pyopneumothorax, while suggestive of a staphylococcic infection, should not be taken as conclusive evidence. The origin of these pneumatoceles is probably explained by abscess formation in the bronchial wall and erosion through the bronchus with direct leakage of air into the parenchyma through a flap-valve defect rather than as the result of a parenchymal abscess with tissue destruction. The delicate bronchial tissues of infants are fairly readily destroyed, even by the less vigorously his-

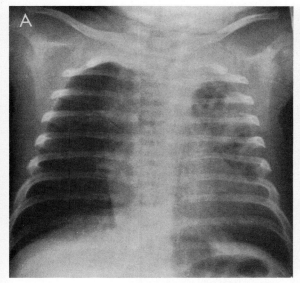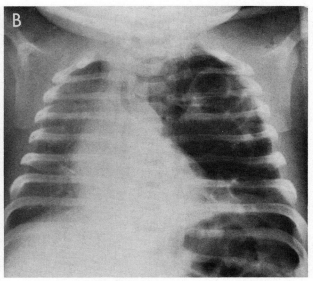

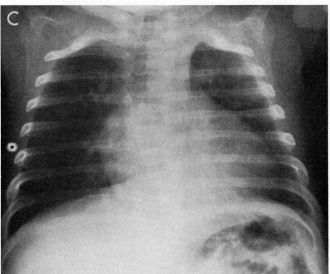

Fig. 32-2.—Staphylococcic pneumonia and tension pneumothorax. **A,** in a profoundly ill infant, the left lung is mottled and numerous small areas of radiolucency can be seen. There is some pulmonary infiltration in both upper lobes. **B,** without having reached very large size, one of the pneumatoceles ruptured into the left pleural cavity. There are tension pneumothorax and displacement of the mediastinum to the right. Although most of the left lung is collapsed and there is a herniation of air across the mediastinum, several of the pneumatoceles remain distended and visible. **C,** tube thoracotomy and negative pressure drainage have expanded the lung and relieved the respiratory embarrassment. The pulmonary infiltration has almost completely disappeared.

tiolytic enzymes of organisms other than the staphylococcus.

TREATMENT.—Massive doses of antibiotics rank first in the treatment of staphylococcic pneumonia. The pattern of resistance of the organisms and effectiveness of antibiotics changes constantly. Currently we employ penicillin G plus one of the penicillinase-resistant penicillins—viz., nafcillin. There is good evidence that a bactericidal antibiotic should also be employed, and penicillin (2-10 million units/day) is used for most patients.

Three principal indications for surgical intervention may be mentioned: (1) *Massive effusion* with respiratory distress, which may occur with astonishing rapidity and require catheter drainage under negative pressure. (2) *Tension pneumothorax,* which is

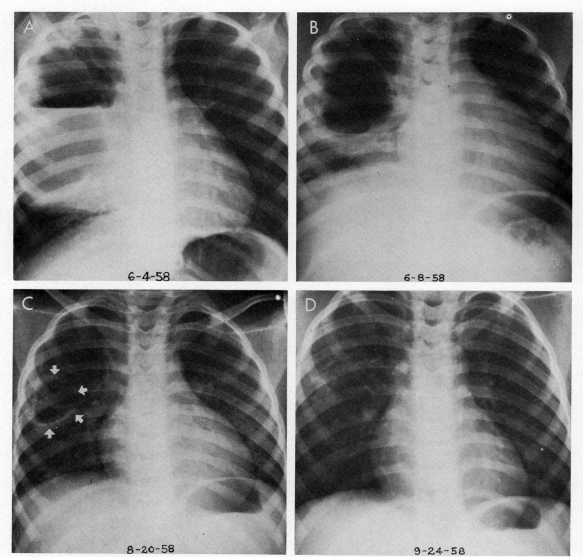

Fig. 32-3.—Staphylococcic pneumonia and pneumatoceles. This infant was admitted with staphylococcic pneumonia. Rapid increase of dyspnea was accompanied by expansion of a previously small pneumatocele which partially filled with fluid. Catheter drainage brought immediate relief and ultimate cure. **A,** the huge pneumatocele occupies most of the right chest; there is a fluid level across its midportion. One might be pardoned for uncertainty as to whether this represented a pneumatocele with fluid level or a pyopneumothorax. The sharp curved outline of the lower portion of the opacity and absence of fluid in the costophrenic sulcus suggest that the air and fluid are in a pneumatocele within the pulmonary parenchyma. **B,** an intercostal catheter has evacuated the fluid. The pneumatocele is decreasing in size and the lower lobe has begun to expand. **C,** the catheter has been removed and the pneumatocele allowed to disappear slowly. **D,** 15 weeks after onset of the pneumonia, the pneumatocele has finally disappeared. It is probable that had the catheter been left in the pneumatocele and negative pressure applied for a longer time, the pneumatocele would have collapsed more rapidly.

treated in the same way. The tension pneumothorax may develop as a more or less anticipated complication of a pre-existing pneumatocele or may result from rupture of a subcortical abscess and a bronchial leak without an obvious pneumatocele. (3) *Rapid expansion of a pneumatocele*, treated by insertion of an intercostal catheter into the pneumatocele and with suction drainage. In occasional sick infants, pneumatoceles form and expand with great suddenness. There is hardly any condition in which hour-to-hour observation and a sense of urgency for immediate treatment is as strongly required as in staphylococcic pneumonia. Pneumatoceles on one side or the other or both may increase in size with great rapidity, causing dyspnea with or without rupture into the pleural cavity and pneumothorax. We have performed as many as five tube thoracotomies in one infant before finally bringing the condition under control. The mere existence of a pneumatocele is not an indication for insertion of a catheter. We reserve this for the very large or rapidly expanding pneumatoceles. Even when the infection itself has been brought under control and when the child is afebrile, comfortable, no longer dyspneic and eating well, the pneumatocele may expand and cause mechanical distress. It is not at all rare for an infant to leave the hospital with a persistent pneumatocele which requires weeks for complete disappearance. At times, such a cyst will begin to expand and require readmission of the child for drainage. Occasionally, an infant is seen in whom the original pneumonia was unremarked at home and whose pneumatocele must now be distinguished from the sac of a congenital lung cyst.[8] If there is any clinical likelihood that the parenchymal air collection represents a pneumatocele, thoracotomy should be postponed for a period of observation to allow the suspected pneumatocele to recede.

Results of treatment.—In the 67 cases previously mentioned, intercostal drainage was employed in 28 (41.8%). In 15 patients, the intercostal catheter was inserted to release a tension pneumothorax following rupture of a pneumatocele. With the frequent use of drainage by an intercostal catheter, rib resection is rarely necessary for open drainage. Such a procedure was employed only once in this series.

Staphylococcic pneumonia may be superimposed upon a severe underlying disease such as cystic fibrosis of the pancreas, congenital biliary atresia or agammaglobulinemia, gravely altering the prognosis of the disease. The 7 patients with such complicating disease died. The over-all mortality in the 60 patients with primary staphylococcic pneumonia was 8%, but in the 25 patients in the first 3 months of life there was a 17% mortality. None of the 14 children over 1 year of age died.

Asp, Pasila and Sulamaa[1] from Helsinki, where staphylococcic pneumonia was still common in 1964, presented a startlingly different therapeutic approach. In 20 very sick children, 3 weeks to 5 years of age with staphylococcic pneumonia and pyopneumothorax, usually under tension, with accompanying mediastinal shift, they performed an immediate open thoracotomy. Pus and fibrin were evacuated, the lung decorticated and bronchial fistulas sutured. All 20 children recovered, although 3 required a second operation. Hospital stay was 1–3 months. This approach is radically contrary to our belief that in staphylococcic empyema, catheter drainage with negative pressure is all that is required and that open thoracotomy should be reserved for the rare failure with catheter drainage.

REFERENCES

1. Asp, K.; Pasila, M., and Sulamaa, M.:Treatment of pyopneumothorax in infants and children, Acta chir. scandinav. 128:715, 1964.
2. Benward, J. H.: Staphylococcus pneumonia and empyema, Journal-Lancet 67:434, 1947.
3. Bloomer, W. E., *et al.*: Staphylococcal pneumonia and empyema in infancy, J. Thoracic Surg. 30:265, 1955.
4. Forbes, G. B.: Diagnosis and management of severe infections in infants and children: Review of experiences since introduction of sulfonamide therapy; Staphylococcal empyema, importance of pyopneumothorax as complication, J. Pediat. 29:45, 1946.
5. Graham, E. A.; Singer, S. J., and Ballon, H. C.: *Surgical Diseases of the Chest* (Philadelphia: Lea & Febiger, 1935).
6. Penberthy, G. C., and Benson, C. D.: A ten-year study of empyema in children, 1926–1936, Ann. Surg. 104:579, 1936.
7. Petersdorf, R. G., *et al.*: Staphylococcal pneumonia: A review of 21 cases in adults, New England J. Med. 258:919, 1958.
8. Potts, W. J., and Riker, W. L.: Differentiation of congenital cysts of the lung and those following staphylococcic pneumonia, Arch. Surg. 61:684, 1950.
9. Ravitch, M. M., and Fein, R.: The changing picture of pneumonia and empyema in infants and children: A review of the experience at the Harriet Lane Home from 1934 through 1958, J.A.M.A. 175:1039, 1961.
10. Riker, W. L.: Lung cysts and pneumothorax in infants and children, S. Clin. North America 36:1613, 1956.
11. Rogers, D. E.: The current problem of staphylococcal hospital infections, Ann. Int. Med. 45:748, 1956.
12. Sabiston, D. C., Jr., *et al.*: The surgical management of complications of staphylococcal pneumonia in infancy and childhood, J. Thoracic & Cardiovas. Surg. 38:421, 1959.
13. Watkins, D. H.: Surgical complications, in the thorax, of staphylococcal pneumonitis, Arch. Surg. 77:508, 1958.
14. Watkins, E., and Hering, A. C.: The management of staphylococcic tension pneumatoceles by intracavitary suction tube drainage, J. Thoracic Surg. 36:642, 1958.
15. Weisel, W., and Gorman, W. C.: Acute thoracic emergencies in infants and children with acute staphylococcic pneumonia, Surgery 45:335, 1959.

M. M. RAVITCH
D. C. SABISTON, JR.

Bronchiectasis

HISTORY.—The pathologic changes in bronchiectasis were well described by Laennec in 1810, a time when this disease in combination with diffuse pulmonary suppuration was uniformly fatal. Jackson in 1905 first demonstrated abnormalities of the bronchial architecture with nebulized bismuth powder. In 1922, Sicard and Forestier introduced iodized oil (Lipiodol). Bronchography in the diagnosis of bronchiectasis was then placed on a firm clinical basis.[2]

Early pulmonary resections were carried out with use of mass ligatures. The mortality rate was in the range of 25% due to exsanguinating hemorrhage from erosion of vessels at the hilus and the frequent development of a bronchopleural fistula with total empyema.

Graham performed the first pneumonectomy for carcinoma in 1933, but pulmonary resection did not achieve a sound technical basis until Churchill and Belsey,[10] later amplified by Blades and Kent,[5] recommended individual ligation and division of the structures at the pulmonary hilus. Jackson and Huber[32] introduced the concept of segmental anatomy, outlined the bronchovascular segments and devised a system of classification that is in current use (Fig. 32-4). Based on this work, Overholt and Langer[40] developed the technique for resection of individual pulmonary segments. Extirpative surgery thus became specific, limiting resection procedures to the area of disease and sparing adjacent parenchyma. As a further refinement of the surgical anatomy of bronchovascular segments, Bloomer *et al.*[7] prepared numerous injection specimens corresponding to the bronchial anomalies, anatomic variations and the various types of bronchopulmonary disease lending themselves to surgical intervention.

In 1948, water-soluble bronchographic media with the advantage of rapid absorption were introduced. Adverse reactions were common and definition was variable. More recently, propyliodine has become popular. The oily form of Dionosil is less irritating and is absorbed in 2-4 days.

Refinements of x-ray technique and anatomic resection have extended the scope and accuracy of surgical intervention. Mortality in partial resection of the lung is close to 1% in capable hands.

PATHOLOGY

Bronchiectasis is a misleading term because it describes only the pathologic state of the peripheral bronchial tree. This dilatation is described as cylindrical, fusiform, saccular or cystic, depending on the configuration observed by mapping the bronchial tree in bronchographic studies. This system of classification has little clinical importance. Early cylindrical change may be reversible and may be seen transiently after acute pulmonary infections. Many asymptomatic patients may have an area of segmental bronchiectasis. The exact mechanism of dilatation of peripheral bronchi is not understood, but from the study of resected specimens it is apparent that destructive changes go on in the walls of the bronchi with a loss of ciliated epithelium. With regeneration, metaplasia occurs, changing from cuboidal to squamous epithelium. In addition, there are loss of elastic tissue within the bronchial wall, thickening and peribronchial fibrosis. It is the involvement of adjacent parenchymal tissue that determines the clinical importance of the disease process. Endobronchial ulceration extends to destroy functioning lung units, gradually replacing

these through waves of infection and healing with fibrous tissue. Multiple abscesses occur with or without bronchial communication. There is a characteristic obstructive endarteritis of the small and medium-sized pulmonary arteries.[48] The segmental nature of bronchiectatic change is well known. The areas most frequently involved are the basal segments of the lower lobes, the right middle lobe and the lingular segments of the left upper lobe. Etiology has much to do with the distribution. The right lower lobe is most frequently involved in foreign body aspiration. Mucoviscidosis is diffuse throughout both lungs. Atelectasis alternates with areas of obstructive emphysema, and the eventual bronchiectasis has a predilection for the upper lobes. With the pronounced hilar lymphadenopathy of primary tuberculosis, the oblique anatomic take-off of the bronchus to the right middle lobe renders it vulnerable to obstructive emphysema, resorption atelectasis and bronchiectatic changes in the peripheral bronchi. Reinfection tuberculosis produces fibrocavitary disease most commonly in segments 2, 1, 6 and 3, in order of decreasing frequency. These inert pools make the patient vulnerable to recurring pneumonitis with each episode of upper respiratory infection.

ETIOLOGY

The most common causes of bronchiectasis in childhood are pulmonary infections, including pneumonia, and in the past complicating pertusis, measles and tuberculosis. These are followed by bronchiectasis secondary to hereditary or congenital disorders and to aspiration or inhalation of foreign bodies. An increasing number of children with cystic fibrosis now survive into the second decade of life through prolonged prophylactic broad-spectrum antibiotic therapy. We are encountering a significant number who require pulmonary resection because of advanced localized bronchiectasis.

The etiology of bronchiectasis in 222 children with bronchiectasis seen at the Children's Hospital Medical Center from 1940 to 1965 is shown in Table 32-3. The etiology of bronchiectasis in the same group of patients arranged in 5-year periods is shown in Figure 32-5. From 1940 to 1945, the leading cause of bronchiectasis was pneumonia, followed by assorted infections, pertussis and the usual causes of bronchiectasis seen today. A similar pattern was seen from 1945 to 1950, when even more children were encountered with advanced, destructive, bilateral lung changes, having survived pulmonary infections in the previous 5-year period. From 1950 to 1955, there was a reduction of the number of cases encountered, plus the virtual disappearance of the postpneumonic form of bronchiectasis and of bronchiectasis following pertussis, attributable to widescale immunization. The period 1955–60 witnessed the further reduction of post-pneumonic bronchiectasis of any bacterial variety and the emer-

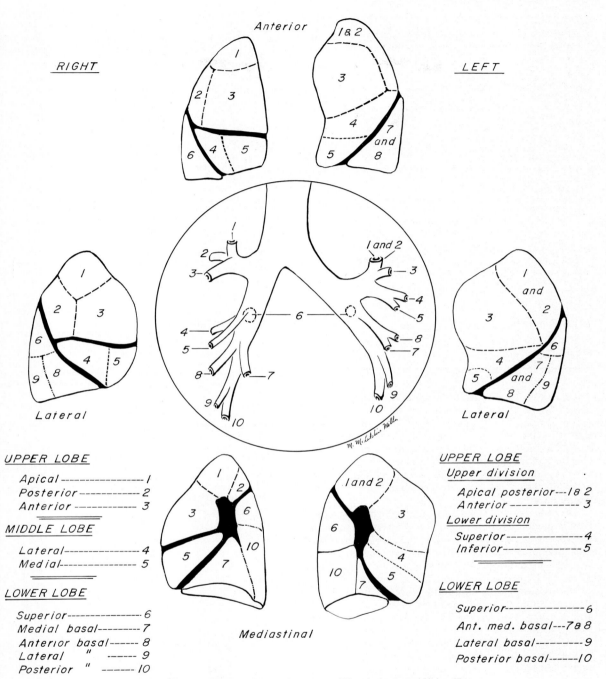

Fig. 32-4.—Pulmonary segmental anatomy. (After Jackson and Huber.[32])

TABLE 32-3.—Etiology of Bronchiectasis in Childhood: Children's Hospital Medical Center; 1940–68

Category*	Cases	%
1. Bronchiectasis secondary to infection	140	49
a) Following pneumonia	71	
b) Associated with nonspecific infection	23	
c) Following pertussis	22	
d) Associated with asthma	16	
e) Complicating tuberculosis	4	
f) Following measles	3	
g) Following scarlet fever	1	
2. Bronchiectasis secondary to cystic fibrosis	78	27
3. Bronchiectasis secondary to hereditary or congenital disorders	37	13
a) Anatomic pulmonary anomalies	15	
b) Kartagener's triad	7	
c) Agammaglobulinemia (congenital)	5	
d) Extrapulmonary cardiovascular anomalies	4	
e) "Congenital" bronchiectasis	3	
f) Alymphothymia	2	
g) Anatomic pulmonary vascular anomalies	1	
4. Bronchiectasis secondary to aspiration	32	11
a) Foreign body	19	
b) Blood	8	
c) Liquid feeding	5	
Total	287	100%

*Classification of Glausser *et al.*[27]

gence of a group of patients with cystic fibrosis, considered to be suitable candidates for palliative resection. In the final period, 1960–65, cystic fibrosis leads the list, with an increased number of cases due to foreign body, congenital anomalies of the lung and hereditary or poorly understood autoimmune disorders that make the individual vulnerable to infections of all types. Various conditions deserve special mention.

Sarcoidosis.—In association with marked regional lymphadenopathy, bronchiectasis is often found with Boeck's sarcoid and with primary pulmonary tuberculosis. Schneid[42] found 1,700 cases in the literature, with 5% in children, the most common age group being 10–15 years. Prednisone appears to control the early lung and extrapulmonary lesions but has little effect on hilar lymphadenopathy or on the residual lung damage that results. The Nickerson-Kveim test is diagnostic of the condition. This is an intradermal test similar to the Frei test, with the antigen obtained from sarcoid tissue. A papule develops in 4–6 weeks. Biopsy shows the typical microscopic appearance in approximately 85% of cases. False positive reactions occur in 4%.

Infection.—The vulnerability of the bronchial system and the destructive lung changes that follow early childhood infection are well known. It is probable that most patients acquire bronchiectasis in the first year of life (80 of 209 in one series, with 75% of pa-

tients under age 5). With aggressive early antibiotic therapy, the postpneumonic group is rapidly shrinking. Ulcerative bronchitis and its sequelae are still seen with pertussis and measles in the relatively small nonimmunized group. Among 1,894 pertussis patients, 87 developed pneumonia with at least transient dilatation of the secondary bronchi.[19] These changes appear to be reversible. Blades and Dugan[6] coined the term pseudobronchitis, particularly

Fig. 32-5.—Changing etiology of bronchiectasis as encountered at Children's Hospital Medical Center, Boston, in 5-year segments from 1940 to 1965. (See also Table 32-3.) From 1940 to 1945, before the availability of antibiotics, the principal cause was primary pulmonary infection in 48 of 61 patients, including 12 with pertussis. From 1945 to 1950, 67 resections were performed. Forty-eight followed pulmonary infection. Following the wider acceptance of specific immunization, there was a reduction in the number of cases due to pertussis. From 1950 to 1955, we observed a dramatic reduction in the number of cases due to pulmonary infection and an increase in the number of children undergoing pulmonary resection for bronchiectasis of diverse causes. Only 6 patients had postpneumonic bronchiectasis and in 4 bronchiectasis followed pertussis. From 1955 to 1960, there was further reduction of bronchiectasis due to pulmonary infection with no cases following pertussis. This era, as medical therapy became more effective, marked the appearance of universal bronchiectasis due to cystic fibrosis. For the first time, children survived long enough to demonstrate total but variable pulmonary involvement. Six of 15 patients with bronchiectasis due to other causes had cystic fibrosis. From 1960 to 1965, bronchiectasis following ordinary bacterial infections remained a rarity. Cystic fibrosis migrated to the head of the list of causes of bronchiectasis, and 12 children were encountered. This trend has continued, and cystic fibrosis is the leading cause of bronchiectasis in our institution. It is estimated that 1/3 of patients with cystic fibrosis will develop bronchiectasis, many requiring resection therapy tailored to their disease and to their pulmonary function. Autopsy study of approximately 40 children a year who have succumbed to the respiratory havoc of cystic fibrosis reveals widespread bronchiectasis and pulmonary suppuration. Selection of patients for resection may be improved by Xenon scans and selective pulmonary artery flow determinations. Most patients have benefited from selective segmental or lobar resection, although the subject remains controversial.

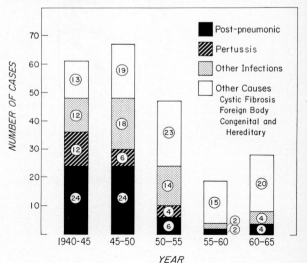

applicable to those children who have transient cylindrical ectasia in 5% of cases.

About 20% of patients with bronchiectasis have associated sinusitis or other evidence of allergy. This is probably not a cause-and-effect relationship. The bronchiectatic focus may serve as the trigger point for recurring attacks of asthma and for persistence of the sinusitis. Following removal of the destroyed pulmonary segment, the asthmatic attacks may be ameliorated and the sinusitis may clear. Aggressive surgical attacks on the maxillary antra are no longer in vogue, although sustained medical treatment may be beneficial before pulmonary resection is undertaken. The poorest results of resection therapy occur in patients with asthma and associated bronchiectasis.

AGAMMAGLOBULINEMA; ALYMPHOTHYMIA. — Agammaglobulinemia has been encountered in 5 patients, all boys, with the congenital form of the disorder and in 1 girl with an acquired deficiency of gamma globulin evident at age 8.[47] All had severe pulmonary disease with repeated episodes of pneumonia, chronic sinusitis and otitis. Two patients underwent pulmonary resection, with a total of five lobes removed; both children were alive at age 17 and 19. The others died between ages 9 and 13. The acquired type should be suspected, identified and appropriately treated much as one would in adults. A new entity, consisting of absence of the thymic gland and severe inadequacy of lymphatic tissue throughout the body, called alymphothymia, is also associated with vulnerability to pulmonary infection and development of bronchiectasis. Two patients with this disorder have been observed, both with moderately advanced bronchiectasis. The condition is fascinating in relation to experimental models that have been constructed in connection with the investigation of antilymphocyte serum (ALS). In both groups, homografted skin will survive for 58 days, in contrast to control survival of 12.6 days.

FOREIGN BODIES. — Grass foreign bodies are difficult to diagnose from the history. They travel in ratchet fashion to the periphery of the right lower lobe, and weeks or months may pass before segmental or lobar suppuration leads to the diagnosis. Bronchial secretions aspirated during diagnostic studies should always be stained and examined for vegetable fibers.[48] Opaque foreign bodies are readily recognized, produce more dramatic initial obstructive symptoms and usually are recovered endoscopically before irreversible lung changes occur.

Vegetable foreign bodies were listed by Gross as the most frequent aspirated foreign bodies leading to pulmonary resection (Fig. 32-6). Of our 8 patients who had inhaled a head of timothy grass (*Phleum pratense*), 7 required lobectomy (Fig. 32-7). With Carter, we[48] have discussed the peculiarities in terms of localization in the right lower lobe and in the intensity of the granuloma reaction. Jackson[21] considered the condition rare. He had only 35 patients among his personal series of nearly 3,000 cases of ingested or inhaled foreign bodies. He was able to remove all of these grass heads by bronchoscopy and no lobectomy was required. This is contrary to our experience. Since our original report in 1948,[48] 3 of 5 additional patients required lobectomy. Wooley[50] added 3 more cases. Seventeen cases of "empyema necessitatus" have been reported with extrusion of the foreign body.[31]

KARTAGENER'S SYNDROME. — We have encountered 7 children with Kartagener's triad of dextrocardia, sinusitis and bronchiectasis (Fig. 32-8). Three have undergone lobectomy. Holmes[30] noted low serum IgA values in 13 patients from eight families. Seven required lobectomy, 4 of them children aged 3, 10, 12 and 14. Holmes described a follicular form of bronchiectasis with prominent lymphoid follicles. In 1962, Kartagener and Straki[35] collected 334 cases, an incidence of 1:8,000; they observed that 20% of patients with situs inversus have bronchiectasis. Nickamin[39] reported the condition in the newborn. The bronchiectasis has no relation to the dextrocardia and seems to be a genetic defect in these individuals with cartilage rings of little stability.

About 12% of children with dextrocardia develop bronchiectasis, but 25% of the siblings of individuals with dextrocardia develop bronchiectasis with the heart in normal position.[17]

Fonkalsrud *et al.*[24] reviewed the manifestations of situs inversus in 37 children seen from 1950 to 1964, 78% of whom had multiple anomalies. Half the patients had major cardiac lesions, tetralogy of Fallot

Fig. 32-6. — Bronchiectasis: foreign body (corn kernel) aspiration. This 5-month-old girl aspirated several kernels of corn. The bronchogram shows complete obstruction of the right lower lobe bronchus. The sharp cut-off of bronchial filling at the level of the most proximal foreign body is well seen; there is complete collapse of the lobe.

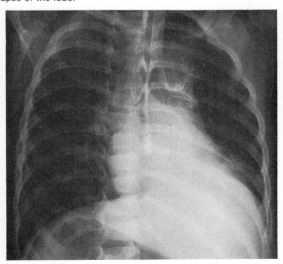

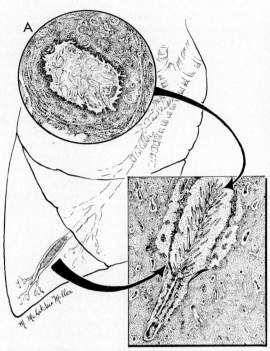

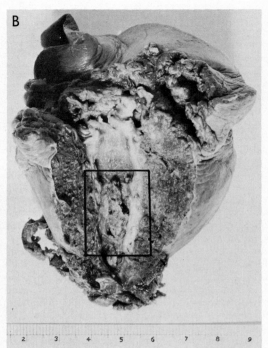

Fig. 32-7. — Bronchiectasis: foreign body (timothy grass head) aspiration. **A,** by ratchet progression, the timothy head advances into the periphery of the right lower lobe. Inset drawings were made from thin section photomicrographs. The grass fibers may at times be seen in stains of material aspirated during bronchoscopy. **B,** resected right lower lobe showing extensive destruction and bronchiectasis. The timothy head is readily seen in the outlined area.

Fig. 32-8. — Kartagener's syndrome in 8-year-old boy. The bronchogram shows complete situs inversus. The left lung is in the right hemithorax, and the lingular branch of the upper lobe, particularly the lower division, is involved in the bronchiectatic process. The left lower lobe in the right hemithorax shows bronchiectasis in all divisions. Sinus films showed pansinusitis. At operation, the basal portion of the lower lobe in the right chest was firm, purple, mottled, and the lingular segment of the upper lobe atelectatic. Lower lobe and lingula were removed. (Courtesy of Dr. M. M. Ravitch.)

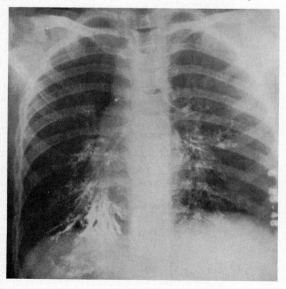

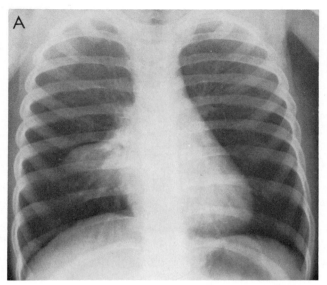

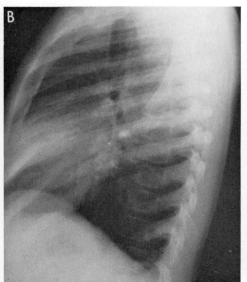

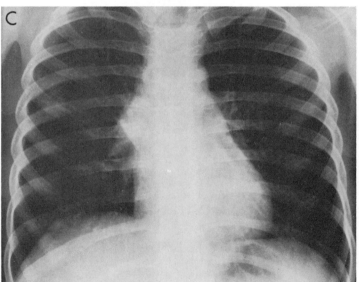

Fig. 32-9.—Right middle lobe syndrome (nontuberculous, postpneumonic). A 6-year-old girl with history of recurring localized pulmonary infection from her first year. **A,** anterior projection, showing typical distribution of the area of absorption atelectasis in middle lobe segments 4 and 5. **B,** lateral view, identifying area of atelectasis. The fissures are now concave, indicating a burned-out process with functional destruction of this lobe. At operation, the middle lobe was shrunken, fibrotic and airless. **C,** roentgenogram 1 month after right middle lobectomy showing residual evidence of hilar dissection. The patient was asthmatic and was substantially improved.

being the commonest. Only 1 patient had Kartagener's triad requiring pulmonary resection. Thirteen of the 37 patients did, however, have pulmonary problems consisting of atelectasis and bronchopneumonia. One patient had a lung abscess that was resected.

MIDDLE LOBE SYNDROME.—In the middle lobe syndrome in children,[15,29] the pneumonitis, bronchial obstruction and ultimate atelectasis (Fig. 32-9) are most frequently due to epibronchitis and extrinsic compression from mediastinal nodes. Congenital anomalies of the bronchi are rare, but when infection is added, there is inevitable development of bronchiectasis (Fig. 32-10). Wilkinson stressed this point in primary tuberculosis in children. In 5 of 20 patients in whom

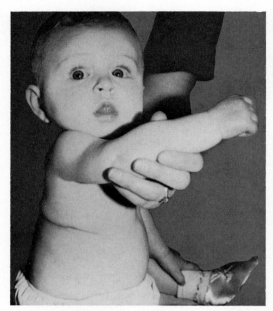

Fig. 32-10.—Photograph after right middle lobectomy for bronchiectasis due to congenital bronchial defect. Operation was performed at 8 months, following a 6-month history of intermittent cough and fever, with a pneumonic infiltrate limited to the middle lobe.

resection was done, evidence was present of a congenital bronchial anomaly in addition to tuberculous disease.

The middle lobe syndrome may occur in children without evidence of tuberculosis. Characteristically, there is a history of pneumonia in early life and density is noted in the medial portion of the right middle lobe (Fig. 32-9). On lateral films, depression of the horizontal fissure and elevation of the oblique fissure are seen. The reverse may be true with check-valve obstruction of these bronchi.

MUCOVISCIDOSIS.—The association of pulmonary mucoviscidosis with cystic fibrosis of the pancreas has become increasingly evident as more patients are brought through the phase of neonatal intestinal obstruction, techniques for maintaining satisfactory nutrition are improved and prophylactic antibiotic therapy protects against recurring pulmonary infection. Many of these children now survive to be followed in special treatment clinics. Williams and O'Reilly[48] reported on 56 patients with bronchiectasis due to cystic fibrosis. This disease is now in first place in the list of etiologic factors. In the nutrition clinic of the Children's Hospital Medical Center, Boston, 920 patients with cystic fibrosis are being followed.[44] Of this group, 140 have survived operation for meconeum ileus, and approximately 270 have pulmonary disease, one-third with clinical and x-ray evidence of bronchiectasis. These patients require antibiotic therapy (tetracycline) for acute episodes of re-

spiratory infection diagnosed by cultures. The youngest patient requiring lobectomy was 10 months old. The histologic picture in resected material is typical of the basic disease, showing a defect of the bronchial glands with mucus defective in quality. Rheometric studies suggest that molecular sodium and chloride content may be an important factor in the increased mucous viscosity. Obstruction by inspissated mucus is present at all levels, with eventual segmental bronchiolar involvement and adjacent parenchymal suppuration. Areas of overdistention alternate with atelectasis, minute abscesses and diffuse bronchial sepsis.[37] Except as a preoperative necessity, bronchography is considered harmful. Lobectomy must be reserved for sharply localized areas of permanent destruction. Pulmonary resection is considered unrewarding in patients under 1 year with this disease. Crossett and Shaw[14] reported resections in 2 infants aged 3 and 5 months; both were dead within 4 months. The usual area of maximal destruction is in the upper lobes (Fig. 32-11). The best theoretical explanation is that the maximal expiratory exchange occurs at the basal portions of the lungs in young children and that relative stasis occurs at the lung apices. The younger the child, the more this is true.

All children suspected of having cystic fibrosis should have a sweat test, which is 99% accurate. The normal average sodium and cloride content of sweat is 59 and 32 mEq/liter respectively. In mucoviscidosis, these figures may rise to 133 and 106. Sodium and chloride values are correspondingly low in bronchial mucus, thought to have much to do with increased viscosity.

In 1949, Katznelson *et al.*[36] reported 5 cases from our hospital of pulmonary resection for bronchiectasis

Fig. 32-11.—Mucoviscidosis: areas of distention alternate with atelectasis. Upper lobes are most commonly involved. Bronchoscopy should be avoided unless there is good clinical evidence that extirpation of an area of maximal involvement may be necessary.

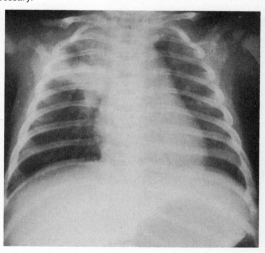

associated with botryomycosis in children with cystic fibrosis. We encountered this situation 7 times in 29 resections for cystic fibrosis performed from 1959 to 1968. In another case, actinomycosis was a complicating factor resulting in death of the patient several months after surgery. The pulmonary fungal overgrowth in these patients must be related to the many years of prophylactic broad-spectrum therapy. On occasion, ordinarily saprophytic fungi convert to pathogenic and destructive form.

Experience with 21 pulmonary resections for cystic fibrosis led Schuster and colleagues[43] to conclude that palliative resection for localized areas of bronchiectasis in carefully selected patients is worth while and should be pursued. There is significant intraoperative and early postoperative mortality from pulmonary resections for this disorder, occurring in 3 of their 21 patients. Patients who have had resections since 1964 have in general done better as a result of careful drying out of the lungs preoperatively, bronchial lavage with N-acetylcysteine,[41] preoperative tracheostomy and operation on the children in facedown position. Four-fifths of patients with disease limited to two lobes and preoperative demonstration of adequate pulmonary reserve will benefit from palliative resection. The etiology of 357 cases of bronchiectasis in children, collected from the literature, is seen in Table 32-4. Cystic fibrosis was more frequently encountered, as in our institution, which is a cystic fibrosis center.

TUMORS. – In children, endobronchial tumors as a rule are benign adenomas which may be attached to a pedicle and intermittently obstruct a lobar bronchus. We relieved a 9-month-old infant of pseudobronchiectasis of the right upper lobe by removing a tumor the size of a golf ball from the right lobe of the thymus.

Neoplasms of the lung as a cause of parenchymal pathology are discussed in Chapter 33. Only 2 of 127 lobectomies for bronchiectasis were associated with neoplasm, both benign bronchial adenomas.

DEFORMITIES. – On occasion, extreme forms of scoliosis, pectus excavatum and deformity produced by somite disturbance (spinomyelodysplasia) may be associated with bronchiectasis. This results from displacement of mediastinal structures, an inefficient thoracic cage and inadequate drainage of the lower lung areas.

In summary, reduction of the number of children with the surgical form of bronchiectasis is the result of a combination of factors: (1) Improved anesthesia methods and adoption of the endotracheal technique for most surgical conditions of the nasopharynx. (2) Adoption of the prone position for tonsillectomy and adenoidectomy has lessened the incidence of septic embolization to the lungs with blood and tissue fragments. Post-tonsillectomy and aspiration bronchiectasis has been largely eliminated through prevention, prompt recognition and treatment with appropriate antibiotics. (3) Rapid antibiotic sterilization of the lung in most pulmonary infections common to childhood has virtually eliminated postpneumonic bronchiectasis of the type described by Field.[21] (4) Recognition that diffuse mild bronchiectasis without localization and without saccular change can be kept under satisfactory medical control, arrested at that stage of the disease or even substantially improved. Not only is there a halt in the bronchiectasis, but pulmonary function studies carried out over a number of years have demonstrated that the medically controlled and asymptomatic group compares favorably with the surgically resected asymptomatic group.[27] Only in advanced symptomatic medical and surgical groups with bilateral disease were test results substantially below normal. The most significant changes occurred in residual lung volume, averaging 147% of the predicted value, and reduced maximal breathing capacity in all but the medically treated group with no residual symptoms.

On the other hand, limitation of spread through prompt bronchographic recognition and resection of advanced lobar or segmental disease has been universally accepted. Pulmonary resection in all groups other than children with cystic fibrosis has a mortality rate close to 1% and very low morbidity. There have been no deaths following lobectomy for bronchiectasis due to conditions other than cystic fibrosis in our institution since 1942.

SYMPTOMS

The commonest complaint in symptomatic bronchiectasis is cough. In "dry" bronchiectasis, paroxysms of coughing occur from irritation of the bronchial passages by temperature change or miscellaneous irritants. In the "wet" variety, cough is associated with production of sputum. Patients with bronchiectasis characteristically have recurring respiratory infections which last 1–2 months. Generally, the sputum is thick and tenacious, yellow-green in color and may vary from a few teaspoons a day to as much as a quart. Coughing is often induced by changes of position. It interrupts children at play and while they sleep, as pools of septic material shift from ectatic

TABLE 32-4. – ETIOLOGY OF BRONCHIECTASIS
IN CHILDHOOD*

CAUSE	CASES
Postpneumonic	127
Mucoviscidosis	70
Pulmonary tuberculosis	53
Foreign body aspiration	31
Congenital bronchovascular defect	26
Allergy (sinusitis-asthma)	18
Exanthems	13
Miscellaneous causes (Kartagener's syndrome; agammaglobulinemia)	13
Undetermined	6
Total	357

*From the literature.

areas into more proximal areas of the bronchial tree, stimulating the cough reflex. Hemoptysis, usually encountered at some stage of the disease, can vary from streaking of the sputum to exsanguinating hemorrhage. This is particularly true with grass foreign bodies that lodge in the right lower lobe. An intense reaction is produced and a very vascular granulation tissue lines the cavity containing the foreign body. Paroxysms of coughing eventually lead to vomiting in younger children. With more extensive disease and sometimes out of proportion to the degree of apparent involvement, many patients have dyspnea. The dyspnea does not appear to be due to a significant decrease of functioning parenchyma but may reflect an associated bronchospasm produced as septic material from the lung base is mobilized. With the disappearance of the hopelessly severe cases of bronchiectasis, we no longer see metastatic brain abscess, empyema and amyloidosis. The incidence of pulmonary osteoarthropathy varies in different series and seems to correlate with the amount of retained secretions. Strang[46] reported it to be as high as 51%. In his series of 209 children, 69 had chest pain, hemoptysis occurred in 54, foul sputum in 51, asthma in 50 and sinusitis in 52. Girls are said to have bronchiectasis more frequently than boys. In Strang's series there were 119 girls and 90 boys. This is of doubtful significance.

DIAGNOSIS

The diagnosis is suggested by a history of major pulmonary disease in early life or by any historical fact or clinical finding pointing to the various causes discussed above. The symptom complex is suggestive, but there seems to be no accurate correlation between the clinical picture and anatomic findings within the lung, either at the time of bronchoscopy or on examination of the resected specimen.

X-RAY EXAMINATIONS. – As a rule, plain anteroposterior and lateral films of the chest are not diagnostic of bronchiectasis. In instances with a specific etiology, such as mediastinal lymph nodes in primary tuberculosis or radiopaque foreign bodies, the findings and distribution may be highly suggestive of the etiology. In most cases, an increase of bronchovascular markings is evident at the hilus. A downward and outward streaking or at times frank segmental or lobar atelectasis may be observed. Any x-ray change in the lower lung fields is suggestive. In all suspected cases, early diagnostic bronchoscopy and bronchography are indicated.

BRONCHOSCOPY AND BRONCHOGRAPHY. – In children under 12, general anesthesia should be employed for diagnostic bronchoscopy. We prefer the Pilling models of the Jackson bronchoscope. In infants, only a 3-mm instrument can be passed. In older children the 4-mm scope can be used. The instrument measures 4 mm in transverse diameter and 7 mm in vertical diameter. It is 30 cm long and permits access

to all of the major bronchi. By shifting the head markedly to the left, it is usually possible to observe the right upper lobe bronchus and, in a more neutral position, the right middle lobe orifice and at least the take-off of the lower lobe bronchus. Secretions should be aspirated into a standard Lukens collector. Specific obstruction should be ruled out. A full range of grasping fenestrated forceps should be available.

When the area of maximal disease has been estimated and appropriate cultures have been obtained, all segments of the bronchial tree should be mapped. Direct aspiration of bronchiectatic cavities should be done before instillation of opaque medium in order to provide better filling and to avoid harmful spill into contralateral bronchi in the various positions that must be adopted to demonstrate all segments. Propyliodine is the most satisfactory medium. The ideal bronchogram should resemble a leafless tree. A good deal of the distribution is accomplished by the patient's own ventilation. The bronchi should not be overfilled to the extent of "putting leaves on the tree." Overfilling of the bronchi, particularly in tiny babies who already have respiratory difficulties, may lead to a dangerous interference with respiration as well as obscure the radiographic features of the instillation. A minimal amount (5-15 cc) of medium instilled under fluoroscopic control allows spot films to capture the bronchographic picture when it is clearest. The water-miscible media have the advantage of being discharged rapidly so that they do not confuse future radiographic examinations, but they are somewhat irritating to the bronchial mucosa. Although some prefer to demonstrate the bronchi in only a single lung at a given examination, we feel that it is usually possible to obtain satisfactory bronchograms of all five lobes at a single sitting. No decision regarding operation should be made without complete visualization and mapping of all lobes and segments.

Pulmonary function studies have limited value in small children. In the case of extensive bilateral disease when a total of as much as one lung in various segmental combinations must be removed to relieve the patient of disease, differential bronchospirometry is advisable.[20] A Carlen catheter is ideal for these studies. Xenon scans and pulmonary artery flow rates now permit highly accurate determinations of total and differential pulmonary function in children of any age.

The anatomic distribution of lung segments resected for bronchiectasis in a collected series is shown in Table 32-5. Bronchiectasis developed in these patients early in life before the advent or appropriate use of antibiotics and contributed to this series between 1940 and 1950.[3,16,21,25,28,46] The emphasis has since shifted from the bronchiectasis of bacterial or unknown origin to that produced by unusual bacterial infections, lesions that obstruct by obturation (foreign bodies, mucoviscidosis and rare endobronchial soft tissue tumors) and anomalies of bronchial origin or

TABLE 32-5.—PULMONARY RESECTION FOR
NONTUBERCULOUS BRONCHIECTASIS IN CHILDHOOD*

OPERATION		CASES
Lobectomy		177
LLL + lingula	65	
LLL	46	
LUL	4	
RLL + RML	28	
RLL	20	
RML	13	
RUL	1	
Pneumonectomy		61
Segmental resection		17
Total		255

*From the literature.

structure. Strang[46] found bilateral disease in 28% of 290 patients. The left lower lobe and lingula, and the left lower lobe alone, are involved more frequently than other areas. This is followed in order of decreasing frequency by right middle lobe and right lower lobe in combination, diffuse involvement of a single lung and involvement of the right lower lobe. In post-pneumonic bronchiectasis, isolated right middle lobe involvement is uncommon but does occur.

Bronchography gives the best anatomic definition of the areas of significant disease (Fig. 32-12). Attempts to read areas as bronchiectatic on body section films (tomography) are unsuccessful. Configuration of the ectatic bronchi, whether they are cylindrical or saccular, seems to have little bearing on the clinical extent of disease and its ability to produce symptoms. Some patients have marked difficulties with minimal bronchographic involvement, and others with focal saccular disease are fully active and without striking symptoms.

BACTERIOLOGY

The flora in bronchiectasis is diverse and constantly changing. Careful culture technique is important at the time of bronchoscopy in order to gain the most information in this regard. One can usually identify normal bacterial flora of the respiratory tract (such as *Neisseria catarrhalis* and nonhemolytic streptococci). In the gram-positive series, pneumococci, hemolytic streptococci and *Staphylococcus aureus* are found in that order. Fortunately, most respond to available antibiotics. In patients who have had prolonged penicillin therapy, gram-negative organisms appear, including *Escherichia coli, Aerobacter aerogenes, H. influenzae,* pseudomonas, *Proteus vulgaris* and on occasion the markedly destructive Klebsiella. If the process has reached the putrid stage, fusospirochetal organisms are added. If broad-spectrum antibiotics have been used over a long period, there is overgrowth of *Candida albicans* probably of little clinical significance even though mycotic nests with active budding may be found within the parenchyma.

With this great range of respiratory tract organisms, it is difficult to chart appropriate antibiotic therapy. Clinical experience has demonstrated, however, that penicillin is the drug of choice in the initial treatment of bronchiectasis.

TREATMENT

NONOPERATIVE MANAGEMENT.—Nonoperative management has its limitations. It has greatly altered the prognosis in patients with extensive bilateral dis-

Fig. 32-12.—Bronchiectasis. **A,** bronchogram with satisfactory filling showing irreversible saccular and cylindrical bronchiectatic changes in the right lower lobe due to recurring episodes of pneumonia. **B,** irreversible changes in the left lower lobe and lingular segment of the left upper lobe following bacterial infection.

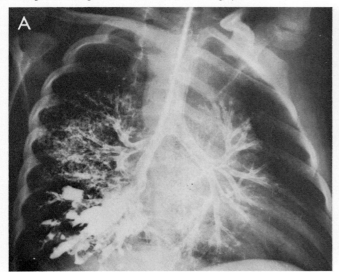
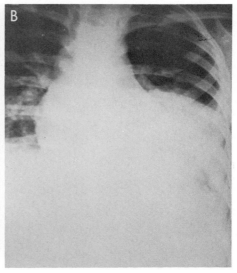

ease, but its long-term value is limited by the development of antibiotic allergy in a certain percentage of patients and by the eventual emergence of resistant organisms. It has great usefulness in preventing destructive bronchopulmonary changes at the time of initial infection. In patients with established bronchiectasis of known anatomic distribution, it can at best be considered a palliative form of therapy. The young patient with adequate pulmonary reserve and without major associated disease should have the advantage of a definitive resection.

PREPARATION FOR OPERATION. — In addition to general supportive care aimed at putting the patient in the best possible condition prior to resection, certain specific steps should be undertaken. All patients will benefit to some degree from postural drainage for 15 minutes three times daily before each meal. In addition, it is advisable to give penicillin as penicillin G, 500,000 units intramuscularly twice a day. If a great number of gram-negative organisms are present, streptomycin may be added. Tetracycline is a broad-spectrum antibiotic of particular value in mucoviscidosis and may be given by mouth in amounts up to 1 Gm a day.

Additional aids in preoperative preparation include the use of Mucomist (acetylcysteine, 1-4 cc of a 10% solution q. i. d. as aerosol). For an expectorant, we prefer glycerylguaiacolate (Robitussin). Preoperative instruction in breathing exercises using all of the muscles of respiration is of great value in children old enough to understand and co-operate.

INDICATIONS FOR RESECTION. — Indications for resection include harassing cough, productive sputum, hemoptysis, toxicity, fever, weight loss and bronchographic evidence of irreversible lung destruction. The age for operation is determined by the time significant symptoms first develop. These children are usually presented for resection at some time between ages 5 and 15, ordinarily before age 10.

AREAS FOR RESECTION. — There is obviously a limit to the amount of pulmonary tissue that can safely be resected. Of considerable importance is the work of Bremer,[9] subsequently supported in pulmonary function studies by Baird *et al.*,[4] that newborn kittens and presumably young children are capable of true pulmonary new growth. Tubular alveolar sprouts form and new functioning pulmonary units are created. This coincides with the universal experience that children can stand extensive pulmonary resection, including pneumonectomy, exceptionally well. In children, the remaining segments are not overdistended to the extent that occurs in adults. Thoracic deformity does

Fig. 32-13 (left). — Bronchiectasis. Bronchogram showing extensive saccular bronchiectasis of left lower lobe with involvement of lingular division of the left upper lobe. Postpneumonic bronchiectasis occurs most frequently in these segments.

Fig. 32-14 (right). — Bronchiectasis. Same patient as in Figure 32-13. Hemisected specimen of resected left lower lobe showing a huge bronchiectatic cavity and parenchymal destructive change throughout the lobe. (MGH #111-56-94.)

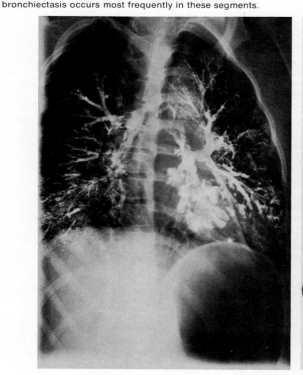

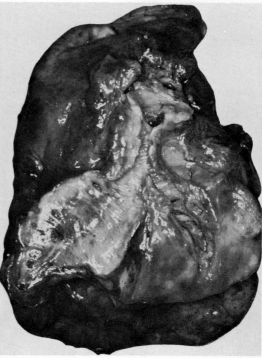

not develop, and in all probability, the younger the patient, the greater is his compensatory ability in this regard. This argues for early resection when clearly indicated. Bilateral procedures are infrequently done at the Boston Children's Hospital and the Mayo Clinic,[13,28] This is consistent with the relatively controlled disease state observed today with aggressive and early medical attention. Reports from Europe still indicate greater exposure or vulnerability to chronic respiratory infection, and bilateral procedures are performed 14 times more often than in the United States.[21,25] The left lung is more often involved than the right, and the estimate of bilateral disease is 30%. The basal segments of the lower lobes are more frequently involved; the superior segments of the lower lobes are usually free from disease except with cystic fibrosis and tuberculosis. With disease of the left basal segment, the lingula is involved in 80% of cases. With diseased basal segments on the right, the right middle lobe is involved in 60%. The usual operative procedure is directed to one side and the segments or lobes most frequently involved. In the event of bilateral disease, one should operate on the worst side first, accepting the remote risk of forced pneumonectomy. Upper lobe segments can often be spared in older children.

The right middle lobe has been called the homologue of the lingular division of the left upper lobe. It is composed of two segments (4 and 5 in the Jackson-Huber system) and is often resected with the right lower lobe with right-sided disease. Postpneumonic bronchiectasis involving the left lower lobe and lingula remains a common indication for pulmonary resection in childhood. An example of this is shown in Figures 32-13 and 32-14.

TECHNIQUE OF PULMONARY RESECTION

LOBECTOMY AND LINGULECTOMY. — Operative exposure is through the right or left seventh interspace, cutting one rib posteriorly if necessary. The incision may be placed somewhat higher if removal of the lingula or right middle lobe is contemplated. Rib resection is not employed in children.

With the patient in the lateral position, an incision is made the entire length of the seventh interspace (Fig. 32-15, A). On occasion, the fifth or sixth interspace may be used. The schematic drawing (Fig. 32-15, B) indicates the segmental distribution of the diseased area as seen in the lateral projection. Figure 32-15, C, shows the arrangement, at each pulmonary hilus, of branches of the pulmonary artery, pulmonary vein and segmental bronchi, which are customarily divided in that order. The line of demarcation between the overinflated dorsal segments of the left upper lobe and the collapsed fibrotic lingula are illustrated in Figure 32-15, D. It is usually more convenient to remove the left lower lobe before lingulectomy. The lower lobe is freed by division of the pulmonary liga-

ment and is drawn superiorly and medially to permit isolation and division of its bronchovascular supply (Fig. 32-15, E). Following removal of the left lower lobe, segmental resection of upper lobe segments 4 and 5 is completed, with preservation of the interlobar vein which serves as an anatomic guide to complete removal of the lingula (Fig. 32-15, F). The bronchial stumps (Fig. 32-15, G) are closed with simple end-on 4-0 silk sutures for the lingula and end-on sutures backed up with several vertical mattress sutures for the left lower lobe. These closures should be made flush with the walls of the parent bronchi without constricting them.

Decision as to the extent of resection is generally made before operation and should be based on bronchographic evidence. Frankly consolidated carneous-appearing pulmonary tissue can be recognized and obviously must be resected, but segments which show gross saccular bronchiectasis radiographically may appear surprisingly normal to inspection and palpation at the time of operation.

POSTOPERATIVE MANAGEMENT

Freedom from complications after pulmonary resection in children depends on careful attention to the maintenance of full expansion of the remaining lobe or segments. This is achieved by constant negative suction through intercostal catheters with 20–40 cm of water negative pressure and replacement of these catheters as indicated by accumulations of fluid and air in the postoperative roentgenograms. X-rays are taken immediately after operation and on the following day. If at this time the child is afebrile and the lung fully expanded, further x-rays need not be taken except on clinical indications. Oxygen tents are seldom required for the postoperative care of children with pulmonary resection, but the maintenance of a moist atmosphere in a Croupette, or with some other vaporizing device, is of the first importance. Children must be strongly encouraged to cough. Intratracheal aspiration should be employed as vigorously as seems required, using fresh sterile catheters for each aspiration. Breathing exercises are resumed as soon after operation as possible. Bronchial suture line leaks are infinitely less common in children, with their soft, pliable, well-nourished bronchi, than in adults. The single most important point in preventing suture line leaks is careful suture of the divided bronchus flush with the surface of its parent stem bronchus. This also prevents the late appearance of distressing symptoms due to infection in an overlong stump. The bronchial stump is further protected because the remaining aerated segments cover the raw area of mediastinal dissection. Tracheostomy will rarely be required, except with cystic fibrosis, if attention is paid to tracheal toilet before, during and after operation. Antibiotics are given for 1 week following operation.

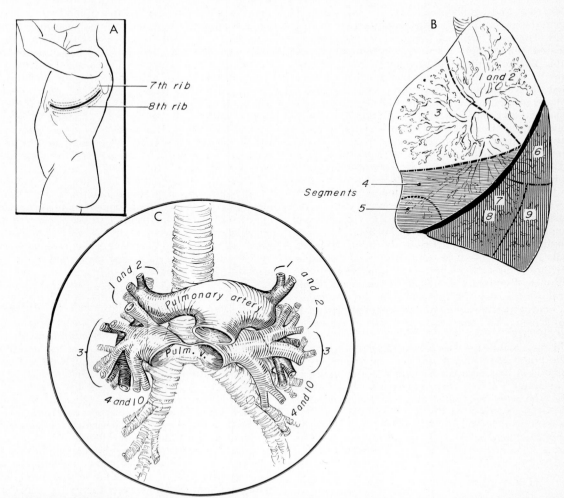

Fig. 32-15.—Technique of left lower lobectomy and lingulectomy, the commonest resection for bronchiectasis (in 85% of cases of left lower lobe bronchiectasis, the lingula is involved). **A,** full posterolateral thoracotomy. Rib section is rarely necessary in children. **B,** segments to be resected in children with unilateral disease. Segmental resection is infrequent, although the superior segment of the lower lobe **(6)** is often uninvolved. **C,** relation of hilar structures. The lingular bronchus arises as the lowest upper lobe bronchus or directly from the main bronchus opposite the bronchus of the superior segment of the lower lobe, as the lingular artery is opposite the artery of the superior segment. (*Continued.*)

RESULTS OF SURGICAL TREATMENT

Cooley *et al.*[13] pointed out that pulmonary resection can be done in children with 1% mortality but that long-term results may be discouraging and the complication rate high in children. In a series of 30 patients, retention of secretions occurred in 18, pleural effusion in 3, bronchopleural fistula in 2 and pneumothorax in 1. New areas of bronchiectasis developed in 5, but the original mapping may not have been accurate. Such an adverse experience with pulmonary resection for bronchiectasis in children is not widely agreed upon, and it is generally believed that operation should be done at any age when there is irreversible bronchial destruction and symptomatic

difficulties are of sufficient degree.[22,50] Lobectomy can be performed in patients under 1 year with a satisfactory low mortality according to Mendez.[38]

Segmental resection has found its place in the operative treatment of young adults with bilateral disease and is used with increasing frequency in this age group because removal of pulmonary tissue can be compensated for only by overdistention. In the younger child, it has its most frequent application in lingulectomy. In 1947, Overholt and Langer[40] reported 100 segmental resections for bronchiectasis. Among them were 85% with multiple segments, 30% bilateral, 60% lingular involvement with left basal segments and 45% with right middle lobe involve-

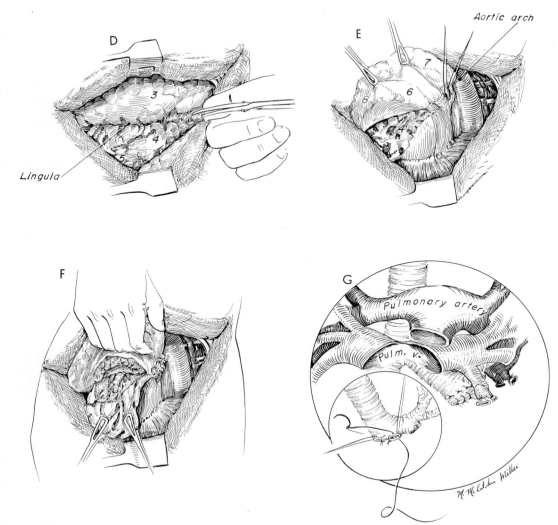

Fig. 32-15 (cont.).—D, the collapsed lingula **(4)** is readily distinguished from the anterior segment **(3). E, F** and **G,** the pulmonary ligament is divided, as succulent nodes are dissected away, the inferior pulmonary vein secured, and the lower lobe bronchus divided serially as the periphery is clamped and the central cut end sutured as it is cut. Inflation of the upper lobe permits separation of the attachment to the lower lobe by sharp or blunt dissection. The lingular artery is secured, the lingular bronchus occluded with a vascular clamp, and the lung inflated to identify the bronchus beyond question. The bronchus is divided and the lingula stripped from the remainder of the upper lobe on the intersegmental plane, bleeders and air leaks being carefully sutured.

ment with right basal segments of both lower lobes. Recent children's series show a reduction of cases of pneumonectomy corresponding to the use of segmental resection with little change in the relative number of lobectomies.

The results of surgical treatment for bronchiectasis at the Children's Hospital Medical Center during the period 1940–65 are indicated in Table 32-6. In that time, 133 lobectomies or segmental resections were performed. Early in the series, extending back to 1934, pneumonectomies were performed in 10 children with an over-all mortality of 40%. The unacceptably high figure is explained by the evolutionary phase of pulmonary resection, primitive anesthesia techniques, the unavailability of antibiotics and the far-advanced bilateral bronchiectasis encountered in that period. Surgical resection was an act of desperation. For many reasons, pneumonectomy for bilateral bronchiectasis is not performed today, and further discussion will be limited to lobectomy and segmental resection in the surgical management of this disorder. Three deaths resulted from lobectomy in chil-

TABLE 32-6.—RESULTS OF LOBECTOMY AND SEGMENTAL
RESECTION FOR BRONCHIECTASIS IN CHILDHOOD:
CHILDREN'S HOSPITAL MEDICAL CENTER*;
1940–65

CATEGORY	NO. OF PATIENTS	NO. OF DEATHS
1. Secondary to infection	45	3†
2. Secondary to hereditary or congenital disorders	17	0
3. Secondary to aspiration	14	0
4. Cystic fibrosis	20	3‡
Total	96	6(6.5%)

*Mortality for 133 resections in 96 patients, 4.5%.
†Operative deaths before 1945.
‡No resections for cystic fibrosis were performed before 1959. There
has been no operative mortality in 112 lobectomies for bronchiectasis
other than cystic fibrosis since 1945.

dren with the postpneumonic form of bronchiectasis. Both occurred before 1945. No resections for cystic fibrosis were performed before 1959, because very few children with advanced pulmonary disease lived long enough to develop the destructive changes as demonstrated by bronchography. We are exploring the advisability and value of pulmonary resection in a limited number of these patients.[43] There is an increased operative mortality in this group, although this is now being reduced through improved selection of patients and surgical innovations mentioned above. The table may be summarized by saying that cystic fibrosis is the commonest indication for pulmonary resection in bronchiectasis in children today. This is followed by bronchiectasis secondary to congenital anomalies of the lobes or bronchi, followed by a group of hereditary disorders that are associated with chronic lung disease. The least frequent indication for resection today is bronchiectasis secondary to aspiration. Permanent changes resulting from the aspiration of vomitus or blood while under anesthesia have disappeared. The importance of immediate extraction of an inhaled foreign body is generally appreciated; this requires a skilled endoscopist. Inhaled foreign bodies most frequently associated with bronchiectasis are the timothy head and peanuts. The former are nearly impossible to remove, and the latter are difficult to remove entirely since the peanuts are usually fragmented and the fragments move peripherally into the bronchial tree. There has been no operative mortality in 112 partial resections for bronchiectasis due to causes other than cystic fibrosis from 1945 to 1968.

Jaubout et al.[33] reported 97 pulmonary resections in children for bronchiectasis with no deaths. Foster et al.[26] reported pulmonary resection in 55 children with only one death, due to cardiac arrest, in 1958. This group included 11 patients with tuberculosis, in contrast to only 4 of 91 patients in our series. Of the 765 patients of all ages with bronchiectasis reviewed by Sealy et al.,[45] 140 underwent resection during the period 1954–64. There was only one death in the postoperative period, in an 11-year-old girl with diffuse, multisegmental disease following the ingestion of kerosine. Seventy patients with localized disease were completely relieved of respiratory symptoms. An equal number of patients had multisegmental disease, and 80% were greatly improved after resection therapy. Bourie and Lichter[8] made a 10-year survey of bronchiectasis in New Zealand during the period 1952–62. Of 125 patients operated on, 91 had unilateral resection and 68 had bilateral resections. Seventy patients had onset of symptoms in the first decade of life, and 45 were operated on. There was only one death following 165 resections. Complications occurred in 93 patients: 39 had collapse, 3 pneumothorax, 2 bronchopleural fistula, 6 empyema and 4 serous effusion. These authors, too, commented on the satisfactory results of resection for bronchiectasis, with 55% classified as excellent and 42% as good. Only 3 patients were not benefited by surgery. Clark[11] surveyed bronchiectasis in Scottish children in the 10 years, 1946-55. There were 116 children, 57 boys and 59 girls, with the categories one would expect in that decade. One hundred and four resections were performed on 80 children with only two deaths. Only 3 children were operated on for cystic fibrosis. No complications were encountered in 47 children. In 42 there was temporary collapse, but 39 of the collapsed lobes and segments were re-expanded following bronchoscopy, and only 3 needed late resections. Pneumothorax occurred in 4 and a sterile effusion in 5. There was only one instance of empyema and one of bronchopleural fistula. Clark concluded that surgery is possible and advisable in 75% of cases of childhood bronchiectasis. In 79 children, repeated bronchograms were made to learn whether bronchiectasis is a progressive disease. In 46 of these children, there was no change. In 27, however, there was increased sacculation, but no new areas were seen. In 6 patients, new bronchiectatic areas developed, all in the upper lobes. This would suggest a chronic aspiration syndrome. This important study negates the statement of Churchill and Belsey[10] that the full extent of the disease is seen at the time of first bronchoscopy. One must assume that complete mapping of all lobes and segments was done on the initial bronchogram and on the follow-up bronchograms performed in this series. Clark concluded that early pulmonary resection is indicated if there is appearance of new disease in the upper lobes.

Antibiotics have radically changed the clinical picture of this disease, the frequency of occurrence and the future of the patients. Adequate medical treatment of pneumonic infection prevents the development of bronchiectasis. The milder grades that do develop are often reversible with continued, carefully selected antibiotic therapy. In the preantibiotic era, the majority of patients died within 15 years of the time of onset. This led Cookson[12] in 1938 to publish a paper entitled "Bronchiectasis, a Fatal Disease." For the patient with advanced bronchiectasis who has had adequate medical preparation, excision offers the best opportunity for a full life and complete rehabilitation. The best prognosis exists in young patients prior to the development of emphysema, loss of compliance, and other aging processes leading to reduction of pulmonary function.

CONCLUSIONS.—It would seem that bronchiectasis is universally treated well surgically. The crop is large and the harvest good, contradicting the prediction in 1950 that the surgical harvest would be small and the crop poor. It is now apparent that the disease does originate in childhood. Although most cases can be kept under medical control for a number of years and may even improve at puberty, medical control thereafter is difficult to sustain as the patient is ravaged by recurring pulmonary infection with gradual loss of pulmonary reserve and compliance. The full symptom complex often reappears in the second and third decades, with worsening bronchographic picture and chronic toxicity. One must conclude that patients do not outgrow this disease and that when it is well localized and well defined in childhood, one should operate at that time rather than risk the loss of additional lung units. Field[23] came to this conclusion in a long-range survey of her material, which extends over the period 1949–61.

If bronchiectasis in the lower lobes is mild and stable without clinical symptoms, a conservative approach may be adopted. The children must, however, be followed carefully, with full awareness that they may not grow out of their disease and will require eventual resection therapy with a less rewarding result than is encountered in childhood.

REFERENCES

1. Adam, R., and Churchill, E. D.: Situs inversus, sinusitis and bronchiectasis, J. Thoracic Surg. 7:206, 1937.
2. Anderson, H. A., and Moersch, H. J.: *Diseases of the Chest* (Springfield, Ill.: Charles C Thomas, Publisher, 1959).
3. Baffes, T. C., and Potts, W. J.: Pulmonary resection in infants and children, Pediat. Clin. North America 1:709, 1954.
4. Baird, G.; Crawford, C., and Rudstrom, P.: Pulmonary function after pneumonectomy and lobectomy, J. Thoracic Surg. 16:492, 1947.
5. Blades, B., and Kent, E. M.: Individual isolation and ligation in pulmonary resection, J. Thoracic Surg. 10:84, 1940.
6. Blades, B., and Dugan, D. J.: Pseudo-bronchiectasis, J. Thoracic Surg. 13:40, 1944.
7. Bloomer, W. E.; Liebow, A. A., and Hales, M. R.: *Surgical Anatomy of the Bronchovascular Segments* (Springfield, Ill.: Charles C Thomas, Publisher, 1960).
8. Bourie, J., and Lichter, I.: Surgical treatment of bronchiectasis: Ten-year survey, Brit. M. J. 2:908, 1965.
9. Bremer, J. L.: The fate of remaining lung tissue after pneumonectomy or lobectomy, J. Thoracic Surg. 6:336, 1937.
10. Churchill, E. D., and Belsey, R.: Segmental pneumonectomy in bronchiectasis: The lingular segment of the left upper lobe. Ann. Surg. 109:481, 1939.
11. Clark, N. S.: Bronchiectasis in childhood, Brit. M. J. 1:80, 1963.
12. Cookson, J. A., and Mason, G. A.: Bronchiectasis, a fatal disease, Edinburgh M. J. 45:844, 1938.
13. Cooley, J. C., *et al.*: Surgical treatment of bronchiectasis in children, J.A.M.A. 158:1007, 1955.
14. Crossett, E. S., and Shaw, R. R.: Pulmonary resection in the first year of life, Surg., Gynec. & Obst. 97:417, 1953.
15. Dees, S. C., and Spock, A.: Right middle lobe syndrome in children, J.A.M.A. 197:8, 1966.
16. Diamond, S., and Van Loon, E. L.: Bronchiectasis in childhood, J.A.M.A. 118:771, 1942.
17. Dickey, L. B.: Kartagener's syndrome in children, Dis. Chest 23:657, 1953.
18. Fadhli, H. A.; James, F., and Derrick, J. R.: Surgery in pulmonary complications of mucoviscidosis, Dis. Chest 49:427, 1966.
19. Fawcitt, J., and Parry, H. E.: Lung changes in pertussis and measles in childhood, Brit. J. Radio. 30:76, 1957.
20. Ferris, B. G.: Studies of pulmonary function, New England J. Med. 262:557, 1960.
21. Field, C. E.: Bronchiectasis in childhood: II. Etiology and pathogenesis—survey of 272 cases, Pediatrics 4:231, 1949.
22. Field, C. E.: Bronchiectasis in childhood: Prophylaxis, treatment and progress, Pediatrics 4:355, 1949.
23. Field, C. E.: Prognosis of bronchiectasis in childhood, Arch. Dis. Childhood 36:587, 1961.
24. Fonkalsrud, E. W.; Tompkin, R., and Clatworthy, H. W.: Manifestations of situs inversus in infants and children, Arch. Surg. 92:791, 1966.
25. Ford, F. J.: The course of bronchiectasis in childhood, Glasgow M. J. 291:19, 1948.
26. Foster, J. H.; Jacobs, J. K., and Daniel, R. A.: Pulmonary resection in infancy and childhood, Ann. Surg. 153:658, 1961.
27. Glausser, E. M.; Cook, C. D., and Harris, G. B. C.: Bronchiectasis: A review of 187 cases in children, with follow-up pulmonary function studies in 58, Acta paediat., supp. 165, 1966.
28. Gross, R. E.: *The Surgery of Infancy and Childhood* (Philadelphia: W. B. Saunders Company, 1951), p. 785.
29. Hatch, H. B., and Buchell, B. C.: Middle lobe syndrome in children, Am. Rev. Tuberc. 76:291, 1957.
30. Holmes, L. B.; Blennerhassett, J. B., and Austen, K. F.: A reappraisal of Kartagener's syndrome, Am. J. M. Sc. 255:13, 1968.
31. Jackson, C.: Grasses as foreign bodies in the bronchus, Laryngoscope 62:897, 1952.
32. Jackson, C. L., and Huber, J. F.: Correlated applied anatomy of the bronchial tree and lungs with a system of nomenclature, Dis. Chest 9:319, 1943.
33. Jaubout, M. deB.; Mollard, P., and Garbit, J. L.: Traitement chirurgical des dilatations des bronches chez l' enfant, Ann. pediat. 41:758, 1965.
34. Kartagener, M.: Zur Pathogenese der Bronchiectasien: Bronchiectasen bei Situs viscerum inversus, Beitr. Klin. Tuberk. 83:489, 1933.
35. Kartagener, M., and Straki, P.: Bronchiectasis with situs inversus, Arch. Pediat. 79:163, 1962.
36. Katznelson, D., *et al.*: Botryomycosis, a complication of cystic fibrosis, Pediatrics 4:53, 1949.
37. Keats, T. C.: Lung changes in cystic fibrosis, Radiology 65:223, 1955.
38. Mendez, F. L., Jr.; Leahy, L. C., and Butsch, W. L.: Some aspects of bronchiectasis in infants, J. Thoracic Surg. 24:50, 1952.
39. Nickamin, S. J.: Kartagener's syndrome in the newborn, J.A.M.A. 161:966, 1956.
40. Overholt, R. H., and Langer, L.: A new technique for pulmonary segmental resection, Surg., Gynec. & Obst. 84:257, 1947.
41. Reas, H. W.: The use of N-acetylcysteine in the treatment of cystic fibrosis, J. Pediat. 65:542, 1964.

42. Schneid, R.: Sarcoidosis: Treatment with ACTH and cortisone, Acta paediat. 45:343, 1956.
43. Schuster, S. R., *et al.*: Pulmonary surgery for cystic fibrosis, J. Thoracic & Cardiovas. Surg. 48:765, 1964.
44. Schwachmann, H.: Personal communication.
45. Sealy, W. C., *et al.*: The surgical treatment of multisegmental and localized bronchiectasis, Surg., Gynec. & Obst. 123:80, 1966.
46. Strang, C.: The fate of children with bronchiectasis, Ann. Int. Med. 44:630, 1956.
47. Suhs, R., *et al.*: Hypogammaglobulinemia with chronic bronchitis or bronchiectasis: Treatment of 5 patients with long term antibiotics, Arch. Int. Med. 116:29, 1965.
48. Welch, K. J., and Carter, M. D.: Bronchiectasis following aspiration of timothy grass: Report of 8 cases, New England J. Med. 238:832, 1948.
49. Williams, H., and O'Reilly, R. N.: Bronchiectasis, clinical and pathologic aspects, Arch. Dis. Childhood 34:192, 1959.
50. Wissler, H., and Hatz, M. L.: Prognosis of bronchiectasis in childhood, Helvet. paediat. acta 12:475, 1958.
51. Wooley, P. V.: Grass "inflorescences" as foreign bodies in the respiratory tract, J. Pediat. 46:704, 1955.

K. J. WELCH

Drawings by
MURIEL MCLATCHIE MILLER

Lung Abscess

HISTORY.—During the period 1930–45, 159 patients with lung abscess were seen at the Children's Hospital Medical Center. At that time, the over-all mortality hovered around 40% with combined medical and surgical therapy. In 1939, Neuhoff and Touroff[5] reported favorable results of aggressive surgical attack and recommended rib resection, saucerization of the abscess cavity and overlying chest wall and packing. Monaldi established the value of intracavitary suction in selected cases. Although these approaches are now considered obsolete, the occasional child will still benefit from application of the basic surgical principles. Suitable candidates might be children with continuing toxicity, active parenchymal disease in other areas of the ipsilateral lung or far-advanced bilateral pulmonary destruction resulting from cystic fibrosis. In 1948, Glover and Clagett[5] demonstrated the value of pulmonary resection, reporting a reduction of mortality to the range of 18%. They also pointed out the ravages and complications resulting from failure to intervene surgically at the appropriate time, with loss of valuable adjacent lung parenchyma. In a significant number of patients, brain abscess developed.

Lung abscess is a destructive, suppurative process in one or more lung segments caused by tissue invasion by pyogenic organisms. The infection is usually polymicrobic, frequently anaerobic and in part fuso-spirochetal.[7]

Much of the recent literature emphasizes that lung abscess is now a combined medical and surgical disease.[1,2,11,13] The apparent conflict in estimate of mortality and morbidity is explained by the fact that lung abscess has a different outlook according to etiology, ranging from excellent when due to aspiration, the so-called nonspecific or primary form of lung abscess, to poor when secondary to malignancy, the air-fluid level in a pulmonary cavity only signalling the presence of the underlying usually fatal disorder. Most adult surgical series are concerned largely with lung abscess deriving from bronchogenic carcinoma and tuberculosis. Most medical reports deal with acute nonspecific or aspiration lung abscess. There is no survey of lung abscess in children in the literature in the decade 1959–69. The statement is made repeatedly in reports of assorted suppurative lung conditions amenable to surgery that no child with lung abscess has been encountered "in the past 5 years." A review of our material reveals that 11 patients were operated upon for lung abscess from 1959 to 1969.

The etiology of lung abscess in children is quite different from that encountered in the adult age group (Table 32-7).

DIAGNOSIS

A history suggesting any of the conditions listed in Table 32-7 is promptly followed by an acute illness with cough production of sputum, chest pain, hemoptysis, fever, leukocytosis, anemia and weight loss. The frequency of specific complaints is listed in Table 32-8. The rule prevails that no physical examination of the chest is complete without good posteroanterior and lateral x-ray study. In the early stage, the condition cannot be distinguished from segmental or lobar consolidation from any cause and is essentially a pneumonic process. Ultimately, confluent lobular infarction results in breakdown of lung parenchyma,

---

TABLE 32-7.—ETIOLOGY AND PATHOGENESIS OF LUNG ABSCESS IN CHILDREN

1. Aspiration abscess
   a) Acute nonspecific
   b) Foreign body
2. Specific pulmonary infections
   a) Staphylococcus
   b) *Klebsiella pneumoniae*
   c) *Mycobacterium tuberculosis*
   d) *Entamoeba histolytica*
   e) Salmonella
   f) Fungi (botryomycosis, actinomycosis, candidiasis)
   g) Protozoa echinococcus
3. Secondary infection of congenital lung cyst or sequestrated lobe
4. Septic infarction
5. Diffuse parenchymatous disease of unknown etiology
   a) Cystic fibrosis
   b) Honeycomb variety of Hamman-Rich syndrome
6. Benign pulmonary neoplasm

TABLE 32-8. – SYMPTOMS IN 70 PATIENTS
WITH LUNG ABSCESS*

SYMPTOMS	NO. OF PATIENTS	%
Cough	61	87
Productive sputum	52	74
Chest pain	36	51
Hemoptysis	36	51
Weight loss	25	36
Fever	25	36
Chills	16	23
Night sweats	11	16

*From Pickar and Ruoff.[10]

and at some point there is sudden communication with the parent bronchus. This is indicated by harassing cough and profuse expectoration. The latter is not evident in children under age 5, who swallow the purulent material. Hemoptysis appears for the first time, and coincident with the evacuation of a septic material there are rapid defervescence and abatement of toxicity. X-ray study now reveals the abscess as a thick-rimmed spherical cavity with a smooth outline and a classic air fluid level. Planigrams are helpful in estimating the thickness of the abscess wall and the maturity of the process, and serial studies reveal the effectiveness of medical therapy over a period of 6–8 weeks. Examination of the copious sputum permits identification of the bacterial offender. Cultures should be planted under aerobic and anaerobic conditions as well as on Sabouraud's medium to rule out fungi. The stained sputum sediment may disclose vegetable fibers inhaled as a foreign body. Infection with acid-fast organisms must be excluded. In younger children, bronchoscopy is helpful at this stage, both for diagnosis and to clear away thick secretions from the parent bronchus. Bronchograpy should be reserved for patients in whom medical therapy has failed and resection is contemplated.

MEDICAL TREATMENT

The mainstay of medical treatment is the intensive use of appropriate antibiotics over a period of several weeks. Penicillin has been effective in 95% of patients with acute nonspecific lung abscess. Weiss and Flippin[12] cured 21 of 25 patients by administering penicillin G on an ambulatory basis, 750 mg orally q. i. d. with calcium carbonate. Only 4 patients required resection. Flavell[4] prefers a combination of penicillin, 2.5 million units a day, and streptomycin, 1.0 Gm/day, with the dose scaled down for children. This regimen requires hospitalization for parenteral administration. Duration of treatment depends on clinical improvement and x-ray evidence of a diminishing cavity. In patients with cystic fibrosis, tetracycline has been the mainstay. These children are kept on a prophylactic regimen for many years, with the dose increased during preparation for surgical intervention

or reinfection. Resistant staphylococci may be encountered and are treated, depending on culture and sensitivity findings, with novobiocin, kanamycin or oxycillin. A valuable adjunct to antibiotic therapy is postural drainage to encourage coughing for three 15-minute periods daily. The positioning of the patient depends on the location of the cavity. The patient is taught to sleep in the appropriate position with the foot of the bed on blocks. Much can be accomplished by the respiratory therapist by encouraging children to cough and by applying cupped percussion over the involved lobe or segments several times a day. Repeat bronchoscopy is of special value in children who remain toxic or are too young to understand the importance of effective coughing. Aerosol antibiotics, expectorants, humidity and mucolytic agents such as acetylcysteine have established value.

Depending on the etiology of the lung abscess and notably successful with aspiration abscess, this program is continued for 6–8 weeks. During this time, fever and toxicity diminish. The sputum measured daily becomes reduced in amount and improved in quality. Coincident with this, the size of the abscess cavity diminishes. A time limit must be placed on medical therapy, usually between 2 and 3 months. Later, the process converts to a chronic lung abscess. The cavity, instead of obliterating, becomes larger, and the walls remain separated and thickened. Ultimately, there is squamous metaplasia with ingrowth of epithelium; these indicate incomplete and unsatisfactory bronchial drainage. Failure to intervene surgically at this point will result inevitably in the late complications of lung abscess (Table 32-9).

TABLE 32-9. – COMPLICATIONS OF CHRONIC LUNG ABSCESS

GENERAL	PULMONARY
1. Bacterial resistance	1. Empyema
2. Resistant anemia	2. Pneumothorax
3. Septicemia	3. Bronchopleural fistula
4. Mediastinitis	4. Bronchiectasis
5. Brain abscess	5. Recurring in situ abscess
	6. Recurring pneumonia, ipsilateral or contra-lateral
	7. Pulmonary insufficiency

VARIETIES OF LUNG ABSCESS

ACUTE NONSPECIFIC ASPIRATION ABSCESS. – The development of aspiration abscess requires one of several conditions: (1) Suppression of the cough reflex that may occur with anesthesia, sedating or narcotizing drugs; a central nervous system lesion such as trauma, neoplasm or epilepsy, or the anoxia associated with semidrowning. (2) Inhalation of septic material, most common in the past, clotted blood and infected tissue associated with nasopharyngeal surgery in children, vomitus or, in a more occult way,

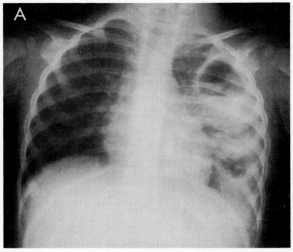

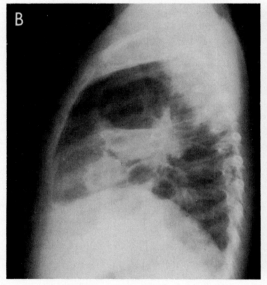

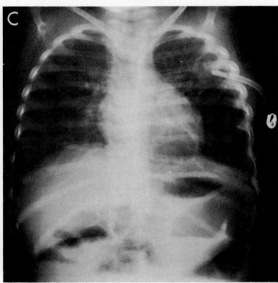

Fig. 32-16.—Lung abscess with diffuse, bilateral staphylococ-cic pneumonia and intrapulmonary cysts. **A,** roentgenogram of a 15-month-old girl with an expanding mature abscess of the left upper lobe that did not respond to antibiotic therapy. **B,** lateral view showing air-fluid level and location of the process in the second apical posterior and anterior segments of the upper lobe. The process was controlled by Monaldi intracavitary suction with obliteration of the cavity and drainage of the septic material, ob-viating the need for pulmonary resection. **C,** roentgenogram 1 month later showing obliteration of abscess cavity and a few unresolved cysts in the lower lung field.

microemboli from carious teeth or chronic sinusitis. (3) Esophageal obstructive disorders that result in overflow of saliva and ingested food and liquids into the airway. This is seen commonly in children who have undergone surgery for esophageal atresia or stenosis, lye burns of the esophagus, achalasia eso-phageal diverticulum and duplication. The most diffi-cult of these conditions to diagnose clinically is the H type of isolated fistula without atresia.

The site of the aspiration abscess is determined by the position of the child at the moment of inhalation.

Thus in a supine patient, the right lung will be in-volved, the material becoming lodged in the apical segment of the right lower lobe. When the patient is on the right side, the posterior segment of the right upper lobe will be maximally involved. With the pa-tient on the left side, the most commonly involved area is the posterior segment of the left upper lobe. If the child is face down at the time of inhaling the for-eign material, as in resuscitation from drowning, the maximally involved areas will be the right middle lobe or the lingular segments of the left upper lobe, being the most anterior. Recovery from anesthesia is a perilous process, and if the patient is unguarded, great havoc may be wrought. The patient is kept on the right side and face down. Heavy sedation is not ordered until the patient has responded sufficiently to understand the spoken voice, and the first word by the recovery-room attendant should be "cough."

Organisms recovered from patients with aspiration abscess are nondescript and ordinary residents of the nasopharynx and upper intestinal tract. Most common are Vincent's organisms and spirochetes followed by E. coli and anaerobic streptococcus. These in combination account for the odor and bad taste of sputum with lung abscess.

LUNG ABSCESS DUE TO SPECIFIC PULMONARY INFECTIONS. — *Staphylococcus.* — Lung abscess due to staphylococcus is the commonest form in infancy (see Fig. 32-16).

Klebsiella pneumoniae. — Friedländer's pneumonia is a virulent, often fatal type of pulmonary infection. It is usually seen in the debilitated infant who has undergone major surgery in the newborn period. This may be an unwanted dividend of the current practice of protecting neonates with multiple antibiotics. Our one example occurred approximately 3 weeks after repair of esophageal atresia with tracheoesophageal fistula in a patient with a variant of D-18 trisomy. An entire lobe is usually involved with massive slough. The responsible organism, *K. pneumoniae,* is recovered from the tracheal secretions at the time of diagnostic and therapeutic bronchoscopy. Streptomycin and kanamycin are the antibiotics of choice, although the usual end-result is lobectomy.

Actinomycosis. — One child has been seen with lung abscess due to *Actinomyces Israelii.* The underlying disease was cystic fibrosis, and he had been treated for several years with tetracycline. This unusually destructive fungus disregards normal tissue barriers and extends uninterruptedly across lung, pleura and chest wall, forming many intercommunicating abscesses and eventual skin sinuses. Diagnosis is possible only by examination of the infected material, which contains sulfur granules. The most effective antibiotic is penicillin, which must be given intravenously in amounts up to 6 million units a day for 6 weeks, then 3 million units for an additional 3 weeks.

Tuberculosis. — The varieties of tuberculosis in childhood are discussed in detail in the following section of this chapter. One child, aged 9, had the reinfection type of tuberculosis with conversion of the right upper lobe to a honeycomb of abscesses of uniform size completely replacing normal lung parenchyma (Fig. 32-17).

Entamoeba histolytica. — The diagnosis of amebic abscess of the lung will not be made unless one suspects the true etiology and pursues the diagnosis with warm stage preparations and cultures of excretions from the gastrointestinal tract and secretions from the lung. The pleuropulmonary complications of amebiasis were presented in the classic paper by De Bakey and Ochsner,[3] who described a hematogenous form of pulmonary abscess with or without liver involvement. Another variety consisted of consolidation of the right lower lobe and bronchohepatic fistula. The clinical symptoms and signs are not specific for the presence of *E. histolytica,* although the sputum characteristically resembles anchovy paste. The infection does not respond to standard antimicrobial agents. The obvious conclusion must be reached that when the etiology of lung abscess cannot be explained, the patient should be given a trial course of emetine or chloroquine. Two cases of left pulmonary amebic abscess without hepatic involvement have recently been described.[9]

Salmonella. — Lung abscess may occur many weeks after clinical salmonellosis. The gastrointestinal symptoms are usually so violent as to require hospitalization because of acute dehydration, blood loss and toxicity. Following mucosal destruction, the organisms spread to the lungs and other organs in a septicemic phase. We have not encountered a child with lung abscess due to salmonella.

Echinococcus. — The disease is seldom seen in the United States, but must now be kept in mind in view of rapid shifts in world populations. It is endemic throughout much of South America. There are curved irregularities within the cavities that can be demonstrated by planigraphy, and a nearly positive diagnosis can usually be made from x-ray examination alone. Treatment consists of enucleation and appropriate pulmonary resection. Our one case, involving the left upper lobe of a 10-year-old boy, is illustrated in Figure 32-18.

SECONDARY INFECTION OF CONGENITAL LUNG CYSTS AND SEQUESTERED LOBES. — Lung abscess may be the

Fig. 32-17. — Lung abscess with reinfection or adult-type pulmonary tuberculosis. Surgical specimen of right upper lobe resected from a 9-year-old boy. Note multiple abscess cavities of uniform size, so-called honeycomb destruction, of the entire lobe. Pulmonary resection for fibrocavitary tuberculosis in our institution has become so rare as to be a curiosity. Only 2 other children had resection for pulmonary tuberculosis in the period 1960–67. They had focal bronchiectasis limited to a lobe or segment without abscess formation.

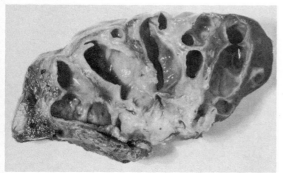

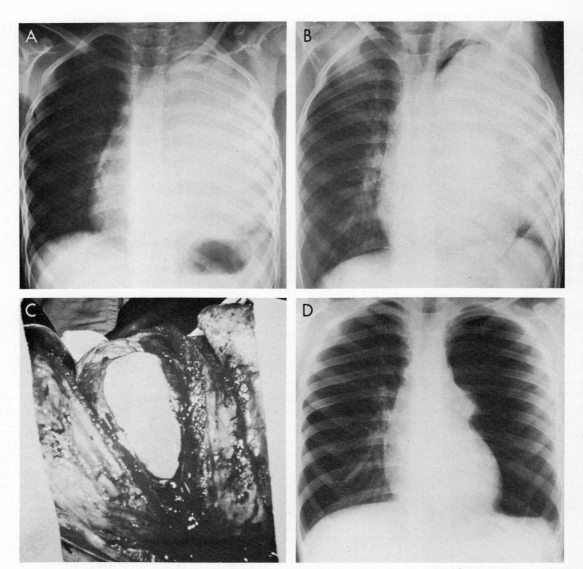

Fig. 32-18.—Hydatid cyst of the lung. Echinococcal disease of the left upper lobe in a 9-year-old Macedonian boy evidenced by cough, chest pain, moderate weight loss and low-grade fever. This disease is infrequently encountered in the New England area. The patient emigrated to the United States from Greece at the age of 9 years. A pleural fluid culture showed no growth. Skin tests for tuberculosis, coccidioidomycosis and histoplasmosis were negative. SK-SD (streptokinase-streptodornase) test was positive, ruling out anergy to tuberculosis with some evidence against sarcoidosis and advanced Hodgkin's disease. The Casoni intradermal test for echinococcus was equivocal (15%). Liver scan was normal and scan of the left lung showed low perfusion. **A,** anteroposterior roentgenogram showing a white-out of the left hemithorax without displacement of mediastinal structures. It could not be determined at this stage whether we were dealing with a primary lung disorder or pleural malignancy. **B,** in order to further define the process, 50 cc of air was injected into the left pleural cavity. The induced pneumothorax clearly defined the intrapulmonary lesion. It also demonstrated the left cardiac border not previously visible. The exact nature of the lesion was still a mystery compounded by negative serum hemagglutination and flocculation tests for hydatid disease (20% of cases). **C,** the left thoracic cavity has been opened widely through an incision in the sixth interspace. This operative photograph (courtesy of Dr. B. McGovern) shows the hydatid cyst as a football-sized unilocular process, marble-white in color. It ballooned outward following division of the moderately thickened visceral pleura. Without further manipulation, the cyst was allowed to deliver itself by repeated positive pressure inflation of the left lung. It was ultimately lifted out intact with insignificant bleeding. There were no macroscopic daughter cysts. The specimen was found to contain a liter of clear fluid and thousands of sandy granules identified microscopically as scolices. Faced with the alternative of in situ ligature of opened branch bronchi with tube drainage or resection of the left upper lobe, we elected the latter approach because there was very little salvageable parenchyma. **D,** postoperative roentgenogram obtained 6 months after operation. There is compensatory emphysema of the left lower lobe. No new lesions have appeared, serial liver scans are negative and the patient is asymptomatic. While the disease is common in South America, the Near East, India and Australia, this is the first patient with hydatid lung abscess encountered in our institution.

ultimate development in undiagnosed and untreated congenital cysts of the lung.

SEPTIC LUNG INFARCTION. – This condition was often observed before the advent of intracardiac surgery, in patients with ventricular septal defect. The jet stream of left-to-right shunting produced an ulceration of the opposite wall of the right ventricular chamber. This was soon followed by the development of ulcerative staphylococcic endocarditis, with seeding of the lungs and the production of multiple pulmonary abscesses. A vegetative colony of *Streptococcus viridans* on the pulmonary artery side of a ductus arteriosus often embolized to the lung but was not capable of a similar degree of parenchymal destruction. Septic lung infarction is seen today as a terminal event in patients with burn septicemia due to *Staphylococcus aureus*. The distribution of the lesions indicates a pyemic spread rather than by inhalation in that they are diffusely scattered throughout both lung fields.

The condition is so much a part of the terminal state of an unsalvageable patient that the pulmonary lesions are largely descriptive.

DIFFUSE PARENCHYMATOUS DISEASE OF UNKNOWN ETIOLOGY. – Cystic fibrosis is a widespread disease

process of unknown etiology affecting primarily the parenchymatous organs, pancreas, spleen, salivary glands and lung, and, to some extent, the entire gastrointestinal tract. Called mucoviscidosis, it represents a disorder of mucus production resulting in high viscosity and high electrolyte content. The pulmonary complications are more fully described in the preceding section on bronchiectasis. On occasion, and in the presence of impaired drainage resulting from cicatricial stenosis of the bronchial supply to a segment or entire lobe, confluent bronchopneumonia, when caused by virulent suppurative bacteria, will convert to a classic lung abscess (Fig. 32-19). Only 1 patient at the Children's Hospital Medical Center has had resection for lung abscess associated with cystic fibrosis, in contrast to 32 patients who have had segmental resection, lobectomy or pneumonectomy for the same disorder. An incidental finding in this patient was botryomycosis of the resected lung tissue, the organism flourishing because of the long period of broad-spectrum antibiotic therapy.

A second form of lung abscess occurring with a widespread pulmonary disorder is the honeycomb variety of the Hamman-Rich syndrome. This consists of diffuse interstitial fibrosis throughout the lungs and

Fig. 32-19. – Lung abscess with cystic fibrosis observed in a 10-year-old boy. Note the diffuse bilateral process with increased bronchovascular markings, areas of overdistention and nodular fibrosis. **A,** anteroposterior roentgenogram showing a large area of homogeneous density. The lesion involved the apical and posterior segments of the right upper lobe with compression of the anterior segment. There was no communication with the parent bronchi. **B,** lateral roentgenogram showing the further limits of the process and the degree of anterior segment displacement.

Pleural symphysis permitted external drainage. The condition has been observed many times but only 1 patient has required resection. With bronchoscopy and vigorous medical and respiratory therapy, most lung abscesses due to cystic fibrosis will eventually evacuate their contents into the tracheobronchial tree. Tuberculoma-like lesions in the mid-lung field can be managed conservatively unless progressive expansion results in atelectasis or air trapping in adjacent lobes or segments.

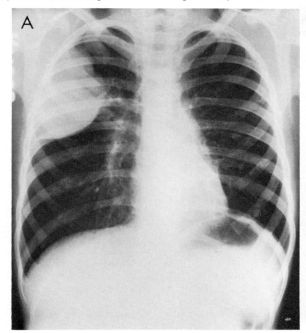
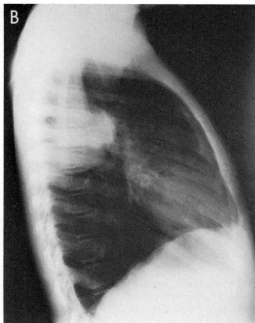

is ordinarily fatal in not more than 6 months. Recently, a group of patients has been encountered who are thought to represent a subtype of the Hamman-Rich syndrome. The disease has a more protracted course, with involvement of all lobes and segments. Resection therapy is contraindicated in such a diffuse process. The x-ray picture is suggestive, and the diagnosis can be made by biopsy via an anterior approach in the seventh interspace to obtain lung tissue from the presenting edge of the lingular segment of the left upper lobe.

SURGICAL TREATMENT

Resection therapy for lung abscess must be considered for the patient who has an unresolved process after more than 2 months of medical and other adjunctive therapy, recognizing that delay will lead to the development of a chronic lung abscess with its known complications. Other clear-cut indications are: life-threatening hemorrhage from an open artery communicating with the tracheobronchial tree; demonstration of bronchial obstruction by bronchography; the association of lung abscess with bronchiectasis in other lobes and segments where additional loss of lung parenchyma adjacent to the abscessed cavity would not be tolerated, and recurrence of the abscess in situ after apparent medical control.

In most instances, lung abscess will be treated by segmental resection or lobectomy. On occasion, with continuing toxicity and rapid expansion of the abscess cavity despite bronchoscopy and medical therapy and with diffuse bilateral pulmonary disease of the chronic type, it may be necessary to stage pulmonary resection according to the method of Neuhoff and Touroff.[8]

This consists of rib resection and the accomplishment of pleural symphysis if this has not occurred spontaneously, followed by saucerization of the intrapulmonary cavity with packing.

REFERENCES

1. Bernhard, W. F.; Malcolm, J. A., and Wylie, R. H.: Lung abscess: A study of 148 cases due to aspiration, Dis. Chest 43:620, 1963.
2. Collins, H. A.; Guest, J. L., and Daniel, R. A: Primary lung abscess, J. Thoracic & Cardiovas. Surg. 47:383, 1964.
3. De Bakey, M. E., and Ochsner, A.: Pleuropulmonary complications of amebiasis, J. Thoracic Surg. 5:225, 1936.
4. Flavell, G.: Lung abscess, Brit. M. J. 1:1032, 1966.
5. Glover, R. P. and Clagett, O. T.: Pulmonary resection for abscess of lung, Surg., Gynec. & Obst. 86:385, 1948.
6. Jensen, H., and Androup, E.: Nonspecific abscess of the lung in 129 cases: Diagnosis and treatment, Acta chir. scandinav. 127:487, 1964.
7. Lindskog, G. E.; Liebow, A., and Glenn, W.: *Thoracic and Cardiac Surgery with Related Pathology* (New York: Appleton-Century-Crofts, Inc., 1962).
8. Neuhoff, H., and Touroff, A. S. W.: Acute putrid abscess of the lung, J. Thoracic Surg. 9:439, 1939.
9. Nunnally, L. C., and Cole, F. H.: Left pulmonary amebic abscess: Two cases, Arch. Surg. 86:621, 1963.
10. Pickar, D. N., and Ruoff, W. F.: Lung abscess: Study of 70 cases, J. Thoracic Surg. 37:452, 1959.
11. Waterman, D. H.; Domm, S. E., and Rudgers, W. K.: Lung abscess—a medicosurgical problem, Am. J. Surg. 89:995, 1965.
12. Weiss, W., and Flippin, H. F.: Treatment of acute nonspecific lung abscess, Arch. Int. Med. 120:8, 1967.
13. Wolcott, M. W.; Coury, O. H., and Baum, G. L.: Changing concepts in the therapy of lung abscess: A twenty-year survey, Dis. Chest. 10:1, 1961.

K. J. WELCH

Pulmonary Tuberculosis

PULMONARY TUBERCULOSIS is caused by inhalation of *Mycobacterium tuberculosis var. hominis* described by Koch in 1882. The organism can persist for weeks in a dry state but is readily killed by moist heat sterilization. The lipid component of its structure accounts for its acid-fast staining property and produces the fibrosis and characteristic cellular response of epithelioid and giant cells forming the tubercle. A protein fraction is probably responsible for the extensive tissue necrosis seen in tuberculous infection in any tissue.

In spite of a steady decrease in the total incidence of tuberculosis, the disease remains prevalent in the lower socioeconomic groups. Three hundred eighty-one cases of primary tuberculosis were registered in Massachusetts from 1960 to 1966—about 5% of adult

cases.[50] It is a common clinical problem in all large municipal hospitals. Approximately 200 new cases of tuberculosis in childhood were encountered at the Boston City Hospital between 1955 and 1961. Among these, 90% were pulmonary and 10% extrapulmonary. The percentage of positive tuberculin reactors of high-school age decreased from 90% in 1930 to approximately 20% in 1960.[47] At the same time, a gradual reduction in the death rate below the age of 15 years has taken place.[31] Fatalities still occur in youngsters under 5 when clinical diagnosis is delayed and appropriate antibacterial therapy is not undertaken. There is also a significant mortality in girls in the adolescent age group. The most virulent and destructive form of the disease due to an apparent lack of resistance is seen in nonwhites (Negroes, Puerto Ricans, American Indians).

Modern chemotherapy suggests the possibility of

controlling, if not sterilizing, and of preventing the known complications of pulmonary tuberculosis. This discussion of the varieties and surgical treatment of pulmonary tuberculosis in childhood may seem an oddity, yet we are seeing this disease with increasing frequency as the consequence of large shifts of rural populations into urban areas. Case-finding must be pursued vigorously in all children's hospitals both for the active treatment of the child and for the protection of members of the hospital family and his community. Pulmonary tuberculosis still ranks near the top of the list of causes of disability and death in children on a global basis.[11,20,26,47] An active and complete tuberculosis registry combined with selective BCG immunization and prophylactic combined antituberculous therapy can break the epidemiologic chain and lead to an over-all decrease in the incidence of this disease.

EARLY DIAGNOSIS.—Symptoms of pulmonary tuberculosis are unreliable. Therefore a routine tuberculin test must be performed on all children with a history of contact and on those over 6 years of age, employing the intradermal Mantoux test, with 0.0001 mg of PPD (purified protein derivative). The test must be repeated annually thereafter.

PREVENTION.—Newborn children of tuberculous mothers must be separated from the source of contact for 12 weeks. If the placenta is involved, these infants must have a tuberculin test and chest x-ray study. If the reaction to the tuberculin test is positive, they must be given isoniazid (INH) for 1 year. Measles immunization is mandatory during antituberculous chemotherapy.[43] If the tuberculin reaction is negative, BCG vaccination is advised.[15,46] Vaccination is also indicated for children living in a household with known tuberculosis at any stage and in certain population groups with a high incidence of tuberculous infection. Rigid conditions are established for BCG vaccination. They include a negative reaction to the tuberculin test by the Mantoux technique and a negative chest film within 2 weeks of the date of vaccination, which is performed by the multiple puncture disk method of Rosenthal using 3 drops of BCG vaccine in the deltoid area after acetone cleansing.[*20] After 12 weeks, both the Mantoux test and chest x-ray survey must be repeated. The tuberculin reaction should now be positive; if not, the vaccination should be repeated. A word of caution must be inserted about major intrathoracic complications that may follow revaccination of an infant or child with a positive tuberculin reaction or initial vaccination without knowledge of the existence of a positive tuberculin reaction. The BCG material creates an antigenic explosion in regional and mediastinal lymph nodes which may perforate into a bronchus with fatal results.

*The material is available through the Research Foundation of Chicago and the Eli Lilly Company, Indianapolis.

Primary Pulmonary Tuberculosis: Childhood Type

Two to 10 weeks after open tuberculosis contact, the previously tuberculin-negative child develops a demonstrable allergy and a characteristic cutaneous reaction following intradermal injection of PPD. At the site of localization, usually in the central or peripheral areas of the lung field, exudation occurs and a tendency to localize the process, shortly followed by enlargement of the regional bronchial, hilar and mediastinal lymph nodes extending to the level of the carina. This pattern has been called the childhood type of tuberculosis. Pulmonary tuberculosis occurring in older children usually represents reinfection from either endogenous or exogenous organisms and has been called the adult, or chronic, type. It is a different pathologic entity, involves the apical and posterior areas of the upper lobes and requires a different surgical approach.

In the childhood type, the spontaneous course of the disease usually is in the direction of control, with healing of the parenchymal lesion and decrease of the mediastinal and hilar lymphadenopathy. Healing of the small primary focus occurs with fibrosis and ultimate calcification, the x-ray stigma of this complex. Hematogenous dissemination is rare today. Occurring either as miliary spread or as meningitis, dissemination under combined antibacterial therapy with or without steroids is less than 0.5%.

Although the tendency in the primary complex is toward healing, other patterns can develop. There may be progressive parenchymal disease with caseation pneumonia. Enlarged caseous bronchial nodes may produce segmental obstruction and on occasion may rupture into the bronchus, producing obturation obstruction or an endobronchial ulcerative process with mechanical sequelae. Massive perforation into the airway has caused fatal asphyxiation.[13]

In a child with a positive Mantoux reaction, asymptomatic primary tuberculosis must be assumed to be in the lungs or hilar lymph nodes. In spite of the relatively good prognosis, it is now recommended that these children be treated for 1 year with isoniazid (INH). They are not considered infectious and are not restricted. They are seen monthly during the period of treatment and annually thereafter. A chest x-ray is obtained at 3 months and at the end of 1 year, with annual chest x-rays from then on. Any child whose tuberculin reaction converts from negative to positive within 1 year should be similarly treated; such conversion is the reason for annual tuberculin-testing of all children. This group must be observed closely at puberty, especially girls. The child over 6 with a positive tuberculin reaction and no known contact can be observed without treatment.[20]

PLEURISY WITH EFFUSION.—Lincoln et al.[24] reviewed 202 consecutive cases of pleurisy with effusion, all with a positive tuberculin reaction. A marked

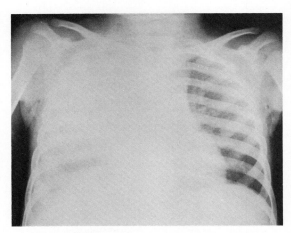

Fig. 32-20.—Pleurisy with effusion. This developed in a 5-year-old boy within 4 months of onset of primary tuberculosis. Diagnostic thoracentesis or aspiration of massive collections may be required, but less than 4% of such instances require decortication.

seasonal incidence of this complication is evident; it is most frequently seen in June and July. These children usually have effusion when first seen, within 3–6 months of the onset of primary tuberculosis. It occurred as late as 41 months in Lincoln's series. Parenchymal calcification is rare and may be masked by the opacity of the hemithorax (Fig. 32-20). It was well established prior to the availability of specific therapy for tuberculosis that no specific treatment was needed for most of these patients and that pleurisy with effusion is not usually associated with a serious prognosis. The effusion generally occurs between age 5 and 9, the "safe period," and is considered a benign self-limited process. Clinical manifestations may be a mild systemic reaction, dyspnea from large effusions or, rarely, high fever and all the evidence of an acute infectious illness. Fibrothorax develops in 4% of untreated patients and decortication is required; 5% later have chronic pulmonary tuberculosis. Of Lincoln's 202 patients, 26 had hematogenous spread, but these patients were seen at Bellevue Hospital before the availability or utilization of modern antimicrobial therapy.

It is now recommended that tuberculous pleurisy with effusion be actively treated with INH and para-aminosalicylic acid (PAS) for 2 years. In addition, prednisone, 1 mg/kg/day in four doses, is given until the effusion clears.[26]

Pleural effusion requires thoracentesis for diagnosis, and on rare occasions repeated taps may be necessary to relieve compression. The effusion usually is absorbed as progress is made in the control and healing of the underlying parenchymal lesion. The rate of disappearance of the effusion is increased markedly by the addition of steroids to conventional antimicrobial therapy.

TUBERCULOUS HILAR LYMPHADENOPATHY.— The node reaction in primary tuberculosis may be massive (Figs. 32-21 and 29-2). Because of the anatomic relation of the segmental bronchi supplying the right middle lobe, this is the lobe earliest and most frequently compromised by nodal matting and constriction. First described by Brock in 1950, the "middle lobe syndrome" has since been reviewed.[27] The early lesion is overinflation (obstructive emphysema) and is followed by resorption atelectasis. If atelectasis persists for several months, the middle lobe fails to re-expand following healing and ultimate disappearance of the hilar mass. In the same way, basal segments of the lower lobes may be involved, but the clinical significance of persisting atelectasis in basal segments is less well established. It is interesting that in 51 resections for tuberculosis in children reported by Webb *et al.,*[49] no isolated middle lobe syndrome was observed. Many young adults with arrested tuberculosis have residual atelectasis at the lung base without clinical evidence of lung disease. The ultimate development of symptomatic bronchiectasis in these areas and additional destruction produced by ordinary pathogens require surgical intervention. Weber reports 25 cases of atelectasis in 235 children with primary tuberculosis. Bronchoscopy relieved the condition within 3 months in 20 patients. Five developed bronchiectasis.[50]

Massive nodal enlargement occurs in 4% of tuberculous patients under 5 and in 11% of older children with the primary complex. Chesterman[7] estimated that less than 0.5% require operation. There is little

Fig. 32-21.—Mediastinal tuberculosis. Massive hilar and mediastinal lymph node reaction with obstruction of the right upper lobe bronchus. In the presence of stridor or evidence of impending perforation, operation should be considered. Steroids may speed up resolution of the process. In this case, under full chemotherapy these nodes completely disappeared in 4 months.

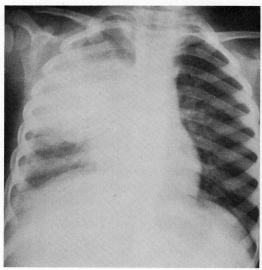

unanimity about surgical intervention to relieve the compression difficulties associated with nodal enlargement.[1,12,14,21] Attitudes vary from nonintervention to aggressive and frequent prophylactic bronchoscopy and attempted evacuation of these nodes by the endoscopic or transthoracic route. Instances are recorded of dramatic asphyxial deaths associated with node perforation. Massive collections of nodes high in the chest may be manifested by stridor or superior caval obstruction. Enucleation of the caseous material in extreme cases seems reasonable without attempting node resection. Such enucleation in conjunction with bronchoscopic maneuvers may open up atelectatic areas and strikingly relieve compression difficulties. Considerable risk attends any extensive mediastinal procedure for the removal of large nodes, and surgeons operating to relieve compression should not be tempted to go beyond that purpose in node exicision or evacuation.

Interesting evidence is available that, in addition to the more rapid clearing of effusion and the healing of endobronchial ulcerations, nodal enlargement may also subside more rapidly under treatment with SM and INH. The use of ACTH and cortisone in these conditions has been recommended.[32,42]

Although there are isolated examples in which nodal resection is indicated, healing and involution occur so consistently that thoracotomy is rarely required. This is the prevailing attitude in the United States. However, the practice is continued with frequency and enthusiasm in the treatment of children with tuberculosis in Wales and England.

ULCERATIVE ENDOBRONCHITIS.—It is not our practice to use the bronchoscope in children with a positive sputum culture. Bronchoscopy is withheld until obstruction occurs, when the lesion may be demonstrated directly or by bronchography. Surgical treatment for this condition is always unsatisfactory and has been used less frequently in recent years as the result of administering prednisone, 1 mg/kg/day for 6–12 weeks during full INH and PAS therapy. The condition is seen as a progression of primary tuberculosis and in the older child with the adult or chronic type of reinfection tuberculosis.

No pulmonary resection procedure should be attempted in the presence of active ulcerative endobronchitis.[25] This process must be followed bronchoscopically to the point of healing. Twelve patients observed healed completely and none required resection. Five additional children with perforation into a bronchus healed without resection.[50] No local manipulation other than removal of obstructing granulation tissue appears to be of significant value.[37] Pulmonary resections attempted in the phase of active endobronchitis are notoriously complicated by the development of bronchopleural fistulas and tuberculous empyema.[40] Late operations may be required because of segmental complications produced by proximal bronchial strictures.[36] Webb[49] pointed out that after several months of therapy, none of 51 preoperative bronchoscopies revealed evidence of endobronchial disease.

BRONCHOESOPHAGEAL FISTULA.—The unusual occurrence of bronchoesophageal fistula was commented on by Danino *et al.*,[9] who referred to 670 cases col-

Fig. 32-22.—Mediastinal tuberculous bronchoesophageal fistula. In this 4-year-old child, the spontaneous fistula followed erosion of caseous mediastinal tuberculosis into the right main bronchus and esophagus. Swallowing resulted in flooding of the right lung. **A,** treatment consisted of gastrostomy and antibacterial therapy without thoracotomy. **B,** chest film after 3 months of antibacterial therapy showing the fistula closed and complete clearing of the right lung with disappearance of most of the enlarged nodes.

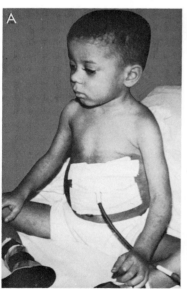
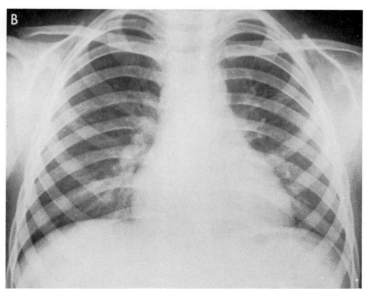

lected by Monserrat, 41 of which were due to tuberculosis. They described a case in a boy of 7 who had a communication between the esophagus and the posterior basal segment of the right lower lobe. He was treated by right lower lobectomy and esophageal suture. We have encountered 3 similar cases. Gastrostomy combined with INH and PAS solved the problem without resort to pulmonary resection or closure of the fistula.

Case history: A boy of 4 developed a bronchoesophageal fistula at the height of the nodal disease and had paroxysms of coughing due to flooding of the right upper lobe (Fig. 32-22). Treatment consisted of gastrostomy and antituberculous therapy. The esophageal perforation healed, the nodes gradually disappeared, the fistula closed and the involved parenchyma of the right upper lobe completely cleared. Biopsy of the enlarged liver at the time of laparotomy for gastrostomy demonstrated tubercles.

ATELECTASIS.—Atelectasis of a pulmonary lobe or segment can result from extrabronchial compression of large reactive hilar nodes. For the same reason, an initial area of atelectasis can convert to obstructive emphysema when there is a check-valve mechanism. Occasionally, this proceeds to perforation of the caseous node into a bronchus. At this stage, therapeutic bronchoscopy has an important role in clearing away the debris and reopening the involved area.

MEDICAL TREATMENT

CHEMOTHERAPY.—Specific antimycobacterial chemotherapeutic agents have radically affected the clinical picture and prognosis of pulmonary tuberculosis. Parenchymal disease can now be treated surgically with the aid of these drugs. Children with mediastinal disease alone and exposed children who have shown tuberculin conversion have a greatly improved prognosis if adequately treated.

Current guides to therapy, in a field changing rapidly as new drugs, new dosages, new schedules and new combinations are tried, are as follows: (1) Combination drug therapy is preferable to single drug therapy. (2) Prolonged therapy is less likely to produce resistant organisms than is interrupted and resumed therapy. (3) In serious complications, a triple drug regimen is used from the outset. (4) All antituberculous drugs now available are potentially toxic.

Streptomycin, isoniazid and para-aminosalicylic acid are the most commonly used drugs and the least toxic of available chemotherapeutic agents. Although a variety of reactions to INH and PAS such as fever, rash and nausea can occur, they are rare. Overdosage with SM may lead to permanent damage to either the auditory nerve or the vestibular branch of the 8th nerve. Dosage schedules must be carefully adhered to. Kanamycin, viomycin and cycloserine are more hazardous, with nephrotoxic and neurotoxic manifestations. They are ordinarily brought into use after interrupted therapy, when organisms emerge that are resistant. Since these drugs may not be tolerated for long, they are best used to cover the period of operative therapy.

The effect of antituberculous therapy on conversion of positive cultures of sputum and gastric washings to negative has been dramatic. In an initial group of treated patients, 30% of positive cultures were reduced to 3% at 3 months and to 1% at 4 months. In untreated controls, positive cultures changed from 20% to 16% at 3 months and increased to 19% at 12 months. Jones and Howard[18] discharged 500 children from institutional care with a readmission rate of only 0.8%. A minimum of 4 months of in-hospital therapy is recommended.

Symptomatic improvement occurs in 3–4 weeks with combined therapy; extension of the parenchymal lesion is rare but x-ray evidence of improvement is slow. Complete clearing occurs in 68% of cases in an average of 6.2 months. Clearing with residual scarring occurs in 32% in an average of 10.6 months.[50] Early and sustained antibacterial therapy has radically altered the course and surgical treatment of pulmonary tuberculosis in childhood.[10,28,48]

Streptomycin sulfate is administered in a dose of 20–40 mg/kg/day or 650 mg/m^2/day. This is given intramuscularly every 12 hours. It is never used alone for the treatment of tuberculosis. Dihydrostreptomycin is never given because of its known propensity for permanently damaging the auditory and vestibular branches of the 8th cranial nerve. Streptomycin sulfate should not be given for more than 1 month and has its principal value in the patient with rapid progression of primary disease, given in combination with INH and PAS as triple therapy. It is also of value in the pre- and postoperative periods in patients requiring surgical resection.

Isoniazid is better tolerated by children than by adults. No known agent will eradicate the tubercle bacillus, but this drug is the mainstay of modern treatment and will arrest the process in most children and eliminate most complications. Neurotoxicity has been reported, consisting of convulsions and peripheral neuritis, thought to be due to an inhibition of pyridoxine metabolism. This has not been commonly reported in children. To prevent this complication, pyridoxine is given with INH (10 mg for each 100 mg of INH) in adolescence. The recommended dosage is 20 mg/kg/day to a maximum of 500 mg, given orally every 12 hours or 300 mg/m^2/day. It is usually combined with PAS, a combination that has produced no failure of therapy and no resistant organisms other than atypical mycobacteria in children. The drug is the keystone of triple therapy in children who have rapid dissemination as evidenced by meningitis, miliary tuberculosis or wildfire pulmonary spread.

Para-aminosalicylic acid competes with INH for acetylation in the liver and allows higher levels of INH to reach infected lung tissue. The recommended dosage is 200 mg/kg/day given orally in 4 doses or 6 Gm/m^2/day.

New antituberculous drugs. — Several drugs under study for the treatment of childhood tuberculosis have limited value and have not had wide clinical applications. Viomycin and cycloserine are derived from a streptomyces subgroup. The former is less potent than and the latter is not as effective as streptomycin sulfate. Furthermore, convulsions have been reported and safe dosage has not been established. Ethionamide has proved toxic for children and safe dosage levels have not been established. Pyrizinamide, although an effective antituberculous agent, has been associated with hepatic toxicity and the emergence of resistant forms of acid-fast bacilli. None of the four drugs have been recommended by the American Thoracic Society.[33] Continuing investigation of these and other new drugs has been stimulated by multiple reports of emerging resistant forms of *M. tuberculosis var. hominis.* Forms resistant to INH have been estimated at 3–16.3% in different studies. Steiner and Cosio[44] commented on the lack of uniform standards defining significant resistance. In their report on the incidence of primary drug-resistant disease in 332 children, this varied with INH from 16.3% using the USPH standard to 6.3% using the Veterans Administration standard. Organism resistance can be encountered in children with initial infection, when it is known as primary drug-resistant infection, and late in the course of the infection, when it is called secondary drug-resistant disease. The implication of this resistance in terms of response to therapy and of threat to others in the community is obvious. The report concludes that the incidence of primary strains resistant to streptomycin and PAS was of a low order (3%). Combined drug resistance was found in only 2 of 101 strains.

The mortality rate in children with active primary disease before the advent of chemotherapy was high, especially in children under 4 years of age. In the experience of Lincoln and Sewall,[26] mortality from tuberculous complications was 24.3%. Miller and Walgren[29] found it to be 35.9% for children from birth to 1 year and 15.6% for children from 1 to 8 years of age. Brailey[4] found the death rate for Negro children infected before age 3 years to be 20.4% within 1 year and 25.9% within 5 years. With an aggressive attitude toward diagnosis, active BCG immunization in selected groups and combined drug therapy for all children with a clear-cut history of contact and evidence of disease, these figures have been reduced to less than 5%. With national awareness on the part of all individuals who deal with children, death from this disorder in the United States should become a rarity.

Surgical Treatment

Pulmonary resection. — Doyen performed lobectomies in growing children with pulmonary tuberculosis in 1939.[26] In 1950, Levitan and Zelman[23] reported pneumonectomy for primary childhood tuberculosis in 4 patients. In 1951, Ross[35] reported 7 lobectomies and 6 pneumonectomies and Botelho *et al.*,[2] 4 pneumonectomies. Rubin and Mishkin[39] in 1952 reported 30 resections, 19 in Negroes, 7 in Puerto Ricans and 4 in white children, with two deaths. The exact indications for resection and the anatomic distribution of the lobes in Rubin's series is not clear.[38,39]

In discussing their experience with 250 pulmonary resections in children, Boyd and Wilkinson[2] stated that 8% were done for tuberculosis (20 cases).

Igini *et al.*[17] reported 25 cases of resection in children with an average age of 11 years, the youngest being 2. Unilateral disease was present in 19. The shortest period of antibacterial therapy prior to resection was 11 months and on the average was 27 months. Leading indications were bronchiectasis developing in basilar lower lobe segments or in segments of the right middle lobe, and cavitary disease in any location (14 patients). Pneumonectomy was performed in 6 patients and lobectomy in 15. The right upper lobe was removed in 7, left upper in 3 and right middle in 5. Segmental resections were done in 4 (apical posterior segments of the upper lobes and basal segments of the lower lobes). There were two deaths in this series, one due to cardiac arrest and one to massive contralateral spread. No bronchopleural fistula developed. Empyema developed in 1 and contralateral spread in 2. From the anatomic distribution of the disease it is apparent that they were dealing with the adult type of tuberculosis in most cases.

Huish,[16] reporting from Dundee in 1956, listed 14 resections for primary tuberculosis; 12 were lobectomies. There were two deaths and two poor late results. The indications were: persistent collapse or consolidation, 9 instances (1 bilateral); symptomatic bronchiectasis, 2; primary cavitation, 1; chronic fibroid lung, 1. In addition, there were two attempted decortications, one abandoned because of caseous pleural disease and the other because of excessively vascular adhesions.

Huish's series included operations in 14 cases of chronic (adult type) tuberculosis. There were 7 lobectomies, with one death, 6 extrapleural pneumonolyses and 1 open intrapleural pneumonolysis. There were poor results in 3 patients, all after extrapleural pneumonolysis. The indications were: residual or very large cavity, 12 instances; tuberculoma, 2.

The brilliant immediate results possible with resection therapy were demonstrated by Webb *et al.*[49] in 51 resections for tuberculosis in 50 children from 1952 to 1960. Ten of the resections were performed for primary tuberculosis and 40 for reactivation tuberculosis. Four of the children were under 6 years. Indications for operation were: in primary tuberculosis, large cavity, 2; persistent tuberculous pneumonia, 4; symptomatic bronchiectasis, 1, and persistent collapse, 3. In reactivation tuberculosis, 18

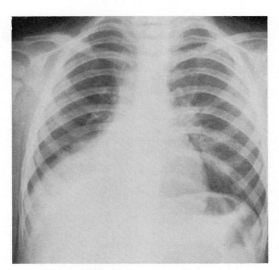

Fig. 32-23.—Mediastinal tuberculosis. Right lower lobe collapse persisting after adequate antibacterial therapy. After 21 months, there are no clinical signs or symptoms of secondary bronchiectasis. Conservatism is recommended in treatment of this lesion.

resections were performed for residual cavities, 11 for destroyed lung or lobes and 10 for residual bronchiectasis. In all, there were 7 pneumonectomies, 28 lobectomies (10 with additional segmental resections) and 16 segmental resections. There were no deaths, no bronchopleural fistulas and no empyema. One child returned with positive sputum and active ulceration in a segmental bronchial stump. On drug therapy, her sputum became negative and she had remained well for 3 years.

Giraud *et al.*[11] operated on 47 children with primary tuberculosis. Resection therapy consisted of 1 pneumonectomy and 32 lobectomies, distributed as follows: right upper lobe, 15; right middle lobe, 7; right middle and lower lobes, 3; left upper lobe, 4, and left lower lobe, 3. In addition, 2 children underwent bronchotomy with evacuation of caseous nodes.

CONSERVATIVE APPROACH.—A conservative medical and surgical attitude was taken by Cameron *et al.*[6] in their experience (1949–55) with 409 patients with primary childhood tuberculosis. Five were ultimately treated operatively: 4 had combined right middle lobe and right lower lobe bronchiectasis, and 1 had a left upper lobe resection occasioned by cicatricial obstruction of the bronchus supplying this lobe. All patients undergoing resection were covered with antimicrobial therapy for 6 weeks preoperatively and 3 months postoperatively. *No node operation was performed in any patient.*

In most cases, the primary tuberculous complex is a self-limited benign disease and the child has spontaneous and individual power to accomplish healing. About 2 years must follow the initial primary infection before the adult type of disease can develop.

During this period, most patients come under full control. Forty-eight of Cameron's patients had suspicious early segmental lesions and were extensively studied by bronchoscopy and bronchography. They could not be classified as having significant residual damage requiring resection. There is no convincing evidence that collapse of basal segments without superimposed mixed-organism bronchiectasis requires resection (Fig. 32-23). It has been estimated that 70% of patients with segmental occlusion will develop some degree of bronchiectasis within 10 years. This does not always progress to clinical disease with suppuration.[37] Repeated bronchoscopy is of value as a prophylactic measure, opening up areas of collapse whenever possible.

Fig. 32-24.—Tuberculoma of right upper lobe. **A,** a round, circumscribed area of opacity with a focus of calcification and immediately beneath it an irregular small cavity **(arrows)**. The rest of the lung field is clear. Acid-fast bacilli were identified in gastric washings. The lesion did not respond to antibacterial therapy. (Courtesy of Dr. R. Overholt.) **B,** x-ray of the resected right upper lobe again shows the tuberculoma-like lesion. It correlates well with the preoperative film **(A).**

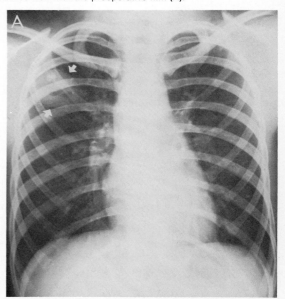

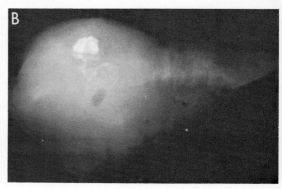

INDICATIONS FOR RESECTION.—Most segmental complications will resolve under medical therapy. Resection is indicated for grossly damaged infected lung tissue especially in the middle and lower lobes in patients who have had the childhood type of tuberculosis. Another indication is total destruction of the chronic fibrosed lung. A very doubtful indication is progressive unilateral disease or spread by contiguity in lower lobe segments. Triple drug therapy is effective in this group.

Tuberculomas often communicate with the adjacent bronchus and should be removed when they can be diagnosed by bronchography and body-section radiography. They are rare in children but do occur, as illustrated by the following case.

H. C., an 8-year-old girl, was found to have a solid, rounded, homogeneous density opposite the second rib on the right (Fig. 32-24, A). The lesion enlarged with evidence of central cavitation. Physical examination of the chest gave negative results. She was asymptomatic and well nourished. Acid-fast bacilli were identified on gastric aspiration studies. The tuberculin reaction was positive. There was no response to SM therapy. The lesion was interpreted as a moderately advanced process resembling a tuberculoma, and right upper lobectomy was done. The x-ray of the resected specimen (Fig. 32-24,B) relates well to the preoperative film and shows an area of calcification in the tuberculoma. The lesion measured 3.5 cm in diameter and contained a single focus of calcification. The adjacent parenchyma contained several areas of scar. There was moderately active tuberculous endobronchitis of the apical segmental bronchus. Operation revealed other caseous nodules in the lower lobe. The rest of the right lung was grossly free from disease.

With careful bronchoscopic mapping of residual segmental disease produced by the primary tuberculous complex, an occasional youngster will be found who will benefit from resection. The decision must be based on more than anatomic evidence of minor degrees of bronchiectasis, for instance, symptomatic difficulty and continuing clinical disease.

The complications of childhood-type primary pulmonary tuberculosis in various age groups occurring within 2 years of onset in 895 untreated patients observed by Lotte *et al.*[28] are shown in Figure 32-25.

Reinfection Pulmonary Tuberculosis: Adult Type

From 2 to 20 years following the original infection, patients may develop the adult type of tuberculosis with typical involvement of the posterior and apical portions of the upper lobes. This occurred in 7% of 622 children with known primary tuberculosis at Bellevue Hospital.[50] The process remains localized because of the altered response of the host. It differs from the childhood disease also, in that there is ultimate fibrocaseous pneumonia with central cavitation, the formation of a fibrous shell and eventual healing. For demonstrated fibrocaseous foci, with or without cavitation, after an adequate period of uninterrupted therapy, resection has much to offer. It has been estimated that 50% of adolescents have upper lobe cavitation. Failure to resect the involved segments in apparently quiescent cases leaves organisms in caseous foci and makes these children vulnerable to reinfection throughout life.

It has been established that, except for resection, operative procedures utilized in adults are not satisfactory when applied to young children. Extrapleural pneumonolysis is ineffective unless the cavities are extremely small (less than 3 cm) and have a thin fibrous rim. The procedure usually fails to accomplish the desired result. Intrapleural pneumonolysis is also unsatisfactory and, when atempted, has been associated with a high incidence of tuberculous empyema. Thoracoplasty procedures are contraindicated below the age of 16 except for extensive bilateral disease and uncontrollable hemoptysis. Medical collapse therapy (pneumothorax and pneumoperitoneum) is obsolete. These procedures are gradually falling into disuse in adults with pulmonary tuberculosis as well.

After a suitable period of chemotherapy and with evidence of unilateral residual cavitary disease, in the absence of endobronchial lesions resection is the procedure of choice. A more conservative policy is favored in children than in adults with comparable degrees of involvement. Resection is seldom indicated less than 3 years from the onset of infection. Webb[49] operated 6-12 months earlier. With undue delay, secondary suppurative bronchiectasis is added, and on occasion severe hemorrhage has occurred. Segmental resection, although theoretically desirable to preserve lung parenchyma, should not be performed in children because it opens up planes of infection, inviting spread in remaining lung tissue, and is associated with a high complication rate, notably, empyema and bronchopleural fistula.[5] For the same reason, there are few indications for wedge resection.

Fig. 32-25.—Pulmonary complications by age groups in 874 untreated patients with primary tuberculosis. (From Lotte *et al.*[28])

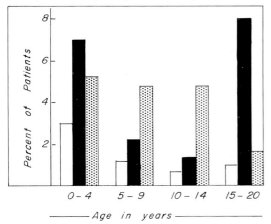

□ —*Compression Atelectasis*

■ — *Parenchymal Involvement*

▦ — *Pleurisy with Effusion*

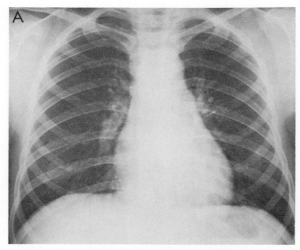

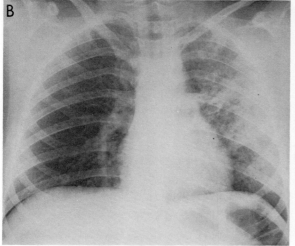

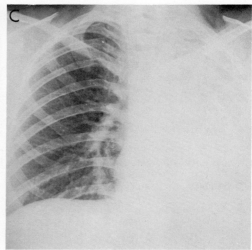

Fig. 32-26.—Tuberculosis of reinfection or adult type, with severe diabetes mellitus. **A,** a small focus of tuberculosis can be identified in the left lung. At this time the patient was 13 years old and had had diabetes since age 10. **B,** 1 year later, the entire left lung is involved by caseous and nodular tuberculosis. There is no evidence of contralateral spread. **C,** left pneumonectomy was performed, after a short period of drug therapy, because of the poor outlook with medical therapy alone. The mediastinum is maintained in relatively good position by a left oleothorax. (Courtesy of Dr. R. Overholt.)

INDICATIONS FOR PULMONARY RESECTION.[41,45]—These include: (1) An open cavity with or without positive sputum after 6 months of combined drug therapy. (2) Residual caseous nodules, fibrocaseous disease or caseous nodose disease. Tubercle bacilli must be considered to be resident in such lesions, and the child is exposed to a high risk of relapse. (3) Irreversible destructive lesions such as bronchiectasis, and bronchostenosis with hemoptysis, a positive sputum and total disorganization of a lobe or segment demonstrated by bronchography. (4) Recurrent or persistent hemorrhage with a life-endangering potential. In the most adverse conditions it may be necessary to do a preliminary tailoring thoracoplasty or utilize subper-

iosteal plombage in one of its various combinations. (5) An unexpandable lobe with chronic encapulated empyema. In this situation, the adjacent lobes are functioning inefficiently, and the surgical treatment usually consists of lobectomy and decortication in continuity. (6) Pulmonary infection due to atypical acid-fast organisms not responding to combined therapy for 4 months and having one or more of the foregoing indications for resection.

CONTRAINDICATIONS TO PULMONARY RESECTION.[41,45]—There are six clear contraindications: (1) Inadequate pulmonary reserve. (2) Extensive bilateral disease. (3) Involvement of an entire lung where active areas will be opened up in a plane of optimal resection. (4) When the risk of resection is greater than the risk of thoracoplasty or plombage. An example is the process that can only be eliminated by pleuropneumonectomy or lobectomy with decortication and a tailoring thoracoplasty. (5) The presence of another fatal disease. (6) Sputum containing organisms resistant to all known drugs. This is not the case with atypical mycobacteria that are notoriously resistant to medication.

At times, the need for operative intervention may be influenced by the presence of other disease. The outlook is poor in diabetic children with the adult form of pulmonary tuberculosis.

H. F., a 13-year-old girl with known severe diabetes since age 10, was found to have a small focus of tuberculosis in the left lung (Fig. 32-26, A). One year later she had total caseonodular involvement of this lung (Fig. 32-26, B) The disease remained unilateral. She had high fever, cough and hemoptysis. Because of the diabetes and the predictable poor survival with standard antituberculous chemotherapy, resection (left pneumonectomy) was elected. Preoperatively, she was given SM and PAS. Bronchoscopy revealed reddening but no true ulceration or diminution of the caliber of any of the visible bronchi. At the time of operation the upper lobe was solid and airless. It could not be inflated. The lower lobe contained air but did not deflate well, and there was extensive nodulation throughout the lower lobe. Following pneumonectomy, the contralateral lung remained clear (Fig. 32-26, C). The resected specimen showed extensive caseonodular involvement with many nodules up to 0.6 cm in diameter.

A distressing but rare complication following resection under chemotherapy is reactivation and dissemination of disease, usually to the opposite side. The presence of bilateral disease ordinarily contraindicates pulmonary resection. In late adolescence, however, a limited thoracoplasty may be necessary on one side with resection on the other. Rivarola et al.[34] reported that 10% of their patients required bilateral surgery, with a mortality of 15%.

There has been a steady increase of the number of patients who undergo resection for reinfection tuberculosis. Operative mortality has fallen to a new low level of 2.1%.[22,45] About 85% of patients followed for 2–5 years have had no reactivation and can be considered to be under satisfactory control.[22,45]

CONCLUSIONS.—In the years since the advent of modern tuberculous antibacterial therapy, we have witnessed the actual disappearance of medical collapse therapy and the virtual disappearance of surgical collapse therapy as definitive treatment for pulmonary tuberculosis. Resection therapy is still indicated for lesions that do not come under medical control, and surgery will ultimately be required by approximately 15% of children with the adult or reinfection form of tuberculosis. Provided the surgical procedure is performed under full antibacterial control, including SM and insistence on preoperative sputum conversion except for the atypical group, pulmonary resection for tuberculosis can be performed with a mortality and complication rate only slightly in excess of that for other suppurative lung conditions. It will always be required for cavernous, nodular, bronchiectatic and carnified residua. As more sophisticated culture techniques are employed, an increasing number of children will be encountered with granulomatous pulmonary lesions due to atypical mycobacteria. The commonest one is *M. kansasii*, which is now the cause of between 3 and 9% of all admissions for acid-fast pulmonary infections. In the face of total resistance to drugs commonly employed, these infections can only lead to widespread lung destruction without resection therapy.[8,19]

Hopefully, with an alert, responsible and pediatric-oriented community, pulmonary tuberculosis will not progress in most children beyond the mild to moderate lesion and resection therapy will rarely be required.[30] This and the preceding sections on bronchiectasis and lung abscess portray an era of great disability for children with suppurative disorders of the lung.

REFERENCES

1. Adler, D., and Richards, W. F.: Consolidation in primary pulmonary tuberculosis, Thorax 8:223, 1953.
2. Botelho, G. H., et al.: Pneumonectomy in the treatment of tuberculosis in children, Dis. Chest 2:642, 1951.
3. Boyd, E. L., and Wilkinson, F. R.: Pulmonary resection in childhood tuberculosis, Dis. Chest 26:442, 1954.
4. Brailey, M. E.: Epidemic Aspects of Harriet Lane Study, in Commonwealth Fund: *Tuberculosis in White and Negro Children* (Cambridge, Mass.: Harvard University Press, 1958), Vol. 2, p. 26.
5. Brewer., L. A.: Tuberculous Empyema and Bronchopleural Fistula in Clinical Tuberculosis, in Pleutae, K. H., and Radner, D. B. (ed): *Clinical Tuberculosis* (Springfield, Ill.: Charles C Thomas, Publisher, 1966).
6. Cameron, J. K.; Hay, J. D., and Temple, L. S.: A critical examination of the role of surgery in the treatment of primary pulmonary tuberculosis in children, Thorax 12:329, 1957.
7. Chesterman, J. T.: The surgery of primary pulmonary tuberculosis in children, Thorax 12:159, 1957.
8. Corpe, R. F., and Liang, J.: Surgical resection in pulmonary tuberculosis due to atypical *Mycobacterium tuberculosis*, J. Thoracic & Cardiovas. Surg. 40:93, 1960.
9. Danino, E. A.; Evans, C. J., and Thomas, J. H.: Tuberculous bronchoesophageal fistula in a child, Thorax 10:351, 1955.
10. Debré, R., and Brissaud, H. E.: Faut-il traiter la tuberculose initiale de l'enfant et de l'adolescent? Presse méd. 62:524, 1954.
11. Giraud, P., et al.: Indications and results of excisional surgery in primary tuberculosis in children, Rev. Tuberc. (Paris) 25:1261, 1961.
12. Giraud, P., et al.: Traitement chirurgical de complications graves de la primo-infection, Pédiatrie 9:557, 1954.
13. Gorgenyi-Gottche, O. G., and Kassay, D.: Importance of bronchial rupture in tuberculosis of endothoracic lymph nodes, Am. J. Dis. Child. 74:166, 1947.
14. Hardy, J. B.; Proctor, D. F., and Turner, J. A.: Bronchial obstruction and bronchiectasis complicating primary tuberculosis infection, J. Pediat. 41:740, 1952.
15. Heimbeck, J.: Vaccination sous-cutanée et cutanée au BCG 1926-1948, Semaine hôp. Paris 25:771, 1949.
16. Huish, D. W.: The surgical treatment of pulmonary tuberculosis in childhood and adolescence, Thorax 11:186, 1956.
17. Igini, J. P.; Fox, R. T., and Less, W. M.: Resection for pulmonary tuberculosis in infants and children, Dis. Chest 37:176, 1960.
18. Jones, E. M., and Howard, W. L.: Treatment of tuberculosis in children, Pediatrics 17:146, 1955.

19. Jones, J. D.: Surgery of Pulmonary Tuberculosis Caused by Unclassified Acid-fast Mycobacteria, in Pleutae, K. H., and Radner, D. B. (ed.): *Clinical Tuberculosis* (Springfield, Ill.: Charles C Thomas, Publisher, 1966).

20. Kendig, E. L.: Tuberculosis, in Gellis, S. S., and Kagan, B. M. (ed.): *Current Pediatric Therapy* (Philadelphia: W. B. Saunders Company, 1968), Vol. 3, p. 779.

21. Laff, H. I.; Hurst, A., and Robinson, A.: Importance of bronchial involvement in primary tuberculosis of childhood, J.A.M.A. 146:778, 1951.

22. Langston, H. T.; Baker, W. L., and Pyle, M. M.: Surgery in pulmonary tuberculosis. Ann. Surg. 164:573, 1966.

23. Levitan, M., and Zelman, M.: Excisional therapy of pulmonary tuberculosis in children, Am. J. Dis. Child. 79:30, 1950.

24. Lincoln, E. M.; Davies, P. A., and Bovornkitti, S.: Tuberculous pleurisy with effusion in children, Am. Rev. Tuberc. 77:271, 1958.

25. Lincoln, E. M., *et al.*: Endobronchial tuberculosis in children, Am. Rev. Tuberc. 77:39, 1958.

26. Lincoln, E. M., and Sewall, E. M.: *Tuberculosis in Children* (2nd ed.: New York: McGraw-Hill Book Company, Inc., 1963), p. 3.

27. Lindskog, G. E., and Spear, H. C.: Middle lobe syndrome, New England J. Med. 253:489, 1955.

28. Lotte, A., *et al.*: The treatment of primary tuberculosis in childhood, Pediatrics 26:641, 1960.

29. Miller, J. A., and Walgren, A.: *Pulmonary Tuberculosis in Adults and Children* (New York: Thos. Nelson & Sons, 1939), p. 173.

30. Mitchell, R. S.: Control of tuberculosis, New England J. Med. 276:842, 1967.

31. Myers, J. A.: Prognosis in treatment of tuberculosis among children, Dis. Chest. 44:27, 1963.

32. Nemir, R. L., *et al.*: Prednisone as an adjunct in the chemotherapy of lymph nodes in bronchial tuberculosis in childhood, Am. Rev. Resp. Dis. 95:402, 1967.

33. Oatway, W. H., *et al.*: *Diagnostic Standards and Classification of Tuberculosis* (New York: American Thoracic Society, 1966).

34. Rivarola, C. H.; Norton, L. W., and Levene, N.: Bilateral resection for cavitary pulmonary tuberculosis, J. Thoracic & Cardiovas. Surg. 50:277, 1965.

35. Ross, C. A.: Pulmonary resection for tuberculosis in children, Thorax 6:375, 1951.

36. Rothman, P. E., and Mapes, R.: Massive unilateral pulmonary fibrosis due to obstructive tracheobronchial tuberculosis, J. Pediat. 17:659, 1940.

37. Rothman, P. E.; Jones, J. C., and Peterson, H. G.: Endoscopic and surgical treatment of pulmonary tuberculosis in children, Am. J. Dis. Child. 99:315, 1960.

38. Rubin, M.: The role of resection for pulmonary tuberculosis in children and adolescents, Am. J. Surg. 89:649, 1955.

39. Rubin, M., and Mishkin, S.: Resection for pulmonary tuberculosis in children and adolescents, Surg., Gynec. & Obst. 95:751, 1952.

40. Seal, R. M. E., and Thomas, D. M. E.: Endobronchial tuberculosis in children, Lancet 2:995, 1956.

41. Sloan, H., and Milnes, R.: Pulmonary Resection for Tuberculosis, in Steele, J. D. (ed.):*Surgical Management of Pulmonary Tuberculosis* (Springfield, Ill.: Charles C Thomas, Publisher, 1957).

42. Smith, M. H. D.: The role of adrenal steroids in the treatment of tuberculosis, Pediatrics 22:774, 1958.

43. Starr, S., and Berkovitch, S.: Effects of measles gamma globulin and vaccine measles on the tuberculin test, New England J. Med. 270:386, 1964.

44. Steiner, M., and Cosio, A.: Primary tuberculosis in children, New England J. Med. 274:755, 1966.

45. Strieder, J. W.; Laforet, E. G., and Lynch, J. P.: Surgery of pulmonary tuberculosis, New England J. Med. 276:960, 1967.

46. Strom, L.: Vaccination against tuberculosis. Am. Rev. Tuberc. 74:28, 1956.

47. *Symposium on Childhood Tuberculosis*, Brit. J. Dis. Chest (London: Baillière, Tindall & Cox, 1960).

48. United States Public Health Service: Tuberculosis prophylaxis trial: Prophylactic effects of isoniazid in primary tuberculosis in children, Am. Rev. Tuberc. 76:942, 1957.

49. Webb, W. R.; Wofford, J. L., and Stauss, H. K.: Resectional therapy for pulmonary tuberculosis in children, Surgery 51:270, 1962.

50. Weber, A. L.; Bird, K. T., and Janower, M. L.: Primary tuberculosis in childhood, with particular emphasis on changes affecting the tracheobronchial tree, Am. J. Roentgenol. 103:123, 1968.

K. J. WELCH

Coccidioidomycosis

HISTORY.—In 1891 Posada[10] first observed an unusual tumor of the skin which he and Wernicke[12] ascribed to a parasite of the protozoan genus of *Coccidia.* Three years later it was recognized that the causative organism, although indeed a protozoan, belonged to the class Sporozoa but because of its resemblance to *Coccidia* the newly discovered fungus was named *Coccidioides.* The most comprehensive and up-to-date bibliography of coccidioidomycosis has been compiled by Fiese.[7] A year-by-year analysis of the entire field is included in the Transactions of the Annual Meetings of the Veterans Administration-Armed Forces Coccidioidomycosis Cooperative Study, beginning with 1956. All cases of coccidioidomycosis in children reported in the literature up to 1956—a total of 99—were collected and reviewed by Christian and his coworkers.[3]

GEOGRAPHIC DISTRIBUTION

Coccidioidomycosis results from contact with *Coccidioides immitis* primarily through inhalation of dust containing spores of this fungus. *Coccidioides immitis* is widespread throughout the Lower Sonoran Zone, but within this climatobiologic region it is limited to areas in which the creosote bush grows. The world's highest concentration of *Coccidioides immitis* is found in the soil of the southern part of the San Joaquin Valley in California and in certain parts of Arizona, particularly around Phoenix. Both regions are considered hyperendemic. Los Angeles and its environs, as well as portions of Nevada and Texas, are hypoendemic areas; that is, the disease is constantly present but with a lower incidence. Incidentally infected individuals scatter throughout the country and the disease, regional in its origin, may be seen anywhere. Coccidioidomycosis is also endemic in the northern part of Mexico, in Argentina (where the disease was discovered), as well as in Bolivia and Paraguay, especially in the Chaco region of these three countries.

INCIDENCE

We estimate that there are annually in the United States more than 10,000 new cases of coccidioidomycosis among children under 14 years of age. Almost everyone born or living in an endemic area will ultimately be infected. Of children who had lived in Kern County, California, less than a year, 25% had a positive coccidioidin reaction, as contrasted with 76% for others who had been residents for 10 years or more.[11]

CLINICAL MANIFESTATIONS

ASYMPTOMATIC PRIMARY INFECTION. — This most frequent form of the disease is discovered only by a skin test. There are no roentgen findings and no pulmonary complications.

SYMPTOMATIC PRIMARY INFECTION. — The clinical manifestations of the symptomatic form of coccidioidomycosis vary from those simulating a mild upper respiratory infection to signs of primary pneumonitis. Cough, one of the commonest symptoms, is often nonproductive and almost always irritative. Fever may be fleeting, or marked and persistent. Duration and height of fever provide a clue to the further course of the disease. In more severe cases, infiltration of the lung parenchyma takes place, and usually a moderate degree of hilar adenopathy is manifest. In addition, there may be cervical lymphadenitis. Pulmonary involvement may regress within a few days or slowly over a number of months or may go on to pleural effusion or cavitation. Cutaneous lesions are common manifestations of primary infection and may take the form of a macular rash simulating measles or urticaria, but the most characteristic skin lesions of acute coccidioidomycosis are erythema nodosum and erythema multiforme. It is noteworthy that in children, erythema nodosum shows no sex predilection, while it has frequently been reported that in adults this skin lesion is twice as common in women as men.

Lesions of this type are not a sign of actual dissemination but are considered to be due to systemic allergic reaction. The same applies to the polyarthritis that is sometimes seen.

DISSEMINATED COCCIDIOIDOMYCOSIS. — Dissemination is the result of reinfection from within and may occur early or late. The most important forms are miliary dissemination and meningitis. In children, meningitis develops rather frequently but usually takes a benign course. In adults, meningitis is often complicated by miliary pulmonary spread and the prognosis is grave.

DIAGNOSIS

Diagnosis of primary infection and prognosis are based largely on laboratory findings. Eosinophilia is almost always present, the eosinophil count ranging from just above normal to 25%. As a rule, the leukocyte count is moderately elevated. The erythrocyte sedimentation rate is elevated in the beginning and returns to normal with recovery. If, upon careful and repeated performance, a previously negative coccidioidin skin test becomes positive after 2 or 3 weeks, it may be regarded as proof of active primary infection. Complement fixation is of greater aid in diagnosis and prognosis than the precipitin test. A strongly positive complement fixation indicates a severe infection, and a persistent high level is a sign of impending dissemination.

A patient with a high titer should be kept under constant observation, because late dissemination is likely to occur several months after recovery from the primary infection.

ROENTGEN FINDINGS. — The first phase of coccidioidomycosis is tracheobronchial and may result in peribronchial thickening.[1] As in tuberculosis, many types of pulmonary changes are seen — mottled bronchopneumonia, pneumonitis (Fig. 32-27) or lobar consolidation. Associated hilar adenitis (Fig. 32-28) may persist for several months. In 5% of cases, chronic residual pulmonary lesions will develop. They may appear as multiple nodular densities (coccidioidomas) or as chronic focalized changes of two different types: thin-walled cavities or thick-walled cavities resulting from a shelled-out coccidioidoma. Roentgen findings in pulmonary dissemination mimic those of miliary tuberculosis (Fig. 32-29).

Fig. 32-27. — Coccidioidomycosis and tuberculosis. Coccidioidal pneumonitis of the right upper lobe with bilateral tuberculous hilar adenitis. Tuberculosis was diagnosed by cervical lymph node biopsy before coccidioidal infection. The patient recovered completely from both diseases.

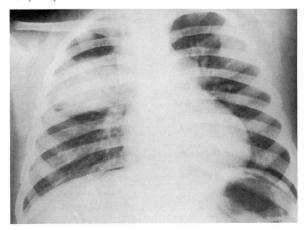

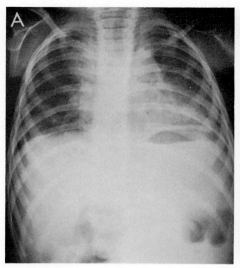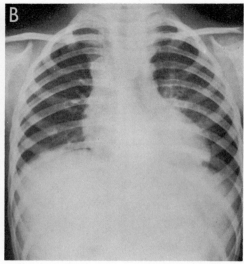

Fig. 32-28.—Coccidioidomycosis. **A,** primary lesion with extreme hilar adenitis. **B,** calcified hilar nodes 19 months later. The patient was well.

DIFFERENTIAL DIAGNOSIS

NONSPECIFIC PNEUMONITIS.—The primary pneumonitis of coccidioidomycosis clinically and roentgenographically simulates nonspecific pneumonitis.

TUBERCULOSIS.—Tuberculosis and coccidioidomycosis present many anatomic, pathologic and diagnostic similarities and the roentgenographic appearances of the two diseases may be almost indistinguishable. The course of coccidioidomycosis is more benign than

Fig. 32-29.—Disseminated coccidioidomycosis. The baby was a white girl of 6 weeks, whose death was proved at autopsy to be due to dissemination of the infection and to coccidioidal meningitis.

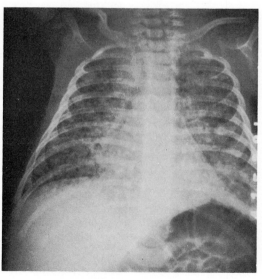

that of tuberculosis and pulmonary cavities and solid lesions are less frequent. A thin-walled cavity with a minimal zone of reaction is suggestive of coccidioidomycosis, but occasionally side by side with these are secondarily infected cavities surrounded by a zone of reaction. Serologic tests are often inconclusive, and at times a definitive differential diagnosis can be made only following surgical intervention or at autopsy.

Coexisting disease creates many puzzling problems. Pulmonary coccidioidomycosis with coexistent tuberculosis has been observed in 24 patients.[5] Of this group, 9 adults treated by pulmonary resection did well. The 8 infants or children in the group not operated on did well and surgical intervention was not necessary.

In children, once a coccidioidal lesion has become focalized, any new infiltrative process should arouse suspicion of tuberculosis. One must also think of coexistent tuberculosis when extreme hilar adenopathy is noted in a child.

LYMPHOMA GROUP.—The hilar lymphadenitis of symptomatic primary coccidioidomycosis has suggested sarcoidosis, lymphosarcoma and Hodgkin's disease. Patients with any one of the lymphomatous diseases show increased susceptibility to infection, and coccidioidomycosis develops frequently. In our series, none of the patients with coexistent lymphomatous disease has been operated on, and most of them died of dissemination of the infection.

MATERIAL FOR STUDY

In all, 3,000 cases of coccidioidomycosis have been analyzed. In every instance, the diagnosis was confirmed by complement fixation test and/or by micro-

TABLE 32-10.—Coccidioidomycosis in 200 Children

COMPLICATIONS	MALE, 104				FEMALE, 96				TOTALS
	WHITE (53)	NEGRO (29)	MEXICAN (18)	OTHER (4)	WHITE (51)	NEGRO (21)	MEXICAN (21)	OTHER (3)	(200)
Acute—									
Pleural effusion	3	2	0	0	5	0	2	1	13
Pericardial effusion	1	0	0	0	0	0	0	0	1
Dissemination {bone	0	17	3	2	2	5	5	0	34
{other	3	0	2	0	2	2	0	0	9
Chronic—									
Fibrosis	0	0	0	0	2	0	1	0	3
Bronchiectasis	2	0	0	0	2	0	0	0	4
Coccidioidoma	2	0	0	0	0	1	0	0	3
Cavitation	3	0	2	0	2	0	2	0	9
Confirmation:									
Skin test positive	35	11	8	1	35	15	15	1	121
Complement fixation positive	40	15	8	0	25	18	14	1	121
Smear and/or culture positive	2	14	2	1	3	7	5	0	34
Spinal fluid positive	1	0	0	0	0	0	0	0	1
Guinea pig positive	0	3	3	0	2	0	0	0	8
Erythema nodosum and/or multiforme	32	0	5	1	29	2	7	1	77
Marked hilar adenopathy	28	6	2	1	13	5	6	0	61
Tuberculosis and coccidioidomycosis	0	2	1	0	0	2	3	0	8
Deaths	2	2	1	0	1	1	0	0	7

scopic demonstration of spherules in the sputum, by culture, animal inoculation or by histopathologic study of specimens obtained at operation or at autopsy. The patients came from the hyperendemic southern part of the San Joaquin Valley and from the neighboring hypoendemic Los Angeles County. Of the 3,000 patients with confirmed coccidioidomycosis, 200 fell into the pediatric group, ranging in age from 3 weeks to 14 years. The distribution as to sex and racial extraction is presented in Table 32-10.

COMPLICATIONS

In the pediatric group, significant complications occur in almost one third of all cases.

Fig. 32-30.—Coccidioidal pericardial effusion. The patient, a white boy of 7½ years, recovered. No spherules were ever found in the fluid.

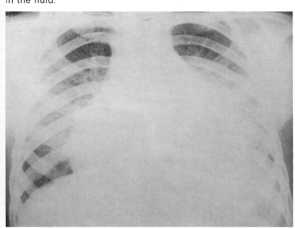

ACUTE COMPLICATIONS.—*Pleural effusion* develops occasionally but as a rule takes a benign course and clears up spontaneously. For massive effusion, repeated aspiration may be necessary. Pleural effusion encountered in coccidioidal lesions already focalized should be assumed to be of tuberculous origin. *Pericardial effusion* (Fig. 32-30) was observed in 1 child. *Dissemination* was the most frequent complication in the pediatric group, developing in 43 children, of whom 7 died. In adults, the death rate is two to three times as high as it is in children. The two most common sites of dissemination are bone and meninges. Invasion of only a single bone or joint is unusual, and no bone or joint is immune. Often a soft tissue abscess is demonstrated in the immediate neighborhood of the bone lesion. We have never seen a case in which a soft tissue abscess secondarily involved the bone. Dissemination to bone is encountered so commonly in coccidioidomycosis that this possibility should always be considered in suspected cases of osteomyelitis or similar bone lesions.[8] The diagnosis of osseous coccidioidomycosis cannot be established on clinical or roentgenologic grounds and is made only by identification of the organism, preferably by the complement fixation test.[2]

In disseminated coccidioidomycosis, the skin is almost always involved except in occasional instances with meningitis. Although cutaneous lesions vary greatly, usually only one type is present in a single patient. Verrucous granulomas, small dermal nodules, indolent ulcers often associated with underlying bone lesions, and subcutaneous abscesses are common manifestations of disseminated disease. Organisms can usually be recovered from such lesions. There is a marked tendency to spontaneous remissions and recrudescences, and in a high but undetermined percentage of patients, ultimate recovery ensues. In extremely rare cases, a solitary cutaneous granuloma may be due to primary skin inoculation, but as a rule all coccidioidal skin lesions are traceable to dissemination.

CHRONIC COMPLICATIONS. — Primary coccidioidomycosis which regresses spontaneously may leave varying degrees of *pulmonary fibrosis*. In our series, it was rarely encountered and, surprisingly, only in females. *Bronchiectasis* occasionally develops in the course of coccidioidomycosis, as it does with other infections of the lung. *Coccidioidoma* is a benign focalized pulmonary granuloma. Over 90% of such residual nodular lesions were located more than 5 cm from the hilar area. Average diameter was 1.3 cm, but the largest in our series was 6 cm in diameter. *Cavitation* occurred in 9 children (4.5%), with complete recovery without operation. Pulmonary resection has been performed in 150 adults. In general, medical management for 1 year is indicated before considering surgical intervention, and it would seem that in children an even longer waiting period might be justified.

TREATMENT

MEDICAL MANAGEMENT. — There is no specific drug therapy for primary coccidioidomycosis. Symptomatic treatment and restriction of activity are advised until sedimentation rate and eosinophil count have returned to normal. In disseminated disease, and most certainly in meningitis, amphotericin B should be tried. This antifungal antibiotic is of relatively low toxicity and may be administered orally or preferably by the intravenous route.[13] How long conservative management should be continued after residual pulmonary coccidioidal lesions have been demonstrated is still a matter of controversy.[9]

SURGICAL MANAGEMENT. — The indications for resection of coccidioidal cavities in adults are well established.[4] In children, conservative management of focalized pulmonary lesions is recommended. All such cavities in our pediatric group healed within a year. It is very unlikely that in this age bracket a solid pulmonary lesion would indicate bronchogenic carcinoma.

Pulmonary resection, however, should be considered when a cavity becomes secondarily infected, or if it grows larger or even if its size remains constant for more than 1 year, and for hemoptysis.[6] Depending on the size of the lesion, lobectomy or wedge resection is indicated. In the latter procedure, a sufficiently wide area must be excised, since the zone of involvement always extends beyond the tissue immediately surrounding the cavity.

REFERENCES

1. Birsner, J. W.: The roentgen aspects of 500 cases of pulmonary coccidioidomycosis, Am. J. Roentgenol. 72:556, 1954.
2. Birsner, J. W., and Smart, S.: Osseous coccidioidomycosis: A chronic form of dissemination, Am. J. Roentgenol. 76:1052, 1956.
3. Christian, J. R., et al.: Pulmonary coccidioidomycosis in a 21-day-old infant: Report of a case and review of the literature, Am. J. Dis. Child. 92:66, 1956.
4. Cotton, B. H., and Birsner, J. W.: Surgical treatment of pulmonary coccidioidomycosis, J. Thoracic Surg. 38:435, 1959.
5. Cotton, B. H., et al.: Coexisting pulmonary coccidioidomycosis and tuberculosis, Am. Rev. Tuberc. 70:109, 1954.
6. Cotton, B. H.; Paulsen, G. A., and Birsner, J. W.: Surgical considerations in pulmonary coccidioidomycosis, Am. J. Surg. 90:101, 1955.
7. Fiese, M. J.: *Coccidioidomycosis* (Springfield, Ill.: Charles C Thomas, Publisher, 1958).
8. Mazel, R.: Skeletal lesions in coccidioidomycosis, Arch. Surg. 70:497, 1955.
9. Melick, D. W. (ed.): *Treatment of Pulmonary Coccidioidomycosis from a Surgical Standpoint*, Proc. Symp. on Coccidioidomycosis, Public Health Service Publ. 575 (Washington, D. C.: U. S. Dept. of Health, Education and Welfare, 1957), p. 69.
10. Posada, A.: Ensayo anatomopatologico sobre una neoplasia considerad como micosis fungoides, An. circ. méd. argent. 15:8, 1892.
11. Thorner, J. E.: Coccidioidomycosis: Relative values of coccidioidin and tuberculin testing among children of the San Joaquin Valley, California & West. Med. 54:12, 1941.
12. Wernicke, R.: Ueber einen Protozoenbefund bei Mycosis fungoides, Zentralbl. Bakt. 12:859, 1892.
13. Winn, W. A.: Coccidioidomycosis, Arch. Int. Med. 106:463, 1960.

B. H. COTTON
J. W. BIRSNER

Tumors of the Lung

33

A NUMBER OF VARIETIES of lung tumor occur in childhood. The total number is so small that their incidence in terms of the occurrence of other tumors in children, or of the occurrence of tumors of the same kind in adults, is without significance. Secondary malignant tumors metastatic from Wilms' tumor, neuroblastoma or osteogenic sarcoma are more common than primary malignancies.

HAMARTOMAS

These tumor-like malformations consisting of an abnormal mixing of the normal components of an organ are obviously congenital in origin and not rare in the lung in adult life. They are seldom discovered in infancy or childhood. Jones[5] reported on a 1,516-Gm premature infant who died 1 hour after birth, having had to be resuscitated during that time. The right upper lobe was replaced by a large spherical mass 3.5 cm in diameter with a peripheral margin of compressed lung. The tumor was composed of bands of fibrous tissue with young fibroblasts, islands of immature cartilage and fetal fat with cleftlike channels lined by respiratory epithelium. Harris and Schattenbergh[2] reported on 2 newborn children with obvious large hamartomas; both died of respiratory distress.

TUMORS OF SMOOTH MUSCLE AND CONNECTIVE TISSUE

Smooth muscle and connective tissue tumors occur and are probably of bronchial origin (Fig. 33-1). Holinger et al.[3] described two leiomyosarcomas, one on the anterior wall of the trachea of a 5-year-old child who indefinitely survived bronchoscopic resection, and the other on the right main bronchus of a 6-year-old girl who died after unsuccessful x-ray treatment. Watson and Anlyan[9] reported three leiomyosarcomas of the lung, one of which was in a 4-year-old boy who had had a cough for 3 months. The right main bronchus was filled with a reddish mass that bled easily and on biopsy was considered to be a spindle cell sarcoma, possibly a myosarcoma. He died during operation, and autopsy disclosed a mass at the right hilus involving the main stem bronchus and complete atelectasis of the right lung. The tumor was polypoid, obliterated the main bronchus and narrowed the tra-

chea, but it was not invasive and could have been cured either by pneumonectomy or by bronchial resection.

Killingsworth et al.[6] saw a 7-year-old girl with repeated cough and fever with a homogeneous shadow in the left chest and, on bronchoscopy, a smooth reddish mass filling the left main bronchus. At operation, the tumor extended into the left atrium, but it was possible to place a clamp beyond it and perform a pneumonectomy. The specimen showed a cellular tumor invading and ulcerating the bronchus and extending also into the pulmonary vein and into the atrium. It was called a low-grade leiomyosarcoma. There were no lymph node metastases. The child was well 2 years later.

Of 8 children with fibrosarcoma of the bronchus collected from the literature by Holinger et al.[4] 4 were under 15 (aged 5½, 13, 13 and 14 years). Two were living and well after operation. One had had an open

Fig. 33-1.—Leiomyoma of the left lower lobe. A 9-year-old girl had had intermittent cough productive of mucoid sputum for 5 years and hemoptysis for 1 month. The large tumor replaced the lower lobe and encroached on the upper lobe bronchus so that pneumonectomy was required. She was well when last seen 10 years after operation and had developed normally. (Courtesy of Dr. R. A. Daniel, Jr., Nashville, Tenn.)

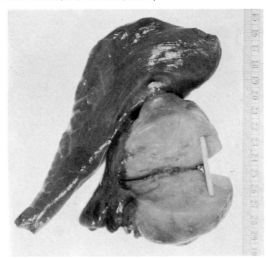

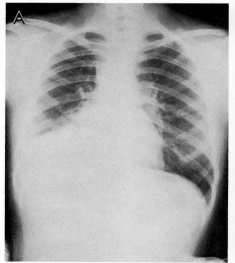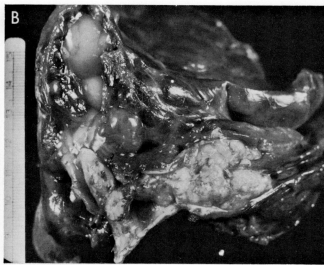

Fig. 33-2.—Bronchial adenoma of the right lower lobe. A 12-year-old girl was subject to repeated attacks of pulmonary infection in the right lower lobe. Bronchoscopic diagnosis of adenoma was made. **A,** roentgenogram showing complete atelectasis of the right lower lobe. **B,** the excised specimen showing the great lobulated polypoid growth dilating and obstructing the bronchus and glairy white retained mucopus in the huge cystic obstructed bronchus. She remained well after the right lower lobectomy.

thoracotomy, another a bronchoscopic resection; 1 died after operation, and 1 coughed up the entire tumor and was living and well. Holinger added a fifth case, of a 5½-year-old boy with cough and fever and repeated attacks of atelectasis of the right lower lobe. The right intermediate bronchus was blocked by a smooth fibrous mass. Right lower and middle lobectomy for the polypoid fibrosarcoma in the right lower lobe bronchus was curative.

Bronchial Adenoma

Bronchial adenoma is occasionally seen in children. Ward *et al.*[7] in 1954 found 8 reported cases in children and added a ninth. Bronchial adenoma begins as an intrabronchial growth, extends through the bronchial wall until the extrabronchial portion may be larger than the portion of the tumor which presents. Atelectasis from obstruction and hemoptysis from the ulcerated intrabronchial tumor are common occurrences. None of the reported adenomas in children are known to have metastasized, although some of the earlier ones were treated only bronchoscopically. On the other hand, the period of follow-up in all of them was short. These tumors in adults have adequately established their capability for ultimate metastasis and should be vigorously treated as malignant tumors for which cure is possible. The importance of bronchoscopy in children with otherwise unexplained chronic coughs cannot be overestimated. We know of 1 child who had been treated for "asthma" from infancy and died in "status asthmaticus"

and was found at autopsy to have a bronchial adenoma obstructing her trachea. Our single experience with bronchial adenoma in childhood (Fig. 33-2) suggests no difference between the lesion in childhood and in adult life.

Carcinoma of the Lung

Epithelial malignancies of the lung in children occur rarely (Fig. 33-3). Cayley *et al.*[1] collected a series of 16 bronchogenic carcinomas of the lung in children, aged 5 months to 14 years. About half of them presented symptoms due to metastasis or to nonspecific evidence of malignancy, and half had symptoms referable to the lungs. The histologic diagnoses vary from squamous cell carcinoma, adenocarcinoma, epithelioid carcinoma to oat-cell carcinoma, small-cell carcinoma and anaplastic carcinoma. One patient[8] was alive 7 years after operation; the others died.

REFERENCES

1. Cayley, C. K.; Kscaez, H. J., and Mersheimer, W.: Primary bronchogenic carcinoma of the lung in children, Am. J. Dis. Child. 82:49, 1951.
2. Harris, W. H., and Schattenbergh, J.: Anlagen and rest tumors of the lung inclusive of "mixed tumors" (Womack and Graham), Am. J. Path. 18:955, 1942.
3. Holinger, P. H.; Slaughter, D. P., and Novak, F. J., III: Unusual tumors obstructing the lower respiratory tract of infants and children, Tr. Am. Acad. Ophth. 54:223, 1950; discussion, p. 233.
4. Holinger, P. H., *et al.*: Primary fibrosarcoma of the bronchus, Dis. Chest 37:137, 1960.
5. Jones, C. J.: Unusual hamartoma of the lung in a newborn infant, Arch. Path. 48:150, 1949.

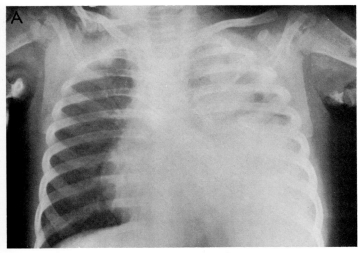

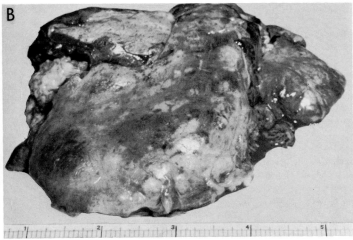

Fig. 33-3.—Embryonal carcinoma of the lung. A 13-month-old child was seen by a physician for anorexia of 5 days' duration, without cough or respiratory symptoms. Sterile fluid was aspirated from the left chest but re-formed. **A,** posteroanterior roentgenogram obtained on hospitalization for operation at age 15 months. There is a dense shadow at the left base extending into the upper lung field, and the heart is displaced to the right. **B,** operative specimen comprising the entire left lung and diaphragm to which it was attached. The surgeon considered the tumor to arise in the lung. Pathologic diagnosis (Dr. Drummond Bowden) was embryonal carcinoma arising in the lung. The child died of diffuse metastases 4 months after operation. Autopsy suggested no other primary source. The ovaries were uninvolved. (Courtesy of Dr. J. E. Lewis, Jr., St. Louis.) Malignant tumors of the lung occur in infants, are sometimes slow-growing and are characteristically bland in initial symptomatology.

6. Killingsworth, W. P.; McReynolds, G. S., and Harrison, A. W.: Pulmonary leiomyosarcoma in a child, J. Pediat. 42:466, 1953.
7. Ward, D. E., Jr.; Bradshaw, H. H., and Prince, T. C., Jr.: Bronchial adenoma in children, J. Thoracic Surg. 27:295, 1954.
8. Wasche, M. G.; Lederer, M., and Epstein, B. S.: Bronchi-ogenic carcinoma of seven years' duration in an eleven-year-old boy, J. Pediat. 17:521, 1940.
9. Watson, W. L., and Anlyan, A. J.: Primary leiomyosar-coma of the lung, Cancer 7:250, 1954.

M. M. RAVITCH

34

Embryology of Anomalies
of the Heart and Great Vessels

DEVELOPMENT OF A mechanism for continuous exchange between each cell and its surrounding fluid has made possible the evolution of single-celled into many-celled organisms. Higher animals have achieved this by a vascular circulatory system and the muscular force of a beating heart. The evolution of this system is repeated in embryonic development. This complex recapitulation, determined by each individual's genes, may be modified by outside influences that change the course of structural development and result in anomalies. An understanding of these variations depends on knowledge of the normal.

To review normal development is beyond the scope of this discussion; for this the reader may refer to other texts. It will suffice to remember that the embryo depends on direct exchange with its environment for only a very short time after the ovum is fertilized. Early in the third week vascular lakes appear in a bilaterally symmetrical mesenchymal net. These soon coalesce into channels radiating from the cardiogenic area at the anterior end of the embryonic disk. As the body folds upward, the heart forms by fusion of paired primordia into a single tube. The endothelium lining the vessels and heart, and the mesenchymal epimyocardial mantle which surrounds the latter differentiate early and by the end of the third week rhythmic contraction waves propel fluid from the heart tube into the surrounding vascular net. Thus circulation is begun. Thereafter, interaction of the evolutionary pattern of growth with the forces of fluid flow determines the form of the cardiovascular system.

With the establishment of circulation at the end of the first month, a period of rapid growth begins during which, within the second month, the heart and great vessels assume their definitive form. It is during this period of buckling and twisting of the growing heart tube and of shifting flow from primitive net

to definitive arterial and venous trunks that the cardiovascular system recapitulates eons of evolution; the result is an efficiently valved four-chambered heart and separate systemic and pulmonary circulations. It is during this period also that most anomalies arise. How they do so is a matter of conjecture based on interpretation of what is known of the normal.

Endless variations are possible and no two are identical. But to the clinician, only those compatible with extrauterine life are important. These are best classified by embryonic origin. Anomalies can usually be assumed to result from a single defect which may result in associated variations. They fall into six categories:

1. *Heterotaxia*. These are the anomalies resulting from abnormal rotation of the primitive heart tube. Concerned primarily with the heart itself, they necessarily are associated also with its vascular attachments.

2. *Arrested development*. Persistence into postnatal life of a normal developmental stage is a common type of anomaly primarily concerned with the internal structure of the heart.

3. *Persistence of normal fetal structures*. Closely related to the above group, but primarily concerned with the great vessels, are the anomalies resulting from persistence into postnatal life of structures which normally involute and disappear.

4. *Involution of structures which normally persist*. This is the reverse of the preceding category. When structures involute which normally remain functional, secondary or compensatory anomalies frequently are present. This type may involve the heart, the great vessels or both.

5. *Abnormal development*. Closely related to the foregoing group are anomalies which result from the development of a normal structure in an abnormal way.

6. *Combinations*. Although many combined anomalies consist of a primary defect with resulting secondary abnormalities, some appear to result from a growth disturbance affecting more than one area undergoing rapid development at the same fetal stage. Others are unexplained.

Cardiac Anomalies

The heart is derived from a single tube which carries blood from the sinus venosus to the aortic sac. Remaining fixed only at these connections with the embryonic body, the central portion becomes detached and lies free in the pleuropericardial coelom, where it buckles and twists as it grows in response to genetic and physical forces. Nearly all anomalies result from arrested development at some stage of this process; a few are due to abnormal development. The heart tube divides into segments: the atriums, the ventricles, and the bulbus cordis. Developmental defects in any of these segments often influence development in other segments. They will therefore be considered together (Fig. 34-1).

HETEROTAXIA

SITUS INVERSUS.—Normally, the primitive heart tube grows into a loop which rotates forward and to the left in association with rapid asymmetrical growth of the liver on the right. In situs inversus, all of the viscera develop in a mirror-image reversal of normal. The heart rotates forward but to the right, and the ventricle on the right forms the apex of the heart. Because the great vessels also develop in reverse of normal, the atrium on the right receives blood from the pulmonary veins, and the ventricle delivers it to a right aortic arch. Similarly, the chambers on the left receive blood from the cavas and deliver it to the pulmonary arteries. The result is a heart which, though abnormal, functions in a normal way.

ISOLATED DEXTROCARDIA.—In this anomaly, the primitive heart tube rotates abnormally to the right, but since the liver develops in normal position, venous drainage through the cavas enters the atrium on the right, and this blood is delivered to the corresponding ventricle which forms the cardiac apex and empties into the aorta. The aortic arch develops normally with a left-sided arch, or the right arch may persist, but in either case the ascending aorta lies anterior to the pulmonary artery and carries venous blood. Correspondingly, the pulmonary venous drainage is into the atrium on the left, and the ventricle on that side passes blood to the lungs.

Life after birth is possible only if an associated defect permits some arterial blood to enter the systemic circulation and some venous blood to enter the pulmonary. Complex associated anomalies are of frequent occurrence. The condition must be distinguished from transposition of the great vessels, which has a different developmental origin but presents a similar clinical picture.

SEPTAL DEFECTS

ATRIAL SEPTAL DEFECTS.—If neither of the two septums which normally fuse to form the atrial septum develops, the result is a *single atrium*. If septum primum fails to form, or if its ostium secundum becomes too large, the normal valvelike structure which closes the foramen ovale at birth is absent, leaving a *patent foramen ovale*. If the superior leaf of septum secundum fails to form, a *patent ostium secundum* will remain. If the inferior leaf is too small or absent and ostium primum in septum primum fails to close, a low, so-called *ostium primum defect* will result. A split aortic leaflet of the mitral valve with a left ventricle to right atrial shunt is frequently present.

Rarely, interatrial communication may result from excessive thinning and multiple perforation of septum primum in place of the normal ostium secundum. A *cribriform septum* results.

ATRIOVENTRICULAR CANAL DEFECTS.—Normally, a narrowing appears in the fifth week between the atrial and ventricular pouches. Through this, atrioventricular canal blood passes from both atriums to both ventricles. The jelly-like mesenchymal mesh that lies between myocardium and endocardium thins out in the atriums but becomes concentrated into two masses, the endocardial cushions at the level of the canal. These meet and fuse, dividing the canal into right (tricuspid) and left (mitral) orifices. Later, ostium primum of atrial septum primum closes by fusion of septum primum and septum secundum with the cushions, and contributions from the latter take part in closure of the interventricular foramen and give rise to the septal leaflet of the tricuspid valve and part of the aortic leaflet of the mitral.

When the endocardial cushions fail to fuse, ostium primum cannot close, an opening remains in the interventricular foramen, and tricuspid and mitral leaflets are incompletely formed. The result is a *persistent atrioventricular canal* that allows blood from both atriums to enter both ventricles.

Fusion of the cushions may occur, but their contribution to the valves or interventricular foramen may be defective. In this way, a *split mitral leaflet* or a *bicuspid tricuspid valve* may result, often associated with an ostium primum defect or a patent interventricular foramen. On the other hand, fusion may progress too far, resulting in *mitral or tricuspid stenosis or atresia*. When this occurs, the corresponding ventricle, deprived of its blood, remains rudimentary and life depends on persisting openings in one or both septa. *Lutembacher's syndrome* is an example of such an anomaly.

VENTRICULAR SEPTAL DEFECTS.—In the fifth week, as the ventricular pouches deepen, a muscular ridge forms between them which is added to from below upward to form the muscular interventricular septum. When this fails to form, a *single ventricle* results which pumps an undivided stream of blood into the bulbus cordis. As a result, the conus ridges may fail to form, resulting in persistent truncus arteriosus,

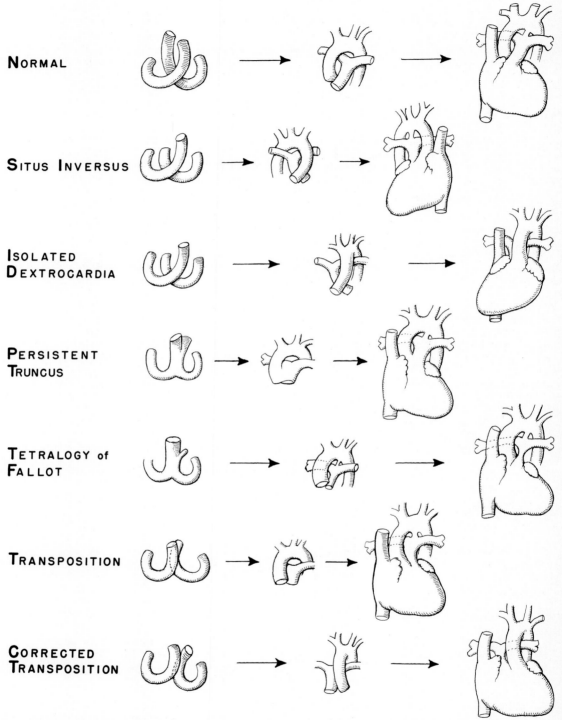

NORMAL

SITUS INVERSUS

ISOLATED DEXTROCARDIA

PERSISTENT TRUNCUS

TETRALOGY of FALLOT

TRANSPOSITION

CORRECTED TRANSPOSITION

Fig. 34-1.—Derivation of the commoner anomalies of rotation and truncus division based on directional streaming from the embryonic ventricular pouches into the bulbus cords. **Left,** inter-relationship of right and left ventricular streams. **Center,** resulting relation of main pulmonary artery to aorta. **Right,** resulting cardiac relationship to great vessels.

or they may form in a straight, rather than spiral, fashion, resulting in transposition of the great vessels (see below). In either case mixed blood enters both systemic and pulmonary circulations.

The muscular ventricular septum does not progress upward as far as the conus ridges but leaves an opening, the interventricular foramen, beneath it. This foramen is later closed by contributions from the endocardial cushions, the conus ridges and the muscular septum to form the membranous portion of the interventricular septum. Any or all of these contributions may fail. A *patent interventricular foramen* will result, the size and location of which will vary with the lacking contribution.

Defects of the muscular septum may also occur. In the third month, formation of ventricular trabeculae and papillary muscles normally takes place by coalescence of bundles of primitive mesenchyme between which are endothelial pouches in the myocardial wall. Abnormal coalescence of these pouches across the interventricular septum may give rise to openings in any part of the septum, or the septum may become a spongelike structure with many openings. Occasionally, this process may result in *false septums*, especially in the right ventricle, sometimes with no single well-defined ventricular cavity.

EBSTEIN'S MALFORMATION. — Here may be another anomaly of trabecula formation. If the coalescing endothelial pouches of the right ventricular wall open above the posterior and septal leaflets of the tricuspid, the attachment of these leaflets would come to lie low in the ventricle, with much of the ventricular wall forming a common chamber with the atrium. Only the outflow tract remains distal to the comparatively small tricuspid orifice, and much of the right atrial blood is diverted through an atrial defect into the left heart.

Bulbus Cordis Anomalies

The bulbus cordis is that part of the primitive heart tube between the ventricular pouches and the aortic sac from which the aortic arches originate. Above the level at which the semilunar valves will develop lies the truncus arteriosus, below it the conus, which is normally absorbed primarily into the right ventricle as the infundibulum. The same plastic mesenchymal mesh which forms the endocardial cushions is present under the endothelium of the bulbus. As the ventricular pouches eject streams of blood at slightly different instants at different angles into the bulbus, these streams spiral upward into the truncus, forming channels in the plastic mesenchyme with intervening ridges. The stream from the left ventricular pouch passes first backward, then to the right and forward into the third and fourth arches; that from the right passes forward and then to the left and back into the sixth arch. The ridges meet and fuse in this spiral, progressing downward to separate the aorta from the pulmonary artery. Ultimately, this process extends below the level of the semilunar valves into

the conus, taking part in the closure of the interventricular foramen, as the conus is absorbed into the right ventricular outflow tract (Fig. 34-1).

CONUS ANOMALIES. — If this process is incomplete, a defect will remain in the interventricular foramen, permitting much of the right ventricular stream to enter the aorta while the conus is incompletely absorbed, resulting in infundibular stenosis. The pulmonary artery, deprived of its normal flow, may remain small or may become atretic. There results a combined anomaly known as *tetralogy of Fallot*. Because the base of the large aorta often straddles or over-rides the muscular edge of the ventricular foramen, it may be that the anomaly is the result of faulty streaming from the ventricular pouches. Part of the blood from the right pouch may be caught in the stream from the left, resulting in unequal division of the whole bulbus and dextroposition of the aorta. When the aorta over-rides a high septal defect but the pulmonary artery is large, the malformation is called an *Eisenmenger complex*.

Conversely, if part of the left ventricular pouch stream is caught in the stream from the right, the bulbus will divide unequally in the opposite way, the aorta will remain small, there may be subaortic stenosis, and a large pulmonary artery will over-ride a high ventricular septal defect. When, in addition, there is transposition of the aortic origin, the anomaly is called a *Taussig-Bing malformation*.

The semilunar valves at the base of the aorta and pulmonary artery form during the development of the truncus and conus ridges. On either side, these leaflets may fuse into a conical diaphragm, resulting in *aortic* or *pulmonary valvular stenosis*. The interventricular foramen may close or may remain patent, giving rise to a clinical picture, in the case of pulmonary stenosis, similar to tetralogy. This resemblance is often enhanced by a secondary muscular hypertrophy of the right ventricular outflow tract (especially the crista supraventricularis) which resembles infundibular stenosis.

Conversely, closure may be incomplete at the semilunar valve level, resulting in *aortic* or *pulmonary insufficiency* associated with a patent interventricular foramen. In extreme cases, a single four-cusped valve remains. With this defect, there may also be failure of the truncus ridges to close above the valves. When this occurs higher, above normally formed semilunar valves, it is termed *aorticopulmonary window*.

TRUNCUS ANOMALIES. — Complete failure of the ventricular pouches to form separate spiraling streams will cause no formation of ridges in the truncus. A *persistent truncus arteriosus* carrying mixed blood to both aorta and pulmonary artery will result. On the other hand, the streams may form but the normal angulation which causes them to spiral may be absent. Parallel streams will enter the truncus, and its ridges will form in a straight, rather than spiral, fashion. Since the right ventricular pouch is anterior, its stream will enter the third and fourth arches, which form the aorta, while the posterior left pouch delivers its stream into the sixth arch and so, ultimately, to the pulmonary artery. Thus the ascending aorta will arise from the right ventricle and the pulmonary artery from the left, a *complete transposition of the great vessels*. As in isolated dextrocardia (see above), extrauterine life is possible only if an associated anomaly permits some arterial blood to enter the systemic circulation and some venous blood to enter the pulmonary.

If the ventricular streams enter the truncus in such a way that they spiral in a direction the reverse of normal (counterclockwise from below instead of clockwise), the right ventricular stream, entering the truncus from the right and progressing posteriorly, would enter the sixth arch, while the left ventricular stream would enter from the left and enter the fourth. The developing truncus ridges would then create an aorta entirely on the left and a pulmonary artery on the right. Although transposed in relation to each other, from a functional standpoint they are normal, giving rise to the term *corrected transposition*.

Vascular Anomalies

Although it might appear that abnormalities of the proximal aorta and pulmonary artery should be considered here, it has been shown (above) that these consist primarily of abnormal development of the primitive heart tube, and so from an embryologic standpoint they are best explained in relation to defects of the heart with which they are so frequently associated. Cardiac and truncus anomalies for the most part are due to arrested development, abnormal development or combinations. Vascular anomalies, on the other hand, are largely due to persistence of fetal structures which normally involute, to involution of structures which normally persist or both.

Arterial Anomalies

THE AORTA AND ITS BRANCHES. — Early in evolution, water-breathing vertebrates developed a respiratory system by pumping blood forward from the heart through a single ventral aorta or truncus arteriosus, around gill cleft openings in the pharynx to a pair of dorsal aortas, which joined caudally into a single dorsal aorta. Man, like all air-breathing vertebrates, in his embryologic development repeats this phylogeny. Though never used for breathing, gill clefts are developed by the embryo between which symmetrical branchial vascular arches pass from the ventral aortic sac to the paired dorsal aortas. The latter then fuse from the tail toward the head to form the dorsal aorta. Unlike fish, the human embryo's arches are never equally developed. Blood flow shifts progressively posteriorly from arch to arch by a series of developments and involutions that end with the head being supplied by remnants of the third arch,

the body by remnants of the fourth arch, and the lungs by outgrowths of the remnant of the sixth arch (Fig. 34-2).

By the fifth week, the first and second arches have involuted, the main flow of blood is shifting from the third to the fourth arches and the sixth arches have appeared, with precursors of the pulmonary artery growing toward the lung buds. The fifth arches appear later and involute promptly. At the end of the sixth week, the head, neck and chest are developing rapidly, drawing the third arches upward, while the fourth and sixth move downward into the chest. The portions of the dorsal aortas between the third and fourth arches involute, leaving the third arches as the innominate and common carotid arteries, while the right fourth arch between the origin of the subclavian and its junction with the dorsal aorta falls behind in growth and eventually disappears. The left fourth arch carries the main flow and will become the aortic arch, while the right, losing its attachment to the dorsal aorta, will become the proximal right subclavian.

Variations in this pattern are numerous. If the left, instead of the right fourth arch involutes below the subclavian origin, the result will be a *right aortic arch*, with the proximal fourth arch persisting as an almost horizontal vessel anterior to the trachea, giving rise to the left carotid and subclavian, as a so-called left innominate artery. This abnormality alone causes no symptoms. If the involution of the right fourth arch progresses to involve the aorta at its junction, or the left also fails to grow between this point and the ductus arteriosus, the result will be a narrowing or *coarctation of the aorta*. If both arches persist and grow equally, a *double aortic arch* will be present.

In the latter event, with downward growth of the heart and upward shift of the fourth arch junction, a *complete vascular ring* will be present encircling the trachea and esophagus. This may cause pressure symptoms on the trachea, esophagus or both. Vascular rings will also result from other anomalous development of the fourth arches. The left fourth arch may partially involute between the ductus and subclavian origins to produce a coarctation proximal to the ductus, or it may completely involute with persistence of the right arch, leaving a cordlike remnant between "left innominate" and descending aorta. If the ductus (see below) remains patent in the presence of a right-sided arch, an *incomplete vascular ring* may result. A similar result will follow involution of the left arch between the origins of carotid and subclavian, with persistence of the right. In this event, the ductus or ligamentum arteriosum will appear to join the left subclavian at or just above its aortic origin.

If the left arch involutes between its carotid and innominate origins, with persistence of the right, there will be no ring unless a cordlike remnant persists, whereas if it merely fails to keep pace with vascular development, and the right arch involutes nor-

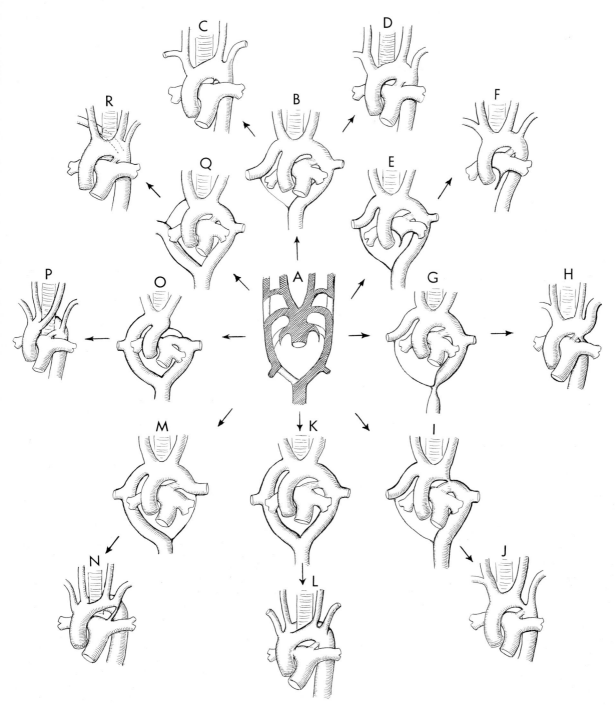

Fig. 34-2.—Origins of various anomalies of the aortic arch from anomalous involution of the embryonic branchial arch complex. **A,** diagram of third, fourth and sixth branchial arch pattern; normally persisting vessels are shaded. **B-C,** normal intermediate and final relationships. **B-D,** persistent patent ductus arteriosus. **E-F,** pulmonary atresia with compensatory patent ductus. **G-H,** coarctation of aorta, "adult type." **I-J,** coarctation of aorta, "infantile type." **K-L,** double aortic arch (complete vascular ring). **M-N,** right aortic arch with left innominate (no ring). **O-P,** right aortic arch without innominate (incomplete ring). **Q-R,** dysphagia lusoria (partial ring).

mally, a coarctation of different origin will result. The descending aorta of these fetuses is supplied by the ductus arteriosus. Because this malformation often results in death in infancy, it is termed *infantile coarctation.*

When the right fourth arch involves between its subclavian origin and its ventral junction with the third arch (which becomes the innominate), while its distal portion persists between the subclavian and its dorsal junction with the left arch to form the descending aorta, there will be no innominate artery, the right subclavian artery will appear to arise from the descending aorta and it will pass behind the esophagus to the apex of the right chest. Because, in these circumstances, the symptoms (if any) are those of esophageal compression only, the anomaly has been called *dysphagia lusoria.*

PULMONARY ARTERY.—As already described, the left sixth branchial arch soon develops branches which supply the lung buds. These branches become the right and left pulmonary arteries. The right sixth arch soon involutes along with the right fourth arch. On the left, the arch persists until birth as a functional vessel, the ductus arteriosus, which carries much of the right ventricular output into the descending aorta. Closure, which should occur soon after birth, may be incomplete or absent; a *patent ductus arteriosus* results. Altered pressure relations between pulmonary and systemic circulations following expansion of the lungs cause the direction of blood flow through the ductus to be reversed when it does not close after birth. Such flow has a deleterious effect in proportion to its volume, unless other defects are present such as isolated dextrocardia or transposition of the great vessels (see above), in which case it may be physiologically compensatory. Its presence may also form a part of an incomplete vascular ring anomaly (see above).

It is interesting to note that even when truncus division is so abnormal that *complete atresia of the pulmonary trunk* results, the branches of the pulmonary artery, since they arise from the sixth arch distal to the aortic sac and truncus, are usually patent and the lungs are perfused through the ductus arteriosus as long as it remains patent. *Localized stenosis of the pulmonary artery* above the valve, or of its branches, often at the point of pericardial reflection, may occur. For these lesions there is no evident developmental reason.

Anomalies of position of a main branch or major secondary branches of the pulmonary artery in relation to the trachea and bronchi presumably result from an abnormal relation of the developing lung bud to the vessel. Accompanying anomalies of the lung are frequent, the commonest being abnormal segmentation and congenital cystic disease. Pressure from an anomalous vessel may be associated with incomplete or absent tracheal or bronchial cartilage

rings with consequent respiratory obstruction. Another cause of obstruction is the rare *retrotracheal right pulmonary artery* apparently resulting from growth of the lung buds ventral rather than dorsal to the developing vessel.

Pulmonary arteriovenous fistula, like peripheral hemangiomas and fistulas, is related to faulty vascularization at the early vascular lake stage. Since it is a peripheral lesion, it does not properly come within this discussion; it is mentioned only because the accompanying murmur and cyanosis may cause confusion with central congenital lesions.

CORONARY VESSELS.—The developing epimyocardial mantle is supplied soon after regular myocardial contractions begin with a fine network of vessels running between the truncus, the cardiac chambers and the sinus venosus. At the time of truncus division, buds appear just above the semilunar valves and join this capillary net. As development proceeds, these are consolidated into the coronary arteries which arise from the anterior aspect of the truncus and so develop an aortic origin, the coronary veins which develop a drainage system into the left duct of Cuvier which becomes the coronary sinus, and the thebesian vessels which retain their primitive netlike arrangement with multiple openings into the cardiac chambers.

Anomalous coronary artery origin from the pulmonary trunk may accompany other anomalies of truncus division (see above) or may occur singly. Since coronary vessels anastomose freely, origin of one of them from the pulmonary artery will have a physiologic effect similar to that of a *coronary arteriovenous fistula,* which may occur as an accompanying lesion. Unlike all other arteriovenous fistulas, the flow and hence the murmur in these is maximal in diastole. The symptoms are those of myocardial ischemia.

ANOMALIES OF VENOUS RETURN

CAVAL ANOMALIES.—When circulation first begins in the fourth week, blood returns to the heart from vitelline, umbilical and common cardinal venous plexuses, all of which drain into the sinus venosus. As the heart tube grows and twists, the sinus venosus moves upward and to the right in relation to it. In the fifth week, the cardinal veins empty through the right and left ducts of Cuvier into the sinus, which is beginning to be absorbed into the right atrial sac. A venous plexus joins the ducts ventrally above the heart and from this develops the left innominate vein. By the fourteenth week, this vein carries most of the venous drainage from the left subclavian and jugular veins across the midline to enter the atrium as the superior vena cava. As a result, the left duct of Cuvier falls behind and usually disappears, except for its proximal portion which remains as the coronary sinus. At the same time, the left cardinal venous system, which becomes the lumbar and azygos, crosses dorsally into the right to empty into the superior vena cava as the main azygos vein.

If the left innominate develops poorly or not at all, the left duct of Cuvier persists as a *left superior vena cava*. This drains into the coronary sinus, which may be considerably larger than normal and may retain a common opening with the inferior vena cava into the right atrium. *Anomalies of azygos drainage* may accompany this condition, as well as those of pulmonary drainage (see below).

The upper portions of the umbilical veins decline and disappear early, while their branches which connect with the vitelline plexus within the liver become major vessels. Meanwhile the hepatic portion of the inferior vena cava is forming and the umbilical channel into it, the ductus venosus, which is joined by the portal system. With closure of the umbilical vein and ductus venosus at birth, the portal vein may also become obstructed, giving rise to *congenital obstruction of the portal vein*. The upper portion of the vitelline plexus remains as the hepatic veins.

ANOMALOUS PULMONARY VENOUS DRAINAGE.— In the fifth week, blood from the developing lung buds drains into the sinus venosus through a rich capillary plexus. Small venous channels thread in all directions through the loose mesenchyme. Some enter the atrium, some enter the ducts of Cuvier and some enter even lower into the inferior cava or vitelline (hepatic) veins. Normally, a definitive path develops as a single vessel which enters the left atrium to the left of septum primum. This vessel is then absorbed into the growing left atrium so that first its two primary branches and finally its four secondary branches enter the left atrium separately.

Many variations of anomalous drainage may occur as a result of abnormal channeling in the pulmonary venous plexus. *Total anomalous pulmonary drainage* will follow if the definitive channel enters to the right of the atrial septums. Survival will then depend on a persistent interatrial communication. It will also follow if the definitive channel enters the left duct of Cuvier instead of the atrium. In this case, *pulmonary drainage into the coronary sinus* may follow. If the sinus becomes separated from the left superior vena cava, there will be *total anomalous pulmonary drainage into a left superior vena cava*, which then drains upward into the left innominate vein, then downward through the right superior vena cava into the right atrium.

If no definitive single channel forms, *partial anomalous pulmonary drainage* may take many forms. Both right pulmonary veins may enter the right atrium, while both left pulmonary veins enter the left. The right superior pulmonary vein may enter the superior vena cava; the right inferior pulmonary vein may enter the inferior vena cava, or both may enter the hepatic vein. All of these anomalies have been encountered clinically, and many others are possible.

In all instances of anomalous pulmonary venous drainage, oxygenated blood enters the right heart. There is no cyanosis even when a septal defect is present, as is often the case. It is difficult clinically, therefore, to distinguish these anomalies from simple atrial defects.

The great variety and apparent complexity of anomalous development of the heart and great vessels often perplexes the clinician who attempts to make a diagnosis during life. Until operative correction became possible, accurate diagnosis was not vital. Now that many of these lesions can be corrected or alleviated by operation, it has become necessary for the cardiologist to recognize the many possibilities which exist in order to decide whether operative correction is feasible. Since absolute anatomic diagnostic accuracy will often be impossible in the living patient, it is even more essential for the surgeon to be familiar with the unexpected abnormalities that may confront him in the operating room. These he can handle successfully only if he understands their embryonic genesis.

BIBLIOGRAPHY

1. Abbott, M. E.: *Atlas of Congenital Heart Disease* (New York: American Heart Association, 1936).
2. Arey, L. B.: *Developmental Anatomy* (Philadelphia: W. B. Saunders Company, 1954), p. 346.
3. Barthel, H.: *Missbildungen des menschlichen Herzens: Entwicklungsgeschichte und Pathologie* (Stuttgart: Georg Thieme Verlag, 1960).
4. Bremer, J. L.: *Congenital Anomalies of the Viscera* (Cambridge, Mass.: Harvard University Press, 1957).
5. Brock, R.: *Anatomy of Congenital Pulmonary Stenosis* (New York: Hoeber Medical Division, Harper & Row, Publishers, Inc., 1957).
6. Congdon, E. D.: Transformation of the aortic arch system during development of the human embryo, Contrib. Embryol., Carnegie Inst. Washington, 14:47, 1922.
7. deVries, P. A.: The development of the ventricles and spiral outflow tract of the human heart, Contrib. Embryol., Carnegie Inst. Washington, 1961.
8. Edward, J. E., et al.: *An Atlas of Congenital Anomalies of the Heart and Great Vessels* (Springfield, Ill.: Charles C Thomas, Publisher, 1954).
9. Hamilton, W. J.; Boyd, J. D., and Mossman, H. W.: *Human Embryology* (Baltimore: Williams & Wilkins, 1952), p. 135.
10. Humphreys, G. H., and Grant, D.: *Anomalies of the Heart* (motion picture) (New York: E. R. Squibb Co., 1958).
11. Humphreys, G. H., and Grant, D.: *Normal Development of the Heart* (motion picture) (New York: E. R. Squibb Co., 1958).
12. Humphreys, G. H., and Grant, D.: *Anomalies of the Aortic Arch* (motion picture) (New York: E. R. Squibb Co., 1957).
13. Humphreys, G. H., and Grant, D.: *Aortic Arch, Normal Development* (motion picture) (New York: E. R. Squibb Co., 1956).
14. Kjellberg, S. R., et al.: *Diagnosis of Congenital Heart Disease* (2nd ed.; Chicago: Year Book Medical Publishers, Inc., 1959).
15. Lev, M.: *Autopsy Diagnosis of Congenitally Malformed Hearts* (Springfield, Ill.: Charles C Thomas, Publisher, 1953).

16. Lev, M., and Vass, A.: *Spitzer's Architecture of Normal and Malformed Hearts* (Springfield, Ill.: Charles C Thomas, Publisher, 1951).
17. Patten, B. M.; in Gould: *Pathology of the Heart* (2nd ed.; Springfield, Ill.: Charles C Thomas, Publisher, 1960), p. 24.
18. Streeter, G. L.: Developmental horizons in human embryos, Contrib. Embryol., Carnegie Inst. Washington, 119:211, 230, 1942.
19. Taussig, H. B.: *Congenital Malformations of the Heart* (New York: The Commonwealth Fund, 1947).

G. H. HUMPHREYS

Drawings by
ALFRED FEINBERG

35

New Diagnostic Methods in Congenital Heart Disease

THE KEY TO successful cardiovascular surgery is accurate preoperative diagnosis. The foundation of this is the clinical impression based on an adequate history and full physical examination, aided by x-ray and fluoroscopic study of the cardiac shadow and the electrocardiogram.

In recent years, the vectorcardiogram has been achieving prominence in this respect as it comes into wider use. But, while in some hands it appears to give a more accurate guide to hemodynamic assessment than the 12-lead scalar electrocardiogram, in general vectorcardiography has not produced any new information, nor yet provided any help which could not be derived from the conventional electrocardiogram.

When a clinical diagnosis has been made to the best of one's ability on the basis of available information, cardiac catheterization and angiocardiography may be indicated. It is certainly indicated in all cases where there is some doubt as to the diagnosis and in all cases where the hemodynamic assessment of the condition is important from the point of view of postoperative course and long-term prognosis. Thus in children with ventricular septal defect and transposition of the great vessels, the level of pulmonary vascular resistance has an important effect on morbidity and mortality and should be ascertained; when possible, serial studies to determine whether the pulmo-

nary vascular resistance is changing and the direction of that change are of great value. In other instances, where the possibility of associated defects exists, it is important that cardiac catheterization be carried out in as full a manner as possible so that all the pathology of the heart is known before operation. For instance, the knowledge of the presence of anomalous pulmonary veins in a child with an atrial septal defect would alter the surgical approach to the repair of this condition. In tetralogy of Fallot, of importance to the surgeon are the size of the pulmonary artery branches and the capacity of the left atrium and left ventricle.

In our laboratory we have been performing angiocardiography in an increasing proportion of patients having diagnostic cardiac catheterization, so that now 85% of all studies have angiocardiography as an integral part of the examination. We feel that the radiation hazard from properly pulsed and collimated machines with image intensification is small compared to the benefit derived.

Indicator dilution studies in the investigation of congenital heart disease are used in varying amounts in different centers. Although we do use indocyanine green dye and ascorbate dilution curves as well as hydrogen ion curves in the assessment of a few cases, we have not found these methods to be necessarily important parts of our investigation of all cases. The oxygen tension polargraphic catheter has been unsatisfactory in the investigation of congenital heart disease because the response time is much too slow.

The manufacture of a fiberoptic catheter has introduced a new instrument in diagnosis. This is a cardiac catheter, the lumen of which contains approximately 300 linear glass fibers. Light is transmitted down one third of them and is reflected from the blood at the distal end, passing up the remaining two thirds of the fibers. The reflected light beam is then split and passed through photocell assemblies at wavelengths of 660 and 805 mμ and the ratio of the output of these two photocells can be read off directly, as oxygen saturation. This instrument is accurate, and its response is extremely rapid, demonstrating fluctuations in oxygen saturation in each cardiac cycle. Thus a rapid pull-back of such a catheter from the pulmonary artery to the superior vena cava can demonstrate the level at which intracardiac left-to-right shunting is taking place. When such an assembly is provided in a catheter with a lumen for recording pressures simultaneously, or a catheter tip transducer, it will be possible to make a diagnosis extremely expeditiously. However, this is not now available in pediatric sizes.

The same assembly can also be used in recording intracardiac dye curves and, because of its extremely rapid response time, ventricular wash-out curves. Until the extra pressure-sensing facility is provided, the conventional pediatric diagnostic methods of sampling of blood through a cuvette oximeter with subsequent reinfusion and the use of external strain gauges will remain.

An investigative innovation has been introduced by Carr and Wells.[1] A great problem in the investigation of cases of transposition of the great vessels is maneuvering a catheter tip into the pulmonary artery, especially when there is a closed ventricular septum. This can be done by the percutaneous technique first described by Radner[3] and reviewed by Rahimtoola *et al.*[4] Carr and Wells's method depends on the passing of a small polyethylene catheter through a regular catheter with the tip in the left atrium; the small catheter tip is carried by the flow of blood through the left ventricle and out into the pulmonary artery. In cases in which other methods have failed, a pulmonary artery pressure recording can be obtained by this technique. However, the question of pulmonary vascular resistance is not solved by the maneuver because the sample of pulmonary artery blood obtained for Fick-type calculations is almost as invalid as a left ventricular sample, since the admixture of bronchial blood flow is not detected by either method.

The most dramatic step forward in recent years has been the introduction of the balloon septostomy procedure by Rashkind and Miller.[5] In complete transposition of the great vessels in infancy, the basic problem in therapy is to secure an adequate admixture between the two essentially separate circulations. Rashkind suggested that a catheter with a balloon at the tip be advanced into the left atrium through the foramen ovale or small atrial septal defect. He demonstrated that an atrial septal defect could be created by pulling the inflated balloon from the left atrium into the right atrium with a sharp tug. This resulted in a tearing of the septum with equalization of the pressure in both the left and the right atrium and increased mixing between the two circulations.

Although this procedure is not without risk, in our hands this technique has proved successful, with improvement in systemic oxygen saturation ranging from 10 to 30%. The procedure is of definite value in this condition where, in the first few days of life, operative mortality is high. If the improvement of systemic oxygen saturation is but temporary, the procedure can be repeated; however, it is our impression that if this procedure can tide the child over the first few months of life, better long-term results would be obtained by subsequent surgical septectomy, such as the Blalock-Hanlon procedure.

The balloon septostomy technique is also of value in some children with total anomalous pulmonary venous drainage and possibly tricuspid atresia and pulmonary atresia where the opening between the two atriums is inadequate.

Other techniques which give further information about the hemodynamic status before operation include the administration of drugs and the use of exercise in children while they are undergoing cardiac catheterization. Gradients in the left ventricular outflow tract may be increased with exercise and isoproterenol, as may also gradients in the right ventricular outflow tract in tetralogy of Fallot and isolated ventricular septal defect. The administration of oxygen and pulmonary vasodilators to children with pulmonary hypertension has, in our hands, proved a not very satisfactory prognostic tool, as the proportion of children whose pulmonary vascular resistance will change under this short-term stimulus appears to be small.

In the future of hemodynamic assessment and cardiovascular diagnosis lies the computer, possibly in an on-line role. At present, however, accurate diagnosis and correct hemodynamic assessment are based on the measurement of pressure and flows, the calculation of resistances and adequate angiocardiography.

Although relatively safe, cardiac catheterization must be performed meticulously and with careful aseptic technique. When major vessels, such as the femoral artery or vein, are entered directly, one should repair the point of entry with fine silk to ensure adequate hemostasis and patency.

Young children and particularly infants are blessed with relatively extensive collateral communications in both arterial and venous circulations so that a limb will usually survive obstruction or ligation of a major artery or vein. However, the long-term effects of such incidents have not been thoroughly studied, and it is likely that, at least in some cases, alterations in growth or function will occur subsequently if the obstruction is not relieved.

Femoral venous obstruction is probably the most common vascular incident seen following cardiac catheterization. It is more frequent in young infants whose long saphenous vein is small and in whom the femoral vein must be used. Mild to moderate swelling and cyanosis of the leg result, but this will subside in a few hours if the limb is elevated. In older children, if there are signs of severe venous obstruction, one should attempt to repair the vein.

Obstruction of the femoral or brachial artery results in a cold, pale limb and may follow either needle puncture or open arteriotomy. Arterial spasm is occasionally the cause, but this should respond to conservative measures such as allowing the limb to be exposed and slightly dependent while the child's trunk is kept warm. The careful use of epidural anesthesia, nerve block or Priscoline may be of value. If, after 2–3 hours, there is still no pulsation in the vessel below the site of obstruction, one should consider operation. In the operating room, adequate exposure of the affected area of the vessel is necessary. The artery should be opened between arterial clamps and all thrombus removed, using Fogarty catheters if neces-sary, until unimpeded proximal and distal flow is obtained. Inspection of the lumen may reveal an intimal tear, and the artery should be repaired to provide an adequate lumen. Significant arterial spasm can be relieved by forcibly dilating the artery by means of either a Fogarty catheter or injection of saline into segments of the artery that are isolated by clamps.[2] Once the wall of the artery is overstretched, the spasm will usually not return.

REFERENCES

1. Carr, I., and Wells, B.: Coaxial flow-guided catheterization of the pulmonary artery in transposition of the great vessels, Lancet 2:318, 1966.
2. Mustard, W. T., and Bull, C.: A reliable method for relief of traumatic vascular spasm, Ann. Surg. 155:339, 1962.
3. Radner, S.: Extended suprasternal puncture technique, Acta med. scandinav. 151:223, 1955.
4. Rahimtoola S. H.; Ongley, P. A., and Swan, H. J. C.: Percutaneous suprasternal puncture (Radner technique) of the pulmonary artery in transposition of the great vessels, Circulation 33:242, 1966.
5. Rashkind, W. J., and Miller, W. W.: Creation of an atrial septal defect without thoracotomy: A palliative approach to complete transposition of the great vessels, J.A.M.A. 196:991, 1966.

B. S. L. KIDD
G. A. TRUSLER

36

Arterial Anomalies

Patent Ductus Arteriosus

HISTORY.—Patent ductus arteriosus was known to Galen in the 2nd Century A.D. Leonardo Botallo described it in the 17th Century. In 1900, Gibson[10] described a classic machinery murmur, and Munro[22] in 1907 suggested not only operative closure but the surgical approach for it. Strieder and his coworkers[11] in 1938 attempted closure of an infected patent ductus but lost the patient in the postoperative period. In 1938, Gross[12] successfully closed a patent ductus for the first time. Touroff and Vesell[29] soon demonstrated the feasibility of ligation of an infected patent ductus, with cure of the subacute endarteritis. Patent ductus arteriosus, once considered rare, difficult to diagnose, impossible to operate on and of little consequence to the patient in any case, is now readily diagnosed, recognized as a serious threat to life and successfully treated with an extremely small mortality.

ANATOMY

The ductus arteriosus, the distal portion of the sixth left aortic arch, is a thick-walled arterial channel connecting the left pulmonary artery to the aorta immediately distal to the origin of the left subclavian artery. This channel by-passes the lungs during the fetal period and closes spontaneously shortly after birth. It is probably completely closed by the end of the first week.[3] The mechanism of closure is still debated, but it is probable that with onset of respiration, a drop in pulmonary vascular resistance causes a pronounced constriction of the diameter of the ductus.[7] Completion of the closure is probably due to the peculiar nature of the thick-walled fetal ductus. The internal elastic lamina fragments and the smooth muscle project into the lumen.[17] Fibrosis then converts the ductus into the ligamentum arteriosum. In the aortic wall of adults, little evidence remains of the original connection with the ductus.

Persistent patency of the ductus may cause little change in pulmonary histology. In the presence of pulmonary hypertension, however, significant changes may occur (see Chap. 43). The left atrium and ventricle become enlarged over the course of years. When the left-to-right shunt is reversed, the right atrium and right ventricle become enlarged.

INCIDENCE AND ETIOLOGY

Keith *et al.*[19] reported an incidence of 1 to 3,850 in the general population, accounting for 12% of the cases of congenital heart disease. Ekstrom[8] noted a preponderance of females (69%); this sex distribution has been confirmed by others.

Patent ductus arteriosus usually is an isolated defect but occasionally is associated with other cardiac anomalies. Rubella in the first trimester of pregnancy seems to have some influence on ductus closure. In 100 cases of patent ductus, a history of maternal rubella in the first trimester was obtained in 8.[19] Genetic factors may be significant; families with multiple cases of patent ductus have been reported.[18] Respiratory difficulty at birth, particularly in prematures, has been suspected of being a cause of incomplete closure.[25]

HEMODYNAMICS. — High pulmonary vascular resistance is responsible for direction of blood from the pulmonary artery through the ductus and into the aorta in fetal life. After birth, the direction of flow depends on the fall of this resistance. Rowe and James[25] noted that pulmonary artery pressure may remain elevated for 2 weeks after birth. In this situation, one would not expect an immediate reversal of the right-to-left shunt. Certainly from 1 month of age onward, if the ductus is patent, the shunt is from left to right in most cases. If the pulmonary artery pressure is 50-75% of that in the aorta, the shunt may be balanced.[33] In the rare cases in which pulmonary hypertension develops, the shunt is from right to left, either intermittently or constantly (see Chap. 43).

SYMPTOMS AND PHYSICAL SIGNS

The uncomplicated patent ductus in childhood produces no symptoms. Although there is no serious limitation of activity, it is striking how frequently one is told that the child was considered normal before operation but after operation has boundless energy. In infancy, however, serious symptoms develop in at least 10% of patients with patent ductus arteriosus. Failure to thrive and frequent respiratory infections are common complaints. Dyspnea and cardiac failure develop in 15% of the group diagnosed under 1 year of age.

In the infant, the characteristic continuous murmur over the pulmonic area is variable and the thrill is nearly always absent. Even if the murmur is purely systolic, in an acyanotic infant whose heart is enlarging, the diagnosis of patent ductus should always be suspected. In the newborn infant, if the decline of high pulmonary vascular resistance is slow, the volume of shunt from aorta to pulmonary artery may not be great, thus accounting for the absence of a continuous murmur.

In childhood, a precordial systolic thrill in the pulmonic area is present in 75% of patients with patent ductus. Pulsation in the suprasternal notch may be present and may be accompanied by a palpable thrill. The most striking sign is the continuous machinery murmur, first described by Gibson.[10] The murmur is rough and thrilling and increases in intensity at the beginning of the second sound. The development of severe pulmonary hypertension may cause this murmur to disappear. A wide pulse pressure at rest is usually found. In the presence of a complete reversal of flow in a patent ductus, the pathognomonic evidence is afforded by cyanosis in the lower extremities, in the absence of cyanosis in the upper extremities.

ELECTROGARDIOGRAPHY, RADIOGRAPHY AND CARDIAC CATHETERIZATION

In 20% of cases, the electrocardiographic tracing is normal, and in 60% left ventricular hypertrophy is present. Left atrial hypertrophy and incomplete bundle-branch block are occasionally noted. Combined hypertrophy is not uncommon. Radiologically, there is always an increase of lung vascularity (Fig. 36-1), and fluoroscopy shows left atrial enlargement with a good deal of activity of the heart. In infancy, the heart may be greatly enlarged in patients in failure, but the cardiac silhouette is not distinctive. The cardiothoracic ratio exceeds 0.55 in 20% of cases. In doubtful instances, retrograde aortography, either by needle through the brachial artery (Fig. 36-2) or by catheter introduced through the femoral artery and advanced to the arch of the aorta, demonstrates immediate filling of the pulmonary artery and may even outline the ductus. The retrograde catheter may actually pass through the ductus into the pulmonary artery.

A rise of oxygen saturation in the pulmonary artery above that in the right ventricle is significant. Direct passage of the catheter through the pulmonary artery into the ductus is, of course, conclusive. The flow

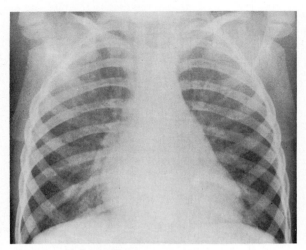

Fig. 36-1.—Patent ductus arteriosus. In this 3-year-old child, the cardiac silhouette is little changed, although the pulmonary artery may be prominent. Most significant is the diffuse increase of pulmonary vascular markings, characteristic of lesions with a left-to-right shunt.

from left to right may be as great as 40% of the left ventricular output.[18] The pressure in the pulmonary artery is usually not raised until the pulmonary vascular changes result in pulmonary hypertension.

CLINICAL COURSE

Untreated patent ductus arteriosus may lead to complications and to premature death in later life. The average life expectancy of 24 years commonly given is probably not accurate, due to its basis solely on selective postmortem material. In children, 90% of deaths from cardiac failure due to patent ductus arteriosus occur under the age of 2. Subacute bacterial endarteritis is a late complication, but may occur in childhood. Since the vegetations tend to proliferate at the pulmonary artery end of the ductus, bacterial emboli into the lung beds may result in a diagnosis of pneumonic infection. The presence of the continuous murmur and positive blood cultures will give the true diagnosis. Treatment with penicillin followed by operative closure will result in a cure.[29]

Aneurysm of the ductus arteriosus may occur. It usually is mycotic in origin in association with a subacute bacterial infection.

DIFFERENTIAL DIAGNOSIS

The continuous murmur in the pulmonic area in an acyanotic, asymptomatic patient is almost pathognomonic of patent ductus arteriosus. Certain other conditions producing a continuous murmur may have to be considered among the diagnostic possibilities.

VENOUS HUM.—A venous hum, at times strident and continuous, may be heard over the base of the heart. Characteristically, it is abolished by compression of the jugular veins, by execution of the Valsalva maneuver or by lateral flexion of the head, and is increased by extension of the head. It may be decreased or abolished by assumption of the recumbent position and exaggerated by assumption of the erect position. It does not reflect any symptom-producing abnormality and the electrocardiogram is normal.

PULMONARY ARTERIOVENOUS FISTULAS.—Pulmonary arteriovenous fistulas may produce a continuous murmur over the site of the fistula in the lung. Severe degrees of cyanosis, polycythemia and clubbing may be seen. Plain films may show opacities in the lungs. Angiocardiography will delineate the lesion precisely. Cardiac catheterization shows no step-up in O_2 saturations from the right ventricle to the pulmonary artery.

AORTICOPULMONARY WINDOW.—Aorticopulmonary window is the lesion most frequently confused with patent ductus arteriosus. It is relatively uncommon. At the Hospital for Sick Children, Toronto, during a period in which 400 patients were treated for patent ductus arteriosus, only 4 were seen with aorticopulmonary window. It may be difficult or impossible to distinguish the two on clinical grounds alone, and aorticopulmonary window is often diagnosed at thoracotomy undertaken for division of a patent ductus. Catheterization of the window directly and visualization by aortography are the certain methods of diagnosis.

OTHER LESIONS.—*Ventricular septal defect and aortic insufficiency* may be difficult to separate from the ventricular septal defect with a patent ductus arteriosus. A rise of oxygen saturation in the pulmonary artery and the use of intracardiac phonocardiography are helpful in arriving at a diagnosis. *Rup-*

Fig. 36-2.—Patent ductus arteriosus. Retrograde aortography (Hypaque-M 75%) through the brachial artery in an infant in whom diagnosis could not be made with certainty on clinical grounds. Filling of the pulmonary arteries from the aorta establishes the patency of the ductus.

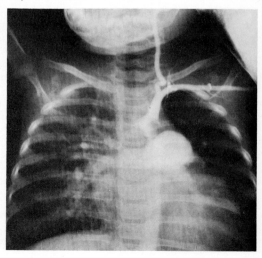

tured sinus of Valsalva usually presents the sudden episode, and here again, the shunt from left to right might be at the right atrial level. *Coronary arteriovenous fistula* produces a left-to-right shunt at the intracardiac level, and retrograde aortography is useful in the differential diagnosis.

ASSOCIATED CONGENITAL CARDIOVASCULAR LESIONS

In pulmonic stenosis, tetralogy of Fallot, pulmonary atresia, tricuspid atresia and single ventricle, the presence of an associated patent ductus is fortunate, and the shunt thus created may be responsible for keeping the child alive. In other associated defects such as coarctation of the aorta and ventricular septal defect, a patent ductus is actually harmful. In infancy particularly, surgical closure of the ductus alone may be life-saving (Fig. 36-3). The records of the Hospital for Sick Children show 12 instances of ventricular septal defect with patent ductus arteriosus in which closure of the patent ductus alone was life-saving. If pulmonary hypertension persists after ligation of the ductus, banding of the pulmonary artery may be necessary.

THE ATYPICAL DUCTUS

In recent years, the patent ductus associated with pulmonary hypertension has become recognized as a clinical entity.[6],[31] Pulmonary hypertension may be due to increased flow, to secondary lesions which are the result of increased flow and, finally, to irreversible alterations in pulmonary vessels.[9] A pressure of 80 mm Hg or over is considered the level of pulmonary hypertension necessary to warrant the label atypical ductus.

In the infant, electrocardiography will show either right or combined ventricular hypertrophy. Cardiac catheterization may reveal high pulmonary artery pressure, and intracardiac phonocardiography may reveal a continuous murmur.[15] These infants are frequently suspected of having a large ventricular septal defect because of the clinical resemblance to the more common lesion of ventricular septal defect and pulmonary hypertension; indeed, at catheterization, occasionally in infants and more commonly in older children, pulmonary incompetence may result in a false rise of oxygen saturation in the right ventricle and thereby contribute to misdiagnosis. In the older child, cyanosis on exertion may be present with a

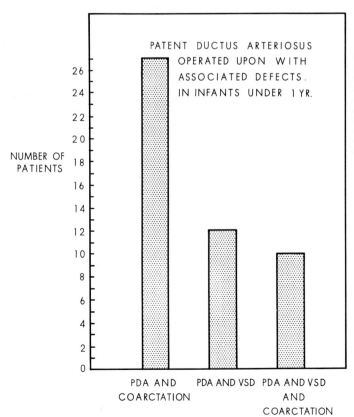

Fig. 36-3.—Patent ductus. Operative experience with patent ductus (PDA) and associated defects at the Toronto Hospital for Sick Children. In cyanotic heart disease, the ductus may be life-saving, but if unrecognized during an open heart operation may cause fatal blood loss. At times, in the presence of a ventricular septal defect (VSD) in a desperately ill infant, ligation of the ductus may assure survival until a transventricular procedure can be tolerated. With coarctation, both lesions are corrected simultaneously.

drop of arterial oxygen saturation demonstrated by oximetry. The murmur may no longer be continuous and the heart may be enlarged. Occlusion of the ductus by a balloon tip catheter[1] while the electrocardiogram and pulmonary artery pressure are being monitored may aid in the decision concerning operation by demonstrating whether the circulation can be maintained with the flow through the ductus interrupted.

TREATMENT

The incidence of patent ductus in children born of pregnancies complicated by rubella in the first trimester is probably not sufficiently high to warrant therapeutic abortion. Protection of exposed mothers with gamma globulin is probably wise. The nonoperative treatment of patent ductus is limited to the temporary treatment of such complications as cardiac failure and superimposed subacute bacterial infection. In the infant, there is some difference of opinion concerning the role of operative and nonoperative treatment of the patent ductus. There is increasing evidence and agreement, however, that surgical intervention in the first year of life is not only advisable but may be required to save life.

In the infant whose heart is enlarging and in whom the ductus has been proved to be the sole cause of cardiac enlargement, or the major contributing cause, the ductus should be interrupted after appropriate

Fig. 36-4.—Patent ductus arteriosus. Results of operation at the Toronto Hospital for Sick Children. Infants under 6 months of age were in cardiac failure. Operation at 6–12 months was undertaken because of borderline failure and repeated upper respiratory infections. At 12–24 months, operation was elective; the ductus was usually large (5–7 mm).

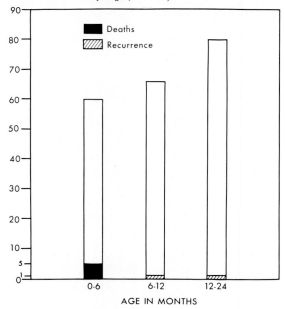

preparation. The optimal age for treatment is under discussion[30] and there is no unanimity of opinion. Experience at the Hospital for Sick Children, Toronto, with 54 infants in heart failure, operated on for otherwise uncomplicated patent ductus arteriosus, has convinced me that the infant withstands the surgical procedure as well as the older child and that there is no justifiable reason for withholding operation.

The optimal age for operation should probably be reduced from the usually stated "preschool" age to the age at which the diagnosis is made.

The ductus closes spontaneously early in infancy or not at all. For the sake of argument, the position might be taken that operation in the asymptomatic infant with patent ductus arteriosus should be deferred until the age of 1, at which time, if the diagnosis is confirmed, operation should be undertaken. The operation is simple, quickly performed and carries a quite low morbidity. Further, early operation eliminates the danger of subsequent development of pulmonary hypertension or subacute bacterial infection.

In the standard operation for ductus operations in childhood, either the anterior or the posterolateral approach may be used. The posterolateral approach provides the best exposure and the greatest freedom of maneuver in the event of operative difficulties. The question of ligation of the ductus versus division has been investigated throughout the world. There are now large series showing the mortality from division versus ligation and the relative recurrence rate. In 1952, Gross[14] reported 525 cases of division with a mortality of 2% and in those with minor symptoms less than 0.5%. Scott,[27] in the same year, reported 273 cases of suture ligation with 7 deaths (2.5%) and 1 recanalization. Waterman *et al.*,[30] in a collected series, found 1,123 cases of ligation with 23 deaths, a mortality of 2%, and 1,659 cases of division of the ductus, with a mortality of 2.1% (34 deaths). Unfortunately, the recurrence rate was not recorded. In our series of 900 cases, the only deaths were in cases of atypical ductus and 1 of a mycotic aneurysm (Fig. 36-4). One proved recurrence and 4 suspect recanalizations are included in this series.

SURGICAL TECHNIQUES.—We have usually preferred the suture ligation technique, introduced by Blalock (Fig. 36-5). Through a posterolateral approach the mediastinal pleura is divided between the phrenic and the vagus nerve. The vagus nerve is retracted either forward or back, to expose the recurrent nerve as it passes behind the ductus. The aorta should be freed sufficiently so that it may be cross-clamped if necessary, to avoid catastrophe in the event of injury to the ductus. Sharp dissection is safer than blunt dissection. Dissection begins close to the aorta and passes toward the pulmonary artery above, below and behind the ductus, dividing the tough connective tissue at a little distance from the ductus and peeling the pericardium back to the pulmonary artery. Blalock used pursestring sutures at either end of the ductus and one or two transfixion sutures in its midportion; the addition

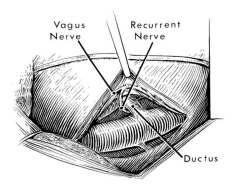

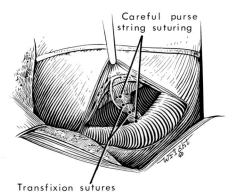

Fig. 36-5.—Patent ductus arteriosus; suture ligation. This technique, advocated by Blalock, is ideal for infants. In older children, many surgeons use this technique routinely, but most

agree that the short wide ductus should be divided. We have abandoned the addition of an umbilical tape in this procedure.

of an umbilical type, as originally described, is unnecessary.

In the child aged 1-3, the operation is simple and effective, with almost no mortality, quite low morbidity and a recurrence rate of less than 1%.

When the ductus is very wide or very short, division and suture is preferable. Potts clamps[24] are applied at the two ends of the ductus (Fig. 36-6), which is divided, and the ends oversewn. In some circumstances, after the ductus has been dissected out and the aorta isolated, it is safest to apply the Potts-Smith clamp around the aorta, occluding the ductus at its origin from the aorta, before the pulmonary end is clamped and the ductus divided. In special instances, hypothermia or hypotensive anesthesia, even with brief periods of inflow occlusion, may be indicated.[28] If pulmonary hypertension is present or suspected, pulmonary artery pressure readings should be taken

while the ductus is temporarily occluded. Maintenance of pulmonary artery pressure, or an elevation of the pressure on occlusion of the ductus, is indicative of inability to withstand interruption of the ductus. In such instances, if the ductus is divided, death from cardiac failure may occur in the immediate postoperative period or later. If, however, a fall of pressure in the pulmonary artery occurs on temporary occlusion of the ductus, one may safely complete the procedure.

POSTOPERATIVE CARE

An intercostal catheter is connected to an underwater seal and removed in 24 hours. Oxygen is not required. Small infants, following intratracheal anesthesia, require a cold, moist atmosphere. Children may be up and about as rapidly as they are able and are usually out of the hospital within a week. The infant in failure usually requires continuation of digitalization after operation. The digitalizing dose is 0.03 mg of Digoxin per pound in three divided doses, with a maintenance dose of 0.06 mg.

COMPLICATIONS

Significant hemothorax is uncommon, having occurred in only 2% of our cases. Injury to the recurrent laryngeal nerve occurs occasionally. Six of our 400 children were found to have a paralyzed left vocal cord after operation, and in 1 of these the paralysis was apparently permanent.

We have had 2 instances of mycotic aneurysm that developed in the ductus 1 month following suture ligation. *Staphylococcus aureus* septicemia apparently developed, resulting in reopening of the ductus. In our first case, the aneurysm ruptured before reoperation was undertaken. Recognizing the serious nature of the lesion, we operated successfully in the second case. The right chest was entered and cardiopulmonary by-pass commenced with cooling to 15 C. The

Fig. 36-6.—Patent ductus arteriosus; division of the ductus. This is ideal for the experienced surgeon. Two Potts clamps, one on the aortic and one on the pulmonary side, in addition to those shown, add to the safety of the procedure. A Potts-Smith clamp encircling the aorta provides an additional safety factor, particularly in the atypical ductus.

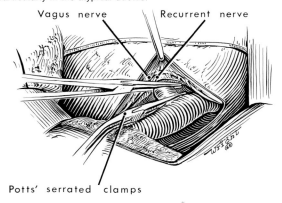

pump was then shut off, the sternum crossed and the aneurysmal sac opened and a communication with the aorta sutured. After 17 minutes of cessation of circulation, the pump oxygenator was restarted and rewarming was begun. The child made a rapid convalescence and 4 years later was perfectly normal. In a child with a preoperative diagnosis of spontaneous aneurysm of the ductus, the same technique was employed with complete success.

PROGNOSIS

After successful closure of the ductus, whether by division or by suture ligation, in the absence of any other cardiac defects, restitution to a physiologically normal state is complete. The incidence of late complications — infection, reopening of the ductus, aneurysm, and so forth — is minute.

REFERENCES

1. Actis-Dato, A., and Tarquini, A.: Evaluation of operability in patients with pulmonary hypertension by catheterization and occlusion of patent ductus arteriosus, Circulation 29:6, 1959.
2. Ash, R., and Rischer, D.: Manifestations and results of treatment of patent ductus arteriosus in infancy and childhood: An analysis of 138 cases, Pediatrics 16:695, 1955.
3. Barclay, A. E., et al.: Radiographic demonstration of circulation through the heart in adult and in fetus and identification of ductus arteriosus, Am. J. Roentgenol. 47:678, 1942.
4. Blalock, A.: Operative closure of the patent ductus arteriosus, Surg., Gynec. & Obst. 82:113, 1946.
5. Burchell, H. B.: Variations in the clinical and pathologic picture of patent ductus arteriosus, M. Clin. North America 32:911, 1948.
6. Dammann, J. F., Jr., and Sell, C. G. R.: Patent ductus arteriosus in the absence of a continuous murmur, Circulation 6:110, 1952.
7. Dawes, G. S., et al.: Changes in the lungs of the newborn lamb, J. Physiol. 121:141, 1953.
8. Ekstrom, G.: The surgical treatment of patent ductus arteriosus: A clinical study of 290 cases, Acta chir. scandinav., Supp. 169, 1952.
9. Gerbode, F., et al.: Atypical patent ductus, Arch. Surg. 72:850, 1956.
10. Gibson, G. A.: Persistence of the arterial duct and its diagnosis, Edinburgh M. J. 8:1, 1900.
11. Graybill, A.; Strieder, J. W., and Boyer, N. H.: An attempt to obliterate the patent ductus arteriosus in a patient with subacute bacterial endocarditis, Am. Heart J. 15:621, 1938.
12. Gross, R. E., and Hubbard, J. P.: Ligation of the patent ductus arteriosus, J.A.M.A. 118:729, 1939.
13. Gross, R. E., and Longino, L. A.: Patent ductus arteriosus: Observations from 412 surgically treated cases, Circulation 3:125, 1951.
14. Gross, R. E.: The patent ductus arteriosus: Observations on diagnosis and therapy in 525 surgically treated cases, Am. J. Med. 12:472, 1952.
15. Gyllensward, A.: Atypical patent ductus arteriosus in infancy, Acta paediat., vol. 48, 1959.
16. Hess et al., quoted in Donzelot, E., and D'Aalaines, F.: *Traité des Cardiopathies Congenitales* (Paris: Masson & Cie, 1954).
17. Jager, B. V., and Wollenman, O. J., Jr.: An anatomic study of the closure of the ductus arteriosus, Am. J. Path. 18:595, 1942.
18. Joyce, J. C., and O'Toole, S. P.: Congenital heart disease: Report on an unusually high incidence in one family, Brit. M. J. 1:1241, 1954.
19. Keith, J. D.; Rowe, R. D., and Vlad, P.: *Heart Disease in Infancy and Childhood* (New York: Macmillan Company, 1958).
20. Keys, A., and Shapiro, M. J.: Patency of the ductus arteriosus in adults, Am. Heart J. 25:158, 1943.
21. Mitchell, S. C.: The ductus arteriosus in the neonatal period, J. Pediat. 51:12, 195.
22. Munro, J. C.: Surgery of the vascular system, Ann. Surg. 46:335, 1907.
23. Mustard, W. T.: Suture ligation of the patent ductus arteriosus in infancy, Canad. M. A. J. 64:243, 1951.
24. Potts, W. J., et al.: Diagnosis and surgical treatment of patent ductus arteriosus, Arch. Surg. 58:612, 1949.
25. Rowe, R. D., and James, L. S.: The pattern of response of pulmonary and systemic arterial pressures in newborn and older infants to short periods of hypoxia (Proc. Soc. Pediat. Res., 1956), Am. J. Dis. Child. 93:13, 1957.
26. Scott, H. W., Jr.: Closure of the patent ductus by suture ligation technique, Surg., Gynec. & Obst. 90:91, 1950.
27. Scott, H. W., Jr.: Surgical treatment of patent ductus arteriosus in childhood, S. Clin. North America 32:1299, 1952.
28. Sirak, H. D., and Humphreys, G. H.: The atypical ductus: Physiologic and technical considerations in its surgical therapy, Surgery 41:112, 1957.
29. Touroff, A. S. W., and Vesell, H.: Subacute *Streptococcus viridans* endarteritis complicating patent ductus arteriosus, J.A.M.A. 115:1270, 1940.
30. Waterman, D. A.; Sampson, P. C., and Bailey, C. P.: Surgery of patent ductus arteriosus, Dis. Chest 29:102, 1956.
31. Welch, K. J., and Kinney, T. D.: The effect of patent ductus arteriosus and of interauricular and interventricular septal defects on the development of pulmonary vascular lesions, Am. J. Path. 24:729, 1948.
32. Young, W. P., et al.: Surgical treatment of atypical patent ductus arteriosus, J. Thoracic Surg. 36:382, 1958.
33. Ziegler, R. F.: The importance of patent ductus arteriosus in infants, Am. Heart J. 43:553, 1952.

W. T. MUSTARD

Drawings by

A. M. WRIGHT

Coarctation of the Aorta

HISTORY. — In 1903, Bonnet[4] described the pathology of coarctation of the aorta and introduced the terms "infantile" and "adult." In the former, the ductus enters below the coarctation and in the latter, above. Abbott[1] carefully documented 200 cases in 1928, and Blalock and Park[3] in 1944 devised an experimental approach to relieve coarctation by turning down the subclavian artery into the aorta distal to the experimental ligation. Before they performed this in man, Crafoord and Nylin[9] and Gross,[11] independently, successfully resected the coarcted segments and anastomosed the aorta with silk sutures. In 1953, Mustard operated successfully on a 12-day-old infant with preductal coarctation and a hypoplastic aorta.[19]

INCIDENCE

The Toronto cardiac registry records coarctation of the aorta in one of every 12,000 children between birth and 15 years of age. Keith[16] found the lesion in 4% of congenital cardiac anomalies and Abbott[2] stated that coarctation is found once in every 1,500-2,000 individuals at postmortem examination. There appears to be no real familial incidence such as has been recorded for patent ductus arteriosus, but we have operated on a coarctation in a boy whose brother was being operated on in an adult hospital at the same time for the same condition. It appears to be more common in males than in females.

PATHOLOGIC ANATOMY

ADULT POSTDUCTAL TYPE.—The site of aortic stenosis in these patients is below the origin of the subclavian artery from the aortic arch and below, or opposite, the ductus or ligamentum arteriosum. It may be directly opposite the origin of the subclavian, in which case there may be no aortic segment between this vessel and the site of coarctation—a matter of some concern to the surgeon. Many patients, however, have a good segment of aorta, 1 or 2 cm below the origin of the subclavian, superior to the coarctation, which renders the anastomosis less difficult. In many patients with coarctation in the usual position, the ductus is closed after the first year of life. The figure of 12% patency of the ductus arteriosus in a large series[7] seems to be a little high. The aorta below the coarctation is invariably dilated. It may be very large in the older child, but in the infant with this type of coarctation the segments may be nearly equal in size. The intercostal vessels arising from the distal aorta are enlarged and thin-walled, gradually increasing in size from infancy to later childhood (Fig. 36-7). The coarctation itself usually presents some form of a diaphragm, the opening of which is somewhat eccentric and more medial than lateral. The diaphragm may be complete or may have an opening 1–2 mm in size. Invariably in this type of lesion the external constriction of the aorta does not reveal the true extent of the narrowing because of the presence of a diaphragm within the lumen. This external constriction of the aorta appears more obvious on the lateral than on the medial wall, and this appearance, which is best seen in vivo, supports the theory that ductal tissue extending into the wall of the aorta causes constriction as this tissue contracts following birth. The left ventricle is enlarged, and bicuspid aortic valves may be present.

PREDUCTAL OR INFANTILE COARCTATION.—In these patients, the actual coarctation is similar to that seen in the adult type, although at operation in our cases the diaphragm is not seen as complete as that in the adult type and there is usually, although not invariably, a hypoplastic segment above the site of the coarctation with considerable variation in diameter and length. This hypoplasia may vary from a slightly smaller aorta than that seen in the adult type of coarctation to a very narrow segment which may extend proximally on the aortic arch to the innominate vessel on the right side. The ductus enters the distal segment and is usually large and widely patent. In the first month of life, the ductus is usually larger than the aorta itself (Fig. 36-7). At operation for preductal coarctation, the ductus was widely patent in all cases, which probably accounts for the cardiac

Fig. 36-7.—Coarctation of the aorta. **Right,** preductal coarctation, with the ductus large and patent. This is almost always fatal in infancy, due, we believe, to associated defects (ventricular septal defect in 33% and transposition of the great vessels in 15% of our series). End-to-end anastomosis is quickly accomplished in the infant because of elasticity of the vessels; sutures in the anterior two thirds should be interrupted to allow for growth. **Left,** postductal coarctation. This may not be discovered until preschool examination. The pathology is almost invariably a pin-point opening in the diaphragm. Surgery should be undertaken between 4 and 6 years.

Preductal

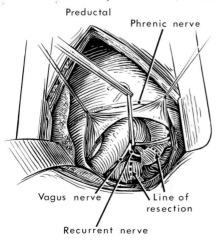

Phrenic nerve

Vagus nerve

Line of resection

Recurrent nerve

Postductal

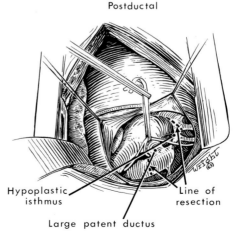

Hypoplastic isthmus

Line of resection

Large patent ductus

failure which brought them to surgery. In these patients, pulmonary hypertension and right ventricular hypertrophy are present invariably, as demonstrated by the electrocardiogram. In a postmortem series of 40 patients, associated defects were common; a ventricular septal defect was found in one third of them. Collateral circulation in the preductal coarctation is notably less at the time of operation than in the postductal type in the first year of life. In fetal life, the flow from the pulmonary artery to the descending aorta is unobstructed and collaterals do not develop. In contrast, in the postductal type, blood passing through the ductus meets the obstruction of the coarctation and collateral circulation develops.

NATURAL HISTORY

Although occasional individuals with coarctation of adult type survive to the fifties or sixties, most of them succumb to cerebral vascular accidents or left heart failure. Gross[13] divided patients with coarctation of the aorta into four groups. One-fourth live a long life with little or no incapacitation, another fourth die of rupture of the aorta, and another fourth from bacterial endarteritis, and the remainder die of cardiac failure or intracranial hemorrhage. If one adds to this group of cases the preductal type, with at least 80% mortality in the first month of life, one can only conclude that coarctation of the aorta is a serious congenital cardiac anomaly.

HEMODYNAMICS

In the adult or postductal type, the ductus arteriosus closes in a large percentage of cases within the first few months of life and places the strain on the left side of the heart. In these cases, the shunt is invariably from left to right if the ductus remains open. In the preductal or infantile type, however, where the ductus is widely patent, one has a different physiologic situation in which the left heart not only is working against an obstruction but also has an overload from the ductus flow to the lungs. Furthermore, owing to the increased flow to the lungs through the widely patent ductus arteriosus, pulmonary hypertension is produced which increases the load on the right side of the heart so that in infants surviving any length of time with preductal coarctation, a biventricular strain is produced. At retrograde aortography through the brachial artery, the pulmonary arteries are seen to fill from the descending aorta, indicating that the shunt, until gross pulmonary hypertension supervenes, is from left to right in preductal coarctation.

DIAGNOSIS

It is necessary to group individuals with coarctation of the aorta not only into preductal and postductal types but also into age groups. Coarctation of the aorta in the first year of life presents clinical features different from those seen in childhood and adolescence.

Preductal Coarctation

CHILDREN UNDER ONE YEAR. — In these infants, dyspnea and cardiac failure are frequently the presenting signs. The classic murmur of a patent ductus may be obscured by accompanying defects. Most will have some enlargement of the heart and liver. As a rule, femoral pulsations are absent, and when gross failure is not present, the pressure is higher in the arm than in the leg. Cyanosis may be present due to associated defects. A plain radiograph is useful to show an enlarged heart with hilar markings indicating congestion. A barium swallow may reveal an indentation in the esophagus due to relative poststenotic dilatation of the aorta compared with the hypoplastic preductal segment, and a retrograde aortogram outlines the hypoplastic segment and the presence of a patent ductus. The electrocardiogram reveals both right and left ventricular hypertrophy, probably due to the associated large patent ductus arteriosus.

Postductal Coarctation of the Aorta

CHILDREN UNDER ONE YEAR. — These infants occasionally are seen because of failure to thrive, but more often are brought in because of cardiac failure. None of the associated defects seen in preductal coarctation of the aorta is present as a rule, and the infant in failure has an enlarged heart and no fem-

Fig. 36-8. — Coarctation of the aorta associated with patent ductus arteriosus. Retrograde injection of 75% Hypaque-M into the brachial artery reveals filling of pulmonary arteries, and collateral circulation of the postductal type of coarctation. At operation for intractable cardiac failure at age 3 months, suture ligation of the patent ductus alone was performed. Ten years later the child was asymptomatic, suggesting that the patent ductus, not the coarctation, was responsible for the cardiac failure.

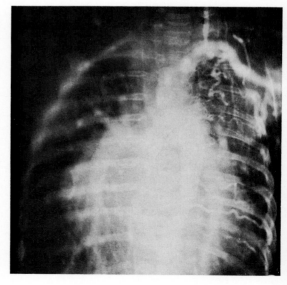

oral pulsations. The electrocardiogram will show left ventricular hypertrophy; in case of doubt, retrograde aortography will confirm the diagnosis (Fig. 36-8).

Coarctation in Children over One Year of Age

These children usually are relatively asymptomatic, and the diagnosis is made on the basis of a soft systolic murmur heard down the left sternal border and transmitted through to the back. Further examination reveals absence of femoral pulses or a disparity in the pressures between the arm and the leg. The blood pressure in the arm invariably is over 120 mm Hg, and the blood pressure in the leg seldom exceeds 100 mm Hg. Our patients have all seemed healthy, although an occasional child has had headaches and eye symptoms, and 1 child of 10 had already had a cerebral vascular accident resulting in hemiplegia. The plain radiograph usually reveals a heart of normal size; in children over 4 years, rib notching may be present, but not before the age of 9 as a rule. Collateral pulsations over the scapulas are felt in the older children. In a good plain radiograph, a poststenotic dilatation may be seen (Fig. 36-9) that can be confirmed by barium swallow. Retrograde aortograms may not be required for diagnosis.

INDICATIONS FOR OPERATION

As experience increases in diagnosis and in medical and surgical management, the optimal time for operation becomes more clearly defined. The infant group must be divided into pre- and postductal types to evaluate the timing for operative intervention.

Fig. 36-9.—Coarctation of the aorta in a 9-year-old boy. Notching of the lower borders of the ribs occurs early and may aid in diagnosis. Although difficult to reproduce in photographs, poststenotic dilatation of the aorta may be recognized in most chest radiographs.

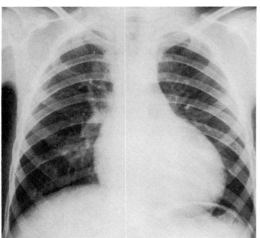

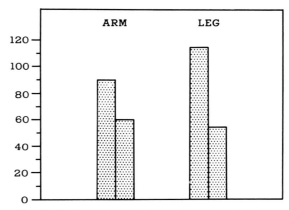

Fig. 36-10.—Coarctation of the aorta, preductal type: cuff blood pressure readings at the time of resection at age 3 months, and at age 8 years.

Preductal Coarctation

CHILDREN UNDER ONE YEAR.—In a postmortem study of 40 cases of coarctation of the aorta in children under 1 year of age, 90% were found to be preductal.[10] This observation alone demands that attention be focused on the group in the first year of life. The infant in failure in the first month of life almost certainly has a preductal coarctation and associated cardiac defects. These infants with proper medical management had a mortality of 87% in our series.[10] This led us to believe that an infant in the first months of life with a diagnosis of coarctation of the aorta should be operated on, a view supported by our experience (Fig. 36-10) and that of others.[6,17,23] In the dying infant with associated defects, simple ligation of the ductus may prove life-saving, and resection of the coarctation can be undertaken at a later date. The large widely patent ductus in these cases, particularly in the presence of a ventricular septal defect, is a contributing factor in death.

Postductal Coarctation

CHILDREN UNDER ONE YEAR.—The infant with postductal coarctation does not appear in failure as early as the infant with the preductal type, despite the fact that almost all of our patients have had a patent ductus arteriosus. Associated defects are not as common, and many of these infants may be relieved of failure and kept in reasonable health on a medical regimen. If the infant does not respond to digitalization and other supportive measures, operation becomes urgent. Repeated bouts of failure despite the use of digitalis are an indication for operation and should lead one to suspect the presence of an associated defect. Endocardial fibroelastosis may be associated with coarctation, possibly as a result of the increased load on the left ventricle.

CHILDREN OVER ONE YEAR.—The exceptional child

with preductal coarctation with or without associated defects may survive infancy and even early childhood without cardiac failure. These patients fall into that rare group in which, with the development of pulmonary hypertension, the flow through the ductus is reversed and the toes become cyanotic. This situation is extremely rare, and we encountered it only once at operation. With the postductal type of coarctation, the children may remain asymptomatic and the coarctation be discovered on routine examination due to the presence of a soft systolic murmur and the difference in pressures between the arm and the leg, or due to absence of femoral pulsations. In 90% of the cases, the ductus has spontaneously closed and the collateral circulation has developed to such an extent that the child is normally active. The time for elective surgery in this group of children has generally been defined as between 8 and 12 years.[13] The rationale behind this elective age is the fear that growth will not occur normally at the anastomotic site.

Coarctation Associated with Aortic Stenosis

Often a bicuspid aortic valve is associated with a coarctation and may cause enough valvular stenosis to warrant division. In 2 of our children, the valvular stenosis was corrected at open operation some years after the coarcted area in the aorta had been resected. Apparently resection of the coarctation did not precipitate cardiac failure, and performance of this procedure first has the added advantage of dealing with a ductus if present, and rendering perfusion through the femoral artery possible at the time of correction of the aortic stenosis.

Coarctation Associated with Ventricular Septal Defect

If a preductal coarctation has been corrected early in life, one third of these patients should be suspected of having a ventricular septal defect. A small defect may close spontaneously or not require operation. When the defect is large, we recommend operation before the age of 6. The occasional postductal or adult type of coarctation in early life with a ventricular septal defect will benefit from resection early and closure of a ductus if patent.

Interruption of the Aortic Arch

A rather rare condition is interruption of the aortic arch below the subclavian artery. The aorta continues as the subclavian and a large ductus enters the descending aorta with no continuity with the arch above. We have operated on such an infant successfully. The syndrome usually is associated with a ventricular septal defect, as in our case.

Growth at the Anastomotic Site

Many experimental studies have been done on growth at the site of an aortic anastomosis in pigs and in puppies. In pigs, which demonstrate 800% increase in growth in 6 months, Johnson *et al.*[15] pointed out that interrupted sutures resulted in slight or no constriction. Brooks[5] and Hurwitt and Rosenblatt[14] showed excellent growth in puppies with interrupted sutures, and Potts and Ricker[20] showed that a continuous suture line will straighten with growth and that growth at the anastomotic site will be limited to the length of the suture. Clatworthy *et al.*[8] demonstrated that in dogs with less than 75% occlusion of the aorta, no collateral changes developed to indicate coarctation of the aorta. A clinical study[18] demonstrated some constriction at the anastomotic site in infants who were operated on in the first 2 years of life and followed from 2 to 4 years. Operating on puppies is difficult and the use of pigs, with their amazing growth, does not parallel the situation in human beings. We were somewhat confused by the conflicting experimental evidence, so did a series of experiments of our own. In order to rule out extrinsic factors, the abdominal aorta below the renal arteries was selected as the site for transection and anastomosis. Puppies under 5 weeks of age have aortas 2–4 mm in diameter and we felt were technically unsuitable for anastomosis, although as Clatworthy[8] demonstrated, a good deal of aortic growth occurs in the first 3 months in puppies. We selected puppies 6–8 weeks of age, in which the abdominal aorta is smaller than that seen in the newborn infant; these puppies were used in a series of experiments to try different suture methods. Twenty-three of these animals survived to adult life

Fig. 36-11. — Coarctation of the aorta: suture technique. To allow for normal growth at the site of anastomosis, suture technique must be meticulous. The continuous mattress suture posteriorly for one third of the circumference should have each suture in close proximity to the next to provide enough suture material to straighten with growth. The anterior two-thirds should be interrupted to allow growth between sutures. Despite the method, a poorly performed anastomosis may not grow adequately.

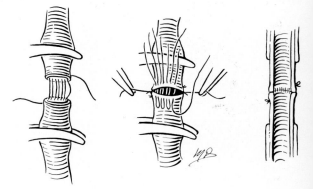

(evident from closure of the epiphyseal plates) and were killed after aortograms had been performed and blood pressures recorded. Normal growth at the anastomotic site was obtained if a continuous mattress silk suture was used in the posterior row and an interrupted mattress suture in the anterior row (Figs. 36-11 and 36-12). Correlating the growth of the puppies with that of children (Fig. 36-13), we found that the aortic growth from the puppy aged 6 weeks to the adult dog paralleled very closely the aortic growth in a 4-year-old child to the age of 16.

With this background of experimental data, we feel that the optimal age for elective operation of the child surviving infancy should be reduced from the 10–14 usually given to 3–5 years (Fig. 36-14). Support for this decision has been illustrated in patients waiting for the so-called optimal age of 10 and over. One child died of mycotic aneurysm as a result of subacute bacterial endarteritis in the poststenotic dilated aorta, and another had hemiplegia. We now believe that surgery for coarctation of the aorta, as an elective procedure, should be performed between 3 and 5 years.

OPERATIVE TECHNIQUE

In the postductal common type of coarctation of the aorta, the technique was well established by Gross.[12] The posterolateral approach is used, with or without resection of the fourth rib. The upper segment is mobilized, and then the distal segment is

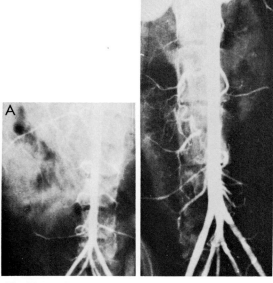

Fig. 36-12.—Coarctation of the aorta: experimental studies. **A,** aortogram of a 5-week-old puppy after transection and resuture of the abdominal aorta below the level of the renal arteries (suture technique as in Fig. 36-10). **B,** aortogram at 12½ months, demonstrating growth at the suture line to have been normal. The epiphyses have closed, and the dog is fully grown.

Fig. 36-13.—Coarctation of the aorta: comparison of growth of aortic diameter in children and puppies in relation to maturation. **Solid line,** after Moss et al.;[18] **broken line,** from the experimental laboratory at the Hospital for Sick Children, Toronto. It is interesting that the 4-year-old child and 2-month-old puppy parallel each other in growth. The aortic diameter of the mature dog equals that of the newborn child.

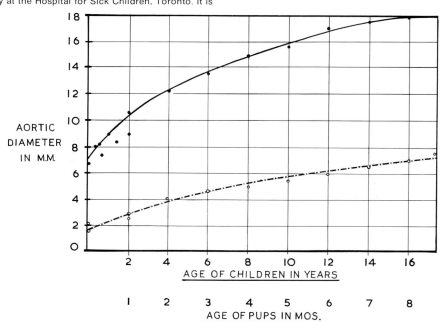

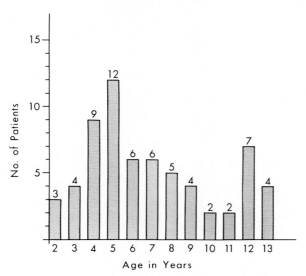

Fig. 36-14.—Coarctation of the aorta: time for elective operation in 64 cases during 3 years at the Hospital for Sick Children, Toronto. The children over 10 years were operated on when first referred.

mobilized to secure enough length for a suitable anastomosis; double ligation of the intercostal vessels is a wise precaution on the distal side because of the danger of displacing a suture during the operative manipulation. Two tragic experiences of complete paraplegia which we felt were due to interruption of the anterior spinal artery and the similar experience of others have led us to spare intercostals whenever possible.

Various methods of excising the coarcted segment are available and various clamps can be used. It has been our practice to suture-ligate the ductus whether it is patent or not and leave the coarcted segment in place, dividing the aorta and bringing the ends together in front of the coarcted segments. Numerous clamps are available. Potts[21] devised an ingenious instrument for use with his serrated toothed clamps to hold the ends stable for suture. The posterior row is completed with a continuous mattress suture of 5-0 silk carried a distance of about one third of the posterior row, and interrupted mattress sutures are placed in the remainder. In the infant, it is wise to place the posterior row of mattress sutures very close together to give a fair length of suture material to allow for growth in this continuous area. In the preductal type of coarctation, the mobilization must be greater to secure a good level for an anastomosis, and we have sacrificed the subclavian and left carotid frequently to secure satisfactory anastomosis, and without resultant hemiplegia (Fig. 36-15). The proximal segment of the aorta should be cut on the bias to give a good length in the suture line. The mobility of the aorta in these infants 1 month of age is often surprising, and despite the fact that there appear to be no collat-

eral vessels, the infant tolerates clamping of the aorta to a remarkable degree. We have used hypothermia as a routine in these cases in order to protect the spinal cord. In the infant, anastomosis must be meticulous and the sutures placed very close to the cut edge of the aorta. The proximal clamp should be removed slowly to avoid the production of sudden hypotension. Following one disastrous experience with wedge resection of a postductal coarctation, we concluded that the aorta should be mobilized completely and divided because of the tension produced at the suture line if one attempts a wedge resection. On two occasions we were forced to use a graft (in the childhood group). Obviously a graft should be avoided because of lack of growth and the unknown ultimate fate of a lifetime use. These facts lend support to early resection because of the mobility and elasticity of the young aorta.

POSTOPERATIVE CARE

Hemostasis must be meticulous and the parietal pleura closed tightly to avoid bleeding into the chest from the chest wall. If a rib has been resected, a tight closure of the intercostal muscles can be effected. In the absence of complications, the postoperative care of these patients is similar to that following other cardiovascular procedures. Blood loss via the chest drainage is usually greater than that following a simple thoracotomy, and for this reason the tube generally is removed on the second or third postoperative day. If drainage appears excessive or the chest x-ray reveals a large collection of blood in the pleural cavity, the chest should be reopened. Although it is rare to find active hemorrhage, the evacuation of clotted blood is very worth while. Antibiotics are adminis-

Fig. 36-15.—Coarctation of the aorta, preductal (infantile) type: technique for anastomosis. The elasticity of the infant's aorta allows end-to-end anastomosis with wide resection. On one occasion, the proximal incision necessitated division of the left common carotid artery, with no neurologic complications.

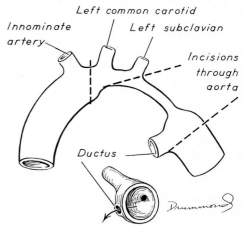

tered prophylactically to reduce the risk of infection. The patients are kept in bed for 10 days, then allowed to go home 2 weeks after operation. Accurate records of blood pressures in both upper and lower extremities are kept.

POSTOPERATIVE COMPLICATIONS

Although the postoperative course most often is benign, many serious complications peculiar to this lesion may develop, ending in disaster if unanticipated. Acute arteritis involving vessels of medium and small size below the anastomosis, first reported by Sealy et al.[22] in 1957, may lead to thrombosis or aneurysm formation with subsequent infarction. Abdominal symptoms must be carefully observed. Abdominal distention may be treated with intravenous fluids and tube decompression. If infarction of the bowel is suspected, one must be prepared to resect seriously involved segments. Coincident with a picture of mesenteric arteritis may be the presence of paradoxical hypertension. This may appear as an early or late development and requires careful attention, as extremely high blood pressures may occur. Should this happen an antihypertensive drug such as Serpasil can be used to prevent the added complications of a cerebral vascular accident or heart failure. With a return to normotensive levels, abdominal symptoms which may have been coexistent commonly subside. Rupture of the anastomosis can occur as an early or late catastrophe and usually indicates excessive tension along the suture line or the presence of infection. If a graft has been used, which is rare in childhood, infection at the anastomosis presents almost unsurmountable difficulties. Severe back pain in the immediate postoperative period suggests dissecting aneurysm from an anastomotic leak and calls for immediate reoperation.

RESULTS OF OPERATION

Figures from the literature give mortality rates including adults; Gross[13] gave 4-5%; in the infant under 1 year of age, the over-all mortality, as collected by Mortenson et al[17] was in the neighborhood of 36%. In the infant group, which includes preductal types, associated defects increase the mortality figures. Statistics from the Hospital for Sick Children are 50% for preductal coarctions and 10% for postductal coarctations in children under 1 year. We have had 2 deaths in some 300 in the childhood group. A marked decrease of the hypertension in the upper extremities immediately following operation does not always occur, which is rather difficult to explain. Over the course of months or a year or so, the pressure falls and remains lower than that in the legs. The heart will decrease in size, and, as far as we can tell, these patients should have a normal life expectancy if they have no associated defect.

REFERENCES

1. Abbott, M. E.: Coarctation of the aorta of the adult type: A statistical study and historical retrospect of 200 recorded cases, with autopsy, of stenosis or obliteration of the descending arch in subjects above the age of two years, Am. Heart J. 3:392, 1928.
2. Abbott, M. E.: Cited by Clagett, O. T., in *Congenital Heart Disease, Nelson's Loose-Leaf Medicine* (New York: Thomas Nelson & Sons, 1951), 4:307.
3. Blalock, A., and Park, E. A.: The surgical treatment of experimental coarctation (atresia) of the aorta, Ann. Surg. 119:445, 1944.
4. Bonnet, L. M.: Cited by Edwards, J. E., and Abbott, M. E.: Sur la lesion dite stenose congenitale de l'aorte dans la region de l'isthme, Rev. méd. 23:108, 1903.
5. Brooks, J. W.: Aortic resection and anostomosis in pups studied after reaching adulthood, Ann. Surg. 132:1035, 1950.
6. Burford, T. H., et al.: Coarctation of the aorta in infants: A clinical and experimental study, J. Thoracic & Cardiovas. Surg. 39:47, 1960.
7. Clagett, O. T., et al.: Anatomic variations and pathologic changes in coarctation of the aorta: A study of 124 cases, Surg., Gynec. & Obst. 98:103, 1954.
8. Clatworthy, W. H., et al.: Thoracic aorta coarctations, Surgery 28:245, 1950.
9. Crafoord, C., and Nylin, G.: Congenital coarctation of the aorta and its surgical treatment, J. Thoracic Surg. 14:347, 1945.
10. Glass, I. H., et al.: Coarctation of the aorta in infants, Pediatrics, 26:109, 1960.
11. Gross, R. E.: Surgical correction for coarctation of the aorta, Surgery 18:673, 1945.
12. Gross, R. E.: Coarctation of the aorta: Surgical treatment of 100 cases, Circulation 1:41, 1950.
13. Gross, R. E.: Coarctation of the aorta, Circulation 7:757, 1953.
14. Hurwitt, E. S., and Rosenblatt, M. A.: Observations on the growth of aortic anastomoses in puppies, Arch. Surg. 70:491, 1955.
15. Johnson, J., et al.: The growth of vascular anastomoses with continuous and interrupted anterior silk suture, Surgery 29:721, 1951.
16. Keith, J. D., et al.: *Heart Disease in Infancy and Childhood* (New York: Macmillan Company, 1958), p. 166.
17. Mortensen, J. D., et al.: Management of coarctation of the aorta in infancy, J. Thoracic Surg. 37:502, 1959.
18. Moss, A. J., et al.: The growth of normal aorta and of the anastomotic site in infants following surgical resection of coarctation of the aorta, Circulation 19:338, 1959.
19. Mustard, W. T., et al.: Coarctation of the aorta with special reference to the first year of life, Ann. Surg. 141:429, 1955.
20. Potts, W. J., and Ricker, W. L.: Study of growth of aortic-pulmonary anastomoses, Surg., Gynec. & Obst. 94:358, 1952.
21. Potts, W. J.: Technique of resection of coarctation of the aorta with aid of new instruments, Ann. Surg. 131:466, 1950.
22. Sealy, W. C., et al.: Paradoxical hypertension following resection of coarctation of the aorta, Surgery 42:148, 1957.
23. Smeloff, E. A., et al.: Coarctation of the aorta in infants and children, Ann. Surg. 146:450, 1957.

W. T. MUSTARD

Drawings by
MARGUERITE DRUMMOND

Vascular Rings Compressing the Esophagus and Trachea

HISTORY.—In 1737, Hommel[8] published the first description of a double aortic arch, and in 1789, Bayford[2] gave an accurate history and autopsy findings in a case of dysphagia lusoria due to an aberrant right subclavian artery. Symptomatic double aortic arch was described by von Siebold[10] in 1836. The surgical significance was noted by Abbott[1] in 1932. Gross[6] in 1945 performed the first successful division of a double aortic arch with relief of symptoms.

Abbott[1] described 5 cases of double aortic arch in 1,000 cases of congenital heart disease. In our records of 3,000 autopsies, there were 22 cases of aberrant right subclavian artery, 3 of double aortic arch and 2 of right aortic arch with ductus arteriosus. In over 600 subclavian pulmonary anastomoses for tetralogy of Fallot, Blalock recorded one instance of double aortic arch and 26 of aberrant left subclavian artery.

VASCULAR ANOMALIES

A description of the embryology of these defects will be found in Chapter 34.

ANOMALOUS SUBCLAVIAN ARTERY.—An aberrant right subclavian artery may arise from the left descending aorta, pass behind the esophagus and trachea to follow its normal course on the right side. The vessel produces an indentation in the esophagus which may be seen on esophagoscopy as a pulsatile

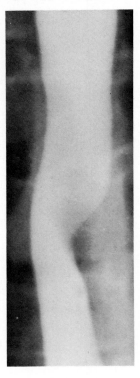

Fig. 36-16.—Aberrant right subclavian artery compressing trachea and esophagus. Roentgenogram after barium swallow. The artery passes obliquely upward and to the left. This is pathognomonic.

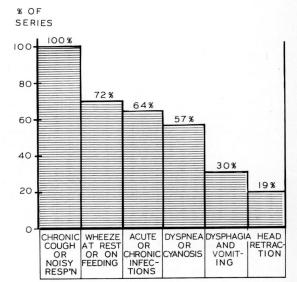

Fig. 36-17.—Vascular rings compressing trachea and esophagus. Clinical findings in 37 cases.

obstruction. The barium swallow demonstrates an indentation passing obliquely up and to the right in the anterior posterior view (Fig. 36-16).

DOUBLE AORTIC ARCH.—A complete vascular ring is formed around the esophagus and trachea in the presence of a double aortic arch. There may be considerable variation in the size of each arch, a fact that is of concern to the surgeon at operation. The anterior arch may be constricted at its junction with the posterior arch. Since this occurs beyond the origin of the left subclavian artery, the decision at operation is simple. At operation or postmortem examination, the constriction of the trachea and esophagus is easily seen, but histologic changes do not occur.

RIGHT AORTIC ARCH.—A complete vascular ring may be formed by a right aortic arch and a persistent ductus arteriosus or ligamentum arteriosum which passes behind the esophagus to reach the aorta on the right side. If the structure is short, a situation will arise similar to that of the double aortic arch and compression of trachea and esophagus will be present.

INNOMINATE ARTERY.—If the innominate artery rises more to the midline than usual, anterior compression of the trachea may occur. This is a common cause of tracheal compression;[5] in 2 years, we have suspended this vessel to the sternum in 30 cases.

Unusual Forms of Vascular Rings

LEFT COMMON CAROTID.—The left common carotid may arise abnormally close to the midline and produce tracheal compression as it passes to the left.

PULMONARY ARTERY.—A left pulmonary artery may arise from the main pulmonary artery, more to the

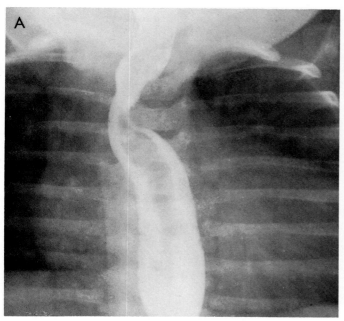

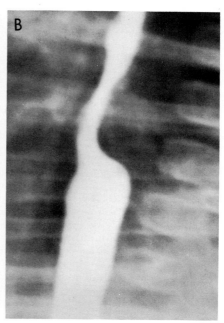

Fig. 36-18.—Double aortic arch compressing trachea and esophagus. **A,** preoperative anteroposterior roentgenogram after barium swallow, demonstrating marked indentation of the esophagus at the level of the 4th vertebra. **B,** lateral view, showing the rounded indentation more clearly. In this infant of 2 months, the small anterior arch was divided where it joined the posterior arch beyond the origin of the subclavian artery. Recovery was slow but uneventful.

right than usual and to reach the left lung pass behind the trachea, between it and the esophagus. We have encountered 1 such case and obtained relief and cure by dividing the ligamentum arteriosum passing from the left pulmonary artery to reach the descending aorta on the left. Others have divided the left pulmonary artery and reconstructed it in front of the trachea.

CLINICAL FEATURES

The mere presence of one of these vascular anomalies is not significant unless compression of the trachea or esophagus or both is produced. The clinical features in 37 patients seen at the Hospital for Sick Children, Toronto, are tabulated in Figure 36-17. An infant with noisy respiration, a wheeze on feeding and some degree of dyspnea should be suspected of having a vascular ring. The neck is often maintained in an almost opisthotonic hyperextension in an effort to relieve the airway. Often after a few gulps of feeding, dyspnea interferes with swallowing. The average age at onset of symptoms in our group was 1.3 months and the age on admission 6.2 months. The barium swallow is most useful in diagnosis and demonstrates the esophagus to be indented posteriorly at the level of the third to fourth dorsal vertebrae in the lateral view and anteriorly just above this level in cases of double aortic arch (Fig. 36-18). Direct vision bron-

Fig. 36-19.—Compression of the trachea by the innominate artery. This is the commonest form of tracheal compression seen at the Hospital for Sick Children, Toronto. Diagnosis is made by bronchoscopy; the typical view of the compression through the bronchoscope is shown on the left. Even with retrograde aortography, we are not certain that the origin of the innominate artery is aberrant.

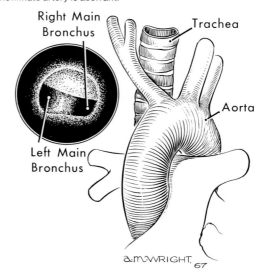

choscopy demonstrates a narrowing of the trachea anteriorly or posteriorly just above the carina by a pulsatile compression. When the compression is anterior, elevation of the tip of the bronchoscope will obliterate the right radial and right carotid pulses in cases of innominate compression[5] (Fig. 36-19). When difficulty in diagnosis arises, intratracheal injection of Lipiodol may be necessary. In the differential diagnosis, one must consider the causes of neonatal respiratory distress and dysphagia such as tracheoesophageal fistula, laryngeal malacia, bronchial web, hiatus hernia and ingestion of a foreign body.

NATURAL HISTORY.—Griswold and Young[5] reviewed 19 cases of double aortic arch: 16 children not operated on died, and of these 16 deaths, 14 were directly attributable to the presence of the vascular ring. Of 38 patients with symptomatic vascular compression in our series, 23 were not operated on, and of these, 5 died. Three of the deaths were attributed to other causes, but in 2 infants death was sudden and directly attributable to the compression. Follow-up studies of 12 of the 18 survivors of vascular compression without additional lesions and without operation, showed that all were doing well from 6 months to 7 years later.

INDICATIONS FOR OPERATION

A good deal of controversy prevails concerning the operative management of these infants. We consider a period of observation in hospital (after the usual investigation) very useful to determine the severity of the symptoms. In our group, only patients with severe symptoms were operated on—a number of them for repeated pulmonary infection. In our experience the infants with the double aortic arch or the right aortic arch with left ligamentum arteriosum are most likely to be in distress and frequently need operative correction (Fig. 36-20). The aberrant left subclavian rarely requires operation, and judgment must depend on the severity of signs and symptoms.

OPERATIVE TECHNIQUE

We favor a posterolateral approach. The decision as to which arch to divide in the case of the double aortic arch is not difficult. Usually the anterior arch will be found to be the larger of the two and to have no constriction where it joins the posterior arch, and the posterior is then the arch to divide although it is less accessible. If the anterior arch is constricted as it joins the posterior arch, division should be performed at the site of this constriction of the anterior arch. Experience has taught us that the dissection around the trachea should be minimal, leaving supporting tissue around it because of the possibility of tracheal collapse with the loss of external support. In cases of innominate compression, the base of the innominate is suspended by heavy silk sutures in the adventitia parallel to the vessel. The sutures are brought through the sternum and tied to suspend the vessel. With a bronchoscope in place, the anesthesiologist is able to confirm relief of compression. In 1 of our cases of double aortic arch and ventricular septal defect with pulmonary hypertension, the posterior arch was divided and at the same time the pulmonary artery was banded to relieve further obstruction of the trachea and to relieve pulmonary hypertension. This infant was well 1 year postoperatively.

POSTOPERATIVE CARE

Some controversy prevails concerning tracheostomy as an elective procedure following, particularly, operation for double aortic arch. Tracheostomies of infants, at least in our hands, invite dangerous complications, and extubation of these infants is difficult, 1 of our patients having to remain in hospital 8

Fig. 36-20.—Vascular rings compressing trachea and esophagus. **A,** the smaller anterior arch should be divided as it joins the posterior arch, and the left common carotid and subclavian arteries allowed to swing upward. Dissection around the trachea should be minimal. **B,** the small posterior arch is divided from the left side by elevating the aorta. **C,** the left ligamentum arteriosum or patent ductus completes the vascular ring and requires division **D,** the aberrant right subclavian artery can be divided at its origin and pushed well over to the right of the esophagus.

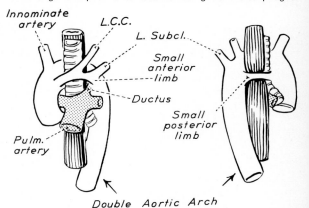

Double Aortic Arch

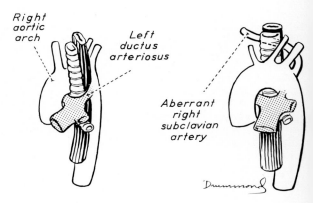

months before extubation could be satisfactorily carried out. Nevertheless some surgeons recommend tracheostomy as an elective procedure at the time of operation. Whether the child has a tracheostomy or not, the postoperative care is as demanding as the actual operative procedure, and a moist atmosphere with careful nursing care is essential.

RESULTS OF OPERATION

The largest series was reported by Gross,[7] with 70 babies having been operated on. Double aortic arches were found in 26 children with 21 survivors; 18 patients with right aortic arch with left ligamentum arteriosum were operated on without a fatality. Operative treatment was carried out with no deaths in 9 patients with anomalous innominate artery, 12 with aberrant right subclavian artery, and 5 with anomalous left common carotid artery. In our series, 57 children were operated on. Among these were 1 child with aberrant right subclavian, 30 with innominate artery compression, 3 with right aortic arch and left ligamentum arteriosum, 1 with aberrant left pulmonary artery, and 22 with double aortic arches. The 3 patients who died had double aortic arch. One infant died during intubation before the chest could be opened and attempts at resuscitation failed; 2 infants died in the postoperative recovery period, 1, we believe, due to obstruction of the tracheostomy tube and the second due to the fact that the tracheal tube was too short and did not support the collapsed trachea.

REFERENCES

1. Abbott, M. E.: *Congenital Heart Disease*, in *Nelson's Loose-Leaf Medicine* (New York: Thomas Nelson & Sons, 1932), 4:155.
2. Bayford, D.: An account of a singular case of deglutition, Mem. M. Soc. (London) 2:275, 1789.
3. Blumenthal, S., and Ravitch, M. M.: Seminar on aortic vascular rings and other anomalies of the aortic arch, Pediatrics 20: No. 5, Part 1, 1957.
4. Fearon, B., and Shortreed, R.: Tracheobronchial compression by congenital cardiovascular anomalies in children, Ann. Otol., Rhin. & Laryng. 72:1, 1963.
5. Griswold, H. E., and Young, M. D.: Double aortic arch: Report of 2 cases and review of the literature, Pediatrics 4:751, 1949.
6. Gross, R. E.: Surgical relief for tracheal obstruction from a vascular ring, New England J. Med. 233:586, 1945.
7. Gross, R. E.: Arterial malformations which cause compression of the trachea or esophagus, Circulation 11:124, 1955.
8. Hommel: Cited by Poynter, C. W. M.: Arterial anomalies pertaining to aortic arches and branches arising from them, Nebraska Univ., Univ. Studies 16:229, 1916.
9. Jacobson, J. H., et al.: Aberrant left pulmonary artery: A correctable cause of respiratory obstruction, J. Thoracic & Cardiovas. Surg. 39:602, 1960.
10. von Siebold, C. T.: Ringformiger Aorten-Bogen bei einem neugeborenen blausuchtigen Kinde, Jahrb. Geburtsh. 16:294, 1836.

W. T. MUSTARD

Drawings by
MARGUERITE DRUMMOND
(FIGURES 36-17 AND 36-20)
A. M. WRIGHT
(FIGURE 36-19)

Aorticopulmonary Window

HISTORY.—A congenital communication between the ascending aorta and the main pulmonary artery is a rare cardiac anomaly. Hektoen[5] described the first case in the American literature in 1900. Maude Abbott[1] encountered 10 lesions of this type in her analysis of 1,000 cases of congenital heart disease. The various descriptive terms which have been applied to the anomaly include aortic septal defect, aortic window, aorticopulmonary window, fenestration, septal defect or fistula. Antemortem diagnosis of this lesion, which closely resembles patent ductus arteriosus clinically and hemodynamically, was not accomplished prior to 1948, when Gross[4] closed an aorticopulmonary window by tape ligation. Successful closure by division and suture was accomplished in 1951,[6] and the advantage of cardiopulmonary by-pass with a pump oxygenator in reducing the risk of surgical closure of these window-like defects was emphasized by Cooley *et al.*[2] in 1957.

ANATOMY

The aortic septum, which ultimately divides the primitive truncus arteriosus into the definitive aorta and pulmonary artery, forms between the fifth and eighth weeks of intrauterine life (see Chap. 34). The failure of fusion of the anlagen of the aortic septum which results in a window-like communication between the aorta and the pulmonary artery above the level of the semilunar valves appears to be a less severe arrest in the development of the primitive septums than that which results in persistent truncus arteriosus. In cases of aorticopulmonary window, unlike persistent truncus arteriosus, the semilunar valves are usually normally formed. The communication between aorta and pulmonary artery is oval or elliptical and most commonly extends from a few millimeters above the pulmonary annulus to a point near the bifurcation of the main pulmonary artery (Fig. 36-21). Defects of smaller size may occur but apparently are less common than the larger ones.

INCIDENCE

The true incidence of aorticopulmonary window is not known with any exactitude. Certainly it is a rare anomaly and very much less common than patent

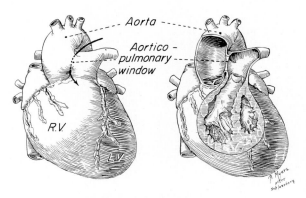

Fig. 36-21.—Aorticopulmonary window.

ductus arteriosus, which it resembles hemodynamically and clinically. In our experience, the anomaly has been verified five times at operation during a period in which over 500 patients with patent ductus were treated surgically. An incidence of 1 patient with aorticopulmonary window per 75–100 patients with patent ductus is a reasonable estimate of frequency.

Symptoms and Signs

The hemodynamic alterations with aorticopulmonary window are essentially identical to those with patent ductus. With the fall of pulmonary vascular resistance which occurs in the first few weeks after birth, oxygenated blood is shunted from the aorta through the window directly into the pulmonary artery. The size of the window and the degree of pulmonary vascular resistance regulate the volume of the shunt. In most instances, a large left-to-right shunt exists and may be accompanied by physical retardation, cardiac enlargement and the development of a precordial bulge. A loud continuous machinery murmur with systolic accentuation and accompanying thrill are frequently present over the base of the heart and may be indistinguishable from those of patent ductus. With aorticopulmonary window, however, the maximal intensity of murmur and thrill is usually in the third or fourth intercostal space to the left of the sternum. A widened pulse pressure and peripheral signs suggesting aortic insufficiency may be present. Cyanosis is characteristically absent. With the existence or development of pulmonary hypertension, the expected continuous murmur may be replaced by a basal systolic murmur of varying intensity with an accentuated and usually split pulmonary second sound. Rarely, with extreme pulmonary hypertension, no murmurs may be audible.

Clinical Course

Untreated aorticopulmonary window tends to cause complications and premature death in a fash-

ion quite similar to patent ductus, but in general the window seems to represent a more severe defect with a poorer outlook. Congestive failure, especially in early life, an increased incidence of respiratory infections, vegetative endocarditis and aneurysmal changes in the great arterial trunks with rupture and the development of severe pulmonary hypertension both individually and in combination serve to limit survival.

Diagnosis

Roentgenograms and fluoroscopy usually show cardiac enlargement, increased pulmonary vascularity and prominence of the pulmonary arterial trunk. Although the electrocardiogram may be normal, it more commonly shows left ventricular hypertrophy or combined left and right ventricular hypertrophy if pulmonary hypertension is present.

Cardiac catheterization is of utmost importance in the diagnosis of aorticopulmonary window and in differentiation from other lesions which it resembles hemodynamically and clinically. As with patent ductus, the oxygen saturation of blood in the main pulmonary artery is elevated. Absence of elevated saturation in right ventricular blood below the pulmonic valve helps to exclude ventricular septal defect. Passage of the tip of the catheter from the pulmonary artery through the aorticopulmonary window into the aorta may differentiate the lesion from patent ductus by virtue of the observed course of the catheter (Fig. 36-22).

Although angiocardiography and dye studies either singly or combined with catheterization may be of help, of considerably greater value in the diagnosis of aorticopulmonary window is contrast aortography with the retrograde injection method.[3] By either a manual method of retrograde injection of contrast material by cannula in the brachial artery (1–1.5 cc/kg) in babies under 2 years, or pressure injection through a catheter passed upward through the femoral artery into the ascending aorta in older patients,

Fig. 36-22.—Aorticopulmonary window. Differentiation from patent ductus by course of the catheter during cardiac catheterization. **A**, patent ductus; **B**, aorticopulmonary window.

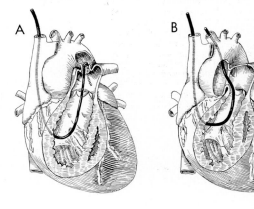

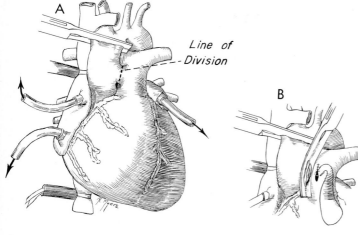

Fig. 36-23.—Aorticopulmonary window. Surgical closure, using a pump oxygenator.

the site of an aorticopulmonary window may be accurately ascertained. The left anterior oblique position and rapid, multiple roentgen exposures are important aspects of this technique. With accurately performed retrograde aortography, the main pulmonary artery is opacified anteriorly near its base if aorticopulmonary window is present, and the absence of patent ductus may be indicated by the smooth outline of the undersurface of the distal aortic arch.

In addition to patent ductus, aorticopulmonary window must be differentiated from ventricular septal defect and true truncus arteriosus. Rarely, aneurysm of the aortic sinuses of Valsalva with aortico-right ventricular fistula, pulmonary arteriovenous fistula and coronary arteriovenous fistula must be considered in diagnostic evaluation. The information provided by cardiac catheterization and retrograde aortography should permit accurate diagnosis in most cases. It is important to reiterate that in many instances, aorticopulmonary window has been found at thoracotomy with a preoperative diagnosis of patent ductus arteriosus.

Treatment

Operative closure of aorticopulmonary window, like patent ductus, is clearly indicated by the nature of the lesion, its hemodynamic effects and its symptomatic manifestations. But closure of an aorticopulmonary window presents a much greater technical challenge than closure of patent ductus. Because of the window-like opening between the two great arterial trunks and the early tendency to aneurysmal weakening and thinning of the adjacent aortic and pulmonary arterial walls, ligation or suture-ligation of the fistula is apt to result in catastrophic tearing of the arterial wall with fatal hemorrhage, and represents a poor principle. Similarly, the division of the fistula between arterial clamps of the Potts type with suture of the narrow vascular cuff as described by Scott and Sabiston[6] is an extremely hazardous undertaking. The use of hypothermia, inflow-outflow stasis and transpulmonary arterial suture of the defect was suggested by Shumway and Lewis[7] in 1956 on the basis of experimental studies, but the technical principle is questionable. In 1957, Cooley *et al.*[2] demonstrated the advantages of cardiopulmonary by-pass with a pump oxygenator in closure of aorticopulmonary window, and this has proved to be the optimal approach to the technical problem of safe closure of this defect.

TECHNIQUE.—A technique for closure of aorticopulmonary window using a pump oxygenator is illustrated in Figure 36-23. Through a median sternotomy incision, the pericardium is widely opened. After eliminating the presence of patent ductus and persistent left superior vena cava, preliminary dissection around the aorta and the pulmonary artery is begun. Cardiopulmonary by-pass is then initiated. The aorta distal to the fistula is cross-clamped and, with tension eliminated in the proximal aorta and pulmonary artery, the dissection is carried around the fistula. The latter is divided and secure closure of aortic and pulmonary arterial openings is accomplished with sutures of fine arterial silk.

Patch closure of the defect through the pulmonary artery has been successfully performed by Trusler[9] and would appear to be the method of choice if the window is very close to a coronary artery.

Closure through the aorta alone has been reported by Wright,[10] and perforation of the patch in balanced shunts has been suggested by Reis *et al.*[6]

PROGNOSIS.—The operative risk is somewhat less than that with closure of ventricular septal defect. If successful closure is accomplished in the absence of other cardiac anomalies, the patient should be restored to a normal status.

REFERENCES

1. Abbott, M. E.: *Atlas of Congenital Heart Disease* (New York: American Heart Association, 1936), p. 60.

2. Cooley, D. A.; McNamara, D. G., and Latson, J. R.: Aorticopulmonary septal defect: Diagnosis and surgical treatment, Surgery 42:101, 1957.

3. Gasul, B. M.; Fell, E. H., and Casas, R.: Diagnosis of aortic septal defect by retrograde aortography, Circulation 4:251, 1951.

4. Gross, R. E.: Surgical closure of an aortic septal defect, Circulation 5:858, 1952.

5. Hektoen, L.: Rare cardiac anomalies: Congenital aorticopulmonary communications, Tr. Chicago Path. Soc. 4:97, 1900.

6. Reis, R. L.; Gay, W. A., Jr., Braunwald, N. S., and Morrow, A. G.: The gradual closure of aortopulmonary septal defects, J. Thoracic Surg. 49:955, 1965.

7. Scott, H. W., Jr., and Sabiston, D. C., Jr.: Surgical treatment for congenital aorticopulmonary fistula, J. Thoracic Surg. 25:26, 1953.

8. Shumway, N. E., and Lewis, F. J.: The closure of experimental aortic septal defects under direct vision and hypothermia, Surgery 39:604, 1956.

9. Trusler, G. A.: Personal communication.

10. Wright, J. S.; Freeman, R., and Johnston, J. B.: Aortopulmonary fenestration. A technique of surgical management, J. Thoracic Surg. 55:280, 1968.

H. W. SCOTT, JR.

Drawings by
R. MYERS

Anomalies of the Coronary Artery

LEFT CORONARY ARTERY RISING FROM THE PULMONARY ARTERY

THIS ANOMALY WAS first described by Abrikosoff in 1911 and clinically defined by Bland, White and Garland.[4] Surgical attempts at correction have not achieved much success, although ligation of the aberrant coronary artery has allowed a few children to live. Keith[9] noted an incidence of 0.5% in his total group of congenital heart disease and pointed out that death occurs usually in the first year of life and in a high percentage of these cases in the first 6 months. Abbott[1] reported in 1927 that a patient had lived to age 64 because of a tremendous collateral circulation through the right coronary artery.

HEMODYNAMICS. — It is definitely established that, because of the difference in pressures in the pulmonary artery and the aorta, the flow is retrograde into the pulmonary artery. Blood samples obtained from the aberrant coronary artery show a higher oxygen saturation than those from the pulmonary artery. It is possible that survival for a month or two is due to the relatively high pulmonary artery pressure which is present in the infant after birth.

PATHOLOGIC ANATOMY. — The left ventricle is grossly enlarged and dilated. At autopsy, a patchy fibrosis is seen over the anterior portion of the myocardium, and this has been noted by us at operation. The left coronary artery rises from the base of the pulmonary artery in a left lateral position.

DIAGNOSIS. — Congestive heart failure appears early in the second month. Radiologic examination reveals an enlarged heart. According to Keith,[9] the electrocardiogram is diagnostic: left ventricular hypertrophy in a Q-R pattern with inverted T in the standard lead I. Confusion may arise in differentiating the endocardial fibroelastosis, but the latter usually occurs at 1 year of age or older.

SURGICAL APPROACH. — It is apparent that even after infarction of the left ventricle has taken place to any extent, it may be possible to save the life of these infants. Early diagnosis within the first month or two is essential for surgical success. Since the flow is retrograde,[3,10] ligation of the aberrant coronary artery may be beneficial. We have attempted this twice; 1 child died some hours after operation, but the other survived.

The surgical approach which we designed is to anastomose a systemic artery to the left coronary artery. The subclavian artery kinks acutely as it crosses over the aorta when one attempts to bring it down to the coronary vessel. For that reason, we have used the internal carotid artery, the diameter of which is equal to that of the coronary. We doubt that hemiplegia will take place in a baby, but this point has not been settled.

Cooley *et al.*[6] have reported successful restoration of the circulation to the aberrant left coronary artery by the use of a graft from the aorta. Their 2 patients were aged 4 and 5, but even in the infant this appears to be the procedure of choice.

CONGENITAL CORONARY ARTERIOVENOUS FISTULAS

Brown and Burnett[5] in 1949 reported the case of a 13-month-old infant thought to have a large patent ductus but autopsy demonstrated the left coronary artery entering the right ventricle. Davis *et al.*[7] reported a successful operation on a 19-year-old patient in which division of the left coronary at its insertion into the right ventricle abolished the continuous murmur. Subsequently, Gasul *et al.*[8] reported successful operation on 3 children.

The diagnosis should be suspected in patients who have a continuous murmur in the pulmonary area. Retrograde aortography may reveal the anomalous correction of either right or left coronary artery. A slight rise of oxygen saturation in the right ventricular outflow tract and a drop on entering the pulmonary artery distinguishes this lesion from patent ductus arteriosus and aorticopulmonary window. Either right or left coronary artery may drain into the coronary sinus, the right atrium, right ventricle or pulmonary artery. The operation consists in ligation of the artery at its insertion and resection of a short segment. We have had 1 such case which was suspected but not diagnosed preoperatively.

It is assumed, but not proved, that collateral circulation will support the myocardium deprived of its blood supply.

REFERENCES

1. Abbott, M. E.: *Congenital Heart Disease*, in *Nelson's Loose-Leaf Medicine* (New York: Thomas Nelson & Sons, 1932), Vol. 4, p. 155.
2. Abrikosoff, A.: Aneurysm of the left ventricle with left coronary artery arising from the pulmonary in a 5-month-old child, Arch. path. Anat. 203:413, 1911.
3. Apley, J., *et al.*: The possible role of surgery in the treatment of anomalous left coronary artery, Thorax 12:28, 1957.
4. Bland, E. F., *et al.*: Congenital anomalies of coronary arteries: Report of unusual case associated with cardiac hypertrophy, Am. Heart J. 8:787, 1933.
5. Brown, R. C., and Burnett, I. D.: Anomalous channel between aorta and right ventricle: Report of a case, Pediatrics 3:597, 1949.
6. Cooley, D. A., *et al.*: Definitive surgical treatment of anomalous origin of left coronary artery from pulmonary artery: Indications and results, J. Thoracic & Cardiovas. Surg. 52:798, 1966.
7. Davis, C., *et al.*: Anomalous coronary artery simulating patent ductus arteriosus, J.A.M.A. 160:1047, 1956.
8. Gasul, B. M., *et al.*: Congenital coronary arteriovenous aneurysm, Arch. Surg. 78:203, 1959.
9. Keith, J. D.: The anomalous origin of the left coronary artery from the pulmonary artery, Brit. Heart J. 21:149, 1959.
10. Sabiston, D. C., *et al.*: The direction of blood flow in anomalous left coronary artery arising from the pulmonary artery, Circulation 22:591, 1960.

W. T. MUSTARD

Congenital Aneurysms of the Aortic Sinuses with Cardioaortic Fistula

THIS INTERESTING LESION was first described in 1839 by Hope *et al.*[1] and the first successful closure reported in 1959 by Lillehei *et al.*[3]

Normally, slight dilations of the aorta are present immediately above the valve cusps. These are the right and left coronary sinuses and the noncoronary sinus. The right coronary sinus projects into the outflow tract of the right ventricle. Rupture of an embryonal dilation produces a cardioaortic fistula between the aorta and right ventricular cavity. The noncoronary sinus projects into the right atrium, and rupture of an aneurysm produces a fistula between the aorta and right atrium (occasionally left atrium). The left coronary sinus lies external to the right ventricle.

The *clinical features* are dyspnea and a continuous murmur along the right and left borders of the sternum in the third, fourth and fifth intercostal spaces.

If a fistula is present, the radiograph shows cardiomegaly with increased vascular markings in the lung. Retrograde aortography may reveal the fistula, and cardiac catheterization discloses a rise of oxygen saturation in right atrium or ventricle, depending on the site of perforation. The average age of rupture was said to be 31 years.[4] Of the cases reported by Kieffer and Winchell,[2] 3 were of children aged 10, 8 and 9 whose fistulas were closed at operation, two successfully. Successful surgical correction can be accomplished with the use of the pump oxygenator.

REFERENCES

1. Hope, J.: *Treatise on Diseases of the Heart and Great Vessels* (3rd ed., 1839).
2. Kieffer, S. A., and Winchell, P.: Congenital aneurysms of the aortic sinuses with cardioaortic fistula, Dis. Chest, 39:79, 1960.
3. Lillehei, C. W., *et al.*: Surgical treatment of ruptured aneurysms of the sinus of Valsalva, Ann. Surg. 146:459, 1959.
4. Sawyer, J. L., *et al.*: Surgical treatment for aneurysms of the aortic sinuses with aorticoatrial fistula, Surgery 41:26, 1957.

W. T. MUSTARD

Aortico-Left Ventricular Tunnel

A RARE COMMUNICATION from the aorta above the anterior aortic sinus to the left ventricle was described by Levy et al.,[1] who successfully closed it on cardiopulmonary by-pass. Since then, other reports have appeared. If the diagnosis is suspected, successful closure should be possible, as in our 1 patient, aged 5.

REFERENCE

1. Levy, M. J., et al.: Aortico-left ventricular tunnel, Circulation 27:841, 1963.

W. T. MUSTARD

37

Anomalous Pulmonary Venous Drainage

HISTORY.—Anomalous communication between the pulmonary and systemic venous systems was first described two centuries ago by Winslow[36] in 1739. Not until 1798 was a case of total pulmonary venous drainage into the right side of the heart described, by Wilson;[35] and Friedlowsky[19] subsequently described this pathologic entity in some detail. In 1942, Brody[4] focused attention on anomalous pulmonary venous drainage in a collective review of reported cases with consideration of the types and location of such anomalies. As recently as 1947, surgical correction of these lesions had not been accomplished when Brantigan[3] suggested that partial anomalous drainage would be benefited by resection of the portion of lung thus drained. For patients with complete anomalous drainage of the entire pulmonary circulation, he speculated that removal of the interatrial septum might be performed or else a major pulmonary vein could be anastomosed to the left atrium.

Muller[27] in 1951 reported successful implantation of an anomalous pulmonary vein into the left atrium by side-to-side anastomosis, and Gerbode[21] reported a similar case. Subsequently, successful repair of partial anomalous drainage involving both left and right lungs was reported.[2,6,24,28] Correction of total anomalous pulmonary venous drainage presented a more difficult technical problem which was ultimately solved with development of the pump oxygenator for temporary cardiopulmonary by-pass. Repair of the type of total anomalous drainage in which pulmonary veins connected directly with the right atrium was reported by Gott et al.[20] They referred to the work of Lewis and his associates,[26] who used hypothermia and cardiac inflow occlusion. Burroughs and Kirklin[5] also were successful in repair of this type of defect using an atrial well technique. Early success with open correction of the supracardiac total anomalous drainage was reported by Cooley and Ochsner[7] in 1957. Subsequent communications from our surgical unit presented additional cases and described modifications of operative technique.[8,11,13] Many recent reports reflect improvements in technique and expansion of cardiac surgery for anomalous pulmonary venous drainage, including correction of the infracardiac type of connection in our center[9] and elsewhere.[30,37]

ANATOMY

1. PARTIAL ANOMALOUS DRAINAGE.—The venous system of the lung itself is normal in this condition, but wide variation occurs in anatomic site of drainage of the anomalous veins. Partial anomalous drainage of the right lung into the right atrium or vena cava is at least twice as common as for the left lung. Only rarely do both lungs have partial anomalous drainage into the systemic circulation.[23] The site of partial drainage from the right lung is, in order of decreasing frequency, to the superior vena cava, the right atrium and to the inferior vena cava.[22] On the left side, the veins usually empty into a persistent left superior vena cava (persistent anterior cardinal vein) and into the innominate vein but rarely enter the coronary sinus posteriorly. In the majority of cases, the partial drainage is accompanied by a patent foramen

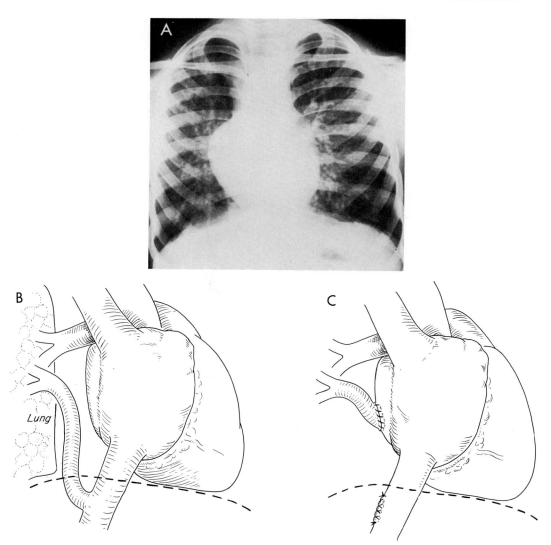

Fig. 37-1.—Anomalous venous drainage. **A,** roentgenogram of the chest of a 6-year-old boy with anomalous venous drainage of the entire right lung into the inferior vena cava, showing partial malrotation of the heart and increased pulmonary vascular markings. **B,** drawing of the anomaly, in which the common pulmon-ary venous trunk entered the inferior vena cava below the diaphragm. **C,** method of repair, consisting of transfer of the pulmonary venous trunk into the left atrium by direct anastomosis and repair of the opening in the inferior vena cava.

ovale or a true atrial septal defect. Indeed, in some cases with a large-volume left-to-right shunt via the pulmonary veins, a septal defect may be a factor in preventing overload of the right heart and provides for adequate left ventricular filling. Occasionally, the lung itself is anomalous, and we have demonstrated abnormal lobulation and pleural reflection in a right lung in which all of the drainage was into the inferior vena cava below the diaphragm (Fig. 37-1, *A*). Anomalous venous drainage of the entire right lung with normal left pulmonary drainage has been observed in 2 of our cases, and in neither instance was a patent

foramen ovale present. The connection of the pulmonary vein with the systemic veins was to the inferior vena cava in both cases. Anomalous drainage of the entire left lung with normal right pulmonary circulation was demonstrated in 1 patient and drainage of only the left upper lobe in another. In both of these patients the connection was to a persistent left superior vena cava (Fig. 37-2, *A*). It is interesting that the foramen ovale was not patent in either case.

Sinus venosus defect.—This unique anomaly is a combination of a high interatrial septal defect and anomalous pulmonary venous drainage of the right

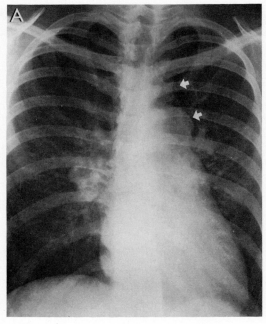

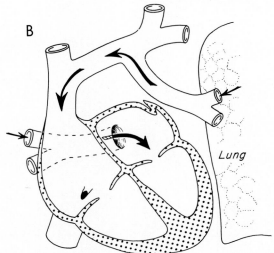

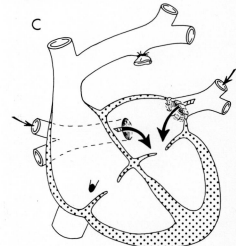

Fig. 37-2.—Anomalous venous drainage. **A,** roentgenogram of the chest of a 29-year-old man with pulmonary drainage of the entire left lung into the left innominate vein, showing a tortuous vein in the left superior mediastinum **(arrows). B,** drawing showing the nature of the anomaly. **C,** technique of surgical repair.

The anomalous pulmonary venous trunk was divided and anastomosed to the left auricular appendage. During the period of venous occlusion, a simultaneous occlusion of pulmonary artery was used to prevent hemorrhagic congestion of the left lung.

upper and sometimes middle lobe veins (Fig. 37-3, *A* and *B*). Although this lesion was described first in 1868,[34] the term sinus venosus defect was suggested only recently by Ross.[29] Characteristically, the sinus venosus defect is located adjacent to the orifice of the superior vena cava, and the superior margin of the atrial septum is missing.[10] The septal defect is located cephalad to the fossa ovalis, which is usually intact.

The point of entry of anomalous veins is at the atrio-caval junction or directly into the superior vena cava at a higher level. In many instances, one or more segmental veins empty separately into the superior vena cava.

2. TOTAL ANOMALOUS DRAINAGE.—Although an atrial septal defect is present in most instances of partial anomalous pulmonary venous drainage, an

interatrial communication must always be present in the total anomalous drainage to permit survival of the patient. The right atrium receives mixed oxygenated and unoxygenated venous blood. Whereas most of this blood enters the right ventricle, some of the mixed pulmonary and systemic venous blood shunts right-to-left to enter the left ventricle and is pumped out into the body, producing cyanosis. Mild cyanosis may or may not be apparent early in life but will always appear later, as the right-to-left shunt increases. Usually, the diameter of the pulmonary artery is

greater than that of the ascending aorta. The left atrium and ventricle may be small in comparison to the right side of the heart, but the left ventricle is usually adequate to provide for complete cardiac outflow. Because of this, surgical correction is possible in a one-stage operation.

Total anomaly of pulmonary venous drainage occurs in several anatomic forms. According to Darling *et al.*,[14] anatomic classification of the types of total anomalous drainage can be based on the level at which the pulmonary veins enter the systemic veins or

Fig. 37-3.—Anomalous venous drainage: sinus venous defect. **A.** typical anatomic configuration of atrial septal defect associated with anomalous pulmonary venous drainage, referred to as the sinus venosus defect. The atrial septal defect is cephalad to the fossa ovale, which is usually intact. **B,** a variation of sinus venosus defect in which segmental veins from the upper lobe drain directly into the right superior vena cava above the atrial

caval junction (*). See text for details of correction of this variant. **C,** recommended technique of repair of sinus venosus defect using Dacron knit prosthesis. **D,** repair of defect in the atrial septum and anomalous drainage by insertion of a Dacron patch. The patch prevents torsion and constriction of the vena cava and pulmonary veins, providing optimal repair of the lesion.

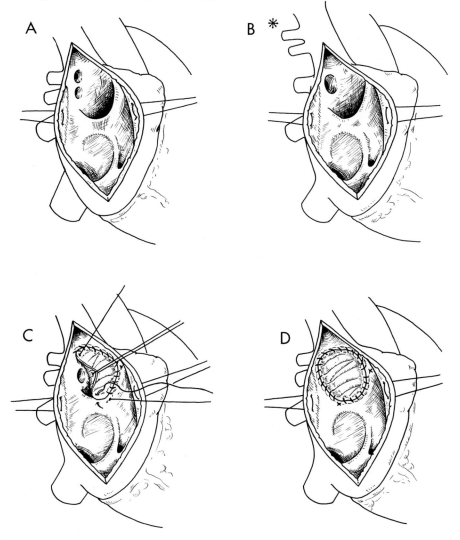

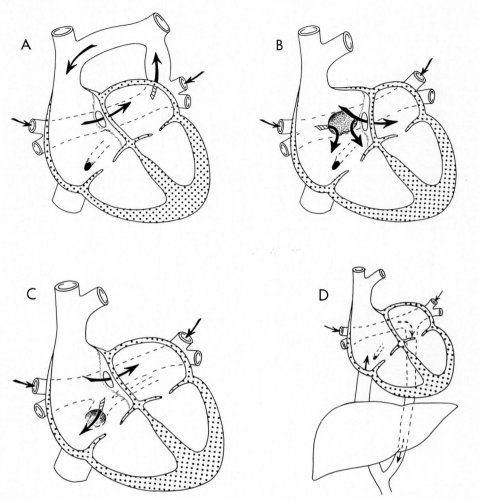

Fig. 37-4.—Total anomalous pulmonary venous drainage: commonly recognized types. **A,** supracardiac type in which a common pulmonary vein carries both right and left pulmonary venous blood into the left innominate vein. **B,** paracardiac type in which both right and left pulmonary veins empty directly into the right atrium. **C,** paracardiac type in which the pulmonary veins empty into the coronary sinus and then into the right atrium. In all cases of total anomalous pulmonary venous drainage, patent foramen ovale or atrial septal defect is also present. **D,** infracardiac type in which pulmonary venous drainage is by the inferior caval system, frequently via the portal vein.

right heart. Thus a supracardiac, paracardiac, infracardiac or a mixed type of communication is possible.

a) Supracardiac type.—This is the most common form. Pulmonary veins drain into the superior vena caval system usually via a persistent left superior vena cava (vertical anomalous pulmonary vein[18]) into the left innominate vein (Fig. 37-4, *A*). Less commonly, the pulmonary venous trunk drains directly into the posterior aspect of the right superior vena cava.

b) Paracardiac type.—In patients with a paracardiac connection, the veins empty directly into the posterior right atrium or into a dilated coronary sinus and then into the right atrium (Fig. 37-4, *B* and *C*).

c) Infracardiac type.—In the rarer infracardiac type, the pulmonary venous blood enters the inferior cava, or ductus venosus (Fig. 37-4, *D*).

d) Mixed type.—In the mixed type, routes of drainage are different for the two lungs. For example, in 1 of our cases the left upper lobe drained into a persistent left superior vena cava while the lower lobe and entire right lung emptied into the posterior aspect of the right atrium.

INCIDENCE

The exact incidence of anomalous pulmonary venous drainage is difficult to estimate since usually the autopsy technique consists of separating the heart and lungs without studying them as a unit. Healy[22] found 1 instance in 251 cadavers (0.4%) and Hughes and Rumore,[23] 2 in 280 autopsies (0.7%). It should be recognized that anomalous drainage of the partial type is relatively common and frequently accompanies atrial septal defect. For example, in 416 cases of atrial septal defect of the septum secundum type corrected by open heart surgery in Baylor University Affiliated Hospitals, anomalous drainage from the right lung was encountered in 33 cases (8%). Fifty-seven patients had sinus venosus type atrial septal defects and 27 (47%) had associated partial anomalous pulmonary venous drainage.[12] If the drainage is of small volume, the lesion is usually not recognized during life.

Total anomalous venous drainage is less common. Healy,[22] in a survey of 147 cases of anomalous drainage, reported 61 complete or total anomalies and 86 partial. In the cases of total anomalous drainage, approximately 39% connected with the superior caval system, usually at the innominate vein region. In 1957, Darling *et al.*[14] collected 80 reported cases of total anomalous drainage of pulmonary veins into the systemic venous circulation. A larger number of such cases has been reported since development of open methods of repair, and our own series of surgically corrected lesions numbers 66 cases.

EMBRYOLOGY

The primordia of the lungs, larynx and tracheobronchial tree are derived by division of the foregut with which the lungs share a common blood supply. The splanchnic plexus drains into the neighboring veins, which are the systemic precardinal and postcardinal veins and the visceral veins of the abdomen, i.e., the umbilicovitelline vessels and associated hepatic sinusoids. Thus initial drainage of the lungs is into the superior vena cava, coronary sinus, innominate veins, portal system, ductus venosus and inferior vena cava, and no direct communication with the heart is present. The developing left atrium must make connection with that portion of the splanchnic bed which is draining the primordial lungs. This it does by developing a "common pulmonary vein" which extends into the dorsal mesocardium.[1] As this junction is taking place, separation of the primary venous connections from the cardinal and umbilicovitelline venous systems occurs. According to Edwards,[17] the underlying cause for anomalous connection is (*a*) failure of connection of the atrial portion of the heart with the pulmonary portion of the splanchnic plexus or (*b*) a secondary obliteration of normally developed communications between the atrial portion of the heart and the pulmonary portion of the splanchnic plexus. This does not provide an adequate explanation for those cases in which the drainage of one or both lungs is into the right atrium directly. An abnormality in development of the atrial septum probably accounts for this anomaly and for the for-mation of the sinus venosus type of anomaly. If the septum develops farther to the left than normal, the outpouching of the left atrium (sinoatrial region) which joins the primitive pulmonary veins may be to the right of the septum, creating a connection with the right atrium. If the atrial septum occupies a position midway between normal and the extreme left position, the sinoatrial pouch could be divided so the left lung drained into the left atrium normally and the right lung into the right atrium.

SYMPTOMS AND PHYSICAL FINDINGS

Partial anomalous drainage of the right lung into the right atrium produces minimal symptoms and findings.[33] Since the vascular shunt is left-to-right, no cyanosis is evident. Usually, right atrial and ventricular enlargement is present, but often no murmur is found. With an associated atrial septal defect of significant size, symptoms of a large-volume left-to-right shunt are evident. The patient has dyspnea on exertion, palpitation and occasional precordial fullness or discomfort. A frail or so-called gracile habitus may be noted, depending on the volume of the shunt and degree of vascular resistance.

Total anomalous pulmonary venous drainage usually causes severe symptoms and striking physical findings. Infants demonstrate signs of severe right-sided failure with cardiomegaly, hepatomegaly and some cyanosis, depending on the size of the interatrial communication. Pulmonary congestion is common because of the excessive pulmonary blood flow. As the heart enlarges, compression of the left lower lobe may occur. Thus the lesion is often mistaken for pneumonia. Left-sided chest deformity develops at an early age because of the tremendous load placed on the right side of the heart. The pulse is usually of small volume during infancy, and blood pressure is low.

The clinical picture in the patient who has survived infancy and childhood is similar to that in patients with other mild forms of cyanotic heart disease. In general, these patients have an interatrial communication of sufficient size to vent the right atrial overload into the left atrium. Often, symptoms in these patients are surprisingly mild; in 1 of our patients who was 35 years old, the symptoms were not disabling and cyanosis was barely evident (see Fig. 37-5, *D*). One should conclude that wide variation in the degree of incapacity results from the number of anatomic variations in the anomalous drainage.

ELECTROCARDIOGRAPHY, RADIOGRAPHY AND CARDIAC CATHETERIZATION

Electrocardiograms demonstrate right axis deviation and right ventricular hypertrophy. If, however, the anomalous pulmonary drainage represents only a small segment of the lung, electrocardiographic

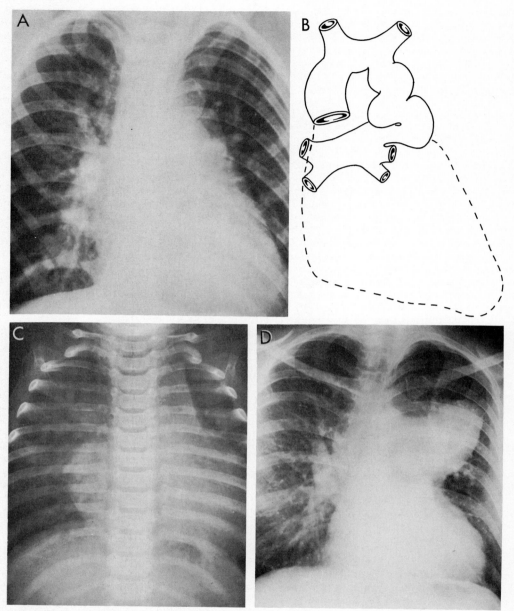

Fig. 37-5.—Total anomalous pulmonary venous drainage into the left innominate vein: roentgenographic features in various age groups. **A,** roentgenogram of a 7-year-old boy showing characteristic superior mediastinal shadow and pulmonary vascular congestion. **B,** diagram made from **A,** showing enlarged left superior vena cava and right superior vena cava producing the mediastinal configuration referred to as "snowman" deformity. **C,** roentgenogram of a 6-month-old infant showing boxlike con- figuration of the superior mediastinum, extreme cardiac enlargement and pulmonary congestion. This picture is not necessarily diagnostic of the anomaly at this age. **D,** roentgenogram of a 35-year-old man showing remarkable dilatation which was mistakenly diagnosed as aneurysm of the aortic arch. Gradual distention of the left and the right superior vena cava produced the unusual appearence of this mediastinum.

changes may be undetectable. In patients with total anomalous drainage, an impressive degree of right atrial enlargement is present.

Roentgenograms of the chest in partial anomalous pulmonary venous drainage reveal right atrial and right ventricular enlargement with dilatation of the main pulmonary artery. Pulmonary vessels in the periphery of the lung field are often prominent, depending on the volume of pulmonary overload. In the sinus venosus type of anomaly, the diagnosis may be suggested by a right hilar bulge at the atriocaval junction. Selective angiocardiography may assist in this diagnosis.[16]

Roentgenograms of the chest in total anomalous pulmonary venous return into the left innominate vein in children reveal an almost pathognomonic cardiac silhouette (Fig. 37-5, *A* and *B*). These findings were clearly described by Snellen and Albers,[31] who described the figure-of-eight configuration of the mediastinum. The upper half of the eight is formed by the ascending or vertical anomalous pulmonary vein on the left, the innominate vein and the prominent right superior vena cava. This same configuration also has been referred to as the snowman and cottage-loaf appearance. A hilar dance is usually demonstrable in the pulmonary vessels on fluoroscopy. Although the above pattern is typical of the total anomaly in children and adults, the appearance in infants may not be characteristic. In infants, cardiac enlargement involving the right ventricle and engorgement of the pulmonary vessels reveals the presence of a large left-to-right shunt. The superior mediastinal shadow may be widened, with a boxlike appearance of the heart due to a somewhat horizontal left border of the heart at its junction with the aortic arch[20] (Fig. 37-5, *C*). In this age group, angiocardiography is useful in delineating the pulmonary venous collecting system (Fig. 37-6).

Cardiac catheterization in all cases of anomalous venous return reveals increased oxygen saturation of right atrial blood when compared to systemic venous blood. These findings are of little value, however, in differentiating partial anomalous drainage from atrial septal defect. Usually, the volume of left-to-right shunt in the anomalous veins is smaller than for atrial septal defect, in which the shunt may be two or three times systemic flow. Dye dilution studies are useful for more precise location of the anomalous drainage and estimation of the volume of shunt. Comparison of right atrial dilution curves is made following injection of indicator solution in right and left pulmonary veins.[35] This reveals the volume of blood which is being recirculated, but the technique does not differentiate in every case the possible sites at which this occurs. Often it is difficult to distinguish anomalous pulmonary venous drainage from atrial septal defect, since in large atrial defects, dilution curves frequently demonstrate a greater degree of anomalous venous drainage to the right atrium from

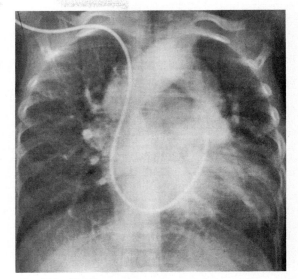

Fig. 37-6.—Total anomalous pulmonary drainage. Representative frame from Elema angiocardiogram of a 10-1/2-year-old girl. Contrast material outlines the vertical anomalous pulmonary vein ("persistent left superior vena cava") connecting the retrocardiac pulmonary venous trunk and left innominate vein.

the right lung than from the left lung due to preferential flow. Nevertheless exploration of the anomalous veins with the catheter combined with use of various injection sites and sampling sites usually will provide adequate diagnostic data for practical purposes.

In total anomalous drainage of pulmonary veins, demonstration of blood oxygen saturation in the right side of the heart which is similar or equal to the saturation in a systemic artery is considered almost diagnostic. Exploration of the superior caval system with the catheter introduced through the left antecubital vein may reveal the connection of the pulmonary venous trunk with the left innominate vein. Passage of the catheter through the anomalous channel into both lungs is occasionally possible. The pressure within the right side of the heart and pulmonary artery is elevated, frequently to a striking degree. Entry into the left atrium from the superior vena cava is usually more difficult than from the inferior cava because of the preferential flow of blood through the foramen ovale from below. Dye dilution studies reveal a shorter appearance time from the atrium than from the right ventricle or pulmonary artery.

PROGNOSIS

Prognosis in partial anomalous pulmonary connection is usually good, and patients frequently have no outward signs of disability. In Brody's series, 76% of patients reached maturity, and Dean and Fox[15] described a patient who lived to 86 years of age. In ordinary circumstances, a single anomalous pulmonary vein without an associated atrial septal defect does not cause symptoms during childhood. Symptoms early in life usually indicate the presence of a large atrial septal defect or anomalous drainage of an entire lung. According to Brody,[4] if less than half of the blood from the pulmonary parenchyma is drained anomalously, the patient may exhibit little disability. When more than half of the pulmonary circulation enters the right side of the heart, evidence of right-sided failure becomes manifest, development is retarded and life span is shortened.

In contrast to partial anomalous drainage, the prognosis in total anomalous pulmonary venous connection is poor. Healy,[22] in a review of reported cases, found the average age at death to be 1.8 years. Patients with total anomalous pulmonary venous drainage rarely survive infancy. The interatrial communication in the usual instance of the malformation is small and may be only a probe-patent foramen ovale. Since the presence of an interatrial communication is vital to survival, the size of the defect may be critical, and those patients surviving infancy and early childhood usually have a sizable interatrial opening which permits right-to-left shunting.

SURGICAL TREATMENT

Repair of anomalous pulmonary venous drainage is recommended in all patients if the volume of shunt is significant and if anatomic findings permit complete correction. The main object of repair is to redirect the pulmonary venous blood into the left atrium.

PARTIAL ANOMALOUS PULMONARY VENOUS DRAINAGE. —Since most patients with anomalous drainage from the right lung have an atrial septal defect, correction is usually accomplished by closing the septal defect laterally and anterior to the rim of the anomalous vein (Fig. 37-7). A patch of synthetic material may be necessary if the atrial septal defect is large. In most cases, a patch graft is not necessary unless the defect is of the sinus venosus type (see Fig. 37-3, *B* and *C*). Direct closure of the defect without a patch should not be attempted in the sinus venosus defect, since tension on the septum could produce stenosis and torsion of the superior caval or pulmonary venous openings.[10] Anomalous upper lobe veins occasionally empty into the superior vena cava cephalad to the atriocaval junction, and transplantation to a more caudad position might produce tension on the veins. In these patients with anomalous veins draining into the superior vena cava, the Dacron patch used to close the sinus venosus atrial septal defect is extended into the superior vena cava and around the ostia of the anomalous veins so that they drain into the left atrium. The incision in the superior vena cava is then closed with a pericardial patch to prevent compromise of its lumen. Occasionally an upper lobectomy may be practical if the anomalous drainage is complicated. If only one pulmonary segment is draining anomalously, this may be left undisturbed since the volume of blood shunted is usually small. In some instances, simple ligation of the segmental vein is possible without producing pulmonary infarction. Indeed, if an anomalous segmental pulmonary vein is an incidental finding at thoracotomy for some other lesions, surgical repair of the vessel is usually not necessary since the lesion has little clinical significance. If the entire left lung is draining into the superior vena cava, this may be corrected by

Fig. 37-7.—Atrial septal defect and anomalous pulmonary venous drainage of the entire right lung into right atrium. **A,** roentgenogram of a 9-year-old girl. The pulmonary arterial segment is prominent, but peripheral lung fields are not engorged, suggesting presence of high pulmonary vascular resistance. **B,** drawing showing the nature of the anomaly. The lesion was corrected by transfer of the atrial septum toward the right with closure of the interatrial septal defect.

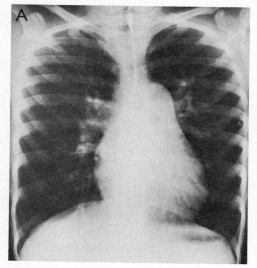

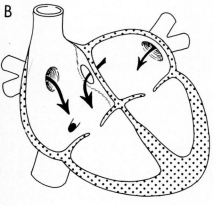

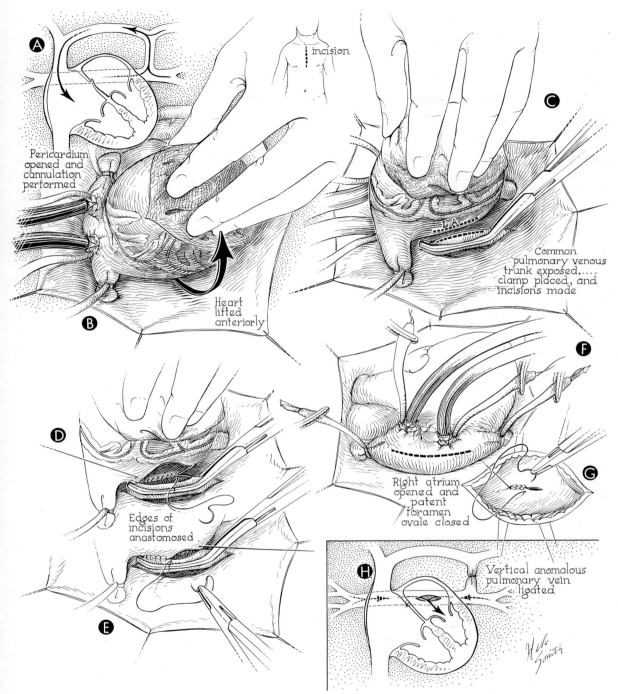

Fig. 37-8.—Total anomalous venous drainage. Technique for correction of supracardiac type with vertical anomalous pulmonary vein ("persistent left superior vena cava"). **Inset,** median sternotomy incision. **A,** pattern of venous connections. **B,** cannulation is done, the ascending aorta clamped, and the heart retracted anteriorly with gauze square or traction suture. **C,** retrocardiac transverse pulmonary venous trunk is dissected and a partial occluding vascular clamp applied. Incision is made in the pulmonary vein and posterior aspect of adjacent left atrium **(broken lines).**

D, edges of incision are united by continuous sutures and posterior row is placed. **E,** anterior row is placed. The heart is returned to the pericardial sac. **F,** longitudinal incision in the right atrium exposes the patent foramen ovale or atrial septal defect. **G,** patent foramen ovale is closed with continuous suture. Clamp is removed and cardiopulmonary by-pass discontinued. **H,** pattern of flow after completion of repair and ligation of vertical anomalous pulmonary vein. (From Cooley and Hallman.[1])

547

transfer of the communicating trunk into the left auricular appendage[6,25] (see Fig. 37-2, *B*). Instances in which the entire right lung drains into the inferior vena cava are corrected by transfer of the common trunk into the left atrium (see Fig. 37-1, *B* and *C*). Tension on the anastomosis should be avoided, since thrombosis of a common pulmonary vein would almost certainly lead to death.

TOTAL ANOMALOUS PULMONARY VENOUS DRAINAGE. —Correction of total anomalous pulmonary connection presents a more complicated technical problem and should always be done using the pump oxygenator for total cardiopulmonary by-pass.[7,8] Each type will be discussed separately.

Supracardiac type. —Operation for the supracardiac type is performed with the patient in the supine position, utilizing a median sternal splitting incision (Fig. 37-8). The technique of cannulation should be varied to avoid inserting a catheter into the superior vena cava until partial cardiopulmonary by-pass has been started. Until this time, the catheter may be allowed to rest in the atrium. Early cannulation of a vena cava that is serving to return pulmonary venous blood to the heart may result in cardiac arrest. The vertical anomalous pulmonary vein is dissected on the left side of the mediastinum and encircled with a silk ligature to which a rubber tourniquet is applied. This vessel may then be occluded during cardiopulmonary by-pass should it become necessary to remove the vascular clamp from the pulmonary vein.

After cardiopulmonary by-pass is begun, the heart is lifted anteriorly by grasping the apex with a gauze square, or a traction suture may be placed in the cardiac apex. The posterior parietal pericardium is incised over the transverse common pulmonary venous trunk, and this structure is dissected sufficiently to allow a partial occluding vascular clamp to be placed transversely along its anterior surface. Complete occlusion of the venous trunk by the clamp is no cause for concern, since the main purpose of the clamp is to prevent pulmonary venous blood from obscuring the operative field. The same end may be accomplished by occluding each extremity of the common venous trunk with tourniquet ligatures. A transverse incision is made within the confines of the clamp and a similar incision made in the posterior wall of the left atrium. These incisions should be as long as the width of the posterior wall of the left atrium. The incisions are then joined by continuous technique, using 4-0 or 5-0 suture. The heart is returned to its bed and a longitudinal incision made in the lateral wall of the right atrium through which the patent foramen ovale or atrial septal defect is closed with continuous suture. The partial occluding clamp is removed from the pulmonary vein and the vascular clamp removed from the ascending aorta. After cardiopulmonary by-pass is discontinued the vertical anomalous pulmonary vein ("persistent left superior vena cava") or communication between the transverse retrocardiac common pulmonary vein and the superior caval system is ligated.

Cardiac type. —Operation is performed with the patient in the supine position and the right chest elevated about 45 degrees (Figs. 37-9 and 37-10). A transverse incision is made through the fourth intercostal space, transecting the sternum but not entering the left pleural cavity. The pericardium is incised longitudinally and suitable cannulations are performed. Through a longitudinal incision in the right atrium, the anatomy of the anomaly is inspected. In patients with drainage of pulmonary veins into the coronary sinus, the portion of atrial septum between the foramen ovale and the large ostium of the coronary sinus is excised (Fig. 37-9). The superior wall of the coronary sinus is then incised, so that blood from it can drain freely into the left atrium. The valve of the foramen ovale is removed. A Dacron patch is sutured to the anterior, superior and posterior walls of the foramen ovale and to the posterior, inferior and anterior margins of the ostium of the coronary sinus. This maneuver closes the interatrial communication and diverts all flow from the pulmonary veins and coronary sinus into the left atrium. The right-to-left shunt that results from diversion of the coronary sinus into the left atrium is unavoidable and of little functional significance.

Patients in whom pulmonary veins enter the body of the right atrium are operated on by the same general approach outlined in the preceding paragraph (Fig. 37-10). Inspection through a longitudinal right atriotomy usually reveals a small recess of the posterior wall of the right atrium into which the pulmonary veins drain. The patent foramen ovale or atrial septal defect is enlarged by excising a major portion of the atrial septum. A Dacron patch is sutured over this defect, carrying the right posterior suture line along the lateral wall of the right atrium anterior to the points of entrance of the pulmonary veins. In this fashion, the interatrial communication is closed and pulmonary venous drainage is diverted into the left atrium.

Infracardiac type. —Patients with an infracardiac type of total anomalous venous drainage are best operated on through a median sternal splitting incision (Fig. 37-11). After institution of cardiopulmonary by-pass, the heart is lifted anteriorly and superiorly. The descending vein is dissected and encircled with a control ligature, but this is not tied initially. The transverse common pulmonary vein is dissected sufficiently to allow the application of a partial occluding vascular clamp, which is placed transversely. A transverse incision is made within the confines of this clamp and a similar incision made in the posterior wall of the overlying left atrium. These two incisions are then anastomosed in a fashion similar to that described for patients with supracardiac type drainage. After removal of the vascular clamp, the descending vein is ligated. The patent foramen ovale

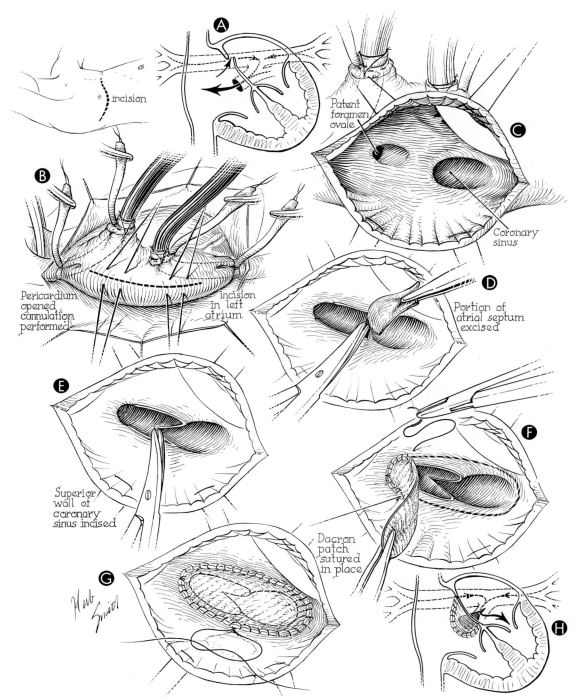

Fig. 37-9.—Total anomalous venous drainage. Technique for correction of cardiac type in which pulmonary veins drain into the coronary sinus. **Inset,** incision in right fourth interspace transecting the sternum. **A,** pattern of venous connection. The common pulmonary vein drains into the coronary sinus. **B,** cannulation is performed, the ascending aorta clamped and traction sutures are placed. The right atrium is then incised. **C,** the ostium of the coronary sinus is greatly enlarged; the foramen ovale is patent but its valve is incompetent. **D,** the atrial septum between foramen ovale and coronary sinus is excised and the valve of the foramen ovale removed. **E,** the superior wall of the coronary sinus is incised so that blood from it can drain into left atrium. **F,** Dacron patch is anchored to margins of the foramen ovale and coronary sinus using continuous suture. **G,** insertion of Dacron patch has been completed. **H,** pattern of venous flow after patch is inserted. All blood from pulmonary vein and coronary sinus drains into the left atrium behind patch. (From Cooley and Hallman.[11])

549

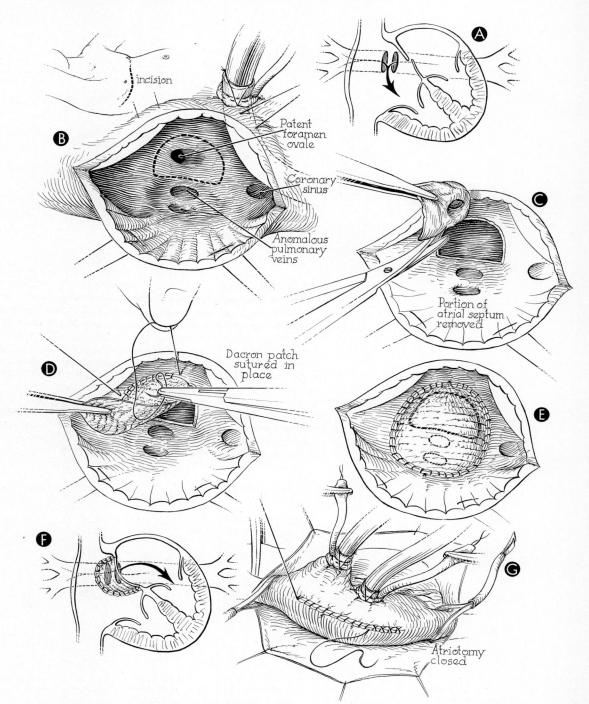

Fig. 37-10.—Total anomalous venous drainage. Technique for correction of cardiac type in which pulmonary veins connect directly to the body of the right atrium. **Inset,** incision in right fourth interspace transecting sternum. **A,** pattern of venous connection. **B,** anatomy of the lesion. **C,** major portion of the atrial septum is excised, including foramen ovale. **D,** Dacron patch is sutured to margins of the defect anteriorly. **E,** suture line is completed. Patch has been sewn to the wall of the right atrium anterior to pulmonary veins. **F,** pattern of flow after patch is inserted. Blood from pulmonary veins drains behind the patch into the left atrium. **G,** atriotomy is closed with two overlapping rows of continuous sutures. (From Cooley and Hallman.[11])

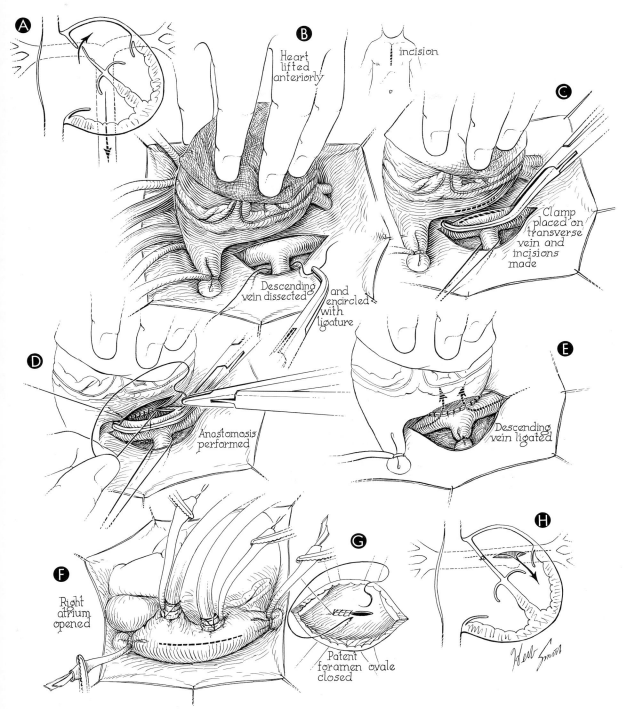

Fig. 37-11.—Total anomalous venous drainage. Technique for correction of infracardiac type. **Inset,** median sternotomy incision. **A,** pattern of venous connection. Retrocardiac pulmonary venous trunk drains via a descending vein that traverses the diaphragm and enters the inferior vena cava, ductus venosus or portal vein **B,** cannulation is performed, the ascending aorta clamped and the heart retracted forward by gauze square or traction suture. The retrocardiac trunk and descending vein are encircled with control ligature. **C,** a partial occluding vascular clamp is applied to the transverse pulmonary vein and an incision made in the vein and in left atrium **(broken lines). D,** incisions in the pulmonary vein and left atrium are joined by continuous suture. A posterior row is placed. **E,** an anterior row is placed, and the descending vein ligated. **F,** a longitudinal incision is made in the right atrium. **G,** foramen ovale is closed with continuous suture. **H,** pattern of flow after repair. (From Cooley and Hallman.[11])

TABLE 37-1.—TOTAL ANOMALOUS PULMONARY VENOUS DRAINAGE: MORTALITY ACCORDING TO AGE GROUPS

AGE	No. OF PATIENTS	No. OF DEATHS	% MORTALITY
12 mo. or less	39	21	54
13–24 mo.	5	2	40
2–10 yr.	17	3	18
11–20 yr.	4	0	0
21 yr. or older	1	0	0
Total	66	26	39

or atrial septal defect is then closed through an incision in the right atrium. The transverse common pulmonary vein is preferable to the descending vein for anastomosis to the left atrium for several reasons. The most important of these is the ability to create a larger communication through which pulmonary venous blood can enter the left atrium. Moreover, the descending vein is usually kinked by turning it forward for an end-to-side anastomosis to the left atrium. Finally, a circular anastomosis between the end of the pulmonary vein and the left atrium is more likely to become stenosed over a period of months or years than is a long elliptical anastomosis between the transverse pulmonary vein and left atrium.

Mixed type.—Patients with a different route of venous drainage from the two lungs are operated on by a combination of the techniques outlined above.

RESULTS OF OPERATION

Operation for partial anomalous venous connection usually is associated with low mortality, which should be less than 2% depending on age and general condition of the patient. Partial drainage lesions occurred in 33 of our 416 patients undergoing repair of atrial septal defect of the ostium secundum type, and death occurred in only 1 patient, who was 48 years old and who had severe pulmonary hypertension. The same rules governing selection of patients for repair of atrial septal defect should apply to patients who

TABLE 37-2.—TOTAL ANOMALOUS PULMONARY VENOUS DRAINAGE: MORTALITY ACCORDING TO TYPE OF CONNECTION

TYPE OF CONNECTION	No. OF PATIENTS	No. OF DEATHS	% MORTALITY
Supracardiac	38	14	37
Right superior vena cava	8	4	50
Left vertical anomalous vein	30	10	33
Cardiac	21	7	35
Body of right atrium	9	3	38
Coronary sinus	12	4	33
Infracardiac	3	1	33
Inferior vena cava	1	0	0
Portal vein	2	1	50
Mixed	4	4	100
Total	66	26	39

TABLE 37-3.—TOTAL ANOMALOUS PULMONARY VENOUS DRAINAGE: CAUSES OF DEATH

CAUSE OF DEATH	No. OF PATIENTS
Pulmonary edema	13
Sudden cardiac arrest	5
Heart block	3
Respiratory insufficiency	2
Renal failure	1
Cerebral edema	1
Intraoperative hemolysis	1
Total	26

have partial anomalous drainage of pulmonary veins. Thus older patients with high pulmonary vascular resistance should not be operated on.

During a 10-year period, 66 patients underwent open heart operations for correction of total anomalous pulmonary venous return. Thirty-nine of the patients were under 1 year of age, and mortality in this group was 54% (Table 37-1). Mortality in older age groups was progressively less, as indicated in Table 37-1.

In 38 patients, venous return was supracardiac via either the right superior vena cava (8 patients) or a left vertical anomalous vein (30 patients) (Table 37-2). Venous return occurred to the body of the right atrium in 9 patients and to the coronary sinus in 12 (cardiac type). In 3 patients, an anomalous trunk descended through the diaphragm to make an infracardiac connection—to the inferior vena cava in 1 patient and to the portal vein in 2. Venous return occurred via a different route from each of the two lungs in 4 patients (mixed type). Table 37-2 indicates that the mortality is approximately the same (33–37%) for each of the types of drainage except the mixed type, in which there were no survivors.

Twenty-six patients died following open heart operations for correction of total anomalous pulmonary venous drainage, yielding a hospital mortality of 39%. The highest mortality occurred among the 39 patients less than a year of age, of whom 21 died (54%) (Table 37-1). The most common cause of death was pulmonary edema, noted in 13 patients. All causes of death are listed in Table 37-3. Our original impression of the cause of pulmonary edema in infants dying after operation was that a small left ventricle was not adequate to handle the volume of blood pumped through the lungs by the hypertrophied right ventricle. We subsequently published data showing a high cardiac output in most such patients, tending to discredit the idea of an inadequate left ventricle.[10] Correlation between physiologic data and surgical mortality indicated that when pulmonary vascular resistance was increased, mortality was high, and vice versa.

REFERENCES

1. Auer, J.: The development of the human pulmonary vein and its major variations, Anat. Rec. 101:581, 1948.

2. Bailey, C.P., *et al.*: Surgical treatment of forty-six inter-atrial septal defects by atrio-septo-pexy, Ann. Surg. 140:805, 1954.

3. Brantigan, O. C.: Anomalies of the pulmonary veins, Surg., Gynec. & Obst. 84:63, 1947.

4. Brody, H.: Drainage of the pulmonary veins into the right side of the heart, Arch. Path. 33:221, 1942.

5. Burroughs, J. T., and Kirklin, J. W.: Complete surgical correction of total anomalous pulmonary venous connection: Report of three cases, Proc. Staff Meet. Mayo Clin. 31:182, 1956.

6. Cooley, D. A., and Mahaffey, D. E.: Anomalous pulmonary venous drainage of entire left lung: Report of case with surgical correction, Ann. Surg. 142:986, 1955.

7. Cooley, D. A., and Ochsner, A., Jr.: Correction of total anomalous pulmonary venous drainage, Surgery 42:1014, 1957.

8. Cooley, D. A., and Collins, H. A.: Anomalous drainage of entire pulmonary venous system into left innominate vein: Clinical and surgical considerations, Circulation 19:486, 1959.

9. Cooley, D. A., and Balas, P. E.: Total anomalous pulmonary drainage into the inferior vena cava: Report of successful surgical correction, Surgery 51:798, 1962.

10. Cooley, D. A.; Ellis, P. R., Jr., and Bellizi, M. E.: Atrial septal defects of the sinus venosus type: Surgical considerations, Dis. Chest 39:185, 1961.

11. Cooley, D. A., and Hallman, G. L.: *Surgical Treatment of Congenital Heart Disease* (Philadelphia: Lea & Febiger, 1966), p. 143.

12. Cooley and Hallman,[12] p. 98.

13. Cooley, D. A.; Hallman, G. L., and Leachman, R. D.: Total anomalous pulmonary venous drainage: Correction using cardiopulmonary bypass in 62 patients, J. Thoracic & Cardiovas. Surg. 51:88, 1966.

14. Darling, R. C.; Rothney, W. B., and Craig, J. M.: Total pulmonary venous drainage into the right side of the heart: Report of 17 autopsied cases not associated with other major cardiovascular anomalies, Lab. Invest. 6:44, 1957.

15. Dean, J. C., and Fox, G. W.: A left pulmonary vein emptying into the left innominate, Wisconsin M. J. 27:120, 1928.

16. Dotter, C. T.; Hardisty, N. M., and Steinberg, I.: Anomalous right pulmonary vein entering the inferior vena cava: Two cases diagnosed during life by angiocardiography and cardiac catheterization, Am. J. M. Sc. 218:31, 1949.

17. Edwards, J. E.: Pathologic and developmental considerations in anomalous pulmonary venous connections, Proc. Staff Meet. Mayo Clin. 28:441, 1953.

18. Edwards, J. E., and Helmholz, H. F., Jr.: A classification of total anomalous pulmonary venous connection based on developmental considerations, Proc. Staff Meet. Mayo Clin. 31:151, 1956.

19. Friedlowsky: Cited by Brody.[4]

20. Gott, V. L., *et al.*: Total pulmonary return: An analysis of 30 cases, Circulation 13:543, 1956.

21. Gerbode, F. L.: Discussion of Scannell, J. G. and Shaw, R. S.: Surgical reconstruction of the superior vena cava, J. Thoracic Surg. 28:163, 1954.

22. Healey, J. E.: An anatomic survey of anomalous pulmonary veins: Their clinical significance, J. Thoracic Surg. 23:433, 1952.

23. Hughes, C. W., and Rumore, P. C.: Anomalous pulmonary veins, Arch. Path. 37:364, 1944.

24. Kirklin, J. W.: Surgical treatment of anomalous pulmonary venous connection, Proc. Staff Meet. Mayo Clin. 28:476, 1953.

25. Kirklin, J. W.; Ellis, F. H., and Wood, E. H.: Treatment of anomalous pulmonary venous connections in association with interatrial communications, Surgery 39:389, 1956.

26. Lewis, F. J., *et al*: Direct vision repair of triatrial heart and total anomalous pulmonary venous drainage, Surg., Gynec. & Obst. 102:713, 1956.

27. Muller, W. H., Jr.: The surgical treatment of transposition of the pulmonary veins, Ann. Surg. 134:683, 1951.

28. Neptune, W. B.; Bailey, C. P., and Goldberg, H.: Surgical correction of atrial septal defects associated with transposition of pulmonary veins, J. Thoracic Surg. 25:623, 1953.

29. Ross, D. N.: Atrial septal defect: Surgical anatomy and technique, Guy's Hosp. Rep. 105:376, 1956.

30. Sloan, H. J., et al.: Open heart surgery in infancy, J. Thoracic & Cardiovas. Surg. 44:459, 1962.

31. Snellen, H. A., and Albers, F. H.: The clinical significance of anomalous pulmonary venous drainage, Circulation 6:6, 1952.

32. Swan, H. J. C.; Burchell, H. B., and Wood, E. H.: Differential diagnosis at cardiac catheterization of anomalous pulmonary venous drainage related to atrial septal defects or abnormal venous connections, Proc. Staff Meet. Mayo Clin. 28:452, 1953.

33. Taussig, H.: *Congenital Malformations of the Heart* (New York: The Commonwealth Fund, 1947).

34. Wagstaffe, W. W.: Two cases of free communication between the auricle by deficiency of the upper part of the septum auricularum, Tr. Path. Soc., London 19:96, 1868.

35. Wilson, J.: A description of a very unusual formation of the human heart, Phil. Tr. Roy. Soc., London 88:346, 1798.

36. Winslow: Cited by Brody.[4]

37. Woodwark, G. M.; Vinve, D. J., and Ashmore, P. G.: Total anomalous pulmonary venous return to the portal vein: Report of a case of successful surgical treatment, J. Thoracic & Cardiovas. Surg. 45:662, 1963.

D. A. Cooley
G. L. Hallman

Drawings by
Barbara Anderson Tuttle
(Figures 37-1, *B*; 37-2 to
37-4, and 37-7)
Herb Smith
(Figures 37-1, *C*; 37-8 to 37-11)

Bulbus Cordis Anomalies

Transposition
of the Great Arteries

HISTORY. — The pathologic anatomy and diagnostic characteristics of transposition were fully described by Taussig[22] in 1938. The first attempt at palliative treatment was creation of an atrial septal defect by Blalock and Hanlon[4] in 1950. In 1953, Lillehei and Varco[14] attempted to transfer the right pulmonary veins to the right atrium and the inferior vena cava to the left atrium. These attempts were unsuccessful. In 1954, Glenn and Patino[10] developed an effective palliative operation for patients with transposition and pulmonary stenosis by anastomosing the right pulmonary artery to the superior vena cava. In 1956, Baffes[3] described transfer of the right pulmonary veins to the right atrium and grafting of the inferior vena cava to the left atrium. By this operation, palliation was achieved in a large number of patients. Various attempts at total correction on the arterial side failed.[11,16] Albert[2] in 1954 suggested complete transfer of the venous side, but this too failed in others' hands.[12,15,25] Senning[20] in 1959 reported atrial transposition in a 9-year-old boy with success. Because of the lethal nature of the lesion in infancy, we devised a two-stage correction, reported in 1964.[17]

INCIDENCE

Transposition is probably more common than statistical surveys indicate. Many babies with this anomaly must die in maternity hospitals, and many probably do not even come to autopsy. However, in one series of cases of cyanotic heart disease that came to autopsy, transposition of the great arteries accounted for 20.2%.[13] Strangely, it is more common in boys than in girls, in a ratio of 2.5:1.[13] The life span without palliation is relatively short, at least 90% dying within the first year of life.

PATHOLOGIC ANATOMY

The simplest explanation for this anomaly is the straight development in the embryo of the conotruncal septum rather than the normal 180° twist.[7] Two functioning ventricles are present, each with a patent atrioventricular valve. The aorta arises from the right ventricle and the pulmonary artery from the left. Associated cardiac anomalies may be present, but for those amenable to surgery there are four groups. In the commonest form of transposition, the ventricular septum is intact and a patent foramen ovale and patent ductus arteriosus are present at birth. The second most common form is that in which a ventricular septal defect is also present. Two relatively uncommon types are associated with left ventricular outflow obstruction with or without a ventricular septal defect.

NATURAL HISTORY

In 243 proved cases of transposition of the great arteries studied by Shaher[21] at the Hospital for Sick Children, Toronto, there were 153 with an intact ventricular septum, and 70% of these patients died within the first month. Of the patients with a ventricular septal defect, 50% survived 1–4 months. When left ventricular outflow obstruction was present, 50% survived 1–5 years. If one includes all types, 90% are dead within the first year of life.

HEMODYNAMICS

In complete transposition of the great arteries, two separate circuits of blood exist: the pulmonary, and the systemic. In the pulmonary circuit, blood flows from the pulmonary veins to the left atrium and ventricle, through the pulmonary artery back to the lungs. In the systemic circuit, blood returns from the venae cavae to the right atrium and ventricle through the aorta to the body. Survival would be impossible if there were no associated defects in the form of a patent foramen ovale, ventricular septal defect or patent ductus arteriosus (Fig. 38-1, A and B). Owing to the separate nature of the two circuits, any shunt that occurs between them has to be bidirectional and equal. In complete transposition of the great arteries, some means of oxygenating the blood in the systemic circuit must exist. This is achieved by exchanging part of the mixed venous blood from the pulmonary circuit through the associated defects. This shunt, therefore, is the effective pulmonary blood flow, since it is the volume of mixed venous blood which, after returning to the right atrium, eventually reaches the pulmonary capillaries.

In the presence of a large ventricular septal defect, the pressure in the left (pulmonic) ventricle is systemic. This results in high pulmonary blood flow and early pulmonary vascular disease. Left ventricular

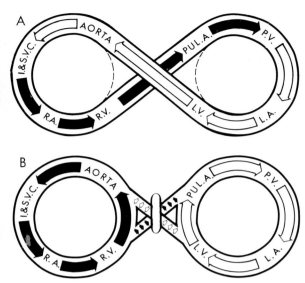

Fig. 38-1.—Circulation in transposition of the great arteries **(B)** compared with normal circulation **(A)**. (From Taussig, H. B.: *Congenital Malformations of the Heart* [Cambridge, Mass.: Harvard University Press, 1960]; by permission.)

outflow obstruction will protect the lung fields from vascular changes.

DIAGNOSIS

INTACT VENTRICULAR SEPTUM.—Within the first week of life, these infants present cyanosis, tachypnea and occasional hypoxia. There may be no murmur, the liver is enlarged, arterial oxygen saturation varies from 20 to 60% and the hemoglobin level is

Fig. 38-2.—Intact ventricular septum. Posteroanterior roentgenogram of an infant 2 weeks old. The heart is egg-shaped and enlarged, and pulmonary vascularity is increased.

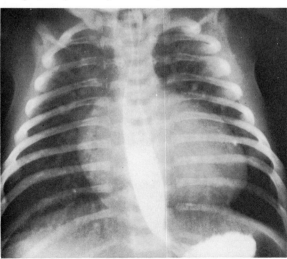

often 20 Gm/100 ml. The heart is typically egg-shaped (Fig. 38-2), and cardiomegaly and increased pulmonary vascularity develop within the first 2 weeks of life. Right heart angiocardiography demonstrates the aorta arising anteriorly, the intact septum and the presence or absence of a patent ductus (Fig. 38-3, *A* and *B*).

VENTRICULAR SEPTAL DEFECT.—The clinical features are similar to those of an intact septum, except for a significant systolic murmur and more pronounced pulmonary vascularity. Right heart angiocardiography will demonstrate the defect (Fig. 38-4), which should be suspected if systemic pressure is present in the left ventricle.

LEFT VENTRICULAR OUTFLOW OBSTRUCTION.—The diagnosis of pulmonary stenosis may be made by angiography or by entering the pulmonary artery during cardiac catheterization. The latter procedure is difficult in the infant, and two techniques have recently been applied. The Radner technique of suprasternal puncture of the pulmonary artery may be useful.[18] Carr[5] has been able almost routinely to enter the pulmonary artery by the introduction of a pre-looped polyethylene tube through a cardiac catheter placed in the left ventricle. We have noted that nearly all cases of pulmonary stenosis have outflow tract obstruction similar to that seen in tetralogy of Fallot (Fig. 38-5).

PALLIATIVE PROCEDURES

INTACT VENTRICULAR SEPTUM.—The creation of an atrial septal defect to enhance pulmonary blood flow has given encouraging results. The Blalock-Hanlon technique (Fig. 38-6) and the inflow occlusion open technique (Fig. 38-7) have a fairly high mortality in the first week or two of life, but in the older infant they are very satisfactory. The advantages of the Blalock-Hanlon technique are the enlargement of both atriums by elimination of the intra-atrial groove and the production of semipartial anomalous pulmonary venous drainage. Dramatic results in the very young infant have been reported with the Rashkind and Miller[19] technique of balloon septostomy, by which a balloon inflated with contrast material is pulled forcibly through the septum, tearing the thin inferior margin (Fig. 38-8). Edwards and Bargeron[9] have transposed the pulmonary veins to the right atrium by a technique similar to the Blalock-Hanlon but without creating an atrial septal defect. This would lessen the pulmonary blood flow but would not increase the effective pulmonary blood flow; that is, the systemic venous return reaching the lungs for oxygenation is not increased. We believe that, if possible, the reduction of pulmonary blood flow and work of the heart may tide a critically ill baby over the newborn period, but that with a closed ventricular septum, an atrial defect should subsequently be created.

VENTRICULAR SEPTAL DEFECT.—A ventricular septal defect large enough to produce systemic or near-systemic pressure in the left ventricle presents a dif-

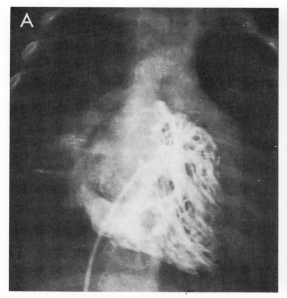
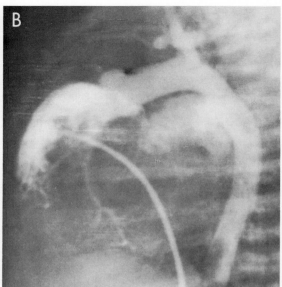

Fig. 38-3.—Intact ventricular septum. **A,** right heart angiogram, anteroposterior view, demonstrating the trabeculated right ventricle giving rise to the aorta. **B,** lateral view, with contrast medium clearly delineating the intact septum, origin of the aorta from the right ventricle, and a large patent ductus.

ferent problem in palliation. Bidirectional shunting may be sufficient to maintain a reasonable arterial oxygen saturation (above 65%), and the creation of an atrial septal defect will not improve the infant's condition.[21] The ventricular septal defect creates a high pulmonary flow with subsequent early pulmonary vascular disease that is irreversible. There is, for palliation, a method of banding the pulmonary artery to protect the lungs. It is difficult to band tightly enough to produce adequate stenosis without having the heart fail. It appears that banding of the pulmonary artery should be accompanied or followed either by the creation of an atrial septal defect or by shifting of the atrial septum, as suggested by Edwards and Bargeron.[9] As the perfusion techniques in infants improve, it may be possible to close the ventricular

Fig. 38-4.—Ventricular septal defect. Right heart angiogram, lateral view, demonstrating the septal defect and transposition of the great arteries. Note also the equal size of the great vessels and absence of left ventricular outflow obstruction.

Fig. 38-5.—Left ventricular outflow obstruction. Left heart angiogram, lateral view; **arrows** indicate the obstruction.

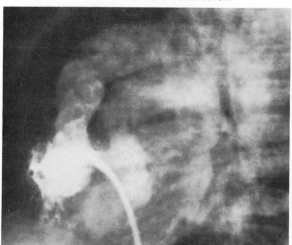
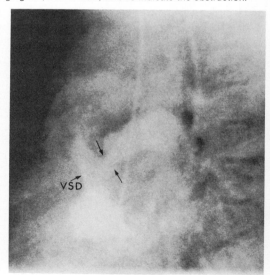

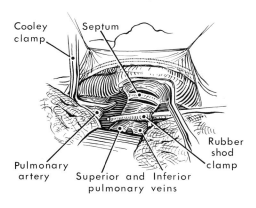

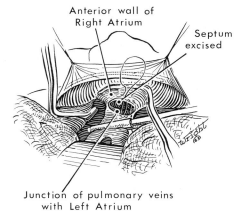

Fig. 38-6.—Creation of atrial septal defect: Blalock-Hanlon technique. When this technique is used, it is important to release the clamp on the pulmonary veins several times to avoid venous engorgement of the right lung.

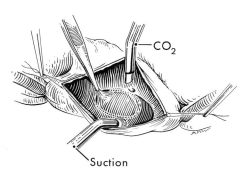

Fig. 38-7.—Creation of atrial septal defect: inflow occlusion open technique. Immediately before a clamp is applied to the right atrium, the anesthesiologist should inflate the lungs to fill the right side of the heart with blood. (From Trusler, G. A., et al.: Canad. M. A. J. 91:1096, 1964.)

Fig. 38-8.—Creation of atrial septal defect: balloon septostomy technique of Rashkind and Miller.[19] The balloon must be pulled forcibly and quickly through the foramen ovale of the left to the right atrium.

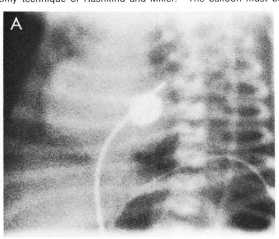

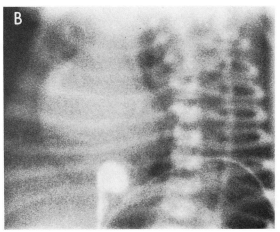

septal defect through the atrium and create an atrial septal defect. Total correction may even be possible, as was reported by Dillard *et al.,*[8] who used deep hypothermia alone. This remarkable surgical feat was, however, performed in an infant with a closed ventricular septum, for which the creation of an atrial septal defect is indicated on the reasonable assumption that the mortality would, in a series of cases, be much less.

PULMONARY STENOSIS. — The infant under 6 months who requires surgery with transposition of the great arteries and pulmonary stenosis must have a shunting procedure to survive. In this age group, the best shunting procedure is that suggested by Waterston[24] of anastomosing the right pulmonary artery to the ascending aorta side-to-side. It is a good procedure because it can be accomplished even with a pulmonary artery of 3 – 4 mm in diameter. In children over 6 months of age, it appears that the procedure suggested by Glenn and Patino[10] of anastomosing the superior vena cava with the right pulmonary artery and ligating the superior vena cava at the caval-atrial junction is the operation of choice. These children develop an oxygen saturation in the high 80's and do very well. It should not preclude total correction at a later date.

TOTAL CORRECTION

Senning[20] reported the first successful total correction in 1959. His technique is very ingenious; the description of the operation will be found in his paper. The principle of the operation is correction on the atrial side. The atrial septum is incised and sewn above the entrance of the left pulmonary veins. The left atrium is incised at the junction of the right pulmonary venous connection, and the medial lip of the right atriotomy is then sutured to the lateral lip of the left atriotomy incision. His first success was in a 9-year-old boy with an ostium secundum defect — a rather rare occurrence. Our concern was that in a small child, the atriums would not be large enough to handle the circulation,[23] and in our experience of 4 cases, the children died postoperatively with low cardiac output and pulmonary edema. These observations led us to develop a two-stage intra-atrial baffle operation[17] based on the original concept of Albert.[2]

INTRA-ATRIAL BAFFLE OPERATION. — Assuming that the child has had a palliative operation in infancy, surgery (Fig. 38-9) is undertaken as early as 18 months or older if the child is doing reasonably well and pulmonary hypertension is not developing.

A median sternotomy provides good exposure. The pericardium is excised, as large a piece as possible, from one phrenic nerve to the other. According to the age of the child, one can gauge roughly the size of this pericardial graft. At 3, 4 or 5 years of age, 4 × 9 cm will suffice. One should not have the baffle too redundant; if the left atrial pressure were higher than

pressure in the right, a redundant baffle might occlude the mitral orifice. The venae cavae are cannulated as caudad and cephalad as possible to ensure adequate exposure through the right atrium, and a curved atriotomy incision is performed (Fig. 38-9, *A*). If a ventricular septal defect is present, one attempts to approach it through the tricuspid valve and repair it by direct suture. If this is not possible, the tricuspid valve is taken down through the annulus of the medial leaflet and either a patch closure or direct closure of the septal defect is performed. If the preoperative pressure in the left ventricle is low (30 – 40 mm Hg), it may be safe to leave the defect. After the atrial septal defect is exposed the remaining portion of the septum is completely excised, with care to suture and endothelialize the entire cephalad surface of the intra-atrial septum. Medially, a portion of the intermuscular septum is left between the mitral and tricuspid valves to avoid damage to the bundle when the baffle is sutured in place. The coronary sinus is generously opened into the left atrium and all tags of the septum are removed to allow as great an area as possible between the left and right atriums to carry both circulations (*B* and *C*). The baffle is sutured in place, commencing at the superior margin of the inferior pulmonary vein on the left, by a double-armed suture (*D*); we prefer to use 3-0 silk. The suturing of the baffle in place must be done extremely carefully to avoid any leaks. It must be quite close to the orifices of the left pulmonary veins to allow adequate flow from the venae cavae to reach the mitral valve. One actually dumbbells in the suturing, excluding the caval cannulas as one comes up along the right atrial wall and down across above the coronary sinus onto the cut edge of the baffle (*E*). Any extra pericardium should be removed; then the tape is removed briefly from the superior vena cava and the superior venal catheter occluded to test the baffle to be sure there are no leaks. The same maneuver is done with the inferior vena cava. The new left atrium is usually enlarged, either by a prosthesis or by pericardial graft which is left over from the removal of pericardium (*F*). As the new left atrium is closed, the right ventricle is vented to allow escape of any trapped air and to prevent overdistention. After completion of the repair of the new left atrium, the superior catheter is removed first, and the inferior catheter withdrawn but not removed in case support is needed. If the heart is taking over very well, it should be removed rather promptly to prevent any inferior caval obstruction. If the flow is annoying during the operation, the temperature can be reduced to 30 C and the flow decreased; temporary occlusion of the aorta to remove the coronary sinus return may be useful to improve the exposure, although we have not found this to be necessary. Venting the ventricle and fibrillating the heart are good safeguards against trapping air, although we do not do this routinely.

Aberdeen and Waterston[1] leave a small portion of

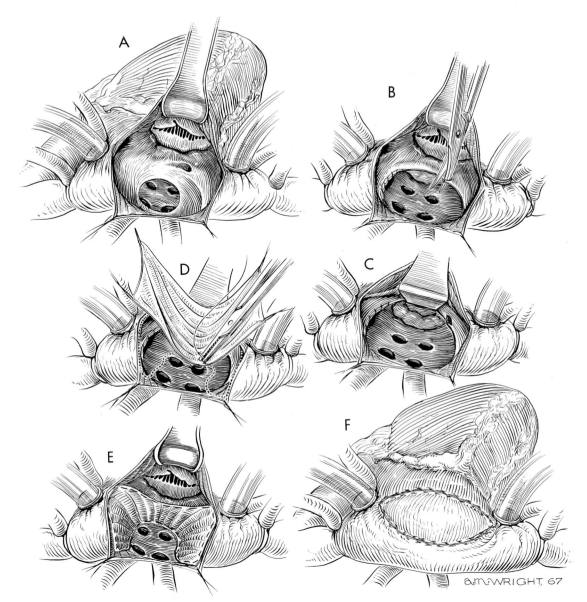

Fig. 38-9.—Total correction by intra-atrial baffle technique. See text for description.

the caudad septum and use this as a pedicle flap hinged on the coronary sinus. The inferior margin of this flap is sutured above the inferior caval catheter and the superior margin to the baffle. There may be some merit in this maneuver since a portion of the baffle is autogenous septum with a good blood supply for future growth.

In the presence of a previous Baffes procedure,[3] we have had gratifying results in 2 children in the older age group. If the pressure in the left ventricle is low, a pericardial baffle may be sutured in place to redirect

the superior vena cava into the left atrium. When one excises the intra-atrial septum, the orifice of the inferior vena cava, by virtue of the position of the graft, is in the center of the posterior wall of the left atrium. To place a baffle in the usual position would almost certainly interfere with left pulmonary venous drainage. Insertion of a pericardial patch and direction of the superior vena cava to the left atrium as one does with partial anomalous venous drainage appears to be safe and simple. The patient is left with pulmonary venous drainage from the left lung into the left atrium. Partial anomalous pulmonary venous drainage with an intact atrial septum may be compatible with longevity.

Postoperative Complications

Apart from the usual complications following a prolonged pump run, certain specific ones follow the intra-atrial baffle operation. An improperly placed baffle may cause caval or pulmonary venous obstruction. With the use of a respirator and proper positioning of the patient, one can hopefully wait for a balancing of the two circulations. We are, however, indebted to Clarke and Barrett-Boyes[6] for drawing attention to severe pulmonary edema caused by mediastinal clot in the postoperative period. Prompt reoperation following recognition of this complication cured their 2 patients. Since their report, we have encountered this on one occasion, with a favorable outcome. Complete heart block is as catastrophic as in other heart operations and must be avoided. Arrhythmias are not uncommon in the postoperative period but generally disappear during the second week. If the heart rate is slow (60 or 65) as the patient comes off by-pass, a temporary pacemaker should be employed.

Results of Surgery

As we gradually recognize that these anomalies in certain children are inoperable, the results are encouraging. In our experience of 30 cases, we would now not attempt total correction in 10 of them. Six patients had systemic pressure in the pulmonary artery and 4 had ventricular septal defects with left ventricular outflow obstruction. The latter condition we now palliate with a superior vena cava-pulmonary artery shunt, which should not preclude eventual total correction. Among the other 20 patients there are 14 survivors, 1 of whom, 5 years after surgery, was doing very well. There were 3 late deaths, 1 due to an improperly placed baffle (3 months after operation), 1 due to the baffle becoming free because of improper suturing and 1 of ventricular fibrillation following a late catheter study. It is gratifying that other centers are having success in the properly selected case with low left ventricular pressure.

REFERENCES

1. Aberdeen, E., and Waterston, D. J.: Successful correction of transposed arteries by Mustard's operation, Lancet 1:1233, 1965.
2. Albert, H. M.: Surgical correction of transposition of the great vessels, S. Forum, p. 74, 1955.
3. Baffes, T. G.: A new method for surgical correction of transposition of the aorta and pulmonary artery, Surg., Gynec. & Obst. 102:227, 1956.
4. Blalock, A., and Hanlon, C. R.: The surgical treatment of complete transposition of the aorta and the pulmonary artery, Surg., Gynec. & Obst. 90:1, 1950.
5. Carr, I., and Wells, B.: Coaxial flow-guided catheterisation of the pulmonary artery in transposition of the great arteries, Lancet 2:318, 1966.
6. Clarke, C. P., and Barrett-Boyes, B. G. The cause and treatment of pulmonary edema after the Mustard operation for correction of complete transposition of the great vessels, J. Thoracic & Cardiovas. Surg. 54:1, 1967.
7. De la Cruz, M. V., and da Rocha, J. P.: An ontogenetic theory for the explanation of congenital malformations involving the truncus, Am. Heart J. 51:782, 1956.
8. Dillard, D. H., et al.: Correction of total anomalous pulmonary venous drainage in infancy utilizing deep hypothermia with total circulatory arrest, Circulation 35 (supp.): 105, 1967.
9. Edwards, W. S., and Bargeron, L. M., Jr.: More effective palliation of transposition of the great vessels, J. Thoracic & Cardiovas. Surg. 49:790, 1965.
10. Glenn, W. W. L., and Patino, J. F.: Circulatory by-pass of the right heart: I. Preliminary observations on the direct delivery of vena caval blood in the pulmonary arterial circulation, Yale J. Biol. & Med. 27:147, 1954.
11. Idriss, F. S., et al.: A new technic for complete correction of transposition of the great vessels, Circulation 24:5, 1961.
12. Kay, E. B., and Cross, F. S.: Transposition of the great vessels corrected by means of atrial transposition, Surgery 41:938, 1957.
13. Keith, J. D.; Rowe, R. D., and Vlad, P.: *Heart Disease in Infancy and Childhood* (New York: Macmillan Company, 1958), p. 472.
14. Lillehei, C. W., and Varco, R. L.: Certain physiologic, pathologic and surgical features of complete transposition of the great vessels, Surgery 34:376, 1953.
15. Merendino, K. A., et al.: Interatrial venous transposition—a one-stage intracardiac operation for the conversion of complete transposition of the aorta and pulmonary artery to corrected transposition: Theory and clinical experience, Surgery 42:898, 1957.
16. Mustard, W. T., et al.: A surgical approach to transposition of the great vessels with extracorporeal circuit, Surgery 36:39, 1954.
17. Mustard, W. T., et al.: Successful two-stage correction of transposition of the great vessels, Surgery 55:469, 1964.
18. Rahimtoola, S. H.; Ongley, P. A., and Swan, H. J. C.: Percutaneous suprasternal puncture (Radner technique) of the pulmonary artery in transposition of the great vessels, Circulation 33:242, 1966.
19. Rashkind, W. J., and Miller, W. W.: Creation of an atrial septal defect without thoracotomy, J.A.M.A. 196:991, 1966.
20. Senning, A.: Surgical correction of transposition of the great vessels, Surgery 45:966, 1959.
21. Shaher, R. M.: Prognosis of transposition of the great vessels with and without atrial septal defect, Brit. Heart J. 25:211, 1963.
22. Taussig, H. B.: Complete transposition of the great vessels, Am. Heart J. 16:728, 1938.
23. Trusler, G. A., et al.: The effect on cardiac output of a reduction in atrial volume, J. Thoracic & Cardiovas. Surg. 46:109, 1963.
24. Waterston, D. J.: Treatment of Fallot's tetralogy in children under one year of age, Rozhl. chir. 41:181, 1962.
25. Wilson, H. E., et al.: Rational approach to surgery for complete transposition of the great vessels, Ann. Surg. 155:258, 1962.

W. T. Mustard

Drawings by
A. M. Wright

Double Outlet from Right Ventricle

AN UNCOMMON LESION is that in which the aorta and the pulmonary artery have their origin from the right ventricle. A ventricular defect is present that allows the left ventricular chamber to empty preferentially into the aorta or pulmonary artery, depending on its location.[4] If pulmonary stenosis is present, differentiation from severe tetralogy of Fallot is difficult. Surgical interest has been stimulated by reports of successful correction by rerouting the ventricular septal defect to the aorta via a tunnel[2,3] (Fig. 38-10, *A*). When the defect is related to the pulmonary artery, it may be possible to correct the condition into a true transposition[1] (*B*) and then perform a total correction by inserting an intra-atrial baffle (see Fig. 38-9).

REFERENCES

1. Daicoff, G. R., and Kirklin, J. W.: Surgical correction of a Taussig-Bing malformation: Report of 3 cases, Am. J. Cardiol. 19:125, 1967 (abst.).
2. McGoon, D. C.: Origin of great vessels from the right ventricle, S. Clin. North America 41:1113, 1961.
3. Redo, S. F., *et al.*: Operative correction of ventricular septal defect with origin of both great vessels from the right ventricle, J. Thoracic & Cardiovas. Surg. 45:526, 1963.

W. T. MUSTARD

Drawings by
E. HOPPER ROSS

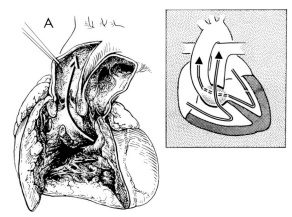 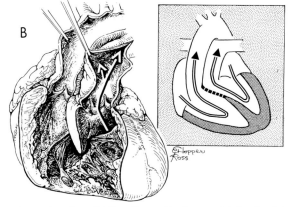

Fig. 38-10.—Double outlet φ from the right ventricle. **A,** when the ventricular septal defect is related to the aorta and there is no fixed pulmonary vascular disease, correction may be accomplished by tunneling the ventricular septal defect to the aorta, using pericardium. **B,** When the ventricular septal defect is related to the pulmonary artery (Taussig-Bing), closure of the defect will create transposition of the great arteries. This can then be corrected with an intra-atrial baffle (see Fig. 38-9).

Single Ventricle

PATHOLOGIC ANATOMY.—In cases of single ventricle, the ventricular septum is not present or is rudimentary and is commonly associated with transposition or corrected transposition of the great arteries. This malformation, which is simply a very large septal defect, may have a muscular band crossing its midportion. A rudimentary septum may arise from the wall of the ventricle.

DIAGNOSIS.—A systolic murmur is heard over the precordium, and usually cyanosis and dyspnea are present. The radiographic patterns are varied, depending on the presence or absence of transposition of the great arteries or of associated defects such as pulmonic stenosis. Because of rotation of the heart, the electrocardiogram reveals a wide range of electrical axis with both left and right ventricular hypertrophy. Cardiac catheterization discloses a rise of oxygen saturation in the common ventricle with systolic systemic pressures. Angiocardiography might be very useful in confirming the diagnosis.

OPERATIVE TREATMENT.—Fortunately for the surgeon, pulmonary stenosis is associated in 25% of the cases. If severe cyanosis is present, palliation may be achieved by anastomosing the ascending aorta to the right pulmonary artery. If the child survives to age $1\frac{1}{2}$–2 years, effective palliation may be obtained by anastomosis of the right pulmonary artery to the superior vena cava. Complete correction using cardiac by-pass had been sporadically reported. Technically, it is a difficult procedure to complete satisfactorily, but in the future may become feasible. We have had experience with 3 patients, 1 of whom survived, but with incomplete closure.

W. T. MUSTARD

Persistent Truncus Arteriosus

Collett and Edwards[1] have classified this lesion into four types. In type I, there is a single arterial trunk giving rise to a single pulmonary artery and ascending aorta. In type II, the right and left pulmonary arteries arise separately from the dorsal wall of the truncus. In type III, one or both pulmonary arteries arise independently from either side of the truncus. In type IV, neither the pulmonary arteries nor the ductus arteriosus is present, and the arterial circulation to the lungs is furnished by the bronchial arteries. The surgeon is interested in types I and II. In infancy and early childhood, banding of the main pulmonary artery in type I or of both in type II might be beneficial and prevent the onset of pulmonary vascular disease. In the absence of pulmonary vascular disease, it is feasible to attempt to reconstruct the main pulmonary artery and close the ventricular septal defect. A valve would be necessary in the reconstructed pulmonary artery. Two unsuccessful attempts were reported by Cooley and Hallman.[2]

REFERENCES

1. Collett, R. W., and Edwards, J. E.: Persistent truncus arteriosus: Classification according to anatomic types, S. Clin. North America 29:1245, 1949.
2. Cooley, D. A., and Hallman, G. L.: *Surgical Treatment of Congenital Heart Disease* (Philadelphia: Lea & Febiger, 1966), p. 185.

W. T. MUSTARD

Aortic Origin of Right Pulmonary Artery

SINCE THE ADVENT of angiocardiography, this rare anomaly has been diagnosed more frequently. Because it is usually fatal in infancy, attempt at surgical correction is indicated. In 1961, Armer *et al.*[1] succeeded in correcting the anomaly in a year-old boy, using a Teflon graft. Several years ago, we attempted to re-anastomose the right pulmonary artery to the main trunk, but the patient died of cardiac arrest on the operating table. Since then, Kirkpatrick and co-workers[2] accomplished this in a 7-month-old infant (Fig. 38-11). This appears to be the logical approach, and on our next attempt we will have a pump stand-by.

REFERENCES

1. Armer, R. M.,*et al.*: Origin of the right pulmonary artery from the ascending aorta: Report of a surgically corrected case, Circulation 24:662, 1961.
2. Kirkpatrick, S. E., *et al.*: Aortic origin of the right pulmonary artery, Circulation 36:777, 1967.

W. T. MUSTARD

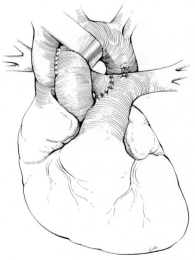

Fig. 38-11.—Aortic origin of the right pulmonary artery; completed surgical repair. The ductus arteriosus has been doubly ligated and divided and the right pulmonary artery anastomosed to the main pulmonary artery behind the aorta. (From Kirkpatrick *et al.*[2])

Pulmonary Atresia and Pulmonic Stenosis with Normal Aortic Root

Pulmonary Atresia with Normal Aortic Root

THIS COMPLEX ANOMALY comprises less than 1% of all congenital heart disease. The atresia usually is at the pulmonary valve with three small ridges marking the site of adhesion of the three partially formed valve leaflets. The pulmonary artery is hypoplastic to a variable extent. The interventricular septum is intact. Frequently, there is marked hypertrophy of the right ventricular myocardium with a very small right ventricular chamber and a small hypoplastic tricuspid valve (Fig. 38-12). In about 15% of cases, the right ventricle has a larger lumen and is less hypertrophied. An interatrial communication is always present. It is usually in the form of a small patent foramen ovale, and as a result there is dilatation of the right atrium with hypertrophy of its wall. All blood entering the right atrium must pass through the interatrial communication to the left atrium and left ventricle and then out the systemic circuit. Pulmonary circulation, and life, are largely maintained by a small patent ductus arteriosus.

CLINICAL FEATURES

Severe cyanosis inversely proportional to the flow through the ductus usually is observed shortly after birth. There are no cardiac murmurs except for those originating in the patent ductus arteriosus. Radiographic examination shows decreased pulmonary vascular markings and a heart that is usually large but may be small. The electrocardiogram demonstrating a left ventricle overloading pattern will distinguish this lesion from tetralogy of Fallot with characteristic right ventricular hypertrophy. In pulmonary atresia and in severe pulmonary stenosis, the venous angiocardiogram shows the filling sequence which is typical of tricuspid atresia as well, and it may be difficult to separate these conditions from one another.

The demonstration of pure left ventricular hypertrophy in the electrocardiogram of a patient with pulmonary atresia suggests that the right ventricle is small. Aside from this, there is no simple way of predicting the size of the ventricle. If a cardiac catheter can be positioned in the right ventricle, selective angiocardiography should clearly indicate ventricular size and demonstrate occlusion of the outflow tract.

TREATMENT

Without treatment, the prognosis is exceedingly poor. Keith *et al.*[10] found that one quarter of the patients died in the first week of life and 78% of the

Fig. 38-12.—Pulmonary atresia with normal aortic root. The drawing **A** of the specimen **B** demonstrates the small right ventricular chamber that almost prohibits surgical correction.

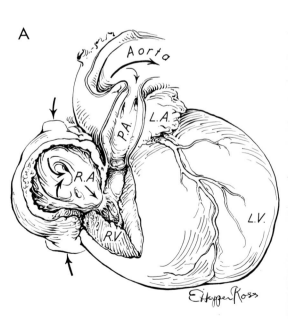
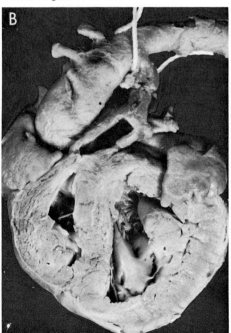

children were dead by 6 months. Frequently, death coincided with closure of the ductus arteriosus. At operation, one must avoid misjudging the size of the right ventricle. The thickness of the right ventricular myocardium sometimes gives the surgeon a mistaken impression of size. The small right ventricular chamber can be suspected if there is an apparent lack of contractility of the right ventricle, a dimple over the lower interventricular sulcus, an anomalous coronary vessel communicating with the right ventricular chamber or a thick, firm feeling to the right ventricle.

When the right ventricle is large, good results should be obtained from pulmonary valvulotomy. When the right ventricle has a small lumen, a systemic-to-pulmonary shunt plus enlargement of the atrial septal defect would seem advisable; we have attempted this unsuccessfully. If the patient with pulmonary atresia with normal aortic root is large enough for a shunt from superior vena cava to pulmonary artery, perhaps this type of right heart bypass would be the procedure of choice. We have not attempted this operation. Unfortunately, no one has reported sufficient cases of pulmonary atresia treated with any of the above methods to allow an accurate estimate of short- or long-term survival.

Pulmonic Stenosis with Normal Aortic Root

Fallot in 1888 separated this malformation from that associated with an interventricular septal defect, and Abrahams and Wood[1] in 1951 introduced the term pulmonic stenosis with normal aortic root.

Fig. 38-13.—Moderate pulmonic stenosis with normal aortic root. **A,** the fish-mouth appearance of the pulmonary valve seen through the incised pulmonary artery at operation with hypothermia and inflow occlusion. Two commissures are seen, one completely and one partially fused. **B,** two incisions between the

Brock[3] and Sellors[14] in 1948 performed the first successful valvulotomies by a transventricular approach, using a valvulotome. Swan[15] introduced the transarterial approach with inflow occlusion and hypothermia in 1954. The open technique with the artificial heart-lung apparatus has been used by a number of surgeons.

INCIDENCE AND PATHOLOGIC ANATOMY

The incidence of pulmonic stenosis appears to be 10% of all congenital heart disease. In all severe forms of pulmonic stenosis, the pulmonary artery is the site of poststenotic dilatation and low pressure. On palpation of the vessel, the valve can be felt projecting into the lumen of the artery like a cervix. A forceful jet through the valve can be eliminated by digital occlusion of the valvular orifice. On inspection, the commissures may be found to be completely fused to the edge of an orifice measuring 2 or 3 mm in diameter. In more moderate pulmonary stenosis, the commissural fusion is less marked, resulting in a larger opening measuring 4–8 mm in diameter. Frequently, the valve is bicuspid and presents a "fish-mouth" appearance (Fig. 38-13). Pure infundibular stenosis must be extremely rare, although Swan *et al.*[16] reported resection in 5 cases. The stenosis in these cases is muscular and located 1 cm below the valve. In our experience with pulmonic stenosis, we encountered only 1 case which had a small ventricular septal defect and therefore did not have a normal aortic root.

commissures to the valve ring give an adequate opening. A sound passed through the valve into the right ventricle encountered no infundibular stenosis. The pressure gradient across the pulmonary valve was reduced from 60 to 20 mm Hg.

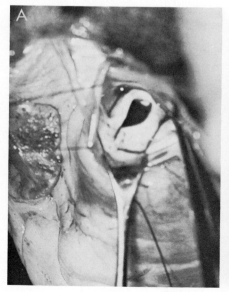
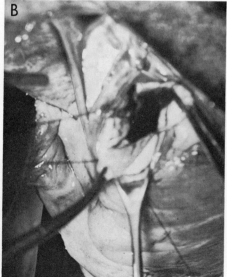

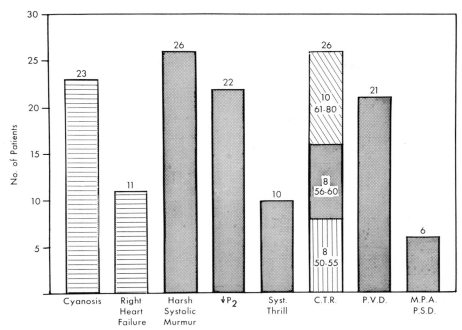

Fig. 38-14.—Pulmonic stenosis with normal aortic root. Clinical and radiographic features in 26 infants in the first year of life. ↓ **P₂**, pulmonary second sound reduced; **C. T. R.**, cardiothoracic ratio; **P. V. D.**, pulmonary vasculature diminished; **M. P. A., P. S. D.**, main pulmonary artery, poststenotic dilatation.

Our experience with childhood lesions leads us to believe that an infundibular stenosis is probably a physiologic hypertrophy of the infundibular area in the presence of a valvular stenosis. Support is lent by Kirklin *et al.*,[11] who proposed resection of the hypertrophied infundibular area since most of their patients were over 15 years of age. As one would expect, right atrial and right ventricular hypertrophy are present and the foramen ovale is usually patent. Occasionally, as in 5 cases in our series, an atrial secundum defect may accompany the pulmonic stenosis. In these children, the valve was only moderately stenosed.

HEMODYNAMICS

In severe stenosis, the right ventricular pressure may be as high as 260 mm Hg. If a patent foramen ovale is present, there may be some degree of cyanosis when the pressure is greater than systemic pressure. Usually in the moderate form of stenosis, pressure in the right ventricle is from 70 to 110 mm Hg. In these cases, in the presence of an open foramen ovale, the shunt is from left to right and the patient is not cyanotic. Oximetry usually yields normal values in patients with pulmonic stenosis except in the more severe forms with a right-to-left shunt.

DIAGNOSIS

In the first year of life, the signs are usually most dramatic. Figure 38-14 illustrates the clinical signs in 26 infants operated on when under 1 year of age at the Hospital for Sick Children, Toronto.

Invariably, a systolic murmur is present over the pulmonary area, usually accompanied by a thrill in severe and in some instances of moderately severe disease. The second heart sound is reduced, and in severe cases there is a precordial heave. In moderate stenosis, the electrocardiogram may be normal, but in the more severe forms, the electrocardiogram shows right axis deviation with a tall R in V₁ (Fig. 38-15). On fluoroscopy, the right atrium may be seen to be enlarged and there is a distinct poststenotic artery

Fig. 38-15.—Pulmonic stenosis with normal aortic root. Height of the R wave in the ECG may be as significant as the pressure recorded in the right ventricle. In this 6-year-old patient, division of the pulmonic valve under direct vision led to dramatic reduction of the R wave 4 years later.

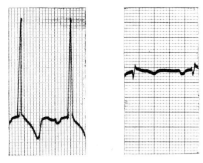

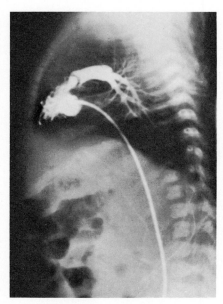

Fig. 38-16.—Pulmonic stenosis with normal aortic root. An-giocardiogram, lateral view, of a 6-week-old infant demonstrates the size of the right ventricle, outline of the stenosed valve and the large pulmonary artery. Selective angiocardiography may aid in diagnosis of severe pulmonic stenosis in infancy.

NATURAL HISTORY

Postmortem studies have indicated 21 years as the average age when death occurs.[4] Severe forms have a graver outlook. Death in the first year of life is not uncommon; of 16 deaths in the first 6 years reported by Keith, 9 were in the first year. Abrahams and Wood[1] expressed the view that patients with severe cases who survive the first year of life die of congestive failure in the second and third decade. Death occurs during anoxic attacks or from right heart failure.

INDICATIONS FOR OPERATION

As in most congenital defects, the indications for operation become more clearly defined as experience is gained by both cardiologist and surgeon. The severity of the lesion must be weighed against the morbidity and mortality of operative intervention. With a mortality of 1% and very little morbidity following valvulotomy, we operate in cases of moderate stenosis when the pressure gradient across the valve is 45 mm Hg or over. In severe cases, particularly in infancy, operation should be undertaken when the diagnosis has been established. The infant in severe distress may present a surgical emergency, as has occurred in several of our cases, particularly in the instance of a 4-day-old infant who was successfully operated on.

bulge. Hilar shadows are reduced; the heart with only moderate stenosis may not be enlarged.

Cardiac catheterization (Fig. 38-16) has proved useful when the diagnosis has been difficult. The withdrawal tracing, if performed carefully, should demonstrate the site of the obstruction. A sharply peaked apex is helpful in distinguishing this defect from tetralogy of Fallot. Cardiac catheterization is very useful to ascertain the right ventricular pressure in cases of moderate stenosis. Furthermore, selective angiocardiography may help to demonstrate the late emptying of the right atrium and right ventricle in severe forms of stenosis.

DIFFERENTIAL DIAGNOSIS

In the infant, pulmonic stenosis with normal aortic root may be difficult to distinguish from aortic stenosis. The cyanotic infant with absence of murmur or a continuous murmur due to a ductus and with left ventricular hypertrophy should lead one to suspect the presence of pulmonary atresia. Hyaline membrane disease with primary pulmonary hypertension may be ruled out by cardiac catheterization. Transposition of the great vessels with pulmonic stenosis may be diagnosed by selective angiocardiography to demonstrate the anteriorly placed aorta. We operated on 1 infant whose findings were typical of pulmonic stenosis only to find a classic Ebstein malformation.

OPERATIVE TECHNIQUE

Valvulotomy through the right ventricle was introduced by Sellors and by Brock and is still performed in some centers. With experience, one should be able to divide a valve reasonably accurately. Perhaps because of our inexperience in earlier cases, we became dissatisfied with this technique and prefer to divide the valve under direct vision. Many of our patients operated on by the blind technique seemed to do well the first few years following division of the valve but subsequently demonstrated an increased right ventricular pressure, indicating perhaps that the stenosis had recurred. At reoperation it did not appear that the valve had been adequately divided, or else the cut edges of the valve had reunited. Whether, when using the transventricular approach, the valve had been inadequately divided or whether the cusps had re-fused will be decided when the long-term results from open valvulotomy are studied. From personal communications, we judge that most surgeons prefer to use hypothermia with inflow occlusion and division of the valve as advocated by Swan. Others, however, still prefer the artificial heart-lung machine with cardiac by-pass. Two main objections can be raised to this procedure. First, the field is not as dry as it is when hypothermia and inflow occlusion are used, necessitating some form of cardioplegia to prevent coronary flow from flooding the field via the right ventricle. Second, the expense and elaborate set-up seem unnecessary. Lam and Raber[12] reported division of the valve with inflow occlusion at normothermic temperatures. Most surgeons prefer to have a greater margin of time.

There are two approaches to the area, one the trans-sternal and one the split-sternal approach. We have used both exposures and indeed have used the trans-sternal approach in the third left interspace, transecting the sternum but not entering the right chest. This gives a fairly adequate exposure but makes taping of the inferior vena cava difficult. With increasing experience with the split-sternal incision, we now use this approach routinely, draining only the mediastinum if the pleural cavities are not entered. There is considerable variation in the actual operative technique in preparation for division of the valve. In early reports, Swan clamped the aorta at the origin of the coronary vessels to prevent air embolism. We no longer consider this necessary, nor is it essential to clamp the pulmonary artery on the distal side of the incision, as the blood seems to pool in the pulmonary artery rather than enter the field. With this background, our present technique consists of taping the venae cavae intrapericardially and incising the pulmonary artery just distal to the valve after application of a curved Potts clamp. Stay sutures at either end of the incision facilitate closure. The length of the incision varies from approximately 2 cm in an older child to 1 cm in the infant.

The caval tapes are closed, the heart is emptied of blood, and the curved clamp removed, allowing the incision in the pulmonary artery to open. The valve is grasped with two forceps, delivered into the incision and inspected to assess the amount of stenosis present and the position of the commissures. In severe forms, where the commissures appear to be completely fused, commissurotomy may be performed. In many cases, however, the commissures appear to be ill-defined, and in many moderate forms it seems that division of the commissures would not produce satisfactory enlargement of the stenosed valve. Since pulmonary incompetence is a relatively benign lesion and adequate relief of stenosis is essential, we have been cutting directly through the valve leaflets to the ring rather than dividing the commissures. An alternative method of dividing the valve may have some merit in lessening incompetence: two commissures are divided to the wall of the pulmonary artery and incisions are extended along the annulus. Only time will reveal the answer to some of these problems, as we do not have a really accurate assessment of pulmonic incompetence in these cases. After division of the valve, a sound of adequate size is passed through the valve to determine the presence of infundibular stenosis and also to assess the size of the right ventricle. In older children, a finger may be put through the valvular orifice. It is possible that in a flaccid heart, one may miss an infundibular stenosis, particularly if it is a physiologic thickening of the muscle and is present only on systole; however, descriptions in the literature of isolated infundibular stenosis in the presence of intact ventricular septum indicate that one could not get a sound or a finger through the obstruction. In our own case, it would have been impossible to introduce even a small sound through the infundibular area. In our experience, right ventricular pressures taken at the time of operation are very unreliable and indeed startling in some cases, although we have recorded a drop of pressure from 125 to 25 mm Hg following valvulotomy in an infant. The drop of pressure in older children may be surprisingly minimal at operation, and in some, the pressure in the right ventricle seems elevated following division of the valve. A drop of pressure which is only slight could be explained on the basis of physiologic hypertrophy of the muscle in the infundibular area due to the valvular stenosis. Engle reported 3 cases with no significant fall of right ventricular pressures of 150 mm Hg after divison of the valve but a year later demonstrated right ventricular pressures of 30 mm Hg. We have felt that the pressure drop is often delayed but is more certain if the patient is under 6 years of age. Johnson,[9] in a study of 75 patients operated on by Brock, found secondary infundibular stenosis present in 51% of those who underwent a closed operation but in 77% following open valvulotomy. There seems to be no adequate explanation for these varying reports. Closure of the incision in the pulmonary artery is effected by a running 5-0 suture, and if neither pleural space has been entered, the mediastinum and pericardial sac are carefully and adequately drained, leaving the pleural cavities intact.

POSTOPERATIVE CARE

These children have an excellent postoperative course. Particularly gratifying are results in the children with severe stenosis, whose improvement over the preoperative state is striking. Oxygen therapy need only be brief. After removal of the drains on the second postoperative day, children of the older age group are usually up within 5 or 6 days of operation. Complications are exceedingly rare beyond the usual ones involved in simple thoracotomy or split-sternal incision. This is no doubt due to the fact that the incision is in the pulmonary artery. Since a fatal air embolus in 1 of our early cases, we have flooded the field with carbon dioxide and released the superior vena cava to cover the foramen ovale with blood prior to closure of the pulmonary artery. In the fatal case of air embolus, autopsy revealed only a patent foramen ovale, and we assumed that the air had entered the left side of the heart via the right ventricle and right atrium.

RESULTS OF OPERATION

Brock reported a mortality of 6% in the last 86 cases treated by his method, and there have been several other reports of good results with the closed technique.[7,8] Some doubt has been cast on these results, notably by Blount et al.[2] With the open technique of Swan, we consider that our results have improved.

REFERENCES

1. Abrahams, D. G., and Wood, P.: Pulmonary stenosis with normal aortic root, Brit. Heart J. 13:519, 1951.
2. Blount, S. G., et al.: Valvular pulmonary stenosis with intact ventricular septum. Clinical and physiologic response to open valvuloplasty, Circulation 15:814, 1957.
3. Brock, R. C.: Pulmonary valvulotomy for the relief of congenital stenosis: Report of 3 cases, Brit. M. J. 1:112, 1948.
4. Campbell, M.: Simple pulmonary stenosis: Pulmonary stenosis with closed ventricular septum, Brit. Heart J. 16:273, 1954.
5. Campbell, M., and Brock, R.: The results of valvotomy for simple pulmonary stenosis, Brit. Heart J. 17:229, 1955.
6. Campbell, M.: Valvulotomy as a corrective operation for simple pulmonary stenosis, Brit. Heart J. 21:415, 1959.
7. Gibson, S., et al.: Congenital pulmonary stenosis with intact ventricular septum, Am. J. Dis. Child. 87:26, 1954.
8. Humphreys, G. H., et al.: Pulmonary valvulotomy. Results of operation in 26 cases, Surgery 35:9, 1954.
9. Johnson, A. M.: Hypertrophic infundibular stenosis complicating simple pulmonary valve stenosis, Brit. Heart J. 21:429, 1959.
10. Keith, J. D., et al.: *Heart Disease in Infancy and Childhood* (New York: Macmillan Company, 1958), p. 388.
11. Kirklin, J. W., et al.: Problems in diagnosis and surgical treatment of pulmonic stenosis with intact ventricular septum, Circulation 8:849, 1953.
12. Lam, C. R., and Raber, R. E.: Simplified technique for direct vision pulmonary valvulotomy, J. Thoracic Surg. 38:309, 1959.
13. Rowe, R. D., et al.: Immediate results of transarterial valvulotomy with notes on the clinical assessment of patients before and after operation, Canad. M. A. J. 78:311, 1958.
14. Sellors, T. H.: Surgery of pulmonic stenosis, Lancet 1:988, 1948.
15. Swan, H., and Zeavin, I.: Cessation of circulation in general hypothermia. Techniques of intracardiac surgery under direct vision, Ann. Surg. 139:385, 1954.
16. Swan, H., et al.: The surgical treatment of isolated infundibular stenosis, J. Thoracic & Cardiovas. Surg. 38:319, 1959.

William T. Mustard
G. A. Trusler
Drawings by
E. Hopper Ross

Tetralogy of Fallot

History.—Although Stensen described the syndrome in 1672,[17] Fallot's[5] report published in 1888 gave the entity of the tetralogy of Fallot its name. The operation developed and described by Blalock and Taussig[2] brought practical importance to the identification of this defect in cyanotic children. Lillehei and associates[10] first achieved complete intracardiac repair of the malformation. Through the observations, experiments and vision of many workers, the patient who has tetralogy of Fallot no longer faces progressing invalidism and death but has a high probability of surviving a corrective intracardiac operation.

Anatomic Features

It is now recognized that tetralogy of Fallot is a specific and unique combination of defects.[15] These include a large ventricular septal defect which is immediately beneath the aortic valve but slightly more anterior than the usual isolated defect in the ventricular septum. The aorta is dextroposed and arises to a variable degree from the right as well as the left ventricle. There is a functionally unimportant minor malformation of the tricuspid valve, and the medial papillary muscle (or papillary muscle of the conus) is absent. There is stenosis of the ostium infundibulum, which alone or associated with additional narrowing downstream to this area offers sufficient resistance to blood flow to result in essentially equal peak systolic pressures in the two ventricles. It is said that tetralogy of Fallot results basically from anterior and upward displacement of the conus septum during embryologic development.

The *ostium infundibulum* is produced by hypertrophy and anterior displacement of the crista supraventricularis. The parietal band (derived from the conus septum) and the septal band are usually hypertrophied and produce additional narrowing at and/or just upstream to the ostium infundibulum. Between the ostium infundibulum and the pulmonary valve is the variably sized *infundibular chamber* (Fig. 38-17). The *orifice of the pulmonary valve*, which may or may not be narrowed, is a little downstream to the attachment of the base of the cusps of this valve to the junctional area between the artery and right ventricle. The level of basal attachment of the cusps is termed the *pulmonary valve ring*. The cusps are also attached at their commissures to the wall of the pulmonary artery. A localized *stenosis* of this area of the main *pulmonary artery* may result from shortening of the free edge of these cusps.

Patients with tetralogy of Fallot have varying degrees of cyanosis because of differences in the severity of the pulmonary stenosis. Neither the location of the ventricular septal defect nor the degree of dextroposition of the aorta apparently has any direct effect on the degree of cyanosis.

A few patients have a lesion similar to that seen in tetralogy of Fallot except for lessened severity of the

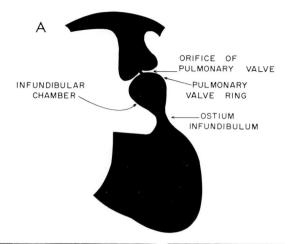

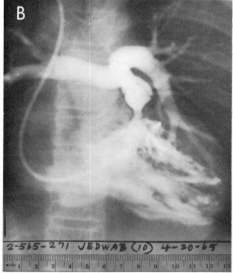

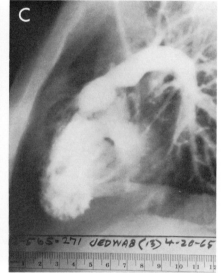

Fig. 38-17.—Tetralogy of Fallot. **A,** schematic representation of the right ventricle and pulmonary artery. **B,** anteroposterior and **C,** lateral angiocardiograms after right ventricular injection of dye. In **C,** dye is seen passing from right ventricle through the ventricular septal defect into left ventricle. There is severe infundibular pulmonary stenosis and a moderate-sized infundibular chamber. The thickened, stenotic pulmonary valve can be seen in profile.

pulmonary stenosis; these patients are acyanotic. The discussion here, however, pertains to patients who are cyanotic.

DIAGNOSIS*

CLINICAL FEATURES.—Cyanosis occurs at or soon after birth in about a third of the patients, before the first year of life in a third, and at any time during the next several years in the remaining third. Since the degree of cyanosis depends on the total amount of

*This discussion was prepared by Dr. P. A. Ongley, Section of Pediatrics, Mayo Clinic.

unsaturated hemoglobin rather than on the arterial oxygen saturation, cyanosis increases as polycythemia develops. Dyspnea depends on the severity of the disease and is increased by exertion or emotional stress. Clubbing of the fingers is rarely noted before 2 years of age and is proportional to the degree of cyanosis. Squatting following exertion is common in younger children when the condition is severe; in older children, however, social consciousness makes them live within their tolerance for exercise, and the need for squatting lessens.

Infants, most often those under 1 year of age, may suffer from attacks of severe anoxia resulting in episodes of unconsciousness that may end fatally. Poly-cythemia develops as a response to the anoxic state and leads to congestive changes in the viscera, with the occasional appearance of epistaxis or hemoptysis. Cerebrovascular thrombosis with deficits of the central nervous system may occur, and cerebral abscesses may develop. Mild albuminuria is common.

PHYSICAL EXAMINATION. — Over-all enlargement of the heart is unusual. The cardiac impulse is dominantly right ventricular in type, with a systolic thrill at the mid-left sternal border in most cases. The first heart sound is normal and is loudest at the apex or lower left sternal border. The second sound is almost always single; it is diminished at the upper left sternal border and is loudest at the middle and lower portions of the left sternal border. This clear single sound almost certainly represents closure of the aortic valve. If a clear-cut splitting of the second sound is noted in a cyanotic patient considered to have tetralogy of Fallot, the accuracy of the diagnosis should be seriously questioned.

The characteristic murmur is systolic in timing and is of variable intensity depending on the severity of the stenosis, being loudest with moderate stenosis and least apparent with severe stenosis. The murmur ends before aortic closure and is rarely more than grade 3 in intensity; occasionally, when the condition is severe, it is no greater than grade 1. During an episode of anoxia, a murmur that usually is grade 2 or 3 may become greatly diminished or even inaudible. Because the pulmonary stenosis is commonly infundibular, the murmur is loudest at the mid-left sternal border, but when valvular stenosis also is present, the murmur may be heard best at the upper left sternal border. Pulmonic diastolic murmurs are rare and, if present, may be associated with congenital hypoplasia of the cusps of the pulmonary valve.

ELECTROCARDIOGRAPHY. — The electrocardiographic findings are dominated by evidence of overwork of the right ventricle. The findings are those of right ventricular systolic overload; this is not so pronounced as that seen in severe pulmonary stenosis with an intact septum but it is perhaps more consistent for a large group of patients. Right atrial hypertrophy is less common and less severe than it is in pulmonary stenosis with an intact septum, but P waves 5 or 6 mm or more in height are encountered sometimes.

ROENTGENOLOGIC ASPECTS. — The roentgenologic picture is dominated by the anatomic structure of the right ventricular outflow tract, but the majority of patients display a typical contour, the so-called coeur en sabot. The heart is normal or even small in size in the posteroanterior projection, with elevation of the apex giving a right ventricular contour. A concavity is present in the region of the right ventricular outflow tract and the main pulmonary artery. The main pulmonary artery and the hilar vessels are diminished in size, and the peripheral vascular shadows in the lungs are less prominent than usual. Moderate enlargement of the right atrium and the aorta is frequent. A right aortic arch occurs in 20–25% of cases, whereas such an anomaly is virtually never present in pulmonary stenosis with an intact septum. Right ventricular hypertrophy is best evaluated in the lateral view, in which it is noted as a forward bulging of the anterior surface of the cardiac silhouette toward the posterior surface of the sternum. When the condition is mild, an infundibular chamber of considerable size may be present and may project as a prominence in the expected region of the main pulmonary artery, thus confusing the picture. The true size of the pulmonary artery is not always obvious from routine studies, and angiocardiography may show a pulmonary artery of reasonable size in cases in which the presence of extreme hypoplasia might be suspected from the usual views and from fluoroscopic observations.

ANGIOCARDIOGRAPHY. — Cardiac catheterization and bi-plane angiocardiography provide the most precise information concerning anatomy. The diagnosis can, of course, usually be made without these special studies. In patients with the severe form of the malformation, angiographic study is useful in identifying associated defects and in planning the operative procedure.

COURSE WITHOUT TREATMENT

Prior to the introduction of operative treatment, the average length of survival in tetralogy of Fallot was about 12 years. Many infants have rapid and early progression of their symptoms and die in the first 2 years of life. Others who have less severe or more slowly progressive symptoms may survive childhood. A very few live past the twentieth year and, rarely, into middle life or beyond.

Congestive cardiac failure is extremely unusual in tetralogy of Fallot. The commonest cause of death during early life is a cerebrovascular accident following severe anoxic episodes, cerebral sinus thrombosis or paradoxical embolism. Many patients dying with tetralogy of Fallot have widespread pulmonary vascular thrombosis. Embolism, endocarditis, cerebral abscess and other intercurrent infections take a constant toll throughout the natural course of the disease.

PALLIATIVE OPERATIONS

Blalock and Taussig[2] in 1945 reported that the cyanosis and polycythemia of patients with tetralogy of Fallot could be decreased by an operation that increased pulmonary blood flow. Numerous publications followed concerning the application of the Blalock-Taussig operation in these patients, and certain variations in surgical technique were explored. Potts and co-workers[13] emphasized the difficulties in making the classic Blalock-Taussig anastomosis in

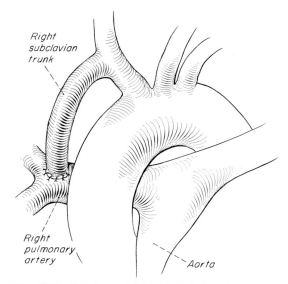

*Right
subclavian
trunk*

*Right
pulmonary
artery*

Aorta

Fig. 38-18.—Tetralogy of Fallot: Blalock-Taussig type of anastomosis (end-to-side junction of subclavian artery to pulmonary artery). An anterolateral incision through the bed of the nonresected right fourth rib is used. Otherwise, the procedure is performed exactly as described by Blalock.[1] The subclavian artery arising from the innominate artery is utilized in making this shunt between the systemic and the pulmonary circulation. When a right aortic arch is present, the anastomosis is made on the left side.

infants and showed the feasibility of accomplishing a direct anastomosis between the side of the upper part of the descending thoracic aorta and the side of the left pulmonary artery.

Shortly after the development of these anastomotic operations, Holmes Sellors[14] performed the first successful closed pulmonary valvotomy in a patient with an intact ventricular septum. Brock[3] soon began to apply a similar procedure to patients with tetralogy of Fallot. Through his efforts, it became evident that at least some patients with this anomaly could be strikingly improved by a direct attack on the pulmonary obstruction, whether this was in the infundibulum or in the pulmonary valve.

On the basis of reports in the literature[12,16] and of follow-up studies in our own cases, it is believed that only a small percentage of patients have the precise relationship between the magnitudes of the right-to-left shunt within the heart and of the left-to-right shunt outside the heart that we consider necessary for a long-term excellent result following the anastomotic operations. Similarly, few patients can be considered to have continuing, truly excellent results after the Brock procedure.[4] Yet many patients, about 60%, are significantly improved for many years after either type of palliative procedure.

The present indication for a palliative operation, at the University of Alabama Medical Center, is the presence of significant and progressing disability in a

patient less than 4 or 5 years old. The palliative procedure of choice is a Blalock-Taussig operation (Fig. 38-18). In infants less than about 1 year of age, the subclavian artery is often too small for this operation. Then a side-to-side anastomosis is made between the ascending aorta and the right pulmonary artery.

OPEN INTRACARDIAC REPAIR

INDICATIONS.—Open operation is recommended as a primary procedure for all patients with tetralogy of Fallot who have reached the age of about 5 years. If a palliative procedure has been performed earlier, complete repair is best done at age 5 or 6.

TECHNIQUE.—Intracardiac repair consists essentially of (1) adequate relief of pulmonary stenosis and (2) complete closure of the ventricular septal defect without the production of heart block.

A median sternotomy incision is made. A disk-type film oxygenator is employed for cardiopulmonary by-pass. A flow rate of 2.2 liters/minute/M² is maintained during cardiopulmonary by-pass. Body temperature is reduced to 30 C and maintained until most of the intracardiac repair has been accomplished. A left ventricular vent is utilized to facilitate removal of the large intracardiac return characteristic of this defect. Intermittent aortic cross-clamping for intervals of 10 minutes allows accurate exposure during the periods of cross-clamping. By use of this method the heart continues to beat. If fibrillation occurs, the heart is immediately defibrillated. In addition to the better coronary perfusion that seems to pertain in the beating heart, an additional advantage seems to be the immediate recognition of heart block if it occurs as the result of any part of the procedure.

If a patent Blalock shunt is present, this is closed before establishment of cardiopulmonary by-pass.[7] When a Potts or ascending aorta-right pulmonary artery anastomosis is present, extracorporeal circulation is established and body temperature is reduced to about 25 C while the aortopulmonary shunt is digitally compressed. Perfusion is then discontinued and during complete circulatory arrest, the stoma is closed with interrupted silk sutures through a pulmonary arteriotomy.[6] The pulmonary artery is closed, body temperature raised to 30 C and the usual intracardiac procedure is begun.

Certain associated defects should be looked for before establishment of cardiopulmonary by-pass. Among these is left persistent superior vena cava, which needs be cannulated if adequate intracardiac exposure is to be accomplished. A patent ductus arteriosus, which in our experience is rare with this defect, should be ligated before by-pass is established. An associated atrial septal defect can be identified by digital examination within the right atrium at the time of placement of the superior vena cava cannula, and should be closed. Occasionally, one may encounter aberrant origin of the left anterior descending cor-

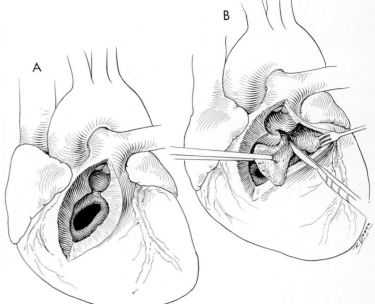

Fig. 38-19.—Tetralogy of Fallot: open intracardiac repair. **A,** in this example, the infundibular stenosis is formed by hypertrophy of the crista, and a large infundibular chamber is present. The ventricular septal defect is immediately below the aortic ring and posterior to the crista. At operation, the aortic cusps can be seen clearly through the septal defect (not shown in this drawing). **B,** resection of the hypertrophied crista supraventricularis is accomplished by sharp dissection; a small sharp retractor is used to elevate the ventricular wall from the hypertrophied limbs of the crista as they are excised on both right and left sides. The margin above the septal defect is largely preserved.

onary artery from the right coronary or a branch of the artery.

A transverse right ventriculotomy is utilized for exposure of the interior of the right ventricle. Those portions of the septal and parietal bands of the crista supraventricularis which offer obstruction to the outflow tract are removed. Further relief of infundibular stenosis is provided by mobilization of the anterior right ventricular wall. Partial resection of the crista itself is done. These maneuvers usually give excellent relief of infundibular obstruction. Pulmonary valvotomy is performed when valvular stenosis is present (Fig. 38-19).

Attention is next directed to repair of the ventricular septal defect. A Dacron or Teflon patch which is slightly smaller than the defect itself is sutured in place in such a way that the crista is pulled dorsally.[9] It appears that this maneuver further enlarges the pulmonary outflow tract. Sutures of 3-0 silk on an atraumatic needle are used in interrupted fashion to secure the patch. One must have excellent exposure and give undivided attention to the placement of each individual stitch if the bundle of His is to be avoided and the aortic valve leaflets are to be left unharmed. After placement of the posterior row of sutures, it is important to check carefully with a small probe for residual defects beneath the suture line. It is sometimes necessary to insert one or two additional sutures at this point to close adequately this important area. Suturing of the remaining portion of the patch is then completed (Fig. 38-20).

The right ventriculotomy is closed, air is aspirated from the heart, and the left ventricular vent is removed. Cardiopulmonary by-pass is discontinued. Adequacy of relief of pulmonary stenosis is now assessed by measurement of intracardiac pressures. If right ventricular pressure exceeds left ventricular pressure, cardiopulmonary by-pass is re-established and a right ventricular outflow patch of pericardium is inserted (Fig. 38-21). As the technique of resection of the pulmonary stenosis has improved, we have found it necessary to use an outflow patch in fewer and fewer patients, with somewhat less than 15% now requiring an outflow patch for adequate relief of stenosis.

POSTOPERATIVE MANAGEMENT

Polyvinyl catheters are brought out from both the left and the right atrium and attached to strain gauge monometers before cardiopulmonary by-pass is established. These are left in place for about 24 hours following operation. Percutaneous insertion of an intra-arterial cannula (usually through the brachial artery) with passage of its tip retrograde into the aorta is utilized for arterial pressure measurements. By means of combined information from atrial and arterial pressure measurements and certain other clinical parameters, an adequate assessment of cardiac output, need for blood replacement and myocardial performance can be obtained.[8] Pulmonary function is best evaluated by observation of the work of breathing and either clinical or laboratory assessment of the blood gas levels.

Left atrial pressure, which usually exceeds right atrial pressure by some 4 to 6 mm Hg postoperatively in patients with tetralogy of Fallot, is maintained at

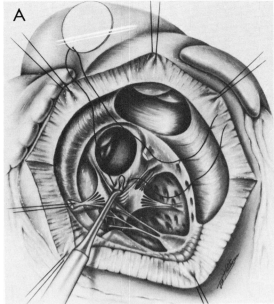

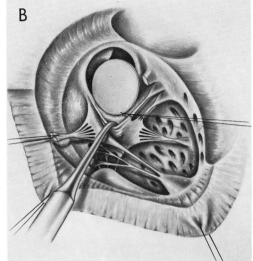

Fig. 38-20.—Tetralogy of Fallot: sutures in intracardiac repair. **A,** the ventricular septal defect is well exposed. The first suture is placed 3–4 mm back from the edge of the defect to avoid damage to the bundle of His. Subsequent stitches along this margin are similarly placed. **B,** the first suture has been tied. The rest of the sutures will also be placed as interrupted stitches.

Fig. 38-21.—Tetralogy of Fallot: reconstruction with pericardium of outflow tract of right ventricle. **A,** measuring calipers are used to determine length and width of patch of pericardial tissue needed to relieve obstruction. **B,** a diamond-shaped patch is fashioned from pericardium. **C,** completed reconstruction of outflow tract after patch of pericardium is sutured to margins of the pulmonary artery and ventriculotomy incision. The previously closed transverse incision just upstream to the ventricular one is not shown.

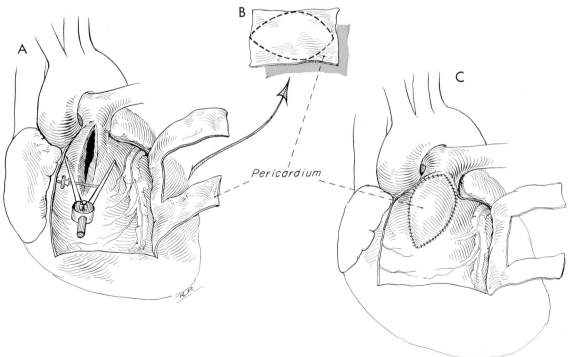

Pericardium

about 15 mm Hg by infusion of blood. The augmentation of blood volume, atrial pressure and thus ventricular end diastolic pressure in most cases increases cardiac output. When appropriate atrial pressure does not result in adequate cardiac output, digitalization is begun if there are no contraindications. Occasionally, severe myocardial depression and acutely falling cardiac output will require an intravenous drip of epinephrine or isoproterenol.

Optimal pulmonary function with minimal work expenditure must be attained in these very sick patients, all of whom have some degree of pulmonary dysfunction. The endotracheal tube is left in place following operation, and intermittent positive pressure breathing is continued until hemodynamics, chest drainage and pulmonary function are under adequate clinical control. Usually, the endotracheal tube is removed within 12–24 hours. In the rare instances in which longer periods of assisted ventilation seem warranted, tracheostomy is done.

In a few patients, particularly older persons who have had previous anastomotic operations, bleeding after operation can be profuse. This bleeding usually diminishes within 4–6 hours after operation. If it continues beyond this time at a rate of more than about 200 ml/M² of body surface per hour, the patient probably should be returned to the operating room. Although a specific bleeding point is often not found, evacuation of retained blood and clots and re-expansion of the lung may be helpful.

Patients are kept in a humid atmosphere with a high concentration of oxygen for 3 or 4 days after operation. Penicillin and streptomycin are given in therapeutic doses for 10 days after operation. During the first 48 hours, only fluids are administered intravenously, the amount being 750 ml of a 5% solution of dextrose in water/M²/ 24 hours.[11] When oral feedings are begun, a diet containing 0.5 Gm of sodium is employed.

Increased venous pressure, hepatomegaly and retention of sodium and water may develop 7–14 days after operation, at the time when the patient's activity is increased. These changes are treated by administration of a diuretic such as chlorothiazide (Diuril) or of digitalis if necessary. These measures, along with the salt-free diet, may be necessary for as long as 6 weeks after operation.

Hospital Mortality

Operative mortality has been progressively lowered (Fig. 38-22) to a point where it is less than 5% (Table 38-1). This has been accomplished in a group of patients, the majority of whom have had the severe form of the disease, and many have had one or more previous operations. It seems likely that with refinement of technique and elimination of human error, the already low mortality can be reduced even further. The incidence of both residual septal defect and permanent heart block has been greatly reduced in recent years as knowledge and technical ability have increased. In the past 3 years, only 1 case of permanent heart block has occurred in our experience. In recent years, reoperation has not been necessary because of residual shunting.

Late Results

The experience of 12 years (to Nov. 1, 1967) in which 604 patients have had complete repair of tetralogy of Fallot has generally been most gratifying. In those patients followed up to 10 years, the long-term results have been excellent in over 90% (Table 38-2).[9] Life expectancy should be normal in this group.

In patients who have required an outflow patch in the right ventricle, some cardiomegaly has persisted. The long-term effect and eventual outcome in these patients is not known. It is felt, however, that use of

Fig. 38-22.—Hospital mortality rate for complete intracardiac repair of tetralogy of Fallot at Mayo Clinic (1955–65) and at University of Alabama Medical Center (1966).

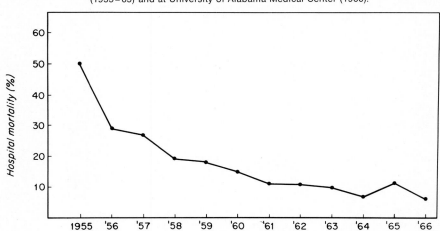

an outflow patch should be avoided, if possible, because of this finding.

REFERENCES

1. Blalock, A.: Surgical procedures employed and anatomic variations encountered in the treatment of congenital pulmonic stenosis, Surg., Gynec. & Obst. 87:385, 1948.
2. Blalock, A., and Taussig, H. B.: The surgical treatment of malformations of the heart in which there is pulmonary stenosis or pulmonary atresia, J.A.M.A. 128:189, 1945.
3. Brock, R. C.: Pulmonary valvulotomy for the relief of congenital pulmonary stenosis: Report of 3 cases, Brit. M. J. 1:1121, 1948.
4. Campbell, M.: Late results of operations for Fallot's tetralogy, Brit. M. J. 2:1175, 1958.
5. Fallot, A.: Contribution à l'anatomie pathologique de la maladie bleue (cyanose cardiaque), Marseille-mèd. 25:77, 138, 207, 341 and 403, 1888.
6. Kirklin, J. W., and Devloo, R. A.: Hypothermic perfusion and circulatory arrest for surgical correction of tetralogy of Fallot with previously constructed Potts' anastomosis, Dis. Chest 39:87, 1961.
7. Kirklin, J. W., and Payne, W. S.: Surgical treatment for tetralogy of Fallot after previous anastomosis of systemic to pulmonary artery, Surg., Gynec. & Obst. 110:707, 1960.
8. Kirklin, J. W., et al.: Factors affecting survival after open operation for tetralogy of Fallot, Ann. Surg. 152:485, 1960.
9. Kirklin, J. W., et al.: Early and late results after intracardiac repair of tetralogy of Fallot, Ann. Surg. 162:578, 1965.
10. Lillehei, C. W., et al.: Direct vision intracardiac surgical correction of the tetralogy of Fallot, pentalogy of Fallot, and pulmonary atresia defects: Report of first 10 cases, Ann. Surg. 142:418, 1955.
11. Lyons, W. S.; DuShane, J. W., and Kirklin, J. W.: Postoperative care after whole-body perfusion and open intracardiac operations: Use of Mayo-Gibbon pump-oxygenator and Brown-Emmons heat exchanger, J.A.M.A. 173:625, 1960.
12. Potts, W. J., et al.: Surgical correction of tetralogy of Fallot: Results in the first 100 cases 6 to 8 years after operation, J.A.M.A. 159:95, 1955.
13. Potts, W. J.; Smith, S., and Gibson, S.: Anastomosis of the aorta to a pulmonary artery: Certain types in congenital heart disease, J.A.M.A. 132:627, 1946.
14. Sellors, T. H.: Surgery of pulmonary stenosis: A case in which the pulmonary valve was successfully divided, Lancet 1:988, 1948.
15. Van Mierop, L. H. S., and Wiglesworth, Frederick W.: Pathogenesis of transposition complexes, Am. J. Cardiol. 12:216, 1963.
16. White, B. D., et al.: Five-year postoperative results of the first 500 patients with Blalock-Taussig anastomosis for pulmonary stenosis or atresia, Circulation 14:512, 1956.
17. Willius, F. A.: An unusually early description of the so-called tetralogy of Fallot, Proc. Staff Meet. Mayo Clin. 23:316, 1948.

J. W. Kirklin
B. W. Hightower

Drawings by
E. Hopper Ross
J. M. Hutcheson (Figure 38-20)

Aortic Stenosis

History. — Bonet[4] collected descriptions of acquired and of probable congenital aortic stenosis, the former by Rayger in 1672 and the latter by Greiselius. Aortic stenosis was recognized as a cause of cardiac enlargement, palpitation and sudden death by Morgagni,[20] who listed Bonet's along with a number of reports of osseous valves. In 1913, Tuffier[27] operated on a patient with aortic stenosis and dilated the stenotic orifice by pressure with a finger through the aortic wall. Bailey[2] described use of a dilator inserted through the left ventricle, a method more useful in adults with calcific stenosis than in children with fibrous stenosis in whom insufficiency is more apt to result.[19] In 1955, Swan and associates[26] and Lewis et al.[17] first incised the fused commissures under hypothermia. Subsequently, an open operation with cardiopulmonary by-pass has been found to be safer and more certain to assure a good result.[11,18,25]

Anatomy

Obstruction between the chamber of the left ventricle and the aorta may occur in any of four places. Most commonly, stenosis is of the valve itself, the cusps being thickened and the commissures partly or completely fused. The commissure between right and left coronary cusps is most frequently affected, and that between the right and noncoronary cusps usually is next most severely involved.

In our experience, subvalvular stenosis occurred about half as frequently as valvular stenosis.[24] The narrowing consists of a fibrous ring 1-3 cm below the valve at or just beneath the membranous portion of the ventricular septum, and usually attached to the mitral valve leaflet. Usually, the fibrous ring is short and almost like a diaphragm, but occasionally there is a long stenotic area, and fibrous tissue may extend up to the aortic cusps, which otherwise are nearly normal.

A muscular hypertrophic subvalvular stenosis occurs more frequently in adults than in children, demonstrated by angiocardiography, pressure measurement and direct observation of bars or bands of hypertrophied muscle 4–5 cm below the aortic valve.[21] Obstruction of this type may be secondary to left ventricular hypertrophy as occurs with systemic hypertension or valvular or subvalvular stenosis;[8] or there may be no other abnormality. In the patients without other abnormalities, the condition may be familial.[3,8]

Least commonly, stenosis may be in the aorta itself at or above the attachment of the aortic leaflets.[23] This may be a thin fibrous membrane, or it may be more extensive, with hypoplasia of the aorta and degeneration and fibrosis of the aortic media.

Compensation for the obstruction occurs by left ventricular hypertrophy. When aortic insufficiency is present, there may also be dilatation. Ordinarily, other portions of the heart are not affected unless ventricular failure occurs. Poststenotic dilatation of the ascending aorta may occur, especially when the stenosis is valvular. Dilatation usually is not seen with the muscular or supravalvular stenosis.

Calcification is rare in aortic stenosis in children, although it is common in adults, some of whom have a mild congenital stenosis on which thrombus, scar and calcification are in time deposited. Our youngest patient with calcification was 18 years old.

INCIDENCE AND ETIOLOGY

Aortic stenosis was present in 39 of the 1,000 cases of congenital heart disease reported by Abbott.[1] Keith *et al.*[15] estimate the incidence as 1 :24,000 in the population from birth to 14 years (compared with 1:16,000 for coarctation of the aorta), and Carlgen[10] found evidence of the condition once in each 2,900 births. It is not a rare defect.

In nearly every child with aortic stenosis, the lesion results from a congenital defect in formation of the aortic cusps, the outflow tract of the left ventricle or the adjacent aorta. Rheumatic heart disease may be an uncommon cause.

SYMPTOMS AND PHYSICAL SIGNS

The clinical picture is determined by the severity of the stenosis and the ability of the left ventricle to compensate for the outflow obstruction. If the stenosis is slight or if compensation by ventricular hypertrophy is adequate, there may be no symptoms, and some individuals lead a normal life with probable mild congenital aortic stenosis.

Irrespective of the type of aortic stenosis, the physiologic effect is the same: interference with ejection of the left ventricle and inadequate blood flow to the body, of which the brain and heart are the most sensitive organs. Fatigue and dyspnea on exertion are the most common complaints. Dizziness—especially on exertion—syncope or convulsions may indicate inadequate cerebral circulation, while anginal pain, substernal tightness or palpitation may indicate coronary insufficiency. The condition always carries the threat of sudden death, usually preceded by some of the above-mentioned symptoms, although sudden death has been described in the absence of pre-existing symptoms or physical activity.

The typical murmur, which may be detected early in life, is harsh, systolic, with crescendo and decrescendo, maximal in the aortic area to the right of the sternum in the second and fourth interspaces and transmitted to the neck. Early in life, it may be maximal to the left. Its intensity varies to some extent with the degree of stenosis. A diastolic murmur of insufficiency is present in about one third of the cases,[14] due to retraction of the scarred leaflets or, in the case of subvalvular stenosis, to downward traction toward the diaphragm. In cases of mild stenosis, the murmur may be the only physical sign, but in the more severe case, the cardiac impulse may be increased in breadth and become heaving with lateral displacement of the apex beat. There may be a low systolic and a narrow pulse pressure. The aortic second sound usually is diminished but need not be. Males are affected two to five times more often than females.

DIAGNOSTIC STUDIES

Left ventricular enlargement may be visible roentgenographically; but usually in children, the heart is of normal size even in symptomatic patients.[6] In over half the patients with significant stenosis, there is poststenotic dilatation of the ascending aorta, which on fluoroscopic examination is seen to be abnormally active.[16]

The electrocardiogram may be normal at rest and in the early stages shows abnormalities only on exertion. Left ventricular hypertrophy, depression of the S-T segment and flat or inverted T waves over the left ventricle indicate clinically significant obstruction. As a rule, the electrical axis is normal.

Catheterization of the right heart may be of value in demonstrating associated conditions, such as ventricular septal defect and infundibular or peripheral pulmonary stenosis, or evidence of left ventricular failure and secondary pulmonary hypertension. Left heart catheterization may be done trans-septally,[22] or a catheter may be passed through the stenotic valve retrograde from the femoral artery and pressure measured above and below it. Occasionally, direct ventricular puncture may be required to estimate the pressure gradient across the valve.[12] When this measurement is combined with cardiac output, the actual size of the orifice can be estimated. Both cardiac output and systolic gradient across the valve are influenced by the degree of cardiac compensation and may be reduced in heart failure. Angiocardiography with injection into the left ventricle and aorta is helpful, but this should be selective into the left side of the heart to avoid obscuration by other chambers.

ASSOCIATED CONDITIONS.—Coarctation of the aorta is the most common additional condition, but endocardial fibroelastosis, patent ductus arteriosus, ventricular septal defect, pulmonary stenosis, left ventricular-right atrial shunt and cystic medial necrosis of the ascending aorta have also been reported. In our experience, congenital aortic stenosis was more frequently associated with other abnormalities in females (7 of 15 cases) than in males (4 of 31 cases).

CLINICAL COURSE

Great variation in disability occurs with aortic stenosis, ranging from long and unlimited life to great disability or sudden death in infancy.[14] The presence of a murmur alone is of little prognostic value, but when easy fatigability, dyspnea on exertion, dizziness, syncope and precordial pain appear, dangerous embarrassment may be present. A healthy left ventricle may compensate for even severe stenosis, but once compensation is inadequate, a vicious cycle may be entered, leading to rapid deterioration. Premonitory symptoms or signs may not appear, even before sudden death or fatal pulmonary edema. Braverman and Gibson[7] reported an 8.2% mortality in children whom they followed before surgical treatment was available.

DIFFERENTIAL DIAGNOSIS

VENTRICULAR SEPTAL DEFECT. — Because of the systolic murmur, left ventricular hypertrophy and cardiac enlargement, ventricular septal defect may resemble aortic stenosis. Cardiac catheterization should distinguish the two if evidence of increased pulmonary vascularity does not.

PULMONARY STENOSIS. — Uncommonly, right axis deviation and right bundle-branch block may suggest pulmonary stenosis, especially in young children. The murmur early in life may also be most prominent to the left of the sternum. When significant obstruction to the right ventricle is present, it usually is evident electrocardiographically. Pulmonary stenosis may also be identified by cardiac catheterization.

OTHER STENOSES. — The commonest question that arises in differential diagnosis is related to the type of stenosis. Distinction between *valvular* and *subvalvular stenosis* may be difficult or impossible. If a good aortic second sound is present, subvalvular stenosis can be diagnosed with fair confidence; if it is absent, the diagnosis rests on the comparative rarity of post-stenotic dilatation in subaortic stenosis or on the shifting character and diffuseness of the murmur. In patients with *supravalvular obstruction*, the murmur and thrill may seem unusually superficial and well transmitted to the neck. Williams and associates[28] described a characteristic facies and mental retardation that may be present in some patients with this condition. *Muscular or functional* aortic stenosis may be suggested by prominence of a systolic thrill and murmur at the apex or lower left sternal border rather than in the aortic area. The thrill may not be transmitted to the carotid region, and usually post-stenotic dilatation is not present. Certain differentiation of these four types of stenosis can be made only by left ventricular angiocardiography or sometimes only on exploration. Hypertrophic subvalvular muscular stenosis may be further identified by the effects of drugs that alter myocardial contractility and peripheral resistance.[21]

TREATMENT

Nonoperative treatment consists simply of digitalis and limiting the patient's activity, as aortic stenosis is one of the few congenital defects in which the patient's symptoms are not an adequate governor for his activities.

Significant symptoms, cardiac enlargement, a pressure gradient across the aortic valve of more than 50 mm Hg and S-T- and T-wave abnormalities in the electrocardiogram are generally considered indications for operation in the typical case. Operation should be undertaken when indications are present, the risk being less than the threat of severe disability or death.

OPERATIVE TREATMENT. — Congenital aortic stenosis of any type is not suitable for treatment by dilatation or with the haste imposed by limitations of hypothermia and circulatory arrest. Cardiopulmonary bypass should be employed and stenosed commissures carefully opened or fibrous stenosis resected.

Median *sternotomy* gives optimal exposure. A single cannula in the right atrium may be used, but individual cannulation of each vena cava allows better control of the circulation. Aspiration of blood through a vent placed in the apex of the left ventricle will assure less blood in the operative area and allow evacuation of air later by tilting the heart up from the pericardial sac. Ischemic arrest of the heart gives a quiet operative field, but we prefer to perfuse the coronary arteries if the aorta is open longer than 12–15 minutes. Moderate hypothermia to around 30 C adds to the safety of this period of ischemia. Incision in the ascending aorta is usually made obliquely, extending into the noncoronary sinus of Valsalva (Fig. 38-23).

The degree of fusion of the individual commissures is variable, but usually the commissure between the

Fig. 38-23. — Valvular aortic stenosis: exposure by incision in the ascending aorta **(A)**. A small knife is best for incision along the commissures, and care should be exercised to stay along the crest **(B)**. In some instances, the commissure between right and left coronary cusps is incompletely formed and should be only partially incised.

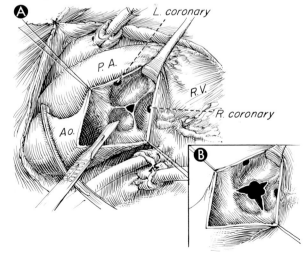

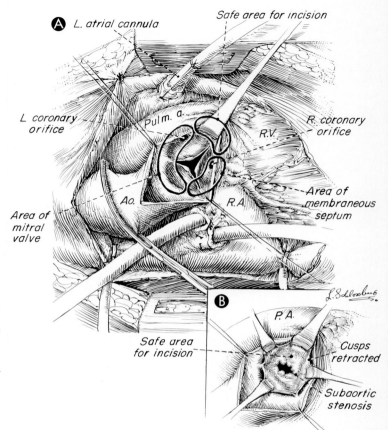

Fig. 38-24.—Subvalvular aortic stenosis: exposure of aortic valve with incision in the ascending aorta under cardiopulmonary by-pass. **A,** structures adjacent to subvalvular stenosis. **B,** if possible, the fibrous constriction should be removed, but growth into adjacent structures may necessitate division of the band only.

right and left cusps is most severely involved. The commissures must be carefully identified and equally carefully incised. If only a rudimentary commissure is present, it should probably be incised little if at all. Incision may be more properly made with a knife than with scissors and should extend back near but not quite to the aortic wall. Wandering off the commissure or making too wide an incision may lead to aortic insufficiency. Calcification is rare except in the older patient with congenital aortic stenosis, but in such instances, removal of calcium deposits may be necessary.

The left ventricle and aorta are allowed to fill with blood as the aortotomy is closed and the aortic occlusion released. If ventricular fibrillation occurs or cardiac action ceases, the left ventricle must be satisfactorily vented when coronary artery flow is resumed until spontaneous rhythm occurs or electrical defibrillation is used. Defibrillation of the overdistended left ventricle is virtually impossible.

When subvalvular stenosis is present, the fibrous ring should be discretely excised. Care must be taken not to injure the mitral valve, the ventricular septum or aortic cusp (Fig. 38-24). As much of the fibrous ring as possible should be removed and the constricting band relieved. More diffuse involvement is the rule in supravalvular stenosis, and a patch of synthetic material may be necessary to enlarge the aortic opening.[23]

There is less consensus about treatment of hypertrophic muscular stenosis, but best results have been obtained by excision of a portion of the hypertrophied muscle.

Typical congenital valvular stenosis can be treated with little risk, the low mortality rate initially reported having been borne out by our subsequent separate experience. Complicating defects add to the danger. Some degree of aortic insufficiency is often produced, but with caution, this should not be severe. Since the valve always remains abnormal, one should aim not for perfection in commissural incision but rather to balance gain by relief of stenosis with possible damage from too generous incision of the commissures. Our liberal indications for operation are dependent on cautious incision and respect for possible regurgitation. With an adequate opening, the pressure gradient virtually disappears, but it may remain partially in patients with badly deformed valves in whom the commissures cannot be satisfactorily opened.

Subaortic stenosis may be more difficult to relieve

completely without damage to adjacent structures. In some cases, a diffuse stenosis and underdeveloped outflow tract preclude complete relief of the obstruction. In many instances, however, since the leaflets are often not involved, a more nearly normal end-result may be obtained than with valvular stenosis.

POSTOPERATIVE CARE. — The postoperative course of patients with congenital aortic stenosis usually is one of the most benign of all those treated with cardiopulmonary by-pass. Pleural drainage, an oxygen tent, limitation of fluids and administration of antibiotics are routine. The most common problem is cardiac failure, which can be treated with digitalis, limitation of fluids, diuretics and oxygen. Failure is particularly apt to appear in patients in whom some aortic insufficiency has been produced or coronary air embolism allowed to occur. The measurement of pressures through a catheter placed in the left atrium at operation[5] has been useful in estimating function of the left ventricle and the limit to which blood replacement can be pushed.

The ultimate fate of patients with surgically opened valves is unknown. It is possible that residual deformity will lead to later thrombosis, scarring and obstruction. For this reason and in spite of a low operative risk, operation is performed at present only when there is evidence of a life-threatening stenosis.

REFERENCES

1. Abbott, M. E.: *Atlas of Congenital Cardiac Disease* (New York: American Heart Association, Inc., 1954).
2. Bailey, C. P.: *Surgery of the Heart* (Philadelphia: Lea & Febiger, 1955).
3. Bercu, B. A., *et al.*: Pseudo-aortic stenosis produced by ventricular hypertrophy, Am. J. Med. 25:814, 1958.
4. Bonet, T.: Sepulchretum sive Anatomia Practica, ex Cadaveribus Morbo Denatis, (a) Sectio XI, Libri Secundi, obs. XXVI, p. 891, (b) Sectio VIII, Libri Secundi, obs. XIII, p. 822, 1700.
5. Boyd, A. D., *et al.*: Estimation of cardiac output soon after intracardiac surgery with cardiopulmonary bypass, Ann. Surg. 150:613, 1959.
6. Braunwald, E., *et al.*: Congenital aortic stenosis, Circulation 27:426, 1963.
7. Braverman, J. B., and Gibson, S.: The outlook for children with congenital aortic stenosis, Am. Heart J. 53:487, 1957.
8. Brent, L. B., *et al.*: Familial muscular aortic stenosis: An unrecognized form of "idiopathic heart disease" with clinical and autopsy observations, Circulation 21:167, 1960.
9. Brock, R. C.: Functional obstruction of the left ventricle, Guy's Hosp. Rep. 106:221, 1957.
10. Carlgen, L. E.: The incidence of congenital heart disease in children born in Gothenburg 1941-1950, Brit. Heart J. 21:40, 1959.
11. Cooley, D. A., *et al.*: Obstructive lesions of the left ventricular outflow tract. Circulation 31:612, 1965.
12. Fleming, P., and Gibson, R.: Percutaneous left ventricular puncture in the assessment of aortic stenosis, Thorax 12:37, 1957.
13. Gorlin, R., *et al.*: Dynamics of the circulation in aortic valvular disease, Am. J. Med. 18:855, 1955.
14. Hohn, A. R., *et al.*: Aortic stenosis. Circulation 32 (supp. 3):4, 1965.
15. *Infancy and Childhood* (New York: Macmillan Company, 1958).
16. Kjellberg, S., *et al.*: *Diagnosis of Congenital Heart Disease* (2d ed.; Chicago: Year Book Medical Publishers, Inc., 1959).
17. Lewis, F. J., *et al.*: Aortic valvulotomy under direct vision during hypothermia, J. Thoracic Surg. 32:481, 1956.
18. Lillehei, C. W., *et al.*: Surgical treatment of stenotic or regurgitant lesions of the mitral and aortic valves by direct vision utilizing a pump-oxygenator, J. Thoracic Surg. 35:154, 1958.
19. Marquis, R. M., and Logan, A.: Congenital aortic stenosis and its surgical treatment, Brit. Heart J. 17:373, 1955.
20. Morgagni, J. B.: *The Seats and Causes of Diseases Investigated by Anatomy* (tr. by Benjamin Alexander) (London: 1769), Leter 23, Article 9.
21. Ross, J., Jr.; *et al.*: The mechanism of the intraventricular pressure gradient in idiopathic hypertrophic subaortic stenosis, Circulation 34:558, 1966.
22. Ross, J., Jr.; Braunwald, E., and Morrow, A. G.: Transseptal left atrial puncture: New technique for the measurement of left atrial pressure in man, Am. J. Cardiol. 3:653, 1959.
23. Shumacker, H. B., and Mandelbaum, I.: Surgical considerations in the management of supravalvular aortic stenosis, Circulation 31 (supp. 1):36, 1965.
24. Spencer, F. C.; Neill, C. A., and Bahnson, H. T.: Treatment of congenital aortic stenosis with valvulotomy during cardiopulmonary bypass, Surgery 44:109, 1958.
25. Spencer, F. C., *et al.*: Anatomical variations in 46 patients with congenital aortic stenosis, Am. Surgeon 26:204, 1960.
26. Swan, H., Wilkenson, R. H., and Blount, S. G., Jr.: Visual repair of congenital aortic stenosis during hypothermia, J. Thoracic Surg. 35:139, 1958.
27. Tuffier, T.: Etat actuel de la chirurgie intrathoracique, Tr. Internat. Cong. Med., London, 1914.
28. Williams, J. C. P., *et al.*: Supravalvular aortic stenosis, Circulation 24:1131, 1961.

H. T. BAHNSON
F. C. SPENCER

Drawings by
LEON SCHLOSSBERG

39

Defects of Septal Closure

Atrial Septal Defect

OSTIUM SECUNDUM

HISTORY. — In 1947, Cohn[5] closed artificially created atrial septal defects in dogs by invaginating the atrial appendage into the defect, sewing it to the rim and then detaching the invaginated wall by a snare technique. In 1948, Murray[20] operated on the first human subject, passing a straight needle through the septum carrying a suture, and circumferentially closing the defect. This ingenious operation was partially successful. Shortly thereafter, Dodrill,[8] Swan et al.[26] and Hufnagel and Gillespie[12] developed ingenious experimental methods which proved unsatisfactory in man. Mustard[22] in 1951 closed iatrogenic septal defects in the dog, using an extracorporeal circulation, and Dennis et al.[7] attempted the first human repair by this method. Bailey[1] in 1952 performed the first successful closure (catheter proved) by his method of atrioseptopexy, using a guiding finger in the atrium. In the same year, Lewis et al.[16] closed an atrial septal defect under direct vision with inflow occlusion and hypothermia. In 1953, Gibbon[10] successfully repaired an atrial septal defect with cardiac by-pass, using an artificial heart-lung machine (the first successful application of the artificial pump oxygenator in man); Gross[11] reported clinical success with his atrial well technique, and Swan[27] reported successful closure under hypothermia. In 1954, Sondergaard[25] reported a method of circumferential occlusion, which was modified by Bjork et al.,[2] who added tactile guidance.

The general trend on this continent is toward open-heart operation with direct suture. Controversy still prevails over the method of cardiac by-pass.

INCIDENCE AND NATURAL HISTORY

Atrial septal defect is the second commonest congenital cardiac malformation met with in adults,[28] and in children the incidence is reported as 7%.[14] The difference in incidence is due to the high mortality from other congenital cardiac anomalies in infancy, childhood and adolescence. In isolated ostium secundum defects, the prognosis is good. Although a few patients die in infancy with pneumonia, the average life span is probably 40–50 years. Roesler[24] in 1934 reported the average age at death to be 36. In a later study, Cosby and Griffith[6] reported the average length of life to be 40 years. Many patients live past 60 and have probably had a misdiagnosis of mitral stenosis. Successful surgical repair has been reported in patients past 60.

PATHOLOGY

Dilatation involves the right atrium, the pulmonary arteries and veins and the right ventricle. The atrial wall is thickened and the right ventricle hypertrophied. The defect may be high, central or low in the

Fig. 39-1. — Atrial septal defect, ostium secundum. If anomalous veins are encountered in the high defect, keen judgment must be exercised. If the vein or veins are not too near the cavaatrial orifice, their inclusion in the closure is not too difficult. If this seems too hazardous, the atrium should be closed and the patient operated on with the pump oxygenator in 1 or 2 weeks. (From Welch, C. E. [ed.]: *Advances in Surgery* [Chicago: Year Book Medical Publishers, Inc., 1965], Vol.1.)

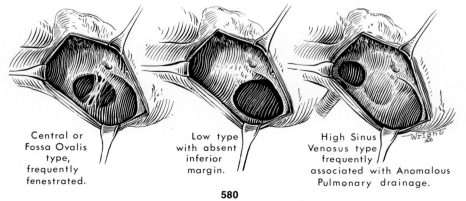

Central or Fossa Ovalis type, frequently fenestrated.

Low type with absent inferior margin.

High Sinus Venosus type frequently associated with Anomalous Pulmonary drainage.

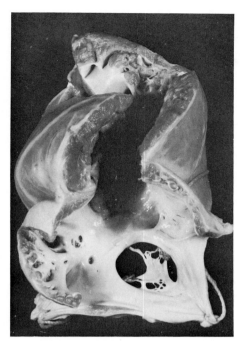

Fig. 39-2. — Atrial septal defect, secundum type. Autopsy specimen of a 2-year-old child with mongolism. Strings tie the superior vena cava on the left and the inferior vena cava on the right. A large, low fenestrated atrial septal defect is present. Note the septal tissue separating the defect from the coronary sinus (above and right) and the tricuspid valve ring (above).

cm. and are often fenestrated (Figs. 39-1 and 39-2). The low defects have no inferior margin, which is important to the surgeon. The central and low defects probably represent degeneration of the septum primum. In one instance of a low defect, we observed a normally closed fossa ovalis superior to the defect.

HEMODYNAMICS

In a small defect, there is a pressure gradient between the left and the right atrium of about 3 mm Hg; if the defect is large (2 cm or more in diameter), there may be no gradient. The shunt in these cases is determined by the size of the respective valvular orifices and the shape of the ventricles. The mitral orifice is smaller than the tricuspid valve, the left ventricle has a long narrow chamber as opposed to the large almost square chamber of the right ventricle. The shunt remains left to right until, with the development of pulmonary hypertension, the right heart fails and the shunt reverses. The right ventricular pressure in children seldom exceeds 50 mm Hg in the secundum type of defect. Pulmonary hypertension in the presence of an atrial septal defect of the secundum type usually develops in early adult life.

DIAGNOSIS

This defect usually is not discovered until preschool age. The murmur is very soft in the younger age group and often considered functional. Our patients have usually been thin, but they did not appear undernourished and as a rule were of average height. The parents considered most of the children to be normally active; but activity, appetite and healthy sleep often increased markedly after complete closure of the defect. From this, we deduce that these children have had a self-imposed limitation of exercise

septum and is separated from the ventricular septum by atrial septal tissue (Fig. 39-1). The high defects measure 1–2 cm in diameter and are almost invariably associated with anomalous pulmonary venous drainage. The central defects vary in size from 1 to 3

Fig. 39-3. — Atrial septal defect, secundum type. **A,** preoperative roentgenogram of an asymptomatic 9-year-old girl with defect proved on cardiac catheterization. **B,** roentgenogram 4 years

after closure of the defect with hypothermia and inflow occlusion. The reduction of heart size emphasizes the benefit of complete closure and need for operation despite absence of symptoms.

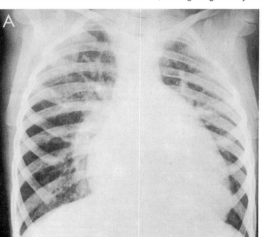

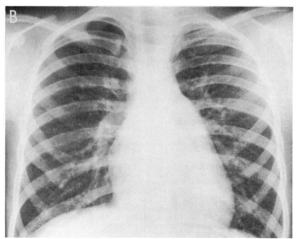

tolerance. Arterial oxygen saturation has been within normal limits in our cases. Very rarely cardiac failure may occur in childhood, with slight cyanosis appearing during the period of failure. An atrial septal defect with pulmonary valvular stenosis may produce cyanosis before cardiac failure.

The right ventricular thrust is nearly always more marked than normal, and in 10% of our cases a thrill was present in the pulmonary area. A grade 2 systolic murmur is almost always present, maximal in the first and second left interspaces. A mild diastolic murmur at the apex is present with most large defects, indicating filling of the right ventricle from an overloaded right atrium. A widely split second sound is always present in the second interspace owing to the greatly increased pulmonary flow (two to five times normal), the pulmonary valve closing after the aortic valve. One third of our patients have slight enlargement of the heart and two-thirds, moderate to gross enlargement. A bulging pulmonary artery and increased hilar shadows are consistent x-ray findings (Figs. 39-3 and 39-4). The electrocardiogram shows right ventricular hypertrophy with a right bundle-branch block, a lengthening of the P-R interval and right axis deviation. The mechanism of the right bundle-branch block has not been satisfactorily explained but may be evidence of right ventricular strain. We have not encountered an isolated secundum type of atrial septal defect with left axis deviation.

CATHETERIZATION.—The cardiac catheter passes through the defect in the majority of cases, and although this is not conclusive, a rise of 2 volumes % in oxygen saturation in the right atrium over that in the superior vena cava aids in diagnosis. The pressure in the right ventricle averages 30 mm Hg in the childhood group and seldom exceeds 50 mm Hg. Pulmonary flow may be increased two to five times normal without development of pulmonary hypertension. A flow of this volume with a ventricular septal defect almost invariably produces a rise of right ventricular pressure due to increased vascular resistance. The explanation usually given is that the jet effect of the ventricular defect is directed to the pulmonary vascular bed, whereas with an atrial defect there is no direct effect since the defect is a considerable distance from the pulmonary valve and the left atrial pressure is low.

ANGIOCARDIOGRAPHY.—Contrast medium injected into the left atrium may outline the defect if the pressure in the left atrium is higher than that in the right. After it leaves the right heart, reappearance of the dye in the left atrium, right atrium and right ventricle demonstrates a left to right shunt at atrial level. Bjork et al.[2] used a balloon-tip catheter to occlude the defect and determine its size.

DIFFERENTIAL DIAGNOSIS

ATYPICAL PATENT DUCTUS ARTERIOSUS.—Patients with a patent ductus and a systolic murmur only, may represent some diagnostic difficulty. Without cardiac catheterization and retrograde aortography, the presence of left ventricular hypertrophy should lead one to suspect a patent ductus. Catheterization in patients with patent ductus arteriosus demonstrates no rise of oxygen saturation at atrial level but a rise of pulmonary artery oxygen saturation and increased pressure in the pulmonary artery.

PULMONARY STENOSIS.—Pure pulmonary stenosis with normal aortic root will not produce the hilar shadows seen when an atrial septal defect is present. Difficulty in diagnosis arises when there is a combination of pulmonic stenosis and atrial septal defect. There is nearly always a functional pressure gradient across the pulmonary valve in pure atrial septal defect, and an occasional stenosis is present which is not severe enough to warrant correction. In such cases, the decision to divide the valve can only be made at operation by direct measurement of the gradient across the valve after the atrial defect has been closed.

ANOMALOUS PULMONARY VEINS.—Total anomalous pulmonary venous drainage may not present a difficult problem in differential diagnosis after catheter studies. Partial drainage into the right atrium or into the coronary sinus in the absence of an atrial septal defect presents obvious hazards in diagnosis. In these

Fig. 39-4.—Atrial septal defect, secundum type. Roentgenogram shows the enlarged right atrium, bulging pulmonary artery, increased hilar markings and slightly enlarged heart. This 11-year-old girl was asymptomatic but had a rise of oxygen saturation of 20% at the right atrial level. With hypothermia and inflow occlusion, the low secundum defect 15 mm in diameter was closed with a running suture. The postoperative course was uneventful and subsequent catheterization showed no shunt.

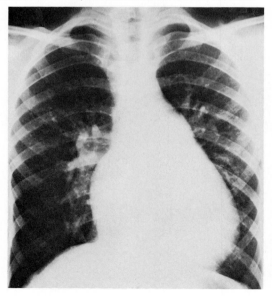

cases, dye injected into the right pulmonary artery may show delayed appearance time, and into the left pulmonary artery may show normal appearance time in the systemic circulation. When partial anomalous drainage is associated with a high atrial secundum defect, direct catheterization of all pulmonary veins may be the only means of diagnosis. Occasionally, the diagnosis can be made only at operation. In any case, at operation for atrial septal defect, anomalous venous drainage would be searched for.

LUTEMBACHER SYNDROME.—Congenital mitral stenosis associated with an atrial septal defect is extremely rare. Clinical diagnosis based on a mid-diastolic mitral murmur is misleading in that it also occurs in atrial septal defect due to rapid inflow of blood into the right ventricle in middiastole. In our primum defect group, we found congenital mitral stenosis twice; the commissures were incised with a fair result.

OSTIUM PRIMUM.—The presence of left axis deviation in the electrocardiogram accompanied by clinical signs of mitral insufficiency should lead one to suspect this diagnosis. The condition is symptomatic in childhood and the hearts are usually larger. In our group of secundum defects, only 1 case was misdiagnosed, and this primum defect was accompanied by an intact mitral valve.

ATRIOVENTRICULARIS COMMUNIS.—The severity of symptoms from this condition in the first 2 years of life is sufficient to indicate the diagnosis. The presence of left axis deviation and a large heart should lead one to anticipate the catheter findings of this condition.

ASSOCIATED ANOMALIES.—The presence of other defects such as ventricular septal defect, patent ductus arteriosus and coarctation of the aorta can usually be ruled out at cardiac catheterization.

PULMONARY HYPERTENSION.—The 4 children in our group of 125 with isolated defects with pressures over 50 mm Hg in the pulmonary artery had an R wave in lead V_1 of 16 mm Hg or over.

INDICATIONS FOR OPERATION

Until recently, the view was taken that asymptomatic patients should not be operated on for septum secundum defects. Significantly lowered mortality rates, lessened morbidity and fewer recurrences after open-heart surgery have led most centers to reconsider this view. Some groups consider a flow to the lungs two times that of the systemic flow as an indication for operation; others operate when the diagnosis has been established, as in patent ductus arteriosus. At the Hospital for Sick Children, Toronto, we operate on secundum defects once the diagnosis has been determined.

OPERATIVE TECHNIQUE

Almost all centers, including those in the Scandinavian countries, are closing ostium secundum defects under direct vision. Some difference of opinion still prevails whether a pump oxygenator should be employed in every case or whether hypothermia with inflow occlusion is satisfactory in the uncomplicated case. In the literature it is difficult to obtain statistics confined to childhood. Swan, and Lewis, using hypothermia, reported remarkably low mortality rates of less than 1% in recent series, even including adults with hypertension. With experienced surgeons employing the heart-lung machine, it appears that the mortality is from 1 to 2%. For the isolated secundum defect, we prefer to use hypothermia because of its inexpensive, unencumbered simplicity. The two operative deaths in our 125 cases were avoidable. One child died as a result of unrecognized postoperative cardiac tamponade and the second, due to a technical error at reoperation for incomplete closure. If one accepts a mortality of 1–2% in the closure of isolated secundum defects, the choice of hypothermia or of the heart-lung apparatus should be the decision of the surgeon.

Operation Employing Hypothermia

At a rectal temperature of 31 C, the chest is opened through a split-sternal incision. The thrill usually present with atrial defects has none of the jetlike quality of pulmonary stenosis if the valve is normal. The defect is felt by invaginating the atrial wall; if it is high, anomalous pulmonary veins are sought at the

Fig. 39-5.—Atrial septal defect, secundum type: operative technique. **A,** double-ended and mattress suture to aid in closure. **B,** carbon dioxide introduced into the right atrium during closure of the defect. (From Mustard, W. T., *et al.*: Surgery 50: 303, 1961.)

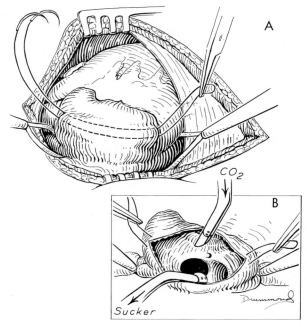

junction of the vena cava with the right atrium. The venae cavae are then taped, and if a left superior vena cava is present, it is also taped. A double line of continuous sutures is placed in the atrial wall (Fig. 39-5, *A*). The suture greatly facilitates closure and is an added safety factor. A Statinsky clamp is placed below the suture in the atrial wall; stay sutures are placed in the edges of the wall to aid in retraction. Carbon dioxide is directed into the field and the table is inclined away from the operator to place the left ventricle in the most dependent position (Fig. 39-5, *B*). The anesthesiologist hyperventilates with oxygen and replaces the usual bottle of citrated blood with heparinized blood. The tapes on the venae cavae are then closed with rubber tourniquets and the heart is emptied by massage. The atrium is opened after a minute and the interior inspected, first for the defect and next for the presence of anomalous veins. In the low defects, the orifice of the coronary sinus and the inferior vena cava are carefully located. Double-0 silk is placed at either end of the defect and a running suture is used for closure. Diversion of the inferior cava into the left atrium must be avoided.[23] The inferior stitch must include the wall of the left atrium in order to seal the left atrium effectively from the opening of the inferior cava. As the last stitch is snugged up, forceps are placed through the defect into the left atrium and the lungs are inflated, expelling the air and carbon dioxide from the left side of the heart. The final suture is tied below the level of blood which wells up from the left atrium. The right atrium is allowed to fill from the superior vena cava, the double continuous suture is elevated and the Statinsky clamp reapplied to the atrial wall. The caval tapes are removed, and one usually sees a hypertensive reactive period with an actual increase of blood pressure as the heart takes over. The atrial wall is then closed with carefully placed running stitches of 4-0 silk. The pericardial sac is left wide open, and plastic catheter underwater drains are placed in the pericardial sac and in the anterior mediastinum and brought through two separate stab wounds below the incision. The sternum is closed by interrupted wire sutures and the skin by subcuticular wire. Warming with hot water bottles and the heating blanket commences when the defect is being closed, and the patient is usually removed to the recovery room when the rectal temperature reaches 93.2 F. If anomalous pulmonary veins are present, we now routinely set up the bag oxygenator with glucose, prime and perform a careful repair on by-pass.

POSTOPERATIVE CARE

We have been impressed by the absence of complications in the postoperative period following correction of atrial septal defects under hypothermia. Oxygen is used sparingly because we believe it tends to thicken bronchial secretions even when moistened. Slight suction is placed on the underwater drains and lost blood carefully replaced. In children, we have not encountered excessive bleeding following hypothermia such as has been reported occasionally in adults. The children are turned frequently and encouraged to cough, and the very young patients have repeated laryngeal suctions by experienced nurses. They are generally kept in the recovery room overnight, and the following day a portable chest film is taken, following which one or both drainage tubes are removed. These patients are up and walking a week after operation and usually discharged from hospital after removal of the wire subcuticular skin sutures on the tenth postoperative day.

RESULTS OF OPERATION

CLOSED METHODS.—Only a few publications have been confined to the childhood group. Older patients with large hearts and pulmonary hypertension obviously affect any statistical survey. Of the blind techniques, that of the atrial well of Gross has been the most effective. The Mayo Clinic group[9] reported 58 children with no deaths and 57 apparently complete closures. The report included 9 cases of partial anomalous pulmonary venous drainage. Using the circumclusion technique of Sondergaard, Bosher[4] reported on 6 children cured by this method.

OPEN METHODS.—Statistics on exclusive series of operations on children are difficult to obtain, but it appears that surgeons experienced in the use of the heart-lung apparatus can close a simple atrial septal defect in a child with a mortality of 1–2%. This figure would apply also to those experienced in the use of hypothermia. With such low mortality figures, which will probably become even lower, the point of interest now is the recurrence or persistence rate. Only time will answer this question.

BIBLIOGRAPHY

1. Bailey, C. P., *et al.*: Congenital interatrial connections: Clinical and surgical considerations with a description of a new surgical technique—atrioseptopexy, Ann. Int. Med. 37:888, 1952.
2. Bjork, V. O., *et al.*: Atrial septal defects: A new surgical approach and diagnostic aspects, Acta chir. scandinav. 107:499, 1954.
3. Blount, S. G., Jr., *et al.*: Atrial septal defect: Clinical and physiologic response to complete closure in 5 patients, Circulation 9:801, 1954.
4. Bosher, L. H., Jr.: Repair of interatrial septal defects by a modified Sondergaard technique (circumclusion), Surgery 41:129, 1957.
5. Cohn, R.: An experimental method for the closure of interauricular septal defects in dogs, Am. Heart J. 33:353, 1947.
6. Cosby, R. S., and Griffith, G. C.: Intraatrial septal defect, Am. Heart J. 38:80, 1949.
7. Dennis, C., *et al.*: Development of a pump-oxygenator to replace the heart and lungs: An apparatus applicable to human patients, and application to one case, Ann. Surg. 134:709, 1951.
8. Dodrill, F. D.: A method for exposure of the cardiac septa: An experimental study, J. Thoracic Surg. 18:652, 1949.

9. Ellis, F. H., Jr., *et al.*: Defect of the atrial septum in the elderly, New England J. Med. 262:219, 1960.

10. Gibbon, J. H., Jr.: In discussion of Warden, H. E., *et al.*: Controlled cross circulation for open intracardiac surgery: Physiologic studies and results of creation and closure of ventricular septal defect, J. Thoracic Surg. 28:343, 1954.

11. Gross, R. E., *et al.*: A method for surgical closure of interauricular septal defects, Surg., Gynec. & Obst. 96:1, 1953.

12. Hufnagel, C. A., and Gillespie, J. F.: Closure of interauricular septal defects, Bull. Georgetown Univ. Med. Center 4:137, 1951.

13. Hull, E.: The cause and effects of flow through defects of the atrial septum, Am. Heart J. 38:350, 1949.

14. Keith, J. D., *et al.*: *Heart Disease in Infancy and Childhood* (New York: Macmillan Company, 1958).

15. Laird, J., and Wegelius, C.: Atrial septal defects in children: An angiocardiographic study, Circulation 7:819, 1953.

16. Lewis, F. J., and Tauffie, M.: Closure of atrial septal defects with aid of hypothermia: Experimental accomplishments and report of one successful case, Surgery 33:52, 1953.

17. Lewis, F. J., *et al.*: The surgical anatomy of atrial septal defects: Experiences with repair under direct vision, Ann. Surg. 142:401, 1955.

18. Lillehei, C. W.: Contributions of open cardiotomy to the correction of congenital and acquired cardiac diseases, New England J. Med. 258:1048, 1958.

19. McGoon, D. C., *et al.*: Surgical treatment of atrial septal defect in children, Pediatrics 24:992, 1959.

20. Murray, G.: Closure of defects in cardiac septa, Ann. Surg. 128:843, 1948.

21. Mustard, W. T., *et al.*: The surgical treatment of atrial septal defects in children, Canad. M. A. J. 84:138, 1961.

22. Mustard, W. T., and Chute, A. L.: Experimental intracardiac surgery with extracorporeal circulation, Surgery 30:684, 1951.

23. Mustard, W. T.; Firor, W. B., and Kidd, L.: Diversion of the venae cavae into the left atrium during closure of atrial septal defects, J. Thoracic & Cardiovas. Surg. 47:317, 1964.

24. Roesler, H.: Interatrial septal defect, Arch. Int. Med. 54:339, 1934.

25. Sondergaard, T., *et al.*: Closure of experimentally produced atrial septal defects, Acta chir. scandinav. 107:485, 1954.

26. Swan, H.; Blount, S. C., Jr., and Virtue, R. W.: Direct vision suture of interatrial septal defect during hypothermia, Surgery 38:858, 1955.

27. Swan, H., *et al.*: The experimental creation and closure of auricular septal defects, J. Thoracic Surg. 20:542, 1950.

28. Wood, P. H.: *Diseases of the Heart and Circulation* (2nd ed.; London: Eyre & Spottiswoode, Ltd., 1956), p. 360.

OSTIUM PRIMUM

HISTORY.—The primum defect in the interatrial septum presents a problem very different from the surgical point of view from that of the secundum defect. Recognition of this fact has been so recent that Blount *et al.*[1] in 1956 were apparently the first to call attention to the differential diagnosis. Edwards[2] in 1948 considered this defect a variant of atrioventricularis communis. Lillehei[4] recognized the necessity for repairing the cleft in the mitral valve when closing the primum defect with the use of the artificial heart-lung apparatus.

INCIDENCE AND NATURAL HISTORY

When one separates this defect from the secundum type and atrioventricularis communis, it is found to be relatively rare. In the cases recorded by Blount *et al.*,[1] there were 5 of ostium primum defects among 85 cases of atrial septal defects of all types. In our surgical series, there was a ratio of 1 ostium primum defect to 6 secundum defects. From published reports, it is difficult to separate the primum defect with both the major cleft in the mitral valve and a minor cleft in the tricuspid valve from atrioventricularis communis.

Keith[5] pointed out that infants with this defect usually survive to 4 years of age and may survive to 30. In his group of 85 cases of atrial septal defects, survival in the 5 documented cases of Blount was 27 months, 28 months, 4 years, 4 years, and 10 years; 3 were confirmed at autopsy, 2 at operation.

PATHOLOGIC ANATOMY

In the literature, there is considerable disparity of criteria in the differentiation of primum defects from atrioventricularis communis. For terms of definition we have taken the view, perhaps incorrectly, that if the mitral and tricuspid valves were fused at the base of the interventricular septum the term ostium primum should be used. If the valves fail to meet, with or without a defect in the interventricular septum, the proper nomenclature should be atrioventricularis communis, partial or complete. The ostium primum defect has no septal tissue between the lateral wall of the defect and the atrioventricular valve ring. Almost invariably (but not in 3 cases of our series), there is an associated cleft in the mitral valve. This cleft in the aortic leaf of the mitral valve may vary from incipient to complete. The edges are composed of nodular fibrous embryonic tissue, and as been pointed out by Blount[1] and Edwards,[2] there may be adventitious rudimentary chordae tendineae. An associated cleft in the tricuspid valve may be present with an underdeveloped septal leaf. In our series, the tricuspid valve has been cleft in 3 cases (Fig. 39-6). The defect in the atrial septum may be small—even smaller than that seen in the secundum defects. On the other hand, there may be no septal tissue discernible at operation. The pathologic anatomy poses an obvious problem to the surgeon. In childhood, there is so little tissue that a prosthesis for the atrial septal defect is almost a necessity.

DIAGNOSIS

In contrast to children with the secundum defect, those with ostium primum defects demonstrate retardation of growth and development. Respiratory infections occur frequently and exercise tolerance is limited early in life. The heart is invariably enlarged, and there is a rough systolic murmur over the second and third left interspaces. A systolic murmur over the apical area should lead one to suspect the mitral insufficiency which almost invariably accompanies this defect.

On fluoroscopic examination, the hilar shadows are

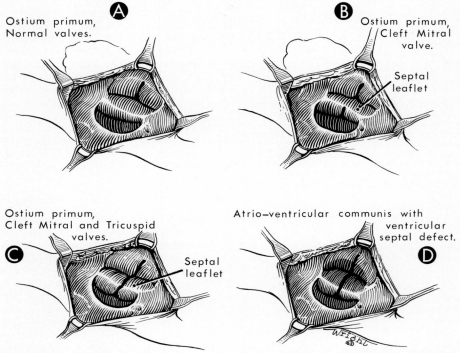

Ⓐ Ostium primum, Normal valves.

Ⓑ Ostium primum, Cleft Mitral valve. Septal leaflet

Ⓒ Ostium primum, Cleft Mitral and Tricuspid valves. Septal leaflet

Ⓓ Atrio-ventricular communis with ventricular septal defect.

Fig. 39-6.—Endocardial cushion defects. The surgeon must familiarize himself with the pathology of these lesions to assure success. It must be remembered that these are diagrams; valves in atrioventricularis communis in an infant a few months old may be hopelessly deformed and repair impossible. Direct suture of the primum type should be avoided; tension on the suture line is prone to reopen the defect, especially in the presence of residual mitral insufficiency. Furthermore, deep sutures in the septum may cause heart block. (From Welch, C. E. [ed.]: *Advances in Surgery* [Chicago: Year Book Medical Publishers, Inc, 1965], Vol.1.)

Fig. 39-7.—Atrial septal defect, primum type. Roentgenogram shows the greatly enlarged heart, prominent right atrium and pulmonary artery and increased lung vascularity. This 3-year-old girl tired easily and had bouts of dyspnea. Catheterization revealed marked rise of oxygen saturation at the atrial level; the ECG showed left axis deviation and a counterclockwise loop in the frontal vector. A cleft mitral valve was repaired and the ostium primum defect closed under direct vision.

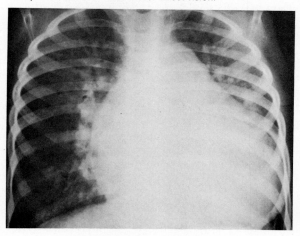

increased and the heart size is greater than that seen in the secundum type of atrial septal defect (Fig. 39-7). The right atrium and right ventricle are enlarged. The electrocardiogram reveals left axis deviation with a counterclockwise loop in the frontal vector (Fig. 39-8). Cardiac catheterization demonstrates a rise of oxygen saturation at the atrial level, seen in any atrial septal defect, and is not very helpful in differentiating these lesions. The absence of a rise of oxygen saturation at the right ventricle level in the atrium primum defect is helpful in differentiating it from atrioventricularis communis. Pulmonary hypertension is unusual in childhood, and in only 2 of our cases was the pulmonary systolic pressure over 50 mm Hg.

OPERATIVE TREATMENT

A proper understanding of the pathology of this defect is imperative in the surgical approach. At present, the use of the artificial heart-lung apparatus is essential for complete correction. Closed techniques are doomed to failure even in the absence of a cleft in either the mitral or tricuspid valve. Hypothermia with inflow occlusion affords inadequate time to correct

FRONTAL

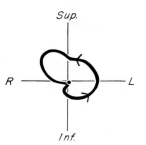

Fig. 39-8.—Atrial septal defect, primum type. Vector cardiography is very useful in differentiating the primum from the secundum type. In the primum type, the loop is counterclockwise above the horizontal in the frontal plane.

REFERENCES

1. Blount, S. G., *et al.*: The persistent ostium primum atrial septal defect, Circulation 13:499, 1956.
2. Edwards, J. E.: *An Atlas of Congenital Anomalies of the Heart and Great Vessels: Pathology of the Heart* (Springfield, Ill.: Charles C Thomas, Publisher, 1953).
3. Flege, J. B., *et al.*: Congenital mitral incompetence, J. Thoracic & Cardiovas. Surg. 53:138, 1967.
4. Kalm, D. R., *et al.*: Long term results of valvuloplasty for mitral insufficiency in children, J. Thoracic & Cardiovas. Surg. 53:1, 1967.
5. Keith, J. D., *et al.*: *Heart Disease in Infancy and Childhood* (New York: Macmillan Company, 1958).
6. Lillehei, C. W.: Contributions of open cardiotomy to the correction of congenital and acquired cardiac disease, New England J. Med. 258:1048, 1958.
7. Mustard, W. T.; Niguidula, F. N., and Trusler, G. A.: Endocardial cushion defects in infants and children: Ten years' surgical experience, Brit. Heart J. 27:768, 1965.
8. Van Mierop, L. H. S., and Alley, R. D.: The management of the cleft mitral valve in endocardial cushion defects, Ann. Thoracic Surg. 2:416, 1966.

W. T. MUSTARD

Drawings by
A. M. WRIGHT
(Figures 39-1 and 39-6)

this defect. The mitral valve should be carefully repaired through the defect, and, as pointed out by Edwards,[2] the adventitious chordae tendineae should be divided to allow adequate valve closure. One must be certain that only adventitious chordae are sacrificed or the cusp will prolapse. In the small heart, finger palpation is difficult, and our experience has led us to err on the side of valvular stenosis rather than leave an incomplete valve. The tricuspid valve is often deficient in its septal leaf. Special prosthetic reconstructive techniques may help overcome this difficult situation. Direct closure of the atrial defect by suture should be avoided, since the valve ring does not allow enough slack for the sutures, which may pull out. A prosthesis (Teflon) should be inserted and great care be taken to avoid the bundle of His as it passes superiorly from the coronary sinus into the interventricular septum. It may be necessary to place sutures very deep to the ventricular septum to avoid the bundle or, if enough tissue is present at the valve level, to place the sutures superficial to the bundle. Repair of the mitral valve may be easy or extremely difficult. From experience, we know that the results of repair of the cleft mitral valve are far from satisfactory. If there is adequate valve tissue and no shortened chordae tendineae, a good result may be obtained by complete closure of the cleft, leaving the child with minimal mitral incompetence.[7] However, certain of the cleft valves are competent and should not be repaired. A preoperative left ventricular angiocardiogram may be useful in assessing the presence or absence of incompetence. Plastic procedures on the grossly incompetent valve may produce greater insufficiency than before the operation due to the closure of the atrial septal defect. Reports of successful relief of incompetence by the use of annuloplasty have appeared in the literature.[3,4] Whatever method one uses, there is no room for complacency, and certain valves should be replaced.[7]

RESULTS OF OPERATION.—The mortality in experienced hands appears to be from 5 to 10%. The degree of completeness of correction has not been statistically evaluated. The mitral valve cannot be considered normal, and subsequent stenosis may develop or regurgitation may persist.

ATRIOVENTRICULARIS COMMUNIS

HISTORY.—In 1875, Von Rokitansky[8] described this defect, and in 1948 Rogers and Edwards[6] clarified the pathologic anatomy. Lillehei[3] in 1954 successfully operated on an infant of 1 year, using the parent donor cross-circulation technique. Among subsequent reports of successful operations is that of Cooley and Kirklin.[1]

PATHOLOGIC ANATOMY

The single atrium and ventricle of the embryo is converted into two chambers by growth of dorsal and ventral partitions called endocardial cushions. The atrioventricular canal is formed by the junction of these two cushions. The septums between these ventricles and atriums form at the same time. The anterior halves of the anterior leaf of the mitral valve and of the septal leaf of the tricuspid valve lie in the ventral cushion and the posterior half of these valves in the dorsal cushion. Failure of fusion of the endocardial cushions results in clefts in the valves and a ventricular and atrial septal defect.

Communications between the two ventricles by fenestrations may be present under the valve ring with fusion of the endocardial cushions. From a clinical point of view we prefer to designate this form partial atrioventricularis communis. In the complete type, the ventricular septal defect may be 1 cm or more in size. Valve tissue, particularly of the septal leaf of the tricuspid valve, may be deficient.

The nomenclature is somewhat confused. Watkins and Gross[10] have preferred the term endocardial cushion defects to include ostium primum and partial and complete atrioventricularis communis. The term persistent atrioventricular canal, according to Wakai and Edwards,[9] includes ostium primum defects.

The right atrium, right ventricle and pulmonary artery are enlarged as a result of the greatly increased left-to-right shunt. Major associated anomalies are not uncommon, and in Keith's series mongolism was present in 37%.[2]

Natural History

A high percentage of infants with this anomaly die in the first year of life, probably as the result of the great flow to the lungs. A few survive to 4 years, and the oldest child we have operated on was 7 years old.

Diagnosis

The infant is usually seen in the first few months of life with dyspnea, tachycardia and failure to thrive. A harsh systolic murmur is present over the precordium and the heart is enlarged. Radiologically, this enlargement of the heart is mainly due to bulging of the right atrium and to some enlargement of the right ventricle (Fig. 39-9). On cardiac catheterization, a rise of oxygen saturation is found in both right atrium and right ventricle. Pulmonary hypertension is the rule and is greater in cases with a true ventricular septal defect. The significant feature on electrocardiography is the axis of the QRS complex, which is usually in the neighborhood of minus 60°. Right ventricular hypertrophy accompanies the left axis deviation.

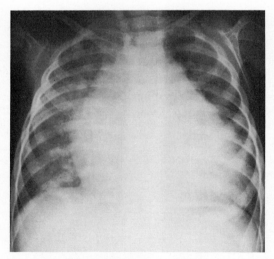

Fig. 39-9.—Atrioventricularis communis. The heart is often tremendously enlarged in infancy, as in this film of a 3-month-old infant whose diagnosis was proved at autopsy. Large interventricular and interatrial septal defects were present with grossly deformed tricuspid and mitral valves which could not have been repaired by present techniques.

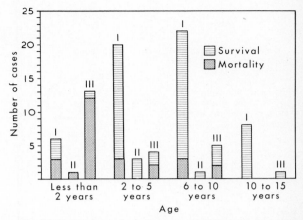

Fig. 39-10.—Atrioventricularis communis. Operative mortality at different ages, of types of atrial septal defects according to classification of Campbell and Missen (Brit Heart J. 19:403, 1957). In this text, **I** is ostium primum; **II**, partial atrioventricularis; **III**, complete atrioventricularis communis. (From Mustard, W. T., *et al.*: Brit. Heart J. 27:768, 1965.)

Indications for Operation

The operative mortality is extremely high in the first year of life (Fig. 39-10). If at all possible, the baby should be carried through this period on a medical regimen, but if it is obvious that the infant is going to succumb, operation must be undertaken. Whether total correction is indicated is a difficult question. We have followed the lead of Muller and Dammann[5] and of Sirak *et al.*[7] in banding the pulmonary artery with some success. If one uses the age of 2 as a minimum for the corrective operation, the natural selection will give better mortality figures. These children usually have small interventricular septal defects and more valve tissue which enables them to survive and thus makes them more amenable to operative correction.

Operative Technique

In the correction of this defect, the use of hypothermia combined with the artificial heart-lung apparatus enables one to use lower flow rates which are more compatible with small cannulas whether the common iliac or the common femoral artery is used. The split-sternal incision gives adequate operative room, and the enlarged right atrium makes it possible to manipulate inside these relatively small hearts. Great care must be taken to rule out fenestrations behind the valves if the endocardial cushions have fused. Occasionally, these fenestrations may be closed by direct suture or deliberately opened to allow one to insert a small Ivalon patch. When the endocardial cushions have not come together, it is obvious that a prosthesis must be inserted. Because the tissue is very muscular and the bundle is passing along its margin, we have preferred to place deep sutures and a patch larger than the actual defect. The mitral valve is first carefully repaired, closing the cleft as completely as possible (we have never produced stenosis). It may be necessary to cut adventitious chordae tendineae in order to allow closure of the valve in systole. The septal leaf of the tricuspid valve usually is somewhat rudimentary, and perhaps one should insert some type of prosthesis to allow the other two cusps to close on the septal leaf. All of our survivors have shown some degree of tricuspid insufficiency. The atrial septal defect is closed with Ivalon or Teflon. Care must be taken to avoid the bundle of His as it passes from the coronary sinus to the rim of the interventricular septum. We have preferred to perform this operation with the heart beating and with careful monitoring with the electrocardiograph to avoid damage to the bundle of His, since our earlier patients developed heart block which terminated fatally.

RESULTS OF SURGERY

Of 15 patients reported by McGoon *et al.*,[4] 3 survived, and since the mortality rate under 3 years was 88% in 8 cases, we presume 1 child at least survived. Heart block and persistent valvular incompetence were the major causes of death. In our series of 16 children under 6 years there were 3 survivors, 1 of whom had some persistent valvular incompetence. If one includes patients operated on in infancy, one must accept a mortality figure of about 80%, and among those surviving, heart block or some degree of mitral or tricuspid insufficiency may persist, probably due to enlarged valvular rings and lack of available valvular tissue or a combination of both. If the valve

rings are greatly enlarged, some attempt at narrowing them may be feasible. On one occasion we carried out this procedure on the tricuspid valve, plicating it over Ivalon buttons in an anteroposterior direction. At present, the outlook for an infant born with a complete atrioventricular canal is gloomy (see Fig. 39-10).

REFERENCES

1. Cooley, J. C., and Kirklin, J. W.: The surgical treatment of persistent common atrioventricular canal: Report of 12 cases, Proc. Staff Meet. Mayo Clin. 31:523, 1956.
2. Keith, J. D., *et al.*: *Heart Disease in Infancy and Childhood* (New York: Macmillan Company, 1958).
3. Lillehei, C. W., *et al.*: The direct vision intracardiac correction of congenital anomalies by controlled cross-circulation: Results in 32 patients with ventricular septal defects, tetralogy of Fallot, and atrioventricularis communis defects, Surgery 38:11, 1955.
4. McGoon, D. C., *et al.*: The surgical treatment of endocardial cushion defects, Surgery 46:185, 1959.
5. Muller, W. H., Jr., and Dammann, J. F., Jr.: Results following the creation of pulmonary artery stenosis, Ann. Surg. 14:6, 1956.
6. Rogers, H. M., and Edwards, J. E.: Incomplete division of the atrioventricular canal with patent interatrial foramen primum (persistent common atrioventricular ostium), Am. Heart J. 36:28, 1948.
7. Sirak, H. D.; Hosier, D. M., and Clatworthy, H. W.: Defects of the interventricular septum in infancy: A two-stage approach to their surgical correction, New England J. Med. 260:147, 1959.
8. Von Rokitansky, C. F.: *Die Defekte der Scheidewände des Herzens: Pathologisch-Anatomische Abhandlung* (Wien: W. Braunmüller, 1875).
9. Wakai, C. S., and Edwards, J. E.: Developmental and pathologic considerations in persistent common atrioventricular canal, Proc. Staff Meet. Mayo Clin. 31:487, 1956.
10. Watkins, E., Jr., and Gross, R. E.: Experiences with surgical repair of atrial septal defects, J. Thoracic Surg. 30:469, 1955.

W. T. MUSTARD

Congenital Mitral Stenosis

ISOLATED congenital mitral stenosis is rare. The first clinically proved case was reported by Bower and associates.[1] Congenital mitral stenosis may occur with other defects such as patent ductus arteriosus and coarctation of the aorta. Angiocardiography and left heart catheterization may be diagnostic, the left atrium failing to empty and demonstrating a marked rise of pressure.

The prognosis is poor; the literature contains few cases of survival of the first year of life. Bower's 2 patients were operated on by valvulotomy, and 1,

aged 5¼ years, appeared to be improved. Experience has been discouraging in the infant or child who fails to survive the postoperative period due to mitral insufficiency. Although occasional success has been reported, the best chance for success seems to be with valve replacement. We have operated on 6 children early in life. Two died of insufficiency and 4 showed some improvement.[2]

REFERENCES

1. Bower, B. D., *et al.*: Two cases of congenital mitral stenosis treated by valvulotomy, Arch. Dis. Childhood 28:91, 1953.
2. Trusler, G. A., and Fowler, R. S.: Congenital mitral stenosis in infancy: Report of a case with open correction, Surgery 58:431, 1965.

W. T. MUSTARD

Congenital Mitral Insufficiency

Isolated mitral insufficiency of congenital origin is uncommon and may be difficult to differentiate from acquired incompetence. The anatomic features have been described by Edwards and Burchell.[1] Although there may be a cleft, elongated or shortened chordae or fenestrations are common. Kahn *et al.*[3] have emphasized that the important therapeutic point is the dilated annulus.

The signs and symptoms range from none to congestive heart failure. With the latter, left atrial and left ventricular enlargement, mitral incompetence (usually severe) and elevated pulmonary artery wedge pressures are present. Left heart angiocardiography reveals the mitral incompetence and large left atrium.

OPERATIVE TECHNIC

The approach is a right thoracotomy. After by-pass is instituted, the left atrium is opened beneath the intra-atrial groove. It is evident from our experience and recent published reports that insufficiency may be caused by a variety of pathologic lesions. Of 13 patients reported on by Flege *et al.*,[2] 3 had a cleft in the septal cusp, 4 lacked chordae to restrain the central portion of the cusp edge requiring repair and 9 required annuloplasty. Nine patients were improved after operation, 3 were not and 1 died. In 9 children followed up by Kahn *et al.*,[3] for 8 months to 8 years, valvuloplasty gave good results. Trusler *et al.*[4] reported that a 14-month-old child was active and well following replacement of the valve with a Starr-Edwards prosthesis (Fig. 39-11).

REFERENCES

1. Edwards, J. T., and Burchell, H. B.: Pathologic anatomy of mitral insufficiency, Proc. Staff Meet. Mayo Clin. 33:497, 1958.
2. Flege, J. B., *et al.*: Congenital mitral incompetence, J. Thoracic & Cardiovas. Surg. 53:138, 1967.
3. Kahn, D. R., *et al.*: Long-term results of valvuloplasty for mitral insufficiency in children, J. Thoracic & Cardiovas. Surg. 53:1; 1967:
4. Trusler, G. A., *et al.*: Mitral valve replacement in a 14-month-old child, Canad. M. A. J. 95:1297, 1966.

W. T. MUSTARD

Fig. 39-11.—Congenital mitral insufficiency. **A,** preoperative anteroposterior roentgenogram of the chest of a 14-month-old child, showing globular enlargement of the heart (cardiothoracic ratio 70%). **B,** anteroposterior view 10 months after operation. with Starr-Edwards mitral valve in place. There were reduction of heart size (cardiothoracic ratio 58%) and dramatic clinical improvement. (From Trusler *et al.*[4])

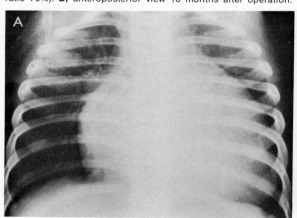
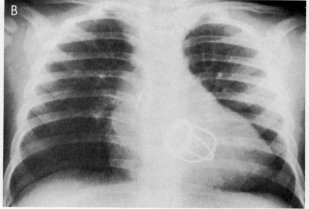

Cor Triatriatum

This rare malformation is essentially a division of the left atrium into two compartments. The upper one is enlarged and probably represents a common pulmonary vein which connects with the true left atrium through a stenotic orifice.[1] The diagnosis is usually congenital mitral stenosis.

Selective angiocardiography will reveal two chambers.[2] A high pulmonary wedge pressure and a relatively normal-sized left atrium should make one reconsider this diagnosis.

The diaphragm is excised through the larger chamber on cardiopulmonary by-pass.

REFERENCES

1. Grondin, C., *et al.*: Cor triatriatum: A diagnostic surgical enigma, J. Thoracic & Cardiovas. Surg. 48:527, 1964.

2. LaSalle, R., *et al.*: Cor triatriatum: Report of a case, with emphasis on cineangiocardiography, Canad. M. A. J. 89:616, 1963.

Ventricular Septal Defects

History.—Roger[31] in 1879 described a harsh systolic murmur to the left of the sternum and indicated the underlying pathology of a ventricular septal defect. Abbott[1] in 1932 correlated the pathology with the clinical findings in a number of cases. Murray[28] in 1948 attempted repair in the human by passing a strip of fascia lata through the defect, and Bailey[2] in 1952 attempted to pull a tube of pericardium through the defect. King[19] modified this technique with tactile guidance. Lillehei *et al.*,[24] using cross-circulation technique and open cardiotomy, successfully closed a ventricular septal defect in a 4-year-old boy.

INCIDENCE AND NATURAL HISTORY

It is difficult to present an accurate picture of the prevalence of ventricular septal defect in childhood. Wood[37] found ventricular septal defect in 8% of congenital heart disease cases and Perry[30] found 35%. Keith[16] reported 25% incidence of isolated ventricular septal defect in 6,600 cases of congenital heart disease. The presence of a ventricular septal defect with other forms of congenital heart disease raised the figure to 50%. In 288 autopsies of children dying of major congenital cardiac anomalies, Zacharioudakis[38] found 23 cases of ventricular septal defect, the second most common cause of death.

An accurate appraisal of the life span of a child born with a ventricular septal defect is difficult to secure. Death in the first year of life from an isolated ventricular defect is not uncommon. In autopsy examination of 50 hearts, Becu *et al.*[3] found isolated ventricular septal defects in 19 children, 12 of them less than 1 year of age.

If an infant survives the first year of life without developing heart failure, or with proper medical management of heart failure, life expectancy should depend on the size of the defect, the volume of flow through it and the pulmonary resistance. There is a relatively large group of infants with low pulmonary vascular resistance and low pulmonary blood flow in whom no sequelae due to the shunt will occur in later life. Indeed, spontaneous closure of a ventricular septal defect has been well documented. Mudd *et al.*[26] observed during a period of 1-9 years that none of 163 patients with pulmonary systolic pressures below 50 mm Hg showed any clinical evidence of progressive deterioration. Forty in this group underwent serial catheterization studies; none showed evidence of progressive pulmonary hypertension and in 2 the de-fect had spontaneously closed. If pulmonary vascular resistance increases, the volume of shunt diminishes, and the child may lead a relatively asymptomatic life until such a time as the shunt becomes bidirectional or from right to left and the patient succumbs in early adult life. In 98 children with catheter-proved ventricular septal defects, Fyler *et al.*[9] found only 1 death after infancy. There were 5 deaths in infancy in this study. Downing and Goldberg[6] made a detailed study (including cardiac catheterization) of 100 patients with ventricular septal defects. There were 23 patients over 15, the oldest being 52. Of the 100 patients, 89 had symptoms and 8 of the remaining asymptomatic patients were below 3 years of age; 71 had shortness of breath, and cardiac failure had been present in 22. It must be concluded that a number of persons survive into adulthood, but it appears that in patients surviving infancy, life expectancy is shortened by half.

PATHOLOGIC ANATOMY

As a rule, the defect in the ventricular septum is in the region of the membranous portion of the ventricular septum; this, as Becu pointed out, is more accurately defined as the area between the papillary muscle of the conus and the crista supraventricularis of the right ventricle. The defects are related to the membranous portion but are not restricted to this membranous portion of the septum. Isolated septal defects produce enlargement of the left ventricle and of the pulmonary artery. At operation, a thrill is palpable over the right ventricle when pressure in the right ventricle is less than the systemic. When the two pressures are equal, no thrill may be present. A white fibrous area occasionally is present opposite the jet stream of the ventricular septal defect on the wall of the right ventricular myocardium. When the defect is above the crista supraventricularis or in the muscular portion of the septum, the rim usually consists of smooth muscle tissue and is circular in outline. When the defect is in the membranous portion of the septum, as it was in 62 of 70 cases studied by us (Fig. 39-12), the shape is usually oval and the superior margin may extend to the aortic valve ring. The inferior margin is most variable, partly muscular and partly fibrous, and is limited by the papillary muscle of the conus (see Fig. 39-16). When the defect is small, 1 cm or less, there may be a well-defined fibrous margin between the septal leaf of the tricuspid valve and the aortic leaf of the mitral valve. When the defect is large, however,

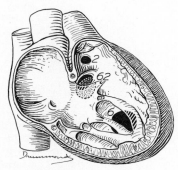

Fig. 39-12.—Ventricular septal defects. Sites of the defect in 70 children operated on, with use of the artificial heart-lung apparatus (From Mustard and Trusler.[29])

the septal leaf of the tricuspid valve occludes the lower third of the defect and the margin then becomes the junction of the aortic leaf of the mitral valve and the septal leaf of the tricuspid valve. Indeed, in large defects the surgeon at operation is faced with a defect whose margins appear to be formed by the aortic ring above and the septal leaf of the tricuspid valve below. Associated defects are not uncommon; in our clinical experience, patent ductus arteriosus was most commonly present. Changes in the pulmonary arterial tree are described in the discussion of pulmonary hypertension in Chapter 43.

Hemodynamics

Because of the difference in pressures between the left and the right side of the heart, the shunt in most cases is from the left to the right ventricle. The volume of this shunt does not seem to be related to the position of the defect or even to its size. A rise of oxygen content of 1 vol% in catheter samples on passing from the right atrium to the right ventricle indicates the presence of a ventricular defect.[17] In our operated patients, the average rise of oxygen saturation was from 10 to 20%. The flow through the pulmonary circulation in patients with ventricular septal defects varies from 1.2 to 5 times systemic,[16] and this flow will be less in cases with increased pulmonary vascular resistance. The estimation of pulmonary blood flow correlated with pulmonary vascular resistance becomes significant in selecting patients for operation and will be further elaborated below.

Diagnosis

A harsh pansystolic murmur in the third or fourth left interspace with a palpable thrill in an acyanotic child is almost pathognomonic of ventricular septal defect. In infants with pulmonary hypertension and high pulmonary blood flow, dyspnea may be present at rest, but in older children, exercise tolerance is remarkable and many lead a normal, active life. In the infant, a classic murmur is present, with a history

of failure to thrive and repeated respiratory infections. Cardiac enlargement is present with increased hilar vascular markings, and the electrocardiogram may demonstrate right ventricular or combined hypertrophy. In the older child, exercise tolerance may be normal or only slightly limited. In appearance, our group of surgical patients were mainly thin, poorly developed, with a bulging precordium. If the defect is moderate or large, a thrust is present over the apex of the heart accompanied by a coarse thrill. On radiologic examination, the heart may be normal in size but often demonstrates some enlargement, particularly of the left atrium, with bulging pulmonary artery, increased hilar shadows and hilar pulsations. Findings on a plain roentgenogram have considerable surgical significance, and increased vascular markings well out into the periphery even in the presence of pulmonary hypertension are considered to indicate increased flow rather than increased resistance (Fig. 39-13). In the older child, the electrocardiogram may be normal, show left ventricular hypertrophy, combined hypertrophy or a moderate degree of right hypertrophy. The axis usually is in the normal range, and right in cases of marked pulmonary hypertension. Cardiac catheterization, although not as useful in the infant, usually demonstrates a rise of oxygen saturation on passing from the right atrium to the right ventricle. Tricuspid incompetence may be reflected in a rise of oxygen saturation in both atrium and ventricle. A further rise on passing through the pulmonary valve into the left pulmonary artery may indicate the presence of a patent ductus arteriosus. Selective angiocardiography may reveal recirculation of the contrast medium through the defect. On some occasions,

Fig. 39-13.—Ventricular septal defect; balanced shunt. Roentgenogram of a 6-year-old boy with catheter-proved isolated defect. Note prominence of pulmonary artery and increased vascular patterns in the lungs. Right ventricular pressure equaled systemic pressure on preoperative catheterization. Oxygen saturation rose 20% as the catheter passed from the right atrium to right ventricle. The ECG demonstrated a deep Q wave in V_6. The defect was closed and postoperative course smooth.

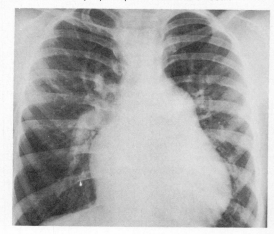

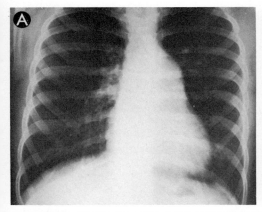
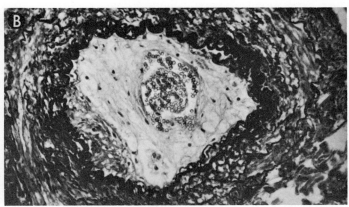

Fig. 39-14.—Ventricular septal defect, with pulmonary hypertension. **A,** anteroposterior roentgenogram of a 15-year-old boy with right ventricular pressure of 100/0. Note the small heart (cardiothoracic ratio 12.5:240) and clear lung fields. He died suddenly 3 days after exploratory thoracotomy. At autopsy, a large ventricular septal defect and vascular lung changes were found. **B,** photomicrograph of a small pulmonary artery from a section of this patient's lung. Note intimal proliferation and medial thickening of the vessel wall.

the defect may be outlined and an indication of its size be obtained.

Estimation of pulmonary blood flow.—Physical examination of children with a large flow will demonstrate an overactive heart with a good systolic murmur and thrill and occasionally an inflow diastolic murmur at the apex. Children who have a low flow with increased pulmonary vascular resistance usually have a soft murmur and no thrill. X-ray examination of patients with a large flow shows the left ventricle to be enlarged, the right ventricle dilated and enlarged and the pulmonary artery and its branches to be well out into the lung fields[7] (Fig. 39-13). In children with a small flow, the left ventricle is not enlarged, the right ventricle is not dilated and lung fields are clear (Fig. 39-14).

Electrocardiogram.—Increased left ventricular work is demonstrated by deep Q waves in leads representing left ventricular potentials; Keith[17] considers these waves to be very significant of increased flow. We have not found lung biopsy to be of much value in distinguishing children who have pulmonary vascular resistance from those who have none. (See Pulmonary Hypertension in Chapter 43.)

Kidd and co-workers[18] set forth six hemodynamic groups in ventricular septal defect and related the electrocardiographic and the vector cardiographic findings to these groupings. In the group with low flow and low resistance, a normal electrocardiographic pattern predominates (54%) and the mean frontal axis is within normal limits and to the left. As the flow and resistance increase, the mean QRS axis shifts around to a point where it is deviated strongly to the right. In this group with high pulmonary resistance and reversal of flow through the defect, a pure right ventricular hypertrophy pattern is found in most cases. The intermediate groups with flows greater than 2:1 and varying degrees of pulmonary vascular resistance have cardiographic patterns that lie between these extremes, with varying left ventricular or combined ventricular hypertrophy and a mean frontal QRS axis between 31 and 146°.

Differential Diagnosis

Pulmonic stenosis.—A pansystolic murmur to the left of the sternum may be confused with the murmur heard in cases of right ventricular and infundibular stenosis and, particularly in the infant, pulmonic stenosis. Right ventricular hypertrophy in the electrocardiogram, the lack of any rise of oxygen saturation on passing a catheter from the right atrium to the right ventricle and an increase of pressure in the right ventricle are useful in the diagnosis of pulmonic stenosis.

Aortic stenosis.—The murmur of aortic stenosis in infancy may be heard over the left precordium. The murmur of aortic stenosis is shorter and comes to a peak in systole, whereas the murmur of a ventricular septal defect is pansystolic.[16]

Atrial septal defect.—Defects of the secundum type with a soft murmur and a widely split second sound in the pulmonary area are not difficult to distinguish. The primum defect and atrioventricularis communis may simulate an isolated ventricular septal defect, and the electrocardiogram with left axis deviation is most useful in differential diagnosis. Cardiac catheterization should show a step-up of oxygen saturation in the right atrium in atrial septal defects.

Combination of defects.—A combination of ventricular septal defect and *patent ductus arteriosus* may be a cause of failure in infancy. The volume of flow through the ductus may be as great as that through the ventricular septal defect. Cardiac catheterization is very useful, particularly if the catheter is passed through the ductus and into the aorta. Ventricular septal defect associated with *aortic insufficiency*, although rare, is sometimes difficult to distinguish from ventricular septal defects associated with patent ductus arteriosus. Wide pulse pressure may be present in both circumstances, and the diastolic murmur of aortic insufficiency with a ventricular septal murmur defect present may be difficult to distinguish from the continuous murmur of a ductus. Left heart catheterization may be necessary to prove the diagnosis, and occasionally the diagnosis can be made only at operation. *Isolated atrial secundum* defect with a ventricular septal defect can be proved on cardiac catheterization. Ventricular septal defect combined with *coarctation of the aorta* is not uncommon; absent femoral pulses or a difference in the blood pressure in the arm and leg are helpful in diagnosis. Children with *tetralogy of Fallot* with normal oximetry may be difficult to distinguish on clinical examination. Cardiac catheterization with a marked pressure differential on passing through the pulmonary valve aids in making the diagnosis.

INDICATIONS FOR OPERATION

The indications for operation have been widely debated and differ from center to center. There is ample evidence of spontaneous closure of small ventricular septal defects. Furthermore, the child with ventricular septal defect and low pulmonary blood flow, normal pulmonary artery pressure and low pulmonary vascular resistance will probably enjoy a normal life span without surgery. Shah *et al.*[32] demonstrated that the risk of subacute bacterial endocarditis is low and in all of their cases was completely curable. Children with the Eisenmenger complex and shunt reversal are obviously inoperable.

AGE.—Most surgeons familiar with the use of extracorporeal circulation take the view that infants tolerate the heart-lung machine poorly. For this reason, encouragement is given the nonoperative handling of these cases until the initial flooding of the lung has passed. During this period, banding of the pulmonary artery[27,33] may tide these infants over until the optimal age for extracorporeal circulation is reached. A heart-lung machine to fill the requirements of an infant may soon be developed, and these infants may be operated on at a young age, as demonstrated by Kirklin.[20] In selecting patients for operation over the age of 1 year, one must be guided by the clinical course and by certain definite signs. If a child is asymptomatic and has the classic murmur of a ventricular septal defect, operation may be deferred for some years. Indeed, we now await the possibility of spontaneous closure of ventricular septal defects with small flows until about age 4. Children with flow ratios less than 2:1 and normal or low pulmonary vascular re-

sistance may never require surgery or until the operative mortality is consistently less than 1%. If, however, the child has an enlarging heart, operation becomes imperative. We have been guided by the use of x-rays, electrocardiogram and cardiac catheterization. If pulmonary hypertension of over 70% systemic is present in an infant over 1 year of age, operation is imperative. If, however, the child is clinically well, the increase of oxygen saturation on passing a catheter from the right atrium to the right ventricle is not large, and the lungs do not show gross plethora, operation may be deferred for some years. We have come to recognize that the child with a ventricular septal defect proved by catheterization and enlargement of the heart and deepening of the Q waves in lead V_6 of the electrocardiogram should be operated on before the age of 6. The development of pulmonary hypertension is always a threat to these children, and although we operate on children whose pressures are identical in right and left ventricles, this always presents some hazard in the postoperative period. The risk of operating on these children is high, and even if they survive the postoperative period, pulmonary vascular disease may progress. In the course of time, the age for elective operation will be more clearly defined, as it has in other defects, as will the inoperability of a patient. At present, we feel that children with a shunt from right to left (demonstrated by oximetry) are inoperable.

TECHNIQUE OF OPERATION

Extracorporeal circulation is necessary for operating on these defects; extracorporeal circulation and hypothermia are discussed in Chapter 43. The presence of a patent ductus arteriosus is very important and makes the surgeon decide whether to use the split-sternal or the trans-sternal approach. If a split-sternal approach is used, the ductus is identified by an extrapericardial dissection over the uppermost part of the bulging pulmonary artery. By retracting the pulmonary artery, the recurrent nerve can be identified as it passes behind the ductus. If the ductus is large, we prefer to use the trans-sternal approach from the left side and, if possible, avoid opening the right chest. We have rarely considered it necessary to divide a patent ductus and have used the suture-ligation technique of Blalock. As a rule, the approach to the ventricular septal defect is through the right ventricle. The incision should be kept high to avoid post operative right heart failure due to the splinting effect on the right ventricle of a long incision, and is directed toward the pulmonary valve ring. Aberrant coronary vessels, particularly in corrected transposition, may pose a problem and alter slightly the line of incision. The coronary sucker placed in the right ventricle will control bleeding until it is placed through the defect into the left ventricle. A left ventricular vent is very useful to secure a relatively dry field. Clamping of the aorta is a matter for the individual

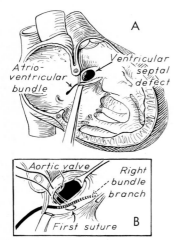

Fig. 39-15.—Ventricular septal defect. Knowledge of the course of the conduction system is important when closing such defects. A suture placed through or around the bundle before division into right and left branches is certain to cause complete heart block. Placement of the sutures on the right ventricular side produces right bundle-branch block which is compatible with normal sinus rhythm. (From Mustard and Trusler.[29])

surgeon; in the presence of aortic insufficiency, it is essential. Cardiac arrest may be used with the awareness that injury to the bundle of His is hindered by any arrest. Most surgeons are using varying periods of anoxic arrest. We have clamped the aorta for 25 minutes with restoration of normal sinus rhythm and recovery. Nevertheless we prefer to use shorter periods (5–10 minutes) and then allow the heart to recover. With experience and careful use of coronary

suction, it is seldom necessary to arrest the heart in the isolated septal defect. By placing the sutures in the right ventricular side of the septum, whatever method of closure is used, one avoids transfixing the bundle of His on the left ventricular side. Sirak *et al.*[33] demonstrated this in 53 consecutive cases of ventricular septal defects without heart block. Lev[23] pointed out that the bundle of His may vary in position but is usually situated on the left side, the center or the right side of the posterior wall of the defect (Fig. 39-15). A full understanding of the pathologic anatomy is necessary, and whether one closes the defect by direct suture or employs some form of plastic material to buttress sutures or uses a plastic patch is determined by the individual surgeon.

In an analysis of our first 70 cases[29] we found 15 children with persistent defects. Ten of these patients were greatly improved and probably will not require reoperation. Two children died, and we considered persistence of the defect to be a contributing factor. Of the 3 who required reoperation, 2 had a successful closure; the third child died. Although most of these defects were closed by direct suture, in the 3 patients who had been reoperated on the defect had been closed with a Teflon patch. The manner in which the patch becomes incorporated in the septal tissue and endothelializes is impressive; it does not appear to act as a foreign body. In each case the patch had lifted at the posterior inferior margin.

As a result of the above observations, we place double-ended sutures of 00 black silk as a mattress stitch in the superior rim and well back from the margin in the inferior rim (Fig. 39-16). If the suture is in muscle tissue, we place the mattress suture through a small pledget of Ivalon. After sutures have

Fig. 39-16.—Ventricular septal defect, membranous type. The technique shown here avoids the main bundle of His and the branch passing to the left ventricle. The key suture is placed through the annulus of the tricuspid valve from the right atrium. Traction on this suture will expose the inferior margin, and

sutures may be placed accurately. Venting of the left ventricle through the apex improves visibility and prevents left heart distention. (From Welch, C. E. [ed.]: *Advances in Surgery* [Chicago: Year Book Medical Publishers, Inc., 1965], Vol. 1.)

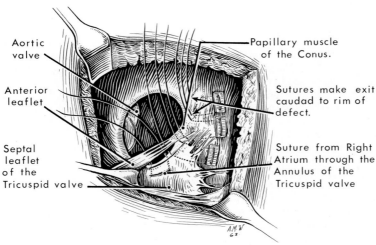

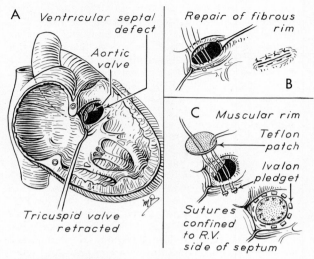

Fig. 39-17.—Ventricular septal defect. Two methods of repair.

thesia to achieve a temperature of 25 C without ventricular fibrillation. A split-sternal approach was utilized and Young's solution injected into the root of the aorta after introduction of 50 cc of arterialized blood. The aorta was cross-clamped after caval occlusion and the ventricular defect repaired in 6–12 minutes! The previously removed arterial blood was warmed and injected into the root of the aorta to resuscitate the heart. Surface warming by immersion resulted in survival of 16 of 18 patients. Although this is a remarkable achievement, it would seem advantageous to lower the temperature to allow more time to close the ventricular septal defect. Hikasa *et al.*[12] reported operating on infants weighing less than 10 kg. The infants were given essential fatty acids and vitamin E for a week prior to surgery. Surface cooling to 20 C was accomplished by deep ether anesthesia with induced cardiac arrest, following Horiuchi's method. Rewarming was performed manually. Later, extracorporeal circulation was used. Of 36 patients operated on for ventricular septal defects, 33 survived.

VENTRICULAR-ATRIAL SEPTAL DEFECT

A rare defect is produced when the opening from the left ventricle in the membranous portion of the septum enters the right atrium through the base of the tricuspid valve. In our single instance, catheterization demonstrated a rise of oxygen saturation at atrial level with the clinical signs of a ventricular septal defect. At operation a jetlike thrill was present over the superolateral aspect of the enlarged right atrium. The defect was easily closed by direct suture through a right atriotomy.

VENTRICULAR SEPTAL DEFECT ASSOCIATED WITH OTHER DEFECTS

PATENT DUCTUS ARTERIOSUS.—It is obvious that the patent ductus arteriosus must be dealt with before any extracorporeal circulation is feasible; if one has not been aware of this diagnosis prior to operation and the heart is open, one is faced with a tremendous flow into the field. The diagnosis should be suspected and a search for a patent ductus arteriosus should always be made. The ductus can be closed through a split-sternal incision if necessary. One should suspect another muscular defect or multiple defects when one closes the interventricular septal defect and red blood continues to well into the right ventricle through the septum (and not from the pulmonary artery).

AORTIC INSUFFICIENCY.—If this diagnosis is not made clear preoperatively, it becomes obvious after right ventriculotomy. Blood from the pump oxygenator passes through the defect because if the incompetent aortic valve. Closure of the defect alone, if the aortic valve is only slightly incompetent, may reduce the incompetence to an acceptable level. If the aortic valve is grossly incompetent, it will not do so, as proved to be the case in one of our children who died

been placed around the rim of the defect, a Teflon patch is shaped to fit the defect and the needles are driven through the rim. The patch is then lowered into the defect and the mattress sutures tied (Fig. 39-17). If a defect is over 1 cm in size and the rim partly muscular, it seems unlikely that direct suture will withstand ventricular contraction and left ventricular pressure. A study of the recurrence rates in a large series of cases will undoubtedly answer this problem. It is possible that the defects which we are operating on are larger than defects which would lend themselves to direct closure at some future time. The left heart is allowed to fill with blood and usually leaks through the patch, following which the right ventricle is closed by a running deep stitch through the entire wall. Hemostasis must be meticulous, as in all open-heart operations, and drainage adequate. The pericardium is left wide open, and it has been our practice to incise the pericardium on the right side posterior to the phrenic nerve, and drain the right chest.

If the right atrium is large enough, the ventricular septal defect may be closed through a right atriotomy. We have closed defects by retracting the medial leaflet of the tricuspid valve, by splitting the valve and by detaching the cusp from the annulus.[14] However, the ventricular approach is the one most surgeons prefer, since it is the customary approach and less tedious than an atriotomy. The value of the atrial approach is undoubtedly the absence of a ventricular myotomy, particularly in the presence of pulmonary hypertension.

Horiuchi *et al.*[13] in 1963 reported operating on a series of infants with a surface-cooling technique at 25 C. The infants had isolated ventricular septal defects with pulmonary artery pressure over 40 mm Hg or more than a 25% left-to-right shunt without pulmonary hypertension. The technique consisted of surface cooling by immersion, using deep ether anes-

postoperatively because of aortic incompetence following successful closure of a ventricular septal defect. If the diagnosis is suspected or made before operation, it is wise to enter the aorta first, repair the aortic incompetence by reefing the adjacent edges of the coronary cusps; then when one opens the right ventricle without aortic occlusion the aortic valves can be inspected for competency. We have had 4 such patients, 1 of whom died without repair of aortic incompetence; 3 had the aortic valve repaired and 1 died. Two are well and have no signs of aortic incompetence or ventricular septal defect.

VENTRICULAR SEPTAL DEFECT WITH ATRIAL SEPTAL DEFECT.—The atrial septal defect is of the secundum type, and closure is effected with a running suture. If the right atriotomy is left open and the ventricular septal defect then closed, both right ventriculotomy and atriotomy can be closed at the same time.

SEVERE PULMONARY HYPERTENSION WITH VENTRICULAR SEPTAL DEFECT.—Controversy still prevails as to the proper approach in cases of pulmonary hypertension. The right ventriculotomy, particularly if it is of any extent, may lessen the function of the right ventricle in patients who have pulmonary hypertension. Exposure through the right atrium may be difficult in children whose tricuspid valves are normal and the right atrium small. If tricuspid incompetence is present, however, or if the atrium is large enough, adequate exposure of the ventricular septal defect can be obtained through the atrium. One may retract the septal leaf of the tricuspid valve or divide it to expose the defect. Repair through the right atrium is more difficult than through the right ventricle, but the immediate postoperative course is less hazardous in a patient who already has pulmonary hypertension and a failing right ventricle. We have employed this approach on four occasions and found it very satisfactory when the tricuspid valve was incompetent or the right atrium of large enough size to effect adequate exposure. But we have also found a ventricular septal defect in the muscular portion of the septum which we were unable to see and identify through a right atrial approach. An advantage of the atriotomy is the feasibility of inspection of the tricuspid valve for incompetence. The question of fenestration of a patch to allow an escape valve mechanism in these cases remains unanswered. Most workers in this field lean toward complete closure of the defect.

VENTRICULAR SEPTAL DEFECT WITH PREVIOUS PULMONARY ARTERY BANDING

Repair of the ventricular septal defect is undertaken at about 4 years of age. Spontaneous closure should not be overlooked; this occurred in one of our cases. Among 14 patients of Hallman et al.,[11] after transection of the band in 4 children the pulmonary artery expanded or could be dilated satisfactorily. In 3, the pulmonary artery was closed transversely; in the rest, reconstruction of the artery was necessary. There were no deaths in the series.

POSTOPERATIVE CARE

For patients who have pulmonary hypertension and whose lungs seem somewhat turgid at operation, it may be wise to perform a tracheostomy and assist them with a ventilator for a few days. Adequate drainage of mediastinal and pleural spaces is imperative, and despite the split-sternal incision we have employed right chest drainage with wide opening of the mediastinal pleura on the right side. Meticulous hemostasis is important, and the use of antiheparin coagulant and antihemophilic globulin plus fresh whole blood is necessary.

COMPLICATIONS

After the initial trials and tribulations of the artificial heart-lung machine have been overcome, there are certain complications peculiar to the treatment of ventricular septal defects.

HEART BLOCK.—The most serious complication is heart block. In a comprehensive survey by Lauer et al.,[22] of 48 patients who developed heart block, 18 died in hospital and 4 of 12 discharged with complete heart block died. The standard treatment is use of the pacemaker and some form of electrode in the myocardium.[35] But essentially the treatment of heart block lies in its prevention, a knowledge of the pathway of the bundle of His and careful monitoring during closure of the defect. For this reason we prefer not to use prolonged arrest, except short periods of anoxic arrest to enable one to see the pathologic anatomy. Our preference is to lower the body temperature with the use of a heat exchanger[4] and lower the flow rate to enable one to see the defect more clearly.

RIGHT VENTRICULAR FAILURE.—Prolonged cardiac arrest produces myocardial necrosis,[36] with arrest induced by potassium citrate producing the greatest damage, reflected in the postoperative period by right heart failure. Short periods of anoxic arrest will lessen the damage to the myocardium.

A short, high right ventriculotomy will lessen the splinting effect of a long incision in the wall of the right ventricle.

In cases of pulmonary hypertension, operation through the right atrium may be of some value in preventing right ventricular failure. An attempt to lessen tricuspid incompetence may be made through the right atriotomy. Supportive measures, such as tracheostomy and use of a ventilator, may be lifesaving.

RECURRENCE OR INCOMPLETE CLOSURE.—Recurrence after complete closure may occur 1 to 2 days postoperatively and is due to sutures pulling out under the strain of the beating heart and left ventricular pressure. Incomplete closure occurred in the early attempts at closure when there were definite hazards in the use of the pump oxygenator. The experience of Kirklin[21] reflects that of most surgeons attempting closure of these defects. The incidence of incomplete closures in the first group of cases was 33%, gradually dropping over the years to 4%.

RESULTS OF OPERATION

Cartmill *et al.*[5] analyzed the results of operation at the Mayo Clinic for the 5 years 1960–65. In 1960, mortality was 14%; in 1961, 12%; in 1962, 4%; in 1963, 2%; in 1964, 2%, and in 1965, 4%. The group was composed of infants over 6 months of age and also those with pulmonary hypertension whose pulmonary flow was greater than the systemic flow. Of 500 patients between 1956 and 1963 analyzed by Hallman *et al.*,[10] 259 with pulmonary artery pressure less than 50% of systemic pressure were operated on with no mortality. In the rest, mortality varied from 9 to 26% depending on the severity of pulmonary hypertension. Kay[15] had 1 death in a series of 100 patients with pulmonary hypertension below 75 mm Hg. Ehrenhaft[8] reported no mortality in 68 patients with isolated ventricular septal defects without pulmonary hypertension. It appears that an isolated ventricular septal defect without pulmonary hypertension can be closed with a mortality rate of less than 5%. The presence of pulmonary hypertension raises this figure to 20%.

REFERENCES

1. Abbott, M. E.: *Congenital Heart Disease,* in *Nelson's Loose-Leaf Medicine* (New York: Thomas Nelson & Sons, 1932), Vol. 4, p. 207.
2. Bailey, C. P., *et al.*: Experimental and clinical attempts at correction of interventricular septal defects, Ann. Surg. 136:919, 1952.
3. Becu, L. M., *et al.*: Anatomic and pathologic studies in ventricular septal defect, Circulation 16:374, 1957.
4. Brown, I. W., *et al.*: Experimental and clinical studies of controlled hypothermia rapidly produced and corrected by a blood heat exchanger during extracorporeal circulation, J. Thoracic Surg. 36:497, 1958.
5. Cartmill, T. B., *et al.*: Results of repair of ventricular septal defect, J. Thoracic & Cardiovas. Surg. 52:486, 1966.
6. Downing, D. F., and Goldberg, H.: Cardiac septal defects, Dis. Chest, 29:475, 1956.
7. DuShane, J. W., *et al.*: Criteria for selection of patients with ventricular septal defects for surgical repair, Circulation 14:929, 1956.
8. Ehrenhaft, I. J., *et al.*: Factors influencing results in the surgical treatment of patients with cardiac septal defects, Circulation 20:689, 1959.
9. Fyler, D. C., *et al.*: Ventricular septal defect in infants and children: A correlation of clinical, physiologic and autopsy data, Circulation 18:833, 1958.
10. Hallman, G. L., *et al.*: Surgical treatment of ventricular septal defect associated with pulmonary hypertension, J. Thoracic & Cardiovas. Surg. 48:588, 1964.
11. Hallman, G. L., *et al.*: Two-stage surgical treatment of ventricular septal defect: Results of pulmonary artery banding in infants and subsequent open-heart repair, J. Thoracic & Cardiovas. Surg. 52:476, 1966.
12. Hikasa, Y., *et al.*: Open heart surgery in infants with aid of hypothermic anesthesia, Arch. jap. Chir., vol. 36, July 1, 1967.
13. Horiuchi, T., *et al.*: Radical operation for ventricular septal defect in infancy, J. Thoracic & Cardiovas. Surg. 46:180, 1963.
14. Hudspeth, A. S., *et al.*: An improved transatrial approach to the closure of ventricular septal defects, J. Thoracic & Cardiovas. Surg. 43:157, 1962.
15. Kay, E. B.: In discussion of Kirklin.[21]
16. Keith, J. D., *et al.*: *Heart Disease in Infancy and Childhood* (New York: Macmillan Company, 1958).
17. Keith, J. D.: Personal communication.
18. Kidd, L., *et al.*: The hemodynamics in ventricular septal defect in childhood, Am. Heart J. 70:732, 1965.
19. King, H., *et al.*: Experimental surgical repair of ventricular septal defects, Surgery 3:1100, 1953.
20. Kirklin, J. W.: Surgical Correction of Ventricular Septal Defects in Infants. Presented before the American Academy of Pediatrics, Chicago, Oct., 1960.
21. Kirklin, J. W., *et al.*: Surgical treatment of ventricular septal defect, J. Thoracic & Cardiovas. Surg. 40:763, 1960.
22. Lauer, P. M., *et al.*: Heart block after repair of ventricular septal defect in children, Circulation 4:526, 1960.
23. Lev, M.: The architecture of the conduction system in congenital heart disease: III. Ventricular septal defect, Arch. Path. 70:529, 1960.
24. Lillehei, C. W., *et al.*: The results of direct vision closure of ventricular septal defects in 8 patients by means of controlled cross-circulation, Surg., Gnynec. & Obst. 101:447, 1955.
25. McFarland, J. A., *et al.*: Myocardial necrosis following elective cardiac arrest induced with potassium cirate, J. Thoracic & Cardiovas. Surg. 40:200, 1960.
26. Mudd, J. G., *et al.*: The natural and postoperative history of 252 patients with proved ventricular septal defects, Am. J. Med. 39:946, 1965.
27. Muller, W. H., Jr., and Dammann, J. F., Jr.: The treatment of certain congenital malformations of the heart by the creation of pulmonic stenosis to reduce pulmonic hypertension and excessive pulmonary blood flow, Surg., Gynec. & Obst. 95:213, 1952.
28. Murray, G.: Closure of defects in the cardiac septa, Am. Surgeon 128:843, 1948.
29. Mustard, W. T., and Trusler, G. A.: Ventricular septal defect: An analysis of 70 cases in childhood surgically treated, Canad. J. Surg. 4:152, 1961.
30. Perry, C. B.: Congenital anomalies of the heart in elementary school children, Arch. Dis. Childhood 6:265, 1931.
31. Roger, H.: Recherches cliniques sur la communication congenitale des deux coeurs, par inocculsion du septum interventriculaire, Bull. Acad. méd. 8:1074, 1189. 1879.
32. Shah, P., *et al.*: Incidence of bacterial endocarditis in ventricular septal defects, Circulation 34:127, 1966.
33. Sirak, H. D., *et al.*: Interventricular septal defects in infancy: A two-stage approach to its surgical correction, New England J. Med. 260:147, 1959.
34. Sirak, H. D., *et al.*: The prevention of heart block in the surgical repair of interventricular septal defect, J. Thoracic & Cardiovas. Surg. 39:229, 1960.
35. Weirich, W. L., *et al.*: Treatment of complete heart block by combined use of myocardial electrode and artificial pacemaker, S. Forum 8:360, 1958.
36. Willman, V. L., *et al.*: Depression of ventricular function following elective cardiac arrest with potassium citrate, Surgery 46:792, 1959.
37. Wood, P. H.: Congenital heart disease: Review of its clinical aspects in light of experience gained by means of modern techniques, Brit. M. J. 2:639, 1960.
38. Zacharioudakis, S. C., *et al.*: Ventricular septal defects in the infant age group, Circulation 16:374, 1957.

W. T. MUSTARD

Drawings by
MARGUERITE DRUMMOND (Figures 39-12, 39-15, 39-17)
A. M. WRIGHT (Figure 39-16)

Ebstein's Anomaly

A RARE CONGENITAL anomaly of the heart described by Ebstein[2] consists primarily of a misplaced tricuspid valve. The valve leaflets are attached near the midportion of the right ventricle and often are incompetent. The right ventricle usually is no larger than a thumb nail, and the portion of the ventricle to the right of the tricuspid valve assumes the thin-walled character of the right atrium. An interatrial communication allows shunting of blood from right to left and leads to progressive cyanosis.

In 1958, Hunter and Lillehei[5] suggested displacement of the line of attachment of the septal and posterior leaflets of the tricuspid valve and plication of the atrialized portion of the right ventricle. Hardy *et al.*[4] successfully applied this technique; they emphasized the need to eliminate the atrialized portion of the right ventricle. Certain patients will require a prosthesis to replace the valve.[1] A palliative procedure was devised by Weinberg *et al.*[6] Three patients were benefited by anastomosis of the superior vena cava to the end of the right pulmonary artery, as described by Glenn.[3]

REFERENCES

1. Barnard, C. N., and Schrire, V.: Surgical correction of Ebstein's malformation with prosthetic tricuspid valve, Surgery 54:302, 1963.
2. Ebstein, W.: A rare case of tricuspid valve insufficiency due to high-grade congenital malformation, Arch. Anat., Physiol. wissench. Med., p. 238, 1866.
3. Glenn, W. W. L., and Patino, J. F.: Circulatory bypass of right heart. I. Preliminary observations on direct delivery of vena caval blood into pulmonary arterial circulation: Azygos vein-pulmonary artery shunt, Yale J. Biol. & Med. 27:147, 1954.
4. Hardy, K. L., *et al.*: Ebstein's anomaly: A functional concept and successful definitive repair, J. Thoracic & Cardiovas. Surg. 48:927, 1964.
5. Hunter, S. W., and Lillehei, C. W.: Ebstein's malformation of the tricuspid valve, Dis. Chest 33:297, 1958.
6. Weinberg, M., *et al.*: Surgical palliation in patients with Ebstein's anomaly and congenital hypoplasia of the right ventricle, J. Thoracic & Cardiovas. Surg. 40:310, 1960.

W. T. MUSTARD

Tricuspid Atresia

PATHOLOGIC ANATOMY

THE PRIMARY LESION in this complex, uncommon congenital anomaly is absence of the tricuspid valve so that a solid wall of myocardium separates the right atrium from the right ventricle. Of necessity, there is an interatrial septal defect, usually of adequate size to empty the right atrium into the left side of the heart. The right ventricle is always diminutive, and usually some degree of pulmonary stenosis or even atresia is present. Pathologic subtypes may be divided into a group in which there is a nonfunctioning right ventricle (Fig. 39-18, *A*) and a group with a functioning right ventricle filled through an interventricular septal defect (Fig. 39-18, *B*), the more common type. Another group has complete transposition of the great vessels, and these are further subdivided into patients with unobstructed pulmonary outflow and others with pulmonary stenosis.

DIAGNOSIS

The cyanotic infant with left heart strain, peaked P waves on the electrocardiogram and a heart of relatively normal size almost invariably will prove to have tricuspid atresia (or stenosis). Cyanosis is moderate, exercise tolerance is conspicuously diminished and spells of unconsciousness are frequent. These children do not squat when fatigued. The loud harsh systolic murmur is heard best at the third intercostal space to the left of the sternum. The liver is often enlarged, and there may be moderate polycythemia.

Roentgenograms of the chest show a heart of normal size or one that is only slightly enlarged. The heart is transverse, with a rounded left border (Fig. 39-19). Vascularity is diminished in the lung fields except for the rare type with transposition of the great vessels and unobstructed pulmonary outflow.

Electrocardiograms invariably show evidence of left ventricular hypertrophy. In infants, this may be represented by absence of the normal right ventricular dominance. In the older child, typical left heart strain with peaked P waves in lead 2 will be found. Angiocardiograms and cardiac catheterization are seldom required to establish the diagnosis. They may be helpful in the doubtful case or to discover associated anomalies.

PROGNOSIS

The outlook for these patients is extremely poor without operation. A majority die during the first few weeks or months of life, presumed frequently to be due to closure of a life-sustaining ductus arteriosus. Relatively few live beyond 3 years of age untreated, and survival into the second decade of life is rare indeed. Death frequently occurs suddenly during an episode of severe hypoxia.

TREATMENT

Conversion of a defective heart to one normal in anatomy and function is always the ideal goal of op-

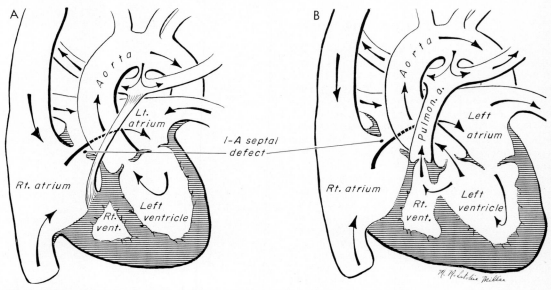

Fig. 39-18.—Tricuspid atresia; pathologic variations. **A,** pulmonary atresia with nonfunctioning right ventricle. **B,** function-ing right ventricle with interventricular septal defect and pulmonary stenosis.

erative correction. In the tricuspid atresias, nothing short of organ transplant could accomplish this. Most efforts have been aimed toward increasing pulmonary blood flow. Enlargement of the interventricular septal defect, if present, and enlargement of the right ventricle and pulmonary outflow tract would be impossible to attain in most cases and would be relatively ineffective. The best that one could produce

Fig. 39-19.—Tricuspid atresia. Roentgenogram demonstrating diminished vascularity of the lung fields, transverse heart of normal size and rounded left cardiac border.

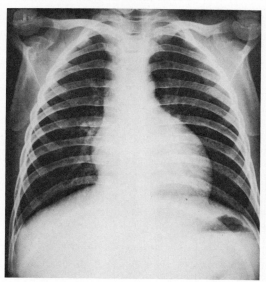

would be a single ventricle complex, the prognosis of which is not good.

The alternative to total correction is the palliative procedure of increasing pulmonary blood flow by some type of shunt. Two types of shunts are in use, anastomosis of the superior vena cava to the distal right pulmonary artery (Glenn procedure) and anastomosis of the pulmonary artery to the systemic arterial circulation, using the aorta or one of its branches.

Excellent results with the superior cava-pulmonary artery shunt have been obtained in older infants and children, since it results in an increased pulmonary blood flow and at the same time diverts 40% of the venous return from the right atrium. This lightens the work load of the right atrium, which formerly had to pump all of the venous blood through the interatrial septal defect into the left side of the heart.

Unfortunately, this type of anastomosis is seldom successful in the small infant, probably because of the poor run-off of blood into a hypoplastic pulmonary vascular bed and the tendency of a small anastomosis to clot when there is slow flow with a relatively small pressure differential between the two vessels being anastomosed.

In the infant below 6 months to a year of age, the preferable shunt is between the aorta and the pulmonary artery, since the high pressure differential and the rapid flow help keep the anastomosis open.

OPERATIVE PROCEDURES

SUPERIOR CAVA DISTAL RIGHT PULMONARY ARTERY ANASTOMOSIS.— This is used on the older infant and child (Fig. 39-20). A right anterolateral incision is

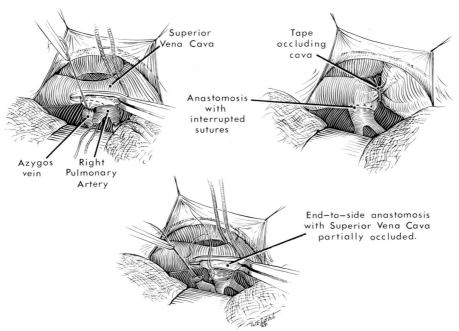

Superior
Vena Cava

Tape
occluding
cava

Anastomosis
with
interrupted
sutures

Azygos
vein

Right
Pulmonary
Artery

End–to–side anastomosis
with Superior Vena Cava
partially occluded.

Fig. 39-20. — Tricuspid atresia: superior cava-right pulmonary artery anastomosis. Anastomosis of the divided end of the pulmonary artery to the side of the superior vena cava may give dramatic relief in selected cases. (From Welch, C. E. [ed.]: *Advances in Surgery* [Year Book Medical Publishers, Inc., 1965], Vol. 1.)

made in the chest, entering the pleural cavity through the fourth intercostal space. The right pulmonary artery, including its major branches, is isolated. The dissection is carried as far as possible toward the main pulmonary branch. The phrenic nerve is dissected free and retracted medially, and the superior cava is freed extensively, from the innominate vein above into the pericardial sac below.

After a short trial occlusion of the right pulmonary artery to be sure the child can tolerate it, the vessel is tied as far proximal as possible, the branches are occluded with temporary ligatures and the artery is divided. A curved, multitoothed Potts-type clamp is applied to the lateral side of the superior vena cava in an area that will be reached easily by the distal end of the right pulmonary artery for anastomosis. This is usually in the region of the stump of the azygos vein, which must be divided. A longitudinal incision or, if possible, a small elliptical excision is made in the lip of cava that has been excluded by the clamp. This opening is made at least as big as the opening in the pulmonary artery stump.

The open, proximal stump of the pulmonary artery is anastomosed to the incision in the cava, using 6-0 cardiovascular silk in an over-and-over stitch. One stitch is started at each end with the knots situated on the outside of the vessels. One of the sutures is used to complete the back row of the anastomosis and the other to finish the anterior portion. The distal ligatures on the pulmonary artery branches

are released and the clamp on the cava is removed.

With a venous pressure monitor in the innominate vein or right jugular vein, a heavy ligature is tightened around the superior vena cava as close to its entry into the right atrium as possible. Total occlusion is the ultimate goal, since this will divert all of the superior caval blood to the right lung. If undue elevation of venous pressure to the anastomosis persists (greater than 25–30 cm of water), a partial occlusion must be accepted.

The pericardium is approximated and the chest closed with tube drainage. The child is kept with the upper part of the body elevated to 45 degrees to minimize the edema and cyanosis above the nipple line that often develops. This usually disappears after a few days.

AORTIC-PULMONARY ANASTOMOSIS. — This is the operation of choice in early infancy. The surgeon sees a majority of the patients with tricuspid atresia during the first few weeks or months of life in precarious condition. Operation cannot be postponed and is performed as an emergency procedure in a desperately ill infant. In these instances, the patent ductus or bronchial arteries may be sustaining life. The keys to success of the procedure are the rapidity of operation and the maintenance of what little blood flow there is to the lung during the anastomosis.

The chest is opened rapidly and the left pulmonary artery and aorta are dissected only as much as is necessary. Completion of the anastomosis as quickly as

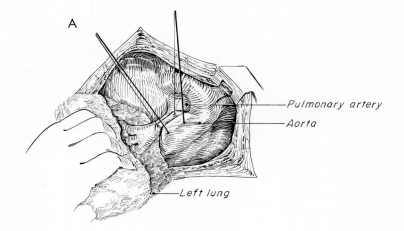

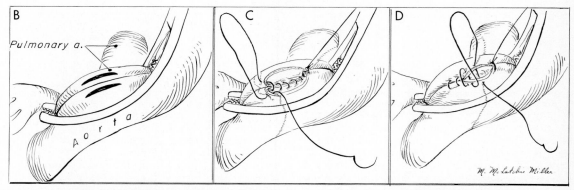

Fig. 39-21.—Tricuspid atresia: aortic-pulmonary anastomosis in the young infant. **A,** traction sutures in the freed pulmonary artery and aorta to pull them up and together. **B,** curved multitoothed clamp applied to occlude and approximate lips of the vessels, **C,** details of suturing posterior portion of the anastomosis with 6-0 silk suture. **D,** completion of anterior portion of the anastomosis.

possible may mean the difference between success and failure. Hypothermia down to the range of 90–93 F may be helpful to tide the patient over the period of severe hypoxia during the anastomosis. The curare type of drugs may help to maintain a quiet operative field during the few minutes of vessel occlusion and anastomosis.

Complete dissection of the aorta and application of the Potts-Smith clamp is time-consuming and may interrupt vital flow to the lung through the patent ductus or bronchial arteries. Even mild traction on the pulmonary artery may cut off the blood flow to the opposite lung, producing anoxia. It is often possible to bare a segment of the aorta near the mobilized left pulmonary artery and catch a portion of both vessels in a curved multitoothed forceps (Fig. 39-21).

The two lips are then incised and the anastomosis is accomplished. Because the four cut surfaces of the vessels are so close together, suturing may be difficult. To avoid this, an alternate approach may be preferred. The curved multitoothed clamp is applied to the aorta alone, and the pulmonary artery occluded and brought over to the ends of the clamp by means of temporary ligatures of 2-0 silk (Fig. 39-22).

The length of the incisions in the vessel lips is kept under 5 mm in the infant patient. The side-to-side anastomosis is made with a continuous over-and-over suture of 6-0 silk amid the asphyxial gasps of the patient, the dire warnings of the anesthesiologist and the ominous slowing of the heart action. Upon release of clamp and ligature at conclusion of the anastomosis, cardiac action improves immediately and the color of the blood becomes less purple.

Enlargement of the interatrial septal defect, especially in the young infant, would be difficult. In a majority of the patients seen at autopsy, the defect seems large enough to carry adequate flow. A normal pink color and continuous murmur immediately after operation is viewed with alarm since it indicates too large a shunt and foretells cardiac decompensation. It is much better to see a residual trace of cyanosis and hear only a systolic murmur during the first few post-

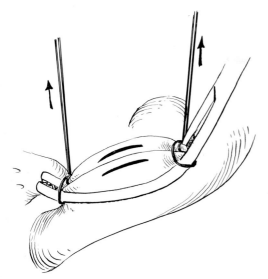

Fig. 39-22.—Tricuspid atresia: aortic-pulmonary anastomosis. A second method—partial occlusion and approximation of pulmonary artery and aorta. A curved clamp is applied to the aorta and ligatures on the pulmonary artery are fastened to the two ends of the clamp.

operative days. In these patients, cyanosis disappears and a ductus murmur becomes audible before discharge from the hospital.

Results of Operation

The experience with the superior cava to right pulmonary artery shunt at Children's Memorial Hospital has been small. Of the 12 patients operated on, 4 were very small infants in the first few weeks of life. All of them died of complications following clotting of the anastomosis. The older children have all done quite well, with loss or marked decrease of cyanosis, improved exercise and tolerance and decrease of liver enlargement.

In 20 years, 110 infants and children with tricuspid atresia or stenosis complex have undergone aortic-pulmonary anastomosis. Of these, 75% survived the operation and left the hospital. During the postoperative follow-up, another 10% died. Evaluation of the surviving 65% indicates that two thirds of these patients can be classified as having good or excellent results.

Loss of cyanosis and increased exercise tolerance are evident, with some increase of heart size and pulmonary vascularity. In a few instances, the anastomosis has grown unduly large, resulting in cardiac failure due to high pulmonary flow. Operative narrowing of the aortic-pulmonary shunt has been necessary in 6 patients. Because of this tendency to enlargement, a confining band of woven Teflon has been left around the anastomosis in recent years.

Although it must be admitted that our present treatment leaves much to be desired, many children are doing reasonably well following these operative procedures. Bold intervention even early in infancy can be rewarding.

BIBLIOGRAPHY

1. Edwards, J. E., and Burchell, H. B.: Congenital tricuspid atresia, A classification, M. Clin. North America 33:1177, 1949.
2. Glenn, W. W. L., and Patino, J. F.: Circulatory bypass of the right heart: 1. Preliminary observations on the direct delivery of vena caval blood into the pulmonary arterial circulation, Yale J. Biol. & Med. 27:147, 1954.
3. Riker, W. L., and Miller, R. A.: Diagnosis and treatment of tricuspid atresia, Surgery 38:886, 1955.
4. Taussig, H. B.: Clinical and pathologic findings in congenital malformations of the heart due to defective development of right ventricle associated with tricuspid atresia or hypoplasia, Bull. Johns Hopkins Hosp. 59:435, 1936.

W. L. Riker

Drawings by
Muriel McLatchie Miller
(Figures 39-18, 39-21, 39-22)
A. M. Wright (Figure 39-20)

40

Congenital Complete Heart Block

HISTORY.—The first report of complete heart block in childhood was published by Schuster[10] in 1896. In 1901, Morquio[7] described a family in which 4 of 8 children died in a manner very suggestive of Stokes-Adams attacks. White and Eustis[13] in 1921 described the first unequivocal case of congenital origin, and in 1929, Yater[14] established the criteria necessary for the diagnosis of congenital complete heart block.

The sinoatrial electrical impulse fails to reach the ventricles, which then contract independently at a slow rate. The diagnosis is confirmed by electrocardiography and its congenital origin by the absence of any history of disease which might have produced the heart block. Increased awareness of the natural history of this condition and improved methods of cardiac pacing have stimulated surgical interest, and there are now a number of reports of pacemaker treatment of congenital heart block.[1,3,6,8,11,12]

INCIDENCE AND ETIOLOGY

Congenital heart block is uncommon, representing less than 1% of congenital heart disease. Both sexes are affected equally, and there are a number of reports of familial occurrence.[2] Heart block may be found as an isolated condition or, less often, in association with other cardiac malformations. It is due to a break of continuity in the conduction system, either within the atrioventricular bundle or between the atrioventricular node and the bundle.[4] There may be fibrosis to suggest prenatal carditis, and in 1 reported case,[5] the bundle was interrupted by an angiomatous tumor.

NATURAL HISTORY

Although most children with congenital heart block are able to lead normal lives, a few may suffer serious or even fatal complications. The most significant prognostic factor is the level of origin of the ventricular impulse as estimated from the electrocardiogram. A QRS interval of 0.10 second or less with a QRS complex which is normally formed, indicates a ventricular impulse arising in the bundle of His. This impulse is relatively stable and shows a good response to exercise, so that these children are usually asymptomatic and rarely suffer Stokes-Adams attacks. In contrast, when the QRS interval is longer than 0.10 second and there is an abnormal QRS configuration (Fig. 40-1), the ventricular impulse originates distal to the bundle of His and is less stable. Children with this type of electrocardiogram usually

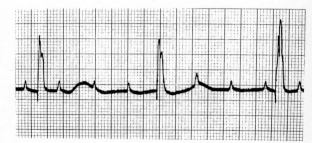

Fig. 40-1.—Complete heart block. Electrocardiogram (lead 2) of a 2-day-old infant. Ventricular rate is 40 and atrial rate 145. The QRS complex is broad (0.12-second duration) with a right bundle-branch block pattern, therefore indicating that the cardiac impulse is arising below the bifurcation of the bundle of His.

are symptomatic and may develop cardiac failure (Fig. 40-2) or Stokes-Adams attacks. The Stokes-Adams attacks represent decreased cerebral blood flow due to sudden ventricular asystole, extreme bradycardia or, in some cases, ventricular tachycardia or fibrillation. These attacks, which may be precipitated by exertion, fear or infection, represent the commonest cause of death.

Of 49 children with congenital complete heart block and no apparent associated cardiac malformations, followed at the Hospital for Sick Children, Toronto, 41 had the first-mentioned, stable type and 8 had the less stable type. All 8 children with the ventricular impulse arising distal to the bundle of His were symptomatic, and 3 required pacemaker therapy.[12]

HEMODYNAMICS

The basic abnormality is a slow ventricular rate usually between 40 and 80 beats per minute. It is increased by exercise, severe physical stress and stimulation of the sympathetic nervous system and decreased by acidosis. Normal cardiac output is maintained by a high stroke volume which also increases with exercise. The high stroke volume depends on increased diastolic filling of the cardiac chambers, and this is reflected in generalized enlargement of the heart. The atrial chambers beat independently, and their normally beneficial effect on ventricular end-diastolic fiber length and closure of the atrioventricu-

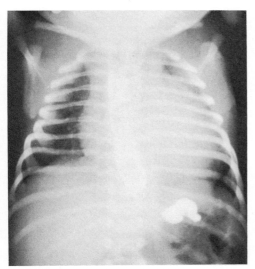

Fig. 40-2. — Congenital heart block. Anteroposterior chest radiograph of 2-day-old infant, showing marked cardiac enlargement with a cardiothoracic ratio of 70%, evidence of severe cardiac failure.

lar valves is lost. When atrial systole occurs during ventricular systole, a large wave (cannon wave) is produced in the jugular venous pulse.

TREATMENT

Asymptomatic children require no treatment. Those children in whom the ventricular impulse is arising below the bundle of His must be followed carefully. Isoproterenol, ephedrine or diuretics may be of value, particularly in times of stress, such as during respiratory infections. Digitalis is seldom useful.

Pacemaker therapy is indicated if Stokes-Adams attacks or cardiac failure develops. Nakamura and Nadas[8] have advocated consideration of pacemaker therapy for any child with congenital heart block who has had two or more Stokes-Adams attacks despite medical treatment. Cardiac failure as a complication of heart block is seen chiefly in the newborn period, at which time pacemaker therapy may be needed urgently. Pacing by means of a transvenous catheter electrode inserted into the right ventricle is conven-

ient for emergency use, but a permanently implanted pacemaker of either standard or radiofrequency type will be necessary subsequently.

Children with congenital heart block in association with other cardiac malformations may benefit from cardiac pacing. Scarpelli and Rudolph[9] have stressed the combined hemodynamic effect of either an obstructive cardiac lesion or a left-to-right shunt in the presence of complete heart block. Once the associated defect is corrected, it may be possible to discontinue pacing.

REFERENCES

1. Ayers, C. R.; Boineau, J. P., and Spach, M. S.: Congenital complete heart block in children, Am. Heart J. 72:381, 1966.
2. Crittenden, I. H.; Latta, H., and Ticinovich, D. A.: Familial congenital heart block, Am. J. Dis. Child. 108:104, 1964.
3. Harris, P. D.; Bowman, F. O., and Griffiths, S. P.: Implantation of a synchronous pacing unit in a 7-month-old infant, J. Thoracic & Cardiovas. Surg. 52:277, 1966.
4. Lev, M.: The anatomic basis for disturbances in conduction and cardiac arrhythmias, Progr. Cardiovas. Dis. 2:360, 1959-60.
5. Linder, E., et al.: Congenital complete heart block: II, Ann. paediat. Fenn. 11:11, 1965.
6. Martin, M. V., et al.: Implantation of Charcack-Greatbatch adjustable rate and current pacemaker in a 4-month-old infant, Pediatrics 37:323, 1966.
7. Morquio, L.: Sur une maladie infantile et familiale caractérisée par des modifications permanentes du pouls, des attaques syncopales et epileptiforme et la mort subite, Arch. med. enf. 4:467, 1901.
8. Nakamura, F. F., and Nadas, A. S.: Complete heart block in infants and children, New England J. Med. 270:1261, 1964.
9. Scarpelli, E. M., and Rudolph, A. M.: The hemodynamics of congenital heart block, Progr. Cardiovas. Dis. 6:327, 1963-64.
10. Schuster: Zur cardialen Bradycardie, Deutsche med. Wchnschr. 22:484, 1896.
11. Taber, R. E., et al.: Treatment of congenital and acquired heart block with an implantable pacemaker, Circulation 29:182, 1964.
12. Trusler, G. A.; Mustard, W. T., and Keith, J. D.: The role of pacemaker therapy in congenital complete heart block: Report of three cases, J. Thoracic & Cardiovas. Surg. 55:105, 1968.
13. White, P. D., and Eustis, R. S.: Congenital heart block, Am. J. Dis. Child. 22:299, 1921.
14. Yater, W. M.: Congenital heart block, Am. J. Dis. Child. 38:112, 1929.

G. A. TRUSLER

41

Acquired Heart Disease

THE SPECTRUM OF surgery for acquired heart disease in children is a narrow one compared with the volume and variety of operations for congenital heart disease. The incidence and death rate of rheumatic heart disease in childhood have decreased greatly in recent years.[4,13] The rate of occurrence of rheumatic heart disease among school children in urban areas of the north temperate zone is 1.3 to 1.8 per 1,000. The mortality rate of acute rheumatic fever and rheumatic heart disease in children ranges from 1.6 to 3.3%.[17] Prophylaxis against rheumatic fever has reduced the threat of progressive cardiac disability. Rheumatic heart disease may no longer be the most common form of heart disease in childhood, but it is still a significant cause of cardiac crippling. Although one-half the children with acute rheumatic fever have evidence of carditis, the majority of them recover from their attack of rheumatic fever without permanent cardiac damage. Only a very few children have severe enough involvement of a valve to threaten life. It is these children who can be helped by operation. The fear that mitral valve surgery in children will reactivate rheumatic fever is unfounded.[5,6,19]

Mitral insufficiency is the most common valve lesion in childhood for which surgical correction is necessary. Mitral stenosis less frequently may become severe enough in children to require an operation. Aortic insufficiency is the second most frequent valve abnormality resulting from rheumatic fever but usually does not cause severe symptoms in childhood. Symptomatic aortic stenosis on a rheumatic basis is extremely rare in children.

Bacterial endocarditis may attack the aortic or mitral valve previously deformed by congenital or acquired disease. With destruction of portions of the aortic valve, such massive aortic insufficiency may occur that valve repair or replacement is necessary.

In spite of the increasing carnage on the highways, blunt trauma to the heart occurs rarely in small children. On the other hand, in the teenage group, deceleration accidents may produce cardiac rupture, myocardial contusion or hemopericardium. Restrictive pericarditis from hemopericardium in childhood does occur. The diagnosis and treatment of these complications of trauma are the same as in the adult. Similarly, penetrating injuries of the heart do occur in children, and, for these, the principles of treatment for adults should be followed.[9,10,18,23]

Mitral Insufficiency

PATHOLOGY

Rheumatic fever is a systemic disease which attacks many parts of the body but seems to cause permanent damage only to the heart. The relationship between rheumatic fever and streptococcic infection is now clearly established. The disease may attack any or all of the cardiac structures. The basic changes consist of edema and proliferative inflammatory reactions in connective tissues. Initially, there are edema of the ground substance, fragmentation of the collagen fibers and infiltration by round cells and scattered polymorphonuclear leukocytes. Scattered through the ground substance are deposits of granular eosinophilic material. The initial reaction is followed by the proliferative phase, in which the characteristic Aschoff body of rheumatic fever develops. This distinctive lesion, a perivascular aggregation of large cells arranged as a rosette around an avascular center of fibrinoid or necrotic protoplasm, has been considered a specific lesion of connective tissue.[11] The concept has been challenged by the suggestion that the Aschoff body is the result of obstruction of the lymphatic channels of the heart.[25] Whatever its etiology, the Aschoff body is believed by many to be related to activity of the rheumatic process, although there seems to be little correlation between the presence of Aschoff bodies in atrial biopsy specimens taken during operation and the results of correction of valve lesions.

The valves of the left side of the heart are involved in rheumatic heart disease more frequently than the valves on the right side, perhaps because they are subjected to higher pressures. The principal lesion is mitral insufficiency, which may occur early in the course of the disease. The precise mechanism which produces insufficiency is uncertain, but it seems related both to direct involvement of the valve structures and the annulus as well as to dilatation of the left atrium and left ventricle. Competence of the mitral valve depends on accurate coaptation of the valve leaflets. Edema of the leaflets and verrucae along the valve margins may prevent the leaflets from sealing. Thickening of the leaflets and shortening of the chordae tendineae increase the insufficiency. Dilatation of the mitral annulus and displacement of the posterior leaflet as the left atrium and ventricle enlarge also increase the incompetence.[16]

CLINICAL PICTURE

Severe mitral insufficiency in the child may cause a significant increase of cardiac size, dyspnea on exertion, poor weight gain and cardiac failure. The seriously ill child may be so orthopneic that he must sit upright to breathe. The signs of cardiac failure are present. There is gross cardiomegaly, and the heart is hyperactive. A left ventricular heave may be present, and a systolic thrill may be palpated over the apex. The principal auscultatory finding is a loud, pansystolic apical murmur. A short mid-diastolic murmur due to the increased volume of blood flowing across the mitral valve in diastole may be heard.

In severe mitral regurgitation, the electrocardiogram reflects enlargement of the left ventricle. Increased QRS voltage, increased R wave voltage and T wave changes are seen in the left chest leads. The P waves may be widened and notched in keeping with the left atrial enlargement. Chest roentgenograms show marked cardiac enlargement. The huge left atrium produces a double density along the right cardiac border and may form part of the cardiac margin. It displaces the esophagus posteriorly and elevates the left main bronchus. The enlarged left ventricle increases the transverse diameter of the heart, with displacement of the apex downward and to the left. The left anterior oblique view shows the posterior projection of the left ventricle over the spine. In the lateral view, the left ventricle projects behind the inferior vena cava. There is congestion in the lung fields.

The pulmonary wedge pressures are elevated. There are high v waves. Mild to moderate pulmonary hypertension is usually present. Left ventricular end-diastolic pressures may be elevated, depending on the severity of the cardiac failure. Contrast studies show the marked reflux of radiopaque materials from the left ventricle into the huge left atrium through the incompetent mitral valve.[8,15]

The indications for repair of mitral insufficiency in childhood are: (1) heart failure uncontrolled by a careful medical regimen; (2) marked enlargement of the left atrium and left ventricle, and (3) atrial fibrillation.

Most children with mitral insufficiency come to the attention of the surgeon after the initial attack of rheumatic fever has subsided and the rheumatic process is no longer in an acute phase. It is of the utmost importance to decide whether active rheumatic myocarditis is or is not present because subsidence of rheumatic activity and the accompanying decrease of heart size may lessen the severity of valvular incompetence and make operation unnecessary. Fur-

thermore, the presence of active myocarditis greatly increases the risk of operation. However, mitral valvuloplasty should be attempted even in the presence of active carditis if it appears that the child may die otherwise.

The differentation of failure due to the mechanical effect of mitral insufficiency from failure due to myocarditis may be extremely difficult. Active rheumatic carditis may be suggested by fever, rash, arthritis, subcutaneous nodules, changing murmurs and a friction rub. Anemia and an elevated white blood cell count may be present. Except in acute failure, the sedimentation rate is usually conspicuously elevated. During the early active phase, the C-reactive protein level is also elevated. A rise or fall of the antistreptolysin titer indicates recent activity.

OPERATION

The patients selected for operation should be those whose lives are threatened by overwhelming mitral insufficiency. Operation must be carried out with the aid of extracorporeal circulation. Although the mitral valve may be approached in several ways, we have preferred a right thoracotomy through the fifth intercostal space with the patient in the lateral position. This approach provides excellent exposure and opportunity to assess valve function after repair.

Because early experience with the repair of congenital mitral insufficiency by annuloplasty was satisfactory,[22] we have used this technique to correct acquired mitral insufficiency. Annular dilatation is a major component of mitral insufficiency in children. The valve leaflets are thickened, but scarring is not pronounced. There may be shortening and adherence of the chordae, or they may appear grossly normal. The valve leaflets are mobile but do not approximate during ventricular systole. Satisfactory closure of the valve can be accomplished by placing annuloplastic sutures at each commissure so that the annulus is narrowed and the posterior leaflet is shortened (Fig. 41-1). Competence of the valve can be tested by allowing the blood-filled ventricle to contract against the valve. Care must be taken to avoid trapping air in the ventricle, and it is advisable to aspirate the aortic root when the valve repair is completed. Insufficiency is rarely abolished, but the remaining insufficiency is usually insignificant (Fig. 41-2).

Other surgeons have replaced the insufficient mitral valve by a prosthesis because they believe correction of mitral insufficiency by annuloplasty has not resulted in long-term improvement.[3] The hazards associated with the use of prostheses, despite their improvements, make it seem unwise to employ prosthetic appliances in children if a more conservative repair, employing the patient's own tissues, can be used. Our own experience shows that with annuloplasty, long-term, satisfactory correction of acquired mitral insufficiency can be achieved. In no child with normal sinus rhythm postoperatively have we seen a systemic embolus.

PRE- AND POSTOPERATIVE CARE

Children requiring repair of mitral insufficiency are often in profound failure before operation. They must be maintained in a sitting position and supported with oxygen. The use of digitalis preparations is necessary, and excess fluid must be removed by diuretics. Although reduction of salt intake and limitation of fluid are desirable, food must be made palatable enough to maintain an adequate caloric intake. Depletion of potassium by diuretics is avoided by giving potassium supplements. The children often have pulmonary infection which must be treated with antibiotics.

Surprisingly, improvement of cardiac function by repair of mitral insufficiency is sufficiently dramatic in most patients so that the postoperative problems of these children are only those of any child undergoing a cardiac operation with extracorporeal circulation. Tracheostomy is necessary only rarely. A strict cardiac regimen must be maintained with digitalis, the use of diuretics and restriction of fluid and salt. Later in the postoperative course, these restrictions can be relaxed as clinical improvement progresses. Antibiotic prophylaxis should be continued.

Atrial fibrillation should be converted to normal sinus rhythm by electric shock or drugs following operation. Normal sinus rhythm both increases cardiac output and decreases the likelihood of postoperative embolic complications. Children need not be given anticoagulants following mitral valve repair unless there is a history of systemic emboli.

OPERATIVE RESULTS

Twelve children required correction of mitral insufficiency alone between 1960 and 1966 at the University of Michigan Medical Center.[14] The patients were between 6 and 18 years of age. Eleven of the patients

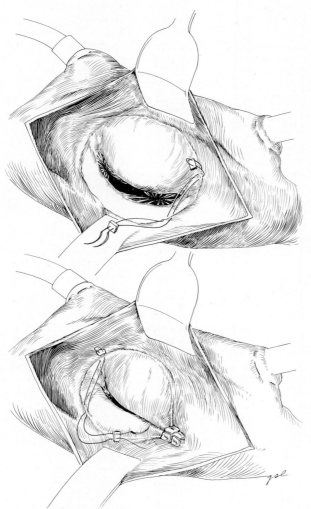

Fig. 41-1. — Mitral insufficiency. Technique of annuloplasty for correction.

Fig. 41-2. — Mitral insufficiency. Left atrial pressures obtained during operation, before and after correction by annuloplasty.

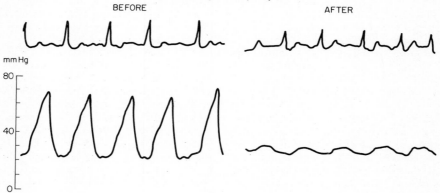

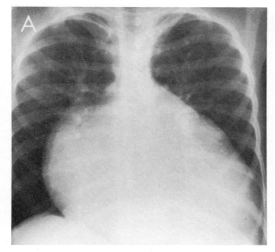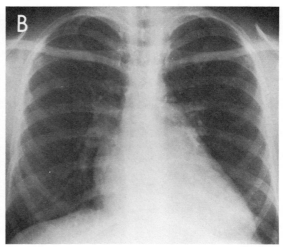

Fig. 41-3. — Mitral insufficiency. Chest roentgenograms of an 8-year-old girl before (**A**) and 4 years after (**B**) correction by annuloplasty.

survived and had been followed from 2 months to 7 years at the time of writing. Seven were asymptomatic and 4 improved. This clinical improvement was accompanied by satisfactory reduction of cardiac size on chest roentgenograms (Fig. 41-3). Most of the patients still had evidence of mild mitral insufficiency, but this was not physiologically important. Seven of the patients had associated minimal aortic insufficiency which persisted.

Progressive symptoms made it necessary to perform a second valvuloplasty for 1 patient 3 years after the first, and improvement was maintained after the second operation. A second patient needed another operation 5 years after the first valvuloplasty, but by this time the valve had calcified and valve replacement was carried out. None of the patients had recurrence of rheumatic fever and all remained on antibiotic prophylaxis.[7] There is no evidence that operation had increased the rate of progression of the valve lesions.

One patient died in heart failure following operation. The decision to attempt repair of mitral insufficiency in the face of myocarditis reflected the severity of the uncontrolled failure. At autopsy, the heart of this desperately ill child showed the histologic stigmas of active rheumatic carditis.

Repair of mitral insufficiency together with repair of major aortic insufficiency or tricuspid insufficiency was attempted in 4 patients. Three of these patients died, 2 with active rheumatic carditis. The presence of multiple valve lesions and active rheumatic carditis greatly increases the risk of operation.

Mitral Stenosis

Mitral stenosis requiring operation does occur in childhood. It has been reported most often in areas with a high incidence of rheumatic fever.[1,5,6,12,19] The clinical picture in these children is essentially that found in adults with mitral stenosis, although the progression of symptoms is more rapid. The mitral valve orifice becomes stenotic because of adhesions between the leaflets at the commissures. This fibrous stenosis can be relieved satisfactorily by either transventricular or open operative techniques,[7] although we now prefer the open technique, believing that a more accurate valvuloplasty can be accomplished and that the risk is no greater. The mitral valves have not yet calcified and in most patients there is not yet significant leaflet destruction or major involvement of the chordae tendineae and papillary muscles.

The initial results from four closed and two open valvuloplasties at the University of Michigan Medical Center in children between age 9 and 18 were excellent. The children had the physical signs of significant mitral stenosis with a diastolic murmur at the apex and an increased second pulmonic sound. Chest roentgenograms showed enlargement of the left atrium and pulmonary congestion. On cardiac catheterization, an increased pulmonary wedge pressure was present with moderate pulmonary hypertension. The electrocardiogram showed right axis deviation and enlargement of the left atrium.

Because stenosis recurred, 1 patient required an open valvuloplasty 6 years following the original closed operation, and another, a valve replacement 9 years later. Again the course of the recurrent stenosis paralleled that seen in adults.

Aortic Insufficiency

Aortic insufficiency of rheumatic origin has not often required operation in childhood, and children tolerate aortic insufficiency moderately well. Subacute bacterial endocarditis occurring on such a damaged valve or on a valve with a congenital abnormality may produce overwhelming aortic insufficiency with massive failure. Correction of aortic insufficiency by cusp replacement or by valvuloplasty has not resulted in long-term improvement. The successful use of aortic prostheses to treat aortic valve disease in children has been reported.[3,21,24] It is possible that the aortic homograft may provide a better means of correcting aortic valve disease in children.[2,20]

REFERENCES

1. Angelino, P. F., *et al.:* Mitral commissurotomy in the younger age group, Am. Heart J. 51:916, 1956.
2. Barratt-Boyes, B. G.: Homograft aortic valve replacement in aortic incompetence and stenosis, Thorax 19:131, 1964.
3. Beall, A. C., Jr., *et al.:* The use of valve replacement in the management of patients with acquired valvular heart disease, Am. J. Surg. 110:834, 1965.
4. Bland, E. F., and Jones, T. D.: Rheumatic fever and rheumatic heart disease: A twenty-year report on 1,000 patients followed since childhood, Circulation 4:836, 1951.
5. Borman, J. B., *et al.:* Mitral valvotomy in children, Am. Heart J. 61:763, 1961.
6. Cherian, G., *et al.:* Mitral valvulotomy in young patients, Brit. Heart J. 26:157, 1964.
7. Collins, H. A., *et al.:* Surgery for mitral valvular disease during childhood and adolescense, J. Thoracic & Cardiovas. Surg. 51:639, 1966.
8. Gasul, B. M.; Arcilla, R. A., and Lev, M.: *Heart Disease in Children* (Philadelphia: J. B. Lippincott Company, 1966).
9. Gibbon, J. H. (ed.): *Surgery of the Chest* (Philadelphia: W. B. Saunders Company, 1962).
10. Goldring, D., *et al.:* Nonpenetrating trauma to the chest, J. Pediat. 68:677, 1966.
11. Gould, S. E. (ed.): *Pathology of the Heart* (2nd ed.; Springfield, Ill.: Charles C Thomas, Publisher, 1960).
12. Gray, I. R.: Mitral valvotomy in the young, Lancet 2:1263, 1958.
13. Joint report by the Rheumatic Fever Working Party of the Medical Research Council of Great Britain and the Subcommittee of Principal Investigators of the American Council on Rheumatic Fever and Congenital Heart Disease, American Heart Association: The natural history of rheumatic fever and rheumatic heart disease: Ten-year report of a cooperative clinical trial of ACTH, cortisone, and aspirin, Circulation 32:457, 1965.
14. Kahn, D. R., *et al.:* Long term results of valvuloplasty for mitral insufficiency in children, J. Thoracic & Cardiovas. Surg. 53:1, 1967.
15. Keith, J. D.; Rowe, R. D., and Vlad, P.: *Heart Disease in Infancy and Childhood* (New York: Macmillan Company, 1967).
16. Levy, M. J., and Edwards, J. E.: Anatomy of mitral insufficiency, Progr. Cardiovas. Dis. 5:119, 1962.
17. Markowitz, M., and Kuttner, A. G.: *Diagnosis and Management of Rheumatic Fever and Rheumatic Heart Disease* (Philadelphia: W. B. Saunders Company, 1965).
18. Naclerio, E. A.: Penetrating wounds of the heart: Experience with 249 patients, Dis. Chest 46:1, 1964.
19. Reale, A.; Colella, C., and Bruno, A. M.: Mitral stenosis in childhood: Clinical and therapeutic aspects, Am. Heart J. 66:15, 1963.
20. Ross, D. N.: Aortic-valve replacement, Lancet 2:461, 1966.
21. Smeloff, E. A.; Cayler, G. G., and Smith, D. F.: The use of valve prostheses in childhood, J. Thoracic & Cardiovas. Surg. 51:839, 1966.
22. Talner, N. S.; Stern, A. M., and Sloan, H. E., Jr.: Congenital mitral insufficiency, Circulation 23:339, 1961.
23. U. S. Army, Medical Department: *Thoracic Surgery* (F. B. Berry, ed.) vol. 2; in "Surgery in World War II" (Washington, D. C.: Office of the Surgeon General, Department of the Army, 1965).
24. Van De Water, J. M.; Wolfe, R. R., and Mulder, D. G.: Total heart-valve replacement in the pediatric age group, J. Thoracic & Cardiovas. Surg. 53:515, 1967.
25. Wedum, B. G., and McGuire, J. W.: Origin of the Aschoff body, Ann. Rheumat. Dis. 22:127, 1963.

H. Sloan
A. M. Stern
S. Vathayanon

Drawings by
Grant L. Lashbrook

42

The Pericardium

Tumors of the Heart and Pericardium

PRIMARY TUMORS OF the heart are rare in adults and very rare in childhood. The majority of the tumors are benign. In an extensive review Prichard[5] found that myxomas comprised 50% of the reported cases, and Bigelow[3] found only 1 proved case of malignant tumor in infancy and childhood.

MYXOMA

With few exceptions the myxomatous tumors arise in the region of the fossa ovalis and project in an intraatrial fashion, 75% into the left atrium. As a rule the tumor is polypoid, often pedunculated, yellow-white in appearance and may be as large as a golf ball. Although a few have been diagnosed clinically, the usual diagnosis is mitral stenosis. A remarkable case in a child was diagnosed with the aid of angiocardiography, the contrast medium demonstrating a polypoid mass in the left atrium.[4] With the aid of extracorporeal circulation, many of these intra-atrial tumors are now being removed successfully.[6]

RHABDOMYOMA

Circumscribed masses in the myocardium which on section appear to be composed of swollen cardiac muscle fibers containing glycogen are generally referred to as rhabdomyomas. The intramural location of these tumors, which are histologically benign, accounts for the fatal outcome usually before the age of 5 years.

We have encountered only 1 patient with tumor, which proved to be an inoperable rhabdomyoma of the right ventricle (Fig. 42-1).

INTRAMURAL FIBROMA

Intramural fibromas arise from the interventricular septum or are located in the myocardium of the left ventricle. The tumor is encapsulated, white and on section is seen to be composed of collagen-filled fibroblasts with scattered strands of cardiac muscle. In most of the cases reported, the tumors occurred in infancy. Valedor et al.[7] reported a fibroma in an 8-month-old infant that arose from the interventricular septum and encroached on the aortic valve. The signs were pallor, coldness, sweating and a systolic murmur at the base of the heart.

SARCOMA

Bigelow et al.[2] in 1954 could find only 1 proved case of malignant tumor in childhood. Engle and Glenn[3] in 1955 described a well-documented case of rhabdomyosarcoma of the right ventricle with secondary deposits in the lungs of a 4-month-old infant. The infant was in failure, with electrocardiographic evidence of coronary occlusion. The correct diagnosis was made before death.

PERICARDIAL TUMORS

Pericardial tumors, which may be mesotheliomas, teratomas, lipomas, fibromas or angiomas, are often malignant. Despite their accessibility to the surgeon, few reports of successful removal are available. Beck's[1] case, reported in 1942, is a notable exception. Benign cysts of the pericardium should present

Fig. 42-1.—Tumor of the heart: rhabdomyoma. Anteroposterior roentgenogram of a 7-year-old child demonstrating an inoperable tumor arising in the right ventricle.

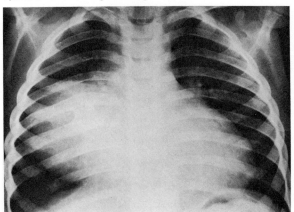

no problem in removal but must be exceedingly rare in childhood.

REFERENCES

1. Beck, C. S.: An intrapericardial teratoma and a tumor of the heart, both removed operatively, Ann. Surg. 116:161, 1942.
2. Bigelow, N. H., *et al.*: Primary tumors of the heart in infancy and childhood, Cancer 7:549, 1954.
3. Engle, M. A., and Glenn, F.: Primary malignant tumor of the heart in infancy: Case report and review of the sub-

ject, Pediatrics 15:562, 1955.
4. Goldberg, H. P., *et al.*: Myxoma of the left atrium: Diagnosis made during life with operative and postmortem findings, Circulation 6:762, 1952.
5. Prichard, R. W.: Tumors of the heart; review of the subject and report on 150 cases, Arch. Path. 51:98, 1951
6. Sanyal, S. K., *et al.*: Right atrial myxoma in infancy and childhood, Am. J. Cardiol. 20:263, 1967.
7. Valedor, T., *et al.*: Fibroma of the heart (case report), Dis. Chest 37:698, 1960.

W. T. Mustard

Pericarditis

History. — Chronic constrictive pericarditis was described satisfactorily by Lower[4] in 1669. Both Weill[10] and Delorme[1] recognized it as a surgical problem in the 1890s. Pericardial resection, however, was first carried out in 1913 by Sauerbruch[8] and Rehn.[6] White's St. Cyre lecture contains an excellent historical review.[11]

PHYSIOPATHOLOGY OF CARDIAC TAMPONADE

Acute cardiac tamponade results in decreased cardiac output, systemic arterial hypotension with a narrowed pulse pressure and venous hypertension; chronic tamponade, in addition, produces peripheral edema, ascites, hepatomegaly, pleural effusion and pulmonary hypertension. Usually associated with the clinical picture are quiet heart sounds, a weak cardiac impulse and frequently a paradoxical pulse. The electrocardiogram tends to reveal low-voltage, elevated S-T segments and T-wave inversion. Though the basic physiopathology has been well understood for years, only recently has the relationship between the site of constriction and the resultant dysfunction been satisfactorily clarified. This information has been derived from findings at operation, from reoperation on patients who were treated initially without cure by either a right- or a left-sided resection, and especially from the experimental studies of Parsons and Holman[5] and of Isaacs, Carter and Haller.[3] It is now clear that constriction of the right side affecting predominantly the venous inflow tract, the right atrium and the right ventricle decreases cardiac output because of reduced cardiac input and results in venous hypertension, hepatomegaly, splenomegaly, ascites and edema. When the constriction affects principally the left side, the cardiac output is also decreased and pulmonary hypertension develops. When the constriction is generalized, all of these features are usually present. Widespread constriction is generally present in clinical cases of acute tamponade, chronic tamponade due to massive effusion and in almost every instance of chronic constrictive peri-

carditis, though in the last-mentioned condition one often finds particularly impressive constriction in one area or another.

ACUTE PERICARDITIS

Not infrequently, acute pericarditis occurs in infancy and childhood as a part of, or secondary to, such general disorders as rheumatic fever, uremia, viral disease, rheumatoid arthritis, tuberculosis, pneumonia and empyema, and osteomyelitis. Only rarely, however, is operation indicated. Its chief applicability relates to pyogenic pericarditis.

The commonest causative agents in acute septic pericarditis are the staphylococcus, streptococcus and pneumococcus. Most cases have been secondary to pneumonia and empyema or to osteomyelitis. The diagnosis is made by the association of fever and the signs and symptoms of acute pericarditis. Among the latter are precordial pain, pericardial friction rub, quiet heart sounds, inactive weak cardiac impulse, increased cardiac dullness and radiologic evidence of increase of the size of the pericardial-cardiac shadow. The electrocardiogram generally shows low-voltage, elevated S-T segments, T-wave inversion, and there may be varying degrees of cardiac tamponade. Pericardial aspiration may be necessary to establish the diagnosis and to provide material for culture of the organism and to ascertain its sensitivity to antibiotics. Aspiration may be life-saving if the effusion is large enough to cause tamponade. Vigorous and prompt specific antibiotic therapy should be instituted. If prompt improvement does not follow administration of appropriate antibiotics and pericardiocentesis as indicated, operative drainage is indicated.

One may encounter cases of tuberculous pericarditis in which the cardiac tamponade increases progressively while general antituberculosis therapy is being carried out in the hope of rendering the process inactive. Since the important contribution of Holman and Willett,[2] it has been evident that such patients are best managed by extensive pericardiectomy and continued antituberculosis drug therapy. Experience has shown that this carries little danger of spreading the

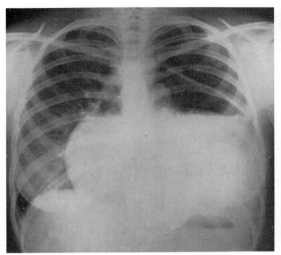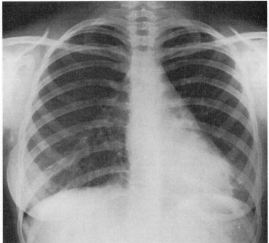

Fig. 42-2.—Pericarditis. Pre- and postoperative roentgenograms of a 16-year-old girl with massive pericardial effusion and cardiac tamponade. The preoperative air-fluid level is due to removal of pericardial fluid and replacement by air.

tuberculous process or of establishing tuberculous sinuses.

MASSIVE PERICARDIAL EFFUSION WITH CARDIAC TAMPONADE

Massive idiopathic pericardial effusion with cardiac tamponade has been observed more commonly in adults than in children but presents the same problem whatever the age group. There develops, usually insidiously, a massive pericardial effusion which persists in spite of repeated pericardiocenteses and is associated with classic symptoms and signs of cardiac tamponade (Fig. 42-2). Low-grade fever may be present at the onset. The pericardial fluid has no characteristic features. Ordinarily, it contains a few leukocytes, and its protein content is in the order of that usually found in serum. It has been successfully managed by thoracotomy and pericardial fenestration but is best treated by extensive pericardiectomy.[5] In such cases, the pericardium is not adherent to the heart and the operation is easy to perform. The procedure not only eliminates the difficulty itself and prevents its recurrence but also removes the diseased pericardium and thus eliminates the possible later development of chronic constrictive pericarditis.

The same type of massive effusion with cardiac tamponade may result from known causes, such as tumor implants in the pericardium and traumatic hemopericardium.

CHRONIC CONSTRICTIVE PERICARDITIS

Chronic constrictive pericarditis occurs far less commonly in children than in adults, but in both age groups it is associated with the same symptoms and signs and is best managed in the same manner.[4] It should be recognized with ease but has often been confused with cirrhosis of the liver or heart failure from intrinsic cardiac disease. The patient usually has dyspnea, orthopnea, ascites and edema. There may be evidence of pleural effusion. As a rule, the characteristic signs and electrocardiographic evidence of cardiac tamponade are present. Fluoroscopic and x-ray studies demonstrate poor cardiac contractions, fixation of the pericardial-cardiac silhouette and often calcification of the pericardium (Fig. 42-3).

Fig. 42-3.—Chronic constrictive pericarditis. Lateral view of a 13-year-old boy, showing calcification of the pericardium. He was cured by extensive pericardiectomy.

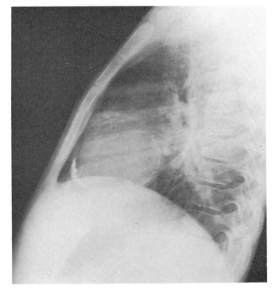

Cardiac catheterization reveals elevated right ventricular and pulmonary artery pressures, increased venous pressure, and the right ventricular pulse wave shows the characteristic diastolic plateau. Cineangiograms demonstrate poor cardiac contractions and sometimes areas of constriction.

The etiology may be obscure. In more than half the cases reported in the pediatric age range, no specific etiologic factor was suggested and the pathologic picture was one of nonspecific inflammatory disease. In a little over one third of the cases, tuberculosis could possibly be implicated on a clinical basis. In only slightly over half of them, however, was tuberculosis established on pathologic study. It has generally been assumed that microscopic demonstration of tuberculosis in the resected pericardium is not necessary to establish the diagnosis in cases in which there was reasonable clinical suspicion. Since tuberculous infection ordinarily leaves tell-tale marks of granulomatous disease, if not of tuberculosis itself, it would appear that the case should be considered one of nonspecific pericarditis when the examination reveals only nonspecific inflammatory disease. Certainly, nonspecific pericarditis is by far the commonest finding.

TREATMENT

INDICATIONS FOR OPERATION.—Some patients can be improved preoperatively by a rigid medical regimen including digitalization, salt restriction and bed rest. If, however, improvement does not follow such a regimen rather promptly, it is not wise to continue it indefinitely. Prompt improvement follows operative resection in such medically refractory cases.

OPERATIVE TECHNIQUE.—The operation can be performed either through a sternal-splitting incision such as is commonly used in open cardiac surgery or by a bilateral interior thoracotomy with sternal transection. While most of my experience has been with the former, and it has proved generally satisfactory, I have also employed the latter incision and have found that it provides very good exposure. Once the pericardium is exposed, a suitable area is selected and carefully incised down to the epicardial surface. It is preferable to begin the resection over the left ventricular area and then to remove carefully all of the pericardium until the entire anterior, lateral and diaphragmatic surfaces of the heart as well as the aorta, pulmonary artery, venae cavae and pulmonary veins are completely freed (Fig. 42-4). This can be accomplished with patience and persistence, and the mortality has proved low. The small shell of pericardium that is left is posteriorly adherent to the vertebral bodies and the heart is freed from this residual pericardium. Extensive near-total pericardiectomy of this kind yields excellent results and reoperation is unnecessary. Most of the patients do well during the postoperative period. An occasional patient, however, may develop alarming heart failure which may require phlebotomy.

RESULTS OF OPERATION.—In a collective review of the literature, including 4 of our own cases,[9] 35 of 68 patients were recorded as having good or excellent results or a cure, and another 12 were improved. Although in this series, 12 patients died at operation, 70% of these children benefited from pericardiectomy. Undoubtedly, the mortality in more recently treated cases is considerably lower and the over-all results far better.

REFERENCES

1. Delorme, E.: Sur un traitement chirurgical de la symphyse cardio-pericardique, Bull et mém. Soc. chir. Paris 24:918, 1898.
2. Holman, E., and Willett, F.: Treatment of acute tuberculous pericarditis by pericardiectomy, J.A.M.A. 146:1, 1951.
3. Isaacs, J. P.; Carter, B. N., II, and Haller, J. H., Jr.: Experimental pericarditis: Pathologic physiology of constrictive pericarditis, Bull. Johns Hopkins Hosp. 90:259, 1952.

Fig. 42-4.—Pericardiectomy: technique. **Dotted line** outlines the approximate extent of residual posterior pericardium after resection has been accomplished.

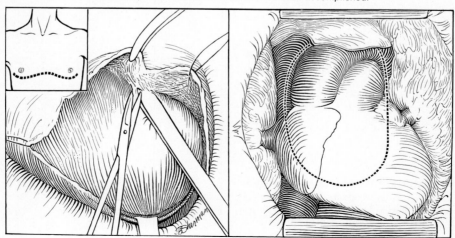

4. Lower, R.: *Fractatus de Corde* (Amsterdam, 1669), p. 104.
5. Parsons, H. G., and Holman, E.: Experimental ascites, S. Forum 1:251, 1950.
6. Rehn, L.: Die perikardialen Verwachsungen im Kindesalter, Arch. Kinderheilk. 63:179, 1920.
7. Roshe, J., and Shumacker, H. B, Jr.: Pericardiectomy for chronic cardiac tamponade in children, Surgery 46:1152, 1959.
8. Sauerbruch, F.: *Die Chirurgie der Brustorgane*, (Berlin: 1925), Vol. II.
9. Shumacker, H. B, Jr., and Harris, J.: Pericardiectomy for chronic idiopathic pericarditis with massive effusion and cardiac tamponade, Surg., Gynec. & Obst. 103:535, 1956.
10. Weill, E.: *Traite' clinique des maladies du coeur chez les enfants* (Paris, 1895).
11. White, P. D.: Chronic constrictive pericarditis (Pick's disease) treated by pericardial resection, Lancet 2:597, 1935.

H. B SHUMACKER, JR.

Drawings by

BETH SHERMAN

Diverticulum of the Left Ventricle

A PULSATING MASS in a congenital epigastric ventral hernia should lead one to suspect the presence of diverticulum of the left ventricle. Angiocardiography will outline the diverticulum (Fig. 42-5) and is helpful in ruling out associated cardiac defects. The diverticula are either tubular or at times almost vermiform, or, as in 1 reported case,[2] frankly saccular but narrower at the neck.

Untreated children with this defect rarely survive infancy, and operation should be undertaken early. The operation is simple; the left ventricle tolerates to an extraordinary degree, cross-clamping of the diverticulum and suturing of the base. Numerous successes have been reported.[1-4]

REFERENCES

1. Mustard, W. T., *et al.*: Congenital diverticulum of the left ventricle of the heart, Canad. J. Surg. 1:49, 1958.
2. Potts, W. J., *et al.*: Congenital diverticulum of the left ventricle, Surgery 33:301, 1953.
3. Roessler, W.: Successful operative removal of an ectopic diverticulum of the heart in a newborn, Deutsche Ztschr. Chir. 258:561, 1944.
4. Skapinker, S.: Diverticulum of the left ventricle of the heart, Arch, Surg. 63:629, 1951.

W. T. MUSTARD

Drawings by

MARGUERITE DRUMMOND

Fig. 42-5.—Diverticulum of the left ventricle. A pulsating mass in the epigastrium of a girl of 10 had been present since birth. Two previous operations were performed for an epigastric hernia. Angiocardiograms: **A**, in systole; **B**, in diastole. She had been asymptomatic since excision of the diverticulum in 1955.

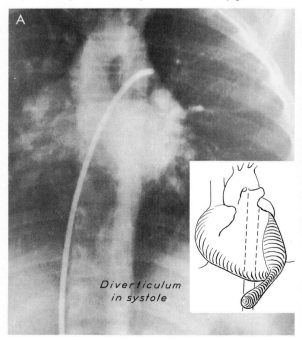
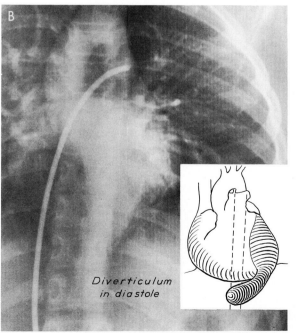

43

<h1 style="text-align:right">Physiologic Considerations</h1>

Pulmonary Hypertension

THE TERM pulmonary hypertension is misleading when used as a criterion for assessing a patient's operability. Pulmonary hypertension may exist when pulmonary blood flow is high and pulmonary resistance only slightly elevated, or it may exist when pulmonary vascular resistance is markedly elevated and flow is normal. Although an equal degree of hypertension may be present in both of these circumstances, the first condition is operable, while in the latter circumstance, operation is inadvisable. Therefore it is not the presence of pulmonary hypertension but rather the magnitude and form of pulmonary vascular resistance that determines operability.

It must be recognized that the vascular system of the lungs, although capacious, is not unlimited. In the normal child, the small pulmonary arteries are large of lumen and thin-walled.[13, 23] They are readily distensible up to the point where further dilatation is prevented by the vessel's fibrous adventitial jacket. The normal child's pulmonary vessels may carry three times the normal blood flow without a significant rise of pressure.[29] When the point of maximal distensibility of the vascular bed is reached, however, an essentially linear relationship between flow and pressure appear.[85] No longer distensible, the system acts more like a series of rigid tubes. For each increment of flow to this system, there must be an added increment of pressure.

Mechanisms of Production

With this concept in mind, several of the mechanisms which may produce pulmonary hypertension become clear. (1) An increase of pulmonary blood flow due to the presence of a left-to-right shunt, if it is of sufficient magnitude to stretch the vascular bed to the limits of distensibility, will produce hypertension.[33,34,83] (2) A reduction of lung tissue, such as follows a pneumonectomy, may reduce the cross-sectional area of the vascular bed to a point where normal pulmonary blood flow is sufficient to raise pulmonary pressure.[4,12,47,54,60,75] (3) Static filling of the pulmonary vascular bed with pooled blood may raise the pressure. A sudden, severe increase of systemic vasomotor tone may shift large volumes of blood from the systemic circulation to the pulmonary circulation with a resultant rise of pulmonary arterial pressure.[71,74] (4) Pulmonary venous obstruction produces an elevation of pulmonary venous pressure and, in order to maintain blood flow through the lungs, pulmonary arterial pressure must rise, although not necessarily by an equivalent amount.[25,28,32,51,52,65,80,84,87,88] (5) In certain individuals it seems probable that an increase of vasomotor tone may be sufficient to raise pulmonary arterial pressure which, in most normal individuals, is of little significance since the muscle mass of the normal pulmonary arteries is small. But when the medial coat of the pulmonary artery is hypertrophied, the effective contraction of the vessel wall resulting from vasomotor stimuli may be sufficient to cause a marked rise of pulmonary artery pressure.[9,15,16,17,42, 44,66,67] (6) Finally, the factor of the time at which stress is placed upon the lungs in the developmental course of the patient is important.

The Fetal and Postnatal Lung

In the partially collapsed and unventilated lung of the fetus, the hypertrophied, constricted and kinked muscular pulmonary arteries are supported by alveolar amniotic fluid and offer strong resistance to the passage of blood.[70] Such vessels are well equipped to withstand stress. Following birth, the extravascular pressure is acutely reduced due to the replacement of alveolar amniotic fluid by air. Tortuous vessels are straightened out by the total increase of lung size secondary to expansion of the chest cage and movement of the diaphragm. The effective transmural pressure (which equals driving pressure minus the sum of wall tension plus extravascular pressure) sharply increases, leading to the rapid dilatation of existing patent vessels and the opening of heretofore closed vessels.[10,11] Pulmonary resistance falls and right ventricular pressure decreases. A decrease of pressure exerted on the walls leads to a decrease of vasomotor tone and eventually to disuse atrophy of the vessels. Thus in essence, the pulmonary vascular bed changes at the time of birth from a high-pressure, high-resistance bed with a relatively small cross-

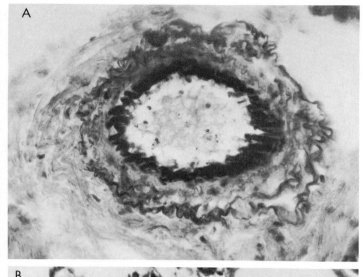

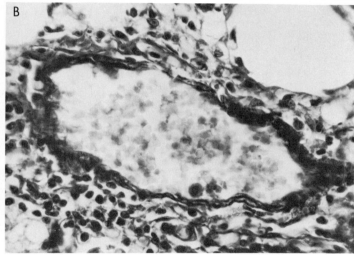

Fig. 43-1.—Pulmonary hypertension. Photomicrographs of a small pulmonary artery: **A,** from a normal newborn baby, and **B,** from a normal 6-year-old child; ×1550.

sectional area and high vasoconstrictive tone, to a low-pressure, low-resistance bed with a large cross-sectional area and low vasomotor tone.[5,26,27,45,58]

The increase of vessel size following birth alters the ability of the vessel to withstand stress. Since the tension required in the wall of a vessel to prevent further dilatation is equal to the intravascular pressure times the square of the radius of the vessel, it is readily apparent that the larger the vessel, the stronger its wall must be or the more susceptible it is to an increase of pressure. Thus the pulmonary vessels are less able to withstand stress after birth not only because the muscular wall has thinned and extravascular pressure has been reduced but also because of the increase of diameter of the vessel (Fig. 43-1). This concept is of major importance in congenital heart disease. The stage of development toward the normal

adult lung at which stress from congenital heart disease is exerted on the lung alters the vascular response.[21] Thick-walled fetal vessels tend to hypertrophy in response to stress. Thin-walled adult vessels are more apt to be injured and develop irreversible intimal change. Fetal vessels tend to remain small, whereas the large thin-walled adult vessels cannot resist stress and dilate further. This difference in the stage of pulmonary vascular evolution at which the lung is subjected to stress explains why there is usually a normal pulmonary artery pressure and a very high flow in the simple auricular defect and yet a somewhat elevated pressure at a much lower flow level in the ventricular septal defect.

We should mention one additional difference between the fetal and the postnatal lung, although it cannot be considered a cause of pulmonary hypertension. In utero, the presence of a large patent ductus with a right-to-left flow and a patent foramen ovale means that the lung is in parallel with other organs. The lung and all other organs can tap off from the main circulation their required blood flow without affecting the rest of the body to any significant degree. Changes of resistance in the lungs, therefore, merely increase or decrease the volume of pulmonary blood flow. After the ductus has closed and the foramen ovale has sealed, however, the lungs assume a position in series with the rest of the body. In these circumstances, a change of resistance in the lungs can directly affect blood flow to the rest of the body. It is this shift of the position of the lung in the circulation which explains the fact that most intracardiac defects are tolerated by the fetus and endanger the newborn only after the circulation has changed.

Pathology

When pulmonary hypertension has been produced by one or more of the factors which have been discussed, what may be expected to happen to the pulmonary vessels? The degree of change in the lungs will depend on the severity and acuteness of the hypertension. Experimental work in our laboratory[19,20,61]

and elsewhere[37,38,39,40] has demonstrated that severe and acute pulmonary hypertension leads to excessive stretch and injury of the vessel wall, passage of fluid and cells into the media and the adventitia, and a secondary acute arteritis. These changes are comparable to those found in the systemic vessels of patients with acute "malignant" hypertension.[69] In the experimental animal, if the stress is removed within a very short time, healing will take place and a relatively normal vascular bed will result, but if the stress is continued, the end-result is obliteration of the vessels with almost complete loss of normal morphology (Fig. 43-2). In contrast, a chronic and moderate rise of pulmonary artery pressure leads to slowly progressive medial hypertrophy of the pulmonary arterial bed, associated eventually with some intimal proliferation. The malignant form is unusual in patients.[53,82] More commonly, early pulmonary hypertension is passive in form. Although pressure is high, the vessels are dilated, and hence vascular resistance is actually subnormal and the pressure drop across the pulmonary vascular bed is decreased. The continued presence of pulmonary hypertension, however, leads to the development of vascular hypertrophy and intimal thickening which in turn increases pulmonary vascular resistance.[24,31,35,49,86] This process may be slow or rapid, depending on the

Fig. 43-2.—Pulmonary hypertension. **A,** photomicrograph of small pulmonary artery demonstrating separation of media and adventitia by hemorrhage following aortic-pulmonary anastomosis in an experimental animal; ×260. **B,** photomicrograph showing end-result of pulmonary arteritis following aortic-pulmonary artery anastomosis in an experimental animal; ×260.

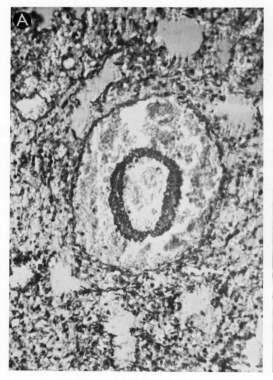
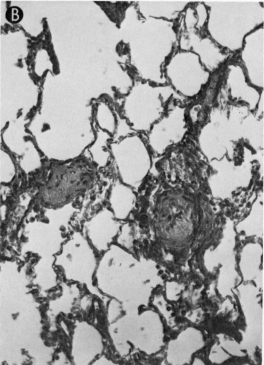

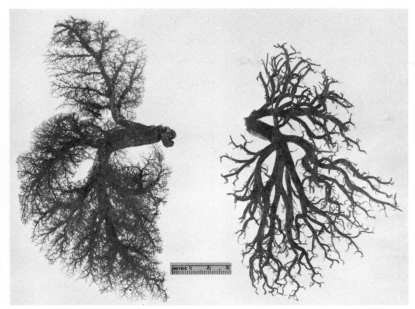

Fig. 43-3. — Pulmonary hypertension. **Left,** plastic cast of the arterial system of the normal lung. **Right,** plastic cast of the arterial system of a 6-year-old boy with a ventricular defect and pulmonary hypertension and balanced flows.

nature of the defect, the time when the defect stresses the lungs (Fig. 43-3), the incidence and severity of pulmonary infections and probably on individual variations in pulmonary vasomotor tone.

When a large high-flow defect is present between the ventricles or great vessels, frequently associated with the signs and symptoms of congestive failure, a gradual increase of pulmonary vascular resistance reduces the work load of the heart by reducing the left-to-right shunt. During this period, the patient improves clinically even to the extent where it would appear that the defect has closed spontaneously. In effect, it has ceased to function physiologically. Patients may remain in this physiologically balanced state for varying periods of time, but eventually additional vascular changes increase pulmonary resistance sufficiently to cause a reversal of shunt, and the patient becomes cyanotic. The progressive development of pulmonary vascular disease may be delayed or may never appear if the defect is small enough so that a systemic pressure does not persist in the pulmonary arteries.

The Role of Surgery

It is of vital importance to the patient that we assess correctly the degree and rapidity of change of pulmonary vascular disease, because the risk of surgical correction becomes progressively greater with the increase of pulmonary resistance.[2,3,30,36,50,57,59] The age when pulmonary vascular disease becomes so severe that the risk of surgery is prohibitive depends in part on the type of defect present. In our experience, children with a ventricular defect and

persistent equal pulmonic and aortic pressures become severe risks by the age of 6. Aortic septal defects or a large patent ductus probably produce irreversible damage at an earlier date. In contrast, defects of the auricular septum may delay the onset of vascular changes until the late teens or may never cause excessive vascular disease.[48] A more careful analysis of the life history of patients with all forms of defects is necessary before we will be able to predict with any assurance the time when severe pulmonary vascular disease will occur.

After pulmonary vascular disease has developed, the question arises as to whether or not the changes may be reversed by corrective operation. The answer to this depends on clarification of at least two important points: (1) Whether or not the original stimulus producing the vascular disease has been totally removed, and (2) whether or not secondary stimuli continue to act after removal of the original stimulus.

When pulmonary pressure can be reduced by elimination of a left-to-right shunt or by relief of pulmonary venous obstruction, there is a good chance that the pulmonary vascular disease may regress. This has been clearly demonstrated in patients after a mitral commissurotomy and after the creation of pulmonary artery stenosis.[62-64]

Concerning the role of secondary stimuli, it must be emphasized that a major part of pulmonary vascular narrowing is due to hypertrophy of the media of the vessel walls. This is particularly true in patients with defects that stress the lungs immediately after birth. There are excellent clinical and laboratory data to indicate that such vessels respond to vasoconstrictor and vasodilator drugs far more than do normal

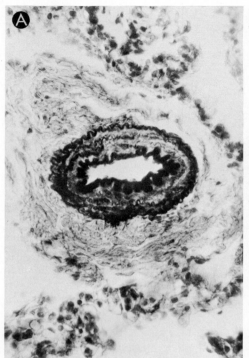 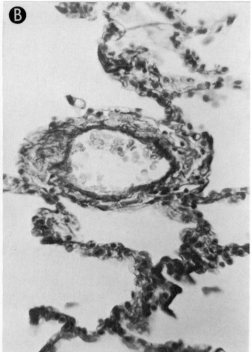

Fig. 43-4. — Pulmonary hypertension. **A,** photomicrograph of small pulmonary vessel obtained from a 22-month-old child during creation of pulmonary stenosis for a ventricular septal defect, pulmonary hypertension and high pulmonary blood flow; ×550.

B, photomicrograph of vessel obtained 6 1/2 years later at the time of total correction of the defect. Note the decrease of wall thickness and increase of lumen size; ×550.

pulmonary arteries.[4,6,9,14,46,55,77,81] In the presence of pulmonary vascular disease, the same stimuli that produce systemic hypertension may alter the pulmonary vasomotor tone sufficiently to continue pulmonary hypertension even after the initiating cause of that hypertension has been removed. This enhanced ability of the pulmonary vessels to respond to stimuli may account for some of the poor results in patients after correction of their primary disease.[56]

Provided the primary stimulus can be successfully diminished and secondary stimuli are not excessive, we believe that pulmonary vascular disease, even though severe, is reversible to some degree.[41,78] Evidence is growing that a change toward normal occurs in the experimental animal in which, first, pulmonary hypertension has been produced by a systemic-pulmonary artery anastomosis and, later, after pulmonary vascular disease has developed, normal pulmonary circulation has been reconstituted.[8] This improvement consists of an increase of lumen size of the small pulmonary vessels associated with varying degrees of wall-thinning and an increase of the total number of vessels seen in any low-power field. This suggests that reduction of pressure by restoring a normal circulation to the affected lung lessens vascular spasm, thus permitting patent ves-

sels to dilate and new vessels to open. In patients, similar changes have been noted after the creation of pulmonary artery stenosis.[22] In each of 6 patients who have undergone corrective surgery a period of years after the creation of pulmonary artery stenosis, a significant improvement in the pulmonary vascular bed has been noted. The most marked improvement occurred in patients with medial hypertrophy alone and in those in whom the time interval between the two operations was the longest.

An example of almost total return to normal is demonstrated in Figure 43-4. The first lung biopsy was done at the age of 22 months in a patient with equal systemic and pulmonary artery pressures and a moderately increased pulmonary blood flow. The second biopsy specimen was obtained at the time the defect was corrected, 6 1/2 years after the initial narrowing of the pulmonary artery.* A less complete return to normal was seen in the second patient, operated on 2 1/2 years after the initial creation of pulmonary stenosis. For reasons not related to her pulmonary vascular disease, this patient failed to survive the second procedure. A cast of her pulmonary arterial circulation is shown in Figure 43-5 and contrasted

---

*We are indebted to Dr. Jerome Kay for the use of his biopsy material.

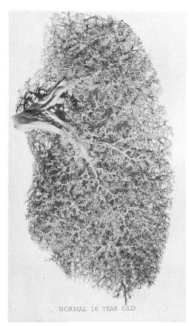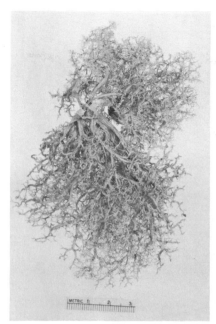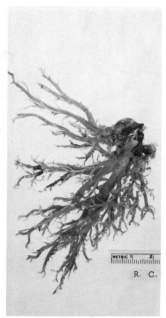

Fig. 43-5.—Pulmonary hypertension. **Left,** cast of the pulmonary arterial tree of a normal lung. **Middle,** cast of arterial tree of a 5-year-old child with atrioventricularis communis and pulmonary hypertension operated on 2 1/2 years after creation of pulmonary stenosis. Arborization of the pulmonary arteries is not completely normal. The number of arteries is decreased, and many are tortuous. **Right,** cast of arterial tree of a 7-year-old boy with pronounced pulmonary hypertension, ventricular septal defect and reversal of flow. There is almost total absence of arborization.

with that of a patient of the same age with marked pulmonary hypertension and with that of a normal patient.

THE BANDING OPERATION

In patients with a large ventricular defect who have already developed marked pulmonary vascular disease, we believe that the creation of pulmonary stenosis may reverse the disease process and permit total correction of the ventricular defect at a later date at much less risk. The first step of narrowing the pulmonary artery has been performed in 3 patients about the age of 10 with large ventricular defects, balanced blood flows and equal pressures. As the second operation will have to wait 2–3 more years, confirmation of our hypothesis is still lacking. The mechanism whereby such patients may be improved is probably twofold. First, placing a resistance in the main pulmonary artery substitutes an operatively removable resistance for a resistance which must be changed by medical means alone. Second, pulmonary artery narrowing reduces the mean pressure only slightly but significantly reduces the systolic peak pressure, which in turn reduces the stretch of the peripheral pulmonary vascular bed. A reduction of stretch should lead to a decrease of vasomotor tone, gradual relaxation and disuse atrophy of the distal pulmonary vessels. A comparable situation in reverse is seen in the occasional patient with coarctation of the aorta[7,68,79] who, following resection, develops acute arteritis distal to the aortic anastomosis. Here, too, the mean pressure in the femoral artery has been changed very little, but a marked increase of the systolic pressure peak has occurred which exerts severe stress on vessels poorly adapted to tolerate high-peak pressures. The result is overdistention, disruption of the intima, loss of fluid into the media and adventitia and subsequent acute arteritis.

OPERATIVE TECHNIQUE. — Appropriate preanesthesia medication is administered. The patient is placed supine on the operating table, and the left side of the chest is elevated to about 15°. If the pulmonary artery is on the right, the right side should be positioned in like manner. After the chest has been prepared and draped, an anterolateral submammary incision is made, and the pleural cavity is entered through the third intercostal space. Division of the third costal cartilage at the sternum facilitates exposure. In the small infant, the thymus gland is usually large and must be reflected from the pericardium. An incision is made in the pericardium beginning over the right ventricle and extending to its reflection on the pulmonary artery superiorly. The pericardium between the pulmonary artery and aorta is incised, and a tape is passed around the artery to facilitate its dissection from the aorta. At this time, pressures are measured in the right ventricle, the distal pulmonary artery and

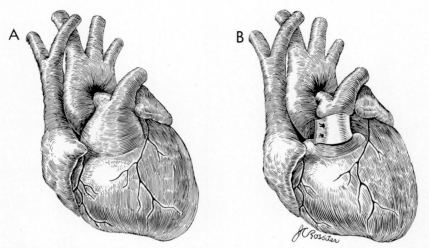

Fig. 43-6.—Pulmonary hypertension; the banding operation. **A**, heart with physiologic single ventricle; the main pulmonary artery is greatly dilated. **B**, the main pulmonary artery has been narrowed to about one-third its original size by a constricting fabric band.

the aorta. A synthetic fabric tape of Dacron or Teflon is passed around the artery and the ends sutured together so that the pulmonary artery is narrowed at lease 50% of its original diameter (Fig. 43-6). Additional sutures are placed below the original ones until the pressure in the distal pulmonary artery is less than one-half that in the right ventricle, preferably 30-35 mm Hg. In some instances, the heart will not tolerate the anticipated degree of constriction of the pulmonary artery, and in these instances, the artery should be released accordingly. Pressures are usually increased in the aorta after constriction of the pulmonary artery. The superfluous ends of the tape are excised, and the pericardium is closed loosely over the pulmonary artery and right ventricle. An incision is made in the pericardium posterior to the phrenic nerve, near the diaphragm, to allow dependent drainage. Pleural drainage through a chest catheter is necessary for about 24 hours. Hypothermia should not be used for this operation, since what appears to be the proper degree of constriction at a reduced temperature may be excessive when a normal temperature is reached, at which time cyanosis may appear.

POSTOPERATIVE CARE.—As yet, the secondary stimuli which may continue pulmonary vascular constriction have not been satisfactorily controlled. The patient with pulmonary vascular disease who is operated on is not to be considered well for many months, because sudden death is not uncommon. Postoperative care must include a rigorous attempt to remove secondary stimuli. Pulmonary infections must be avoided. Excessive emotion which might trigger an increase of vasomotor tone should be prevented when possible or reduced to a minimum. Active treatment with pulmonary vasodilators should be carried out. Our patients who fall into this category are kept on prophy-

lactic antibiotics, given sedation and tranquilizers and instructed in the use of 100% oxygen two to three times a day. If home care is inadequate, an attempt is made to keep the patient in a convalescent home. Normal life is resumed slowly, and full activity is not permitted until there is good evidence of a decrease of pulmonary vascular resistance.

Conclusion

It should be reiterated that the best treatment for pulmonary vascular disease is its prevention. At present, the best method of avoiding pulmonary vascular disease is very careful serial evaluation of the patient.[18] Cardiac catheterization should be performed if there is evidence of a decreasing left-to-right shunt, an increasing pulmonary second sound, a shifting electrocardiogram from predominant left ventricular hypertrophy to predominant right ventricular hypertrophy; and if, in truth, pulmonary resistance has increased, early operation is mandatory. We strongly advise that all patients with congenital heart disease be seen as early as possible and that they be followed at least at yearly intervals. Serial electrocardiograms must be taken and, when possible, serial cardiac catheterization should be carried out. Only in this way will we obtain the necessary understanding of the life history of congenital heart disease and discover the ideal age for repair of the patient's defect.

REFERENCES

1. Adams, F. H.; Lind, J., and Rauramo, L.: Physiologic studies in the cardiovascular status of normal newborn infants: Effect of Adrenalin, Noradrenalin, 10% and

100% oxygen and acetylcholine, Etude Neonatalis, 7:62, 1958.

2. Adams, P.; Anderson, P. A., and Lillehei, C. W.: Physiologic changes with age in ventricular septal defects, Circulation 16:857, 1957.

3. Adams, P., et al.: Significance of pulmonary vascular pathology in ventricular septal defects as determined by lung biopsy, Circulation 14:905, 1956.

4. Adams, W. E., et al.: Significance of pulmonary hypertension as a cause of death following pulmonary resection, J. Thoracic Surg. 26:407, 1953.

5. Adran, G. N., et al.: Effect of ventilation of the fetal lungs upon the pulmonary circulation, J. Physiol. 118:12, 1952.

6. Avioda, D. M.; Ling, J. S. L., and Schmidt, C. F.: Effects of anoxia on the pulmonary circulation: Reflex pulmonary vasoconstriction, Am. J. Physiol. 189:253, 1957.

7. Benson, W. R., and Sealy, W. C.: Arterial necrosis following resection of coarctation of the aorta, Lab. Invest. 5:359, 1956.

8. Blank, R. H.; Muller, W. H., Jr., and Dammann, J. F., Jr.: Changes in pulmonary vascular lesions after restoring normal pulmonary artery pressure, S. Forum 9:356, 1959.

9. Borst, H. G.; Berlund, E., and McGregor, M.: Effects of pharmacologic agents on the pulmonary circulation in the dog, J. Clin. Invest. 36:5, 1957.

10. Burton, A. C.: Relation of structure to function of the tissues of the walls of blood vessels, Physiol. Rev. 34:619, 1954.

11. Burton, A. C.: On the physical equilibrium of small blood vessels, Am. J. Physiol. 164:319, 1951.

12. Carlson, R. F., et al.: Effect of decreasing the amount of lung tissue on the RVP in animals, J. Thoracic Surg. 21:621, 1951.

13. Civin, H. W., and Edwards, J. E.: Postnatal structural changes in the intrapulmonary arteries and arterioles, Arch. Path. 51:192, 1951.

14. Crittenden, I. H.; Adams, F. H., and Latta, H.: Preoperative evaluation of the pulmonary vascular bed in patients with pulmonary hypertension associated with left-to-right shunts: Effect of acetylcholine, Pediatrics 24:448, 1959.

15. Daly, I. DeB.; and Daly, M. DeB.: Observations on the changes and resistance of the pulmonary vascular bed and response to stimulation of the carotid sinus barrel receptors in the dog, J. Physiol. 137:127, 1957.

16. Daly, I. DeB., et al.: Pulmonary vasomotor nerve activity, Quart. J. Exper. Physiol. 37:149, 1952.

17. Daly, I. DeB., and Daly, M. DeB.: Effects of stimulation of the carotid body chemoreceptors on pulmonary vascular resistance in the dog, J. Physiol. 137:436, 1957.

18. Dammann, J. F., Jr., et al.: Anatomy, physiology and natural history of simple ventricular septal defects, Am. J. Cardiol. 5:136, 1960.

19. Dammann, J. F., Jr.; Baker, J. P., and Muller, W. H., Jr.: Pulmonary vascular changes induced by experimentally produced pulmonary arterial hypertension, Surg., Gynec. & Obst. 105:16, 1957.

20. Dammann, J. F., Jr.; Smith, R. T., and Muller, W. H., Jr.: Experimental production of pulmonary vascular disease, S. Forum 6:155, 1956.

21. Damman, J. F., Jr.: The Relationships of Flow to Pressure in Various Types of Congenital Heart Disease, Particularly Those Associated with Pulmonary Hypertension, in Adams, W. R., and Veith, I. (ed.): Pulmonary Circulation (New York: Grune & Stratton, Inc., 1959).

22. Dammann, J. F., Jr.; McEachen, J. A., and Thompson, W. M., Jr.: The regression of pulmonary vascular disease after the creation of pulmonary stenosis, J. Thoracic & Cardiovas. Surg. 42:722, 1961.

23. Dammann, J. F., Jr., and Ferencz, C.: Significance of the pulmonary vascular bed in congenital heart disease: I. Normal lungs, Am. Heart J. 52:7, 1956.

24. Dammann, J. F., Jr., and Ferencz, C.: Significance of the pulmonary vascular bed in congenital heart disease: III. Defects between the ventricles or great vessels in which both increased pressure and blood flow may act upon the

lungs and in which there is a common injectile force, Am. Heart J. 52:210, 1956.

25. Davies, L. G.; Goodwin, J. F., and VanLevven, B. D.: Nature of pulmonary hypertension in mitral stenosis, Brit. Heart J. 16:440, 1954.

26. Dawes, G. S., et al.: Changes in the lungs in the newborn lamb, J. Physiol. 121:141, 1953.

27. Dawes, G. S.; Mott, J. C., and Widdicomb, J. G.: Fetal circulation in the lamb, J. Physiol. 126:563, 1954.

28. Denst, J., et al.: Biopsies of lung and atrial appendages in mitral stenosis: Correlation of data from cardiac catheterizations and pulmonary vascular lesions, Am. Heart J. 48:506, 1954.

29. Dexter, L., et al.: Studies of the pulmonary circulation in man at rest: Normal variations and the interrelations between increased pulmonary blood flow, elevated pulmonary arterial pressure and high pulmonary "capillary" pressures, J. Clin. Invest. 29:602, 1950.

30. DuShane, J. W., and Kirklin, J. W.: Selection for surgery of patients with ventricular septal defect and pulmonary hypertension, Circulation 21:13, 1960.

31. Edwards, J. E.: Advances in pathology of cardiovascular diseases, Tufts M. Alumni Bull., vol. 2, no. 1 and 2, 1952.

32. Edwards, J. E., et al.: Biopsy of the lungs and cardiac catheterization studies in patients treated surgically for mitral stenosis, J. Lab. & Clin. Med. 40:795, 1952.

33. Edwards, J. E.: Functional pathology of the pulmonary vascular tree in congenital heart disease, Circulation 15:164, 1957.

34. Edwards, J. E.: Pathologic Considerations and Adjustments between Systemic and Pulmonary Circulations, in Inter-national Symposium on Cardiovascular Surgery, Henry Ford Hospital (Philadelphia: W. B. Saunders Company, 1955).

35. Edwards, J. E.: Pathology of Pulmonary Hypertension, Proc. Postgrad. Cardiovas. Seminar Florida Heart A., p. 121, 1952.

36. Ellis, F. H., et al.: Patent ductus arteriosus with pulmonary hypertension: An analysis of cases treated surgically, J. Thoracic Surg. 81:268, 1956.

37. Ferguson, D. J.; Miller, F. A., and Varco, R. L.: A study of patent ductus type shunts in the dog using a new technique for measuring gas content of the mixed pulmonary artery blood, S. Forum, 5:74, 1954.

38. Ferguson, D. J.; Berkas, E. M., and Varco, R. L.: Circulatory factors contributing to alterations in pulmonary vascular histology, S. Forum 4:267, 1953.

39. Ferguson, D. J.; Berkas, E. M., and Varco, R. L.: Experimental Methods for the Production of Pulmonary Hypertension, in Adams, W. R., and Veith, I. (ed.): Pulmonary Circulation, (New York: Grune & Stratton, Inc., 1959), p. 130.

40. Ferguson, D. J., and Varco, R. L.: The relation of blood pressure and flow to the development and regression of experimentally induced pulmonary arteriosclerosis, Circulation Res. 3:152, 1955.

41. Ferrer, M. I., and Harvey, R. M.: Etiology of secondary pulmonary hypertension, Bull. New York Acad. Med. 30:208,1954.

42. Fowler, N. O., et al.: Observations on autonomic participation in pulmonary arteriolar resistance in man, J. Clin. Invest. 29:1387, 1950.

43. Goodale, F., et al.: Correlation of pulmonary arteriolar resistance with pulmonary vascular changes in patients with mitral stenosis before and after valvulotomy, New England J. Med. 252:979, 1955.

44. Halmogyi, D., et al.: The role of the nervous system in the maintenance of pulmonary arterial hypertension in heart failure, Brit. Heart J. 15:15, 1953.

45. Hamilton, W. F.; Woodbury, R. A., and Woods, E. B.: Relationship between systemic and pulmonary blood pressures in the fetus, Am. J. Physiol. 119:206, 1937.

46. Harris, P.: Influence of acetylcholine on the pulmonary arterial pressure, Brit. Heart J. 19:272, 1957.

47. Harrison, R. W., et al.: Cardiopulmonary reserve 5 to 15

years following 50% or more reduction in lung volume, S. Forum 7:209, 1956.

48. Heath, D., *et al.*: Graded pulmonary vascular changes and hemodynamic findings in cases of atrial and ventricular septal defect and patent ductus arteriosus, Circulation 18:1155, 1958.
49. Heath, D., and Whitaker, W.: Hypertensive pulmonary vascular disease, Circulation 14:323, 1956.
50. Heath, D., *et al.*: Relation between structural changes in the small pulmonary arteries and the immediate reversibility of pulmonary hypertension following closure of ventricular and atrial septal defects, Circulation 18:1167, 1958.
51. Heath, D., and Whitaker, W.: The pulmonary vessels in mitral stenosis, J. Path. & Bact. 70:291, 1955.
52. Henry, E. W.: The small pulmonary vessels in mitral stenosis, Brit. Heart J. 14:406, 1952.
53. Hicks, J. D.: Acute arterial necrosis in the lungs, J. Path. & Bact. 65:333, 1953.
54. Hurst, A.; Dressler, S. H., and Denst, J.: Relationship between pathologic changes in blood vessels in resected lobes and lungs as correlated with pulmonary artery pressure; changes recorded during cardiac catheterization, Dis. Chest 24:41, 1953.
55. James, L. S., and Rowe, R. D.: The pattern of response of pulmonary and systemic arterial pressures in newborn and older infants to short periods of hypoxia, J. Pediat. 51:5, 1957.
56. Kattus, A. A., and Muller, W. H., Jr.: A follow-up note on a previously reported patient with surgical closure of patent ductus arteriosus with reversal of flow, Ann. Surg. 146:178, 1957.
57. Kirklin, J. W., and McGoon, E. C.: Evaluation and current applications of open heart surgery in congenital and acquired heart disease, Progr. Cardiovas. Dis. 1:66, 1958.
58. Lind, J., and Wegelius, C.: Human fetal circulation: Changes in the cardiovascular system at birth and disturbances in the postnatal closure of the foramen ovale and ductus arteriosus, Cold Spring Harbor Symp. 1954.
59. McGoon, D. C., *et al.*: Atrial septal defect: Factors affecting the surgical mortality rate, Circulation 19:195, 1959.
60. Mendelsohn, H. J.; Zimmerman, H. A., and Adelman, A.: A study of pulmonary hemodynamics during pulmonary resection, J. Thoracic Surg. 20:366, 1950.
61. Muller, W. H., Jr.; Dammann, J. F., Jr., and Head, W. H.: Changes in the pulmonary vessels produced by experimental pulmonary hypertension, Surgery 34:363, 1953.
62. Muller, W. H., Jr., and Dammann, J. F., Jr.: Results following the creation of pulmonary artery stenosis, Ann. Surg. 143:6, 1956.
63. Muller, W. H., Jr., and Dammann, J. F., Jr.: Surgical significance of pulmonary hypertension, Tr. Am. S. A. 70:199, 1952.
64. Muller, W. H., Jr., and Dammann, J. F., Jr.: Treatment of certain congenital malformations of the heart by the creation of pulmonic stenosis to reduce pulmonary hypertension and excessive pulmonary blood flow: A preliminary report, Surg., Gynec. & Obst. 95:213, 1952.
65. Parker, F., Jr., and Weiss, S.: The nature and significance of the structural changes in the lungs in mitral stenosis, Am. J. Path. 12:573, 1936.
66. Patel, D. J., and Burton, A. C.: Active constriction of small pulmonary arteries in the rabbit, Circulation Res. 5:620, 1957.
67. Patel, D. J.; Lange, R. L., and Hecht, H. H.: Some evidence for active constriction in the human pulmonary vascular bed, Circulation 18:19, 1958.
68. Perez-Alvarez, J. J., and Oudkerk, S.: Necrotizing arteriolitis of the abdominal organs as a postoperative complication following correction of coarctation of the aorta: Case report, Surgery 37:833, 1955.

69. Pickering, G. W.; Wright, A. D., and Heptinstall, R. H.: The reversibility of malignant hypertension, Lancet 2:952, 1952.
70. Reynolds, S. R. M.: Pulmonary vascular changes and hemodynamic changes at birth, Anat. Rec. 121:414, 1955.
71. Sarnoff, S. J.: Massive pulmonary edema of central nervous system origin: Hemodynamic observations and the role of sympathetic pathways, Fed. Proc. 10:118, 1951.
72. Sarnoff, S. J., and Sarnoff, L. C.: Neurohemodynamics of pulmonary edema: The role of sympathetic pathway in the elevation of pulmonary and systemic vascular pressures following the intracisternal injection of fibrin, Circulation 6:51, 1952.
73. Sarnoff, S. J., and Berglund, E.: Pressure volume characteristics and stress relaxation on the pulmonary vascular bed of the dog, Am. J. Physiol. 171:238, 1952.
74. Sarnoff, S. J., and Farr, H. W.: Spinal anesthesia and the therapy of pulmonary edema: A preliminary report, Anesthesiology 5:69, 1944.
75. Schilling, J. A., *et al.*: Extensive pulmonary resection in dogs: Altitude tolerance, work capacity and pathologic-physiologic changes, Ann. Surg. 144:635, 1956.
76. Semler, H. J.; Shepherd, J. T., and Wood, E. H.: The role of vessel tone in maintaining pulmonary vascular resistance in patients with mitral stenosis, Circulation 19:386, 1959.
77. Shepherd, J. T., and Wood, E. H.: The role of vessel tone in pulmonary hypertension, Circulation 19:641, 1959.
78. Silver, A. W., *et al.*: Regression of pulmonary hypertension after closure of patent ductus arteriosus, Proc. Staff Meet. Mayo Clin. 29:293, 1954.
79. Singleton, A. O.; McGinnis, L. M. S., and Eason, H. R.: Arteritis following correction of coarctation of the aorta, Surgery 45:665, 1959.
80. Smith, R. C.; Burchell, H. B., and Edwards, J. E.: Pathology of the pulmonary vascular tree: IV. Structural changes in the pulmonary vessels in chronic left heart failure, Circulation 10:801, 1954.
81. Swan, H. J. C.; Burchell, H. P., and Wood, E. H.: Effects of oxygen on pulmonary vascular resistance in patients with pulmonary hypertension associated with atrial septal defects, Circulation 20:66, 1959.
82. Symmers, W. St. C.: Necrotizing pulmonary arteriopathy associated with pulmonary hypertension, J. Clin. Path. 5:36, 1952.
83. Welch, K. J., and Kinney, T. D.: Effect of patent ductus arteriosus and of interauricular and interventricular septal defects on the development of pulmonary vascular lesions, Am. J. Path. 24:729, 1948.
84. Werko, L., *et al.*: Pulmonary circulatory dynamics in mitral stenosis before and after commissurotomy, Am. Heart J. 45:477, 1953.
85. Williams, M. H.: Relationships between pulmonary artery pressure and blood flow in the dog lung, Am. J. Physiol. 179:243, 1954.
86. Wood, P.: Pulmonary hypertension, Mod. Concepts Cardiovas. Dis., vol. 28, no. 3, 1959.
87. Wood, P., *et al.*: The effect of acetylcholine on pulmonary vascular resistance and left artial pressure in mitral stenosis, Brit. Heart J. 29:279, 1957.
88. Yu, P. N. G., *et al.*: Studies of pulmonary hypertension: IV. Pulmonary circulatory dynamics in patients with mitral stenosis at rest, Am. Heart J. 47:330, 1954.

J. F. DAMMANN, JR.
W. H. MULLER, JR.

Drawings by
J. C. ROSSITER

Treatment of Cardiac Arrest

HISTORY.—The introduction of anesthesia (1842-1846) was soon followed by the recognition of cardiac arrest as an anesthetic complication. As early as 1848, 4 fatalities from cardiac arrest during operations under anesthesia were reported. The first successful cardiac resuscitation by direct massage was performed by Igelsrud in 1901,[6] 7 previous attempts by other surgeons having been unsuccessful. The treatment of ventricular fibrillation by electrical defibrillation was developed in physiology laboratories by Wiggers and by Hooker and Kouwenhoven, and the first successful clinical defibrillation was reported by Beck in 1947.[6]

CLINICAL FEATURES

The frequency of cardiac arrest varies from approximately 1 per 1,000 to 1 per 3,000 operations.[6] Myocardial ischemia with the combination of inadequate oxygenation and carbon dioxide retention is the most common cause. Operations on the heart are associated with a high incidence of cardiac arrest, partly because diseased hearts are very susceptible to ischemia. Anesthetic agents, especially cyclopropane, can cause cardiac arrest from the direct action of the anesthetic agent on the myocardium. Cardiac arrest may be precipitated by vagal stimulation induced by manipulation of the trachea or esophagus as occurs during intubation, extubation, endotracheal suction or insertion of a nasogastric tube; but experimental evidence indicates that neurogenic reflexes alone will not cause cardiac arrest unless myocardial injury from anoxia or cardiac disease is already present. Ventricular fibrillation is much less frequent than cardiac arrest. It occurs most commonly during operations under hypothermia, during cardiac catheterization or following administration of excessive amounts of quinidine or digitalis.

As a rule, cerebral function is impaired first by circulatory arrest; irreversible neurologic injury may occur if cerebral circulation is stopped more than 4–6 minutes. The conscious patient immediately becomes unconscious, with absent respiratory or cardiac activity. The anesthetized patient with cardiac arrest undergoes a similar immediate loss of respiratory and cardiac action. The diagnosis can be made simply by noting the absence of a pulse (usually best detected by palpating the carotid or femoral arteries), absence of heart sounds, absence of respiratory activity and loss of consciousness. Time is so important that the diagnosis should be made within less than a minute, after which the patient should be treated for cardiac arrest until it can be proved to be absent or corrected. Diagnostic procedures which require longer periods of time should be rejected. The electrocardiogram, although helpful in identifying ventricular fibrillation, is definitely not a reliable guide for excluding circulatory arrest, since electrical complexes can be recorded from a heart which is not propelling blood.

TREATMENT

The first step in treatment is to establish adequate respiration since, without it, attempts at cardiac resuscitation are futile. If an endotracheal tube is not readily available, ventilation is best begun in the majority of patients by direct mouth-to-mouth or mouth-to-airway insufflation.[4] No special equipment is needed for this, and the method is much more effective than artificial respiration by intermittent compression of the chest.[5]

CARDIAC MASSAGE.—If cardiac massage can be started within 4 minutes after the onset of cardiac arrest, most patients will recover without neurologic injury. In 90% of the survivors of 1,200 collected cases of cardiac arrest, massage was started within 4 minutes after the beginning of cardiac arrest.[7] External cardiac massage (Fig. 43-7) has been used extensively at Johns Hopkins Hospital since 1960 and seems to be applicable to most patients.[2] It

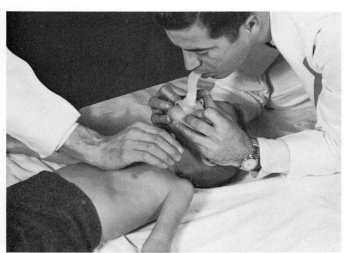

Fig. 43-7.—External cardiac massage. The heart is compressed intermittently between sternum and vertebral column. The heel of the operator's hand presses the sternum against the vertebral column 60-80 times a minute. An assistant provides mouth-to-double-ended-airway insufflation. The chin is held well up, the nostrils closed. In infants, only puffs of air are delivered. In older patients, the operator may require two hands for effective sternal compression. Effective compression should produce easily palpable peripheral pulse. If no pulse is felt, the chest must be opened at once and the heart compressed directly. (Courtesy of Dr. J. R. Jude.)

is most easily applied in children, whose chest wall is more readily compressed than adults'. In brief, the method consists of forceful intermittent pressure with both hands to compress the lower sternum against the vertebral column, thereby compressing the heart and propelling blood. The rate of compression is 80-100 times per minute for children. The effectiveness of the compression should be constantly monitored by palpating a peripheral pulse during massage. A systolic blood pressure of at least 70-80 mm Hg should be obtained. External massage is of particular value when cardiac arrest occurs outside the operating room and also as a preliminary trial before opening the chest for direct massage.

If external massage is not immediately effective, thoracotomy through the left fourth or fifth interspace should be performed and direct massage begun. Thoracotomy should not be delayed until special instruments are obtained. A knife blade is all that is required, as bleeding from the wound will not occur until cardiac activity is restored. The intercostal incision can be quickly made, the ribs manually separated and massage begun while additional instruments are obtained. Regardless of the method by which massage is done, a peripheral pulse should be monitored to make certain that massage is effectively propelling an adequate amount of blood. Excessive force is not required and can cause myocardial injury or rupture.

How long massage should be continued if the heart fails to beat is a difficult question. Most successful cardiac resuscitations occur with only a few minutes of massage. Massage should be continued for an hour or longer if there are no signs of severe neurologic injury and if there are no indications of irreversible myocardial injury. On one occasion, we used cardiac massage for 2 1/2 hours with complete recovery; the patient had developed intractable ventricular fibrillation while under hypothermia and required prolonged massage before defibrillation was effective.

Epinephrine (2-5 cc, 1:10,000 concentration) and calcium chloride (2-5 cc, 10% solution) are the drugs most useful in stimulating cardiac contractility. If cardiac massage does not result in a prompt return of cardiac activity, either or both of the drugs should be used and injected directly into the right or left atrium. As blood volume deficiency often is present, the rapid infusion of 500–1,000 cc of blood may be indicated. A vasopressor drug may be given to increase central aortic pressure and concurrently coronary and cerebral blood flow; similarly, when accessible, the descending thoracic aorta may be clamped briefly in order to increase coronary perfusion during massage. Sodium bicarbonate (50–100 mEq) intravenously has been useful in treating metabolic acidosis in patients in whom massage has been ineffective. Other drugs, such as digitalis, atropine and cardiac stimulants, have seldom proved of benefit.

VENTRICULAR DEFIBRILLATION.—Ventricular fibrillation may be treated by external defibrillation if a

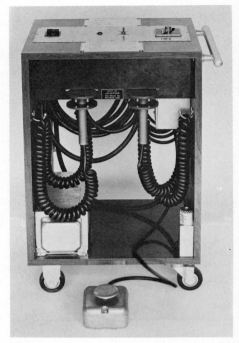

Fig. 43-8.—External cardiac defibrillator. Basic parts are: (1) selector switch for voltage desired (240 v for children, 480 v for adults); (2) timer for regulating current duration (recommended duration 0.25 second); (3) isolation transformer; (4) foot switch; (5) two-hand electrodes, each 9 sq. in. in area, one applied at the suprasternal notch, the other at the left midclavicular line at the level of the xiphoid.

diagnosis can be made without thoracotomy[3] (Fig. 43-8). As, unless a thoracotomy is performed, the diagnosis can be established only by electrocardiography, the usefulness of an external defibrillator is limited to patients in whom an electrocardiogram is immediately available. In such instances, fibrillation can be stopped by an external defibrillator. An external defibrillator has been of particular value in the cardiac catheterization laboratory, where the electrocardiogram is routinely monitored in patients undergoing cardiac catheterization.

Ventricular fibrillation commonly develops during attempts at resuscitation of cardiac arrest by cardiac massage. Electrical defibrillation can almost always be accomplished if the myocardium has not been seriously injured and is well oxygenated by massage before defibrillation is attempted. Massage should be vigorously performed, usually supplemented by intracardiac injections of calcium or epinephrine, until the myocardium is red and "firm." Attempts to defibrillate a cyanotic, flabby heart are usually futile. A second cause of ineffective defibrillation is inadequate contact between the electrodes and the surface of the heart. The electrodes should be moistened with saline and one firmly applied near the apex of the left ventricle, the other on the opposite side of the heart.

When firmly applied to a fibrillating heart that is well oxygenated, a single shock of 120-200 volts for 0.1 second will defibrillate most hearts. When an adequate current is passed through the heart, it contracts vigorously and fibrillation stops. If fibrillation stops but begins again, either the heart has not been adequately oxygenated or it has not recovered from the insult initially causing fibrillation.

CARE FOLLOWING
CARDIAC RESUSCITATION

The chest incision should be closed in the ordinary manner after insertion of an intercostal tube for drainage. It is surprising how rarely infection occurs, even after a nonsterile emergency thoracotomy for cardiac massage. Following closure of the chest incision, the prognosis can be closely correlated with the severity of the neurologic injury. Cerebral injury is rare when massage is begun within 4 minutes after cardiac arrest but increases progressively in severity after this time. A review of 25 patients resuscitated from cardiac arrest at Johns Hopkins Hospital over a period of 30 months showed 13 survivors, a recovery rate of 52%. Six patients without neurologic injury recovered; only 7 of 19 with such injury survived.[1]

It has been observed that the neurologic injury from anoxia becomes more severe in the hours following cardiac resuscitation, presumably because of the development of cerebral edema. Prevention and treatment of the cerebral edema have materially increased the survival rate in patients with neurologic injury. For several years, hypothermia has been used in all patients with cerebral injury after cardiac resuscitation. Of 7 patients with neurologic injury who were treated before hypothermia was employed, only 1 survived: in contrast, 6 of 12 treated by cooling recovered.[8] Similarly, in the laboratory the survival rate of dogs subjected to 10 minutes of circulatory arrest was raised from 25 to 57% by the use of hypothermia (Table 43-1).[9] The favorable effect of hypothermia is probably related to the prevention of cerebral edema, although other beneficial effects may exist. Patients are cooled with a refrigeration blanket or with chipped ice around the body until the temperature has decreased to 34 C, after which the temperature will drift to 31–32 C. More extreme cooling is avoided because of lack of experimental evidence of additional benefit as well as the fact that cardiac arrhythmias are more common at the lower temperatures. Hypothermia is continued for 2–4 days unless signs of recovery occur; a beneficial effect beyond this time has not been observed. Once hypothermia is begun, it is easily maintained by placing a refrigeration blanket beneath the patient and by administering chlorpromazine or promethazine as necessary to prevent shivering. No harmful effects have been observed from the use of hypothermia in this manner.

Cerebral edema can be reduced also by strict limitation of fluids and by the use of osmotic diuretics. Fluids should be limited for 2-3 days to 600–800 cc/M^2 of body surface area /24 hours. Intravenous infusions of urea (20-40 Gm of a 40% solution) cause a profuse osmotic diuresis and may effectively reduce cerebral edema. A tracheostomy usually is performed in comatose patients. This facilitates the removal of bronchial secretions and also avoids respiratory obstruction during the convulsions which commonly occur in these patients.

PROGNOSIS

The recovery rate from cardiac arrest is between 40 and 60%. The widespread use of external massage may increase this rate because of its applicability in situations where thoracotomy has been attempted too late or not at all. The vigorous treatment of cerebral edema by hypothermia, fluid restriction and osmotic diuretics may increase the recovery rate of patients with neurologic injury from 10–15% to 40–50%.[1] Fortunately, surviving patients usually recover completely from the neurologic injury. None of our patients who recovered after neurologic injury had any significant residual damage.

REFERENCES

1. Benson, D. W., *et al.*: The use of hypothermia after cardiac arrest, Anesth. & Analg. 38:423, 1959.
2. Kouwenhoven, W. B.; Jude, J. R., and Knickerbocker, G. G.: Closed chest cardiac massage, J.A.M.A. 173:1064, 1960.
3. Kouwenhoven, W. B., *et al.*: Closed chest defibrillation of the heart, Surgery 42:550, 1957.
4. Safar, P.; Escarraga, L., and Elam, J.: A comparison of the mouth-to-mouth and mouth-to-airway methods of artificial respiration with the chest-pressure arm-lift methods, New England J. Med. 258:671, 1958.
5. Safar, P.: The failure of manual respiration, J. Appl. Physiol. 14:84, 1959.
6. Stephenson, H. E.: *Cardiac Arrest and Resuscitation* (St. Louis: C. V. Mosby Company, 1958), chap. 1 and 2.
7. Stephenson, H. E.; Reid, L. C., and Hinton, J. W.: Some common denominators in 1200 cases of cardiac arrest, Ann. Surg. 137:731, 1953.
8. Williams, G. R., and Spencer, F. C.: The clinical use of hypothermia following cardiac arrest, Ann. Surg. 148:462, 1958.
9. Zimmerman, J. M., and Spencer, F. C.: The influence of hypothermia on cerebral injury resulting from circulatory occlusion, Forum 9:216, 1958.

F. C. SPENCER
H. T. BAHNSON

TABLE 43-1.—EFFECT OF HYPOTHERMIA ON CEREBRAL INJURY RESULTING FROM 10 MINUTES OF CIRCULATORY OCCLUSION

THERAPY	No. OF DOGS	NEUROLOGIC RECOVERY RATE, %	SURVIVAL RATE, %
None	12	17	25
Hypothermia (31–33 C, 24–48 hours)	14	79	57

Hypothermia
for Cardiac Surgery

HISTORY.—Claude Bernard[4] in 1876 reported cooling guinea pigs to body temperatures of 18-20 C with successful rewarming. Horvath[26] in 1881 discovered that hibernating animals could be rewarmed from temperatures as low as 0 C. Benedict and Lee[3] in 1938 reported oxygen consumption of only 3-10% of normal in deep hibernation. Fay[18] in 1940 investigated the use of hypothermia of 30 C for treating patients with malignancies. Bigelow *et al.*[5] in 1950 showed that if shivering was controlled, oxygen consumption fell consistently with reduction of temperature to 18 C in the dog. Interruption of the circulation for periods of time exceeding those at normothermic temperatures was investigated experimentally by Bigelow *et al.*,[6] who first suggested the use of hypothermia with inflow occlusion for intracardiac procedures. Lewis and Taufic[29] performed the first operation on a human subject, using hypothermia with inflow occlusion to close an atrial septal defect under direct vision. Hypothermia induced by cooling circulating blood was investigated independently by Delorme[16] and Gollan[20] in 1952. The combined use of hypothermia and a pump oxygenator with low flow rates was introduced by Peirce[38] and Sealy[40] in 1956. Profound hypothermia (10–20 C) was investigated experimentally by Niazi and Lewis[35] and combined with a pump oxygenator by Gollan[21] in 1954. Niazi and Lewis[36] cooled a patient with advanced carcinoma to 9 C rectal temperature and cardiac standstill of 1 hour, with immediate recovery. Sealy[40] cooled patients as low as 9 C, combining hypothermia and extracorporeal circulation. Profound hypothermia with autogenous oxygenation was introduced by Drew and Anderson[18] in 1959. Selective cooling of the heart to produce cardioplegia has been reported by Urschel and Greenberg.[44]

Moderate Hypothermia

Lowering of the body temperature by artificial means to an esophageal temperature range of 25-32 C is accomplished by surface cooling and is generally termed moderate hypothermia.

Surface cooling is performed by using a blanket through which cold fluid is circulated or by immersing the patient in ice water. Infants and children have a relatively larger body surface than adults and have a low heat production, especially during anesthesia. In the first year of life, infants are virtually poikilothermic, but temperature regulation stabilizes during the second year and remains labile throughout childhood;[41] thus the hypothermic state is much more readily produced in children than in adults.

METHOD.—In our series of over 700 patients, a Therm-O-Rite blanket has been used as a simple, safe and satisfactory means. Neonates and infants will cool rapidly while merely lying on a cold blanket with perhaps an adjacent ice-bag. Children weighing up to 75 lb. cool readily when ice-bags are placed over the axillary and inguinal areas and they are then wrapped in the blanket (Fig. 43-9). Above this weight, ice may be added sparingly to the skin surface to accelerate the onset of hypothermia.

The use of ice and ice baths for infants and children has been discontinued because of the difficulty in reversing the rapid falls of temperature that ensue. As an example, 1 infant was removed from an ice bath at 35 C and then continued to cool to 28 C despite all efforts at rewarming.[10] At temperatures below 33 C, movement of the patient should be minimized to avoid undue stimulation of a hypothermic heart.

TEMPERATURE.—In the early development of hypothermia, rectal temperatures were considered an adequate guide to body temperature. It is well recognized now that when cooling or rewarming proceeds rapidly, the rectal and pharyngeal temperatures may lag 1–3 degrees behind that of the esophagus. In man and animals, the esophageal temperature at heart level is the most reliable index of heart and blood temperature.[13] In pediatric hypothermia, it is essential that both rectal and esophageal sites be monitored as temperatures may alter readily. If desired, deep thigh muscle temperatures provide a helpful forecast to the temperature course, and pharyngeal temperatures approximate cerebral temperatures.[33]

Temperature drift.—A drift of temperature after

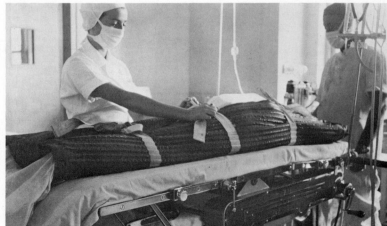

Fig. 43-9.—Hypothermia. The anesthetized child is surrounded with ice in cellophane bags, then wrapped in a Therm-O-Rite blanket.

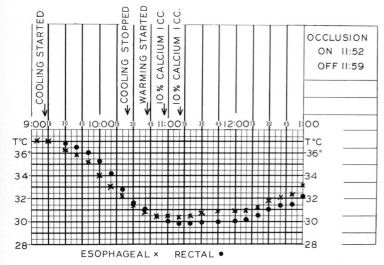

Fig. 43-10.—Hypothermia. Temperature chart of a 10-year-old child undergoing operation for correction of an atrial septal defect of secundum type.

ESOPHAGEAL ×   RECTAL ●

cessation of cooling depends on (1) the size of the patient, (2) degree of muscle tone, (3) amount of peripheral vasodilation, and (4) ambient temperature and humidity. Considerable individual variation exists, and the best indication of subsequent temperatures is the slope of the temperature curve. As the slope grows steeper, cooling should cease at higher temperatures because the drift will be greater. It appears wiser to cool a patient more slowly and thus retain more control over the temperature.[10] An actual temperature chart is illustrated in Figure 43-10.

Rewarming.—A late model of the Therm-O-Rite machine has one solution at 0 C (32 F) and a second separate solution at 40.5 C (105 F). By turning a valve, one can alternate the circulation fluid as desired. In our early experience the rewarming solution was kept at 110 F., but 1 patient received a slight first-degree burn. Rewarming is hastened by the use of hot-water bottles. When all temperatures have reached 33 C or more, the child is allowed to awaken and is taken to the recovery room.

Physiologic Considerations of Moderate Hypothermia

INITIAL RESPONSE.—The initial response of a patient to hypothermia mimics that of intense sympathetic stimulation due to any stress.[19] Shivering occurs, vasoconstriction is profound, oxygen consumption increases tremendously, the respiratory rate is accelerated, pulse rate is increased, blood pressure is elevated, and there is a significant increase of cardiac output. As hypothermia proceeds, a gradual depression of physiologic function occurs, with a fairly direct relationship to the degree of cooling.

METABOLISM.—Bigelow[5] believed that if oxygen demand was decreased by lowering the body temperature, the brain could survive prolonged circulatory occlusion, allowing intracardiac surgery under direct vision. His experiments showed a reduction of oxygen consumption almost linear with body temperature. There is disagreement whether the relationship is linear or exponential, but there is general agreement that a 6–7% fall of oxygen consumption occurs with each degree of lowering of body temperature. The tissue oxygen requirement is reduced,[12] but the oxygen supply remains adequate, as indicated by analysis of arteriovenous differences at various temperatures.[5] Shivering must be prevented or the metabolic rate and oxygen consumption will be greatly elevated. During hypothermic anesthesia, gross shivering is uncommon in children before puberty, but increased muscle tone is constant.[10]

CIRCULATION.—Following the initial stimulation, the pulse rate, blood pressure and cardiac output gradually fall with cooling. In the range of moderate hypothermia, bradycardia will respond to atropine and the blood pressure shows a minimal fall but may be difficult to obtain due to vasoconstriction.

The electrocardiogram shows prolongation of the P-R interval, lengthening of the QRS complex and an increased Q-T interval. The delayed interventricular conduction is directly related to body temperature[15] and produces prolonged systole and isometric contraction. At temperatures below 28 C, there is frequent occurrence of such arrhythmias as nodal rhythm, premature ventricular extrasystoles, A-V block and even ventricular fibrillation. Many factors influence cardiac irritability, and the risk of ventricular fibrillation limits the range of hypothermia using surface cooling.

BLOOD.—Hypothermia causes a shift of body water into the cells, reducing blood volume and increasing the viscosity. These changes conserve body heat by keeping blood away from the skin and reducing the available water for insensible heat loss and evaporation.[41] The hemoconcentration results in increased red cell counts and high hematocrit, but the leukocytes and platelets show a marked reduction. Of greater significance is the intravascular agglutination of red cells that has been shown to occur during hypothermia.[31]

Hypothermia produces a slight decrease of serum sodium levels. Most reports indicate a considerable reduction of serum potassium levels.[2,43,46] A rise of potassium or sudden shifts in electrolyte concentrations have been blamed as the main cause of ventricular fibrillation.[23] From our studies,[10] hypothermic anesthesia with circulatory occlusion appears to produce minimal changes in serum sodium, serum chloride and blood urea nitrogen values. Following occlusion, serum potassium decreases and blood glucose rises. Hyperglycemia also occurs with shivering but may persist because of failure to metabolize glucose at temperatures of 30 C and below.[47,48]

RESPIRATION.—A slowing of respiration occurs with hypothermia,[45] and an increase of the anatomic and physiologic dead space due to bronchodilation has been reported.[34] No agreement has been reached regarding the adequacy of spontaneous respiration. It has been stated that hypothermia does not produce acidosis but does produce pH changes due solely to increased carbon dioxide solubility with cooling.[24] The pH of arterial blood does decrease[43] and carbon dioxide solubility does increase with hypothermia. Metabolic acidosis is also said to occur.[8] In clinical practice, such factors as shivering, circulatory occlusion, shock, transfusion, anesthesia and hypoventilation are able to produce acidosis to some degree.

CENTRAL NERVOUS SYSTEM.—Cerebral oxygen consumption decreases with hypothermia. At 25 C, the oxygen uptake is reduced to one-third that at normal temperatures, which allows a maximal occlusion period of 15 minutes.[32] Children readily regain consciousness at 28 C, so that moderate hypothermia does not greatly affect cortical functioning. There is no striking evidence that 25–30 C per se produces any permanent defect in memory, intelligence or other psychologic functions.[14] Amplitude of the electroencephalogram is decreased with cooling, and delta waves of large amplitude appear at 30 C.[13] A slight reduction of brain volume and spinal fluid pressure also occurs. Although the spinal cord is more resistant to inadequate circulation than the brain, it too is endangered by prolonged circulatory or aortic occlusion. With hypothermia of 30 C., however, the incidence of paraplegic symptoms following aortic occlusion is reduced.[1] Afferent peripheral nerve conduction is slightly reduced to 25 C, but stimulation may provoke an increased central response as the cortical thresholds are lowered. Central threshold stimuli are said to be able to provoke a convulsive reaction during hypothermia, but this has not occurred in our experience.

VISCERA.—With a fall of temperature and blood pressure, reduction of renal flow and glomerular filtration occurs.[37] Urine volumes are only slightly diminished, however, because tubular reabsorption is decreased due to cold.

Reduced liver function is important because the detoxification of drugs is thereby retarded. For example, the half-life of morphine increases from 3.7 minutes at 37 C to 94 minutes at 24 C, a 23-fold increase in the time necessary for the liver to conjugate free morphine.[39]

The initial stress of hypothermia activates the adrenal cortex,[19] but later there is depression of the pituitary and secretion of ACTH and adrenal corticoid secretions.[28] During moderate hypothermia, the body remains extremely responsive to stress, as evident from the great release of catecholamines during the postocclusion period.[11]

COMPLICATIONS.—Inadequate myocardial contractility or ventricular fibrillation may occur in poor-risk patients at esophageal temperatures below 28 C. In other pateints, ventricular fibrillation may occur spontaneously when the period of inflow occlusion exceeds 6–8 minutes. The hypothermic heart deprived of coronary flow at levels of 28 C is susceptible to irregularities and fibrillation because of interference with the conduction system. With careful massage and surface rewarming of the heart with normal saline solution, no real difficulty in restoring normal sinus rhythm has been encountered. An increased bleeding tendency was present in only 1 patient in whom heparinized blood was not immediately neutralized. Gross shivering is seen only in children past puberty, but increased muscular tone is constant. Mild degrees of metabolic acidosis probably occur even with short occlusion, moderate hypothermia, and light anesthesia with hyperventilation. Children apparently can compensate for mild degrees of acidosis, but no complete biochemical studies have been undertaken.

Thermal burns have been noted in 4 patients despite vigilant attention, but frostbite has not occurred even when ice has been placed directly on the skin. One infant exhibited firm subcutaneous lumps that were suggestive of frozen fat tissue early in the series when low temperatures and ice were used for infants.

Moderate hypothermia has been employed extensively for short-term intracardiac operations. We have consistently used temperatures of 30 C with inflow occlusion times up to 8 minutes in the operative treatment of interatrial septal defects of the secundum type and for pure pulmonary valve stenosis. Moderate hypothermia at 32–34 C is a helpful adjunct to lower metabolism during the operation during shunting procedures in cyanotic children. In correction of coarctation of the aorta, such temperatures will protect the spinal cord from possible ischemia and resulting lower limb paralysis.

Anesthesia for Hypothermia

Patients are thoroughly examined the day before operation and the cardiovascular system is examined in detail. In the presence of complicating factors, particularly an upper respiratory tract infection, or a hemoglobin level below 10 Gm, operation is deferred. Premedication consists of atropine 0.12 mg (1/500 gr) /10 lb. and, over 1 year, pentobarbital 1 mg/lb. and Demerol 0.6 mg/lb. given intramuscularly 1 hour preoperatively. In older children, morphine sulfate 1 mg/10 lb. is substituted for Demerol. This premedication produced a sleepy acquiescent patient without depression.

INDUCTION. — For induction, a sleep dose of 2.5% thiopental sodium (1-2 mg/lb.) is slowly injected through a 25-gauge needle, to be followed by succinylcholine 1 mg/3 lb. The patient is ventilated with nitrous oxide and oxygen 5:3 until spontaneous respiration returns, when 0.5-1% halothane is added.

Immediately after intubation, the esophageal stethoscope and thermister probe are inserted, followed by the muscle and rectal thermister probes and the needle electrodes for electrocardiograph and electroencephalograph. An 18-gauge needle with stylet is inserted in the right saphenous vein at the ankle to provide a "spare" venous entrance. A cut-down is started in the left saphenous vein and a blood pump administration set connected. A graduated bag is used to measure fluid in 10-cc increments for infants weighing under 20 lb. A Y-connector is inserted next to the cut-down to allow direct injection of drugs.

COOLING. — Coolant at 0 C is pumped through a Therm-O-Rite blanket on which the patient lies, protected only by a thin sheet. All bolsters used for positioning the patient are placed beneath the cooling mattress to ensure maximal contact with the mattress. For weights under 10 lb., skin preparation ensures a temperature drop; 10-40 lb., use one ice-bag/10 lb.; over 40 lb., use six ice-bags plus one for each additional 10 lb. Ice-bags may be removed and skin preparation commenced when the esophageal temperature approximates 33 C. If cooling is very rapid or very slow, the temperature may be altered by 1 C.

The temperature usually desired for a 7-minute period of cardiac venous inflow occlusion is 30-31 C in the esophagus. When the desired temperature has been reached, about 30 minutes before circulatory occlusion, the blanket is connected to the heating tank (set at 105 F), to avert further drift and ensure rapid rewarming after restoration of the circulation.

Anesthesia having been established with nitrous oxide, oxygen and halothane 0.5-1%, the halothane is decreased to 0.5% and succinylcholine 2 mg/10 lbs. given to facilitate controlled respiration shortly before the skin incision is made. In children under 20 lb., hyperventilation is maintained by using an Ayre T-piece system, and a Waters canister of appropriate size in larger children. This technique ensures adequate oxygenation and carbon dioxide elimination while maintaining a light plane of anesthesia.

Halothane is nonexplosive, reduces oxygen consumption, prevents shivering, decreases peripheral and pulmonary vascular resistance and does not depress the cardiac musculature or cardiac output. Furthermore, halothane does not cause metabolic acidosis or cardiac arrhythmia other than bradycardia. Nitrous oxide is the least toxic inhalation anesthetic agent. Its ability to prevent shivering is probably due to its analgesic action.

DRUGS. — Certain drugs must be immediately available. The normal heart rate at different ages is set out in Table 43-2. Bradycardia is always treated by stopping any manipulation, by oxygenation, by withholding succinylcholine and halothane and by giving atropine (0.2-0.6 mg intravenously) to reduce vagal tone.

Paroxysmal tachycardia unrelated to hypovolemia or hypoxia is treated by injection of prostigmine. It is administered in doses of 0.1 mg intravenously, repeated every 5 minutes until the heart rate slows.

Transient arrhythmias may occur, particularly when the heart is manipulated and when the tapes are placed around the venae cavae. Ventricular fibrillation may occur with marked blood loss, with air embolism or for no obvious reason. After full oxygenation and removal of the precipitating factor, a single shock at 60 v for 1/10 second from the electrical defibrillator usually restores sinus rhythm.

Rarely, the cardiac output needs to be increased. Epinephrine 1:250,000 is preferred in infants because its positive inotropic effect directly increases the force and rate of the heart. The solution is given from a bottle graduated in 10 cc and the rate of flow titrated to maintain blood pressure over 75 mm Hg. If cardiac arrest occurs and the tone of the heart is diminished, 1-2 cc of 1:10,000 epinephrine may be injected into the heart and massage continued until electrical defibrillation can be performed. During hypothermia, epinephrine maintains its activity down to at least 25 C, though the response is diminished and delayed. In older children, methoxamine (Vasoxyl) is given intravenously in doses of 1–2 mg every 5 minutes to increase blood pressure.

When large amounts of citrated blood are rapidly tranfused, 1 cc of 10% calcium gluconate is administered intravenously by a separate route for each 100 cc of blood given. This preserves normal cardiac contractility. Calcium must be used with caution in a digitalized patient. Digitalis is rarely necessary in hypo-

TABLE 43-2. — NORMAL HEART RATE ACCORDING TO AGE

Age	Under 1 yr.	1-5 yr.	5 yr.+
Rate	120-160	100-140	80-120

Hypothermia at 30 C reduces the heart rate by 20%.

thermia, and although its action may be potentiated by cold, it should not be withheld preoperatively when indicated. The digitalizing dose of digoxin is 0.03 mg/lb. in 24 hours for ages from 1 to 24 months. Under 1 month, this dose is halved; and over 50 lb. 0.02 mg/lb. is given for 24 hours. Initially, half the digitalizing dose is given intravenously or intramuscularly, followed by one quarter of this dose in 6 hours and the final quarter 8 hours later. The daily maintenance dose usually is one fifth of the digitalizing dose. Digitalis toxicity is treated by slow infusion of 10 cc of 10% potassium chloride in 250 cc of 5% dextrose until coupling toxic effects such as bigeminal rhythm are abolished. Isopropylarterenol (Isuprel) may also be used to strengthen cardiac contractility and increase cardiac rate. It is especially suitable for patients with complete heart block: 1 cc of a 1:50,000 solution may be injected every 5 minutes until the desired effect is observed.

MANAGEMENT BEFORE AND AFTER OCCLUSION.—*Before occlusion* of the circulation, the following measures are taken. (1) The table is tilted to the left to facilitate exposure and to avoid trapping of air in the left atrium. (2) Blood loss is replaced with citrated blood; 500 cc of heparinized blood is available to replace the large losses which may occur from an atriotomy in order to avoid citrate intoxication in the hypothermic patient. The heparin given may be neutralized by an equal dose of Polybrene. (3) Halothane is turned off and the lungs hyperventilated with oxygen for 1 minute. (4) Carbon dioxide, 3 liters/minute is allowed to flow from an ether hook placed at the edge of the incision. As the carbon dioxide is heavier and more soluble in blood than in air, it is hoped that it will displace air from the wound and left atrium so that any gas trapped in the left heart will be dissolved and not cause air embolism. (5) Succinylcholine 2.0 mg/10 lb. is given to abolish diaphragmatic movement during the occlusion. (6) The anesthesiologist times the duration of occlusion and notifies the surgeon at the end of 5 minutes.

During occlusion, the gas escape valve is opened and the lungs allowed to collapse. Electroencephalogram tracings are completely flattened within 20 seconds of circulatory occlusion and usually return to their previous pattern within 4 minutes of restoration of adequate flow. Even in instances in which EEG restoration has been delayed for up to an hour, no after-effects have been discernible.

After occlusion, there is a rapid rise of both systolic and diastolic blood pressure, even reaching 230/30 mm Hg in 5 minutes, owing to release of catecholamines. The blood pressure then gradually returns to normal over the next 15-40 minutes. This transient hypertension is not seen if blood replacement is inadequate or if there is inadequate cardiac action. If ventricular fibrillation occurs, the surgeon should assume that air has entered the coronary artery system. Air may actually be seen in the coronary arteries and

massage should be started immediately. While massage is carried out, warm saline should be instilled in the pericardial sac. Cross-clamping of the aorta for short periods during massage[27] may assist in driving the air through the heart. When the heart is warm, defibrillation by electrical shock usually restores normal sinus rhythm.

Once normothermia has been achieved, the postoperative care is that for any thoracic operation. Patients recover more quickly and with less evidence of disturbance than after employment of cardiopulmonary by-pass.

Profound Hypothermia

For purposes of definition, the term profound hypothermia will be used for the lowering of general body temperature below 20 C measured at esophageal level. At varying levels below this temperature (16-18 C), the heart goes into asystole. To reach this low temperature, surface cooling or "core" cooling with a pump and heat exchanger may be employed.

Fig. 43-11.—Hypothermia. Brown and Harrison heat exchanger. **A,** the heat exchanger assembled. **B,** end-on view of thin-walled stainless steel tubes through which blood passes.

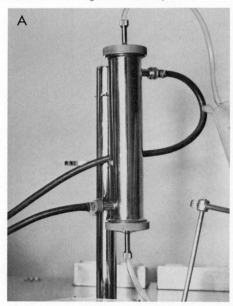

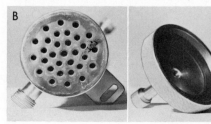

SURFACE COOLING.—The basic problem in achieving extremely low temperatures in larger animals and human beings is the rate of cooling. Although small animals, such as the rat, may be surface-cooled to levels of cardiac asystole and rewarmed with survival, larger animals and man, because of the slow rate of cooling due to the larger mass to be cooled, develop cardiac irregularities and fibrillation before temperatures are reached which allow for inadequate circulation. If some method could be devised for supporting the circulation without the use of an extracorporeal circulation, simple surface cooling to cardiac asystole in man might prove practical for intracardiac surgery. Bigelow and associates for a number of years have been investigating the hibernating gland of the ground hog, searching for the mechanism by which a ground hog maintains a circulation sufficient for its metabolic needs at temperatures in the area of 4 C. In our laboratory, we have been interested in some method of maintaining a warm heart while surface cooling to profound levels. Our experimental efforts have been unrewarding. The immature animal and infant appear to tolerate low levels of hypothermia better than the mature animal or human. Surface cooling to temperatures of 15 C or lower may yet prove feasible in the infant.

PROFOUND HYPOTHERMIA WITH EXTRACORPOREAL CIRCULATION.—Rapid cooling of patients to temperatures below 20 C with a heat exchanger in the circuit can be achieved by the use of a pump and artificial oxygenation or a pump and autogenous oxygenation.

HEAT EXCHANGER.—Early mechanisms for cooling the circulating blood consisted of coils of tubing in water baths. This method of cooling was not efficient and control of temperature relatively inaccurate. Brown et al.[9] in 1958 described an amazingly simple and efficient heat exchanger (Fig. 43-11) which, when incorporated in the pump oxygenator circuit, allowed precise control of the body temperature. This heat exchanger consists of an outer cylindrical stainless steel jacket through which 24 thin-walled steel tubes run longitudinally. Oxygenated blood is passed through the tubes which are surrounded by either hot or cold water passing through inlet and outlet openings in the side of the steel cylinder. There have been many modifications of this type of heat exchanger which proved to be safe and efficient. Surprisingly enough, hemolysis is not increased by the introduction of multiple thin-walled steel tubes in the circuit.

PROFOUND HYPOTHERMIA WITH A PUMP AND AUTOGENOUS OXYGENATION.—By-passing the heart but utilizing the patient's own lung as an oxygenator is obviously more physiologic than using artificial oxygenation. This technique, employing a heat exchanger to cool and rewarm the blood rapidly, has been successfully employed on patients[17] and in the laboratory.[42] The technique makes use of two pumps, one for the right side of the heart and one for the left. Blood is removed from the right atrium and pumped into the

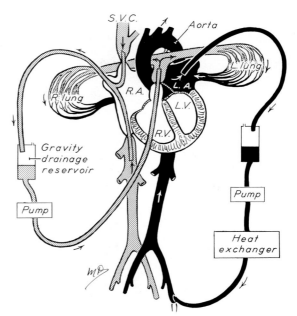

Fig. 43-12.—Profound hypothermia. Autogenous oxygenation and use of a pump and heat exchanger.

pulmonary artery, which is cannulated through the right ventricle. Blood is removed from the left atrium and pumped through a heat exchanger into a systemic artery (Fig. 43-12). When the desired temperature is obtained (15-18 C), the pump is shut off, the cavae clamped and the intracardiac operation performed. At the conclusion of the operation, the cannula is replaced in the pulmonary artery, all air is removed from the heart and the pumps started with the heat exchanger warming to the desired level. The obvious physiologic advantage of autogenous oxygenation must be weighed against the disadvantages of cannulating the pulmonary artery and the left atrium. It is not always possible to get adequate return from the left atrium, particularly in infants. Using this method, Drew and Anderson[17] reported that 3 children survived periods of by-pass of 40 minutes at a temperature of 15 C.

PROFOUND HYPOTHERMIA WITH PUMP AND ARTIFICIAL OXYGENATOR.—Gollan et al.[21] demonstrated that in dogs, cardiac arrest for 1 hour at 0 C was possible with the use of an artificial heart-lung apparatus to support the circulation. Sealy et al.[40] operated on patients at temperatures from 3 to 22 C, employing an artificial heart-lung machine and a heat exchanger (Fig. 43-13). These patients were placed on partial by-pass until heart action was ineffectual and then placed on complete by-pass. Flow rates of 15–25 cc/kg of body weight/minute were used for patients above 30 kg; below this weight, rates of 35–50 cc/kg minute were employed.

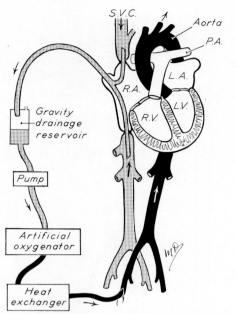

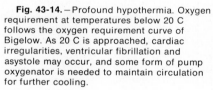

Fig. 43-13. — Profound hypothermia. Artificial oxygenation and use of a pump and heat exchanger.

oxygen consumption is 50% of normal, 25% at 22C and 3% at 6 C (Fig. 43-14). Based on the assumption that 50% reduction of oxygen consumption doubles the safe period of circulatory arrest, they concluded that at a temperature of 10 C, a period of 64-80 minutes of circulatory arrest could be tolerated.

Hikasa and associates[25] have revived interest in deep hypothermia for the correction of certain lesions in infants. On the premise that hibernating animals store liquids, the Japanese group administered essential fatty acids and vitamin E for 1 week before operation. Under deep ether anesthesia surface cooling to 20 C allowed circulatory arrest for an average of 37 minutes. Rewarming using extracorporeal circulation resulted in survival of 40 of 43 infants under 10 kg who were operated on.

METABOLIC EFFECTS OF PROFOUND HYPOTHERMIA. — No significant changes in metabolic responses should be observed if flow rates and arterial and venous pressures are carefully monitored. Gordon *et al.*[22] recorded normal arterial and venous pH, CO_2 content, lactic acid and pyruvic acid in two patients cooled to 10 C. The pH determinations must be run at the same temperature at which the blood is drawn. While the pH entered the acidotic range during rewarming, all metabolic determinations were normal 8 hours postoperatively.

BLOOD ELEMENTS. — Shields and Lewis[42] recorded a slight rise of plasma hemoglobin and a slight depression of the white blood cell and platelet counts in the experimental animal.

DIFFERENTIAL HYPOTHERMIC CARDIOPLEGIA. — There are many advantages in operating upon a heart in cardiac arrest. Decrease of blood loss and clear view of

The venous oxygen saturation was kept well above 70% and a normal arteriovenous difference maintained. The electroencephalogram becomes silent below 20 C, and cardiac asystole occurs between 20 and 10 C. Gordon *et al.*[22] studied oxygen consumption at low temperatures and concluded that at 29 C,

Fig. 43-14. — Profound hypothermia. Oxygen requirement at temperatures below 20 C follows the oxygen requirement curve of Bigelow. As 20 C is approached, cardiac irregularities, ventricular fibrillation and asystole may occur, and some form of pump oxygenator is needed to maintain circulation for further cooling.

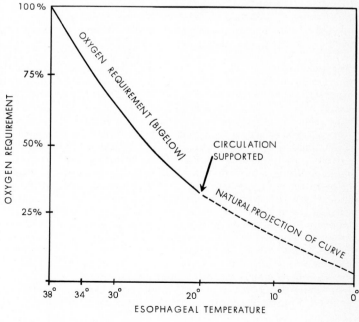

the defect at the time of repair are two important considerations. The arrested heart has basic oxygen requirements which become significantly reduced with lowering of the myocardial temperature. At temperatures below 16 C, the heart goes into asystole without the use of cardioplegic drugs.[23] To achieve this temperature in the myocardium while the rest of the body is at much higher temperatures, differential cooling of the heart must be carried out. Cannulating the coronary arteries and perfusing with cold blood or with Ringer's solution at 2 C [44] or the topical application of cold saline or ice will achieve a low temperature and arrest of the heart. Numerous reports of clinical successes are now appearing in the literature describing the use of a variety of techniques to achieve cardiac temperatures of 16 C and asystole.

REFERENCES

1. Beattie, E. J., et al.: Refrigeration in experimental surgery of the aorta, Surg., Gynec. & Obst. 96:711, 1953.
2. Beavers, W. R., and Covino, B. G.: Relationship of potassium and calcium to hypothermic ventricular fibrillation, J. Appl. Physiol. 14:60, 1959.
3. Benedict, F. C., and Lee, R. C.: *Hibernation and Marmot Physiology* (Washington, D.C.: Carnegie Institution, 1938), Pub. no. 494.
4. Bernard, C.: *Leçus sur la chaleur animale* (Paris: Baillière, 1876).
5. Bigelow, W. G., et al.: Oxygen transport and ulitization in dogs at low body temperatures, Am. J. Physiol. 160:125, 1950.
6. Bigelow, W. G., et al.: Hypothermia, Ann. Surg. 132:849, 1950.
7. Bigelow, W. G.: Hypothermia, Surgery 43:683, 1958.
8. Brewin, E. G., et al.: An investigation of problems of acid-base equilibrium in hypothermia, Guy's Hosp. Rep. 104:177, 1955.
9. Brown, I. W., Jr., et al.: An efficient blood heat exchanger for use with extracorporeal circulation, Surgery 44:372, 1958.
10. Conn, A. W., et al.: Anesthesia with hypothermia for closure of atrial septal defects in children, Canad. Anaesth. Soc. J. 6:327, 1959.
11. Conn, A. W., and Millar, R. A.: Postocclusion hypertension and plasma catecholamine levels, Canad. Anaesth. Soc. J. 7:443, 1960.
12. Cooper, K. L., and Ross, D.: Preface in *Hypothermia in Surgical Practice* (London: Cassell & Co., Ltd., 1960).
13. Cooper, K. L., and Kenyon, J. R.: A comparison of the temperatures measured in the rectum, esophagus and on the surface of the aorta during hypothermia in man, Brit. J. Surg. 44:616, 1957.
14. Cooper, K.: Physiology of hypothermia, Brit. J. Anaesth. 31:96, 1959.
15. Covine, B. G., and Hegnauer, A. H.: Ventricular excitability during hypothermia and rewarming in dogs, Proc. Soc. Exper. Biol. & Med. 89:659, 1955.
16. Delorme, E. J.: Experimental cooling of the blood stream: Preliminary communication, Lancet 2:914, 1952.
17. Drew, C. E., and Anderson, I. M.: Profound hypothermia in cardiac surgery: Report of 3 cases, Lancet 1:748, 1959.
18. Fay, T.: Observations on prolonged human refrigeration, New York J. Med. 40:1351, 1940.
19. Fisher, E. R., et al.: Stressor effect of hypothermia in the rat, Am. J. Physiol. 188:470, 1957.
20. Gollan, F., et al.: Exclusion of the heart and lungs from circulation in the hypothermic closed-chest dog by means of a pump-oxygenator, J. Appl. Physiol. 5:180, 1952.
21. Gollan, F., et al.: Consecutive survival of open-chest hypothermic dogs after prolonged bypass of heart and lungs by means of a pump-oxygenator, Surgery 35:88, 1954.
22. Gordon, A. S., et al.: Open-heart surgery using deep hypothermia without an oxygenator, J. Thoracic & Cardiovas Surg. 40:787, 1960.
23. Gordon, A. S., and Jones, J. C.: The mechanism of ventricular fibrillation and cardiac arrest during surgery, J. Thoracic & Cardiovas. Surg. 38:618, 1959.
24. Gordon, A. S.: Post Graduate Assembly in Anaesthesiology: Session on Hypothermia by Perfusion, Dec., 1960.
25. Hikasa, Y., et al.: Open heart surgery in infants with aid of hypothermic anesthesia, Arch. jap. Chir., Vol. 36, July 1, 1967.
26. Horvath, A.: Einfluss verschiedener Temperaturen auf die Winterschläfer, Verhandl. phys.-med. Ges. Warzb. 15:187, 1881.
27. James, T. N., et al.: Electrocardiographic manifestations of air in coronary arteries in dying and resuscitated hearts, Am. Heart J. 46:215, 1953.
28. Khalil, H. H.: Effect of hypothermia on hypothalamic-pituitary response to stress, Brit. M. J. 2:733, 1954.
29. Lewis, F. J., and Taufic, M.: Closure of atrial septal defect with the aid of hypothermia, Surgery 33:52, 1953.
30. Little, S. M.: Hypothermia, Anesthesiology 20:242, 1959.
31. Lofstrom, B.: Induced hypothermia and intravascular aggregation, Acta anaesth. scandinav., Supp. 3, 1959.
32. Lougheed, W. M., and Kohn, D. S.: Circumvention of anoxia during arrest of cerebral circulation for intracranial surgery, J. Neurosurg. 12:226, 1955.
33. Lucas, B. G. B.: Application of hypothermia to surgical procedures, Proc. Roy. Soc. Med. 49:345, 1956.
34. Miles, B. E., and Churchill-Davidson, H. C.: Effects of hypothermia on renal circulation of dog, Anesthesiology 16:230, 1955.
35. Niazi, S. A., and Lewis, F. J.: Tolerance of adult rats to profound hypothermia and simultaneous cardiac standstill, Surgery 36:25, 1954.
36. Niazi, S. A., and Lewis, F. J.: Profound hypothermia in man, Ann. Surg. 147:214, 1958.
37. Page, L. B.: Effects of hypothermia on renal function, Am. J. Physiol. 181:171, 1955.
38. Peirce, E. C., II, et al.: Reduced metabolism by means of hypothermia and the low-flow pump-oxygenator, Surg., Gynec. & Obst. 107:339, 1958.
39. Rink, R. A., et al.: Effect of hypothermia on morphine metabolism in isolated perfused liver, Anesthesiology 17:377, 1956.
40. Sealy, W. C., et al.: A report on the use of both extracorporeal circulation and hypothermia for open-heart surgery, Ann. Surg. 147:603, 1958.
41. Selle, W. A.: *Body Temperature* (Springfield, Ill.: Charles C Thomas, Publisher, 1952).
42. Shields, T. W., and Lewis, F. J.: Rapid cooling and surgery at temperatures below 20 C., Surgery 46:164, 1959.
43. Swan, H., et al.: Cessation of circulation in general hypothermia, Ann. Surg. 138:360, 1953.
44. Urschel, H. C., Jr., and Greenberg, J. J.: Differential cardiac hypothermia for elective cardioplegia, Ann. Surg. 152:845, 1960.
45. Virtue, R. W.: *Hypothermic Anesthesia* (Springfield, Ill.: Charles C Thomas, Publisher, 1955), p. 23.
46. Waddell, W. G., et al.: Improved management of clinical hypothermia, Ann. Surg. 146:592, 1957.
47. Wynn, V.: Electrolyte disturbances associated with failure to metabolize glucose during hypothermia, Lancet 2:575, 1957.
48. Wynn, V.: The metabolism of fructose during hypothermia in man, Clin. Sc. 15:297, 1956.

A. W. CONN
W. T. MUSTARD

Drawings by
MARGUERITE DRUMMOND

Hyperbaric Oxygenation

HISTORY.—Medical interest in the therapeutic potential of increased environmental air pressure dates back over 125 years, and followed Tiger's development of the caisson in 1841 as an aid to underwater construction work. In that era, pressure chambers became fashionable in many European cities for the treatment of patients with pulmonary tuberculosis and other chronic infections, with uniformly disappointing results. A second wave of interest in pressure therapy developed in 1878 following the investigations of the French physiologist, Paul Bert, who published the first scientific treatise on the effects of oxygen and inert gas breathing under hyperbaric conditions. The next year, Fontaine, an anesthesiologist, observed that the administration of low concentrations of nitrous oxide and oxygen under pressure resulted in excellent abdominal relaxation along with a superior degree of patient oxygenation. Fontaine's plan was to construct an operating theater within a pressure chamber to permit administration of nitrous oxide to patients undergoing abdominal surgery. However, this ingenious scheme never reached fruition.

Progress in hyperbaric medicine was hampered by the high incidence of "bends" and air embolism which followed too rapid decompression after deep and prolonged dives. When, however, Haldane formulated the concept of staged decompression and assembled the first decompression tables (1907), diving and experimental work under pressure were finally placed on a firm foundation. In 1932, Albert Behnke, a U.S. Naval medical officer, began a study of oxygen inhalation in volunteers during dry dives in a compression chamber.[27] This classic work, carried out in the laboratories of Cecil Drinker and Louis Agassiz Shaw, using a pressure tank in the Harvard School of Public Health, established the maximal tolerance of man for 100% oxygen breathing at pressures of 15, 30 and 45 lb./in.² gauge (psi g).

In recent years, clinical investigations utilizing hyperbaric oxygenation have been undertaken by Illingworth and Smith[16, 25, 26] in Glasgow and Boerema's group[7] in Amsterdam. These scientists treated small groups of patients with carbon monoxide poisoning, anaerobic gas-forming infections and peripheral arterial occlusive disease, using pressures of 15–30 psi g. Reports of their work revived interest in this subject in both Europe and the United States.

A symposium published by the Division of Medical Science, National Research Council, is an excellent introduction to the subject of hyperbaric medicine and is recommended reading for all interested students and investigators.[6]

Since 1962, numerous medical scientists and engineers have clamored for the widespread construction of hyperbaric facilities in this country. Fortunately, recognition of the dangers of acute oxygen toxicity and the expense of hyperbaric equipment have led to reasonable restraint within the medical community. The wisdom of this action has become increasingly apparent, since little evidence has been generated in the succeeding 5 years to indicate that hyperbaric oxygenation is superior to the usual methods of oxygen administration in many of the clinical situations for which benefit has been claimed.

Reasons for this disappointing development are suggested by a review of the factors that affect tissue oxygenation in addition to arterial oxygen tension. These include: the oxygen-carrying capacity of the blood, the presence of adequate arterial, venous and capillary circulations, and the individual oxygen requirements of specific organ systems. Disease may affect one or all of these components simultaneously, resulting in hypoxic tissue damage despite arterial oxygen tension (Po_2) values in the range of 1,000–2,000 mm Hg.

The ability to elevate the arterial oxygen tension alone, during high-pressure oxygen breathing, depends on the existing cardiopulmonary dynamics. For example, if a cardiac defect in the form of a right-to-left shunt is present, all oxygen physically dissolved in the fully saturated pulmonary venous blood is rapidly combined with the reduced hemoglobin of the systemic venous return. In such a situation, the effect of increasing environmental pressure would be merely to achieve a more complete saturation of the circulating red cell volume rather than to obtain supersaturation of the plasma and extracellular fluid. Similarly, extensive pneumonitis or severe pulmonary congestion can result in persistent hypoxemia, despite a high alveolar oxygen tension, if scattered segments of the lung are adequately perfused but poorly ventilated.

OXYGEN TRANSPORT IN MAN

At ambient pressure, ventilation with 100% oxygen increases the tension and concentration of the alveolar gas approximately fivefold. In these circumstances, if the environmental pressure is then elevated, an additional rise of alveolar oxygen tension takes place rapidly. At 3 atm of pressure (30 psi g.), the arterial Po_2 in normal animals and man approaches 2,000 mm Hg.

Since hemoglobin is almost fully saturated when a man breathes air at sea level, the capacity for increasing the quantity of oxyhemoglobin is limited. Therefore any additional oxygen present in arterial blood under hyperbaric conditions must enter into physical solution in the extracellular fluid. Because oxygen is a relatively insoluble gas, the plasma content rises only 3 vol% with each 1,000 mm Hg increase of alveolar oxygen tension. Nevertheless sufficient oxygen in excess of normal tissue demands can be forced into solution during hyperbaric exposure to supply all of the tissue requirements.

In order to improve tissue oxygenation, oxygen in both blood and extracellular fluid must be delivered to the site of utilization. Because this gas diffuses only a fraction of a millimeter beyond the nutrient capillaries, the prime requirement for any method of increasing the concentration of oxygen at the cellular level is homogeneous perfusion of tissue.[23]

Physiologic data accumulated both in experimental animals and in man indicate that 100% oxygen ventilation under increased environmental pressure decreases cardiac output and increases peripheral vascular resistance.[30] Fortunately, a small "reservoir" of oxygen (produced by hyperoxia) is available for intracellular metabolic needs and compensates for the apparent decrease of peripheral blood flow. The importance of this observation must be emphasized, since oxygen is the most flow-limited of substrates needed for intermediary cellular metabolism.

Evidence in support of the "oxygen reservoir" concept may be found, first, in the increased content and tension of oxygen in systemic venous blood which are demonstrable under the hyperbaric conditions. Second, following total interruption of blood flow to an organ, normal function persists for slightly longer intervals if the animal or patient has been hyperoxygenated prior to circulatory arrest. In such experimental conditions, however, the central nervous system is protected from hyperoxic damage for only slightly longer than in a normothermic, normobaric environment.

Oxygen Toxicity

In recent years, histopathologic changes attributed to high oxygen tension have been demonstrated experimentally in the eye, central nervous system and lung. Pulmonary oxygen toxicity, characterized by progressive dyspnea, hypoxemia and hypercapnia, has been produced in a variety of laboratory animals. At autopsy, the findings consist of pulmonary congestion and edema, segmental atelectasis, occasional hyaline membrane formation, alveolar cell hyperplasia and hypertrophy as well as pulmonary arteriosclerosis.[21,28] It is of interest that changes similar to these can be induced in laboratory animals exposed to 100% oxygen at ambient pressure.

Although it is recognized that man's resistance to pulmonary oxygen toxicity exceeds that of most animals, respiratory symptoms have been described in human beings exposed to 100% oxygen at sea level for 24 hours. Pratt[22] noted proliferation of alveolar capillaries and interstitial fibrosis in the lungs of patients subjected to prolonged periods of oxygen inhalation prior to death. In addition, at least one fatality has been attributed to pulmonary oxygen toxicity in a patient exposed to hyperbaric oxygen.[13]

The ocular lesions produced by oxygen inhalation at increased environmental pressure are of three types. (1) A proliferation of retinal vessels (retrolental fibroplasia) can develop in premature infants exposed to a high oxygen concentration for many days. (2) Selective necrosis of the visual cell layer of the retina has been produced in rabbits by 4-hour exposure to oxygen at 30 psi g. This necrosis is followed by degeneration of the outer layer of the retina. (3) Segmental degeneration of axons in the ganglion cell layer of the retina has been produced in dogs following extended periods of oxygen breathing at the same high pressure (30 psi g.). In some of these experiments, necrosis of retinal ganglion cells was also observed.[20]

Although retinal lesions are one of the major hazards of prolonged exposure to hyperbaric oxygen, no permanent oxygen-induced ocular damage, other than retrolental fibroplasia, has been noted in man. High oxygen tensions do, however, produce retinal vasoconstriction and reversible constriction of the visual fields.

Oxygen toxicity involving the central nervous system, in both man and animals, is manifested by the onset of grand mal seizures. Despite wide differences in individual thresholds to convulsions, seizures are most likely to develop during oxygen ventilation at pressures of 30 psi g. and higher. Although no permanent neurologic deficits or central nervous system lesions have been recorded in man, selective neuronal necrosis and permanent paralysis have been produced in experimental animals by a number of investigators.[1,10,17,24]

According to investigations by Chance, Jamieson and Williamson,[8] oxygen appears to be injurious at the cellular level because it inactivates essential enzyme systems. Their studies indicate that excessive concentrations of oxidized pyridine nucleotides occur in the tissues of animals exposed to increased oxygen tensions. Oxidative phosphorylation proceeds in a normal fashion, but the mitochondria appear to be unable to transfer hydrogen to available acceptor systems. Thus an inhibition of energy transfer may be the ultimate mechanism of acute hyperbaric oxygen poisoning.

It is apparent that many features of oxygen toxicity are ill-defined. Accordingly, investigations to elucidate mechanisms of normal and abnormal cell metabolism contain the hope for future advantageous application of hyperbaric oxygenation in medicine.

Factors to Be Considered during Hyperbaric Exposure

Ventilation with 100% oxygen at an environmental pressure of 30 psi g. (3.0 atm abs) should not be maintained longer than 2 hours if acute oxygen toxicity is to be avoided. This same restriction applied to hyperbaric research personnel as well as patients, although the former are not subject to oxygen toxicity since their breathing mixture consists of compressed air. Unfortunately, inhalation of an inert gas (nitrogen) under hyperbaric conditions results in absorption of the gas by tissues in direct proportion to the increased blood gas tension. In the case of air breathing (containing approximately 80% nitrogen), central nervous system depression (narcosis) can occur, along with the development of decompression sickness (bends) if the decompression period is inadequate. The potential damages, familiar to divers for many years, may occur in mild forms, including arthralgia and transitory dermatitis, or the bends may be manifested as a major neurologic injury, producing paralysis, coma and death.

Fortunately, exposure to increased environmental pressure for biomedical research purposes can be virtually free from the serious sequelae of decompression sickness. This demands conservative application of decompression schedules and prompt recompression if symptoms do appear. In general, patients have been spared these problems since they breath oxygen and denitrogenate their tissues continuously during hyperbaric exposure.

TABLE 43-4.—SURGICAL RESULTS IN 120 INFANTS WITH CYANOTIC CONGENITAL HEART DISEASE

DIAGNOSIS AND OPERATION	PATIENTS No.	Surviving	
Transposition of great vessels			
Operation: atrial septal defect, pulmonary artery banding or systemic PA shunt*	54	48	(89%)
Tetralogy of Fallot			
Operation: systemic PA shunt	39	35	(90%)
Tricuspid atresia			
Operation: systemic PA shunt	16	11	(66%)
Pulmonary atresia (intact ventricular septum)			
Operation: Brock procedure or atrial septal defect plus a shunt	8	3	(38%)
Ebstein's anomaly			
Operation: systemic PA shunt	2	0	0
Mitral atresia			
Operation: atrial septal defect	1	1	(100%)
Total	120	98	(82%)

*Shunt = ascending aorta to right pulmonary artery anastomosis.

Blalock-Hanlon procedure for the following reasons. (1) A large segment of the atrial septum can be excised under direct vision, including portions of the septum primum and septum secundum overlying the pulmonary veins, (2) Brief periods (1–2 minutes) of inflow occlusion are well tolerated by these patients when the arterial oxygen tension is transiently elevated to the 40–50 mm Hg range, (3) Temporary interruption of the circulation prevents the development of intrapulmonary hemorrhage (occasionally noted after a Blalock-Hanlon operation) because the pulmonary and bronchial arterial blood flow are eliminated simultaneously, and the right pulmonary veins do not need to be occluded.

In addition to placement of tourniquets around the superior and inferior venae cavae, the aorta and pulmonary artery are also clamped during atriotomy. This is necesssary to prevent air embolism. After completion of the septectomy, air is evacuated from the heart by flooding the atriotomy incision with physiologic saline solution followed by inflation of the lungs to force blood from the pulmonary veins into the left atrium and through the septal defect.

When required, pulmonary artery banding can be carried out through the same right lateral thoracotomy incision. The main pulmonary artery is constricted sufficiently to reduce the mean arterial pressure distal to the band by approximately 50%.

Rashkind has advocated atrial septostomy produced by means of a balloon catheter. Passage of the catheter through a patent foramen ovale, followed by forceful withdrawal of the inflated balloon, tears the thin septum and has resulted in immediate improvement of right atrial mixing. This ingenious technique may ultimately replace direct excision of the atrial septum, so that the definitive operation, which can be carried out at about 2 years of age, need be the only surgical procedure. However, a number of balloon septostomy failures have occurred (in 4 of 8 patients in the limited experience at the Children's Hospital), so that the surgeon's responsibility in this desperate clinical situation has not been completely relinquinished.

TETRALOGY OF FALLOT AND TRICUSPID ATRESIA

Fifty-three infants with marked arterial unsaturation secondary to a right-to-left shunt and diminished pulmonary blood flow were operated on at an environmental pressure of 30 psi g. (3.0 atm abs). The precompression arterial oxygen tension in these babies ranged from 15 to 35 mm Hg, and increased by an average of 25 mm Hg following hyperventilation with 90% oxygen-10% nitrous oxide at pressure. Nine infants died 12 hours to 6 months following operation; 7 of these had diminutive subclavian arteries which contributed to an inadequate Blalock anastomosis. Two others died of pulmonary congestion on the second and third postoperative days because of an excessively large flow through a potts aorticopulmonary shunt (see Table 43-4).

For several years, the Blalock and Potts shunts have not been used in most patients under 1 year of age. Instead, a side-to-side, intrapericardial anastomosis has been created between the posterior wall of the ascending aorta and the right pulmonary artery, as described by Waterston[29] and Cooley and Hallman.[9] This operation is performed through a right lateral thoracotomy incision, entering the pleura through the fourth intercostal space. In the presence of a right aortic arch (20% of patients), exposure of the right pulmonary artery was achieved by elevation of the superior vena cava following division of the azygos vein. This aorticopulmonary shunt has proved to be extremely satisfactory for the following reasons.(1) An anastomosis is created between the largest systemic artery available (ascending aorta) and the intrapericardial portion of the right pulmonary artery. The diameter of this segment of the vessel is invariably greater than that of the more distal portion of the artery present at the hilus of the lung. (2) A side-to-side anastomosis should grow with the infant and provide a satisfactory increase of pulmonary blood flow during the interval of maximal growth and development. (3) Since this operation is always performed through a right thoracotomy incision, other operative procedures such as creation of an atrial septal defect and pulmonic valvulotomy may be carried out at the same time, if necessary. (4) Closure of the surgically produced fistula at the time of total repair of tetralogy of Fallot can be accomplished without undue difficulty since the anastomosis is located just above the sinuses of Valsalva in the ascending aorta.

PULMONIC VALVULAR ATRESIA

The ideal operation in patients with pulmonic valvular atresia and an intact ventricular septum should achieve continuity between the blind end of the right ventricle and the small, but patent, main pulmonary artery. This procedure is possible only if the obstruction is in the form of a relatively thin membrane rather than a fibrous thick cord. Such an operation was successfully accomplished in 3 of 4 surviving patients (among nine attempts) by direct incision of the obstructing membrane during inflow occlusion of 1–2 minutes. Dilating instruments were passed through the incision to enlarge the opening initially created with an iridectomy scalpel. Inflow occlusion was well tolerated by these patients even though the arterial oxygen saturation remained low (50–65 %) at high atmospheric pressure. The fourth surviving infant was treated by creating an atrial septal defect to decompress the hypertensive right ventricle (with tricuspid regurgitation) and by establishing an ascending aorta-to-right pulmonary artery shunt.

AORTIC AND PULMONIC VALVULAR STENOSIS

In a previous series of infants with aortic stenosis, operation consisted of open aortic valvulotomy utilizing cardiopulmonary by-pass. Half of these patients died of progressive respiratory insufficiency within 24 hours. To avoid this pump-induced syndrome of pulmonary interstitial hemorrhage and atelectasis, valvulotomy was accomplished in a second group of patients by use of inflow occlusion and moderate hypothermia (30–32 C). In each instance, ventricular fibrillation developed just before or during the 2–3 minute interval of circulatory interruption. Electrical defibrillation of the cold myocardium was unsuccessful.

The difficulties encountered in the management of cardiac arrhythmias in the hypothermic infant prompted evaluation of a third method for the production of temporary circulatory arrest. Previous laboratory studies indicated that venous inflow occlusion was permissible for 3–5 minutes at 37 C during oxygen ventilation at a pressure of 30 psi g. An arterial Po$_2$ of 1,500 mm Hg was obtained, resulting in approximately 5.0 vol % of oxygen dissolved in the plasma.

Twelve infants underwent open aortic valulotomy by this method (Table 43-5). Ten were improved and subsequently discharged from the hospital. In the immediate postoperative period, there were 2 deaths, attributed to previously undetected mitral stenosis in 1 patient and to infantile coarctation of the aorta in the other.

In babies with severe pulmonic valvular stenosis and an intact ventricular septum, cyanosis, cardiomegaly and congestive failure were frequently noted. Arterial unsaturation produced by a right-to-left shunt through a patent foramen ovale resulted in arterial oxygen tension in the range of 20–40 mm Hg. Twenty consecutive patients who underwent open pulmonic valvulotomy during inflow occlusion under increased environmental pressure are alive and well. One patient required a second operation at 3 years of age (utilizing cardiopulmonary by-pass) to resect a residual subvalvular muscular obstruction.

Operations for either aortic or pulmonic stenosis were performed through a median stenotomy incision. The stenotic aortic or pulmonic valve was incised with a knife in two diametrically opposed sites in the region of the commissures. A straight vascular clamp was passed into the ventricular cavity to estimate the size of the opening created and to eliminate the possibility of a residual subvalvular obstruction. Prior to closure of the aortotomy incision, the lungs were inflated by the anesthesiologist to fill the left side of the heart with blood and evacuate air from the left ventricle.

MISCELLANEOUS CONDITIONS

Thirty patients with ventricular septal defects, common atrioventricular canal or complicated forms of coarctation of the aorta and 3 babies with anomalous left coronary artery are included in this group (Table 43-6). The rationale for operation in a hyperbaric facility in these cases was (1) to maintain the arterial oxygen tension in the normal range (70–90 mm Hg) if compromised alveolar diffusion had resulted in arterial unsaturation, and (2) to facilitate cardiac resuscitation and defibrillation in the presence of severe arrhythmias, often encountered in infants with severe left ventricular failure and pulmonary hypertension.

During the postoperative period, 4 of these gravely ill babies died. Two infants with complicated coarctation of the aortic died of digitalis intoxication and aspiration pneumonia during the first week. A third infant, with common atrioventricular canal, died suddenly 24 hours after pulmonary artery banding. The fourth infant, with a large myocardial infarction secondary to anomalous left coronary artery originating from the pulmonary artery, died after ligation of

TABLE 43-5.—SURGICAL RESULTS IN INFANTS WITH ACYANOTIC CARDIAC DEFECTS

DIAGNOSIS AND OPERATION	PATIENTS No.	Surviving
Valvular aortic stenosis		
Operation: valvulotomy	12	10 (83%)
Valvular pulmonic stenosis		
Operation: valvulotomy	20	20 (100%)
Total	32	30 (93%)

TABLE 43-6.—SURGICAL RESULTS IN 33 MISCELLANEOUS
CONDITIONS

DIAGNOSIS AND OPERATION	PATIENTS No.	Surviving
Ventricular septal defect, pulmonary hypertension		
Operation: pulmonary artery banding*	20	20 (100%)
Common atrioventricular canal, pulmonary hypertension		
Operation: pulmonary artery banding	5	4 (80%)
Coarctation of aorta, ventricular septal defect, patent ductus arteriosus		
Operation: resection of coarctation, division of patent ductus, pulmonary artery banding	5	3 (60%)
Anomalous left coronary artery from pulmonary artery		
Operation: ligation of left coronary artery	3	2 (66%)
	33	29 (87%)

*Pulmonary artery banding sufficient to reduce pressure by 50%.

the anomalous vessel due to intractable left ventricular failure.

METABOLIC ALTERATIONS IN INFANTS WITH CYANOTIC CONGENITAL HEART DISEASE

In the first weeks of life, a number of compensatory mechanisms can be activated to maintain tissue homeostasis temporarily in the presence of severe oxygen deprivation. A quantity of reserve phosphate bond energy (adenosine triphosphate and creatine phosphate) is available for cellular metabolism, and the hypoxic state per se serves as a stimulus for the anaerobic production of additional adenosine triphosphate by conversion of glucose to lactate. Unfortunately, anaerobiosis is poorly tolerated in man, resulting in a rapid rise of hydrogen ion concentration, progressive cardiac decompensation, reduced tissue perfusion and, finally, cell death.[14,15]

Certain infants with transposition and poor arteriovenous mixing and others possessing a diminished pulmonary blood flow and right-to-left intracardiac shunt characterize the type of hypoxic, acidemic patient who may be presented to the surgeon in a moribund state. Among the 54 patients with transposition operated on in our hospital, the most serious metabolic disturbances developed in those with poor mixing and a Po_2 in the range of 18–35 mm Hg. The arterial pH in 25 of 35 infants who underwent atrial septectomy alone ranged between 6.8 and 7.30. Carbon dioxide retention, with Pco_2 of 50–80 mm Hg, was noted

in 10 babies, and this intensified the acidemia produced by anaerobic metabolism. Thirty-five of the 53 infants in this category exhibited a significant base deficit which, if untreated, might have precipitated cardiac arrest and death during operation.

Sixty-three babies with tetralogy of Fallot, tricuspid atresia and pulmonary atresia (intact septum) were treated by a variety of palliative operative procedures. The arterial Po_2 in these patients during hyperventilation with 90% oxygen 10% nitrous oxide ranged from 15 to 40 mm Hg. Assisted ventilation resulted in respiratory alkalosis in 31 patients (pH 7.45–7.60 and Pco_2 18–35 mm Hg); the other 32 infants sustained a metabolic acidosis of varying severity. Blood pH in these ranged between 6.68 and 7.30, with Pco_2 30–50 mm Hg. Three patients with pulmonary atresia and an intact ventricular septum and others with tetralogy of Fallot developed hypercapnia during the operative procedure (Pco_2 50–90 mm Hg).

ACID-BASE DISTURBANCES IN ACYANOTIC BABIES

Of 12 infants with valvular aortic stenosis and severe left ventricular decompensation, 6 had both metabolic and respiratory acidosis at the time of surgery. Arterial blood pH ranged between 7.15 and 7.30, with carbon dioxide tensions in the range of 54–72 mm Hg. Preoperative studies of pulmonary ventilation in 6, all with pulmonary congestion and edema, revealed markedly reduced pulmonary compliance, indicated by CL values of 0.5–1.0 ml/cm H_2O/kg.* Normal values for compliance in infants range between 1.5 to 3.0 ml/cm H_2O/kg.[12]

Severe pulmonic valvular stenosis in 20 patients was associated with disturbance of acid-base metabolism if a right-to-left shunt through the foramen ovale existed. Five of these infants were severely hypoxic, with arterial Po_2 of 20–30 mm Hg. They had severe lacticacidemia with arterial pH of 7.10–7.25.

The 33 patients grouped in the miscellaneous category exhibited pulmonary congestion, pulmonary venous hypertension and left ventricular failure. Inadequate diffusion of carbon dioxide and oxygen across damaged alveolar membranes was demonstrated in 15 babies whose arterial Po_2 was 50–65 mm Hg with Pco_2 tensions of 45–60 mm Hg. Nine of them later developed severe respiratory acidosis with a pH of 7.05–7.30 and greatly elevated Pco_2 (55–80 mm Hg). Measurement of pulmonary compliance in five representative patients of this group also indicated a pronounced reduction of elasticity of the lungs (CL of 0.7–1.2 ml/cm H_2O/kg).

TREATMENT OF ACID-BASE DISTURBANCES DURING OPERATION.—Changes in acid-base equilibrium during surgery were measured by obtaining serial arterial

---

*CL=lung compliance in ml/cmH_2O; Vt=tidal volumes; ΔP=pressure change measured via an intraesophageal catheter. CL=Vt/ΔP.

blood samples from the exposed ascending aorta. If acidemia was detected, treatment was initiated by the administration of sodium bicarbonate (1.8 mEq/kg of body weight) or Tris buffer (THAM; 150 mg/kg) administered in a concentrated (0.6 M) solution.[18, 19] The latter, an organic hydrogen ion acceptor, proved to be an invaluable buffering compound since it is capable of modifying both intracellular and extracellular pH. In addition, its buffering effect does not depend on normal alveolar diffusion, and therefore it can be used effectively in the presence of hypercapnia encountered during the operative procedure. In most instances, when the palliative operative procedure is completed, the increase of pulmonary blood flow or improvement of arterial-venous mixing eliminates the potentially lethal problem of carbon dioxide retention. Tris buffer given the critical portions of the operative procedure can effectively stabilize arterial pH until the critical portion of the operation has been completed.

The original quantity of buffer administered to an acidotic patient amounted to 1.25 mM/kg. Additional THAM and sodium bicarbonate were infused if indicated by repeated estimation of blood gases and pH. All plasma and whole blood used during operation was buffered to a normal pH (7.35–7.45) to compensate for the elevated hydrogen ion concentration (lactic acid) present in both.

SUMMARY

One hundred and eighty-five patients less than 1 year of age have undergone a variety of palliative cardiovascular surgical procedures in a hyperbaric facility between January, 1963, and July, 1967. There were 157 survivors (84%). Twenty-eight patients died from 12 hours to 6 months after operation.

Hypoxic cardiac arrest was eliminated completely as the cause of death in this series. Although ventricular fibrillation occurred during operation on a number of occasions, cardiac resuscitation was uniformly successful.

Severe alterations in acid-base metabolism occurred in 52% of the cases and was managed by the administration of sodium bicarbonate and Tris buffer through an indwelling caval catheter. In addition, all blood and plasma used at the time of operation was buffered to a normal pH prior to use.

Our investigations indicate that several factors are important in achieving satisfactory surgical results in critically ill babies. These include (1) establishment of an accurate anatomic diagnosis prior to operation, (2) skillful anesthetic management, (3) detection and treatment of disturbed acid-base equilibrium and (4) performance of a technically accurate surgical operation. Addition of a fifth factor, improved tissue oxygen availability provided by a hyperbaric environment, also seems warranted.

NOTE.—These studies were supported by research grants from the National Heart Institute, National Institutes of Health, U.S. Public Health Service; American Heart Association; the Greater Boston Chapter of the Massachusetts Heart Association, and the John A. Hartford Foundation, Inc.

REFERENCES

1. Bean, J. W.: Alterations in CNS associated with chronic motor disabilities induced by O_2 at high pressure, Proc. Soc. Exper. Biol. & Med. 58:20, 1945.
2. Bernhard, W. F.: Current status of hyperbaric oxygenation in pediatric surgery, S. Clin. North America 44:1583, 1964.
3. Bernhard, W. F., and Tank, E. S.: Effect of oxygen inhalation at 3.0 to 3.6 atmospheres upon infants with cyanotic congenital heart disease, Surgery 54:203, 1963.
4. Bernhard, W. F.; Danis, R., and Gross, R. E.: Metabolic alterations noted in cyanotic and acyanotic infants during operations under hyperbaric conditions, J. Thoracic & Cardiovas. Surg. 50:374, 1965.
5. Bernhard, W. F., et al.: The feasibility of hypothermic perfusion under hyperbaric conditions in surgical management of infants with cyanotic congenital heart disease, J. Thoracic & Cardiovas. Surg. 46:651, 1963.
6. Brown, I. W., Jr. (ed.): Proceedings of the Third International Conference on Hyperbaric Medicine, National Research Council publ. 1404 (Washington, D. C.: 1966).
7. Brummelkamp, W. H.; Boerema, I., and Hoogendijk, J. L.: Treatment of clostridial infections with hyperbaric oxygen drenching, Lancet 1:235, 1963.
8. Chance, B.; Jamieson, D., and Williamson, J. R.: Control of Oxidation-Reduction State of Reduced Pyridine Nucleotides in Vivo and in Vitro by Hyperbaric Medicine, in Brown,[6] p. 15.
9. Cooley, D. A., and Hallman, G. L.: Surgical Treatment of Congenital Heart Disease (Philadelphia: Lea & Febiger, 1966), p. 127.
10. Dickens, F.: Toxic Effect of Oxygen on Nervous Tissue, in Elliot, K. A. C., et al. (ed.): Neurochemistry: The Chemistry of Brain and Nerve (Springfield, Ill.: Charles C Thomas, Publisher, 1962). p. 851.
11. Downing, S. E.; Talner, N. S., and Gardner, T. H.: Influences of arterial oxygen tension and pH on cardiac function in the newborn lamb, Am. J. Physiol. 211:1203, 1966.
12. Drorbough, J. E., and Fenn, W. O.: A barometric method for measuring ventilation in newborn infants, J. Pediat. 16:81, 1965.
13. Fuson, R. L.: Clinical hyperbaric oxygenation with severe oxygen toxicity, New England J. Med. 273:415, 1965.
14. Greene, N. M., and Talner, N.S.: Blood lactate, pyruvate and lactate-pyruvate ratios in congenital heart disease, New England J. Med. 270:1331, 1964.
15. Huckabee, W. E.: Relationships of pyruvate and lactate during anaerobic metabolism: I. Effects of infusion of pyruvate or glucose and of hyperventilation, J. Clin. Invest. 37:244, 1958.
16 Illingworth, C. F. W., et al.: Surgical and physiological observations in an experimental pressure chamber, Brit. J. Surg. 49:222, 1961.
17. Jamieson, D., and Van den Brenk, H. A. S.: Measurements of oxygen tensions in cerebral tissues of rats exposed to high pressures of oxygen, J. Appl. Physiol. 18:869, 1963.
18. Moore, D., and Bernhard, W. F.: Efficacy of 2-amino-2-hydroxy-methyl-1, 3-propanediol (Tris buffer) in management of metabolic lacticacidosis: Accompanying prolonged hypothermic perfusion, Surgery 52:905, 1962.
19. Moore, D.; Bernhard, W. F., and Kevy, S. V.: Method for control of hydrogen ion concentration in stored heparinized blood prior to use in cardiac surgery, Ann. Surg. 158:1000, 1963.
20. Noell, W. K.: Effect of High or Low Oxygen Tension on Visual System, in First International Symposium on

Submarine and Space Medicine (New London, Conn.: 1958).

21. Penrod, K. E.: Nature of pulmonary damage produced by high oxygen pressures, J. Appl. Physiol. 9:1, 1956.
22. Pratt, P. C.: Pulmonary capillary proliferation induced by oxygen inhalation Am. J. Path, 34:1033, 1958.
23. Saltzman, H. A., *et al.*: Hyperbaric Oxygenation, in Monograph in Surgical Science Vol. II, p. 1, 1965.
24. Schaefer, K. E. (ed.): *Environmental Effects on Consciousness* (New York: Macmillan Company, 1958), p. 3.
25. Smith, G., and Sharp, G. R.: Treatment of carbon-monoxide poisoning with oxygen under pressure, Lancet 2:905 and 922, 1960.
26. Smith, G., *et al.*: Treatment of coal-gas poisoning with oxygen at 2 atmospheres of pressure, Lancet 1:816, 1962.

27. Behnke, A. R., Shaw, L. A., Shilling, C. W., Thomson, R. M., and Messer, A. C.: Studies on the effects of high oxygen pressure, Am. J. Physiol. 107:13, 1934.
28. Van den Brenk, H. A. S., and Jamieson, D.: Pulmonary damage due to high pressure oxygen breathing in rats: I. Lung weight, histological and radiological studies, Australian J. Exper. Biol. & M. Sc. 50:37, 1962.
29. Waterston, D.: Personal communication.
30. Whalen, R. E., *et al.*: Cardiovascular and blood gas responses to hyperbaric oxygenation, Am. J. Cardiol. 15:638, 1965.

W. F. BERNHARD

Extracorporeal Circulation

HISTORY.—In 1932 Gibbon began work on a pumpoxygenator to by-pass the heart and lungs and allow work within the cardiac cavities. After considerable refinement and enlargement, this work culminated in 1953 in the first successful correction of an intracardiac defect with cardiopulmonary by-pass.[13] The apparatus used was complex and expensive. Lillehei and his associates[21] used simpler apparatus with controlled cross-circulation in which a fixed, relatively small volume of blood was pumped from a healthy adult donor to a child patient. Despite the risk to 2 individuals in order to improve the lot of 1, the procedure was used in a number of cases and clearly demonstrated that complicated congenital cardiac defects could be surgically corrected. Following these successes, equipment was refined and pumps and oxygenators of various types were developed, so that open-heart surgery is now widely practiced with a pump oxygenator for treatment of both congenital and acquired defects.

REQUIREMENTS

The aim during cardiopulmonary by-pass is to supply the body with volumes of blood and oxygen equal to those used by the body normally under conditions of the operation. Normal cardiac output during thoracotomy is between 2 and 2.5 liters/M² of body surface area/minute, and oxygen consumption is between 110 and 120 ml/M²,[2,18] Eighty to 90% of this volume of carbon dioxide must be removed, but because of the greater diffusibility of carbon dioxide than of oxygen, adequate oxygenation almost invariably includes adequate release of carbon dioxide.

Successful intracardiac surgery is possible when less than the optimal amount of blood and oxygen is supplied to the patient. Warden and associates[21] made an important contribution by demonstrating that a patient could survive a short period of strikingly low cardiac output. There are, however, important physiologic effects of this vascular starvation, most easily reflected in development of metabolic acidosis because of tissue ischemia and hypoxia. With equipment available adequate to supply needs even for a large adult, the low-flow principle as applied to cardiopulmonary by-pass is largely of historical interest.

EQUIPMENT

THE OXYGENATOR.—The oxygenator first used clinically by Gibbon consisted of stainless steel screens over which blood flowed by gravity. This method is efficient in terms of volume of oxygen added per volume of blood required to fill the oxygenator but requires a recirculating system so that the film over the screens, once obtained, is not lost (Fig. 43-17).

One of the most commonly used oxygenators was devised by Bjork and Crafoord and later modified by Kay and Cross (Fig. 43-18).[2,9] This consists of a series of disks revolving and dipping in a pool of blood beneath an atmosphere of oxygen. Simplicity of operation has much to recommend this oxygenator, although it is not as efficient as some other types.

The bubble oxygenator has been extremely popular, particularly that used at the University of Minnesota in a large number of clinical perfusions[11] (Fig. 43-19). It is one of the most efficient oxygenators since an enormous oxygen-blood interface can be obtained by the use of relatively small bubbles. Success of the bubble oxygenator depends on use of a silicone antifoam compound which is relatively innocuous to the

Fig. 43-17.—Screen oxygenator. Blood is distributed along the top of the screens and a film obtained by mechanical wiping. Once obtained, the film must be maintained by recirculating a constant volume over the screen.

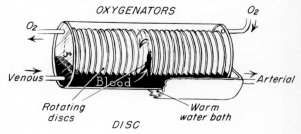

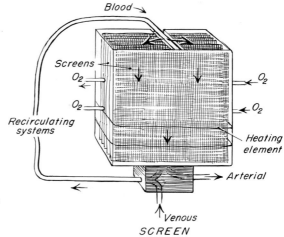

Fig. 43-18. — Disk oxygenator. A constantly changing blood film is formed by dipping the rotating disk in blood. Oxygenation can be increased by acceleration of disk speed.

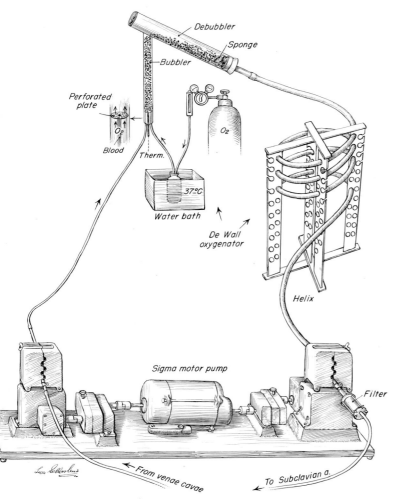

Fig. 43-19. — Bubble oxygenator and Sigmamotor pump. Oxygenation occurs from bubbles introduced into the blood. A large blood-gas interface is easily obtained. Bubbles are made to coalesce and rupture by an antifoam compound.

patient, and a reservoir in which bubbles that have not coalesced and have been removed chemically rise and separate from the blood. A packaged and disposable bubble oxygenator, primed with 5% dextrose, has been extensively used, notably by Cooley and associates.[8] For emergency operations this is especially useful, but it has also allowed rapidly working surgeons to perform more extensive operations.

In an effort more nearly to duplicate nature's method of respiration, an oxygenator in which blood and gas are separated by a membrane has been intensively studied, aiming toward a disposable package which would rival the normal lung in efficiency.[7] Problems of construction have been surmounted and a practical unit developed by Bramson *et al.*[4] Some of the attraction of separating blood and gas phases is lost if one must, as is commonly done, aspirate blood from the heart and pericardium during the cardiotomy, since in these circumstances gas and bubbles are mixed with blood and must be removed chemically or by allowing them to rise and separate.

It is likely that a small-volume highly efficient oxygenator rivaling the natural one will be developed, but none is yet so efficient that air can be used in its ventilation. The five fold increase of partial pressure of oxygen with an atmosphere of oxygen is needed in order to oxygenate adequately. Carbon dioxide diffuses more readily, and except in the bubble oxygenator, 2–4% of carbon dioxide is added to the ventilating gas to prevent washing out.

Sporadically, interest in the use of the patient's own lung as an oxygenator is revived. This technique combined with hypothermia was advocated by Drew.[12] Additional cannulations are required to bypass each ventricle separately; it is probable that, as equipment is further simplified and improved, total by-pass will remain as the preferred method.

THE PUMP.—There has been less evidence of imaginative design in mechanisms for pumping than for oxygenating. If there were conclusive evidence that any parameter should be met in the pump, it could almost surely be readily accomplished. Unfortunately, there is no decisive evidence that anything other than a means of atraumatic propulsion of blood is necessary. In a sense, most of the pumps in clinical use have not followed nature's example, and most are nonpulsatile or only mildly pulsatile. The body is un-

doubtedly adapted to a pulsatile flow, and it is impossible to imagine any other type in the living system, which must intermittently rest. Wesolowski[22] found no difference in survival, or the volume of blood required to assure it, between animals perfused with a pulsatile and a nonpulsatile flow. Work by Ogata[19] demonstrated that during by-pass, animals perfused with nonpulsatile flow took up a greater volume of blood in maintaining the same pressure, probably indicating that the control and reflex systems in the body are more sensitive and attuned to a pulsatile flow. Whether or not the ideal pump will be similar to present models, clinical perfusion can be satisfactorily accomplished with any of several pumps now available. Gibbon selected the DeBakey roller pump, and most people in this country have followed his lead. It is simple in design, easily controlled, relatively atraumatic to blood and presents no problem in cleaning (Fig. 43-20). The Sigmamotor finger pump used by Lillehei was commercially available and ideally suited for controlled cross-circulation for which Lillehei originally used it, but it is cruder and a little more damaging to formed elements of the blood than the carefully constructed roller pump which has largely supplanted it.

The pump which is least traumatic to the blood employs two alternately filling chambers working in parallel with proper valves.[10] Filling and ejection can be regulated to prevent rapid pressure changes and consequent hemolysis. Such a pump is a little more complicated in design and has not found wide usage. It can easily be altered to give a pulse of considerable amplitude if desired.

CANNULATION

The superior and inferior venae cavae are cannulated for removal of venous blood, and constricting tapes around them effectively seal the general venous return from the heart during by-pass (Fig. 43-21). The cannulas must be large so that blood can be extracted through them with relatively little negative pressure, but at the same time they must not be so large that normal flow is unduly obstructed in the time between cannulation and commencement of the by-pass. Arterial blood from the machine, which in initial clinical experience was introduced through the subclavian artery, is now more commonly returned through a

Fig. 43-20.—Pumps commonly used in cardiopulmonary by-pass. **A**, De Bakey roller pump. **B**, Sigmamotor finger pump. **C**, intermittent pulsatile pump with external valves.

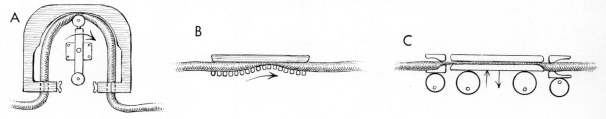

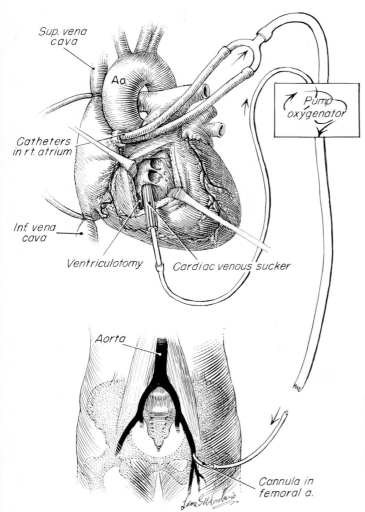

Sup. vena
cava

Ao.

Catheters
in rt. atrium

Inf. vena
cava

Ventriculotomy   Cardiac venous sucker

Aorta

Pump
oxygenator

Cannula in
femoral a.

Fig. 43-21. — Extracorporeal circulation; by-pass plan. Blood is aspirated from each vena cava and led by siphon drainage to the pump oxygenator, where it is oxygenated and pumped back to the arterial system through the femoral or other available artery. Gentle suction and siphon are used to aspirate blood from the heart; after separation of the froth, the blood is returned to the circulation.

femoral or iliac artery. The ascending aorta may be cannulated either directly or through a tubular prosthesis sutured to it. How the blood enters the arterial tree makes no apparent difference to the body.

Some cardiac venous blood (which may be very great in amount in patients with cyanotic congenital heart disease), as well as bronchial flow through the lungs, returns to the heart when the cavae are constricted around the cannulas and must be aspirated during cardiotomy by gentle suction; the gas and blood mixture can be passed over antifoam compound, the air allowed to rise out of the blood and the blood returned to the by-pass circulation.

Controls

Considerable diversity of practice is evident in the means used to control by-pass flow. Fixing the flow is

possible if relatively low flows are used. In such circumstances, when only a portion of the normal venous return is by-passed, the venous pressure will rise, great veins will be constantly distended and blood will be available for aspiration. If there is too much restriction of flow, metabolic acidosis develops, so that current practice involves drawing off the complete venous return into the by-pass. When the venae cavae are thus kept emptied, a temporary reduction of venous return will lead to sucking of the vein walls into the cannula and injury to them if strong suction is applied, as by a fixed-volume pump. Gentle suction can be applied by siphon or gravity drainage. As flow increases through the tubing in such a system, more of the pressure is lost to resistance, and self-regulation is to some extent obtained.

During by-pass, the volume of blood in the apparatus must be kept constant either automatically or by manual control so that the patient is neither bled into the machine nor transfused from it. A by-pass flow of about 1.6 liters/M² at normal body temperatures is necessary to prevent the development of metabolic acidosis or a decrease of general oxygen consumption;[1] the usual resting flow under the conditions of anesthesia and thoracotomy is closer to 2.3–2.5 liters. Should the flow fall below this level, transfusion may be required to increase it. Kirby and associates[17] have shown that the volume of blood required to fill the vascular system is greater at high than at low flows. To increase the flow, the vascular system must be slightly distended.

Arterial pressure often falls during cardiopulmonary by-pass, but this does not appear to be detrimental provided an adequate flow is maintained. Venous pressure must not be allowed to rise significantly, as this is an important indicator of restricted flow. Care must be taken that the cannulas are not obstructed or kinked. Some groups attempt to maintain a fixed arterial pressure, transfusing the patient if necessary from a reservoir. Our experience has been that provided an adequate flow of 2 liters or more per M² is maintained, the level of arterial pressure is of little consequence. The venous pressure is more important in assuring that by-pass is proceeding adequately.

Clark[6] presented a nomogram which defines the volume of by-pass flow required to maintain mixed venous oxygen saturation at about 50% and thus ensure that tissue oxygenation does not fall below an adequate level. This may give a valuable guide to the required level of flow, although in our practice we have simply kept the flow at least around 2.5 litters/M² for the noncyanotic patient and up to 3 liters for the cyanotic one in whom allowance must be made for the increased bronchial flow.

Conduct of the Operation

Operative exposure is determined to some extent by the requirements of venous and arterial cannulation. Median sternotomy gives adequate exposure for most operations in children and is the ideal exposure for ventricular septal defect, tetralogy of Fallot and aortic stenosis. Neither pleural cavity need be entered unless it is desired at the end of the operation to drain the pericardium into one side to avoid accumulation of blood in the pericardial sac. When only the atrium is to be entered, we prefer a right anterolateral exposure through the fourth interspace; access to the mitral valve, as in a patient with an atrioventricular canal, is better, and the caval cannulas may be inserted in an area more out of the operative field.

Normally during operation we monitor the arterial and central venous pressures on strain gauges connected to catheters inserted into the femoral vessels. Direct measurement of arterial pressure is required because during by-pass the amplitude of the pulse of the arterial pump is so small that blood pressure can-

not be obtained by the cuff method. Oxygen saturation and pH of the arterial blood are intermittently measured to make sure of the adequacy of perfusion. Because of the large shifts of blood volume possible during by-pass, some estimate of adequacy of final blood volume is desirable at the completion of the by-pass. Measurement of central venous pressure and especially its changes in response to small transfusions has been a simple, effective indicator of regaining balance.

Citrated blood, preferably no more than 1–2 days old, to which heparin and calcium are added, may be used to prime the machine. Dilution of the priming volume with 5% dextrose has been widely used. The patient is given heparin 2–3 mg/kg of body weight. We fear the dangers of deficient heparinization much more than of any excess, as the heparin can be adequately counteracted with protamine, a specific heparin antagonist. On the other hand, if the blood is inadequately anticoagulated, widespread thrombosis may deplete the body of clotting substances and lead to afibrinogenemia. For this reason and since it can be demonstrated that heparin is metabolized during the by-pass, we give additional heparin every 30 minutes, 1mg/kg for the first dose and 0.5 mg/kg each half-hour thereafter. Meticulous hemostasis is required to prevent postoperative hemorrhage in the patient who has been heparinized. There is more bleeding after a by-pass procedure than after other thoracic operations, but it should not be excessive. Formed elements of the blood, including white blood cells and platelets, usually diminish during cardiopulmonary by-pass. Invariably some hemolysis occurs, the exact amount in clinical perfusions being difficult to measure because of continued removal of free hemoglobin by the body.

In the repairing of complicated defects, it is helpful to have the heart relatively quiet. The method which has proved most satisfactory in our experience has been intermittent occlusion of the ascending aorta, usually for 4–5 minutes, followed by resumption of coronary flow until cardiac action returns to normal. When coronary flow is shut off, vision is better and intracardiac work easier in the absence of coronary venous return. The heart slows but usually does not stop in the 4–5 minute period. Experimentally there is minimal subsequent depression of ventricular function with this method. When the occluded aorta is released, the ascending aorta and left ventricle must be vented carefully to avoid entrapment of air and subsequent coronary air embolism.

Hypothermia.—Hypothermia was used regularly as a means of accomplishing open-heart operations before cardiopulmonary by-pass was found to be safe.It was only natural then that the two modalities should be combined. By reducing the needs of the body for oxygen and flow, the demands on the by-pass machine can be diminished—an important advantage when oxygenators of limited capacity are used.[5, 14]

Drew[12] advocated profound hypothermia to 16 C with extracorporeal cooling, by-pass of each ventricle and perfusion of the patient's own lung for oxygenation. At the low temperature the by-pass and blood flow can be stopped so that a completely dry and bloodless field is obtained. On the basis of clinical results, there does not seem to be a great advantage over more thoroughly tested methods at normal temperature.

Moderate degrees of hypothermia, 24–30 C, are used frequently to diminish the needs of the body for blood and oxygen during periods when coronary flow is interrupted, as in patients with aortic stenosis, tetralogy of Fallot and ventricular septal defect. Moderate hypothermia adds some benefit without incurring the disadvantages of a deeper level.

Selective hypothermia has been used to cool the heart alone. Cooling can be induced by perfusion of cold blood into the ascending aorta, or the heart can be bathed in cold Ringer's solution in the pericardial sac to the point of cardiac arrest. Selective cooling and induced arrest allow a longer safe period of aortic occlusion and facilitate the repair of intracardiac or aortic valvular defects. On the other hand, our results have been much better with careful perfusion of the coronary arteries when the aorta must be occluded for more than 10–15 minutes.

The risk of cardiopulmonary by-pass is quite low, of the order of 1% or less. By-pass must be unhurried and long enough to allow proper correction of the defect being treated. This is amply demonstrated in treatment of the tetralogy of Fallot where, unless the obstruction to outflow from the right ventricle is relieved, the mortality rate is greatly increased. Similarly, if a ventricular septal defect is not completely repaired or recurs, the persistent defect added to the insult of operation is often more than can be tolerated by the patient. In short, as was amply demonstrated in the shunt operation for tetralogy of Fallot, if the patient is not helped, he is hurt by operation.

The treatment of individual lesions is discussed elsewhere in this book.

Postoperative Care

Postoperative care is unusually important because of the magnitude of the surgical insult and the vital nature of the cardiorespiratory system which has been insulted. Rest in an atmosphere of high humidity and oxygen is essential. Fluids should be restricted, as there is added to the normal antidiuresis the effect of a heart damaged by a cardiotomy. Kirklin,[18] Sturtz and associates[20] outlined a satisfactory regimen of fluid administration in the early postoperative period.

Except for the simpler procedures, the intratracheal tube is left in place and a mechanical ventilator used to assist respiration until the patient has fully recovered from the anesthesia, and sometimes overnight. Tracheostomy may be needed the following day if ventilation is not adequate as estimated by arterial blood gases and pH. Adequate blood volume must be maintained; venous pressure is a useful guide.

If disturbance of the conducting mechanism of the heart has been produced, electrical pacemaking may be life-saving. In the presence of heart block such as might be caused from the trauma of repair of a septal defect, the heart does not respond to increased demands by the proper increase of rate, and an accelerated rate must be maintained electrically between 80 or 90 for adults and 120 for young children. With improvement of cardiac function and after the initial stress of the postoperative period, the normal conducting mechanism often recovers and the pacemaker wire may be removed.

In our experience, it has been helpful to have studies of oxygen saturation of blood from the pulmonary and femoral arteries, with samples obtained through small plastic catheters left in place at the time of operation.[3] A fall in saturation of the femoral arterial blood may indicate the need for improvement of ventilation by tracheostomy or respirator. A fall in pulmonary arterial saturation indicates reduced cardiac output and may focus increased vigilance on measures to improve it by blood replacement, relief of cardiac tamponade, use of digitalis, further restriction of fluids or use of diuretics.

Cardiac tamponade must be watched for after operation. There is some increased tendency to bleed, even in the absence of demonstrable clotting defects. Catheters are left in the pericardial sac for drainage, but these may seal off and tamponade occur. Widening of the mediastinal shadow in the roentgenograms, fall of arterial and rise of venous pressure and low cardiac output may point to the cause for cardiac decompensation and indicate immediate thoracotomy and relief.

Blood pH is a good indicator of adequate circulation in patients undergoing open-heart operations. Metabolic acidosis may develop because of decreased flow during by-pass or, in the postoperative period, poor cardiac function.[16] In the absence of such diminished flow, acidosis should not appear. The body normally compensates for metabolic acidosis, but once acidosis has developed, a vicious cycle may be entered from which the patient can be extricated only by giving alkali. In such circumstances, sodium bicarbonate intravenously (2 mEq/kg) may be life-saving.

REFERENCES

1. Anderson, M. N., and Senning, A.: Studies in oxygen consumption during extracorporeal circulation with pump-oxygenator, Ann. Surg. 148:59, 1958.
2. Bjork, V. O.: Brain perfusions in dogs with artificially oxygenated blood, Acta chir. scandinav. 96:137, 1948.
3. Boyd, A. D., et al.: Estimation of cardiac output soon after intracardiac surgery with cardiopulmonary bypass, Ann. Surg. 150:613, 1959.
4. Bramson, M. L., et al.: A new disposable membrane oxygenator with integral heat exchanger, J. Thoracic & Cardiovas. Surg. 50:391, 1965.

5. Brown, I. W., *et al.*: Experimental and clinical studies of controlled hypothermia rapidly produced and corrected by a blood heat exchanger during extracorporeal circulation, J. Thoracic Surg. 36:497, 1958.

6. Clark, L. C., Jr.: Optimal Flow Rate in Perfusion, in Allen, J. G. (ed.): *Extracorporeal Circulation* (Springfield, Ill.: Charles C Thomas, Publisher, 1958), p. 150.

7. Clowes, G. H. A., Jr., and Neville, W. E.: The Membrane Oxygenator, in Allen, J. G. (ed.): *Extracorporeal Circulation* (Springfield, Ill.: Charles C Thomas, Publisher, 1958).

8. Cooley, D. A.; Beall, A. C., Jr., and Grondin, P.: Open-heart operations with disposable oxygenators, 5 per cent dextrose prime, and normothermia, Surgery 52:713, 1962.

9. Cross, F. S., *et al.*: Evaluation of a rotating disk type reservoir-oxygenator, Proc. Soc. Exper. Biol. & Med. 92:210, 1956.

10. Crafoord, C.; Norberg, B., and Senning, A.: Clinical studies in extracorporeal circulation with a heart-lung machine, Acta chir. scandinav. 112:220, 1957.

11. DeWall, R. A.; Warden, H. E., and Lillehei, C. W.: The Helix Reservoir Bubble Oxygenator and Its Clinical Application, in Allen, J. G. (ed.): *Extracorporeal Circulation* (Springfield, Ill.: Charles C Thomas, Publisher, 1958).

12. Drew, C. E., and Anderson, I. M.: Profound hypothermia in cardiac surgery: Report of three cases, Lancet 1:748, 1959.

13. Gibbon, J. H.: Application of a mechanical heart and lung apparatus to cardiac surgery, Minnesota Med. 37:171, 1954.

14. Gollan, F., *et al.*: Hypothermia of 1.5 C. in dogs followed by survival, Am. J. Physiol. 181:297, 1955.

15. Helmsworth, J. A., *et al.*: Myocardial injury associated with asystole induced with potassium citrate, Ann. Surg. 149:200, 1959.

16. Ito, I.; Faulkner, W. R., and Kolff, W. J.: Metabolic acidosis and its correction in patients undergoing open-heart-operation, Cleveland Clin. Quart. 24:193, 1957.

17. Kirby. C. K., *et al.*: Simple automatic method of blood volume control during cardiac bypass for open-heart surgery, Arch. Surg. 78:193, 1959.

18. Kirklin, J. W.; Patrick, R. T., and Theye, R. A.: Theory and practice in the use of a pump-oxygenator for open intracardiac surgery, Thorax 12:93, 1957.

19. Ogata, T., *et al.*: A comparative study on the effectiveness of pulsatile and nonpulsatile blood flow in extracorporeal circulation, Arch, japan. Chir., vol. 29, no. 1, 1960.

20. Sturtz, G. S., *et al.*: Water metabolism after cardiac operations involving a gibbon-type pump-oxygenator, Circulation 16:988, 1957.

21. Warden, H. E., *et al.*: Controlled cross-circulation for open intracardiac surgery, J. Thoracic Surg. 28:331, 1954.

22. Wesolowski, S. A.; Sauvage, L. R., and Pinc, R. D.: Extracorporeal circulation: The role of the pulse in maintenance of the systemic circulation during heart-lung bypass, Surgery 37:663, 1955.

H. T. Bahnson
F. C. Spencer

Drawings by
Leon Schlossberg

Abdomen

SECTIONS ONE-THREE

PLATE IV

A. Omphalocele. A large omphalocele measuring 8 cm in diameter. The sac contained small intestine and a portion of the liver. The sac and a large Meckel's diverticulum were excised, and the wound was closed by undermining the skin flaps widely as a first-stage procedure.

B. Meckel's Diverticulum. Meckel's diverticulum communicating with a persistent vitellinic duct and presenting as an umbilical fistula in a 4-week-old infant. Diverticulectomy and excision of the vitellinic duct and the umbilical fistula resulted in an uneventful recovery.

C. Patent Omphalomesenteric Duct, with Complete Eversion of Proximal and Distal Loops of Bowel. The Y-shaped mass presents a mucosal external surface. In this 23-day-old child the fecal discharge came entirely from one arm of the "Y." The stem of the "Y" had room within it for both the afferent and efferent loops of bowel and for a knuckle of bowel which was herniated up into the serosa-lined cavity. A small incision around the umbilicus allowed the bowel to be reduced, the omphalomesenteric persistence to be amputated and the bowel to be closed. This is the most complete form of persistence of an omphalomesenteric duct: at one end, it leaves a Meckel's diverticulum and, at the other, no more than a tuft of mucosa in the umbilicus.

D. Umbilical Hernia with Rupture and Protrusion of Omentum. In this 1-year-old baby an intact and uninfected umbilical hernia ruptured during a crying spell. Large umbilical hernias cannot be expected to repair themselves spontaneously; they should be corrected operatively.

E. Lymphosarcoma of the Small Bowel. The tumor was easily palpable through the abdominal wall of this 4-year-old child who had vague symptoms. The U-shaped loop at the left is diffusely replaced by tumor, so that its lumen is a mere slit. There is an obvious disproportion between the proximal dilated bowel (*left*) and the distal collapsed bowel (*lower center*), but the child had no obstructive symptoms. Although the involved segment of bowel was resected, the numerous enlarged mesenteric nodes precluded an operative cure.

F. Irreducible Ileoileo Intussusception. Irreducible ileoileo intussusception secondary to an inverted Meckel's diverticulum in a 2-year-old infant. Resection and primary anastomosis were performed. Ectopic gastric mucosa was found at the base of the Meckel's diverticulum.

PLATE IV

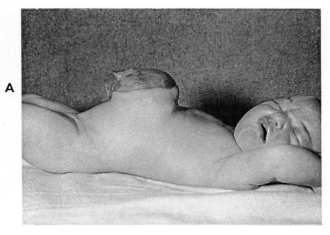

A

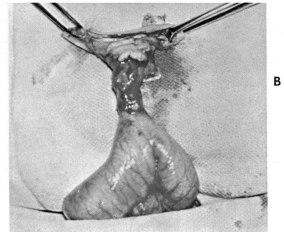

B

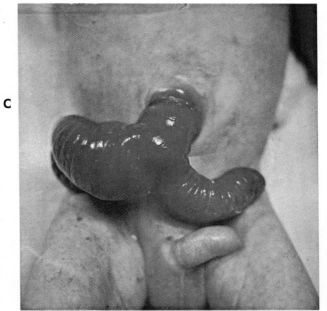

C

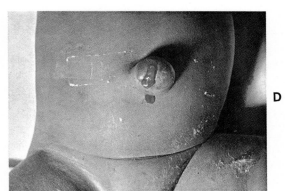

D

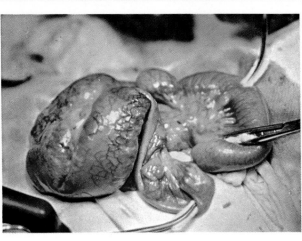

E

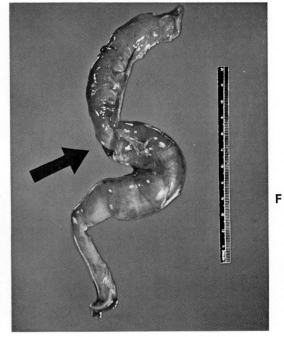

F

44

Miscellaneous Conditions of the Abdominal Wall

The Abdominal Parietes

THE ABDOMINAL PARIETES contain and protect the abdominal viscera. Since abdominal conditions constitute a major part of pediatric surgery, it is essential that the surgeon have a sound knowledge of the anatomy of the abdominal wall and of the methods of performing a laparotomy. Once having performed a successful intra-abdominal procedure, nothing is more disheartening than to have the results nullified by a catastrophic evisceration and a subsequent fatal peritonitis.

EMBRYOLOGY

The muscles of the abdominal wall have a segmental origin, arising from the thoracolumbar somites. Although this primitive arrangement of myotomes is soon lost, the segmental nature of the spinal nerves supplying the muscles is retained throughout life. Muscle fibers arise posteriorly and run parallel to the long axis of the body, but early in embryonic life an anterior and downward migration occurs. A fusion of the myotomes takes place anteriorly to form the rectus abdominis muscles. Tangential splitting also occurs so that the abdominal wall becomes laminated. The direction of fibers of individual muscles then changes to assume the final pattern as seen in adult life. The last step in the embryonic process is a fibrous replacement of portions of the myotomes to form aponeuroses.

ANATOMY

The abdominal wall is a laminated structure. Laterally, from within out, the layers consist of: peritoneum, properitoneal fat, fascia transversalis, transversus, internal oblique and external oblique muscles, superficial fascia, subcutaneous fat and skin. As the muscle layers extend anteriorly they become aponeurotic and then fuse to form the anterior and posterior sheaths of the rectus abdominis muscles. In the lower abdomen, below the arcuate line, the aponeuroses of all three lateral muscles contribute to form the anterior sheath, so that posterior to the muscle belly there is only fascia transversalis and peritoneum. In the midline, all aponeurotic fibers fuse to form the linea alba. Below the umbilicus, the linea alba is truly linear in character, but above the umbilicus the medial borders of the rectus muscles may be separated.

The attachments of the rectus abdominis muscles are to the fifth, sixth and seventh costal cartilages and to the pubic bone. The bulk of the muscles is fleshy but becomes tendinous just above the attachment at the pubis. Three, and sometimes more, transverse tendinous intersections occur, usually at the levels of the umbilicus, the costal margin and the xiphisternum. Their adherence to the anterior sheath prevents wide separation of the muscle bellies when a transverse incision is made.

In infants and children, the superficial fascia is a well-defined layer. This is particularly true in the lower abdomen, where the fascia has on occasion been mistaken by the inexperienced surgeon for the aponeurosis of the external oblique muscle.

Skin tension (Langer's) lines for the most part run in a transverse direction across the anterior abdominal wall. In infants and children, definite skin creases are easily seen in the lower abdomen. While the cosmetic appearance of healed incisions on the abdominal wall is perhaps not of major importance, transverse skin incisions heal with almost invisible scars. It is my impression that they heal faster and with fewer complications than do vertical incisions.

BLOOD SUPPLY.—The blood supply to the lateral

abdominal wall is segmental, with paired arteries originating from the aorta. Anteriorly, the area above the umbilicus receives its blood supply from the superior epigastric, musculophrenic and lower intercostal arteries. Below the umbilicus, the blood supply is from the inferior epigastric, superficial epigastric, superficial circumflex iliac and superficial external pudendal arteries.

Venous drainage accompanies the arterial supply.

LYMPH DRAINAGE.—The lymphatics of the abdominal wall are divided into two general groups. Those in the supraumbilical region drain to nodes in the axillas, while those in the infraumbilical area drain to the superficial inguinal nodes.

NERVE SUPPLY.—Incisions in small children are often of necessity relatively longer than are comparable incisions in the adult. Because of this, there is a danger that nerves will be severed or injured with resulting weakness. A knowledge of the location and course of the nerves will in most instances prevent this complication.

The anterior branches of the lower six thoracic nerves extend from the posterior flank to the anterior abdominal wall, between the transversus and internal oblique muscles. The anterior ramus of the first lumbar nerve divides in two—the iliohypogastric and the ilioinguinal nerves. Laterally, these nerves course between the transversus and internal oblique muscles, but in about the line of the anterior superior iliac spine they pierce the internal oblique muscle. They then run anteriorly between internal oblique and the aponeurosis of the external oblique, hence they are readily seen during operations for inguinal hernias.

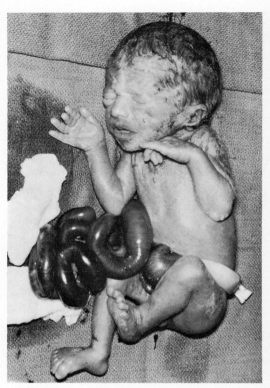

Fig. 44-1.—Premature infant with extensive gastroschisis.

CONGENITAL ABNORMALITIES

Congenital abnormalities involving the umbilicus are common and are considered in another section.

Diastasis of the upper rectus abdominis muscles is frequently observed in infants and in children. Usually the condition is of no significance unless accompanied by a small ventral hernia with protrusion of properitoneal fat.

Agenesis of the muscles of the abdominal wall occurs rarely. In the cases reported by Silverman and Huang,[7] an extreme deficiency of the musculature rather than a complete absence was present. Males are much more commonly affected than females. Associated abnormalities of the urinary tract are almost invariably found. In these children, death occurs as a rule from urinary or respiratory infection.

Treatment is directed to provide external support of the abdominal wall and early surgical correction of urinary tract abnormalities and prevention of urinary and respiratory infections.

Gastroschisis occurs when there is improper closure of the body wall in the midventral line (Fig. 44-1). There is no covering sac. Berman[1] reported a high incidence of associated intestinal atresias. Treatment consists of correction of the associated abnormality, replacement of viscera into the abdominal cavity and closure of the midline defect as in cases of omphalocele.

If, because of extensive evisceration and a disproportionately small abdominal cavity, skin or layer closure of the defect is impossible, then an artificial peritoneal covering may be constructed. Dacron-reinforced Silastic membrane is sutured to the edges of the enlarged defect as a bag covering the exposed viscera (Fig. 44-2). Antibiotics are injected regularly into the bag to minimize infection, and by gradually reducing the size of the bag over a period of several days the viscera can be returned to the enlarging abdominal cavity. A primary repair of the abdominal defect can then be performed without tension.

TRAUMA

Injury to the abdominal wall of children is by no means uncommon.

Most nonpenetrating injuries are minor and require no treatment. Rarely, a hematoma may have to be evacuated. In more serious injuries, trauma to the abdominal wall is of secondary consideration to more lethal damage within the abdomen.

With penetrating wounds in which there is a doubt

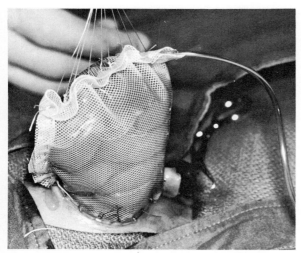

Fig. 44-2.—Extensive gastroschisis treated by sewing dacron-reinforced Silastic membrane bag to edges of defect, thus permitting gradual return of viscera to the abdominal cavity.

as to whether or not the peritoneal cavity has been entered, the wise surgeon explores the abdomen through a short laparotomy incision adjacent to the wound. If the peritoneum has not been penetrated, this small incision is easily closed. If, however, intra-abdominal injury has been sustained, the incision may be enlarged and definitive surgery performed.

INFECTIONS

Infections of the abdominal wall for the most part are essentially similar to superficial infections occurring elsewhere.

Metastatic abscesses are not uncommon in septicemia. The usual offending organism is *Staphylococcus aureus*, and treatment consists primarily of the indicated antibiotic, hot compresses, with incision and drainage of localized fluctuant collections of pus.

Synergistic gangrene, also known as chronic progressive cutaneous gangrene, may complicate operations for purulent conditions of the peritoneal cavity. It is caused by a micro-aerophilic nonhemolytic streptococcus in combination with an aerobic hemolytic staphylococcus. It and other unusual infections are fortunately rare in pediatric patients.

Omphalitis or infections occurring in the region of the umbilicus in the newborn require prompt and intensive treatment. The common infecting pathogens are the streptococcus and *Staph. aureus*. Because of the extensive lymphatic drainage and the persistence of patent vascular channels leading to the porta hepatis, rapid dissemination of the infection commonly occurs. Not only is septicemia an immediate serious problem, but peritonitis may occur. Thrombosis of the portal vein with subsequent development of portal

hypertension is a frequent and serious complication.

When abdominal surgery is performed on a newborn baby, omphalitis may be prevented by excising the cord remnant and by leaving the umbilical stump exposed. If it should become moist, applications of 70% alcohol will dry the area.

Omphalitis is treated by intensive systemic antibiotic therapy, the local application of antibiotic powders or ointments and with hot foments. Early intensive treatment usually prevents the development of complications.

ABDOMINAL INCISIONS

An ideal abdominal incision gives direct access to the viscus being treated, good exposure for the performance of the operation and, when repaired, a strong closure of the abdominal wall. The choice of incision depends on the location of the intra-abdominal pathology and on the estimate of the extent of exposure required.

Although long incisions usually heal well and without complications, in general the shorter the incision and the more layers used in wound closure, the better is the healing and stronger is the abdominal wall. Thus, when the preoperative diagnosis is known with considerable certainty, a limited abdominal incision is preferred.

GRIDIRON INCISIONS.—In cases of acute appendicitis, and in some cases of intussusception, that is, when there is doubt as to whether or not barium enema reduction has been complete, a modified McBurney[4] (Davis or Rockey) incision is employed (Fig. 44-3). The skin incision is transverse and, because the cecum of a child usually lies relatively high, it is made at a level above the anterior superior iliac spine. Each muscle layer of the abdominal wall is split in the direction of its fibers. Fascia transversalis and peritoneum are opened in a transverse direction. After removal of retractors, this wound practically closes by itself, and following suture of the layers, a very strong closure is obtained.

This incision having been made, if exposure proves inadequate, the incision may easily be extended. Partial cutting of anterior and posterior rectus sheaths with medial retraction of the rectus muscle will give additional exposure (Weir's extension). If still further medial exposure should be required, the wound may be extended as a transverse incision across one or even both rectus muscles. If a more lateral exposure is needed, the incision may be extended into the flank by cutting across fibers of internal oblique and transversus muscles.

The Robertson[5] muscle-splitting incision is used in cases of hypertrophic pyloric stenosis. The skin incision is made transversely one finger-breadth below the right costal margin. The external oblique, internal oblique and transversus muscles are split in the direction of their fibers. On opening the peritoneum in a transverse direction, the liver is found to extend be-

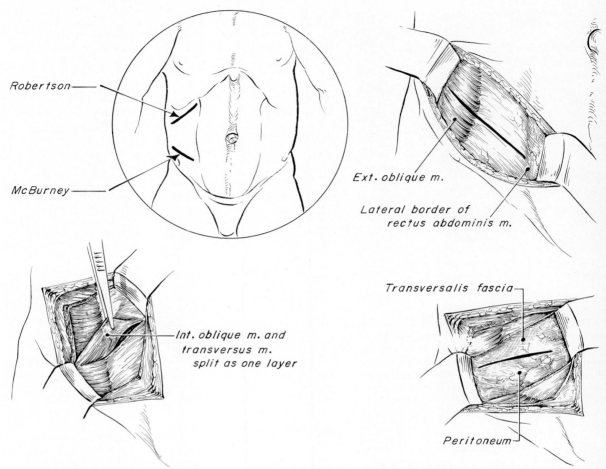

Fig. 44-3.—Gridiron muscle-splitting incisions, used in cases of pyloric stenosis (Robertson) and acute appendicitis (Mc-Burney). The skin incisions follow Langer's lines in a transverse direction. Muscle layers are split individually in the direction of their fibers. The peritoneum is opened transversely.

low the level of the incision. During the performance of the pyloromyotomy, the liver is gently retracted upward. When the retractor is removed, the liver reassumes its normal position. It then acts as a convenient buffer, preventing herniation of intestinal loops and omentum during closure of the peritoneum.

If greater exposure is ever needed, this incision can easily be extended medially across one or even both rectus abdominis muscles.

TRANSVERSE INCISIONS.—Because these incisions follow the lines of skin and maximal abdominal wall tension, they are ideal for most laparotomies (Fig. 44-4). A limited incision across one rectus muscle above or below the level of the umbilicus may be made initially. After determination of the extent of the intra-abdominal lesion and the exposure required, the incision may be extended to either one or both sides of the abdomen. Lateral to the rectus sheath, the wound is

extended by splitting the muscle layers in the direction of their fibers, with care taken to avoid damage to nerves. In this manner, the incision may extend across both rectus muscles and out into each flank, a very wide exposure thus being obtained. These incisions invariably heal well, and danger of subsequent wound dehiscence or evisceration is minimal.

Lateral transverse muscle-cutting incisions are also employed. For splenectomy (Fig. 44-5), the child is positioned with the left flank hyperextended. The incision is made just below the costal margin and extends through all layers of the abdominal wall from the flank to the lateral margin of the left rectus muscle. The nerves are identified and are retracted out of harm's way without compromising the exposure. Though this incision is quite short, even a large spleen can be freed from its diaphragmatic and lateral abdominal wall attachments to be easily delivered

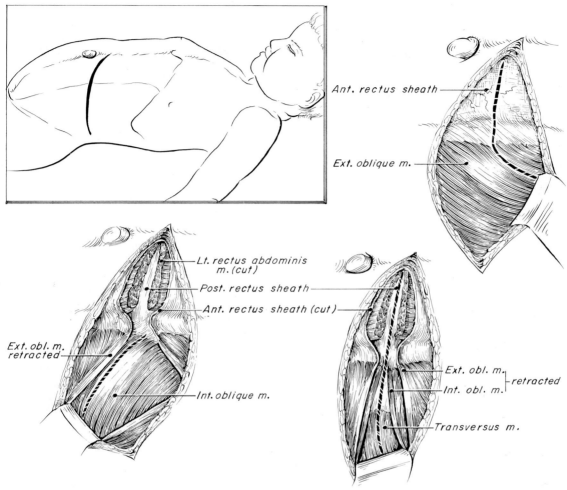

Ant. rectus sheath

Ext. oblique m.

Lt. rectus abdominis m. (cut)

Post. rectus sheath

Ant. rectus sheath (cut)

Ext. obl. m. retracted

Int. oblique m.

Ext. obl. m. ⎤
Int. obl. m. ⎦ *retracted*

Transversus m.

Fig. 44-4.—Left transverse rectus incision. The wound is extended into the flank by dividing muscle layers in the direction of their fibers. The incision may be extended across the right rectus muscle and out into the right flank to obtain a very wide exposure.

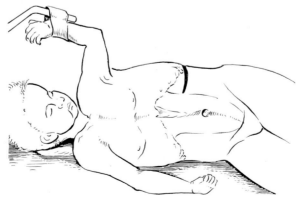

Fig. 44-5.—Subcostal transverse muscle-cutting incision, used for splenectomy.

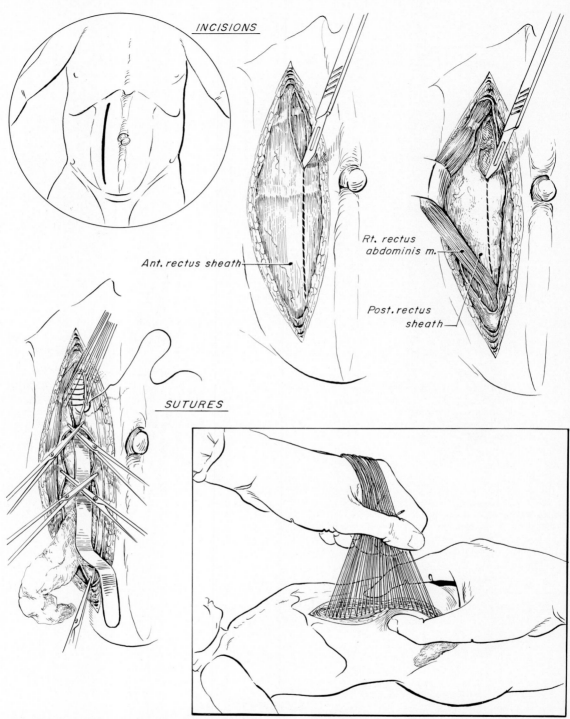

INCISIONS

Ant. rectus sheath

Rt. rectus abdominis m.

Post. rectus sheath

SUTURES

Fig. 44-6. — Vertical incision. The right rectus muscle is retracted laterally. When closure is difficult, interrupted sutures of 4-0 silk are inserted; when these are drawn up, closure of the perito- neum and posterior rectus sheath is achieved by distributing the tension to all strands.

into the wound. The gastrosplenic ligament and the pedicle of the spleen can then be dealt with under full vision and with complete control.

Combined transverse and oblique incisions may be used to advantage on occasion. For bowel resection in aganglionic megacolon, Hiatt[3] recommended a transverse incision across the left and across part of the right rectus muscles. The incision is then extended obliquely up into the left flank by splitting the external oblique in the direction of its fibers and by cutting internal oblique and transversus muscles. This approach gives good access to the pelvis and to the left colon, and to a considerable extent reduces the need to pack the small intestine out of the operative field. The incision is also used when performing an abdominoperineal anoplasty.

The Pfannenstiel incision has a limited application in pediatric surgery. In certain cases of intersex, however, when exploration is required to ascertain the nature of the internal genitalia, the incision gives sufficient exposure and has the advantage of healing quickly with an almost invisible scar. If the patient is a newborn, the baby can be discharged from hospital at the same time as the mother leaves the maternity center. The information obtained from the operation, coupled with other criteria of sex determination, will usually indicate beyond doubt the sex of rearing.

VERTICAL INCISIONS.—Many surgeons use a vertical incision when an exploration of the intra-abdominal contents is indicated. The incisions are easy to make and to close, give good exposure and are extended upward or downward with facility. However, they cross lines of maximal abdominal tension and therefore predispose to evisceration and to postoperative wound complications to a greater extent than do transverse incisions.

If a vertical incision is to be employed on an infant or a child, the *paramedian incision*, in which the rectus muscle is retracted laterally, is preferred (Fig. 44-6). A limited incision at about the level of the umbilicus is first made. Once the extent of the abdominal lesion has been ascertained, the wound is extended either upward or downward. The anterior rectus sheath is incised in the midline of the rectus muscle belly. Then by sharp dissection and with gentle traction on the medial edge of the sheath, this portion of the sheath is freed to the midline from the underlying muscle and its tendinous intersections. The muscle belly is then retracted laterally, and the posterior sheath and peritoneum are opened in the same line as the anterior sheath incision. When this wound is closed, the belly of the rectus muscle falls back in place and becomes interposed as a strong buttress between anterior and posterior sheaths.

Rectus muscle-splitting incisions sever nerve fibers and produce weakness of the medial muscle segment. For these reasons, they should not be used in pediatric surgical practice except when the incisions are very short, as in a colostomy or a feeding gastrostomy.

Medial rectus-retracting vertical incisions (Battle) cause extensive nerve damage with paralysis and should never be used.

Midline vertical incisions have a limited use in pediatric surgery. Because of the paucity of the blood supply and the fusion of the layers into one at the linea alba, they are easily made. Repair, however, depends on only one layer and, should infection occur, evisceration or wound hernia is almost inevitable.

Short lower abdominal midline incisions are used for exposing the bladder in suprapubic cystotomy and when an anterior approach is required for excision of posterior urethral valves.

Thoracoabdominal incisions (Fig. 44-7) are ideal for extensive procedures in the upper abdomen or lower mediastinum. The incision is made either on the right or left and extends obliquely through the lower chest wall in the eighth or ninth intercostal space. The costal margin is cut and the wound extended into the abdomen as an oblique muscle-cutting incision. The periphery of the diaphragm is split and, with a rib spreader inserted, a very wide exposure is obtained. If further abdominal exposure is required, the incision is easily extended medially in a transverse direction across the rectus muscle.

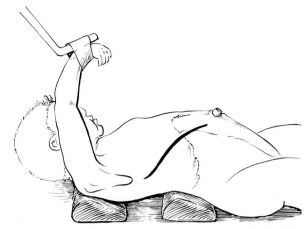

Fig. 44-7.—A thoracoabdominal incision gives a very wide exposure.

DRAINAGE

Considerable diversity of opinion prevails among pediatric surgeons as to when and when not to insert a drain. My own experience has been that when in doubt, it is better to drain than to take the chance of having to perform a secondary drainage procedure. With a gridiron incision, the drain is brought out through the wound, but when other incisions have been used, it is best to place the drain through a separate stab wound.

Either a Penrose or a cigarette drain is most commonly employed. If one anticipates copious postoperative drainage, as from a bile or pancreatic fistula, a sump drain should be inserted.

In obese children with acute purulent appendicitis, at least the subcutaneous tissue should be drained.

Wound Closure

In most patients, closure of the abdominal wound is accomplished without difficulty. A continuous 3-0 chromic catgut suture is used for the peritoneum and fascia transversalis. Interrupted sutures of 4-0 black silk are employed for closure of muscle and aponeurotic layers. The superficial fascia is similarly closed as a separate layer. A few buried subcutaneous sutures will help prevent spreading of the scar once skin sutures have been removed. Skin edges are approximated by either continuous or interrupted sutures of 5-0 silk. If the wound is contaminated, interrupted sutures of 3-0 chromic catgut instead of silk are used for all deep layers.

In the presence of intestinal distention or when the abdominal cavity is disproportionately small compared to its contents, as for example omphalocele or diaphragmatic hernia, great difficulty in closure may be experienced.

With intestinal distention, much may be accomplished by the use of intestinal tube suction preoperatively and during the procedure. If, despite this, loops remain grossly distended, an aspirator should be inserted into the lumen through a purse-string suture in the bowel wall. Gas and intestinal fluid are removed with gentle suction. While this procedure may potentially contaminate an otherwise "clean" operation, it can be accomplished without spillage and without fear of subsequent infection. Decompression performed in this way changes a difficult and traumatic operation into one which is simple and where wound closure is made easy.

In cases without gross intestinal dilatation, yet where layer closure of the wound is difficult, it is on occasion possible to close only the skin. A difficult secondary repair of the ventral hernia then lies ahead. In the majority of cases of this type, however, with gentle perseverance on the part of the surgeon and the judicious use of muscle relaxants by the anesthesiologist, a primary layer closure of the abdomen may be accomplished. A thin moist gauze spread over protruding intestines like a fishnet is of great help in replacing intestinal loops into the peritoneal cavity. Closely spaced interrupted sutures of 4-0 black silk are then inserted through peritoneum and fascia transversalis. When these are all simultaneously drawn tight, thus distributing tension to all strands, individual sutures may be tied without cutting through the delicate tissues. Suture of other layers may be carried out in a routine fashion.

Tension or stay sutures are rarely required, but in very difficult situations they may be inserted as additional insurance against evisceration. Through-and-through sutures of 2-0 silk are used and are placed through short segments of rubber tubing to prevent cutting of the skin.

Unlike the situation in an adult, when an ileostomy or a colostomy is performed on an infant, it is necessary to suture the exteriorized bowel wall to the peritoneum. If this is not done, loops of small intestine are very likely to herniate through the wound with disastrous consequences.

FACTORS INFLUENCING WOUND HEALING. – As in all aspects of pediatric surgery, closure of abdominal wounds must be accomplished by gentle, meticulous technique. Aggressive blunt dissection, pulling, tearing, forceful retraction and ligation of large tissue masses must be avoided. Anemia, hypoproteinemia, edema, tissue necrosis, malnutrition, vitamin deficiency and infection all contribute to poor wound healing. Proper preoperative preparation and intensive postoperative care are essential in preventing or correcting these abnormal body states.

WOUND DEHISCENCE. – With better preoperative and postoperative care, with greater attention to technique and with better control of infections by antibiotic therapy, wound disruptions in the pediatric surgical patient are now much less frequent than was the case 15–20 years ago. Gross and Ferguson[2] reported the following incidence of evisceration and associated mortality rates. During the years 1931–35, the incidence of evisceration in pediatric patients was 1.31%, with a mortality rate of 55%. From 1936 to 1940, the incidence of dehiscence was 1.65%, with mortality of 45%. From 1941 to 1945, evisceration occurred in 0.61% of major abdominal wounds, with a mortality rate of 46%. In their most recent figures, for the years 1946–50, the incidence of evisceration had dropped to 0.39%, with an accompanying drop of mortality to 27%. Snyder[3] in 1962, in a study of 2,035 cases, found dehiscence in 7, an incidence of 0.35%, with 1 death, or a mortality rate of 14.3%.

Even though skin sutures may remain intact, disruption is invariably accompanied by the appearance of serosanguineous fluid on the abdominal dressing and demands immediate inspection of the wound.

At one time, if a partial disruption through only the deep layers of the incision occurred, it was the practice to apply an abdominal binder and to hope that the situation would not become worse. A secondary repair of the resultant hernia was then performed. While this policy of watchful waiting was successful in some instances, in others operative intervention became necessary because of eviseration or intestinal obstruction. Often the intervention had to be performed at a time when the patient's condition had deteriorated. For this reason, in the presence of a partial disruption it is advisable to reoperate on the child as soon as possible and to perform a resuture of the abdominal wall. In these circumstances, through-

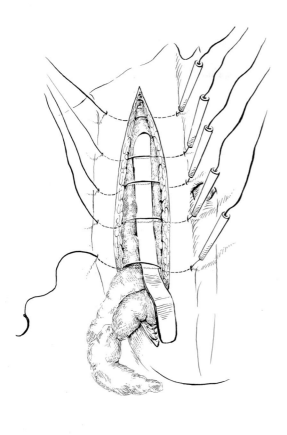

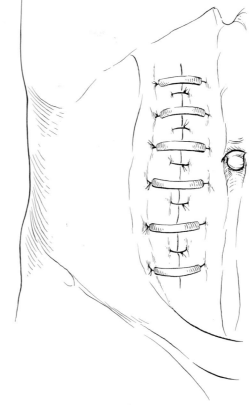

Fig. 44-8.—In cases of wound disruption, through-and-through sutures of 00 black silk are used. Threading the sutures through segments of rubber tubing prevents cutting of the skin. Intervening stitches accurately approximate the skin edges.

and-through sutures of silk are inserted and are tied over short segments of rubber tubing (Fig. 44-8).

If evisceration with protrusion of intestinal loops through the wound has occurred, the exposed bowel should be immediately covered with sterile warm saline-soaked pads, and a sterile binder applied. Large doses of antibiotic are given, and the infant or child is prepared for reoperation as soon as possible. In the operating room, using general anesthesia and with sterile precautions, the viscera are held up out of the way and the skin of the abdominal wall is cleansed with pHisoHex or aqueous Zephiran chloride 1:1,000 solution. The exposed viscera are then returned to the abdominal cavity and, as in partial disruption, the wound is resutured with through-and-through sutures.

These patients are frequently very ill and require every available support, which will include gastric or intestinal suction, parenteral alimentation, oxygen and continued intensive antibiotic therapy. Fortunately, in most cases, uneventful wound healing will occur and the through-and-through sutures may be removed on the tenth to fourteenth postoperative day.

VINYL DRAPES

These plastic drapes are particularly useful in the pediatric surgical patient. They permit good view of the operative site, diminish the possibility of wound infection by skin contamination, effectively seal off contaminated areas of the abdominal wall, i. e., colostomy, and, as reported by Roe, Santulli and Blair,[6] help prevent heat loss in infants during anesthesia and operations.

REFERENCES

1. Berman, E. J.: Gastrochisis, with comments on embryologic development and surgical treatment, Arch. Surg. 75:788, 1957.
2. Gross, R. E., and Ferguson, C. C.: Abdominal incisions in infants and children: A study of evisceration, Ann. Surg. 137:349, 1953.
3. Hiatt, R. B.: Surgical treatment of congenital megacolon, Ann. Surg. 133:321, 1951.
4. McBurney, C.: The incision made in the abdominal wall in cases of appendicitis, with a description of a new method of operating, Ann. Surg. 20:38, 1894.
5. Robertson, D. E.: Congenital pyloric stenosis, Ann. Surg. 112:687, 1940.

6. Roe, C. F.; Santulli, T. V., and Blair, C. S.: Heat loss in infants during general anesthesia and operations, J. Pediat. Surg. 1:266, 1966.
7. Silverman, F. N., and Huang, N.: Congenital absence of the abdominal muscles associated with malformation of genitourinary and alimentary tracts: Report of cases and review of literature, Am. J. Dis. Child. 80:91, 1950.

8. Snyder, W. H.: Personal communication.

C. C. FERGUSON

Drawings by
MURIEL MCLATCHIE MILLER

Omphalitis

OMPHALITIS IS BECOMING less frequently seen as a result of improved methods of care of the newborn and the use of antibiotic drugs. In the early weeks of life, however, inflammation of the umbilicus may be a very serious problem, since open pathways often exist from the umbilicus to distant sites of possible infection.

ETIOLOGY

Cord contamination occurs most frequently when the cord is severed after birth or during subsequent changes of the stump dressing. Even tetanus occasionally occurs as a result of contamination of the stump. The cord may become contaminated even before birth if the membranes rupture prematurely or if numerous vaginal examinations are made before delivery. Wilson and Armstrong[3] studied frozen sections of the umbilical cord of 104 infants born 24 hours or more after fetal membranes had been ruptured and compared these with cords of 92 control infants. Amnionitis was associated with cord inflammation, as would be expected. However, according to this study, most instances of cord inflammation in infants born after prolonged rupture of fetal membranes occurred without apparent clinical infection in either mother or infant. Some inflamed cords were not associated with amnionitis, and in 14 instances of clinical amnionitis, the cords were normal on microscopic examination. The most frequent organisms are *Staph. aureus*, hemolytic streptococci and *Escherichia coli*, in this order. Babies with omphalitis caused by anaerobic organisms may have an extensive undermining type of massive ulceration.

The anatomic peculiarities of the umbilical area explain the complications which develop secondary to omphalitis. The two umbilical arteries pass through the abdominal wall and then descend as the hypogastric vessels. These vessels pass between the transversalis fascia and the peritoneum, joining the internal iliac arteries in the pelvis. These vessels usually become obliterated soon after birth, but the lumen may remain for a number of weeks. An infection which begins at the umbilicus might readily pass through or along these open channels in such a way as to cause infection of the lower abdominal wall, septicemia or peritonitis.

The umbilical vein passes inward at the edge of the falciform ligament. It branches and communicates with the portal veins and with the vena cava by way of the ductus venosus, which usually atrophies about the time of birth. It is therefore possible for bacteria to reach either the portal system or the general circulation via the vena cava from the umbilicus. Umbilical vein thrombosis secondary to omphalitis extending to the portal vein causes extrahepatic portal obstruction, probably the most common causative mechanism.

Infection from the umbilicus may spread by the lymphatic system as well as by the blood vessels. This lymphatic drainage, as regards the superficial channels, is in the direction of the inguinal lymph nodes. The deeper lymphatics drain superiorly and spread out over the area of the lower chest. Severe infection of the umbilicus spreading by way of the lymphatics results in extensive cellulitis which may involve the lower abdominal wall or the upper abdominal wall and lower thoracic area. Omphalitis may be secondary to infection in a patent urachus or to a patent connection with Meckel's diverticulum.

CLINICAL FINDINGS

The clinical findings in omphalitis vary from the most minor type of infection at the umbilicus to extensive cellulitis, abscess, necrotizing lesions producing sloughing, peritonitis and even septicemia.

If there is only a simple omphalitis, there will be local swelling associated with redness and tenderness around the umbilicus. There may be a small amount of seropurulent discharge from the area. A small area of granulation tissue harboring some infection may persist in the umbilicus for some time after the cord has disappeared.

More extensive cellulitis usually signifies that the infection has spread by way of the lymphatics. In such cases, tenderness, redness and swelling may be found in the epigastric area and even over the lower chest since the deeper lymphatics travel in this direction. There may also be some tenderness, redness and swelling over the lower abdomen extending toward the inguinal regions. In some instances, an abscess forms, or ulceration with tissue necrosis and undermining of the edges of the ulcer may develop.

The most serious complications of omphalitis are

those which result from an invasion of the blood stream by way of the vascular channels of the umbilicus. A high fever and severe toxicity are symptoms of septicemia. These patients have a tendency to infection at distant sites as a result of the infection in the blood stream. If peritonitis occurs, in addition to fever and evidence of toxicity, marked abdominal distention, vomiting and consequent dehydration are usually present.

TREATMENT

The granulation tissue which frequently presents as a small area of infection in the umbilical area after the cord has fallen away, may be successfully managed with one or two applications of silver nitrate. Mild cellulitis often responds to such local measures as meticulous care of the umbilical area plus the application of warm boric acid compresses. In general, omphalitis which shows evidence of anything more than the mildest type of infection should be managed with wide-spectrum antibiotic therapy combined with moist warm compresses and gentle

mechanical cleansing of the umbilical area. An abscess should be drained, and a draining sinus should be carefully unroofed in order to provide adequate drainage. The necrotizing ulcerations of the abdominal wall which occur secondary to anaerobic infections require militant treatment. Necrotic tissue must be removed and undermined edges elevated or clipped away to open the wounds widely. Care must be taken to maintain an adequate hemoglobin level and proper fluid and electrolyte balance. Antibiotic therapy should be used.

REFERENCES

1. Gross, R. E.: *The Surgery of Infancy and Childhood* (Philadelphia: W. B. Saunders Company, 1953).
2. Potter, E. L.: *Pathology of the Fetus and Infant* (2nd ed.; Chicago: Year Book Medical Publishers, Inc., 1961).
3. Wilson, M. G., and Armstrong, D. H.: Inflammation of the umbilical cord and neonatal illness, Am. J. Obst. & Gynec. 90:843, 1964.

HARWELL WILSON

Umbilical Remnants

ANATOMICALLY, the umbilicus marks the point of insertion of the umbilical cord into the abdominal wall, and embryologically, it marks the junction of several nutritional pathways vital to the developing fetus. At parturition, function of these pathways ceases and involutional changes begin. The umbilical arteries, vein and the urachus come to be represented by ligamentous remnants. The omphalomesenteric duct and vitelline vessels normally disappear by the sixth fetal week, and at the time of birth there is no evidence of their having existed. The failure of any of these structures to undergo proper involution results in various troublesome conditions ranging from minor inconvenience to life-threatening complications.[1, 2]

UMBILICAL GRANULOMA AND POLYP

Weeks or months after birth, long after the umbilicus should have healed, there may persist a lesion which early is represented by a small, rounded, cherry-red mass 2-10 mm in diameter (Fig. 44-9, *A*). The mass is composed of granulation tissue and usually disappears with one or two applications of silver nitrate. Untreated, it may heal spontaneously but tends to develop into a troublesome granuloma that is the seat of a low-grade chronic infection. Constant

cleanliness, and cauterization with silver nitrate on repeated occasions, may be necessary to bring about healing of the lesion, with rare resort to surgical excision. If the lesion fails to heal after 2 or 3 weeks of conservative management, or if there is persistent recurrence after apparent healing, a patent omphalomesenteric sinus or fistula or a patent urachus must be suspected.

A lesion similar in appearance to the umbilical granuloma is the umbilical polyp. It consists of intestinal mucosa and secretes mucus. It is not affected by astringents or responds only temporarily. Failure to demonstrate an opening in the polyp helps to differentiate the lesion from a patent vitelline duct or sinus. Surgical excision is necessary, preferably performed as the primary procedure on a correctly diagnosed lesion.

Small epithelial tags at the umbilicus are not uncommon and for the most part are of no importance other than being cosmetically undesirable. If the stalk is very slender (1-2 mm in diameter), these lesions may be eradicated on an outpatient basis by simple ligation of the stalk. Should the pedicle be larger (3-5 mm in diameter), it may contain large vessels capable of serious hemorrhage. Such problems are best dealt with in the operating room, where the vessels can be identified and ligated after excision of the lesion at its base. The umbilical granuloma may become epithelized and persist as a small rounded mass in the umbilicus. Unless they are pedunculated or cosmetically disturbing, they need not be excised.

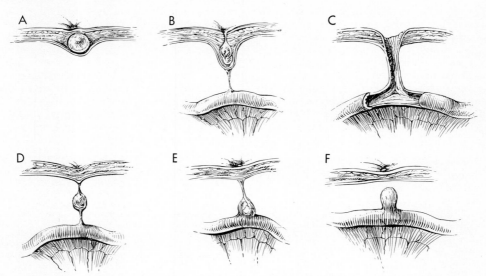

Fig. 44-9.—Umbilical remnants. **A,** subumbilical cyst. **B,** omphalomesenteric duct sinus with cordlike remnant of vitelline duct. **C,** patent omphalomesenteric duct through which ileum can prolapse. **D,** cordlike remnant of an omphalomesenteric duct with cystic dilation. **E,** persistence of ileal end of omphalomesenteric duct (Meckel's diverticulum) with attachment to anterior abdominal wall. **F,** Meckel's diverticulum.

Persistent Omphalomesenteric Band

Normally, obliteration of the omphalomesenteric duct is completed during the fifth to seventh fetal week and no evidence of the structure may be found postnatally. Incomplete or total failure of this process of obliteration results in several possibly troublesome lesions (Fig. 44-9, *B-F*). Usually, the complications that arise as a result of this anomalous development are manifest during the first few weeks of life but may not appear until months or years later.

Obliteration of the lumen of the duct but persistence of its muscular wall results in a fibrous band which extends from the umbilicus to the ileum or to the base of the mesentery. An associated opening or mucosal bud at the umbilicus may or may not be present. While it is quite possible to go through life without difficulty from this condition, it is nevertheless a potential hazard that allows looping or twisting of varying lengths of intestine around the band, producing a mechanical small bowel obstruction. The patient vomits bile-stained material and the abdomen becomes severely distended. When such a situation arises in the newborn period, lesions such as malrotation, congenital megacolon and stenotic or atretic lesions of the small bowel must be considered in the differential diagnosis. Because of the tendency of the bowel to become strangulated by this form of obstruction, early surgical intervention is mandatory. Blood in the stool of such an infant or child is indicative of strangulation and calls for emergency surgery. Once the abdomen is opened, the problem usually is readily apparent. Division of the band and reduction of the hernia or volvulus is curative except when nonviable

bowel is present. In the latter situation, resection of the nonviable intestine and end-to-end anastomosis should be performed. Any coexisting abnormality of the umbilicus should be corrected at the time of surgery.

Omphalomesenteric Duct Cyst

Cystic dilatations at any point along this remnant may be present and occasionally become so large as to present as an abdominal mass (Fig. 44-9, *D*). Operative investigation is indicated, and the removal of the cyst and band are curative.

Omphalomesenteric Duct Sinus and Fistula

Patency of the distal part of the duct with a discharge of mucinous material at the umbilicus is the condition known as omphalomesenteric duct sinus. Usually, there is a small, rounded, red protrusion of mucous membrane in the umbilicus. The tract may be delineated by injecting radiopaque material through a small polyethylene catheter introduced into the lumen of the sinus. X-ray films in at least the posteroanterior and lateral projections are obtained. The radiopaque material will outline the course of the sinus tract which may extend for only a few millimeters or may proceed for several centimeters. In some instances, a communication with the small intestine (patent omphalomesenteric duct) will be demonstrated (Fig. 44-9, *C*). The latter problem is managed in a manner similar to the treatment for Meckel's diverticulum.

The patent vitelline sinus will become infected occasionally and if such is the case, cultures are obtained, hot compresses are applied and treatment with the appropriate antibiotic is instituted. Surgical drainage is established if the lesion becomes fluctuant. Elective repair of this anomaly should not be undertaken if there is any inflammatory process present.

Usually the sinus may be excised without entering the peritoneal cavity. A subumbilical curvelinear incision is made and dissection carefully carried through the subcutaneous tissue and fascial layers until the sinus is identified. A small probe or catheter previously inserted into the sinus will aid in its identification. The sinus should be removed in its entirety, and if there be any doubt about the adequacy of removal or any evidence that there is a connection to the bowel or mesentery, the peritoneum should be opened in order to obtain adequate exposure. The coexisting mucosal bud in the umbilicus should be excised at the same time.

Patent Omphalomesenteric Duct

When there is a communication between the umbilicus and the small intestine, the structure is known as a patent omphalomesenteric duct (Fig. 44-9, C). This is assumed to be present when there is fecal drainage at the umbilicus. Confirmation is obtained by roentgenographically demonstrating the passage of contrast material into the small intestine from the umbilical opening.

Surgically, a patent omphalomesenteric duct is managed at its junction with the small intestine in a manner similar to that recommended for excision of Meckel's diverticulum. The duct is clamped across its base, excised and the enterotomy closed with two layers of interrupted 5-0 Atraumatic silk sutures. It is rarely necessary to resect any of the small bowel in order to remove the fistula.

Urachal Remnants

PATENT URACHUS. — Whereas the discharge of fecal material from an umbilical fistula is indicative of a communication with the intestine, the discharge of urine from such a fistula is indicative of a persistent urachal remnant with communication to the bladder. Positive identification of the tract is made only with x-ray studies *after* any existing inflammatory process is brought under control. Lower urinary tract infection in such cases is prevented, or controlled if already present, only by eradication of the abnormal pathway from the outside. The surgical attack is similar to the excision of the vitelline duct remnant, and care is taken to preserve the umbilicus. The umbilical opening is circumferentially excised and through an infraumbilical incision, the patent urachus is traced through the subcutaneous tissues and fascial layers

to its midline extraperitoneal position. Insertion of a malleable probe into the sinus tract will aid in its identification. Occasionally, a short midline extension of the incision toward the pubis gives additional valuable exposure. The fistula should be traced to its junction with the bladder and there doubly ligated with 3-0 or 4-0 chromic catgut and excised. The incision is reapproximated with fine silk and the skin closed with 5-0 silk. The incision in the umbilicus need not be closed.

A word of caution is interjected at this point to emphasize care in handling the obliterated hypogastric arteries. Although of rare occurrence, these vessels may be patent in the infant and major hemorrhage may result from cutting across one of the vessels. Blood loss in these cases is otherwise insignificant and transfusions should not be necessary.

URACHAL CYSTS AND SINUSES. — Closure of the umbilical end of the urachus with patency beyond may result in a cystic dilatation superior to the bladder and may occasionally be associated with lower urinary tract infection secondary to stasis of urine in a urachal cyst. When small, the cysts are asymptomatic, especially if there is adequate drainage into the bladder so that stasis and infection do not occur. Larger cysts of the urachus may present as a lower abdominal midline mass. A cystogram performed with radiopaque material will nearly always fill the cyst, and oblique or lateral films help demonstrate the configuration of the anomalous structure. Cystoscopy is of little help in identifying such a lesion and should not be employed as the primary diagnostic procedure. Surgical removal of a urachal cyst is best accomplished through a lower abdominal transverse extraperitoneal approach. The cyst should be removed flush with the bladder and the defect inverted and closed with a double layer of Atraumatic 4-0 chromic catgut. A persistent cyst without either umbilical or vesicle connection is unusual. Even though asymptomatic, such cysts should be removed to make certain that the mass is not an otherwise unsuspected malignant lesion.

INFECTED URACHAL CYSTS. — The urachal cyst that becomes infected and results in a large abscess cannot be removed as in the case of the sterile cyst. Incision and drainage, curettage of the lining and marsupialization of the cyst by packing with gauze was reported to be a satisfactory method for the management of these lesions.[3]

COMBINED OMPHALOMESENTERIC-URACHAL REMNANTS. — For the most part, urachal remnants and vitelline duct remnants occur as individual lesions but may occasionally present as a combined lesion. This is not often detectable on the x-ray examination. The chance that one or the other of the remnants may not fill with contrast material must be kept in mind, and the surgeon should be prepared to deal definitively with both lesions when this combination is unexpectedly encountered.

Infections of the Umbilicus

Inflammatory processes that involve the healing umbilicus constitute a major threat to the infant. Fortunately, these lesions are much less common in this age of improved postnatal care and at the same time are effectively controlled with modern antibiotic therapy when they do occur. Omphalitis may range from minimal redness and edema around the umbilicus to fulminating cellulitis of the abdominal wall. Should the infectious process involve the umbilical vein and spread to the portal system, frank septicemia may occur. An equally serious situation may arise as a result of thrombosis of the portal vein with consequent extrahepatic portal obstruction associated with ascites and bleeding from esophageal varices. Since the advent of antibiotics, the inflammatory process is no longer associated with a high mortality but can still be lethal without adequate treatment. Continuous warm, moist compresses together with adequate antibiotic therapy bring most of these infections under control before they become seriously advanced.

Relation of the Umbilicus to Incisional Infections

Many surgeons consider the umbilicus one of the dirtiest areas of the body and certainly of the abdomen. This is especially true of the deep umbilicus that is difficult to clean. Amazing and unsuspected amounts of debris, not to mention foreign bodies, may be harbored in this innocent-appearing dimple of the abdominal skin. Preparation of the abdomen for surgery should perforce include an evacuation and thorough cleansing of the umbilicus and its subsequent exclusion from the operative field by adequate draping. This cleansing project is readily accomplished with cotton-tipped applicator sticks and an antiseptic soap. Any indifference to this detail may result in serious incisional infections.

REFERENCES

1. Cresson, S. L., and Pilling, G. P.: Lesions about the umbilicus in infants and children, Pediat. Clin. North America 6:1085–1116, 1959.
2. Fox, P. F.: Uncommon umbilical anomalies in children, Surg., Gynec. & Obst. 92:95, 1951.
3. Trimingham, H. L., and McDonald, J. R.: Congenital anomalies in the region of the umbilicus, Surg., Gynec. & Obst. 80:152, 1945.

C. D. Benson
Drawings by
ROBERT MOHR

Conjoined Twins

Conjoined twins vary from two symmetrical well-developed individuals separated by a minor superficial connection to monsters represented only by portions of the body attached to each other or to a more completely developed host. Symmetrical attached twins are a rarity and offer a novel and complex problem. In the past, surgical separation was not often accomplished because of superstitions attached to such phenomena, lack of medical knowledge or the fact that most were stillborn or died in the immediate neonatal period. Success of separation has depended on the extent of conjoining and whether vital organs were shared. Most cases of long survival have been those joined by a band at the upper abdomen. There are only a few instances of both twins surviving separation.

History.—The earliest known conjoined twins were the Biddenden Twins, born in 1100 in England, who lived 34 years with a single pair of upper and lower extremities and a common rectum and vagina. A bas-relief in the church of La Scala depicts the Florentine Twins, born in the 14th Century, with three upper and lower extremities. The Scottish Brothers lived 28 years in the 15th Century joined from the waist down. Possibly the most famous pair of conjoined twins in the past were the Hungarian Sisters, born in Szorny in 1701. They were objects of great curiosity and were shown in many countries. They were joined back to back in the lumbar region and had a common anus and vagina. There were several other such twins in history. The best-known recent pair were Chang and Eng Bunker of Siam, born in 1811, who lived most of their lives in the United States. The term Siamese twins as a synonym for attached twins originated with this pair. They lived eventful lives to the age of 63 but were advised against operation by the physicians of their day because of shared liver tissue. Luckhardt[39] documented their lives and physiology in complete detail. Aird[2] in 1954 documented 36 cases of attached twins that survived and developed after birth, and in 1959, he[1] listed additional known British cases. Voris *et al.*[68] listed known cases and Robertson[52] compiled a list of 117 conjoined twins. The tabulation of operative cases by Kiesewetter[31] showed types and survival to 1963.

Classification

Symmetrical twins are classified according to the parts of the bodies which are joined or shared. They are usually similar in structure, two out of three are females, and they are attached at the same anatomic location. Scammon[56] in 1926 made a very complete classification of types. Using this and one prepared by Wilder[70] in 1904, Potter[49] presented an enlarged and rearranged classification of free and conjoined twins, symmetrical and asymmetrical. The following conjoined types would be of concern to the surgeon.

SYMMETRICAL.—Each component of the twins is complete or nearly so.

Thoracopagus, xiphopagus or *sternopagus,* and *omphalopagus.*—The connection is in or near the sternal region, usually median, and the individuals are face to face. The internal anatomy varies, with each twin usually having separate organs except for the liver, which may be partially united unless the attachment is superficial. If the area of attachment is wide, the possibility of sharing heart or parts of the digestive system is increased. The ileum in the region of the attachment of the yolk sac may be shared.

Pygopagus.—The connection is back to back and usually at the pelvis. Usually, the sacrum and coccyx are common and the digestive tubes join in a common rectum and anus with one urethra attached to one bladder. There may be multiple kidneys, uteri and vaginas and usually four adrenal glands and gonads.

Craniopagus.—The connection is by the heads, usually median, although the union varies and may be in the region of the vertex, occiput or lateral parietal areas. As a rule, the brains are separate or only lightly fused despite union of soft tissues and bones.

Ischiopagus.—The connection is in the lower pelvic region, the bodies being fused in the region of the pelvis up to the common umbilicus. Above this point, the bodies are normal and separate. The lower ends of the spines are abnormal, with single sacrum and pelvis. Two legs extend at right angles from each lateral surface with vaginal, urethral and anal orifices between each pair. If only one pelvis is present, the legs on the opposite side are only rudimentary.

ASYMMETRICAL.—One individual is smaller and dependent. One individual may be normal or nearly so and the other incomplete and attached as a parasite. Terminology in the literature varies from parasites to double monsters. Differentiation from teratomas (which are not true twins) and tumors is sometimes difficult.

Foetus in foetu is a term applied to cases in which one or more parasitic twins are found within the bearer.

ETIOLOGY

Various theories of embryologic deviations, mechanisms and patterns resulting in conjoined twins or double monsters have been discussed in detail by numerous investigators.[25,42,47,49,56,62,71,75] In general, double monsters seem to be structurally related to monozygotic twins. Fission of the embryo is a commonly accepted theory, the place of splitting determining the type of conjoining. Peterson and Hill[48] believed that a defect in the primitive streak or the degree of propinquity existing between two developing embryonic axes on a single embryonal disk might be factors favoring conjoining. Witchi[75] suggested that the cause of human conjoining is aging of the ovum. Dragstedt[12] pointed out that environmental factors may be involved since many congenital abnormalities are not due to genetic factors but may be caused by impairment of growth and nutrition of the embryo because of infection or deficient blood supply. Scammon[55] supported environmental factors as possibly influencing malformation from animal experimentation in which retardation of the growth of the embryo in early stages was produced by reducing temperature or oxygen concentration. Environmental factors affecting circulation or growth of one twin in utero may cause uneven development and eventually dependence of one twin on the other. According to Jenkins *et al.,*[30] twins might be joined by fusion of some other epithelial surface with the underlying mesodermal masses. O'Connell *et al.*[46] pointed out that conjoined twins are believed to result from the development of two overlapping areas on one blastocyst or from a bifurcation of a single embryonic axis. Eades and Thomas'[14] diagram of the similarity of the embryonic development between identical and conjoined twins indicates that conjoining is determined by the end of the second week of fertilization. Willis[71] has emphasized the early stage of malformation, stating that it can be produced only by disturbance of the embryo prior to the establishment of its axis.

PREOPERATIVE PROCEDURES

The extent of the preoperative studies to be carried out before one attempts the separation of conjoined twins will depend largely on the type and extent of the joining between the twins. A number of special examinations may be indicated in addition to the routine preoperative studies. This requires co-operative planning with various medical disciplines.[5,13,24] Surgical management has been discussed in detail, with emphasis on the value of detailed preoperative planning and study.[14, 34, 46, 48, 73] At separation, two surgical teams (one for each twin) need to be ready to work simultaneously. The surgeon bears the ultimate responsibility of leadership and decision and must keep in mind the fact that there may be anomalies which are not readily apparent. When the twins are joined at the skull, plain x-ray films will be desired as an early step in the examination. In addition to these studies, pneumoencephalograms, ventriculograms and electroencephalograms may provide helpful information in planning procedures to be used. In certain cases, arteriograms may give further, more definite data concerning the intracranial state of the joined twins.

Extensive preoperative studies are usually indicated in those conjoined twins united in the thoracic and abdominal areas. Anomalies in the cardiopulmonary system may be so extensive as to make separation impossible. Cardiac catheterization may now be added to the plain film studies which have been routinely carried out in such cases. One must weigh the value to be gained from such a procedure against the risk which it entails. Studies of the gastrointestinal tract with a thin radiopaque material will prove helpful in confirming or ruling out anomalies of the gastrointestinal tract. In addition to such studies, one twin may be given charcoal or indigo carmine and the stools carefully observed to see whether such material is evacuated from one or both twins. Intravenous pyelography has proved helpful in studying the urinary tract of such twins.

Radioactive isotopes have been used in an attempt to study the extent of circulatory exchange between the twins. Tagged red cells injected into one individual may be followed with the Geiger counter in order to measure the length of time for complete equilibrium to develop between the joined individuals. Peterson and Hill[48] used this method and found in the twins which they separated that approximately 29 minutes passed before complete equilibrium was reached. They also sought to ascertain the exact site of the greatest transfer of blood by using the scintillator but were unable to gain additional information from this part of the study.

Before proceeding with the actual separation, the surgeon should have a cannula secured in the ankle vein of each twin so that blood and electrolytes may be infused as needed. The management of this part of the procedure is very important, since untoward results might easily occur either from giving too much or too little fluid.

With craniopagus patients, careful attention must be given to planning methods of closing the defect in the scalp which may follow separation. A delayed bucket-handle flap of the type used in the craniopagus twins separated by Murphey may prove helpful.[73] It may be wise to create such a delayed flap and to advance it at the time of separation, covering the secondary defect with a split graft from the separated twin or in certain instances using a homograft temporarily from one of the parents. Baldwin and Dekaban[4] used tissue supplied by the Tissue Bank of the U.S. Naval Medical Center.

Closure of the defect in the abdominal wall may also offer difficulty and requires a staged procedure, as in the case of the twins separated by Wilson.[73] After the separation had been completed in this case, it was noted that a muscle and facial closure could not be satisfactorily accomplished at the same time. The subcutaneous tissue and skin were simply closed and the ventral hernias which resulted were repaired with no difficulty some 2 months later. The subsequent correction needed for limb realignment, as in the cases of Spencer,[61] Eades and Thomas[14] and Solerio,[59] must also be planned and evaluated in terms of the initial separation.

SURGICAL SEPARATION

According to the literature, the first attempted separation of conjoined twins was that of two sisters born in 1495 and joined at the heads. They lived to the age of 10, when one died and was "cut off" from the other. The second did not survive. There is also mention in the literature of separation attempted without success in 1689 by Farius of Basle. Scammon[56] cited the separation in 1902 of the Radica-Doodica sisters; one died of tuberculosis, and the other survived as the first known instance of successful separation. Ischiopagus twins were separated in 1912 at Portsmouth, England. One twin died at 4 months of pneumonia, while the other was living a normal life in 1958.[1] With advances in anesthesia, diagnostic procedures, antibiotic therapy and surgical techniques, especially vascular, an increasing number of successful separations are appearing.

THORACOPAGUS.—Conjoined twins joined at the chest face to face frequently present bizarre cardiac findings which create an interdependence of circulation incompatible with separate life.

One of the conjoined twins of Kano survived. These twins were joined by a bridge which extended from the sixth costal cartilage to the umbilicus. The preoperative and operative procedures were discussed in detail by Aird.[1, 2] In 1958, Jenkins et al.[30] described the problems encountered in separating thoracopagus twins who were joined at the anterior chest wall and upper abdomen, sharing a common pericardial sac and profoundly bizarre heart. There was a single liver with ramifications of two different biliary systems. The liver was divided externally only by a peritoneal curtain. Separation was performed after the death of one twin. The other survived only 6 hours because of the bizarre heart. Robertson and MacKenzie[53] reported on nonseparable thoracopagus female twins found to have differing first arch defects. The two hearts, enclosed in one large pericardial cavity, were completely fused, but the cavities of the common ventricle did not communicate and the septum between the common atriums was intact. The livers were also fused. Riker and Traisman[51] reported three cases of thoracopagus twins with bizarre hearts incompatible with life. Fine et al.[17] in 1964 described male twins with complete and independent viscera except for a common three-chambered heart located in the connecting soft tissue.

In Oregon, Peterson and Hill[26, 48] successfully separated twins joined from above the nipple line to the common umbilicus and reported in detail the preopera-

---

Fig. 44-10.—Xiphopagus twins, joined from manubrium to umbilicus, were born with a large omphalocele and died 2 days after closure. Drawings show diagrammatically the findings at autopsy. **A,** from the distal duodenum to terminal ileum there is a common small intestine. One twin had strictures at the ureteropelvic junctions. **B,** there are a separate single atrium and ventricle for each infant; the third ventricle, common to both infants, communicates with the pulmonary veins of infant **I** and the aorta of infant **II** (dotted outline). The inferior vena cava of both infants opens into the atrium of infant **I**. **Arrow** indicates the ventricular septal defect between the ventricle of infant **II** and the common third ventricle. (From Wilson and Storer.[73])

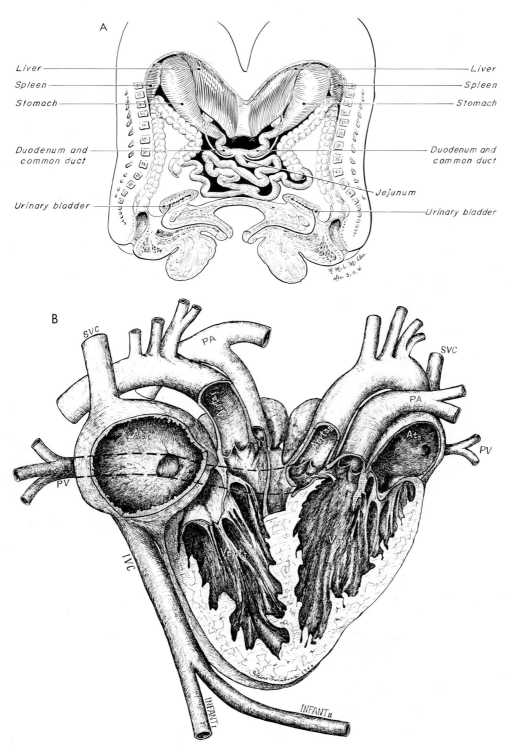

Fig. 44-10.—See legend on facing page.

tive procedures used. Another successful separation was accomplished by Kiesewetter[31] in 1966. These twins were 12-day-old females joined from approximately the fourth interspace for 13 cm just below a common umbilicus with shared liver, diaphragm and septum pericardium. Kiesewetter and Wijthoff[39] have summarized in detail the literature and surgical management of this type of conjoined twin.

XIPHOPAGUS.—In 1927, Holm[28] in Minnesota performed a successful separation on 7-week-old twins joined from the xiphoid cartilage to the umbilicus, an area about 9 cm long. Fluoroscopic studies had demonstrated separate gastrointestinal tracts. A common peritoneum was found at the site of fusion but no organs were involved. The abdominal hiatus created in each twin by the separation was closed under some tension and both twins did well. A similar case in Nigeria was reported by McLaren[40] in 1936 as successfully separated. Reitman's[50] patients, joined by a band, were successfully separated on the day of delivery. In 1957, Dragstedt[12] succeeded in separating female xiphopagus twins from Siam joined in the upper abdomen in the same manner as the original Siamese twins. The tissue bridge contained a band of liver about 7 cm in diameter, and there was a common peritoneal cavity. The conjoined twins born in 1953 and reported by Wilson and Storer[73] were joined from the manubrium to the umbilicus but survived

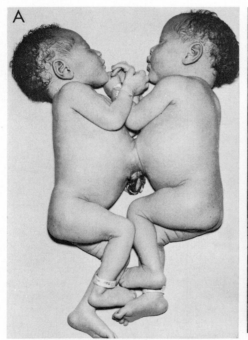

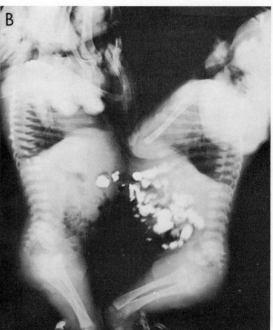

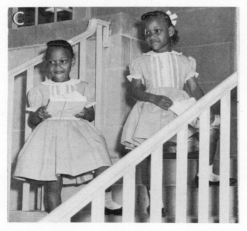

Fig. 44-11.—Xiphopagus twins. **A,** before separation. A bridge of tissue joins them from the lower body of the sternum to the umbilicus. **B,** gastrointestinal series of one twin shows intestinal herniation into the abdominal cavity of the other, but no communication between the intestinal tracts of the two. **C,** 5 years after separation. The abdominal walls were closed incompletely and under tension, and the resultant hernias were closed readily when the twins were 4 months old. The connecting bridge between them consisted of skin, fascia, cartilage joining the sternums and a small mass of liver. The peritoneal cavities communicated freely. (From Wilson and Storer.[73])

only two days following repair of omphalocele. Autopsy revealed a common small intestine from the distal duodenum to the terminal ileum. One twin had strictures at the ureteropelvic junction bilaterally (Fig. 44-10, A). These anomalies were compatible with life, but the cardiovascular system was so anomalous as to be incompatible with life and separation. There was a single inferior vena cava and only two atriums and three ventricles in a partially shared heart (Fig. 44-10, B).

We[73,74] successfully separated another set of xiphopagus twins at the University of Tennessee in Memphis in 1955. The twins had a bridge of tissue which joined them from the lower body of the sternum to the umbilicus (Fig. 44-11). The roentgenogram taken after one twin had been given barium by mouth showed that the intestine of one herniated into the abdominal cavity of the other, but no communication between the twins' intestinal tracts could be demonstrated. Separation was performed when the twins were 5 1/2 weeks old, using procaine locally supplemented by ether inhalation for closure of the abdominal wall. The connecting bridge consisted of skin and fascia, cartilage joining the sternums and a small bridge of liver which was divided between clamps. Centrally, a common peritoneal system was present so that, in separation, one twin received the peritoneal covering, which resulted in a widely opened peritoneal cavity of the other. Closure of the fascial defects in both was accomplished under some tension. The resulting ventral hernias were repaired when the twins were 4 months old. Both have grown normally since then. Holgate and Ikpeme[27] 1 also reported successful separation of xiphopagus twins.

Wooley and Joergensen[76] in 1963 separated a pair of twins joined from the midthorax to a point below the midabdomen, one of whon died 2 1/2 days after separation. Their report includes a detailed review of preoperative evaluation, operative technique and postoperative care of xiphopagus twins.

OMPHALOPAGUS TWINS.—From Capetown, South Africa, Cywes and Block[10] in 1964 described the separation of omphalopagus twins presented as an emergency with ruptured omphaloceles. One twin was stillborn with a large ruptured omphalocele and evisceration of liver and most of the gastrointestinal tract. The live twin was successfully separated. Two examples of conjoined twins with unruptured omphaloceles were reported in 1957. The twins described by Wilson and Storer[73] had the omphaloceles repaired but died before separation was attempted, and those reported by Roddie[54] did not survive.

In 1964, we[58] separated thoraco-omphalopagus female twins with common liver and diaphragm and many circulatory abnormalities. Prior to separation the circulation balance was compatible with life, but both twins died in the early postoperative period of cardiac failure due to anomalies of circulation incompatible with separate existence.

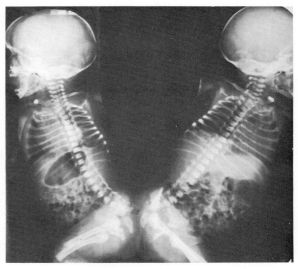

Fig. 44-12.—Pygopagus twins. Although this film shows no bony fusion between the twins, they were firmly attached at the level of the sacrum and had to be cut apart with a knife. The periosteum covering the two bony areas was one layer. (From Koop.[34])

PYGOPAGUS.—The incidence of pygopagus twins is small. Dawson[11] described postmortem findings in a pair in 1944. Ochsner[43] separated such a pair in 1957, documented in a motion picture.[44] A lay magazine mentioned a case in 1955 and 1956.[64,65] Koop[34] described in detail the separation in 1957 of 9-day-old females with separate colons emptying into a common anus (Fig. 44-12). The smaller twin had a cardiac arrest following separation due, it was thought, to a disproportionate share of the blood volume going to the larger twin. Heart beat was re-established. Later, when reaching 12 lb in weight, this twin developed cardiac failure which was controlled with digitalis. Cardiac studies in 1960 established a diagnosis of tetralogy of Fallot. At age 8 1/2, this twin died of unexplained cause following a Blalock procedure.[33]

The successful separation of a set of 6 1/2-year-old pygopagus girls has been described by Salerio.[59] The area of joining included the osseous structures of the sacrococcygeal vertebral column from the third sacral vertebra to the apex of the coccyx and the entire extent of the pelvic floor.

Both Koop[34] and Solerio[59] have discussed the surgical management of pygopagus twins in detail.

CRANIOPAGUS.—The successful separation of craniopagus twins depends on the presence of separate brains with independent vascular systems. The famed Brodie twins, reported in 1953 by Grossman[23] and Sugar[63] and their associates, represent the first recorded survivals of more than a few hours after craniopagus separation. One of these patients died a month later; the other survived 11 years. Earlier at-

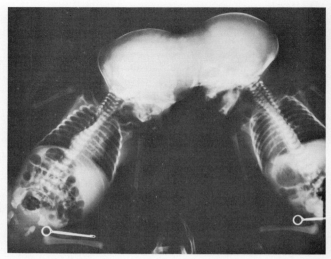

Fig. 44-13. — Craniopagus twins, brow to vertex union. Pneumoencephalography shows separate brains with a small communication. Separation was accomplished after preliminary elevation of skin flaps. One twin survived only 5 hours; the other lived. (From Wilson and Storer.[73])

tempts at separating craniopagus twins had been made by Cameron[7] in 1928, Leiter[36] in 1932 and Barbosa[6] in 1949.

We[73] separated craniopagus twins with a brow to vertex union in 1954. Pneumoencephalography before operation indicated separate brains with a small communication through the common septum (Fig. 44-13). A week before separation, a preliminary elevation of skin flaps in both was done so that temporally attached bucket-handle flaps would be available to cover the anticipated defect. Cranial separation was carried out by Dr. Francis Murphey. One twin survived only 5 hours after separation. The other was developing normally at the time of writing. Voris[68] reported the first known recorded case of long-term survival of both craniopagus female twins after surgical separation. These twins were separated in 1954 at the age of 8 1/2 months. Voris described the thorough preoperative studies, visualization techniques and operative procedures used. One twin had a skull defect repaired,[66] and recently was said to be normal and doing well in school.[67] The other was extremely retarded.

In 1956, Baldwin[4] and Hall[24] and their associates successfully separated 3-month-old twins joined at the brow; both survived. When it was discovered that the dual connections were extensive, the separation was done in two stages. At the second operation, a connection with the right frontal lobe was uncovered which included a sharing of the right anterior cerebral artery. The wounds were closed with dual grafts over which homografts of skin were placed. A detailed follow-up report in 1965[3] indicated that their condition continued to be satisfactory. In 1962 and 1964, O'Connell[45,46] analyzed in detail two pairs of twins, one set of males and the other females, in which one member of each set survived separation. The radiologic[13] and anesthesiologic[5] aspects of the operative procedure have also been reported on these 2 cases, as well as the pediatric care.[19]

ISCHIOPAGUS. — Ischiopagus twins are further classified according to the number of lower extremities present: ischiopagus bipus with no lower extremities on one side,[70] ischiopagus tripus with a single composite limb on one side[18,20,41,57] and ischiopagus tetrapus with continuous longitudinal axis, the lower extremities at right angles to the axis of the common trunk. Ischiopagus twins are also rare and offer a dramatic challenge because of the many organs involved and the complexities of anatomic findings.[8,16] Eades and Thomas[14] documented the cases known in the literature; few have been considered for surgical separation.

When one or more vital organs are shared, division into two viable organisms is impossible, although it may be possible to save one by giving him the shared organ, as in the dramatic ischiopagus tetrapus case reported by Spencer[61] in 1956. These twins were joined at the lower abdomen and pelvis (Fig. 44-14). The separation was made 18 hours after birth because the smaller twin's deterioration was influencing the viability of the larger one. The surviving twin had "a complete gastrointestinal tract with Meckel's diverticulum and a malrotation; two kidneys, normal to palpation, each draining into a separate bladder; two uteri with four tubes and four ovaries and three vaginas. . . " and was growing normally. In December, 1964, she was attending school, but her legs were badly rotated externally.[60]

The first successful separation of ischiopagus twins was reported and analyzed in detail in 1966 by Eades and Thomas,[14] with emphasis on preoperative and operative procedures and anatomic detail. These twins were females, 7 months of age. The lower extremities were at right angles to the axis of the common trunk with union of each small bowel in a

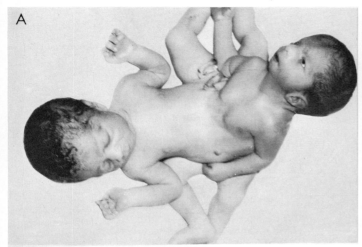

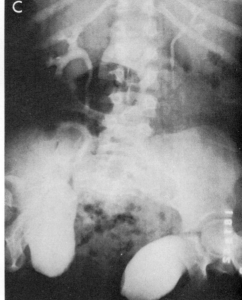

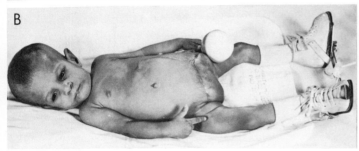

Fig. 44-14.—Ischiopagus twins, operated on by Spencer. **A,** the twins were joined at the lower abdomen and pelvis. Although there were eight extremities and two heads and chests, one twin seemed more complete than the other. **B,** in a remarkable undertaking, the stronger twin was salvaged when the small one began to deteriorate. The survivor grew normally and had "a complete gastrointestinal tract, with Meckel's diverticulum, and a malrotation; 2 uteri with 4 tubes and 4 ovaries and 3 vaginas." (**A** and **B** from Spencer.[61]) **C,** roentgenogram obtained at age 9 1/2 years, showing two bladders. There were no symptoms in any organ system. The legs are badly rotated externally, but the child goes to school. (Courtesy of Dr. R. Spencer.)

common cecum and essentially shared pelvic viscera.

ASYMMETRICAL ANOMALIES.—Varieties of asymmetrical conjoined twins, parasites and other anomalies have been outlined in detail by Potter,[49] Willis[71] and others.[42,56,62,70] The differentiation of teratomas, tumors and *foetus in foetu* is difficult because of overlapping borderline features.[37] Teratoma, though it may contain highly organized structures, is a neoplasm which arises from embryonic pleuripotential cells with benign or malignant propensities, according to Willis, and are not included monsters or malformed twins.[71,72] Lewis[37] in 1961 reported a *foetus in foetu* and retroperitoneal teratoma with a review of theories regarding teratomas.

Foetus in foetu.—Rare instances of one or more fetuses found within the body of its bearer (usually in the retroperitoneal region of the upper abdomen) have been reported. Willis[71] distinguished *foetus in foetu* from teratoma by the presence of a vertebral axis and the appropriate arrangement of other organs and limbs with respect to the axis. The pathogenesis of foetus in foetu has not been clarified. It is thought to be a monozygotic twin developing from a single ovum with early retarded growth and anatomic confinement, later becoming dependent for blood supply on its bearer (twin) without developing a heart and circulation of its own. Lord,[38] Lewis[37] and Janovski[29] have written comprehensive reports concerning this anomaly.

In most cases, only one intra-abdominal fetus has been found.[9,15,29,37,39,77] Gross and Clatworthy[22] reported finding twin fetuses in fetu, and Lee[35] in 1965 reported finding three fetuses of various stages of development in a single sac with well-formed skeletal, intestinal and nervous parts, each having an umbilical cord attached to the host. Kimmel *et al.*[32] had earlier described a cerebral tumor containing what was thought to be five human fetuses.

In many instances, the parasitic twins can be surgically removed with survival of the host.

PRENATAL CONSIDERATIONS

We have discussed here only those cases diagnosed and treated after birth. Diagnosis is rarely made before delivery. It is conceivable that diagnosis during pregnancy could be established to assure maximal care in delivery. Gray *et al.*[21] presented the following criteria for prenatal diagnosis of conjoined twins: (1) heads are at the same level; (2) usually there is backward flexion of the spines and (3) unusual proximity of the spine, and (4) there is no change of relative position.

Fine and associates[17] described with diagrams, suggested maneuvers for vaginal delivery of intact conjoined twins and such delivery of a set of thoracopagus twins. However, with the reliability and safety of cesarean section, when conjoined twins are suspected, consideration should be given to cesarean delivery as the method of choice.

REFERENCES

1. Aird, I.: Conjoined twins—further observations, Brit. M. J. 1:1313, 1959.
2. Aird, I.: The conjoined twins of Kano, Brit. M. J. 1:831, 1954.
3. Baldwin, M., and Dekaban, A.: Cephalopagus twins seven years after separation, J. Neurosurg. 23:199, 1965.
4. Baldwin, M., and Dekaban, A.: The surgical separation of Siamese twins conjoined by the head (cephalopagus frontalis) followed by normal development, J. Neurol., Neurosurg. & Psychiat. 21:195, 1958.
5. Ballatine, R. I., and Jackson, I.: Anesthesia for separation of craniopagus twins, Brit. M. J. 1:1339-1340, 1964.
6. Barbosa, A.: Tentativa cirurgica em um caso de craniopagos, Rev. brasil. cir. 18:1047, 1949.
7. Cameron, H. C.: A craniopagus, Lancet 1:284, 1928.
8. Chan, D. P. C., and Lee, M. M. C.: A report of a case of ischiopagus tetrapus, Singapore M. J. 5:125, 1964.
9. Curtis, E.: Physiological anomaly (a study of fetus in fetu), New England J. Med. & Surg. 15:31, 1826.
10. Cywes, S., and Block, C. E.: Conjoined twins, South African M. J. 38:1817, 1964.
11. Dawson, H.: Pygopagus twins: Report of dissection of thorax, abdomen and pelvis, Am. J. Dis. Child. 68:395, 1944.
12. Dragstedt, L. R.: Siamese twins, Quart. Bull. Northwestern Univ. M. School 31:359, 1957.
13. DuBoulay, G. H.: Radiological examination of two pairs of craniopagus twins, Brit. M. J. 1:1337, 1964.
14. Eades, J. W., and Thomas, C. G., Jr.: Successful separation of ischiopagus tetrapus-conjoined twins, Ann. Surg. 164:1059, 1966.
15. Farris, J. M., and Bishop, R. C.: Surgical aspects of abnormal twinning, Surgery 28:443, 1950.
16. Ferris, Henry W.: Ischiopagus tetrapus, Arch. Path. 61:390, 1956.
17. Fine, E.; Lewis, P. L., and English, T. J.: Maneuver for vaginal delivery of intact conjoined twins, Obst. & Gynec. 24:554, 1964.
18. Fox, J. L., and Barnes, B.: Siamese twins: Case report, Delaware M. J. 22:132, 1950.
19. Franklin, A. W.: Pediatric care of craniopagus twins, Brit. M. J. 1:1342, 1964.
20. Gemmill, J. F.: An ischiopagus tripus with special reference to the anatomy of the composite limb, J. Anat. Physiol. 36:263, 1902.
21. Gray, C. M.; Nix, H. G., and Wallace, A. J.: Thoracopagus twins, Radiology 54:398, 1950.
22. Gross, R. E., and Clatworthy, H. W., Jr.: Fetuses in fetu, J. Pediat. 38:502, 1951.
23. Grossman, H. J., *et al.*: Surgical separation in craniopagus, J. A. M. A. 153:201, 1953.
24. Hall, K. O.; Merzig, J., and Norris, F. H., Jr.: Separation of craniopagus: Case report, Anesthesiology 18:908, 1957.
25. Hamilton, W. J.: A note on the embryology of twinning, Proc. Roy. Soc. Med. 47:682, 1954.
26. Hill, A. J., Jr., *et al.*: Conjoined thoracopagus twins: Pre- and postoperative considerations, J. Pediat. 58:59, 1961.
27. Holgate, J., and Ikpeme, B. J.: Conjoined twins, Brit. J. Surg. 43:626, 1956.
28. Holm, H. H.: Siamese twins: Report of delivery and successful operation, Minnesota Med. 19:740, 1936.
29. Janovski, N. A.: Fetus in fetu, J. Pediat. 61:100, 1962.
30. Jenkins, E. W.; Watson, T. R., and Mosenthall, W. T.: Surgery in conjoined twins, Arch. Surg. 76:35, 1958.
31. Kiesewetter, W. B.: Surgery on conjoined (Siamese) twins, Surgery 59:860, 1966.
32. Kimmel, O. L., *et al.*: A cerebral tumor containing five human fetuses: A case of fetus in fetu, Anat. Rec. 106:141, 1950.
33. Koop, C. E.: Personal communication.
34. Koop, C. E.: The successful separation of pygopagus twins, Surgery 49:271, 1961.
35. Lee, E. Y. C.: Foetus in foetu, Arch. Dis. Childhood 40:689, 1965.
36. Leiter, K.: Ein cranopagus parietalis vivens, Zentralbl. Gynäk. 56:1644, 1932.
37. Lewis, R. H.: Foetus in foetu and the retroperitoneal teratoma, Arch. Dis. Childhood 36:220, 1961.
38. Lord, J. M.: Intra-abdominal foetus in foetu, J. Path. & Bact. 72: 627, 1956.
39. Luckhardt, A. B.: Report of the autopsy of the Siamese twins together with other interesting information concerning their life: A sketch of the life of Chang and Eng, Surg., Gynec. & Obst. 72:116, 1941.
40. McLaren, D. W.: Separation of conjoined twins, Brit. M. J. 2:971, 1936.
41. Mortimer, B., and Kirshbaum, J. D.: Human double monsters (so-called Siamese twins), Am. J. Dis. Child. 64:697, 1942.
42. Newman, H. H.: *Multiple Human Births* (New York: Doubleday & Company, Inc., 1940), chap. 5, p. 60.
43. Ochsner, A.: Discussion of paper by Wilson and Storer[73], Ann. Surg. 145:725, 1957.
44. Ochsner, A.: "Pygopagus Twins" (motion picture, Ochsner Foundation).
45. O'Connell, J. E. A.: Surgical problems in the separation of craniopagus twins, J. Neurol., Neurosurg. & Psychiat. 25:392, 1962.
46. O'Connell, J. E. A., *et al.*: Surgical separation of 2 pairs of craniopagus twins, Brit. M. J. 1:1333, 1964.
47. Patten, B. M.: *Human Embryology* (2nd ed.; New York: McGraw Hill Book Company, 1953).
48. Peterson, C. G., and Hill, A. J.: The separation of conjoined thoracopagus twins, Ann. Surg. 152:375, 1960.
49. Potter, E. L.: *Pathology of the Fetus and Infant* (2nd ed.: Chicago, Year Book Medical Publishers, Inc., 1961).
50. Reitman, H.; Smith, E. E., and Geller, J. S.: Separation and survival of xiphopagus twins, J. A. M. A. 153:1360, 1953.
51. Riker, W., and Traisman, H.: Conjoined twins: Report of three cases, Illinois M. J. 126:450, 1964.
52. Robertson, E. G.: Craniopagus parietalis, Arch. Neurol. & Psychiat. 70:189, 1953.
53. Robertson, G. S., and McKenzie, J.: Thoracopagus twins with differing first arch defects, Brit. J. Surg. 51:362, 1964.
54. Roddie, T. W.: A case of conjoined twins, Brit. M. J. 1:1163, 1957.
55. Scammon, R. E.: Fetal Malformations, in Abt, I A. (ed.): *Pediatrics* (Philadelphia: W. B. Saunders Company, 1926).
56. Scammon, R. E.: The Surgical Separation of Symmetri-

cal Double Monsters, in Abt, I. A. (ed.): *Pediatrics* (Philadelphia: W. B. Saunders Company, 1926).

57. Schlumberger, H. G., and Gotwals, J. E.: Ischiopagus tripus: Report of two cases, Arch. Path. 39:142, 1945.

58. Sherman, R. T.; Wilson, H., and Pate, J. W.: Separation of thoraco-omphalopagus "Siamese" twins: Case report, Ann.Surg. 161:390, 1965.

59. Solerio, L.: Separation of pygopagus twins, Panminerva med. 8:153, 1966.

60. Spencer, R.: Personal communication.

61. Spencer, R.: Surgical separation of Siamese twins: Case report, Surgery 39:827, 1956.

62. Stockard, C. R.: Development rate and structural expressivity: Experimental study of twins, double monsters and single deformities, and interaction among embryonic organs during their origin and development, Am. J. Anat. 28:115, 1921.

63. Sugar, O., *et al.*: The Brodie craniopagus twins, Tr. Am. Neurol. A., p. 178, 1953.

64. *Time* (news magazine): 65:58, June 6, 1955.

65. *Time* (news magazine): 68:34, July 30, 1956.

66. Voris, H. C.: Cranioplasty in a craniopagus twin, J. Neurosurg. 20:145, 1963.

67. Voris, H. C.: Personal communication.

68. Voris, H. C., *et al.*: Successful separation of craniopagus twins, J. Neurosurg. 14:548, 1957.

69. Wijthoff, J. P.: The conjoined twins of Molenend, Friesland, Arch. chir. neerl. 9:13, 1957.

70. Wilder, H. H.: Duplicate twins and double monsters, Am. J. Anat. 2:387, 1904.

71. Willis, R. A.: *The Borderland of Embryology and Pathology* (London: Butterworth & Co., Ltd., 1962.)

72. Willis, R. A.: *Pathology of Tumours* (2nd ed.; London: Butterworth & Co., Ltd., 1953).

73. Wilson, H., and Storer, E. H.: Surgery in Siamese twins: A report of three sets of conjoined twins treated surgically, Ann. Surg. 145:718, 1957.

74. Wilson, H.: "Surgery in Siamese Twins" (motion picture, American College of Surgeons Film Library).

75. Witschi, E.: Appearance of accessory "organizers" in over ripe eggs of the frog, Proc. Soc. Biol. & Med. 31, 1934.

76. Wooley, M. M., and Joergensen, E. J.: Xiphopagus conjoined twins, Am. J. Surg. 108:277, 1964.

77. Young, G. W.: A case of a foetus found in the abdomen of a boy, M. & Chir. Tr. 1:234, 1809.

Harwell Wilson

Drawings by
Susan H. Wilkes (Figure 44-10, *A*)
Shiro Turukawa (Figure 44-10, *B*)

45

Hernias of the Abdominal Wall Other Than Inguinal

There are rare and potentially fatal failures of development in and around the umbilicus. These include the omphalocele, which is a failure of closure of the abdominal wall at the umbilical cord, with herniation of the abdominal structures into the cord; gastroschisis, which is a defect beside the umbilical cord structures without any hernial sac; and vesicointestinal fissure, which is a defect of the lower abdominal musculature in which there is extrusion of the end of the small and large bowel and bladder. New techniques of treatment have been introduced which, when appropriately employed, contribute to a low mortality rate.

In addition to these three severe neonatal lesions, there are lesser problems of the abdominal wall in the midline. Among them are diastasis recti and epigastric hernia. Inguinal hernia is discussed in Chapter 46.

Embryology

Much has been written about the embryology of the anterior abdominal wall. This was reviewed by Duhamel[6] in relation to the congenital defects seen, summing up the work of previous authors. His terminology does not entirely coincide with that of American authors.

The factors which are agreed on are that there are four tissue folds which come together in the region of the umbilicus. One fold is from above, one from below, and one from each side. Normally, these should close as the intestinal tract re-enters the abdomen from the umbilical coelom. This re-entry and closure leave the normal-appearing umbilicus, with the umbilical vessels protruding through it. It is assumed that infants with omphalocele have suffered a failure of the return of the viscera from the umbilical coelom

and at the same time a failure of closure of the umbilical ring. Inasmuch as the gastroschisis defect is actually an opening beside the umbilical cord, and is without a sac, the failure of development here must be due to some other mechanism. There has been speculation as to the origin of this defect, but no adequate explanation seems to have been agreed upon.

Diastasis Recti

A CERTAIN NUMBER of children are seen in whom the rectus muscles are spread wider than usual, leaving the fascial connection between them without a muscular component. When either distended or straining, these children have a bulging area between the two rectus muscles extending from the xiphoid down to the umbilicus. This condition is known as diastasis

recti. We have not seen clinical problems from this abnormality. The bulge is smooth on the anterior abdominal wall. It has no small neck which could strangulate tissue, and it causes no discomfort.

Presumably this redundant area could be excised and the edges could be brought together for cosmetic purposes. However, we have never seen the necessity for doing this.

A. H. BILL, JR.

Epigastric Hernia

A FEW INDIVIDUALS will be seen with a small mass presenting subcutaneously in the midline of the abdomen between the xiphoid and the umbilicus. Such a mass may be painful on straining, although it may be asymptomatic. Usually it is 1–2 cm in diameter. It may or may not be reducible through an opening.

As a rule, exploration discloses a small nubbin of fat protruding through a defect in the fascia and peritoneum, lying in the midline between the rectus muscles. Although we have not seen it in our own patients, such a hernia undoubtedly has the capacity of becoming infarcted.

SURGICAL REPAIR.—When these lesions are found, their surgical repair is quite simple provided one precaution is followed. As a preliminary to surgery, the position of the small mass must be located by a

scratch mark on the skin before the patient is anesthetized. Otherwise the mass of fat may return through its neck after the anesthetic is given, and the problem of finding the defect may be surprisingly difficult. Once the location of the mass is marked and the anesthetic administered, a transverse incision is made through the skin directly over the mass or the defect in the fascia. The sac is dissected free and the edges of the opening in the fascia are identified. The peritoneal sac can then be opened, trimmed off and closed in the normal manner. A fascial repair is then done as circumstances indicate. Depending on the axis of the defect, closure is accomplished either in a transverse or in a longitudinal direction. The edges are brought together, using mattress sutures of fairly heavy silk. Usually 3-0 silk is adequate. The subcutaneous tissue is then closed with 4-0 silk, and the skin with interrupted silk.

A. H. BILL, JR.

Omphalocele

MOORE[15] HAS DESCRIBED an omphalocele as being "a herniation of viscera into the base of the umbilical cord, with a covering membranous sac or its remnants present, and the umbilical cord inserted into the

sac." As would be anticipated from their embryologic derivation, there are many variations in the size and content of omphalocele sacs (Fig. 45-1). At its greatest extent, an omphalocele may contain liver and spleen, in addition to part of the intestinal tract. At its smallest extent, an omphalocele may be represented merely by a slight enlargement of the base of the

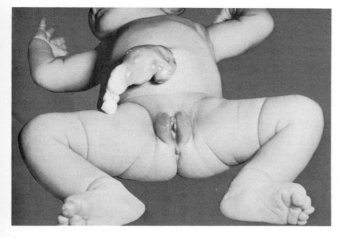

Fig. 45-1.—Omphalocele. A relatively small sac that was closed in one procedure.

umbilical cord, which may contain only a loop of small intestine. These small defects may be mistaken for a thickened umbilical cord, and the unwary obstetrician may clamp and divide the protruding bowel with the cord structures.

When the defect is large, and when it contains liver and a large portion of the intestinal tract, one must expect the intestinal tract to have the defect known as nonrotation. This will mean that the entire midgut from the duodenum back to the midtransverse colon is suspended on a single pedicle, which includes these two segments of bowel, together with the superior mesenteric vessels. Because of the lack of a broad attachment of this portion of intestine, it is subject to volvulus or obstruction of the duodenum. If the bowel has returned farther into the abdomen, there may be a partial degree of malrotation and failure of attachment.

Associated Anomalies

Each infant seen with a true omphalocele should be suspected of having associated congenital abnormalities (Table 45-1). Of the 12 patients with apparently true omphalocele observed during 1955–67 in

---

TABLE 45-1.—Associated Anomalies in 6 of 12 Cases of Omphalocele (1955–67): Children's Orthopedic Hospital and Medical Center, Seattle

Anomaly	No.
Severe cardiovascular	2
Macroglossia and organomegaly	2
Inguinal hernia	1
Cryptorchidism	1
Defect of right clavicle	1
Diaphragmatic hernia	1
Atresia of duodenum	1
Malrotation	3
Prematurity	2

---

our hospital, 2 are known to have had severe congenital defects of the heart. Two other infants had the syndrome which includes macroglossia and generalized organomegaly of the liver and pancreas. One had a defect of the right clavicle. In the severe defects, there was assumed to be some degree of malrotation or nonrotation of the bowel. This was not usually investigated unless at autopsy. In 1 case there was a diaphragmatic hernia, in 1, cryptorchidism, and in 1, atresia of the duodenum. Other defects may be present and unrecognized in infants who have survived. The anomalies listed in Table 45-1 all occurred in 6 of the 12 infants.

Treatment

Three basic forms of treatment may be used for omphalocele. In the one-stage repair, the contents of the omphalocele are reduced and the abdominal wall is brought together in layers. This is suitable when the proportion of the abdominal viscera which is out in the sac is relatively small. In the two-stage repair, skin flaps from either side of the abdomen are brought over the intact omphalocele sac as the first stage. Subsequently, the rectus muscles are brought together in a second-stage procedure. This may be facilitated by the use of pneumoperitoneum. Lastly, there is the so-called expectant treatment, in which the intact omphalocele sac is protected by various means until it is covered by an eschar. Beneath the eschar, the skin of the abdominal wall will grow over the sac with astonishing speed. During the process of this growth, the size of the herniation will diminish rapidly until almost normal configuration of the abdomen is attained. This form of treatment is essential for the huge sacs that cannot be covered by skin flaps, and may be used for the smaller ones as well.

GENERAL PRINCIPLES.—The problems faced in the treatment of some of these infants are serious. One important factor is that one cannot severely overcrowd the abdominal cavity and expect the patient to

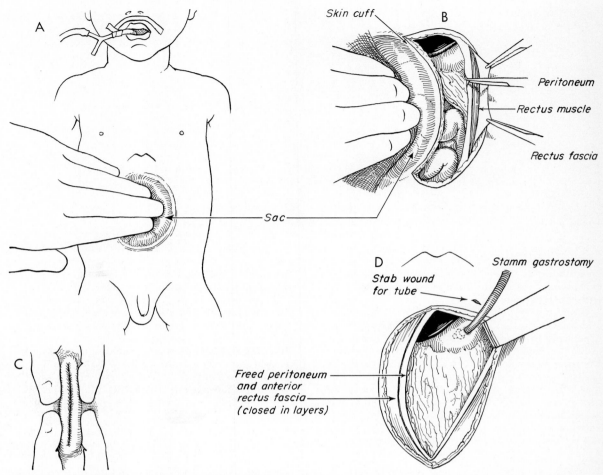

Fig. 45-2.—Omphalocele: technique of one-stage closure. **A** and **B**, with infant anesthetized and stomach empty, an attempt is made to reduce the contents of the sac within the peritoneum. If this can be done, primary closure of the abdominal wall is undertaken. **C**, the sac is trimmed off at skin level, freshening the medial edges of the rectus muscles. The umbilical vessels are divided and secured. **D**, with the abdomen open, a mushroom catheter is placed through the anterior wall of the stomach beneath two purse-string sutures and is brought out through a stab wound in the left upper quadrant. The abdomen is then closed in layers with fine suture material.

survive. If the contents of the abdomen are replaced under too much tension, the force on the abdominal contents is transmitted upward to the diaphragm, with consequent diminution of the already small vital capacity of these infants. This will lead to atelectasis and, at times, death. The pressure likewise is transmitted posteriorly to the inferior vena cava. This results in failure of return flow of venous blood from the lower body, with pooling of blood away from the heart. This may lead to circulatory failure and death. Because of these possibilities heroic abdominal closure under pressure should be avoided.

For practical purposes, when one finds a small herniation, the primary closure should be done within the first day or so. When the defect is very large, with a large herniation which contains liver, the surgeon will at times have the choice between immediate coverage with skin flaps and the expectant treatment. Some defects are so huge that skin coverage is obviously impossible, and the expectant treatment is mandatory.

Excellent results have been reported from use of the expectant treatment. Therefore this method is being used with increasing frequency, especially when there is any doubt about the possibility of success of an early operation.

Technique of One-Stage Repair

When the infant is first seen, the omphalocele sac is covered with gauze sponges moistened with antibiotic solution and the abdomen wrapped in a sterile towel. Gastric suction is instituted, and the infant is taken to surgery as soon as arrangements can be completed. In the operating room, an inlying catheter is placed in a vein. The omphalocele sac and abdomen are cleansed and draped. An attempt to reduce the contents of the sac is made after the anesthesia has been induced (Fig. 45-2). If the entire viscera can be placed in the abdomen and the edges approximated, complete closure of the abdomen should be planned.

The incision is carried around the base of the sac through the skin. The umbilical vessels are secured and divided, and the sac and its rim of skin are then removed.

A Stamm gastrostomy may then be performed for postoperative control of the patient. This is done by placing a no. 18 mushroom or Malecot catheter through the anterior wall of the stomach. This is in-

verted beneath two purse-string sutures of silk. The catheter is brought out through the left upper quadrant of the abdominal wall, and the stomach is sutured to the peritoneum around the catheter.

Next, the intestinal tract is inspected for any failure of rotation. If there are bands present which should be divided, this is accomplished. An appendectomy may be performed. If there is complete nonrotation, this should be stabilized (see later, under "Gastroschisis").

Following this, the abdominal wall is closed in layers in the usual fashion. An attempt to duplicate an umbilicus should be made at the lower end of the incision by bringing the skin together with transverse and up-and-down sutures, to leave a cruciate, puckered type of closure.

Postoperative care of these infants includes decom-

Fig. 45-3.—Omphalocele: first stage of repair. **A,** large omphalocele over which skin could be brought to cover the intact sac as first stage of repair. **B,** the skin has been dissected laterally and the edges are being approximated. **C,** completed first-stage closure of abdomen. The rectus muscles were brought together at age 1 year.

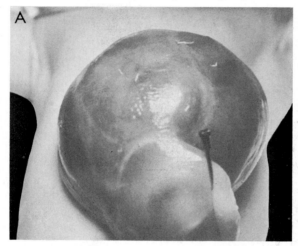

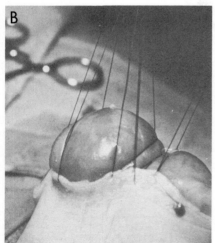

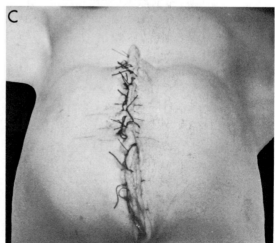

pression of the intestinal tract via the gastrostomy tube until evidence of intestinal motility is shown by the passage of one or two stools. The infant should be maintained in a heated incubator with adequate moisture. Intravenous fluids are used until the intestinal tract starts to function.

Technique of Two-Stage Operation

This procedure, starting with skin coverage, was popularized by Gross[9] in 1948. It is said to have been first suggested by Olshausen[17] in 1887. It should be attempted only when it seems likely that the skin flaps can be brought over the omphalocele sac without undue tension (Fig. 45-3). In addition, one should consider carefully the possibility that the omphalocele sac has been exposed for too long a period of time with consequent surface infection. If there is likelihood of severe tension on the skin flaps, or of infection, in all probability the conservative method should be used.

The procedure, as described by Gross (Fig. 45-4), includes first a thorough cleansing of the omphalocele sac and surrounding skin, following which the umbilical stump is excised. Following this, the rim of skin is excised from the membrane around the base of the sac, taking care to leave the membrane intact. Dissection of the skin and subcutaneous tissue is carefully carried out toward each flank, and yet not upward on the epigastrium. The latter precaution is necessary, since upward dissection may allow the liver to angulate over the chest wall. If this occurs, a later secondary repair will often be extremely difficult.

When the lateral dissections have been carried out, the raw surfaces are brought together over the intact sac, and the edges are closed with vertical mattress sutures of monofilament Nylon. The abdomen is wrapped in a firm binder, which is kept in place for 14 days, when the sutures are removed. Compression of the abdomen is then maintained by means of an elastic bandage.

The second-stage closure of the fascial planes may

Fig. 45-4.—Omphalocele: technique of first stage of two-stage abdominal repair. **A**, after thorough cleansing of the sac and surrounding skin, the stump of the umbilical cord is excised. **B**, the cuff of skin at the base of the sac is incised in a circumferential direction. The small rim of skin attached directly to the sac is removed. **C**, skin and subcutaneous tissue are dissected laterally only as far as necessary to bring the skin edges together. Too much dissection will do harm to blood supply. Dissection must not be carried up over the chest. **D**, the skin edges are approximated with everting mattress sutures. Closure is supported with a firm circumferential dressing.

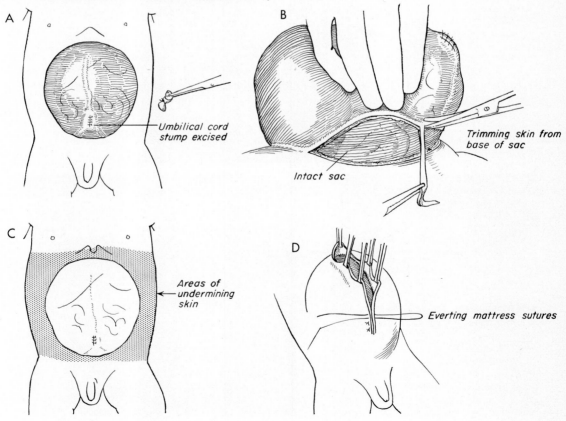

A — Umbilical cord stump excised

B — Trimming skin from base of sac / Intact sac

C — Areas of undermining skin

D — Everting mattress sutures

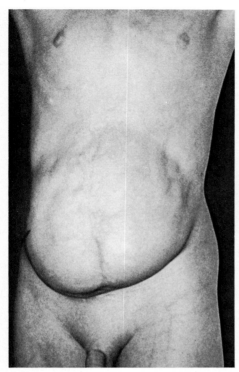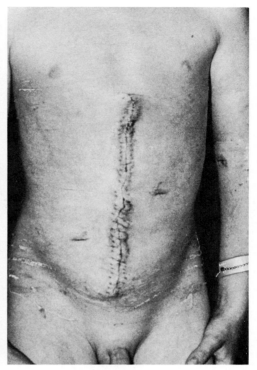

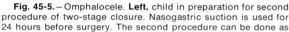

Fig. 45-5.—Omphalocele. **Left,** child in preparation for second procedure of two-stage closure. Nasogastric suction is used for 24 hours before surgery. The second procedure can be done as early as 1 year of age. **Right,** after approximation of rectus muscles and skin. Note small incisions where drains were placed.

be undertaken within the first year. Prior to undertaking the closure, it may be advisable to use pneumoperitoneum, as suggested by Ravitch.[18] He now advocates the insertion of a small polyethylene catheter into the peritoneum, with its position checked by x-rays after injection of 2 cc. of Hypaque into the tube. The tube is then left in place, and air is injected to the point of distention. Reinjections are carried out until it is felt that the abdominal wall is stretched sufficiently for closure. For 1 day prior to the secondary closure, the patient should be put on nasogastric suction.

After these preliminaries, the child is taken to surgery, and the redundant skin and sac are removed. The bowel should be checked for malrotation or nonrotation, and this should be repaired if necessary. A gastrostomy may be advisable. The abdominal wall is then closed in layers in the usual manner (Fig. 45-5).

Conservative Treatment

The conservative treatment of intact omphaloceles has been used increasingly in the past decade. Its first use is attributed to Ahlfeld[1] in 1899. In his case, he used repeated applications of alcohol to form an eschar. Grob[7] reported the conservative management

of the sac in 1957, and in 1963, he[8] described its use in 16 patients who had intact sacs. Three died, 2 of midgut volvulus and 1 of pneumonia. Wollenweber and Coe[24] described a successful case in 1959. In 1963, Drescher[5] from Poland described the use of the method in 12 cases. Seven patients survived. Four of the 5 deaths were said to be due to congenital heart disease. Bozek[3] (cited by Drescher) is said to have reported 2 successful cases in Poland in 1953. Soave[22] described its use in 6 cases without a failure.

Our own experience includes 2 successful cases, which indeed could not have been treated successfully in any other way. One was reported by Wollenweber and Coe.[24] The more recent case was of an infant girl with an enormous sac which could not conceivably have been covered by skin flaps. In addition, there was a small tear in the side of the sac, evidently incurred at birth. After an unsuccessful attempt to repair this tear, the entire sac was covered by Dacron cloth which was sutured to the skin. This was kept sterile by the repeated use of a Neosporin spray. After a month, the Dacron was removed, and healing of the skin continued over the sac beneath an eschar. Healing was complete at the end of 8 months.

We have not seen a report of rupture of the sac during use of the expectant treatment.

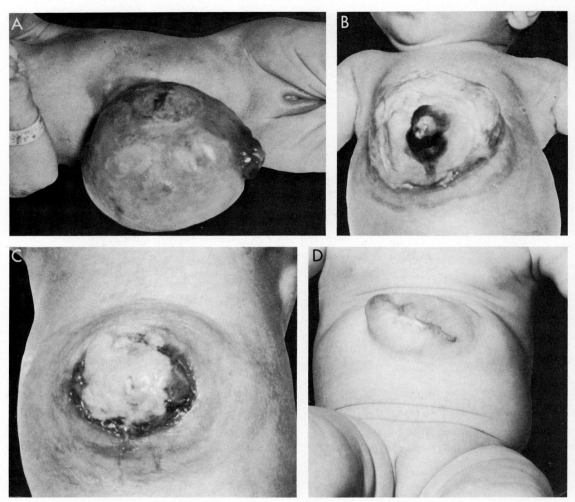

Fig. 45-6.—Omphalocele: conservative treatment. **A,** in a 6-day-old infant, the sac was so large that skin could not be brought across it. The sac was cleansed daily with aqueous Zephiran and protected with sterile polyethylene film. **B,** at age 7 weeks, note relative decrease of size of the sac and growth of skin. **C,** at age 10 weeks, the sac has thickened and been further covered by skin. **D,** the skin has come together. (See same case in Fig. 45-7.) (Figs. 45-6 and 45-7, from Willenweber and Coe.[24])

The method of management and the course of healing, as described by Grob[7], follows (Figs. 45-6 and 45-7). The cord is trimmed close to the sac. The sac is then painted with 2% tincture of mercurochrome every 4–6 hours. A thick crust develops over the sac within a few days. At this point, the frequency of use of mercurochrome is decreased. The infant is kept on his back, and if necessary the sac is supported by a doughnut type of dressing. The skin grows up and over the sac beneath the eschar. The eschar peels off as the skin grows beneath it. As this growth takes place, the sac decreases in size and flattens, and the viscera are slowly pushed back into the abdomen.

Although this method of management is said to offer the disadvantage of long hospitalization, we found it possible to let our 2 patients go home at the end of 2 months, without ill effects.

The possibility of midgut volvulus must be kept in mind. Grob lost 2 patients to this event. In 1 further case treated in our hospital, expectant treatment was tried for a month. At the end of this time, the baby began to vomit. He was explored and found to have a midgut volvulus, which was repaired. At this time the defect, which was relatively small, was closed primarily.

A. H. BILL, JR.

Drawings by
KNUTE BERGER, M.D.

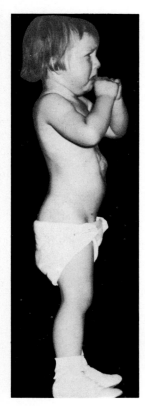

Fig. 45-7.—Omphalocele; patient shown in Figure 45-6 at age 2 1/2 years. Note how little protrusion of the defect is now present.

Gastroschisis

THIS ENTITY has been clearly differentiated from ruptured omphalocele relatively recently. Moore and Stokes[16] defined it in 1953 as being an "extraumbilical abdominal wall anomaly, in which there is a normal cord insertion, and without a sac or a sac remnant." To this we should like to add "and with nonrotation of an abnormally short midgut."

Careful inspection of these cases will show that the differentiation is a valid one. Whereas the omphaloceles all have sacs which are in the base of the umbilical cord, the gastroschisis defect is always *beside* the insertion of the cord. In our experience, it has been on the right of this structure. While many of the omphalocele patients have other anomalies, the babies with gastroschisis rarely do so. This would suggest a different time of teratogenesis.

The entity was well described by Bernstein[2] in 1940, and by others.[3,14,23] In many of the studies of neonatal umbilical defects, gastroschisis has been described as "ruptured omphalocele."

Rickham[19] in 1963 described 13 cases of gastroschisis occurring during a period when he also recorded 48 cases of omphalocele. Izant *et al.*[11] found 4 cases of gastroschisis and 39 of omphalocele. However, they listed nine of the omphaloceles as "ruptured prenatally." A critical review of 36 cases of neonatal umbilical defects at the Children's Orthopedic Hospital and Medical Center in Seattle between 1955 and mid-1967 disclosed 12 to have been omphaloceles and 24 to have been gastroschises. We are at a loss to explain the discrepancy between our figures and those reported elsewhere.

PATHOLOGIC FINDINGS

This lesion is characterized by the presence of the bowel supplied by the superior mesenteric vessels, from the duodenum to the midtransverse colon, protruding out of the abdominal cavity through a defect beside the umbilical cord. There is no sac. In our experience and that of Rickham, the defect has been to the right of the cord. As a rule, the bowel is grossly thickened and edematous. It may have a grayish exudate on its surface. The fascial defect is characteristically about 2 cm in diameter. It may be larger. Its usual small size probably accounts for the edema of the bowel. When the bowel lies kinked over the edge of the defect before birth of the baby, there is partial obstruction of the venous and lymphatic return from the bowel wall. Irritation of the serosal surface of the bowel by exposure to the amniotic fluid very likely accounts for its frosted appearance and for some of the swelling.

Critical inspection of the mass of bowel will reveal the characteristic configuration of nonrotation of the bowel. The duodenum extends to lie parallel to the mesenteric vessels, closely bound together with them and with the midtransverse colon. These three structures, duodenum, transverse colon and vessels, form a tightly circumscribed single pedicle from which are suspended the rest of the small bowel and the ascending colon. The duodenum may be compromised by the surrounding serosal covering, and the whole mass of midgut bowel is susceptible to volvulus. Autopsy studies have shown that the bowel of the midgut is considerably shorter than the bowel of an infant of comparable size with an intact abdomen. We have never seen the liver or spleen protruding through such a defect. Some of our patients had the stomach and the descending colon out of the abdomen. We have also similarly encountered the bladder and the uterus.

Emphasis has been placed in other writings on the presence of a strip of skin between the cord structures and the defect. In our experience, this strip of skin is not always present or else may be so narrow as to be negligible.

ASSOCIATED ANOMALIES

Examination of Table 45-2 will show that in the 24 cases which we have studied, there were few other anomalies recorded. There were 2 cases of atresia of the small bowel. These, and the 1 poorly described

TABLE 45-2.—Association of Anomalies in 24 Cases of
Gastroschisis: 1955–67, Children's Orthopedic
Hospital and Medical Center, Seattle

Anomaly*	No.
Nonrotation of intestine	24
Short small intestine	24
Prematurity	10
Atresia of small bowel	2
Hypoplasia of left kidney	1
Duplication of small intestine	1

*It will be seen that *all* patients had some degree of malrotation and
shortening of the bowel. These, then, should be part of the definition of
the entity. Ten patients were premature. There were three cases of other
bowel anomaly, each of which may have been mechanically induced by
the main lesion.

instance of "duplication," may have been caused by
mechanical kinking of the misplaced bowel. There
was 1 instance of hypoplasia of one kidney recorded
in an autopsy protocol. Prematurity was recorded for
10 of the 24 patients. Each of the patients had the
typical finding of nonrotation of the bowel. We regard
this as an integral part of the anomaly.

Moore[15] in 1963 reviewed 31 cases collected from
the literature and from his own experience. In this
group, he found 3 instances of atresia of the bowel.
Rickham[19] reported 2 "gross abnormalities" among his
13 cases. Ten of his patients were premature.

TREATMENT

One reason for the relatively scanty literature on
gastroschisis may have been the almost universally
fatal outcome following treatment. A few instances
of survival have been recorded following primary closure or the use of skin flaps directly over the bowel.
The first of these that we have found was reported by
Watkins[23] in 1943. Others have recorded survivals as
well.[4,10,11,15,19,21]

Until recently, the possible methods of treatment
included: closure either directly or by skin flaps; removal of the peel from the bowel and then closure,
and partial resection of the bowel with abdominal
closure. From the last method we have seen no reports of success. The reports of success with the first
two methods have been scanty.

In the fall of 1964, Schuster[21] presented a talk de-

TABLE 45-3.—Survivals among 24 Cases of
Gastroschisis: 1955–67, Children's Orthopedic
Hospital and Medical Center, Seattle

Period	No. of Cases	Survival No.	%
1955 to mid-1964	14	2	14
Mid-1964 to mid-1967*	10	7	70

*The notable improvement in survivals occurred beginning in mid-
1964, when we started to use polyethylene film reinforced with Dacron
as a temporary covering for the irreducible, edematous bowel.

scribing the use of a temporary plastic covering for
the irreducible portion of the bowel. Since that time
we have used a modification of his method of treatment. Before then, from 1955 through mid-1964
(Table 45-3), we had treated 14 patients in our institution with only 2 survivors. Since the use of Schuster's
principle, we have treated 10 patients, with 7 survivors. Two of the survivors were treated with primary
closure, and 5 by means of a temporary covering of
thin polyethylene held in place by Dacron cloth. Complete closure was accomplished as a second stage.
One of the 3 deaths was from atelectasis and menin-
geal hemorrhage in a premature. One was from complete absence of effective peristalsis at age 4 weeks,
but without infection or adhesions, following abdominal closure in two stages. Ganglion cells were present
in the bowel. The third was from perforation of the
intestine through the use of polyethylene which was
too thick and therefore had firm, traumatic edges
against the bowel.

As stated earlier, until recently the infants with
this lesion usually died. This was so because of two
factors: the edematous bowel generally harbors pathogenic organisms on its surface by the time the baby
receives surgical care. In addition, the bowel is so
thickened that in most instances it will not fit within
the peritoneal cavity. This combination generally precluded primary closure of the whole abdominal wall
or successful coverage by skin flaps.

Technique of Two-Stage Repair

The infant with gastroschisis should be brought for
definitive surgical care as soon as possible. Sponges
soaked in antibiotic solution should be wrapped
around the bowel, and the whole trunk should be
wrapped in a sterile towel during transportation.

STAGE 1.—Surgery should be carried out as soon as
it can be arranged (Fig. 45-8). A heating pad is placed
under the infant on the operating room table. An
intravenous cannula is inserted into an ankle vein.

After thorough preparation of the exposed bowel
and abdominal wall, the area is draped. The cord structures are then removed by individually ligating and
dividing them at the level of the peritoneum. It will usually now be found that the defect is too small for replacement of any of the bowel or for performance of a
gastrostomy. The defect is therefore extended upward
by means of a midline incision.

The stomach will now come into view, and a
Stamm gastrostomy is performed, using a no. 18 Malecot or mushroom catheter. The tube is brought out
through a stab wound in the left upper abdominal
wall, and the anterior wall of the stomach is sutured
to the peritoneum around the catheter.

The operator's attention should now be directed to
the base, or pedicle, of the bowel which lies outside
the defect (Fig. 45-9, *A*). The duodenum can be traced
as it enters this pedicle on the right, and the trans-

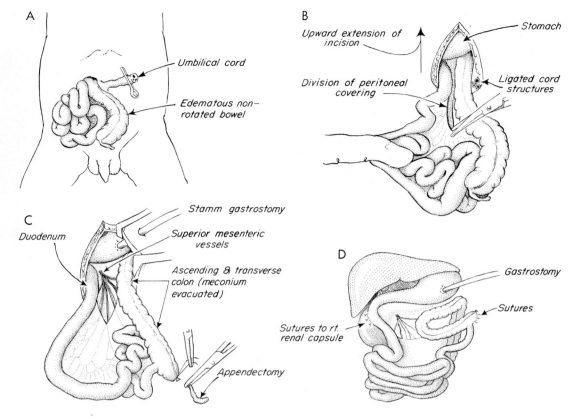

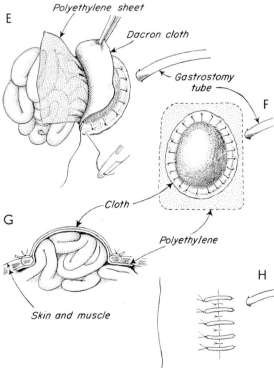

Fig. 45-8.—Gastroschisis: technique of two-stage repair. **A,** diagram showing complete nonrotation of shortened midgut, edema of bowel and thickened serosa. The umbilical cord enters the abdomen at the rim of the defect on the left. **B,** the defect is first enlarged upward. The cord is removed. The serosal covering of the pedicle of the nonrotated gut is divided on the side away from the superior mesenteric vessels. Meconium is expressed from the colon via the anus. **C,** the duodenum and transverse colon have been gently separated to give a broad base to the mesentery. This helps prevent volvulus. A Stamm gastrostomy and appendectomy are performed. **D,** method of stabilization of bowel. A few sutures are placed between the duodenum and capsule of the right kidney. The cecum may then be stabilized to the left abdominal wall or to the stomach. **E,** the edematous bowel cannot usually be wholly returned to the abdomen. To cover the excess temporarily, an "annex" is made of thin polyethylene held in place by Dacron fabric. In practice, it is best to sew the Dacron almost all of the way around and then to reduce the bowel with its polyethylene covering. The last few sutures are then put in place to hold the Dacron. **F,** anterior view of the finished "annex" sutured in place. The gastrostomy tube is also shown. **G,** cut-away diagram to show final relationship of the fabric and polyethylene film to the abdominal wall and bowel. Monofilament Nylon mattress sutures are used to hold the fabric. **H,** second-stage closure. After a week, edema of the bowel will have subsided and feedings commenced by gastrostomy. Under anesthesia, the fabric and polyethylene are removed. The abdominal wall is then closed with through-and-through heavy Nylon and individual sutures to the skin.

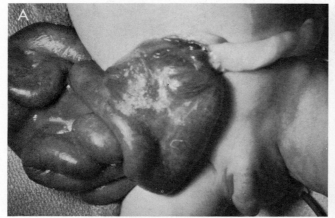

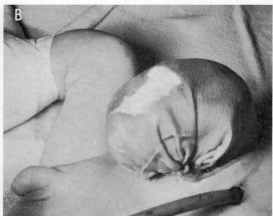

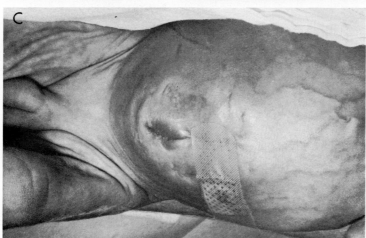

Fig. 45-9.—Gastroschisis: two-stage repair. **A,** the thickened, edematous bowel represents the entire midgut from duodenum to midtransverse colon. The cord comes from the left margin of the defect, which has no sac. **B,** infant after the initial operation. The nonrotated bowel has been stabilized. Bowel that could not be replaced is covered by thin polyethylene held in place by Dacron fabric sutured to the margins of the enlarged defect. **C,** infant after closure of the abdominal wall, done at 1 week of age, after initial edema of the bowel had subsided.

verse colon will be found to emerge from it on the left. These two portions of bowel lie closely apposed and anterior to the superior mesenteric vessels. All of these structures are bound together by a serosal covering which extends outward for some distance. The serosal covering should be divided on the antimesenteric border. The duodenum should then be dissected gently from the colon until these two lie separated anteriorly, and attached posteriorly by the spreading mesenteric branches.

An appendectomy should be performed so that acute appendicitis will not develop later with the appendix in an unusual position.

Attention should next be directed to evacuating the meconium from the colon in order to give as much space as possible within the abdominal cavity. This is done by expressing the meconium gently from the bowel out through the anus. When this has been done, the mesentery may be stabilized by tacking the duodenum to the posterior peritoneum over the right kidney and by securing the cecum to the left, either to

the stomach or to the left lateral peritoneal wall (Fig. 45-8, *D*). This then gives a broad attachment of the mesentery which prevents volvulus.

With these simple measures completed, an attempt is made to place the bowel into the abdomen and to close its wall. In most cases, the abdominal wall cannot be closed primarily. In these instances, a piece of sterile, thin, pliable polyethylene film is placed over the protruding bowel, and its edges are tucked within the peritoneum (Figs. 45-8, *E–G*; 45-9, *B*). It is important that the film be pliable and soft. Since this film will not hold sutures, a suitable fabric, such as a piece of sterile Dacron or cotton fabric, is then secured to the edges of the defect with interrupted Nylon sutures. This fabric can be of the ordinary type, bought from a department store. This holds both the polyethylene and the bowel in place.

Postoperatively, the gastrostomy tube is placed to straight drainage until peristalsis is established. Until then, the infant is maintained on intravenous fluids. Wide-spectrum antibiotics are administered in the intravenous fluids during this period. The infant is kept in an incubator with adequate heat and humidity. The cloth covering and the abdomen are sprayed with Neosporin solution at intervals.

STAGE 2.—At the end of 7–10 days, the infant will usually have established normal feeding. Infection, if any, will be under control. At about this time, the sutures holding the fabric to the rim of the abdominal defect will have begun to give way. Pressure on the protruding mass of bowel within the "annex" of polyethylene and cloth will show that it can be compressed down to the level of the abdomen.

After 12 hours without feeding, and with the gastrostomy tube to drainage, the infant is returned to the operating room. Under anesthesia, the fabric and polyethylene are removed. The edges of the defect are trimmed and then closed in one layer, using interrupted through-and-through 3-0 Nylon sutures (Fig. 45-8, *H*). The skin is protected by running these through short lengths of plastic intravenous tubing as the sutures cross the incision. The skin edges are accurately approximated with fine sutures.

Following the second procedure, the infant is again maintained on intravenous fluids and decompressed via the gastrostomy tube. As a rule, his intestinal function will soon return, and he will begin to gain weight with an intact abdomen.

SUMMARY

1. Gastroschisis is an abdominal defect beside the insertion of the umbilical cord. There is no sac. Through it projects the nonrotated, short, midgut segment of bowel, which is usually grossly edematous.

2. Infants with this defect are frequently premature, yet they rarely have other congenital anomalies.

3. Until recent years, the surgical treatment of this defect has been largely unsuccessful.

4. The principle suggested by Schuster has greatly improved the outlook for survival. He suggested the temporary covering of the edematous bowel with thin plastic, held in place by fabric, until the edema subsides. Abdominal closure is then carried out at the end of a week.

REFERENCES

1. Ahlfeld, F.: Der alkohol bei der beihandlung inoperabeler bauchbrücher, Monatschr. Geb. Gynäk. 10:124, 1899.
2. Bernstein, P.: Gastroschisis, a rare tetratological condition in the newborn, Arch. Pediat. 57:505, 1940.
3. Bozek, J.: Observations concerning the treatment of umbilical hernia, Pediat. pol. 28:1125, 1953.
4. Cavenaugh, C. R., and Welty, R. F.: Gastroschisis: Report of four cases, Northwest Med. 64:33, 1965.
5. Drescher, E.: Observations on the conservative treatment of exomphalos, Arch. Dis. Childhood 38:135, 1963.
6. Duhamel, B.: Embryology of exomphalos and allied malformations, Arch. Dis. Childhood 38:142, 1963.
7. Grob, M.: *Lehrbuch der Kinderchirurgie* (Stuttgart: Georg Thieme Verlag, 1957).
8. Grob, M.: Conservative treatment of exomphalos, Arch. Dis. Childhood 38:148, 1963.
9. Gross, R. E.: A new method for surgical treatment of large omphaloceles, Surgery 24:277, 1948.
10. Hutchin, P.: Gastroschisis with antenatal evisceration of the entire gastrointestinal tract, Surgery 57:297, 1965.
11. Izant, R.; Brown, F., and Rothmann, B. F.: Current embryology and treatment of gastroschisis and omphalocele, Arch. Surg. 93:49, 1966.
12. Johnson, A. H.: Omphalocele and related defects, Am. J. Surg. 114:279, 1967.
13. Koons, F. W.: A case of embryonal ectopia intestinalis, J. Kansas M. Soc. 35:136, 1934.
14. Krauss, F.: Zwei seltene Missbildungen, Deutsche med. Wchnschr. 62:258, 1936.
15. Moore, R. C.: Gastroschisis with antenatal evisceration of intestines and urinary bladder, Ann. Surg. 158:263, 1963.
16. Moore, T. C., and Stokes, G. E.: Gastroschisis, Surgery 33:112, 1953.
17. Olshausen, R.: Arch. Gynäk. 29:443, 1887.
18. Ravitch, M. M.: Giant omphalocele, J.A.M.A. 185:42, 1963, and personal communication.
19. Rickham, P. P.: Rupture of exomphalos and gastroschisis, Arch. Dis. Childhood 38:138, 1963.
20. Sauvage, L. R., and Bill, A. H., Jr.: The congenitally malformed: III. Omphaloceles and gastroschisis defects, Northwest Med. 64:672, 1965.
21. Schuster, S. R.: A new method for the staged repair of large omphaloceles (preprint from the author).
22. Soave, F.: Conservative treatment of giant omphalocele, Arch. Dis. Childhood 38:130, 1963.
23. Watkins, D. E.: Gastroschisis, Virginia M. Month. 70:42, 1943.
24. Wollenweber, E. J., and Coe, H. E.: Conservative management of eventration in the newborn, with survival, Am. J. Surg. 97:769, 1959.

A. H. BILL, JR.

Drawings by

KNUTE BERGER, M.D.

Umbilical Hernia

AN UMBILICAL HERNIA results from incomplete closure of the fascia of the umbilical ring through which intra-abdominal organs can protrude. Skin covers the area.

ETIOLOGY.—By the tenth week of embryonic life, the abdominal cavity is large enough to admit extruded viscera into the abdominal cavity proper. The particular anatomy of the umbilical cord at birth explains in part the cause of hernia at this location. The cord at birth is a firm structure and the umbilical ring is closed by vascular structures present and by Wharton's jelly. As involution takes place in these structures, a defect of varying size can occur.[1]

Premature infants have a high incidence of umbilical hernia, varying from 84% in newborns weighing 1,000 – 1,500 Gm to 20.5% in those weighing 2,000 – 2,500 Gm.[3] Woods[5] found an increased incidence of umbilical hernia in infants weighing 3,200 Gm or more at birth. He held the view that the persistent defect may be due to the huge size of the cord. A definite familial tendency has been noted by a number of authors, but any condition such as chronic cough, constipation and ascites which increases the intra-abdominal pressure may be the cause of the umbilical hernia. Diseases such as cretinism, mongolism and gargoylism are often associated with umbilical hernia.

Incidence. — There is a very high incidence of umbilical hernia in Negroes. Crump[2] reported that in Negro infants under 1 year of age the incidence was 41.6%; this decreases steadily to 15.9% at the age of 4 years and is essentially zero after 8 years of age. Until the true natural history of umbilical hernia is properly evaluated, not only in infancy and childhood but into adulthood, there will be confusion as to the proper time for operative cure.

Diagnosis. — In the infant and child there is obvious fullness at the umbilical region with an excessive amount of loose skin over the defect, and when the child cries or strains this protrusion of viscera into the hernial sac becomes more apparent. Small bowel entering the hernial sac is easily reducible by palpation and is accompanied by a gurgle. The size of the defect in the fascia varies from 0.5 to 3-4 cm. In infancy, the extent of protrusion of the umbilical hernia is much more pronounced in colored infants than in white. In a small percentage of patients, there is a diastasis recti which may be confined to the first inch above the umbilical ring but can extend along the midline to the ensiform.

Treatment

The incidence of incarceration or strangulation is very rare in infants and children, and I have seen only 3 patients who had to be operated on because of a true incarceration of small bowel in the hernial sac. At operation, the small bowel was cyanotic, but when the umbilical ring was enlarged and hot packs were applied to the bowel wall, the color returned to normal within a few minutes. The operative closure of the defect was successful.

Much has been written about strapping the umbilical hernia in infants. No doubt strapping relieves the anxiety of the mother but appears to be of little benefit to the infant in hastening closure of the ring. The umbilical ring normally shows a progressive contraction during the first 18 months of life. The good results attributed to strapping probably would have happened without strapping. Furthermore, the use of adhesive tape is not successful because the adhesive slips after a few days even though the skin is painted with tincture of benzoin. The skin easily becomes excoriated and the hernia does not remain reduced. During the past 10 years we have used no strapping of any type. The process of umbilical ring contracture should be explained to the parents, because our patients have all been more comfortable without strapping.

The indications for surgical repair of an umbilical hernia must be evaluated on an individual basis. Only in those infants under 18 months of age who have evidence of partial small bowel obstruction by reason of the small bowel entering the hernial sac which has a neck of 2 cm. or less in diameter, or those in whom the hernia is associated with abdominal cramps, especially after meals, should surgical repair be advised. There is no unanimity of opinion as to the ideal time for elective repair of an umbilical hernia in infants and young children. Until the natural history of umbilical hernia is known, we can recommend a general rule for elective surgical repair: If there is protrusion and the fascial defect measures 1.5 cm or larger at the age of 24 – 36 months, we believe surgical repair is warranted. If an umbilical hernia exists in a female infant at 3 years, surgical repair seems indicated because of a possibility of a recurrence during pregnancy or in later life when many of these women become obese and the abdominal wall has been stretched, and when the threat of a strangulating umbilical hernia can evolve into a lethal lesion. We have seen incarceration of a uterine fibroid during pregnancy, necessitating emergency surgical repair in the eighth month of pregnancy.

Operative Technique

The surgical repair of umbilical hernia in infants and children is illustrated in Figure 45-10. The incision is placed on the inferior border of the neck of the protrusion and superiorly if there is an associated diastasis recti which can also be easily repaired. The umbilicus should always be preserved and can be in infants and children. There is no indication for its removal, as is sometimes done in the repair in adults. The fascial defect can be closed longitudinally or transversely. If silk sutures are placed closely, recurrence is a rarity. The dressing applied in the operating room consists of a sterile ball of cotton which is kept in place by an Elastoplast dressing. This approximates the loose umbilical skin to the underlying fascia and eliminates the collection of serum. The entire dressing is not disturbed for 1 week, at which time the operative wound is nicely healed. Most of these patients can be discharged from the hospital the day after operation, and they are not restricted in their normal activities.

In Gross's[4] series (1940 – 51), a total of 439 umbilical hernias were operated on with no deaths and only 1 recurrence, which was secondarily repaired satisfactorily. In the Clinic at the Children's Hospital of Michigan, approximately 350 patients a year are seen with umbilical hernia.

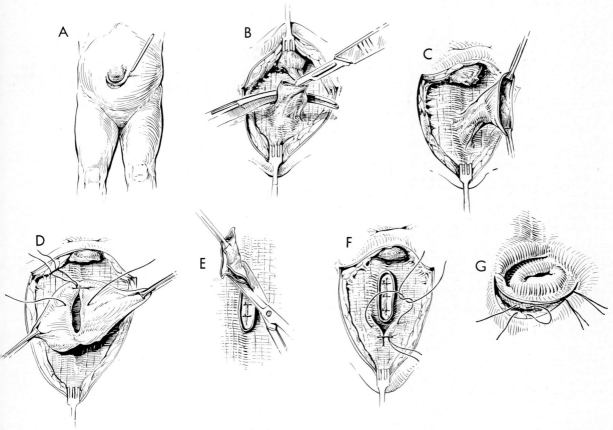

Fig. 45-10.—Umbilical hernia: technique of repair. **A,** curved incision of inferior margin of the umbilicus. **B,** sac is freed from attachment to the skin. **C,** the sac is opened and cleared of overlying fat. **D,** the peritoneum (hernial sac) is closed by interrupted 3-0 chromic catgut sutures. **E,** excess sac is excised. **F,** edges of rectus sheaths are approximated by 4-0 silk sutures. **G,** skin edges are approximated by subcuticular 4-0 plain catgut sutures.

During the past 5 years, 241 patients have been operated on for umbilical hernia, with 1 recurrence which was subsequently repaired. One boy, aged 7 years, had a rupture of an existing umbilical hernia following trauma to the abdomen. The small intestine immediately protruded through the umbilicus, requiring an emergency laparotomy and umbilical herniorrhapy. There was no operative mortality in this entire group.

REFERENCES

1. Cresson, S. L., and Pilling, G. P.: Lesions about the umbilicus in infants and children, Pediat. Clin. North America 6:1085, 1959.
2. Crump, E. P.: Umbilical hernia: Occurrence of the infantile type in Negro infants and children, J. Pediat. 40:214, 1952.
3. Evans, A. G.: The comparative incidence of umbilical hernias in colored and white infants, J. Nat. M. A. 33:158, 1941.
4. Gross, R. E.: *The Surgery of Infancy and Childhood* (Philadelphia: W. B. Saunders Company, 1953).
5. Woods, G. E.: Some observations on umbilical hernia in infants, Arch. Dis. Childhood 28:450, 1953.

C. D. Benson

Drawings by
Robert Mohr

46

Inguinal Hernias

HISTORY.—Galen in 176 A. D. stated: "The duct descending to the testicle is a small offshoot of the great peritoneal sac in the lower abdomen (*processus vaginalis*)."[108] Paré, in about 1540, stated that in children an operative cure may be achieved according to "the first intention" without infection, but after childhood this is not possible.[99] During the 18th and 19th Centuries in over 500 carefully studied infant autopsies, a 56% incidence of potential hernia or patent processus vaginalis was found (Table 46-1). From these studies has developed a rational means of management and cure for this developmental anomaly.

A present-day operation for repair of hernia in childhood was advocated by Banks[5] in 1884, and Felizet[38] in France in 1894 reported on 51 children from 5 weeks to 6½ years of age operated on by this technique. In 1889, Hamilton Russell[102] strongly defended the saccular theory of hernia against scathing opposition of the leading anatomist of the day[63] and favored the simple operative approach. MacLennan[78] and Hertzfeld[54] in England and Coles[22] in the United States avoided repair of the posterior wall of the canal and were content with high ligation of the sac.

In 1950, Potts, Riker and Lewis[93] gave strong support to the principle of simple ligation and removal of the sac for routine repair of hernias in pediatric patients. Many are following in their footsteps. The pendulum has swung between early and late repair, and now, repair when the hernia appears is generally advocated.

EMBRYOLOGY, ANATOMY AND PATHOLOGY

During the third month, when the embryo is about as long as a thumb, the peritoneum lining the abdominal wall protrudes outward at the internal ring to form a pocket or diverticulum or sac, the processus vaginalis.[1] This little sac follows into the scrotum the course of the gubernaculum, which is a small cord of tissue extending from the base of the testicle. At this time, the testicle is within the abdominal cavity. In the female, the processus vaginalis is called the canal of Nuck and follows the round ligament which extends from the ovary to the labia. In the male, the processus vaginalis rarely extends to the scrotum unless followed by the testis.[58] The processus is in open communication with the abdominal cavity during intrauterine development of the baby. Even at the time of birth, it remains open in 80–94% of examined bodies[16,96,103] (Tables 46-1 and 46-2). Closure takes place with increasing frequency during the ensuing year. Even at the end of the first year, the processus vaginalis was open or partly open in 57% of the bodies examined by Sachs.[103] Contralateral exploration at the time of repair of unilateral hernia by Minton and Clatworthy,[80] Kiesewetter[66] and others[21,57,77,85,101,113] have confirmed the earlier observations as applied at least to children who already have a hernia on one side. Although the open processus vaginalis provides the congenital defect which is the basis of hernia in childhood, a hernia does not exist until some part of the abdominal contents is pushed into the open sac.[127] This is a point that is difficult to explain to parents.

When or if the open processus will close unaided by surgery is another matter. It is true, however, that a completely or partly open processus vaginalis has been found in adult autopsy sepcimens without clinical evidence of hernia in from 15 to 37% of several

TABLE 46-1.—PROCESSUS VAGINALIS IN INFANCY, FROM AUTOPSY SPECIMENS

AUTHOR	No. OF BODIES*	AGE	OPEN† No.	%
Campers, 1785	17	0	16	94
Engel, 1857	100	0–14 days	90	90
Zuckerkandl, 1877	100	0–3 mo.	37	37
Fére, 1879	146	0–18 mo.	62	42
Sachs, 1885	155	0–1 yr.	88	57
Cricks	32	0–2 yr.	17	53
Total	550	0–2 yr.	310	56

*Includes number of bodies with either one or both sides involved.
†Partial or complete.

TABLE 46-2.—PROCESSUS VAGINALIS IN INFANCY FROM AUTOPSY SPECIMENS—H. SACHS[103]

No. OF BODIES	AGE	OBLITER- ATED, *%	PARTLY OPEN, %	COM- PLETELY OPEN, %	OPEN OR PARTLY OPEN, %
27	0–10 days	20	19	61	80
40	10–20 days	50	32	18	50
15	20–30 days	47	23	30	53
25	1–2 mo.	36	34	30	64
22	2–3 mo.	36	39	25	64
13	3–4 mo.	65	16	19	35
13	4 mo.–1 yr.	69	27	4	31
155	0–1 yr.	43%	29%	28%	57%

*Refers to bodies with either one or both sides involved.

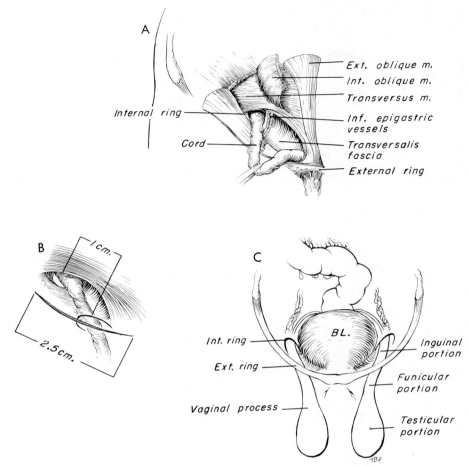

Fig. 46-1.—A, the inguinal canal of the older child is similar to that of the adult. Shown are the internal ring, the oblique nature of the canal, the opened fascia of the external oblique, the transversalis fascia forming the posterior wall and the cord in normal position. **B,** in early infancy. the internal and external rings are as marked and the distance between them is only 1 cm (about 1/2 in.) This is the full length of the canal. Often the external ring lies directly over the internal ring, so that the length of the canal is identical with the thickness of the body wall. The length of the skin incision is shown for comparison. **C,** drawing of a photograph of a young baby, from Sachs.[103] The processus vaginalis is seen as an extension of the abdominal cavity surrounding the testes, which are in the scrotum. Peristence of this processus is the congenital basis for complete inguinal hernia. Lack of obliquity of the canal and close proximity of the bladder to the internal ring are clearly shown.

hundred specimens (Engel,[36] 37% in 100 bodies; Ramonéde,[96] 15% in 215 bodies; Morgan and Anson,[82] 20% in 100 half-bodies.

The processus vaginalis always lies in an anterior medial position in relation to the spermatic cord or round ligament. As it passes through the abdominal wall and along the inguinal canal, the muscular and fascial coats from the transversus muscle and the internal oblique surround it, forming the so-called inguinal bursa. The muscle slips from the internal oblique form the overlying cremaster, which is the first layer to be dissected away in exposing the sac. The close intimacy of the sac and its coverings with the cord and the vas deferens requires care and delicacy in the separation of the sac, so that the all-important vessels and vas will not be injured.

The detailed anatomy of the inguinal canal is familiar to the surgeon and will not be discussed further (Fig. 46-1, A). It is important to emphasize, however, that in infancy the canal is extremely short and has not developed an oblique direction through the abdominal wall (Fig. 46-1, B and C). The external ring is almost directly over the internal ring.[22,59,62] It averages 12 mm (1/2 in.) in length.[12] Many surgeons used the Mitchell-Banks operation with excellent results. This technique depends on the anatomic fact that the canal is short and straight and that the sac can be pulled out through the external ring without

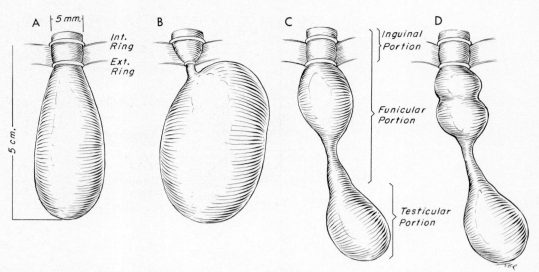

Fig. 46-2.—Processus vaginalis; various forms, from postmortem dissections of young infants by Sachs. **A,** locations of the internal and external rings are indicated. Length of the entire processus vaginalis is about 5 cm. **B,** obliteration of the proces-sus just distal to the external ring will result in a large hydrocele. **C** and **D,** obliteration of the processus in its midportion will result in potential incomplete hernia (the usual type of inguinal hernia).

Fig. 46-3.—Development of hernias and hydroceles. **A,** extension of the peritoneal cavity to the base of the testicle through the internal and external rings of the inguinal canal. This is the processus vaginalis, which ordinarily is completely obliterated except for its distal portion, which surrounds the testicle as the tunica vaginalis. **B,** the process of obliteration. **C,** obliteration of the processus vaginalis just distal to its junction with the peritoneum and again obliteration just proximal to the testis. This re-sults in hydrocele of the cord. **D,** partial obliteration of the major portion of the processus, with fluid passing from the peritoneal cavity into the dilated distal portion of the processus, forming a communicating hydrocele. **E,** obliteration of the processus just proximal to the testis. The opening, in this instance, allows for passage of intestinal contents into the processus vaginalis, re-sulting in the usual type of hernia.

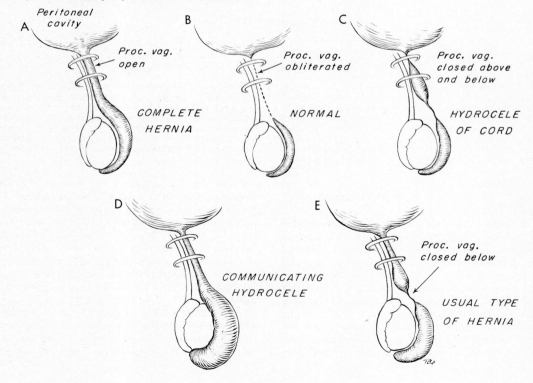

dividing the ring, so that a high ligation of the sac can be obtained by this method. As the child grows and becomes a few years old, however, the canal lengthens, and this technique becomes less desirable on an anatomic basis, as pointed out by Turner[117] in 1912.

Much study has been given the mode of natural *obliteration of the processus vaginalis,*[89] but the initiating causes, the key to which may at some future time eliminate the need for the surgeon's knife, have not been found. A study of the steps (Figs. 46-2 and 46-3) in the process of obliteration does provide an understanding of (1) the complete or scrotal hernia, (2) the formation of the tunica vaginalis of the testis, (3) the encysted hydrocele, (4) the communicating hydrocele, and (5) the most frequent and usual type of inguinal hernia (called incomplete or funicular, or just inguinal).

The *content of the hernial sac* in infancy is usually small intestine and rarely omentum, but the testis, and the overy, tube and uterus[2,4,12,32,44,50,67,71,100, 105,114,118,121,124] are not infrequent occupants. Emphasis on the sliding nature of the last-mentioned type of hernia would seem to be important, as described by Goldstein and Potts,[50] Swenson,[114] and others.[18,44] The presence of the cecum[26,54,95] and even the acutely inflamed appendix[31,84] and Meckel's diverticulum[3,68,76,121] has been reported several times. The older literature contained reports[54,78] of bright yellow, tiny bodies in an occasional sac which on microscopic section were found to be adrenal rests. Tuberculosis of the sac in association with tuberculous peritonitis was fairly common in the past[43,78,121] but now is not mentioned. Chamberlain[18] reported certain other rare conditions. Among these was a cyst

lined with epithelium surrounded by smooth muscle extending from the internal ring. Studies by J. L. Bremer proved this to be the remnant of a müllerian duct.

INCIDENCE

Herniorrhaphy is the operation most frequently performed on infants and children by the general surgeon. Its performance is exceeded in frequency only by tonsillectomy. When the incidence of hernia is tabulated by decades, peaks come in the first and third 10-year periods with a lowered frequency in the second decade.[127] When the age of patients with hernia admitted to a pediatric hospital is recorded (Fig. 46-4), it is obvious that the largest number appear in the first year of life. In further considering only those which occur in the first year of life, if the age at which the hernia was first noted is recorded (Fig. 46-5), it is evident that the greatest number occur during the first month, and that 80% have been noted by the end of the third month. These statistics are taken from Fraser's book, *Surgery of Childhood*, written in 1926.[43] We can find no such extensive observations in the literature before or after the printing of this book. Parenthetically, it should be noted that the evidence provided here is good that these hernias are congenital, that is, they are present at birth or at least potentially present, and that the major proportion of them can be repaired during the first 3 months of life.

The actual incidence of hernia in the childhood population has been recorded variously from 0.8%[88] to 4.4%.[64] The former figure was derived from a study of 130,243 patients under 5 years of age at the Hospital for Sick Children, Great Ormond Street, London,

Fig. 46-4.—Age at herniorrhapy in 1,794 patients from five series,[20,30,33,67,72] representing a wide distribution of hospitals and size of series and giving a composite picture. One series with

several years included in one figure was averaged. Patients over 12 were excluded (possible calculated error, 2%).

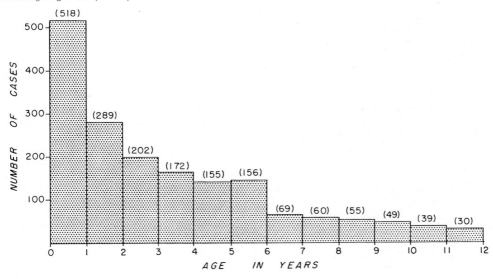

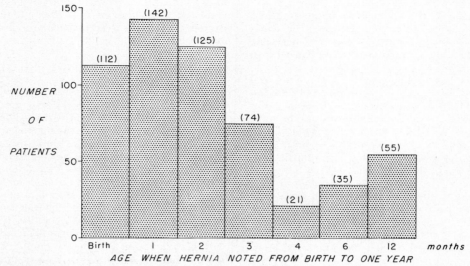

Fig. 46-5.—Age of occurrence of 564 inguinal hernias during the first year of life (from Fraser[43]). Between birth and the end of 1 month, 254 (45%) hernias were noted. This is more than 10 times the number occurring in the fourth month. By the end of the third month, 453 (80%) of the hernias had been noted.

and the latter was estimated by Sir Arthur Keith. Herzfeld,[54] studying 16,250 new cases in the outpatient department, found an incidence of 13% of inguinal hernias. In McLaughlin's[77] study of 24,000 admissions, there were 521 inguinal hernias, or a little over 2%. Recent estimated incidence varies slightly from those of the past.[69] The over-all incidence of inguinal hernias in *prematures* is recorded as 4.8% in the largest series that could be found in the literature.[48] Additional studies of prematures are certainly indicated.

The influence of *sex* in the incidence of hernia is obvious from Table 46-3, which shows that boys are afflicted about nine times more frequently than girls. Of each 100 hernias, about 90 will be in boys and 10 in girls. The adverse influence of the descending testis on the closure of the processus vaginalis may explain the increased susceptibility of the male to hernia. In this regard it is interesting to note that when infants are separated from older children, there are 14 times as many boys as girls,[30] whereas among older children there are only five times as many boys as girls.

The more recent series of children's hernias reported give the frequency according to *side*. Some of the larger series have been combined in Table 46-3. In contrast, in reports of adult hernias, the side is infrequently mentioned, yet this information is important in answering the question regarding repair of the contralateral side in a child with a unilateral hernia. The rough formula for sides in children is 60-25-15, that is, 60% right-sided, 25% left-sided and 15% bilateral. Further refinements are necessary in dealing with the problem of the sides in females and in prematures. There is some evidence that bilateral hernias are considerably more frequent in girls.[48] The largest series of Gross[52] and that of Goldstein and Potts[50] show an incidence of bilaterality of 17.5 and 21% respectively. In *prematures*, bilaterality was 47.7% in one series[20] and 19% in another.[49]

DIAGNOSIS

Inguinal hernia is recognizable at birth as a bulge in the groin which may occur with the first cry or may not appear until weeks, months or years later. In the groin of a child, a mass which comes and goes with straining must be a hernia. Increased abdominal pressure from coughing, a tight phimosis and meatal stricture are other instigating causes. The hernial bulge has a tendency to be absent in the morning and to appear during the day. The majority are recognized by the parent, the pediatrician or attending physician. Rarely, an actively retractile testis drawn upward to the external ring may mistakenly be considered to be a hernia by the mother or unwary physician. The surgeon confirms the presence of the mass when the child cries or strains or by gentle pressure on the abdomen. When the child is older the hernia can usually

TABLE 46-3.—Sex and Side from Birth through 12–15 Years: Compilation of Statistics from 12 Authors*

		Male	Female	Right	Left	Bilateral
No. of cases	6,025	5,322	703	3,558	2,658	809
Per cent	100	88	12	59	28	13

*From ref. 15, 20, 21, 27, 28, 30, 33, 72, 77, 86, 87, 105.

be made to come down by activity or lifting. At times, however, it is necessary to base the diagnosis on a reliable history alone, for the dangers of delay in repair may outweigh the possibility of error. At the same time that a diagnosis of hernia on one side is made, the other side should be carefully examined, and if none is found the mother is so informed.[92]

Symptoms referable to hernia, such as evidence of pain, irritability, colic or incarceration, were present in 24% of the infants and 13% of the older children studied by Potts, Riker and Lewis.[93] The hidden or suspected hernia in infancy[106] may explain many a feeding problem or the cause of irritability in a child.

The first part of the *physical examination* should be a careful inspection of both groins, exposed so that any slight prominence of one side can be seen. In the very well-nourished infant, the eyes may be better than the hands in recognizing a small lump beneath a thick layer of adipose tissue. On palpation, thickening of the cord or the sensation of silk rubbing together when the examining finger is rolled over the cord in the region of the external ring[52] may aid the astute clinician in making the diagnosis. Statistically, however, palpation has not proved reliable even in expert hands.[48]

It can be difficult and even impossible to differentiate between *hydrocele* and hernia in a small baby, and repeated examinations may be necessary. Usually, however, an oblong, nontender, nonreducible, asymptomatic, light-transmitting mass along the cord or a collection around the testicle can be easily recognized as a hydrocele.[92] Of course, both hernia and hydrocele may be present at the same time. The differentiation is important. Hydrocele should not be operated on until the child is at least 4 months old, since it may disappear spontaneously.[70] If the mass is reported to enlarge during the day, or when the baby cries, even though the mass transmits light, it is a hernia of the communicating type[22] and should be operated on. Aspiration should *not* be used to differentiate the two in any circumstance because of the danger of perforating the bowel and producing peritonitis. Hydroceles of the cord or around the testicle are found in 15%[52] or more[20] of groin operations on pediatric patients. Hydroceles around the testicle almost always[20,22,93] are of the communicating type and coexist with a hernia, although at times no communication can be demonstrated.[20,27]

Femoral hernia, though rare, must be looked for. Many reported series of hernias in children[27,47,54,72] contain at least one example or more; therefore the pediatric surgeon must not exclude it from his mind. With the child standing, it is best demonstrated as a protrusion beneath the inguinal ligament. It can be missed in infants at operation unless one is wary.[79] *Direct hernias* tend to be large, with a palpable defect at Hesselbach's triangle. They do not descend into the scrotum. They are infrequently encountered although reported in many series, often in association

with exstrophy of the bladder and other anomalies.[15,23,28,61,87,105] Fonkalsrud *et al.*[42] reported on 25 patients with femoral and inguinal hernias, with a correct diagnosis made in only 8.

In male patients with suspected hernia, it is always important to check the scrotum for an absent or *undescended testis*, which occurs in about 6% of patients with hernia (Table 46-4). The testis at the external ring may be mistaken for an incarcerated hernia. The surgeon must know and inform the parents before operation whether or not he must also deal with a maldescended testis. Furthermore, the undescended testis is more subject to torsion of the cord than the normally placed one. The condition and torsion of an appendix testis may be difficult to differentiate from an *incarcerated hernia*.

In girls, a hernia may be discovered as a small nubbin the size of a marble at the external ring. It is often not reducible but still is not tender and causes no symptoms unless efforts are made to reduce it.[9] These findings provide a presumptive diagnosis of incarcerated hernia and require early operation. It is also important to remember that what may seem to be an ovary in the hernial sac of an otherwise normal-appearing girl, on rare occasions at operation may represent testis[24,46,50,120] (see later discussion under Inguinal Hernia in Girls).

TABLE 46-4.—INCIDENCE OF UNDESCENDED TESTES IN HERNIAS OF CHILDHOOD

AUTHOR	HERNIAS, No.	UNDESCENDED TESTES No.	%
Bonner	201	16	8
Duckett	380	15	3.9
Herzfeld	894	32	3.2
Kurzweg	100	4	4
Snyder & Chaffin	1,987	134	6.7
Total	3,562	201	5.6

TREATMENT

The main problems of treatment center on the *infant* with a hernia. If the baby is ill or under par and not gaining weight, or is premature, many surgeons consider a truss useful. In such circumstances, operation probably should be deferred until the condition is corrected or unless an emergency in relation to the hernia arises. The local anesthesia should be considered in repair, using 1/4 of 1% xylocaine sparingly. With these exceptions, all other hernias should be repaired when they are noted, regardless of age. This statement would have been radical according to the standards of 1940[91] and would have been very bold in 1950.[6,61]

It is true that Ladd[73] in 1941 stated that he operated on hernias when they came to him; however, neither he nor Gross specifically made this recommendation in their textbook of that time.[74] From a review of the current literature, most surgeons and pediatricians seem to agree with our statement today and would advise operation when the diagnosis is made. Furthermore, the parents of these little children suffer as much or more than the child. They will be glad of the change in the attitude of the profession. There may be some who would operate on the newborn child or premature infant before he begins to gain weight and others who would still prefer to delay operation on the tiny infant. Even we would agree with the latter attitude, unless the surgeon and anesthesiologist have had considerable experience with the surgery of infancy. As Chamberlain[18] stated, "only rarely is this procedure as easy to carry out as it sounds, sometimes because the neck of the sac is large and sometimes because the sac is firmly adherent to the spermatic cord, but most often because of the extreme fragility of the wall of the sac." There will surely be a rebound to the present enthusiasm for early operation unless it is performed by an experienced team.

TRUSS. – In most centers, the use of trusses has been given up entirely[97] and perhaps should not even be mentioned in an up-to-date book on pediatric surgery; there are, however, situations in which the infant cannot be admitted to the hospital. In these circumstances, when a hernia is bothersome or has been temporarily incarcerated, especially when the patient is a newborn before weight gain has begun, or is premature, or is ill, he may be benefited by a truss which may tide him over until he can be admitted to the hospital for operation. The disadvantages of skin irritation and pressure, false sense of security[6] and the occurrence of incarceration even while the truss is in place[75] have convinced most physicians that it is an unsatisfactory means of managing hernia. Several forms of trusses have been devised.[91] The solid or inflatable rubber horseshoe type was widely used in England.[6,14,109] The yarn truss is readily available. It is formed by taking a skein of yarn about 1 in. thick and encircling the baby's waist with it. A knot is then made with another piece over the area of the hernia, and this piece brought between the legs and fastened posteriorly so that pressure is applied over the internal ring, just lateral to the pubis. This must be kept snugly in place at all times and changed only as necessary for cleanliness.

CORRECTION OF INSTIGATING CAUSE OF HERNIA. – As a rule, crying and straining cannot be prevented. It is important, however, to check for the existence of phimosis or meatal stricture because their correction is possible and necessary.[49,54,93] Boland[10] cited the case of a baby seen in World War I with massive bilateral bulging hernias and extreme phimosis treated by circumcision alone. Twenty years later, a picture and letter confirmed the fact that this child, now free of hernias, had grown to manhood without operation for hernia having been performed. The benefits may be overstretched in this case, but the importance of phimosis and meatal obstruction as instigating causes of hernia is real.

Operative Repair

PREPARATION FOR OPERATION. – Although the operation has been performed as an outpatient procedure in over 1,000 consecutive cases[54] with only 1 death, admission of the child to the hospital the day before operation is advisable. Complete examination and routine laboratory studies are performed. If there is any suggestion of an upper respiratory tract infection or premonitory signs of disease, the child is sent home for a later appointment.

OPERATION. – The anesthetic agents and methods used depend on the experience and skill of the anesthesiologist. Whatever is used, relaxation is essential to safe repair in most instances. Drop ether,[112] safe and satisfying for many years, has been replaced by intratracheal anesthetic gases in many centers.

As stated by Russell[102] in 1899, the principle involved in the operation is ligature and removal of the sac. Actually, ligation and excision of a portion of the sac is satisfactory. This concept is based on the belief that the defect to be repaired is the open sac. When high ligation of the sac is accomplished, the defect is closed by this means and the hernia repaired. The close proximity of the transversalis fascia to the neck of the sac soon fills in whatever additional defect other than an open peritoneum there may be, and recurrences are not a problem. The infrequent massive or direct hernias require repair of the abdominal wall defect, and here closure of the transversalis fascia and the conventional hernia repairs used in adult surgery may be necessary. For the routine case, however, repair of the posterior wall of the inguinal canal, by the Bassini technique, is considered to be unnecessary. Still widely used is the Ferguson technique,[40] which leaves the cord undisturbed and closes and reinforces the posterior wall with the attachment of the internal oblique and conjoined tendon to the inguinal ligament over the cord and under the fascia of the external oblique[52,97,114] Potts and his co-workers[93] deserve much credit for emphasizing the satisfactory results of the simplified technique for the benefit of the present generation of surgeons.

CONTRALATERAL REPAIR. – This topic is of current interest. The basis of the proposal for repairing the opposite side when a unilateral hernia exists, especially a left hernia, is the frequency with which observers[21,48,65,77,85,101,119] have noted persistence of the processus vaginalis when the other side is explored. An additional reason is the appearance of a second hernia at a later time after one side has been repaired. Studies made thus far,[15,20,21,27,28,56,75,77,87] when tabulated, have indicated that after 3,026 hernia repairs, 142 patients (5%) have returned for repair of the other side. In one series, patients were followed up to 20 years[75] and in another series 3–5 years.[28] A comprehensive study of this sort was made by Clausen *et al.*[21] of 97 patients followed 10–28 years. In this group, 16% returned for repair of a second side. In 1959, Kiesewetter and Parenzan[66] reported

237 cases of infants with unilateral hernia followed for 9 years; of these, 77 (31%) became bilateral. A report by Santulli and Shaw[104] in 1961 indicated the incidence of involvement of the other side to be 12% in a large, carefully followed series. Further studies are indicated to clarify the actual risk of involvement of the contralateral side. A final reason for repairing the other side is that if it is not involved by young adulthood, it may be later in life. Complete statistics on this point are not obtainable. In a study of 500 hernias at all ages, but mostly in adults, McVay[79] found that bilateral hernias, including the 5% with previous unilateral repair, accounted for only 20% of the group. In an earlier study, Erdman[37] found 26% bilateral. Clausen *et al.* found that 24.2% of 1,000 indirect *adult* hernias were bilateral and that 4% of these had their inception in childhood. Furthermore, they studied 100 patients with indirect inguinal hernias who were *more than 60 years of age*; 33 had bilateral involvement but none had had a previous operation in childhood.

At this point we, if not the reader, have become burdened with statistics. The position which seems most tenable today is that in an *infant*, unless there is evidence that the other side is involved either from the history or by the finding of a second hernia on examination, it is best to repair only the side with the hernia. DeBoer and Potts[29] added further weight to this position with an excellent review of 100 personal cases of infants under 2. Nine per cent required contralateral surgery in a 10-year follow-up.

Gilbert and Clatworthy[48] threw real doubt on the success of predicting which groins will contain a patent processus vaginalis on the basis of thickening and the "silk test." Furthermore, even if the surgeon finds a patent processus vaginalis at operation, this does not mean that a hernia will develop because of patent processus vaginalis is present in 57% of normal babies up to 1 year of age (Table 46-2). Even granting the high incidence of involvement of the other side found by Kiesewetter and Parenzan, it would mean that 3 infants would have to have a bilateral repair in order to prevent 1 infant from having a second side operated on. In the hands of the average surgeon, including us, increasing the length of anesthesia, subjecting many infants to an unnecessary procedure with minimal but certain definite hazards (see Complications) does not seem justified as a routine.

Technique for Repair of Infant Hernia and Hydrocele

A transverse incision 2–4 cm long is made over the lowest flexion crease of the abdomen. The medial end of the incision is begun at a point above and just lateral to the pubic spine (Fig. 46-6, *A*). The incision is made as long as is necessary to give good exposure. It is longer in chubby babies and older children, and it will become shorter as one gains experience. The subcutaneous tissue is transected and the bleeding

points ligated. The superficial layer of fascia (Scarpa's) has more substance to it relatively than it does in adults. It must not be mistaken for the fascia of the external oblique. The latter fascia is incised and the external ring exposed just lateral to the pubic spine. The fibers which form the boundaries of the ring (pillars) and the anterior margin of the ring itself are easily exposed with the blunt end of the knife as the edges of the wound are gently pulled away with retractors. An incision is then made in the fascia of the external oblique. This is most safely accomplished by inserting a small blunt hemostat under the fascia beneath the anterior margin of the ring (Fig. 46-6, *B*). Care should be taken to avoid injury to the ilioinguinal nerve as it lies just beneath the fascia. In small babies, we open the fascia of the external oblique in the direction of its fibers for a distance of 1/2 in. (1 cm) starting on the anterior margin of the external ring, which gives ample exposure of the internal ring. By some surgeons[27,70,93] in all patients, and by us in older infants and young children, the external ring is left intact and the incision in the fascia of the external oblique made just above the ring (Fig. 46-6, *C*). In either event, the cord and the coverings over the sac are exposed without further mobilization. The fibers of the cremaster muscle overlying the sac and the underlying spermatic fascia can be separated from the surface of the sac (Fig. 46-6, *D*). The sac always lies on top of the vas deferens and to its lateral side. By picking up the sac with a small hemostat, it can be separated by delicate sharp and blunt dissection from the cord and vas without damage to either. Special care must be taken not to injure either the vas with its tiny blood supply or the small blood vessels in the cord. When the sac is freed, a small hemostat can be placed on either side and the sac transected (Fig. 46-6, *E*).

The distal end is now examined. If a *hydrocele* is present, it can be delivered into the wound and widely opened. It is believed that this is important, although ignored by some.[22] In the presence of a large hydrocele, it may be necessary to aspirate some of its fluid content before it is brought into the wound. The bottle operation, or sewing the edges of the hydrocele behind the testicle, is not used. If the distal portion of the sac is narrow, as in a communicating hydrocele, the sac is opened down to the testicle and a portion of the sac excised. The entire sac is not usually removed unless it is small, and thus far we have not encountered postoperatively recurrent or persistent hydroceles, although Duckett[33] saw such an occurrence when the entire sac was not removed.

Final attention is directed to the proximal portion of the sac. Several clamps are placed on the margin of the sac and it is lifted upward (Fig. 46-6, *F*), and with fine scissors or with a knife its remaining attachments with the cord are separated. We have not twisted the sac as an aid to its separation from the cord, as suggested by Potts, Riker and Lewis. This method, however, can be utilized, especially when the

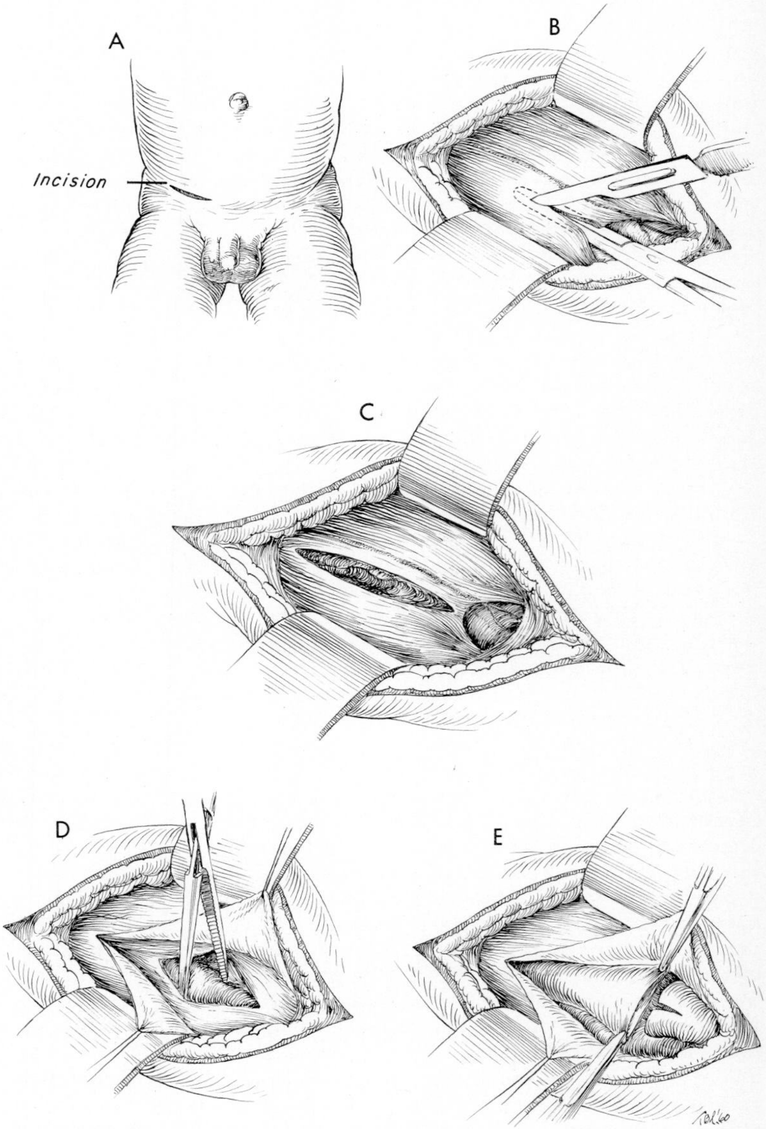

Fig. 46-6.—Inguinal hernia and hydrocele: techniques of repair. **A,** the incision in the distal flexion crease of the abdomen is 2-4 cm long and extends laterally from a point just above the pubic spine. **B,** the superficial fascia has been incised and the external oblique exposed. A small hemostat has been inserted under the anterior aspect of the external ring. Fascia of the external oblique is being incised in the direction of its fibers for a distance of 1 cm. The inguinal nerve, seen just above the hemostat, is carefully avoided. We use this technique in young infants. **C,** the external oblique has been excised. The incision in its fibers is made proximal to the external ring, leaving it intact. The incision gives adequate exposure of the hernial sac and cord. This technique is especially applicable in older infants and children. **D,** the external oblique fascia is turned back, exposing the cremaster muscle and internal spermatic fascia overlying the sac and cord. The sac is being exposed by separating these two covering layers. **E,** the sac extending through the canal and external ring has been separated from the cord below. It has been transected. The distal end has been partly opened. The proximal end will be ligated high in the neck of the sac. (*Continued.*)

sac is narrow. When the yellowish fat overlying the bladder comes into view on the medial aspect of the sac, seen best when the sac is open one is assured that he has secured a high point in the sac for ligation. Beyond this level, however, the bladder may be damaged. The sac is ligated with two stick ties of 4-0 arterial silk ligatures. The excess is trimmed off, but a little less than a 0.5 cm stump is left to prevent the ligature from slipping. The sac is dropped back, the fascia of the external oblique closed with 4-0 silk or chromic catgut sutures exactly as it was, so that the external ring will not be too tight (Fig. 46-6, *G*).

The wound is carefully checked for bleeding points, especially along the cord. One or two interrupted 4-0 chromic catgut sutures close Scarpa's fascia, and the skin is closed with 5-0 chromic subcuticular sutures. We prefer these even to white silk because they are absorbed and so far have never needed removal (Fig. 46-6, *H*). A tiny dressing is preferred to collodion.

Preperitoneal approach.—This approach has been utilized by Shandling and Thomson[107] and is an application of the Cheatle-Henry procedure to the repair of hernias in infants and children. In their hands, it has been very satisfactory.

Results of repair of reducible inguinal hernia.—The over-all results in all series, large and small, are excellent. The mortality is almost zero. The only deaths in this group would be from the in-

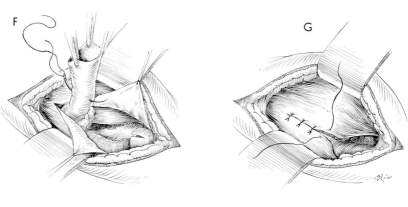

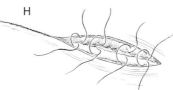

Fig. 46-6 (cont.).—F, the proximal end of the sac has been lifted up. The retroperitoneal fat pad, which is always present and indicates a proper point for high ligation, is shown. A 4-0 silk suture is passed through the neck of the sac under direct vision to avoid inclusion of any abdominal content. After the suture is tied around the neck of the sac, a second suture is placed just distal to the first to ensure permanent ligation. **G,** the fibers of the external oblique are closed with 4-0 silk sutures exactly as they were before incision. **H,** 5-0 chromic catgut sutures are placed in the subcuticular sutures, resulting in hairline approximation. Knots are tied on the undersurface to prevent extrusion into the incision.

herent dangers of any anesthetic and the exceedingly rare possibility of an overwhelming infection. Complications in expert hands are rare. The known recurrences of hernia have averaged less than 1%.

Complications

Because the sac is thin and friable, it can be torn so that the ligation is incomplete. This is especially true in incarcerated hernias and justifies delay for 24–48 hours after successful conservative reduction of such hernias before instituting a definitive repair. Incomplete ligation of the sac may result in recurrence. Damage to the arterial supply of the testis by injury to the internal spermatic artery or artery to the vas deferens may result in atrophy.[65,81,122] The vas deferens must be protected from injury at all times during the operation because transection or clamping may result in sterility on the operated side. In infants, the bladder is high and may overlap the internal ring, as pointed out by Campers in 1785. Its close proximity makes incision into it an ever-possible, though infrequent, complication. The dangers from such an accident, if it occurs, can be eliminated almost completely by recognition and careful vesical closure. Wound hemorrhage and hemorrhage extending into the scrotum with a scrotal hematoma can be avoided almost completely by meticulous ligation of all bleeding points at the time of operation. Wound infections do occur but can be kept at an absolute minimum by rigorous aseptic technique.

Respiratory complications are infrequent. In a series of 942 reducible hernias analyzed by Wiklander [123] they constituted 4%. In 183 patients less than 1 year of age the rate was 8%. None of these infections was serious, and the real and potential danger of in-

carceration offsets the increased susceptibility to respiratory trouble. Operation safely eliminates the distress to the child, anxiety to the mother and dangers of strangulation and infarction of the testis. Today, therefore, it is nearly the unanimous opinion that in the healthy child, with experienced anesthesiologists and surgeons, operation should be performed when the diagnosis is made.

INGUINAL HERNIA IN GIRLS

A separate discussion of this aspect of hernia in childhood is warranted.[2,32,44,50,121,124] Many reports have been made of the presence of adnexa and uterus in the hernial sac[4,12,35,51,105] (Fig. 46-7. *A*). In a study at the Childrens Hospital of Los Angeles,[71] it was found that the incidence of incarceration among 351 hernias in females was 14%, which is considerably higher than the incidence among males (3.7%) in this institution. The contents of the sac at operation in 51 girls with incarceration are indicated in Table 46-5. Although the adnexa were badly damaged in some cases and in one the ovary actually appeared black, all were returned to the abdomen. There was no mortality. For actual unequivocal gangrene, excision would be necessary[31,67,90] but we agree with Donovan and Stanley-Brown[32] that the need for it is certainly rare.

One aspect of female hernias recently stressed is the *sliding nature* of many of them. In about 25%,[28,44,50] the broad ligament or vascular pedicle actually makes up part of the wall of the sac. Lateral incisions are made through the wall of the sac on either side of the vascular pedicle and this tongue of tissue turned into the abdomen, so that high ligation of the sac may be accomplished,[18,44,50] or the sac is ligated below the

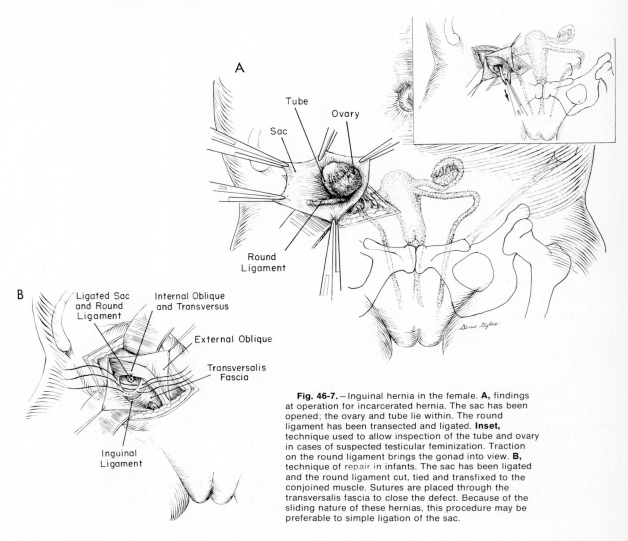

A

Tube

Sac

Ovary

Round
Ligament

B

Ligated Sac
and Round
Ligament

Internal Oblique
and Transversus

External Oblique

Transversalis
Fascia

Inguinal
Ligament

Fig. 46-7.—Inguinal hernia in the female. **A,** findings at operation for incarcerated hernia. The sac has been opened; the ovary and tube lie within. The round ligament has been transected and ligated. **Inset,** technique used to allow inspection of the tube and ovary in cases of suspected testicular feminization. Traction on the round ligament brings the gonad into view. **B,** technique of repair in infants. The sac has been ligated and the round ligament cut, tied and transfixed to the conjoined muscle. Sutures are placed through the transversalis fascia to close the defect. Because of the sliding nature of these hernias, this procedure may be preferable to simple ligation of the sac.

sliding portion and then turned in with a multiple purse-string suture[114] or simply ligated distal to the sliding portion, the excess of the sac removed and the stump dropped back and the transversalis fascia closed snugly with interrupted sutures (Fig. 46-7, *B*). At the Childrens Hospital of Los Angeles, the last method has been used with 1 known recurrence in 351 female pediatric patients with hernia.[71]

TESTICULAR "FEMININIZATION."—This is an uncommon condition occurring once or twice in every 100 "girls" with an inguinal hernia.[45,60] The external genitalia are entirely female and the vagina is normal or slightly shortened; the cervix, uterus and fallopian tubes are, however, absent and the gonad is grossly and histologically a testis. Estrogen secretion is entirely adequate for a most desirable feminization at puberty. Normal marital relations are to be antici-

pated. Menstruation and fertility, of course, are not to be expected. Inguinal hernias are present in 80% of the patients with testicular feminization.[53] The surgeon therefore has the opportunity and responsibility of occasionally making the diagnosis. In some centers,[45] buccal smears are taken as routine before operation, and if chromatin bodies are not found, the condition can be predicted.[125]

Examination of the external genitalia shows no ambiguity whatever. In about 19%, a gonad can be palpated in the labia.[53] It may be possible by rectal examination to demonstrate that the uterus is not present. A vaginal examination is often not feasible except under anesthesia, but this or a vaginogram will reveal absence of the cervix. This history of sterile aunts is confirmed in many cases but usually not until the condition has been discovered.

TABLE 46-5.—Incarcerated Inguinal Hernia in Female Infants and Children: Childrens Hospital of Los Angeles*

	Cases	
Content of Sac	No.	%
Ovary only	28 ⎫	
Ovary and tube	16 ⎬	94.0
Ovary and small bowel	4 ⎭	
Small bowel only	1	2.0
Omentum	1	2.0
Organs (not described)	1	2.0
Total	51	

*From Kristiansen and Snyder.[71]

At operation, the diagnosis can be made if a testicle, confirmed by biopsy, is found in the inguinal hernia sac, as stated by de Quervain[94] in 1923. If the gonad is not present in the sac, it can usually be brought into view by gentle traction on the round ligament (Fig. 46-7, A). If either a tube or an ovary is found, testicular feminization is ruled out.

When the diagnosis is made at the operating table, in our opinion, the gonad should be returned to the abdomen and the hernia repaired. It is our practice to delay gonadectomy until after feminization has occurred.[8] Endocrine function is then provided artificially. Gonadectomy is indicated to prevent carcinoma in the retained testis (8% in collected series).[53,83]

IRREDUCIBLE HERNIA

An incarcerated hernia is one in which the contents of the sac are held or retained outside the abdomen. It does not refer to changes in the blood supply of the retained part nor to the intestinal obstruction usually produced. A *strangulated* hernia is one that is tightly constricted and has become or is likely to become gangrenous. In pediatric patients, in contrast to adults, incarceration unrelieved almost always leads to death from gangrene of the part[115] or from intestinal obstruction.[15] Incarceration in adults often is tolerated for years. Thus, according to the definition in pediatric patients, almost all incarcerated hernias will become strangulated. At what point in their progress the term strangulation is to be applied varies with the author, from the presence of actual gangrene[115] to beginning vascular changes.[19,110] Evidence of vascular change, that is, strangulation, includes cyanosis, edema and ecchymosis of the bowel wall and mesentery. Deep red or black discoloration of the bowel wall also is considered evidence of strangulation whether or not the color returns sufficiently to avoid the need for resection. With this interpretation, about one half of the surgical cases[19,110] fall into this classification.

The *diagnosis* of an irreducible hernia, incarcerated or strangulated, is usually evident because of the sudden appearance of a mass in the groin or scrotum that does not reduce spontaneously, is tender and often painful. Aspiration of such a mass is contraindicated because of the possibility of perforating the bowel wall and thus increasing the likelihood of infection. Nausea and vomiting appear in about 50% of the patients. Some children show distention of the abdomen and x-rays may indicate dilated loops of intestine in the abdomen and at times in the scrotum.[19] The *differential diagnosis* includes diarrhea and vomiting of unknown cause, intestinal obstruction and pyloric stenosis. Incarcerated hernia is by far the most common cause of intestinal obstruction from the end of the first week of life until the fourth month, being much more common than intussusception during this period.[36] In addition, acute lymphadenitis of the groin must be considered occasionally, but an evident source of infection and the usual lateral position of the nodes help make the differential diagnosis. Torsion of the testis and appendix testis may rightly be confused, because pain and swelling are common in both conditions. Actually, a hidden small incarcerated hernia may accompany torsion or infarction of the testis.[7] Abscess of the scrotum, although rare, must be considered.[28]

The *frequency* of incarceration in childhood is surprisingly great. Potts, Riker and Lewis[93] found that of 38 infants admitted below 4 months of age, 26% had or had had incarceration. When the entire pediatric age group is considered, the incidence varies from 1.6 to 18% (Table 46-6). When the patients are grouped by years,[110] 24% occur in the first year, and when by month, 59% in the first 3 months[98,115] (Table 46-7). These facts strongly support the present trend toward repairing hernias when they are diagnosed, regardless of age. Not all incarcerations can be prevented, however, by this aggressive approach as incarceration may be the first manifestation of hernia in from 21% of the cases according to Wiklander[123] to 50% according to Clatworthy et al.[20]

TABLE 46-6.—Irreducible Hernia: Incarceration, Strangulation

	No. with Hernia	Irreducible		Reduced by Suspension when Used	Males	Gangrene	Mortality from Irreducibility
		No.	%	%	No.	%	%
Thorndike and Ferguson	1,740	106	6	75	96	4.7	2.8
Gross	3,874	63	1.6				
Clatworthy	940	134	14.2	50	96	1.4	.7
Rendle-Short		45			98		11.0
Smith	546	50	9.1	75	96	4.7	2.0
Wiklander	1,053	111	10.4		98	0	0
Fevre		164		50	91	3.7	1.2
DeBoer	2,110	379	18.0	83		.8	.3

TABLE 46-7.—INCIDENCE OF ALL HERNIAS WHICH BECAME IRREDUCIBLE IN EACH AGE GROUP

AGE IN YEARS	No. CASES*	IRREDUCIBLE HERNIA		AGE IN MONTHS	IRREDUCIBLE HERNIA No. Cases†	
		Cases	%			%
0 - 1	121	29	24	1-2-3	53	59
1 - 2	85	7	8.2	4-5-6	22	25
2 - 3	101	6	6.0	7-8-9	12	13
3 - 4	49	2	4.2	10-11-12	3	3
4 - 5	41	3	7.3			
5 - 6	32	1	3.0	Total for first		
				12 mo.	90	100

*From Smith.[110]
†From Thorndike and Ferguson[115] and Rendle-Short.[98]

MANAGEMENT.—Incarceration means the sudden appearance of a hernia that does not reduce by ordinary means. It may reduce while the patient is being brought to the hospital or after he has been given the proper dose of morphine or a barbiturate by rectum. It may slip back when he is placed with his head down on a bed at about a 20° angle and held there by a loose hitch of muslin around his ankles. It is also well to place a cold pack over the hernia for an hour or two. Following this regimen, reduction may take place when a little gentle and never forceful pressure is applied, or the hernia may be reduced only after the patient is given an anesthetic before surgery begins, or it may not be relieved until the surgeon's knife frees the constriction at the external or internal ring. At operation, if the intestine slips back before it can be examined and its viability assessed, it may be necessary to explore the abdomen, depending on the severity of the findings. This can be accomplished by extending the hernia incision laterally and incising the transversalis fascia and peritoneum, or by the LaRoque maneuver. This is simply performed in the infant and leaves the internal ring intact. (See Cryptorchism in Chapter 76.)

A second incision can be made, but this is usually not necessary or advisable. If the intestine is bluish or black and does not recover after release and after 5–10 minutes of observation, resection of the damaged bowel and end-to-end anastomosis is necessary. In 106 cases reported by Thorndike and Ferguson,[115] resection was necessary in only 4. A similarly low incidence of resection was reported by Smith.[110] A black or bluish testis or ovary is not necessarily an indication for resection (see Infarction, below). Return of the ovary to the abdomen and the testis to the scrotum is the rule.

Some of these incarcerations are violent from the start. The little patient whines, whimpers, cries or screams, and the crying may be almost continuous. This suggests a tight constriction. If examination discloses in addition to the lump or scrotal mass considerable edema and redness of the tissues, if there is a history of vomiting and if distention is present, or x-ray evidence of dilated loops, if there is blood in the stool[87] or if any of these findings are sufficiently convincing, it is essential, after preparation of the child, to proceed with operative relief without delay. Even then, most surgeons are willing to utilize conservative methods of reduction, as mentioned above, concomitantly with preparation for operation. We found no reported deaths when conservative reduction was induced with the above methods, regardless of the duration of symptoms.[19,28,41,52,98,110,115,123] In most cases, it would not be wise to utilize more than an hour for gastric suction and administration of fluids and electrolytes before operation is undertaken. Two or 3 hours can be safely used in most cases of incarceration.

Because of the occasional presence of an acutely inflamed appendix[31,75,84] or Meckel's diverticulum[3,126] in the sac as a part of the incarceration, and also for fear of reducing gangrenous bowel, some surgeons[75,77] do not favor conservative measures. But we concur with most writers on the subject who utilize the aforementioned methods in the majority of cases. The difficulties due to the edematous friable tissues make one shy away from operation without such a trial in most cases in view of the excellent results obtained with the above regimen.

An elective herniotomy should be performed within 48 hours after conservative reduction. If there is any doubt that the hernia has been reduced, if the scrotum or testicle or lower abdomen remains tender after apparent reduction, operation had better not be delayed.[98]

Infarction of the Testicle

That incarcerated hernia can produce infarction of the testis without torsion of the cord has long been mentioned in the literature.[7,17,28,74,92,116] In 1951, Wiklander[123] reported an incidence of severe irreversible circulatory impairment of the testis in 12% of 111 cases of incarceration. Sloman[109] in 1958 reported 8 infarctions in 53 patients (15%) with incarcerated hernia under 2 years of age. Evidence of infarction is obtained at the time of operation when the testis is severely discolored or black and from follow-up examination that reveals atrophy. That atrophy is due to the incarceration per se is evident from the findings at operation and from the fact that atrophy is rare after operation for reducible hernia.[28,65,122,123]

In the main, management at the time of operation is replacement of the testis in the scrotum. Except in unusual circumstances[14] this seems safe, and ordinarily it is not necessary or wise to remove the testicle. Several patients handled in this way have done well, and a few have not even shown atrophy in the ensuing years.[28,92,109,123] Again, early operation can be expected to eliminate this condition in at least one-half the cases.[123] It will be difficult to eliminate if the first manifestation of hernia is an episode of incarceration.

RESULTS.—Strangulated and incarcerated hernias are serious and without treatment death is certain. Under the regimen described here the mortality varies from 0.3 to 11% (Table 46-6). About 3 out of 4 can be reduced by nonoperative means so that a safer operative procedure can be performed 24–48 hours later. Bowel resection or removal of the testis or adnexa is seldom required, but the morbidity in terms of increased distress, lengthened hospital stay, increased incidence of infection and hazards of recovery is greatly increased. The incidence of testicular infarction with resulting atrophy is considerable.

REFERENCES

1. Arey, L. B.: *Developmental Anatomy* (5th ed.: Philadelphia: W. B. Saunders Company, 1946).
2. Arnheim, E. E., and Linder, J. M.: Inguinal hernia of the pelvic viscera in female infants, Am. J. Surg. 92:436, 1956.
3. Baillie, R. C.: Incarceration of a Meckel's inguinal hernia in an infant, Brit. J. Surg. 46:459, 1959.
4. Bancroft, P. M.: Inguinal ectopia of the ovary, J. Pediat. 26:489, 1945.
5. Banks, W. M.: *Notes on Radical Cure of Hernia* (London: Harrison & Sons, 1884).
6. Barrington-Ward, L.: The hernia problem in children, Practitioner 159:376, 1947.
7. Bennett-Jones, M. J.: Strangulation of the testicle by a hernia in infancy, Liverpool M. -Chir. J. 45:121, 1937.
8. Blizzard, R. M., and Money, J.: Discussion of article by Gans, S. L., in Gellis, S. S. (ed.): *Year Book of Pediatrics, 1963-64* (Chicago: Year Book Medical Publishers, Inc.).
9. Blomquist, H. E.: Hydrocele of canal of Nuck simulating strangulated hernia, Nord. med. 41:651, 1949.
10. Boland, W. K.: In discussion of Schiebel and Freeman.[105]
11. Bonner, R. A., Jr.: The hernia problem in children (a review of 236 hernias treated in two Waterbury hospitals), Connecticut M. J. 16:160, 1952.
12. Boothroyd, L. A.: Strangulated adnexa in infantile hernia, Canad. J. Surg. 2:311, 1959.
13. Brayton, D.: Personal communication.
14. Browne, D.: Abdominal hernia in childhood, Brit. M. J. 2:1144, 1952.
15. Bruton, O. C., and Seeley, S. F.: The surgical treatment of inguinal hernia in infants and children, U.S. Armed Forces M. J. 2:1075, 1951.
16. Campers, P.: *Kleinere Schriften* (Leipzig: Siegfried Crusius, 1785).
17. Cedermark, J.: Infarction of testis, Acta chir. scandinav. 78:447, 1936.
18. Chamberlain, J. W.: Anomalies and accidents complicating repair of inguinal hernias in infancy and childhood, Boston M. Quart. 7:23, 1956.
19. Clatworthy, H. W., Jr., and Thompson, A. G.: Incarcerated and strangulated, inguinal hernia in infants: A preventable risk, J.A.M.A. 154:123, 1954.
20. Clatworthy, H. W., Jr.; Gilbert, M., and Clement, A.: The inguinal hernia, hydrocele and undescended testicle problem in infants and children, Postgrad. Med. 22:122, 1957.
21. Clausen, E. G.; Jake, R. J. and Brinkley, F. M.: Contralateral inguinal exploration of unilateral hernia in infants and children, Surgery 44:735, 1958.
22. Coles, J. S.: Operative cure of inguinal hernia in infancy and childhood, Am. J. Surg. 69:366, 1945.
23. Coley, B. L., and Hoguet, A.: *The Encyclopedia of Medical and Surgical Specialties* (Philadelphia: F. A. Davis Company, 1939).
24. Cook, J.: Testes as contents of hernial sacs in two "female" children, Brit. J. Urol. 22:211, 1950.
25. Cricks: Cited by Hessert.[55]
26. David, V. C.: Sliding hernias of the cecum and appendix in children, Ann. Surg. 77:438, 1923.
27. Davis, C. E., Jr.: The surgical treatment of inguinal hernia in infancy and childhood—changing concepts, Virginia M. Month. 80:431, 1953.
28. DeBoer, A.: Inguinal hernia in infants and children, Arch. Surg. 75:920, 1957.
29. DeBoer, A., and Potts, W. J.: Inguinal hernias in children, Arch. Surg. 86:1072, 1963.
30. de C. Pinto, V. A.: Inguinal hernia in infants and children, J. Internat. Coll. Surgeons 17:729, 1952.
31. Dodson, H. C., Jr., and Burnett, H. A.: Unusual strangulated hernias in infants, J. Oklahoma M. A. 42:243, 1949.
32. Donovan, E. J., and Stanley-Brown, E. G.: Inguinal hernia in female infants and children, Surg., Gynec. & Obst. 107:663, 1958.
33. Duckett, J. W.: Treatment of congenital inguinal hernia, Ann. Surg. 135:879, 1952.
34. Dunavant, W. D., and Wilson, H.: Inguinal hernias in infants and children, J. Pediat. 44:558, 1954.
35. Duren, N., and Frank, S. R.: Herniated ovary in an infant, J. Pediat. 31:227, 1947.
36. Engel: Einige Bemerkungen über Lageverhältnisse der Baucheingeweide im gesunden Zustande, Wien. med. Wchnschr. 39:705, 1857.
37. Erdman, S.: Inguinal hernia in the male, Ann. Surg. 27:171, 1923.
38. Felizet, G.: *Les hernies inguinales de l'enfance* (Paris: G. Masson, 1894).
39. Fére, C.: Études sur les orifices herniaires et sur les hernies abdominales des nouveau-nés et des enfants à la Mamelle, Rev. men, méd. chir. 3:551, 1879.
40. Ferguson, A. H.: Oblique inguinal hernia: Typical operation for its radical cure, J. A. M. A. 33:6, 1899.
41. Fevre, M.: Hernies étranglées chez l'enfant, in *Chirurgie infantile d'urgence* (Paris: Masson & Cie, 1958).
42. Fonkalsrud, E. W.; deLorimier, A. A., and Clatworthy, H. W., Jr.: Femoral and direct inguinal hernias in infants and children, J.A.M.A. 192:101, 1965.
43. Fraser, J.: *Surgery of Childhood* (New York: William Wood Co., 1926), Vol. 2 chap. 32.
44. Gans, S. L.: Sliding inguinal hernia in female infants, Arch. Surg. 79:109, 1959.
45. Gans, L. S., and Rubin, C. L.: Apparent female infants with hernias and testes. Am. J. Dis. Child. 104:114, 1962.
46. Gaspar, M. R.; Kimber, J. H., and Berkaw, K. A.: Children with hernias, testes and female external genitalia, Am. J. Dis. Child. 91:542, 1956.
47. Gatti, G.: *L'ernia inguinale nell'infanzid* (Bologna: L. Cappelli, 1920).
48. Gilbert, M., and Clatworthy, H. W., Jr.: Bilateral operations for inguinal hernia and hydrocele in infancy and childhood, Am. J. Surg. 97:255, 1959.
49. Goldberg, S. L., and Rambar, A. C.: Strangulated inguinal hernia in premature infants, Am. J. Surg. 32:475, 1936.
50. Goldstein, I. R., and Potts, W. J.: Inguinal hernia in female infants and children, Ann. Surg. 148:819, 1958.
51. Graves, G. Y., and McIlvoy, D. B.: Hernia of uterus, ovaries and tubes in a six-week-old infant, Am. J. Dis. Child. 81:250, 1951.
52. Gross, R. E.: *The Surgery of Infancy and Childhood* (Philadelphia: W. B. Saunders Company, 1953).
53. Hauser, G. A.: Testicular Feminization, in Overhizer, C. (ed.): *Intersexuality* (New York: Academic Press, Inc., 1963).
54. Herzfeld, G.: The radical cure of hernia in infants and

young children, Edinburgh M. J. 32:281, 1925.

55. Hessert, W.: The frequency of congenital sacs in oblique inguinal hernia, Surg., Gynec. & Obst. 10:252, 1910.

56. Hoag, B. M.: Inguinal hernia in childhood, S. Clin. North America 21:425, 1941.

57. Holcomb, G. W., Jr.: Routine bilateral inguinal hernia repair, Am. J. Dis. Child. 109:114, 1965.

58. Hutchinson, C., and Koop, C. E.: The relationship of testis and processus vaginalis testis in the infant, Anat. Rec. 124:310, 1956.

59. Iason, A. H.: Hernia in infancy and childhood, Am. J. Surg. 68:287, 1945.

60. Jagiello, G., and Atwell, J. D.: Prevalence of testicular feminization. Lancet 1:329, 1962.

61. Jarrett, J. T., and Bradford, B., Jr.: Inguinal hernia in infancy and early childhood, West Virginia M. J. 48:253, 1952.

62. Keeley, J. L.: Hernias and hydroceles in infants and children, Illinois M. J. 105:1, 1954.

63. Keith, A.: The "saccular theory" of hernia, Lancet 2:1398, 1906.

64. Keith, A.: On the origin and nature of hernia, Brit. J. Surg. 11:455, 1924.

65. Kiesewetter, W. B.: Hernias and hydroceles, Pediat. Clin. North America 6:1129, 1959.

66. Kiesewetter, W. B., and Parenzan, L.: When should hernia in the infant be treated bilaterally? J.A.M.A. 171:287, 1959.

67. Kirchoff, A.: Strangulated hernia with adnexa in infancy and childhood, Zentralbl. Chir. 81:2011, 1956.

68. Kline, H. A.: Incarceration of Meckel's diverticulum in an inguinal hernia, J. Pediat. 53:479, 1958.

69. Knox, G.: Incidence of inguinal hernia in Newcastle children, Arch. Dis. Childhood 34:482, 1959.

70. Koop, C. E.: Inguinal herniorrhaphy in infants and children, S. Clin. North America 37:1675, 1957.

71. Kristiansen, C. T., and Snyder, W. H., Jr.: Inguinal hernia in female infants and children, West. J. Surg. 64:481, 1956.

72. Kurzweg, F. T.: Inguinal and umbilical hernias in infancy and childhood: Contrast in the management, South. M. J. 51:961, 1958.

73. Ladd, W. E.: Hernia in infancy and childhood, Nebraska M. J. 26:235, 1941.

74. Ladd, W. E., and Gross, R. E: *Abdominal Surgery of Infancy and Childhood* (Philadelphia: W. B. Saunders Company, 1941).

75. Larsen, R. M.: Inguinal hernia in childhood, J. Kentucky M. A. 53:123, 1955.

76. Lind, S. C.: Littré's hernia – a Meckel's diverticulum in a hernia sac with report of a case, Ohio M. J. 29:549, 1933.

77. McLaughlin C. W., Jr., and Kleager, C.: The management of inguinal hernia in infancy and early childhood, Am. J. Dis. Child. 92:266, 1956.

78. MacLennan, A.: The radical cure of inguinal hernia in children with special reference to the embryonic rests found associated with the sacs, Brit. J. Surg. 9:445, 1922.

79. McVay, C. B.: In discussion of Mueller and Rader.[85]

80. Minton, J. P., and Clatworthy, H. W., Jr.: Incidence of potency of the processus vaginalis, a study based on 600 bilateral operations for inguinal hernia, Ohio M. J. 57:530, 1961.

81. Mixter, C. G.: Undescended testicle, Surg., Gynec. & Obst. 39:275, 1924.

82. Morgan, E. H., and Anson, B. J.: Anatomy of region of inguinal hernia: IV. The internal surfaces of the parietal layers, Quart. Bull. Northwestern Univ. M. School 16:20, 1942.

83. Morris, J. M.: The syndrome of testicular feminization in male pseudohermaphrodites, Am. J. Obst. & Gynec. 6:1192, 1962.

84. Morton, T. V., Jr., and Carter, O. B.: Hernia of the vermiform appendix, J. M. Soc. New Jersey 54:372, 1957.

85. Mueller, C. B., and Rader, G.: Inguinal hernia in children, Arch. Surg. 73:595, 1956.

86. Nip, G. H.: The management of incarcerated hernias in infants and children, Hawaii M. J. 15:30, 1955.

87. Packard, G. B., and McLauthlin, C. H.: Treatment of inguinal hernia in infancy and childhood, Surg., Gynec. & Obst. 97:603, 1953.

88. Paterson, D., and Gray, G. M.: An investigation into the incidence of hernia in children, Arch. Dis. Childhood 2:328, 1927.

89. Pellacani, P.: Der Bau des menschlichen Saamenstranges, Arch. f. microscop. Anat. 23:305, 1883-84.

90. Pender, R.: Report on inguinal hernias in female childrens, Clin. Proc. Children's Hosp., Washington, D.C. 7:113, 1951.

91. Potts, W. J.: Truss for inguinal hernia in infants, J.A.M.A. 117:1440, 1941.

92. Potts, W. J.: Inguinal hernia in infants, Pediatrics 1:772, 1948.

93. Potts, W. J.; Riker, W. L., and Lewis, J. E.: The treatment of inguinal hernia in infants and children, Ann. Surg. 132:566, 1950.

94. de Quervain, F.: Ein Fall von Pseudohermaphroditis masculinis, Schweiz. med. Wchnschr. 53:563, 1923.

95. Rack, F. J., and Webb, E. A.: Sliding hernia: Experiences with 33 cases with report of two cases in infants, Ohio M. J. 50:441, 1954.

96. Ramonéde, L.: *Le canal péritoneo-vaginal et la hernie péritoneo-vaginale étranglée chez l'adulte* (Paris: Thèse, 1883).

97. Ravitch, M. M.: Personal communication.

98. Rendle-Short, J., and Havard, C.: Incarcerated and strangulated inguinal hernia in the first year of life, Brit. M. J. 1:680, 1954.

99. Rhead, A.: Description of the Body of Man, in *An explanation of the Fashion and Use of Three and Fifty Instruments of Chirurgery Gathered out of Ambrosius* (London: Printed for Michael Sparks, 1634).

100. Roberto, A. E.: Unusual inguinal hernia in infancy, New York J. Med. 53:3044, 1953.

101. Rothenburg, R. E., and Barnett, T.: Bilateral herniotomy in infants and children, Surgery 37:947, 1955.

102. Russell, R. H.: The etiology and treatment of inguinal hernia in the young, Lancet 2:1353, 1899.

103. Sachs, H.: *Untersuchungen über den processus vaginalis peritonei als Prädisponirendes* (Dorpat: Moment für die äussere Leistenhernie, Inaugural Dissertation, 1885).

104. Santulli, T. V., and Shaw, A.: Inguinal hernia: Infancy and childhood, J.A.M.A. 176:110, 1961.

105. Schiebel, H. M., and Freeman, W. H.: The treatment of inguinal hernia in infants and children, South. M. J. 43:605, 1950.

106. Schneck, H., and Leider, S.: Hernia as cause of colic in infancy, New York J. Med. 55:1467, 1955.

107. Shandling, B., and Thomson, S.: The Cheatle-Henry approach for inguinal herniotomy in infants and children: The Hospital for Sick Children, Toronto, Canad. J. Surg. 6:484, 1963.

108. Singer, C.: *Galen on Anatomical Procedures* (London: Oxford University Press, 1956).

109. Sloman, J. G.: Testicular infarction in infancy: Its association with irreducible inguinal hernia, M. J. Australia 45:242, 1958.

110. Smith, I.: Irreducible inguinal hernia in children — gangrenous bowel in a 25-day-old infant, Brit. J. Surg. 42:271, 1954.

111. Snyder, W. H., Jr., and Chaffin, L.: Inguinal hernia complicated by undescended testes. Am. J. Surg. 90:325, 1955.

112. Snyder, W. H., Jr., Snyder, M. H., and Chaffin, L.: Cardiac arrests in infants and children: Report of 66 original cases, Arch. Surg. 66:714, 1953.

113. Sparkman, R. S.: Bilateral exploration in inguinal hernia in juvenile patients, Surgery 51:393, 1962.
114. Swenson, O.: *Pediatric Surgery* (New York: Appleton-Century-Crofts, Inc., 1958).
115. Thorndike, A., Jr., and Ferguson, C. F.: Incarcerated inguinal hernia in infancy and childhood, Am. J. Surg. 39:429, 1938.
116. Tow, A.: Threatened gangrene of testicle in 3-month-old infant due to incarcerated inguinal hernia, Arch. Pediat. 55:254, 1938.
117. Turner, P.: The radical cure of inguinal hernia in children, Proc. Roy. Soc. Med. 5:133, 1912.
118. Wakeley, C. P. G.: Hernia of the ovary and fallopian tube, Surg., Gynec. & Obst. 51:256, 1930.
119. Wansbrough, R. M.: In discussion of Mueller and Rader.[85]
120. Ward-McQuaid, J. N., and Lennon, G. G.: Inguinal hernias, absence of the uterus and pseudohermaphroditism, Surg., Gynec. & Obst. 90:96, 1950.
121. Watson, L. F.: *Hernia* (5th ed.: St. Louis: C. V. Mosby Company, 1948).
122. Welch, K. S.: Cited by Kiesewetter.[66]
123. Wiklander, O.: Incarcerated inguinal hernia in childhood, Acta chir. scandinav. 101:303, 1951.
124. Wiley, J., and Chavez, H. A.: Uterine adnexa in inguinal hernia in infant females, West. J. Surg. 65:283, 1957.
125. Wilkins, L.: *Endocrine Disorders in Childhood and Adolescence* (2nd ed.: Springfield, Ill.: Charles C Thomas, Publisher, 1960).
126. Wolgast, G. F., and Hilz, J. M.: Littré's hernia: Strangulation of Meckel's diverticulum in a femoral hernia and an inguinal hernia, Am. Surgeon 28:741, 1962.
127. Zimmerman, L. M., and Anson, B. J.: *Anatomy and Surgery of Hernia* (Baltimore: Williams & Wilkins Company, 1953).
128. Zuckerkandl, E.: Über den Scheidenforsatz des Bauchfelles und dessen Beziehung zur äusseren Leistenhernia, Arch. klin. Chir. 20:215, 1877.

W. H. SNYDER, JR.
E. M. GREANEY, JR.

Drawings by
TED BLOODHART (Figures 46-1 to 46-6)
DENIS DYKES (Figures 46-7 and 46-8)

47

Abdominal and Thoracic Injuries

TRAUMA IS an increasing problem in the pediatric age group. Accidents cause one third of all deaths in children up to age 14 years. In the United States approximately 13,000 children are killed annually and another 50,000 seriously injured.[18] In Canada in 1965, accidents caused more deaths in children than all other causes combined, with a rate of 29.5 per 100,000.[19] Berfenstam *et al.*[5] reported 25,000 major injuries to the children of Sweden in 1 year. Of these, 463 were injuries to thoracic or abdominal viscera. In all countries there is an alarming rise in deaths due to vehicular accidents.

During the period 1952–68, 418 children were admitted to the Pediatric Surgical Service of the Boston City Hospital with abdominal, thoracic or genitourinary injuries. Of these, 391 (93%) were due to blunt trauma, and only 27 (6.5%) were penetrating or perforating wounds. This is in marked contrast to adult experience.[32,62,100] Stalowsky[80] came to the same conclusion on reviewing a large group of German children with abdominal injuries.

Of our group, 326 patients were boys (78%) and 92 (22%) girls. Ages ranged from the neonatal period to 14 years, with a peak incidence at 8 years (Fig. 47-1). At this age, youngsters in a crowded metropolitan area begin to escape parental supervision and extend their range into dangerous accident-producing situations. The accidents occur nearby, and the children are brought promptly to the hospital for evaluation and treatment. To a large extent, this accounts for any success we may have had in terms of ultimate mortality and morbidity. Fifty-seven per cent sus-

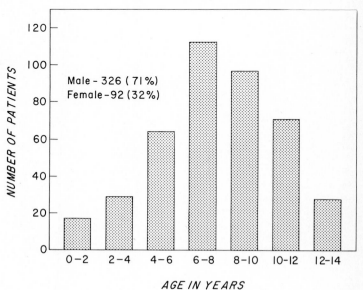

Fig. 47-1.—Age and sex distribution of 418 children with abdominal and thoracic injuries treated at Boston City Hospital, 1952-68.

Male – 326 (71%)
Female –92 (32%)

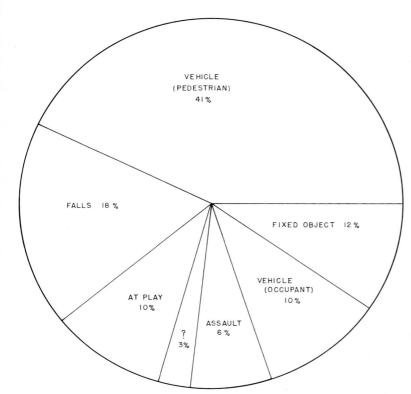

Fig. 47-2. — Etiology of abdominal and thoracic injuries.

tained complicating craniocerebral, thoracic and/or musculoskeletal injuries of major importance. The various patterns of organ damage, isolated or in combination, indications for surgical intervention or nonintervention, and aspects of technical management in each category of visceral injury comprise the basis for the following dicussion.

ETIOLOGY

Forty-one per cent of the patients were involved as pedestrians in motor vehicle accidents. Another 30% fell from a height or against a fixed object. Others were occupants of motor vehicles or injured at play or by direct assault. The last category is of great importance because it is not suspected, especially in the younger children (and see Chap. 8). The incidence of assault in this series was 6%. It is the responsibility of every physician to uncover such unprovoked attacks on helpless small children by adults. The epidemiology is probably typical of any area where substandard communities are served by a large municipal hospital (Fig. 47-2).

MANAGEMENT

Children with massive, multisystem injuries should be admitted to a general or pediatric surgical service and should remain under the close supervision of individuals familiar with the variables of diagnosis and the complex pattern of organ injury in closed abdominal trauma. Such an administrative plan is not difficult to inaugurate and execute if one is realistic and prompt in obtaining the assistance of appropriate specialty services.

Initial management consists of a carefully taken history, because it tells much about the type of injury that can occur, and an orderly physical examination. Extra-abdominal injuries may be unrecognized and appear later to complicate the phase of operative management. Vital signs are recorded on a close time schedule and blood is drawn at the time of the cutdown for appropriate laboratory study and typing and cross-matching. Hourly records of urinary volume provide a useful guide to effective circulating blood volume. For this reason, a Foley catheter is inserted in the bladder.

Certain lesions are capable of producing profound blood loss. It is not hydraulically possible to replace large amounts of blood in a short period of time through a single cut-down site. With evidence of rapid exsanguination, notably in liver, pelvic and combined abdominal and thoracic injuries, a central venous pressure line should be established and kept at 10–15 cm of water. Concealed pancreatic injury is more common that has been recognized. For this reason, the serum amylase content is measured to serve as a base line and is repeated on the third and fifth days. A nasogastric tube is inserted and the gastric contents are examined.

Anteroposterior and lateral chest films should be obtained routinely. Seven cases of hemopneumothorax complicating matters below the diaphragm have been encountered. Flat, upright and left lateral decubitus projections of the abdomen are taken. Additional exposures of the skull and extremities are obtained as needed. Renografin (1 cc/kg to 40 cc) is injected intravenously in all cases of abdominal injury whether or not hematuria is observed. A cystourethrogram is obtained in all cases of pelvic fracture or predominantly lower abdominal findings. Selective transfemoral retrograde arteriography performed by the percutaneous Soldinger technique is valuable in cases of pelvic crush, renal injuries and traumatic hemobilia.

Repeated examination at intervals by a skilled observer is the best guide we have in the management of these patients. It is the regression or progression of signs from hour to hour that in large part indicates the severity of injury and the need for exploration.

Abdominal Contusion

The diagnosis of abdominal contusion has been reserved for the 172 patients who gave a history of injury to the abdomen with subsequent development of abdominal pain, tenderness and rigidity with or without vomiting. Bowel sounds often were not present, and most patients had pronounced leukocytosis

Fig. 47-3.—Abdominal contusion. Unconscious patient with superficial left upper quadrant abrasion and perineal laceration.

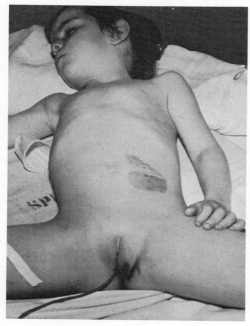

with a shift to the left. Many had multiple contusions and abrasions or injuries outside the abdominal cavity to complicate this interpretation (Fig. 47-3).

Recent reports of abdominal injury recognize this category as one that can closely mimic major visceral injuries. This is a distinct entity and in all probability represents injury to the muculature of the abdominal wall or at times retroperitoneal bleeding. One cannot rule out minor contusions of the abdominal viscera, such as subserosal hemorrhagic infiltrates and subcapsular bleeding of the liver or spleen. The clinical effect is maximal within a few hours, and there is pronounced improvement of this situation under a few hours of observation. In a very dramatic way, an apparently rigid abdomen suggesting an abdominal catastrophe is converted to a soft abdomen with return of peristalsis and tenderness localized to some area of the abdominal wall.

It is impossible to diagnose contusion with exactness. We ultimately explored 12 patients (7%). In 5, minor findings were encountered in the peritoneal cavity; in 7, the laparotomy was nonrevealing. There was no mortality in this group. Two patients had significant pancreatic enzyme elevations on the third and fifth days. All of these patients are hospitalized for 5 days and are allowed some ambulation prior to discharge from the hospital. Acute gastric dilatation occurred in 6 patients. The great concern in the management of this group is that an important injury may be overlooked. This is apparent from two reviews of nonpenetrating abdominal injury. Morton et al.[60] reported that autopsy on 9 patients disclosed surgically correctable lesions. In a series of 230 patients, Allen and Curry[1] encountered 18 who died without laparotomy and were found to have abdominal visceral injuries. Presumably many of these fall into the multiple-injury group. It must be emphasized that, when in doubt, we do not hesitate to perform an exploratory operation on any patient tentatively classified in this group.

Ruptured Spleen

Seventy-one patients had splenectomy for traumatic rupture (Fig. 47-4). All spleens but one were previously normal; the exception was oversized on the basis of leukemia. Nearly all were operated on within 24 hours of injury. There were only 2 instances of delayed rupture, an incidence of 3%. This is the lowest among recent reports, most series averaging about 15%. Shirkey et al.[76] reported delayed rupture in 12 of 64 patients with blunt splenic injury. Watkins[92] reported 8 instances of delayed rupture in a group of 56. Bollinger and Fowler[10] collected 248 cases of splenic rupture and found a delay incidence of 21.5%. The over-all mortality in this group was 15%.

There were 2 deaths in our consecutive series. Both children had extra-abdominal injuries that were untreatable by today's techniques. One had a grossly lacerated brain, and the other, a torn-apart pelvis

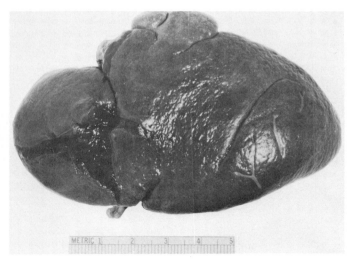

Fig. 47-4.—Splenic rupture. Gross specimen shows one of many patterns of anatomic injury.

with complex pelvic vascular injury. This low mortality rate is not unusual for isolated or combined splenic injury in children. Boley *et al.*[9] reported 33 consecutive splenectomies for trauma in children with no deaths. A similar experience was reported by Eraklis, Tank and Gross,[25] who performed splenectomy for trauma in 55 children without a fatality. Two factors permit a higher salvage rate than is achieved in adults. The first is the relative ease of diagnosis of splenic rupture in children, permitting earlier intervention, and the second is the anatomic fact that the spleen in young children can be literally avulsed without exsanguinating hemorrhage. The small, muscular splenic artery and its branches are capable of contracting and forming a life-saving thrombus. In 1 instance, the spleen was found free in the pelvis and the vessels were completely shut off at the time of operation. The incidence of multiple combined injury is about the same in children and adults and is the most important factor in determining survival. Seven patients had associated pancreatic injury, and 19 had renal contusion. Five had perforation of the antimesenteric surface of the small bowel, and nearly two thirds of the patients had injuries in addition outside the abdominal cavity.

The diagnosis of splenic rupture depends on the usual history of a relatively minor blow over the left upper quadrant or lower chest. The classic example is the sledding accident. The impact is immediately followed by pain, pallor, collapse and occasional vomiting. After the initial insult, there is gradual improvement. Physical examination reveals tenderness of the left upper quadrant and moderate rigidity. Many patients have referred pain to the crest of the left shoul-

Fig. 47-5.—Splenic rupture. Three patients admitted in a 1-week period. The boy on the left had associated left hemopneumothorax and a complex knee fracture. The girl had multiple deep abrasions and fracture of the left femur. The boy on the right had a cerebral contusion and hematuria. The left paramedian rectus-splitting incision is preferred.

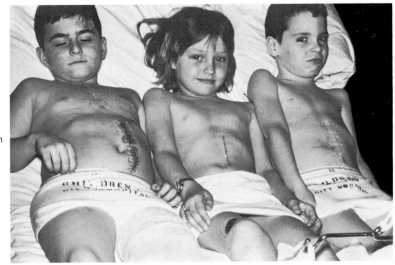

der on bimanual compression of the left upper quadrant (Kehr's sign). At the time of hospitalization, these children are not in shock in the supine position. Systolic blood pressure is usually over 100 and pulse rate is in about the same range. The hematocrit is over 30, although there may be a drop of several points in serial hematocrit readings over a period of several hours. Abdominal taps are performed in quadrants in borderline cases if the decision has been made not to operate. They are of particular value in unconscious patients and others with multi-system injuries.

Average age of our patients was 8.4 years. The youngest was a newborn infant. Sieber and Girdany[78] reported splenic rupture in the newborn period, thought to be due to sharp, lateral flexion of the spine and often associated with breech extraction.

X-ray examination of the abdomen was helpful in establishing an accurate diagnosis of splenic rupture in only 5 cases (14%). This is explained by the short interval between the time of injury and surgical exploration in this series. Wang and Robbins[87] described the cardinal x-ray signs of splenic rupture. In order of frequency they are: loss of splenic outline, increased size of splenic shadow, loss of renal outline, loss of psoas shadow, and serration of the greater curvature of the stomach with medial displacement. Rib fractures lend support to the diagnosis, as does fixation of the diaphragm on fluoroscopy. Scoliosis has been described, but review of our films, even in retrospect,

revealed no such evidence. The spleen in a child is essentially a thoracic organ. It is small, and if one can see the sharp outline of a small or normal spleen, there is little likelihood of splenic rupture. But even this rule is not infallible. Zachary,[103] Storsteen[82] and their associates, among others, have noted splenosis following splenic rupture. We make every effort to recover all of the splenic fragments. This is most easily accomplished through a long left paramedian incision which permits exploration of all four quadrants of the abdomen (Figs. 47-5 and 47-6).

The technique of splenectomy for rupture, which is similar for children and adults, is shown in Figure 47-7.

There is an apparent vulnerability to sepsis following splenectomy in some situations. In two series,[46,50] the patients had been operated on for a primary hematologic disorder. Eraklis and his colleagues[24] reached the same conclusion after reviewing several hundred cases of splenectomy for miscellaneous conditions. The incidence of postsplenectomy sepsis was highest in patients with Cooley's anemia. No problem was encountered in patients who had splenectomy for trauma or whose spleen was incidentally removed, regardless of age of the child. A follow-up of all of our patients revealed that none had had recurring major sepsis up to 15 years after splenectomy. This experience coincidences with that reported by MacKinnon,[52] who studied 26 children who survived splenectomy for rupture. It would seem that this problem, which is real enough, is more directly related to a primary hematologic disturbance than to removal of a normal spleen.

Genitourinary Injuries

Injuries of the genitourinary tract fall in third place in order of frequency in trunk trauma. The reader is referred to Chapter 65 for full discussion of the problem.

In 1965, I[96] reviewed 78 cases of genitourinary trauma in children 14 years or younger from the clinical and pathologic records of the Boston City Hospital and the Children's Hospital Medical Center. The two hospitals contributed 47 and 31 cases respectively. This material, though a duplication of effort, is presented here in abbreviated form because genitourinary injuries constitute a large segment of the total picture with intraperitoneal solid or hollow organ injuries and, at times, with injuries involving the ipsilateral hemithorax. An arbitary system of classification based on the seriousness of injury was devised; thus all renal injuries are referred to as class I, A to D (Table 47-1).

RENAL INJURIES

Subcutaneous damage to the kidney is the commonest form of genitourinary injury. Sixty patients fell in this category; all had blunt or closed trauma.

Fig. 47-6.—Splenic rupture; optimal position and incision for surgery. Thorough exploration of the abdomen can be carried out, and the incision is equally valuable for dealing with commonly associated injuries of the pancreas and left kidney. Arching of the back facilitates exposure. A similar right rectus incision is used for suspected injury of the liver, duodenum and right kidney.

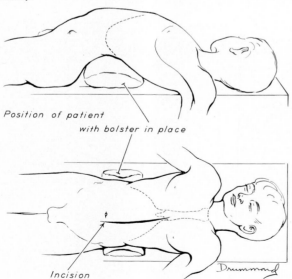

Position of patient

with bolster in place

Incision

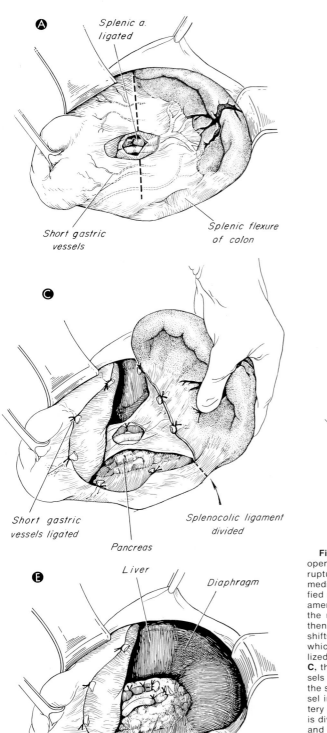

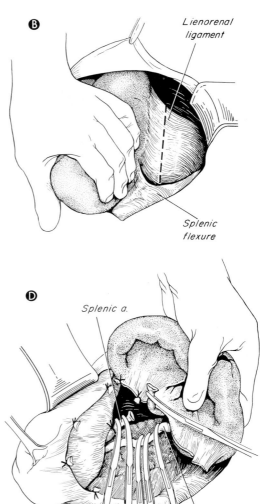

A

Splenic a. ligated

Short gastric vessels

Splenic flexure of colon

B

Lienorenal ligament

Splenic flexure

C

Short gastric vessels ligated

Pancreas

Splenocolic ligament divided

D

Splenic a.

Splenic v.

E

Liver

Diaphragm

Pancreas

Splenic flexure

Fig. 47-7.—Technique of splenectomy. **A,** the abdomen is opened through a long left paramedian rectus incision and the ruptured spleen immediately identified. The stomach is retracted medially with a Babock clamp, and the splenic vessels are identified at the superior border of the pancreas in the gastrolienal ligament. This is opened vertically and a 2-0 silk tie placed around the renal artery to control significant bleeding. **B,** the surgeon then sweeps his hand over the superior pole of the spleen and shifts the organ medially. This discloses the lienorenal ligament, which is divided. The splenic flexure of the colon may be mobilized in the process and displaced inferiorly to avoid injury to it. **C,** the splenocolic ligament is divided and the short gastric vessels are ligated. A transfixion suture should be used, grasping the seromuscular coat of the stomach and incorporating the vessel in the ligature. **D,** attention is now directed to the splenic artery and vein proximal to their branching at the hilus. The artery is divided first between double clamps, and an additional ligature and transfixion suture are placed to provide secure hemostasis. An identical technique is used in dividing, ligating and transfixing the splenic vein. Blunt dissection must be used to separate both structures from the tail and superior surface of the pancreas to avoid pancreatic injury and creation of a fistula. **E,** the raw bed is inspected for additional bleeding, and an empty Penrose drain is brought out through a posterolateral stab wound.

TABLE 47-1.—Genitourinary Injuries

Classification	No. of Patients	Assoc. Injuries	Treatment	No. of Patients	Compl.	Alive	Dead
I. Renal Injuries							
A. Shattered kidney	11	4	Nephrectomy	11	3	9	2
B. Shattered pole	4	2	Heminephrectomy	4	3	4	
C. Lacerated; impaled	9	4	Suture laceration	3	3	9	
			Explored only	2			
			Expectant	4			
D. Renal contusion	35	25	Expectant	35	0	35	
II. Pelviureteral injuries							
A. Lacerated pelvis	1	1	Repair	1	0	1	
B. Transected ureter	1	1	Anastomosis	1	0	1	
III. Bladder injuries	6	3	Repair	5	3	5	1
			Combined (2)				
			EP* (3)				
			Hemicystectomy	1			
IV. Urethral injuries							
A. Prostatomembranous rupture	4	4	Cystostomy and Foley Traction	4	4	2	2
B. Laceration-contusion; instrument perf.	5	2	Catheter Splint and Cystostomy	5	2	5	
V. Penis-scrotum	2	1	Orchiectomy Repair (1)	1	1	1	1
Total	78	47			19	72	6

*Extraperitoneal repair.

Shattered kidney requiring nephrectomy was encountered 11 times (Fig. 47-8). Impalement of the kidney on the end of a fractured eleventh rib occurred twice.

This review re-emphasized the several axioms regarding undisclosed kidney anomalies, notably double kidney, solitary kidney, horseshoe kidney and congenital ureteropelvic obstruction. Unsuspected retroperitoneal malignancy, Wilms' tumor, was encountered twice.

The first step on the road to mismanagement is failure to establish the diagnosis. For this reason, intravenous pyelography is ordered in all cases of abdominal trauma and, when indicated, cystography,

retrograde pyeloureterography and retrograde selective renal arteriography. The practical value of selective arteriography in patients with renal infarct (encountered twice) is demonstrated in Figure 47-9. Two weeks previously, the patient had had a ruptured spleen removed. He did not have an intravenous pyelogram or other urologic studies at the time of injury. When removed, the kidney had the classic butterscotch-yellow appearance of the total infarct.

Although most authors extol the virtues of conservative management of kidney injuries, and certainly this is the rule with renal contusion, we have been impressed by the unfortunate problems created

Fig. 47-8.—Shattered kidney.
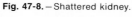
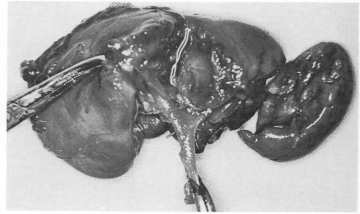

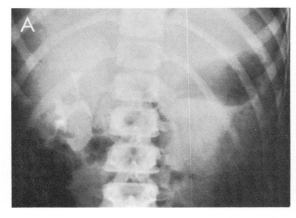

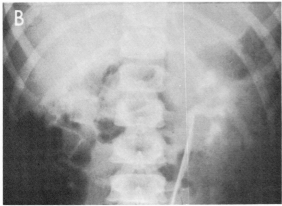

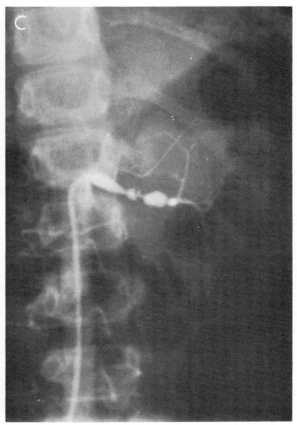

Fig. 47-9. — Infarct of left kidney due to unrecognized laceration of the left renal artery. **A,** intravenous pyelogram showing normally functioning right kidney, with no function up to 12 hours of the left. **B,** left retrograde pyelogram showing normal ureter and pyelocalyceal architecture of the nonfunctioning left kidney ap- proximately 10 days after removal of a ruptured spleen. **C,** selective left renal arteriogram employing the Seldinger technique. This shows the site of renal artery injury; just beyond this, a false aneurysm. Only a few capsular vessels fill with dye. At operation, a butterscotch-yellow totally infarcted kidney was removed.

through failure to document and treat lacerations of the renal artery (2 cases) and pulverization of one pole of the kidney (4 cases).[26,56,74] The great tragedy of removing a solitary kidney for trauma was found 11 times in the literature and was well discussed by Anderson and Harrison.[2] Infarct of a solitary kidney has also been reported.[22] The 35 patients with renal contusion in our series were managed conservatively. Only 2 had any recognizable change from normal in a routine intravenous pyelogram taken 6 weeks after injury. In none of these children has hypertension developed. Considerable illness and morbidity resulted from failure to carry out surgical debridement of a shattered single pole, with resultant hemorrhage, sepsis and the formation of a urinary pseudocyst.

PELVIURETERAL INJURIES

Isolated injuries of the pelvis and ureter without damage to adjacent renal parenchyma are extremely rare and were encountered only twice in this review. These are thought to be caused by extreme lateral flexion with avulsive traction.[31] The ureter usually parts in the upper third or at the ureteropelvic junction. Once again, the intravenous pyelogram suggests the diagnosis because of the intact parenchyma and retroperitoneal extravasation of the opaque medium. If the situation is unclear, retrograde studies are indicated, with plans made to explore the site of injury under the same anesthesia. Repair by end-to-end ureteral anastomosis in 1 patient and dismembered pyeloureterostomy in another, successfully salvaged the kidney in these 2 patients.

BLADDER INJURIES

Six children had isolated bladder injuries. Three involved the dome with intraperitoneal rupture. All had combined repair with catheter drainage. One patient had re-perforation at the same site. One had

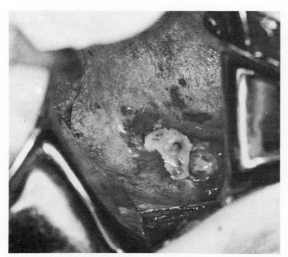

Fig. 47-10.—Bladder burn. This 12-year-old boy sustained an electrical burn of the bladder base from a resectoscope. The double ureteral ostiums are seen, brought into relief through the coagulation necrosis. The burn extended through the bladder wall, communicating with the iliac artery. Massive transfusions were required, and the problem was finally solved by hemicystectomy and nephroureterectomy of the complete duplex system.

delayed recognition of perforation with coma and profound electrolyte derangement due to peritoneal self-dialysis. A similar case has been reported by Kwang Wook-Ko *et al.*[48] Three patients had extraperitoneal rupture. One died because of extensive pelvic and lumbar vascular injuries plus a shattered pelvis. Two had satisfactory extraperitoneal repair with cystostomy and tube drainage. One child underwent hemicystectomy because of an electrical burn of the bladder base resulting from an attempt to fulgurate a ureterocele associated with duplex kidney and ureter (Fig. 47-10). One infant with posterior urethral valves sustained a bladder perforation at the time of cystoscopy. Four injuries were due to blunt trauma.

URETHRAL INJURIES

Nine patients sustained urethral injuries. Two had complete transection of the prostatomembranous urethra as a result of a massive shearing force that tore the pelvis apart, avulsing arterial and venous roots and converting the retroperitoneum to an arteriovenous marsh that defied surgical control. Surgical intervention became mandatory in 2 patients because of a pulseless lower extremity. Two patients had exsanguination arrest and died on the operating table after multiple resuscitative efforts and blood volume replacement times 4. The 2 patients surviving prostatomembranous disruption had re-establishment of continuity by cystostomy and Foley traction.[45] In 1, an unyielding stricture developed. For this reason, repair of the severed prostatomembranous urethra by

the combined approach recommended by Seitzman[75] may have some virtue in the child in reasonably good condition without complicating multisystem injury.

Five patients had lacerations or perforation of the anterior urethra. One was self-induced, 2 were iatrogenic and 2 were due to blunt trauma. All responded well to urethral catheter splint with cystostomy. In none did a stricture develop.

PENIS AND SCROTUM

Avulsive injuries to the penis and scrotum and scrotal contents are rare in children. Only 2 examples were recorded in this series. One was incidental to multiple injuries to the pelvis, bladder and great vessels. Contusion and minor lacerations are very common as straddle injuries (not included here). They seldom require hospitalization or, at the most, perineal care and a short period of urethral urinary diversion.

To summarize, 78 cases of genitourinary injuries were briefly reviewed to indicate some of the problems in management (see Table 47-1). Attention has been called to the significant mortality associated with ruptured bladder, transection of the posterior urethra and shattered pelvis.[70]

Gastrointestinal Injuries

Twenty-eight patients had injuries of the gastrointestinal tract (Table 47-2). Perforation may occur after the most trivial blow or may be combined with extensive trauma to the solid abdominal organs. Typical of the first group is the 4-year-old youngster who goes out to play after a large noon meal and presumably has an overdistended subparietal segment of the jejunum. He receives a slight blow in the central area of the abdomen. This area is unprotected because of inadequate development of the rectus muscles, and the jejunum is ruptured 2 or 3 ft. beyond the ligament of Treitz (Fig. 47-11). Eight ruptures fell in this cate-

TABLE 47-2. — NONPENETRATING GASTROINTESTINAL INJURIES

		CASES
Rupture in continuity		17
Jejunum	8	
Ileum	5	
Duodenum	2	
Stomach	1	
Colon	1	
Transection		2
Jejunum	1	
Ileum	1	
Mesentery and blood supply		6
Obstructing intramural hematoma		3
Duodenum	2	
Ileum	1	
Total		28

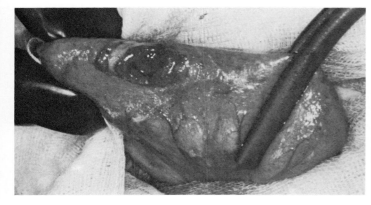

Fig. 47-11.—Traumatic perforation of the jejunum. Such injuries typically involve the antimesenteric surface and present a pouting mucosal layer with no tendency to spontaneous closure. This patient was unconscious for 4 days; laparotomy was performed on the seventh day after injury because of a subhepatic abscess.

gory. Rupture of the ileum in continuity was encountered 5 times. Usually, this was an unexpected finding on examination of the small bowel after recognition and treatment of a second injury in the upper abdomen. Duodenal rupture occurred twice, both involving the second portion; 1 patient was operated on with a diagnosis of appendicitis, only to find a normal appendix and green staining of the retroperitoneum. The single example of gastric rupture was impressive in that the laceration involved several inches of the greater curvature. The single colon rupture was small and was treated by primary suture within 6 hours of injury. Rupture with loss of continuity occurred twice, once in the proximal jejunum and once in the terminal ileum, actually an amputation of the terminal ileum and cecum (Fig. 47-12). Both injuries were treated by primary interrupted silk anastomosis with satisfactory outcome. All 19 patients with rupture of the gastrointestinal tract survived.

Injury to the mesentery or superior mesenteric vascular axis occurred in 6 patients. One patient, a 23-month-old boy, was technically not admitted to the hospital, having been moribund when brought to the accident room. There was an alleged history of a kick to the central area of the abdomen by a parent. Autopsy disclosed the abdominal cavity full of blood and a devitalized segment of ileum with rupture of the mesenteric root (Fig. 47-13). There were no other injuries within the abdomen or elsewhere, thus representing a fatality from injury to the small intestine.

Avulsion of the mesentery, as reported by Penberthy,[62] can be fatal either because of immediate exsanguinating hemorrhage or because of subsequent necrosis and perforation of the devitalized segment. The 5 other patients in our series with tears of the mesentery survived. In 2, it was necessary to resect a segment of the adjacent intestinal wall.

Contusion of the retroperitoneal portion of the duodenum and/or proximal jejunum with resulting intramural obstructing hematoma occurred 3 times. This tamponade obstruction usually occurs in the fixed or retroperitoneal portion of the duodenum or in the relatively fixed first segment of the jejunum. Mestel et al.[57] reported 19 cases of small bowel hematoma with obstruction, 16 of them in the pediatric age group. Other cases were reported by Robart.[71] In our patients, it was possible to evacuate the intramural clotted blood, ligate or fulgurate bleeding points and reconstruct the duodenum.

Ultimately, these hematomas would subside and patency of the intestinal tract would be restored spontaneously. To shorten this period of obstruction with its attendant dangers, an early laparotomy is indicated. These lesions should be treated by conservative

Fig. 47-12.—Avulsed cecum. Such injuries are rare and occur adjacent to fixed points such as the ligament of Treitz and the ileocecal angle.

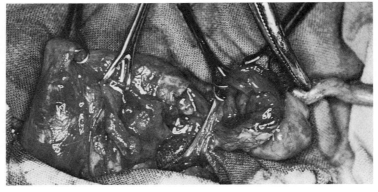

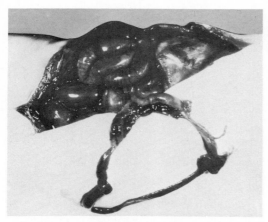

Fig. 47-13.—Avulsion of the small bowel mesentery (ileum) due to assault. This child was kicked in the abdomen and died of exsanguinating hemorrhage and gram-negative septicemia, without operation.

means as outlined above, and one should not be tempted to resect the grossly deformed and discolored segment. Gastrostomy and passage of a splinting Levin tube 1 or 2 ft. beyond the ligament of Treitz for feeding purposes have been useful. The proximal end of the tube is brought out through a no. 26 Malecot catheter. The Levin tube is removed in 1 week, and the gastrostomy tube after a period of clamping and barium studies indicate normal transit through the duodenum and proximal jejunum.

The most important isolated injury to the gastrointestinal tract is avulsion of its major blood supply. Direct repair of arterial injuries of the mesenteric veins is possible. Ulvestad[95] reported successful repair of a lacerated superior mesenteric artery, and I, too, have repaired a lacerated and skeletonized superior mesenteric artery in 1 patient. On initial inspection, the injury was obscured by a large hematoma and the entire midgut was cyanotic. Repair of a 1.5 cm longitudinal laceration restored bowel circulation to normal. In addition, the patient had a pulverized pancreatic body and a completely divided jejunum 15 cm beyond the ligament. The management of injuries to the major intestinal veins is less satisfactory, if not impossible, because of the low pressure normally carried in this circuit.

In conclusion, blunt injuries of the gastrointestinal tract were encountered in 28 patients, thus falling in third place in order of organ system involvement. Twenty-seven patients survived operation. One death on arrival occurred because of delay in diagnosis, hemorrhage and gram-negative septicemia.

Traumatic Pancreatitis

Pancreatitis in the acute or chronic form is a common disease in adults. The etiology is poorly understood in most cases, but less than 4% are thought to be due to direct injury. Kinnaird[47] reviewed 1,973 cases of pancreatitis in adults and found that 56 were due to trauma.

In contrast, pancreatitis is uncommon in childhood. It may occur in small infants after protracted vomiting and in association with severe dehydration. Rarely, it is due to a viral infection. Of the known causes, the commonest is direct injury to the central portion of the pancreas as it crosses the vertebral column. The only other etiologic agent noted with frequency is obstruction of the pancreatic duct by roundworms. Blumenstock *et al.*[8] collected 36 cases of pancreatitis in childhood; 7 were due to trauma. Our attention was directed to this entity in the postoperative management of certain youngsters who had removal of a ruptured spleen. Some convalesced exceptionally well and others had a protracted course with ileus, back pain and fever. A chance amylase evaluation in 1 of the early cases revealed 560 Somogyi units. This child subsequently had formation of a pseudocyst, as did 3 others.

Serum amylase levels are measured routinely on the first, third and fifth days in all patients admitted with the diagnosis of abdominal trauma. Twenty patients have had serum amylase levels in excess of normal, that is, over 200 Somogyi units.[23] Six were excluded as not meeting the criteria for diagnosis of traumatic pancreatitis because of considerable postoperative ileus, vomiting or an open lesion in the gastrointestinal tract. Direct absorption of enzymes by the peritoneal surface or a condition resulting in an increase of intraduodenal pressure will cause elevations of the serum pancreatic enzyme levels.[12] We did not agree that levels twice normal or more represent simple stress and ran a control group of 30 patients: 10 had exploratory laparotomy for other cause, 10 had severe isolated craniocerebral injury, and 10 had peripheral major musculoskeletal injuries. All had levels within the normal range for our laboratory (80–140 Somogyi units/100 cc of blood). This is in agreement with findings of Howard *et al.*[40] in a study of combat casualties during the Korean conflict. Most elevations occurred the first day; others did not peak until the second or third day. Nardi and Lees[61] suggested that serum trypsin levels more actively reflect the transudation of pancreatic enzymes, but this test has not yet been accepted for clinical use. Ekengren and Soderlund[21] described the radiologic features in 17 children with pancreatic trauma. Edema with duodenal atony in the acute stage was uniformly encountered with or without organ displacement. All 14 of their patients who had drainage survived. No resections were performed. A pseudocyst developed in 6.

Laboratory data were supportive in 11 cases proved by operation. Three patients were not explored but had classic symptoms that responded to colloid, antibiotics, nasogastric suction and atropine derivatives. Operative treatment, in addition to complete exposure

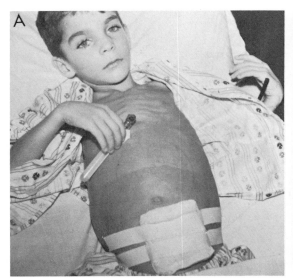

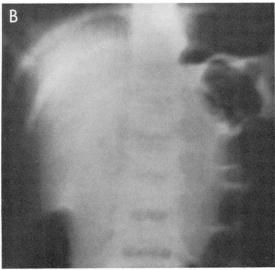

Fig. 47-14.—Pancreatic pseudocyst. **A,** in this 10-year-old boy, a pseudocyst developed after nonpenetrating abdominal injury. He also had chylous ascites and severe malnutrition. After cyst-jejunostomy, the ascites promptly disappeared. **B,** abdominal film of this patient. (See also Fig. 47-15.)

of the pancreas by wide opening of the lesser sac, consisted of sump and multiple slip drainage. Distal pancreatectomy was performed twice. Up to 50% resection of the pancreas for trauma has the support of several reports of resection in children.[34,84,94]

Pancreatic pseudocysts following trauma in children are being reported with increasing frequency.[36,64,89,97] We believe they should be operated on when diagnosed, usually about 2 weeks after injury, often associated with amylase levels above 1,000 Somogyi units. Waiting for the cyst to mature results in severe inanition because of progressive interference with gastrointestinal function. Four children with pseudocysts had the following treatment. One had external drainage with a Malecot catheter. When drainage is less than 1 oz. a day, the tube is clamped. If this is tolerated for 2 weeks and if the cavity is obliterated, the catheter can be removed.[90] Two patients had posterior cyst-gastrostomy, a large opening being made and the margin run with a lock chromic suture. The fourth had cyst-jejunostomy (Figs. 47-14 and 47-15). An unusual feature in this patient was the association with massive chylous ascites, which disappeared dramatically after drainage of the pseudocyst. Chylous ascites is the rarest of all abdominal injuries; in a review of the literature, Hoffman[39] was able to find only 4 cases due to trauma, and 2 additional cases of traumatic chylous ascites have recently been reported.[81,86] Both of the latter involved laceration of the drainage ducts; neither was associated with a pancreatic pseudocyst.

Occasionally, it may be possible to resect the pseudocyst with incidental splenectomy. Roux-en-Y drainage is mentioned to be condemned. Primary repair of the duct of Wirsung is indicated only with complete division of the duct to the right of the mesenteric vessels, and anastomosis must be carried out over a Silastic splint brought to the surface at a distance through the jejunal wall after division of the sphincter of Oddi.[84]

Multiple-organ injury occurred in 7 patients, in

Fig. 47-15.—Pancreatic pseudocyst; artist's conception of the pseudocyst in Figure 47-14. A segment of jejunum was firmly attached to the cyst wall, permitting direct anastomosis. Posterior cyst-gastrostomy would be optional in this instance.

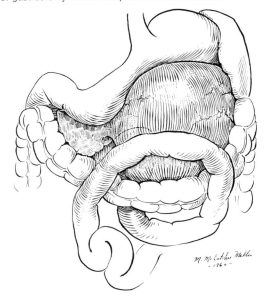

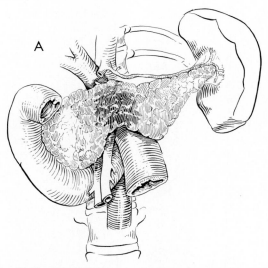 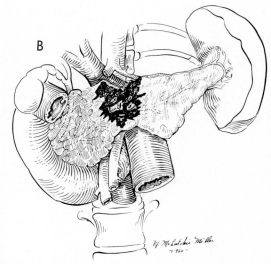

Fig. 47-16.—Pancreatic injuries. **A**, contusion of the body of the pancreas as it crosses the vertebral column. The lesser peritoneal sac should be opened and the degree of injury estimated by direct inspection. **B**, anatomic transection of the pancreatic body. Such injuries should be treated by distal pancreatectomy with splenectomy and sump drainage.

contrast to Ekengren and Soderlund's[21] report of isolated pancreatic injury, usually due to fall from a bicycle, in 17 children. Reports of experience in adults stress the greater frequency of penetrating injuries.[42,83] In general, the principles of surgical management are the same in any age group. A disturbing note was added by Warren and Wagner[91] after a study of long-term results of nonpenetrating pancreatic trauma. Twenty patients followed 2–28 years had a high incidence of chronic pancreatitis, ulcers and recurrent cysts.

Because of the unexpected high incidence of traumatic pancreatitis in this series (4%), it would seem important to open the lesser peritoneal cavity in every patient undergoing exploration for abdominal injury. There may be only a diffuse contusion, or there may be anatomic transection of the body (Fig. 47-16). In the latter instance, one should not hesitate to perform a distal pancreatectomy and close the stump with nonabsorbable sutures after ligation of the pancreatic duct. Failure to remove this damaged segment by distal pancreatectomy results in a prolonged illness and eventual reoperation for removal of the necrotic material or treatment of a pseudocyst.

Medical management of pancreatitis due to trauma is substantially the same as that of other forms of the disease and consists of gastrostomy and administration of anticholinergic drugs, colloids and antibiotics.

Liver Injuries

Liver injuries have been said to be second only to injuries of the head in autopsy material and are rap-idly fatal.[59] They are more common in children than in adults. These injuries involve the right lobe in 80%; convex surface injuries are about twice as common as other types. One of our patients sustained a right lobe injury apparently related to birth trauma; Potter[68] described 22 such cases in her series of 2,000 autopsies. The reader is referred to Chapter 7, Birth Trauma, and to Giedion's able review.[33]

Of our 21 patients who sustained hepatic rupture, 4 died. These injuries fall into four anatomic groups (Fig. 47-17): *A*, convex surface and dome. This injury is usually not evident when the abdomen is first opened. *B*, anterior surface and margin, left or right lobe. *C*, inferior or concave surface, usually the right lobe and most likely to be associated with injuries to the extrahepatic bile duct. *D*, posterior surface or contrecoup, usually the right lobe; with *A*, these account for most cases of traumatic hemobilia.[72]

Hepatic rupture is a major unsolved problem in the management of nonpenetrating wounds of the abdomen. Mikesky *et al.*[58] in 1956 analyzed 300 consecutive cases, with a review of the literature, and found a striking improvement in the management of penetrating liver wounds, with mortality in the range of 15%. In contrast, there had been no progress in the management of blunt hepatic rupture in this century. Of 596 patients, 67% died following hepatic rupture. In their own series, 17 of 24 (71%) of these injuries were lethal. The problem is all the more acute in children (Fig. 47-18). Mortality was 40% for all types of liver injury in the age group up to 10 years. This is higher than for any other age decade, including patients aged 60 or older.

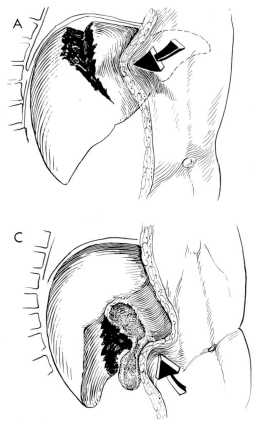

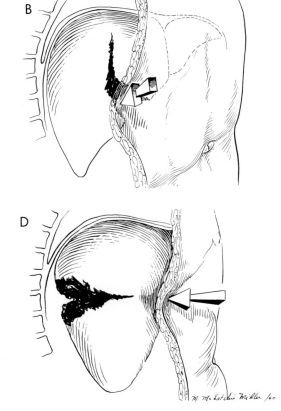

Fig. 47-17.—Mechanisma of hepatic rupture. Right lobe and convex surface injuries account for 80% of these cases. Prompt and courageous debridement of all liver tissue lateral to the trau-matic defect is advocated to avoid late sepsis, hemorrhage and hemobilia. Adjunct hypothermia has been found useful in such cases.

Review of the problem after 10 years shows no definite reduction of mortality from the more extensive liver injuries resulting from blunt trauma, although a favorable trend was indicated by Longmire,[51] who had a mortality rate of 39% in 90 cases. Success or failure would seem to be primarily a matter of the location and extent of liver injury. Some are superficial lacerations of the liver that ordinarily can be dealt with by simple surgical techniques and are not of themselves lethal.

Four of our 21 cases of hepatic injury were fatal. One youngster fell from a bicycle and the handlebar caused a massive tear of the right lobe. With delay of hospitalization she became exsanguinated and at autopsy was found to have a liver rupture. Another patient, a 22-month-old boy, was allegedly kicked in the abdomen by an adult baby sitter. The insult produced a rupture of the liver and perforation of the ileum. He was brought to the hospital 9 hours later in combined septic and exsanguination shock and died in the accident room within minutes of his arrival. No operation was performed. Autopsy disclosed hemoper-itoneum, liver rupture and a free perforation proximal to the ileocecal valve. Similarity in the appearance of these 2 youngsters at the time of hospitalization has led us to believe that one can suspect hepatic rupture with exsanguination by exclusion in the absence of a fractured pelvis.

SURGICAL MANAGEMENT

When the diagnosis of suspected hepatic rupture is made, the following protocol is suggested. The largest possible intravenous line is established by catheter or cut-down in one upper extremity and the opposite lower extremity. A central venous pressure line is established in the neck, and blood is drawn for typing, cross-matching and estimation of peripheral values, blood gases and pH. The always-present hypovolemic shock is treated initially with 5% albumin, single-donor AB plasma or Plasmanate. Within 10 minutes, a reliable cross-match can be obtained, and with fresh whole blood in citrate phosphate dextrose solution (CPD), transfusion is started as soon as possible,

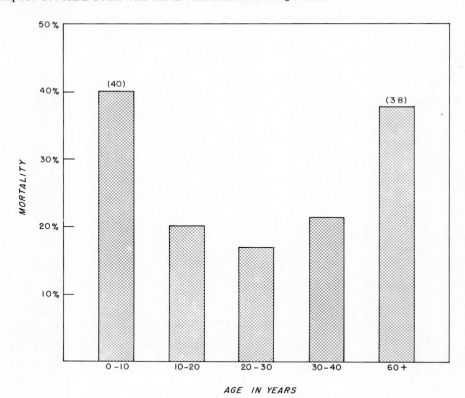

Fig. 47-18. — Age and mortality in hepatic injuries.

using a warming coil. Citrate intoxication is less of a problem with CPD blood, and availability of ionized calcium is assured by adding 0.5 Gm of calcium as calcium gluconate for each unit of whole blood administered. More important than either of the foregoing considerations is the accurate monitoring of pH, with Tris buffering when indicated. As in all low perfusion states, anoxic lactic acidosis should be anticipated and treated.[14]

One must plan on replacing the total calculated blood volume in the first hour. This calculation is based on kilogram weight. Estimates of blood volume range from 5% of the total body weight in older children to 8% in younger ones. Thus a 30-kg youngster has approximately 2,500 cc of total blood volume.

At this point, the child is intubated and, with succinylcholine, lightly anesthetized to prevent shivering, then placed on a cooling mat (Davol) and ice is added to reduce body temperature as rapidly as possible to the range of 90 F (31 C). Bernhard[7] demonstrated that hepatic cellular activity as measured by glucose, glycogen and lactose metabolism ceases at 85–88 F (27–30 C). For this reason, hypothermia has been proposed as an adjunct to extensive hepatic resection. Wangensteen[88] showed that intermittent clamping of the blood supply to the liver could be carried out for periods up to 15 minutes without causing hepatic ne-

crosis. At normothermic levels, however, occasional and unpredictable liver necrosis has occurred with this period of clamping. With the protection of hypothermia, the period of clamping can probably be safely doubled in quinidinized children with a previously normal liver. It is essential to accomplish homeostasis during the period of temperature reduction. A cold heart combined with any degree of anoxia due to uncorrected shock or anesthesia will result in extreme irritability and probable fibrillation. We have not encountered this problem, but Howland *et al.*[41] showed that hypothermic patients are particularly vulnerable to cardiac irregularities with massive whole blood replacement. For this reason, electrocardiographic monitoring is essential.

The scene now moves to the operating room, where anesthesia is induced with cyclopropane. The cyclopropane is then washed out, continuing with fluothane to permit electrofulguration and dissection. The abdomen is entered through an exploratory midline incision extending from the manubrium to the umbilicus, removing the xyphoid (Fig. 47-19). In younger children, a paramedian incision is preferable. The hand is passed across the surface of the liver, and if a rupture is identified, the incision is carried around into the sixth interspace as a lateral T. Depending on the location of the injury, and particularly with in-

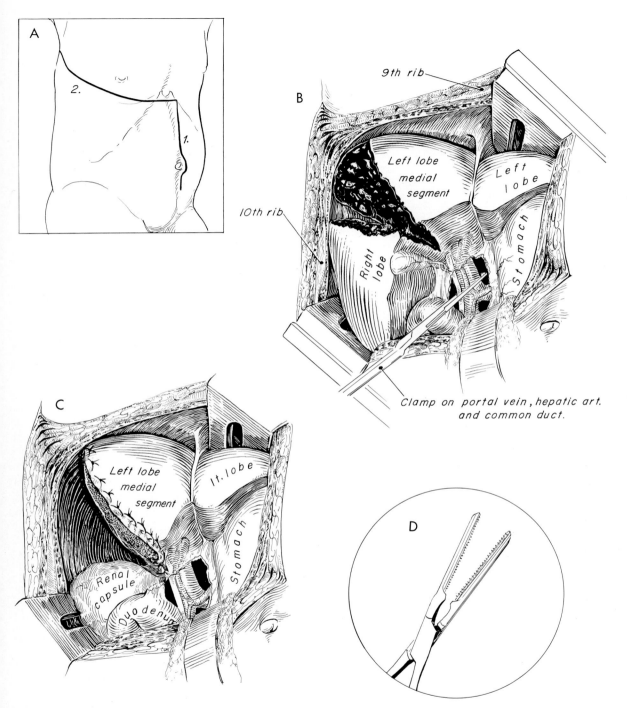

Fig. 47-19.—Technique of right hepatic lobectomy for traumatic rupture. Inflow and outflow occlusion is accomplished by crossclamping the structures in the hepatoduodenal ligament and ligating the right hepatic vein from above after dividing the diaphragm. A T-tube should be left in the common duct in older children and drains should be placed in the lesser sac, above and behind the medial segment of the left lobe. A soft sump drain should lead out from the upper pole of the kidney. The detailed surgical anatomy of such a resection is indicated in Figure 47-20.

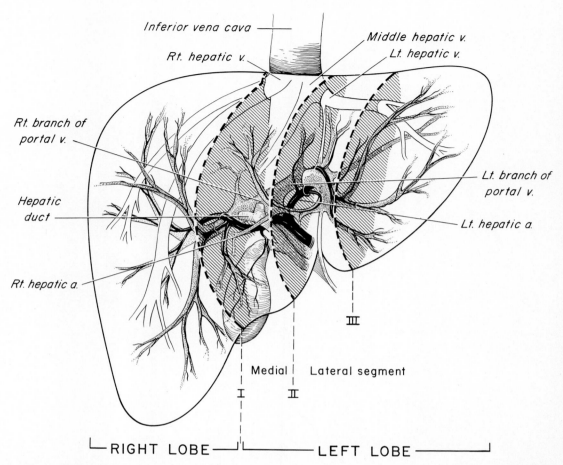

Inferior vena cava

Rt. hepatic v.

Middle hepatic v.

Lt. hepatic v.

Rt. branch of portal v.

Lt. branch of portal v.

Hepatic duct

Lt. hepatic a.

Rt. hepatic a.

Medial | Lateral segment

I   II   III

└─RIGHT LOBE─┘ └──── LEFT LOBE ────┘

Fig. 47-20.—Surgical anatomy of the liver. In addition to the three planes for lobar segmental or subsegmental resection, this drawing shows in detail the distribution and course of the hepatic artery, portal vein and the hepatic veins. The hepatic ducts are intimately associated with the branches of the portal vein and have been left out for purposes of clarity. More accurate knowledge about the internal architecture of the liver in children will be forthcoming from injection studies now in progress.

juries extending across the convex surface near the falciform ligament, better exposure is obtained by a slightly higher incision, cutting the diaphragm down to the vena cava. During this phase, control of respiration must be taken over by the anesthesiologist, to avoid the definite possibility of air embolism through the raw liver surface by ligating the right hepatic vein. Air embolism and further bleeding can be greatly reduced by manual compression of the liver. A Greene comb clamp is then applied to the common duct, portal vein and hepatic artery, incorporating all of the structures in the hepatoduodenal ligament, and the time is noted. Then, as rapidly as possible, all liver tissue lateral to the injury is debrided, and the vessels and bile ducts exposed on the liver surface are ligated with nonabsorbable transfixion sutures. Interlocking deep sutures of 0 silk are placed peripherally in the

manner indicated. Three periods of clamping not in excess of 20 minutes are permissible during the course of right lobe resection. Bleeding during this phase is minimal. In this patient, a 9-year-old girl, the rupture extended to within 3 mm of the portal vein. In addition to the liver injury that required right lobectomy, the patient had right hemopneumothorax, a severely lacerated right kidney that remained a problem long after liver healing was complete, a double fracture of the pelvic girdle and a plateau fracture of the right tibia. Except for the long period of intermittent hematuria, this youngster had an exceedingly smooth postoperative course and was discharged from the hospital on the twenty-sixth postoperative day.

Many materials have been proposed for covering the extensive raw liver surface following hepatic lobectomy. A plasma coagulum has been used,[73] and

Ivalon sponge has been recommended.[43] Freese *et al.*[29] advocated the use of acrylic adhesive; there has been some experience with this in Viet Nam casualties. McDermott and Ottinger[54] suggested a practical technique of detaching the falciform ligament from the anterior abdominal wall and applying it to the raw liver surface; in effect, retroperitonealizing. In view of the many methods that have been tried and the many that have failed, it would seem that there is obligatory bile peritonitis and continued raw surface bleeding after liver injury. For this reason, we routinely decompress the biliary tract with a T-tube in older children and with tube cholecystostomy in younger ones. An operative cholangiogram is then obtained to rule out undisclosed injury to the ducts. Multiple soft drains are placed in the subdiaphragmatic and subhepatic spaces and in the lesser sac. At least one of these is brought out posteriorly. The chest is left on water-seal drainage for 48 hours.

DISCUSSION

The two most frequent and best indications for hepatic resection are hemangioma and trauma, both common in children. We should like to enter a plea for more accurate reporting of resection for trauma. The present view of liver anatomy (Fig. 47-20) suggests that the right hepatic lobe includes 70% of the tissue to the right of the falciform ligament and always to the right of the portal vein and vena cava. Resection of the medial segment of the left lobe will only rarely be successful in trauma. Resection of the lateral segment of the left lobe may be total or subsegmental. We have pioneered in the use of hypothermia and did report the first instance of its successful use in resection of the entire right lobe for trauma.[98] Madding and Kennedy,[43] have commented on the role of hypothermia in liver injuries.

Of our 21 cases of nonpenetrating liver injury, the 2 that were fatal without operation were described earlier. Two patients died despite heroic efforts along the lines outlined above. In the 17 patients who survived hepatic injury or laceration due to blunt trauma, the severity of injury was considered to be average. Two additional patients survived operation for penetrating injury. Although the total experience is small in comparison to adult series, there is a trend toward improved management of this condition.[55] In all probability, deep ruptures involving the segment of the left lobe that is medial to the portal vein and centered on the vena cava—so-called no man's land—are rapidly fatal. Selective arteriography is of little help in planning or executing hepatic resection for trauma, but it can be of value in the management of traumatic hemobilia.[28]

INJURIES OF THE EXTRAHEPATIC BILIARY TRACT

Extrahepatic duct injuries in children have been reported sporadically for many years.[4,37,38,49,93,99] These can occur without associated liver injury, but for a surgeon to miss a ruptured gallbladder or divided hepatic or common duct at the time of laparotomy for trauma is unforgivable. Our 1 patient had an avulsed gallbladder removed by simple ligation of the cystic duct and artery. The gallbladder is electively removed in right hepatic lobectomy. Hartman and Greaney[35] have once again called attention to the syndrome of anorexia, weight loss, biliary ascites, jaundice and acholic stools. They reported on 5 children aged 2–7 years. Two patients had transection of the left hepatic duct, 1 had a split at the junction of the hepatic ducts, 1 had complete division of the common duct at the duodenal wall, and 1 had a perforated gallbladder. All injuries were due to blunt force, once again in contrast to adult experience. Dietrich *et al.*[17] reported on 61 adults with biliary tract injuries, only 6 of them due to blunt trauma. Direct repair of such injuries at the time of initial laparotomy is obligatory. The technique of repair will vary.

HEMOBILIA

Traumatic hemobilia is a rare complication of liver injury. The term was coined by Sandblom[72] in 1948, although Owing[65] described the condition a century before. The condition is largely iatrogenic because of failure to resect pulverized tissue. It can occur, however, with rupture of the central convex surface of the medial segment requiring suture. The main clinical features are biliary colic followed by hematemesis and melena. The presence of a T-tube permits prompt recognition but adds little to treatment. Selective hepatic arteriography by the Seldinger technique may be helpful in locating the site of bleeding and cavitation.[102] Surgical treatment consists of resection or extensive debridement; ligation of a major hepatic artery branch, or intracavitary ligation and packing.

We have encountered 3 cases in children. The first patient was untreated and died of exsanguination (Fig. 47-21). The second patient survived following a right hepatic artery ligation.[77] The third had a frivolous "blind gastrectomy" after "negative gastric and duodenal exploration."

More than 70 cases of hemobilia due to blunt trauma, many in children, have been reported. For this reason, it behooves surgeons to be aware of the condition and the several methods of successful treatment in order to improve the survival rate following this complication of liver injury.

In summary, we have outlined our program for the general and operative management of liver injuries. Hypothermia is a valuable adjunct, and is particularly applicable in children whose temperature can be brought to 30–31 C in 30 minutes. It has been suggested that attempts be made to achieve hypothermic levels through a peripheral circuit employing a pump oxygenator with an incorporated heat exchanger. Valuable additional measures would be circulatory

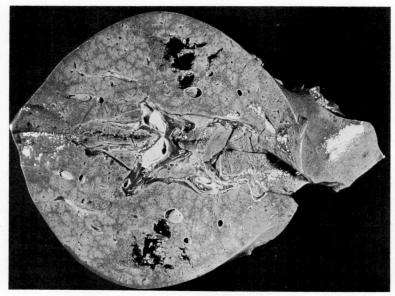

Fig. 47-21.—Hemobilia.

Fig. 47-22.—Traumatic hernia. **A,** anteroposterior chest film shows right traumatic diaphragmatic hernia extending to the fourth interspace, containing stomach and liver. **B,** lateral view. The child was operated on immediately, and the blood supply of the stomach was found to be seriously compromised. A laceration of the dome of the liver was repaired, as was the diaphragmatic defect. The concept of urgent operation is supported by the findings in this case.

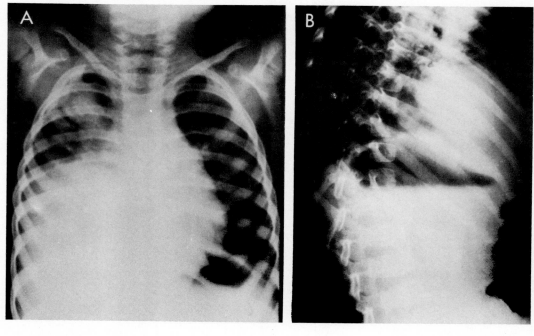

TABLE 47-3.—PENETRATING INJURIES OF THE ABDOMEN

INJURY	No. OF PATIENTS	OPERATION	MORTALITY
Parietes	8	8	0
Small bowel	5	5	0
Large bowel	3	3	0
Stomach	2	2	0
Liver	2	2	0
Spleen	1	1	0
Total	21	21	0

assistance via an auxiliary ventricle plus a means for constant monitoring of blood gases and blood pH on the arterial side.[27]

Traumatic Hernia

Four cases of traumatic hernia were encountered, 3 involving the diaphragm and 1 the ventral abdominal wall[101] (Fig. 47-22). Opinions differ on the need for immediate exploration of patients with diaphragmatic hernia.[11,13,15] According to Bugden et al.,[11] 90% of strangulated hernias are traumatic in origin. We favor early exploration in children, particularly on the right side, where there is likely to be torsion and strangulation of the stomach or interference with return of blood to the right side of the heart because of a dislocated liver. The possibility of associated injuries to these structures must be ruled out.

Penetrating Injuries of the Abdomen

Twenty-one children (5%) had penetrating injuries of the abdomen, a very low incidence in comparison to the 378 with blunt trauma. In this respect, children differ from adults, whose experience is about equally divided between open and closed trauma.[100] Stalowsky[80] made a similar observation in a large series of German children. As would be expected, all of our patients were explored. In 8, the parietes were involved (Table 47-3). In 10, the bowel was lacerated; 3 had lacerations of the liver or spleen.

Nonpenetrating Thoracic Injuries

HEMOPNEUMOTHORAX

Seven patients had hemopneumothorax complicating the diagnosis and management of the abdominal

TABLE 47-4.—NONPENETRATING CHEST INJURIES

INJURY	No. OF PATIENTS	OPERATION	MORTALITY
Hemopneumothorax	7	7	1
Diaphragmatic hernia	3	3	0
Crushed chest	2	0	2
Fat embolism	1	0	0
Total	13	10	3

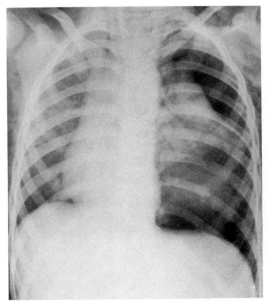

Fig. 47-23.—Traumatic hemopneumothorax associated with splenic rupture. Failure to recognize the combined injury may seriously compromise anesthetic and surgical management of these patients. Closed intercostal drainage with water seal should be established before induction of anesthesia and laparotomy.

injury (Table 47-4). In the first case, a preoperative chest film was not obtained, and during laparotomy, the anesthesiologist suddenly was faced with a blood-filled trachea (Fig. 47-23). The situation was recognized and a closed thoracotomy established, with uneventful recovery. In the second case, the hemopneumothorax was diagnosed but the abdominal signs were misinterpreted, and exploratory laparotomy was carried out with a preoperative diagnosis of ruptured spleen. No intra-abdominal injury was identified. This child had posterior rib fractures on the left. Intercostal blocks may permit correct interpretation of abdominal signs. Abdominal taps and selective arteriography may also be useful in this situation. The third and fourth patients had correct diagnosis and management. Both had left traumatic hemopneumothorax and abdominal contusion; laparotomy was not performed. The fifth patient had an associated massive rupture of the right lobe of the liver. Combined blunt thoracoabdominal injuries are especially troublesome in left-sided cases when there is overlap with the problem of splenic rupture. Economy et al.[20] reported 4 cases in a series of 48 splenectomies, an incidence of 8.3%. The sixth patient had renal impalement on the proximal end of a fractured eleventh rib, and the seventh had a ruptured spleen. In 5 patients, the left hemithorax was involved and in 2, the right; this is considered a random incidence.

Failure to recognize hemopneumothorax may lead

to serious anesthetic difficulties. It greatly alters upper abdominal physical findings on which the decision for surgical intervention largely depends. Hemopneumothorax as an isolated entity, if properly managed, should not add to the mortality of these combined injuries, and in our experience, there is prompt return of the pleural cavity to normal in about 2 weeks. Hemothorax is somewhat more rare and can be diagnosed only in an upright or lateral chest film. Failure to diagnose this condition will result in incarceration of the lower half of the involved lung. Pace *et al.*[66] reported on 76 patients with this condition. In their series, no mortality was associated with pneumo- or hemopneumothorax as isolated injuries. The over-all 20% mortality was based on multiple injuries outside the thoracic cavity.

OTHER NONPENETRATING CHEST INJURIES

Bilateral crushed chest, often without rib fractures, is usually lethal within 12 hours in spite of efforts to preserve functioning lung parenchyma. The child usually has been run over by a vehicle and has only minimal contusion and abrasions of the chest wall. We encountered this twice, and both children died. Fat embolism occurred once in an obese 10-year-old boy with bilateral proximal femoral fractures and fat necrosis of the thighs and buttocks. Management of this condition is the same as in adults. Ours is believed to be the youngest patient on record with documented bilateral pulmonary lesions and fat-positive urine and sputum.

Our experience with nonpenetrating chest injuries is shown in Table 47-4.

Penetrating Injuries of the Chest

Six patients had penetrating thoracic injury. One had multiple lacerations of each lung caused by a knife. Three injuries were caused by projectiles, two

TABLE 47-5.—PENETRATING CHEST INJURIES

INJURY	No. OF PATIENTS	OPERATION	MORTALITY
Lung	5	5	0
Multiple	1	1	0
Total	6	6	0

discharged from a pistol and one by a ten-penny nail thrown at high velocity by a rotary power mower. The nail struck an 8-year-old girl as she was bicycling past the mower some 50 ft. away. The missile entered her right chest, pierced the diaphragm and lodged in the right lobe of the liver. A patient with a self-inflicted injury is shown in Figure 47-24. All 6 patients survived operation (Table 47-5).

Conclusion

A 15-year experience with abdominal, genitourinary and thoracic injuries in 418 children has been described (Table 47-6). Management of patients with multiple injuries and treatment of isolated and combined-organ injury has been outlined. The spectrum is complete except for the rarest of all injuries in childhood—rupture of the cardiac septum or valve leaflets, or both.[6]

TABLE 47.6.—SUMMARY OF ABDOMINAL AND THORACIC INJURIES, 1952–67 (418 PATIENTS)

INJURY	No. OF PATIENTS	OPERATION	MORTALITY
I. Nonpenetrating of abdomen	378	160	12
II. Penetrating of abdomen	21	21	0
III. Nonpenetrating of chest	13	10	3
IV. Penetrating of chest	6	6	0
Total	418	197	15 (3.6%)

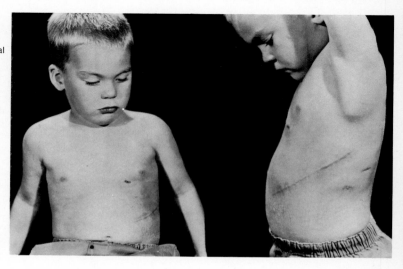

Fig. 47-24.—Penetrating thoracoabdominal injury. This 7-year-old boy shot himself with a 38-caliber revolver. The bullet passed through the left lung, diaphragm, stomach and spleen. The wounds of entrance and exit are readily seen. Only 6% of abdominal injuries were due to penetration.

TABLE 47-7.—NONPENETRATING INJURIES OF THE ABDOMEN

INJURY	NO. OF PATIENTS	OPERATION	MORTALITY
Contusion	172	12	0
Ruptured spleen	71	71	2
Genitourinary*	47	11	0
Gastrointestinal	28	28	1
Vascular (pelvic fracture)	24	7	5
Liver	21	21	4
Pancreas	14	9	0
Ventral hernia	1	1	0
Total	378	160	12 (3.2%)

*BCH cases only.

Nonpenetrating abdominal injuries accounted for 378 of the 418 cases (Table 47-7). Over-all mortality for this group was 3.2%. In the patients requiring laparotomy, mortality was 6.6%. The highest mortality (21%) was encountered in patients with extensive vascular injury associated with torn-apart pelvis,[74] followed by blunt hepatic rupture (19%). Abdominal contusion is considered an important surgical-clinical entity in children and accounts for the high over-all salvage rate.

Promptly recognized and treated penetrating or nonpenetrating wounds of the thorax and penetrating injuries of the abdomen have a conspicuously low mortality—long recognized in adult experience.

In this series, blunt or closed trauma accounted for 93% of cases, and multiple systems were involved in 56%. Both figures are adverse for survival.

REFERENCES

1. Allen, R. B., and Curry, G. J.: Abdominal trauma. A study of 297 consecutive cases, Am. J. Surg. 93:398, 1957.
2. Anderson, E. E., and Harrison, J. H.: Surgical importance of the solitary kidney, New England J. Med. 273:683, 1965.
3. Bailey, W. C., and Akers, D. R: Traumatic intramural hematoma of the duodenum in children, Am. J. Surg. 110:695, 1965.
4. Benson, C. D.: Traumatic injury to the liver, gallbladder and biliary tract, S. Clin. North America 33:1189, 1953.
5. Berfenstam, R., et al.: Accident cases in Stockholm in 1955, Svenska läkartidn. 54:1950, 1957.
6. Berman, R. W., et al.: Traumatic nonpenetrating ventricular septal defects: Recovery under conservative management, J. Pediat. Surg. 1:275, 1966.
7. Bernhard, W. F.: Feasibility of partial liver resection under hypothermia, New England J. Med. 253:159, 1955.
8. Blumenstock, D. A.; Mithoefer, J., and Santulli, T. V.: Acute pancreatitis In children, Pediatrics 19:1002, 1957.
9. Boley, S. J.; MacKinnon, M. P., and Marpel, J.: Rupture of the spleen in children Surg., Gynec. & Obst. 109:78, 1959.
10. Bollinger, J. A., and Fowler, E. F.: Traumatic rupture of the spleen with special reference to delayed splenic rupture, Am. J. Surg. 91:561, 1956.
11. Bugden, W. F.; Chu, P. T., and Delmonico, J. E.: Traumatic diaphragmatic hernia, Ann. Surg. 142:851, 1955.
12. Byrne, J. J., and Boyd, T. F.: Serum amylase levels in experimental intestinal obstruction, New England J. Med. 256:176, 1957.
13. Chamberlain, J. M.: Diaphragmatic hernia produced by indirect violence, S. Clin. North America 33:1505, 1953.
14. Clowes, G. H., Jr.; Vucinic, M., and Weidner, M. G.: Circulatory and metabolic alterations associated with survival or death in peritonitis, Ann. Surg. 163:866, 1966.
15. Desforges, G., et al.: Traumatic rupture of the diaphragm, J. Thoracic Surg. 34:799, 1957.
16. Devroede, G. J., et al.: Intramural hematoma of the duodenum and jejunum, Am. J. Surg. 112:947, 1966.
17. Dietrich, E. B., et al.: Traumatic injuries to the extrahepatic biliary tract, Am. J. Surg. 112:756, 1966.
18. Dietrich, H. F.: Accidental injuries in childhood, J.A.M.A. 156:929, 1954.
19. Dominion Bureau of Statistics: Death from Selected Causes, 1-14 Years (Ottawa, Canada: 1965).
20. Economy, D.; Koucky, C., and Novack, R. L.: Nonpenetrating injuries to the spleen, Am. J. Surg. 99:646, 1960.
21. Ekengren, K., and Soderlund, K.: Radiological findings in traumatic lesions of the pancreas in childhood, Ann. radiol. 9:279, 1966.
22. Elighov, H. E.; Boichis, H., and Eden, E.: Traumatic infarction in a solitary kidney J. Urol. 90:16, 1963.
23. Elman, R.; Arneson, N., and Graham, E. A.: Value of blood amylase determinations in the diagnosis of pancreatic disease, Arch. Surg. 19:943, 1929.
24. Eraklis, A. J., et al.: Hazard of overwhelming infection after splenectomy in childhood, New England J. Med. 276:1225, 1967.
25. Eraklis, A. J.; Tank, E., and Gross, R. E.: Abdominal Injuries in Childhood, Presented at the Annual Meeting, American Association for the Surgery of Trauma, Chicago, 1967.
26. Fock, G.; Stenstrom, R., and Lindfors, O.: Subcutaneous kidney ruptures in children; Ann. chir. et gynaec. Fenniae 55:112, 1966.
27. Folkman, M. J.: Personal Communication
28. Fowler, R., and Hiller, H. G.: Selective hepatic arteriography in the management of traumatic hemobilia, J. Pediat. Surg. 2:253, 1967.
29. Freese, P.; Heinrich, P., and Hinze, M.: Care of traumatic liver wounds with acrylic adhesives, Chirurg 36:483, 1965.
30. Frey, C., et al.: Use of Arteriography as Adjunct to Diagnosis of Hemorrhage from Blunt Abdominal Trauma. Presented before the Society for Surgery of the Alimentary Tract, Chicago, June 25, 1966.
31. Fruchtman, B., and Newman, H.: Upper ureteral avulsion secondary to nonpenetrating injury, J. Urol. 93:452, 1965.
32. Griswold, R. H., and Collier, H. S. Blunt abdominal trauma: Collective review, Surg., Gynec. & Obst. 112:309, 1961.
33. Giedion, A.: Die geburtstraumatische Ruptur parenchymatöser Bauchorgane (Leber, milz, nebenniere und niere) mit massivem Blutverlust und ihre radiologische Darstellung, Helvet. paediat acta 18:349, 1963.
34. Hannon, D. W., and Sprafka, J.: Resection for traumatic pancreatitis, Ann. Surg. 91:552, 1956.
35. Hartman, S. W., and Greaney, E. M.: Traumatic injuries to the biliary system in children, Am. J. Surg. 108:150, 1964.
36. Hendren, W. H., Jr.; Greep, J. M., and Patton, A. S.: Pancreatitis in childhood. Experience with 15 cases, Arch Dis. Childhood 40:132:1965.
37. Hicken, N. F., and Stevenson, V. L.: Traumatic rupture of the choledochus associated with an acute hemorrhagic pancreatitis, Ann. Surg. 128:1178, 1948.
38. Hicks, J. H.: A case of traumatic perforation of the gall-

bladder in a child of three years, Brit. J. Surg. 31:305, 1944.

39. Hoffman, W.: Collective review: Free chyle in the acute abdomen, Surg., Gynec. & Obst. 98:209, 1954.

40. Howard, J. H., *et al.*: Plasma amylase activity in combat casualties, Ann. Surg. 141:338, 1955.

41. Howland, W. S., *et al.*: Physiologic alterations with massive blood replacement, Surg., Gynec. & Obst. 99:478, 1955.

42. Jones, R. C., and Shires, G. T.: The management of pancreatic injuries, Arch. Surg. 90:502, 1965.

43. Jones, T. W.; Nyjus, L., and Harkins, H. N.: Formalinized polyvinyl alcohol (Ivalon) sponge in repair of liver wounds, Arch. Surg. 76:583, 1958.

44. Judd, D. R., and Moore, T. C.: Right hepatic lobectomy for massive liver trauma. Case report, Ann. Surg. 163:149, 1966.

45. Kaiser, T. F., and Farrow, F. C.: Injury to bladder and prostatomembranous urethra associated with fractures of the bony pelvis, Surg., Gynec. & Obst. 120:99, 1965.

46. King, H., and Schumacher, H. B., Jr.: Susceptibility to infection after splenectomy performed in infancy, Ann. Surg. 136:239, 1955.

47. Kinnaird, D. W.: Pancreatic injuries due to nonpenetrating abdominal trauma, Am. J. Surg. 91:552, 1956.

48. Kwang, Wook-Ko; Randolph, J., and Fellers, F.: Peritoneal self dialysis following traumatic rupture of the urethra, J. Urol. 91:343, 1961.

49. Ladd, W. E., and Gross, R. E.: *Abdominal Surgery of Infancy and Childhood* (Philadelphia: W. B. Saunders Company, 1941).

50. Laski, B., and MacMillan, A.: Incidence of infection in children after splenectomy, Pediatrics 24:523, 1959.

51. Longmire, W. P., Jr.: Hepatic surgery: Trauma, tumors and cysts, Ann. Surg. 161:1, 1965.

52. MacKinnon, M. P.; Boley, S. J., and Marpel, J.: Susceptibility to infection following spenectomy for rupture, Am. J. Dis. Child. 98:710, 1959.

53. Madding, G. F., and Kennedy, P. A.: *Trauma to the Liver* (Philadelphia: W. B. Saunders Company, 1965).

54. McDermott, W. V., Jr., and Ottinger, L. W.: Elective hepatic resection, Am. J. Surg. 112:376, 1966.

55. McLelland, R. N., and Shires, T.: Management of liver trauma in 259 consecutive patients, Ann. Surg. 161:248, 1965.

56. Merz, H. O.: Injury of the kidney in children, J. Urol. 69:39, 1953.

57. Mestel, A. L., *et al.*: Acute obstruction of small intestine secondary to hematoma in children, Arch. Surg. 78:25, 1959.

58. Mikeskey, W. E.; Howard, J. M., and DeBakey, M. E.: Collective review: Injuries of the liver in 300 consecutive patients, Surg., Gynec. & Obst. 103:323, 1956.

59. Moritz, A.: *Pathology of Trauma* (Philadelphia: Lea & Febiger, 1954).

60. Morton, J. H.; Hinshaw, J. R., and Morton, J. J.: Blunt trauma to the abdomen, Ann. Surg. 145:699, 1957.

61. Nardi, G. L., and Lees, C. W.: A new diagnostic test for pancreatic disease, New England J. Med. 258:797, 1958.

62. Nation, E. F., and Massey, B. D.: Renal trauma, experience with 258 cases, J. Urol. 89:775, 1963.

63. Nusbaum, M., *et al.*: Demonstration of intra-abdominal bleeding by selective arteriography, J.A.M.A. 191:389, 1965.

64. Oeconomopolous, C. T., and Lee, C. M.: Pseudocysts of the pancreas in infants and young children: Report of four cases, Surgery 47:836, 1960.

65. Owing, H. K.: Case of lacerated liver, London M. Gaz. 7:1048, 1848.

66. Pace, W. G.; Passaro, E., and Klassen, K. P.: Experience with intrathoracic injury following automobile accidents, Am. J. Surg. 99:827, 1960.

67. Penberthy, G. C.: Avulsion of mesentery with adjacent necrosis, S. Clin. North America 33:1179, 1953.

68. Potter, E. L.: Fetal and neonatal deaths: A statistical analysis of 2,000 autopsies, J.A.M.A. 115:996, 1940.

69. Poulos, E.; *et al.*: Traumatic hemobilia treated by massive liver resection, Arch. Surg. 88:596, 1964.

70. Quimby, W. C., Jr.: Fracture of the pelvis and associated injuries in children, J. Pediat. Surg. 1:353, 1966.

71. Robart, F. H.: Traumatic Intramural Haematoma of the Proximal Jejunal loop. Presented at the Annual Meeting of the British Association of Pediatric Surgeons, Edinburgh, 1957.

72. Sandblom, P.: Hemorrhage into the biliary tract following trauma: "Traumatic hemobilia," Surgery 24:571, 1948.

73. Sano, M. E., and Holland, C.: Coagulum technique in traumatic rupture of the liver in dogs, Science 98:524, 1943.

74. Scott, R., Jr., *et al.*: Initial management of nonpenetrating renal injuries: Clinical review of 111 cases, J. Urol. 90:535, 1963.

75. Seitzman, D. M.: Repair of the severed prostatomembranous urethra by the combined approach, J. Urol. 89:433, 1963.

76. Shirkey, A. L., *et al.*: Surgical management of splenic injuries Am. J. Surg. 108:630, 1964.

77. Shohl, T.: Hepatic artery ligation for massive hemobilia, Surgery 56:855, 1964.

78. Sieber, W. K., and Girdany, B. R.: Rupture of the spleen in newborn infants, New England J. Med. 259:1074, 1959.

79. Spencer, R.: Injuries of the Spleen and Liver in Children. Presented at the Clinical Congress, American College of Surgeons, Atlantic City, 1965.

80. Stalowsky, H. J.: Stumpfes Bauchtrauma und Darmruptur in Kindesalter, Chirurg 36:4, 1965.

81. Stormo, A. C.: Traumatic chylous ascites, Arch. Surg. 92:115, 1966.

82. Storsteen, K. A., and Remine, W. H.: Rupture of the spleen with splenic implants, Ann. Surg. 137:551, 1953.

83. Sturim, H. S.: Surgical management of pancreatic injuries, Surg., Gynec. & Obst. 122:133, 1966.

84. Sulamaa, M., and Vitanen, I.: Treatment of pancreatic rupture, Arch. Dis. Childhood 39:187, 1964.

85. Ulvestad, L. E.: Repair of laceration of superior mesenteric artery acquired by nonpenetrating injury of the abdomen, Ann. Surg. 140:752, 1954.

86. Vollman, R. W.: Keenan, W. J., and Eraklis, A. J.: Post-traumatic chylous ascites in infancy, New England J. Med. 275:875, 1966.

87. Wang, C. C., and Robbins, L. L.: Roentgenologic diagnosis of ruptured spleen, New England J. Med. 254:445, 1956.

88. Wangensteen, O.: *Cancer of Esophagus and Stomach* (New York: American Cancer Society, Inc., 1951).

89. Warren, K. W., *et al.*: Surgical treatment of pancreatic cysts: Review of 183 cases, Ann. Surg. 163:886, 1966.

90. Warren, K. W.: Personal communication.

91. Warren, K. W., and Wagner, R. B.: Long term results of nonpenetrating pancreatic trauma, Lahey Clin. Bull. 16:218, 1967.

92. Watkins, G. L.: Blunt trauma to the abdomen, Arch. Surg. 80:187, 1960.

93. Waugh, G. E.: Traumatic rupture of the common bile duct in a boy six years old, Brit. J. Surg. 3:685, 1916.

94. Weitzman, J. J., and Swenson, O.: Traumatic rupture of the pancreas in a toddler, Surgery 57:309, 1965.

95. Welch, C. E.: Abdominal surgery, New England J. Med. 275:1291, 1967.

96. Welch, K. J.: Genitourinary Injuries in Children: Report of 78 Cases. Presented at the Clinical Congress, American College of Surgeons, Atlantic City, 1965.

97. Welch, K. J.: Traumatic pancreatitis in childhood, Newton-Wellesley M. Bull. 11:22, 1959.

98. Welch, K. J.: Right Hepatic Lobectomy for Blunt trauma with Adjunct Hypothermia (nonpenetrating Abdominal

Injuries in Children). Presented at the Annual Meeting, American Association for the Surgery of Trauma, San Diego, Calif., October 5, 1960.

99. Westland, J. C.; Greaney, E. M., and Snyder, W. H., Jr.: Experience with abdominal trauma in childhood, West. J. Surg. 63:609, 1955.

100. Williams, R. D., and Zollinger, R. M.: Diagnostic and prognostic factors in abdominal trauma, Am. J. Surg. 97:575, 1959.

101. Williams, R. D., and Yurko, A. A., Jr.: Controversial aspects of diagnosis and management of blunt abdominal trauma, Am. J. Surg. 111:477, 1966.

102. Wilson, T. H., Jr.: Traumatic hernia of abdominal wall, Am. J. Surg. 97:340, 1959.

103. Wright, P. W., and Orloff, M. J.: Traumatic hemobilia, Ann. Surg. 160:42, 1964.

104. Zachary, R. B., and Emery, J. L.: Abdominal splenosis following rupture of the spleen in a boy aged 10 years, Brit. J. Surg. 46:415, 1959.

K. J. WELCH

Drawings by

MURIEL MCLATCHIE MILLER

PAMELA BERGLUND

MARGARET DRUMMOND

SECTION THREE

48

Liver and Biliary Tract

Obstructive Jaundice

OBSTRUCTIVE JAUNDICE in infancy presents a surgical challenge, not only in the differential diagnosis of cases amenable to surgical correction as opposed to those of hepatocellular origin, but also to improve the persistently low salvage rate obtained even for the correctable lesions. Surgery should be undertaken before 3 months of age, and preferably by 2 months of age, to prevent the ravages of prolonged obstruction, namely, cirrhosis, portal hypertension, liver failure and death. Thus there is only a short time between the appearance of the jaundice at 4–6 weeks of age and the optimal time for surgical intervention.

NEONATAL JAUNDICE

Hyperbilirubinemia in the first few days to 2 weeks of life is usually characterized by elevation of the unconjugated bilirubin fraction, signifying problems involving hemolysis that cause an increased production of bilirubin or a delayed development of the glucuronide conjugation. Formerly, this was known as physiologic jaundice. In addition to the obvious problems of hemolysis, including RH and type incompatibility persistent hyperbilirubinemia of a nonobstructive nature may be due to congenital familial deficiency of glucuronal transferase, as in the Crigler-Najjar syndrome, to excretion deficiencies similar to the Dubin-Johnson syndrome or to other rare and unusual inborn errors in the conjugation and excretion phenomena.

More confusing perhaps are the infants who become jaundiced after the immediate neonatal period on the basis of sepsis, reflecting such conditions as congenital syphilis, a problem again on the increase on the national scene, viral disease such as cytomegalic inclusion disease, hereditary galactosemia and, finally, neonatal hepatitis with giant cell transforma-

tion of the hepatic parenchyma. Most of these conditions are not truly obstructive from the anatomic standpoint, but they mimic obstructive disease and must be differentiated by appropriate tests. The differentiation is necessarily urgent, as the clinical observations to follow will indicate. Survival of patients whose obstruction is relieved after 3 months of age is rare, and many of those operated on before this time have a severe morbidity or even mortality due to the ravages of cirrhosis and later portal hypertension.

LABORATORY DIFFERENTIATION

Differential diagnosis in cases of obstructive jaundice is important. The surgical correction of biliary atresia is urgent because of the early development of cirrhosis secondary to atresia. It will be shown that surgical correction is not synonymous with surgical salvage unless the operation is undertaken before 3 months of age, preferably by 8 weeks.

The laboratory is useful in the differentiation of early hemolytic disease and hyperbilirubinemia due to nonobstructive causes from those enumerated in the obstructive field. Laboratory investigation aids in identifying obstructive disease by demonstrating an increase of the conjugated fraction of the bilirubin, decrease of bilirubin in the stool, increase of bilirubin in the urine, decrease of urine urobilinogen and the indirect reflection of hepatic obstruction in the numerous liver function tests, such as alkaline phosphatase, thymol turbidity and the various flocculation tests. The true differentiation of obstructive disease that has an anatomic basis from that caused by hepatocellular disease or neonatal hepatitis with giant cell replacement cannot be made from laboratory data. Studies of serum transaminase patterns have been advocated by Kove *et al*[12] repeatedly, but few other authors have found them to be of value as a distinguishing feature. Serum transaminase activity (measured as glutamic oxalacetic transaminase) in the extremely high range very early in the disease tends to indicate infectious origin, but most of the problems fall into the middle range of transaminase values that are not diagnostic. Color in the stool is not diagnostic, since studies with tagged bilirubin by Schmid[17] have proved that bilirubin may cross the intestinal membrane in both directions. The use of I[131]-labeled rose bengal[2] is helpful in detecting minute amounts of excretion, but has no further significance in the differentiation of the hepatocellular vs. the anatomic obstructive group. In the face of the urgency in making the diagnosis and lack of assistance from the laboratory, differential diagnosis must be accomplished by radiologic examination of the extrahepatic biliary system in combination with demonstration of the histopathology of the liver.

SURGICAL PROCEDURE

Once the jaundice in the infant has been proved to be on an obstructive basis, one should proceed to procure an operative cholangiogram to demonstrate the status of the extrahepatic biliary system.

Preparation of the patient for surgery is important. Liver function deficiencies should be corrected if possible. Administration of vitamin K is indicated when prothrombin function is decreased, and transfusion to correct anemia. The choice of anesthetic agent is important. Smith[21] noted that the child with biliary atresia without extensive hepatocellular damage seems to tolerate open-drop ether anesthesia quite well, but he advocated the use of cyclopropane with the attendant high oxygen flow for a child who may have considerable hepatocellular damage. Other anesthetic agents should be evaluated in the light of their hepatocellular toxicity; probably most agents will be discarded in favor of the two mentioned here.

The child should be placed on oxygen and gastric suction with intravenous replacement for 12 hours before operation. This decompresses the small intestine, allowing for easier and less traumatic exploration and a shorter procedure. Under general anesthesia with the proper intravenous support, a right upper quadrant incision can be made, exposing the liver and the porta hepatis. A generous and adequate liver biopsy specimen can be taken under direct vision and hemostasis adequately established. Superficial exploration will either demonstrate or show the lack of an extrahepatic biliary tree. Should a gallbladder be visible, a fine polyethylene tube can be sewed into the lumen of the gallbladder and the extrahepatic tree irrigated with 20–30 cc of normal saline solution so that artifacts due to inspissation of the bile or collapsed biliary tree will not be present in the x-ray film to follow. Then, after injection of a suitable contrast medium of low viscosity, a cholangiogram can be made, and within a very few minutes the interpretation can be obtained from the department of radiology. If a normal extrahepatic biliary tree is demonstrated (Fig. 48-1), the procedure is terminated. The

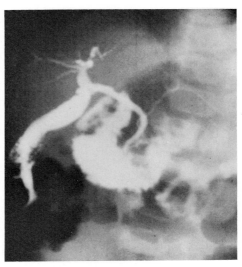

Fig. 48-1.—Normal operative cholangiogram. A liver biopsy specimen showed a picture compatible with hepatitis.

procedure is short, the answer is definitive and no permanent damage should be done. The interpretation of the liver biopsy and the subsequent course of the patient will determine the outcome. Surgery in such a case offers nothing more than a diagnosis.

If a defective extrahepatic biliary tree (Figs. 48-2 and 48-3) is demonstrated, further exploration to correct this defect or to estimate operability is undertaken.

In the child whose extrahepatic biliary tree is not totally demonstrated or in whom a gallbladder cannot be found for such cholangiography, meticulous exploration of the porta hepatis and its contents with demonstration of all the normal structures can be carried out. It is most important that unidentifiable structures encountered should not be transected, since there are many examples in the literature of small accessory or hypoplastic biliary ducts developing after what has previously been reported as unsuccessful surgical exploration with eventual survival of a non-jaundiced patient. Adequate anesthesia, good exposure and meticulous dissection with the demonstration of the anatomic structures should reveal a remnant of hepatic, cystic or common duct, when present, that can be anastomosed to the intestinal tract. Such a remnant may be well up within the substance of the liver or under an edge of an enlarged organ with obvious biliary cirrhosis.

When one encounters such a suspected remnant, cautious aspiration with a small-bore needle will show whether it is vascular or biliary in nature. Should one achieve a bile-stained return from the aspiration, anastomosis to the intestinal tract can be carried out. Whether one uses a Roux-en-Y technique as advocated by Koop or direct anastomosis to the

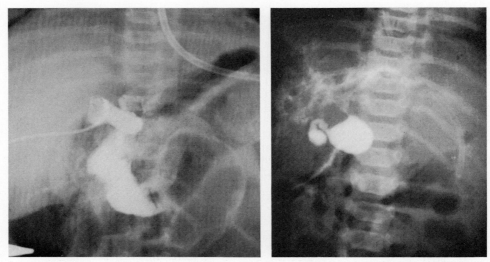

Fig. 48-2 (left).—Operative cholangiogram showing patency of the gallbladder, cystic duct and common duct but no evidence of hepatic ducts. Further exploration revealed inoperable atresia of hepatic ducts.
Fig. 48-3 (right).—Operative cholangiogram showing cystic dilatation of the common duct with no communication to the intestine. Anastomosis of the duodenum to this cystic remnant relieved the obstructive jaundice and led to total recovery.

duodenum as advocated by Gross[7] and Swenson[26] depends on the anatomy at the site, the duration of the operation and the technical preference of the surgeon.

It is important to remember that these children are not good candidates for prolonged anesthesia should the search for the remnant be a long one or the remnant be discovered at the end of a long anesthesia. It may be wiser to sew a tube or catheter into this remnant and exteriorize it to create an external biliary fistula until secondary repair several weeks after the baby has recovered from the anesthesia and the biliary obstruction has been decompressed. This procedure has been most helpful in several cases in which the prolonged anesthesia for anastomosis might have been fatal to a child already debilitated.

POSTOPERATIVE MANAGEMENT.—Whether the anastomosis is of an isolated loop as in the Roux-en-Y technique or a direct anastomosis, the most important factor is an adequately wide anastomosis to prevent obstruction. Ascending cholangitis has been a com-

Fig. 48-4.—Pre- and postoperative bilirubin levels in a 6-week-old infant with cystic dilatation of the common duct and recovery after anastomosis to the duodenum. (Courtesy of Dr. W. J. Waters.)

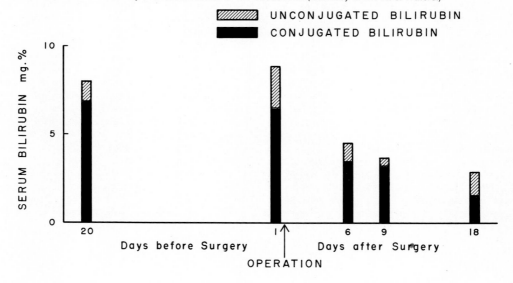

mon problem in the postoperative phase in those whose defect has been successfully corrected. This seems to be a factor of relative obstruction rather than the reflux of stomach or intestinal contents into the biliary tree. An anastomosis that is widely patent seems to tolerate the presence of intestinal contents within the biliary tree as long as there is no obstruction to free flow of this material back into the duodenum. Since the structure with which one is dealing is tiny, it is advocated that the child be kept on some broad-spectrum antibiotics for some time postoperatively and that they be used intermittently for 6 months should there be any indication of repeated cholangitis. Permanent biliary tract damage from such an insult is probably as responsible for the poor postoperative results as is the long delay before operation.

Choleretics such as dihydrocholic acid are also very useful. In babies with repeated jaundice and fever following anastomosis, a combination of broad-spectrum antibiotics plus the hydrocholeretic seems to promote the flow of dilute bile and protects liver substance. Subsidence of postoperative edema results, and growth corrects the relative obstruction.

No one method can be advocated over another, the choice depending on the anatomic situation one encounters and one's technical preference. If the anastomosis is a direct one, many prefer to anastomose over a small piece of rubber catheter or plastic tube to ensure patency. An inner layer mucosa-to-mucosa anastomosis reinforced by an outer layer for strength without turning in too great a cuff of tissue has been found to be adequate. A fine nonabsorbable suture material such as 5-0 silk or Dacron should be used.

Figure 48-4 shows the expected results in terms of bilirubin levels following successful anastomosis of a biliary remnant to the intestinal tract. Jaundice should disappear in several days, but total return of bilirubin levels to normal may take 3–4 weeks.

TYPES OF BILIARY ATRESIA

Figure 48-5 indicates the commonly encountered types of biliary atresia, both inoperable and operable. The largest single review of the results of surgery for biliary atresia was made by members of the Surgical Section of the American Academy of Pediatrics in a 10-year survey from 1954 to 1964.[11] The records of 1,025 cases of obstructive jaundice were examined, 843 of which were documented cases of biliary atresia. Of the 843 cases, 102 were classed as correctable with patent remnants of biliary tree in continuity with the liver. This correctability rate of 12% (102 cases) agrees with many reports in the literature of the previous two decades. Most alarming, however, was the report that only 53 of the 102 patients were alive at the time of the survey. Thus, of a total of 1,025 patients, 1 of every 10 who are explored will have a correctable lesion, but only 1 of 20 with correction at exploration will survive. This series is from the United States, Canada, Puerto Rico and Mexico. A report from Finland gives comparable statistics on 41 cases of biliary atresia.[25] Twelve patients had a remnant of hepatic duct available for anastomosis; only 6 of these 12 had satisfactory bile drainage postoperatively and all died. A study from Japan by Shiraki *et al.*[18] between 1959 and 1965 detailed 62 cases of con-

Fig. 48-5.—Common types of atresia of bile ducts. **Upper row,** inoperable; **lower row,** correctable.

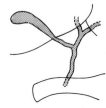

Gallbladder
and Extrahepatic Bile Ducts

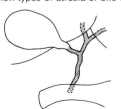

Extrahepatic Bile Ducts

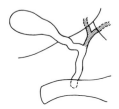

Common Hepatic Bile Duct

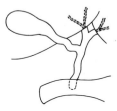

Intrahepatic Bile Ducts

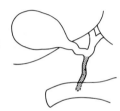

Common Bile Duct

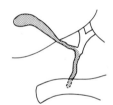

Gallbladder
and Common Bile Duct

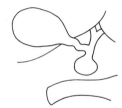

Distal Common Bile Duct

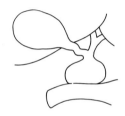

of Common Bile Duct

genital bile duct atresia with successful establishment of biliary drainage to the intestinal tract in only 4 of the 11 patients who were deemed operable. These authors also stated that their follow-up study of prolonged jaundice indicated that progressive hepatic fibrosis is the principal cause of death; the 4 patients who survived were all operated on before 3 months of age. These figures were compared to the long-term survival of children with so-called neonatal hepatitis. Seventy-five cases were studied: only 12 patients (16%) died, 4 of hepatic failure, 3 of cirrhosis, 3 postoperatively following diagnostic laparotomy and 2 were reported to have died of pneumonia after discharge. Other survival figures for nonsurgical conditions mimicking atresia may be found in the literature, but few have been studied as completely as the Japanese series. In another publication, the same group[19] reported a study of histologic changes in congenital biliary atresia in relation to age and concluded that in both correctable and noncorrectable types of biliary atresia, the number of giant cells was increased in the younger age group. Further, there was an increase of the amount of bile duct hyperplasia in the younger age group. It was also evident that the degree of hepatic fibrosis had increased with age of the individuals studied by biopsy. The significance of these observations is discussed later under Etiology.

OTHER CONDITIONS CAUSING OBSTRUCTION

In the Academy of Pediatrics survey of 1,025 cases of obstructive jaundice, 182 were reported to be due to causes other than biliary atresia. Eighty of these were classified as inspissated bile. This condition, originally described by Ladd and since described by many others, including Benson *et al.,*[1] is characterized by obstructive jaundice relieved by irrigation of the extrahepatic biliary tree with subsequent resolu-

Fig. 48-6.— A, on the left, operative cholangiogram before removal of inspissated biliary material; on the right, relief of obstruction and relatively normal cholangiogram. **B,** the biliary material that was removed; ×9. (Courtesy of Dr. C. D. Benson.)

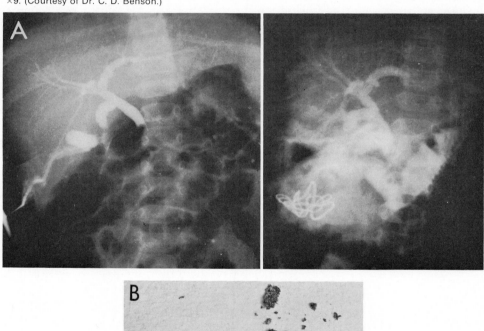

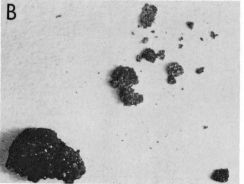

tion of the jaundice. The term inspissated bile was used in the past to refer to cases that showed resolution of jaundice after laparotomy. Many of these since have been considered to be cases of neonatal hepatitis with giant cell transformation or replacement. Benson referred to 5 cases in which true common duct obstruction was relieved by irrigation. Rickham and Lee[16] mentioned 3 similar cases. Figure 48-6 is an example of one of Benson's cases. Infants who have had a severe hemolytic disease in the newborn period with or without exchange transfusion often after initial clearing of the jaundice may again become jaundiced, this time with evidence of obstruction. This is the only known cause of inspissation or common duct plugs, i.e., hemolysis. All other cases may represent sequelae of hepatitis. Histologic studies on these livers may prove useful.

Among the 182 cases without biliary atresia, 49 were noted to have hypoplasia of the intrahepatic bile ducts. Longmire[14] has described 5 patients with extrahepatic bile duct hypoplasia. The same picture was described in 1959 by Krovetz,[13] who called the condition intrahepatic atresia. The tiny size of the extrahepatic ducts was felt by many to be atrophy of disuse in association with the intrahepatic ducts rather than a primary hypoplasia of an embryonal nature.

In the syndrome of biliary hypoplasia observed by Longmire in his cases and in 10 cases seen by us over 15 years, a paucity of intrahepatic ducts accompanies hypoplasia of the extrahepatic region. Most of these children have intermittent jaundice, splenomegaly, elevated cholesterol levels with severe pruritus, and xanthomatous skin lesions noted on biopsy to be made up largely of cholesterol. Many of these children improve with age, although repeated liver biopsies, as noted by Tidrick,[27] show progressive diminution of the number of intrahepatic ducts.

Full understanding of this syndrome of hypoplasia will come with further study. Smetana et al.[20] relate this condition to a place in the spectrum of liver response manifested by giant cell replacement: " . . . it is proposed that there is a strong suggestion of a pathogenic linkage between the various forms of extrahepatic and intrahepatic biliary atresia, giant cell transformation and combinations of these anomalies of the biliary passages as causes of persistent clinical obstructive neonatal jaundice." The importance in recognizing hypoplasia has been mentioned. There is no surgical correction for this condition, and most children will survive for some time.

The other causes of obstruction in the survey by the American Academy of Pediatrics include 36 cases of choledochal cyst (discussed later in this chapter), several cases of lymphatic obstruction and inflammation in the porta hepatis, 1 instance of pancreatic inflammation and 1 of common duct stone.[11] Other series have reported neonatal jaundice secondary to malignancies or hemangiomas of the port of hepatis. None were noted in this series of 1,025 cases.

OTHER DIAGNOSTIC APPROACHES

It is evident from the number of individuals who undergo operation and are found to have essentially hepatocellular disease, that other methods of diagnosis prior to surgery have been attempted. Percutaneous cholangiography has been advocated but found to be impractical, with no satisfactory studies other than sporadic reports in the literature that it provided absolute differentiation, thus avoiding surgery. Percutaneous liver biopsy has been more satisfactory than percutaneous cholangiography. The safety and usefulness of percutaneous liver biopsy were emphasized by Walker et al.,[28] who performed 210 biopsies without a serious complication. Of these, 21 were done for diagnosis of obstructive jaundice, and valuable information contributing to the diagnosis was obtained in 18.

In a careful evaluation of the three standard procedures used in differentiation between biliary atresia and neonatal hepatitis, Hays et al.[8] demonstrated the effectiveness and accuracy of the percutaneous needle biopsy as compared to open operative hepatic biopsy. The accuracy of these two methods was quite similar, with approximately one third of the specimens obtained by either method failing to offer distinguishing evidence. They found that operative cholangiography invariably led to the proper operation or surgical management, but one fifth of the interpretations of the films suggested a diagnosis ultimately found to be incorrect. Their studies further indicated that several infants appeared to show evidence of both conditions, i.e., biliary atresia and neonatal hepatitis, each appearing during different phases in the course of the illness. Since percutaneous liver biopsy offers no absolute answer to the diagnosis of obstructive jaundice, in that it cannot be relied on for either adequacy of specimen or accuracy of diagnosis, a combination of open biopsy, with a guaranteed adequacy of size of specimen, and operative cholangiography is recommended as the ideal approach to the obstructed child.

OTHER SURGICAL APPROACHES

In view of the rather dismal outlook for children with biliary atresia, it is not surprising that numerous other surgical approaches for salvage of these unfortunate individuals have been undertaken. Prominent among these is the work of Sterling,[22] who introduced the use of artificial bile ducts to create internal biliary fistulas in the hope of prolonging the lives of patients otherwise deemed inoperable. Though Sterling feels that this has prolonged the lives of some of these infants, no one else using the technique has experienced the same degree of success. Most authors observe that one must create a mucosa-to-mucosa anastomosis to ensure patency and longevity.

Fonkalsrud et al.[6] have employed a method of anastomosing the lymphatic channels in the porta hepatis to the intestinal tract, since it has been shown that serum bilirubin levels will drop with copious lymphatic drainage immediately postoperatively. Such attempts have not proved satisfactory. In a similar attempt to divert lymphatic drainage, a different method has been tried in Japan by Sugura *et al.*,[24] connecting the thoracic duct to some portion of the intestinal tract, the floor of the mouth, the esophagus or pharynx. With an exteriorized thoracic duct, the serum bilirubin level will drop precipitously. Unless one is able to make a satisfactory communication between the thoracic duct and the intestinal tract, which so far has been impossible, the improvement is short-lived and the fate of these youngsters has been uniformly poor. Many years ago, Longmire and Sanford[15] introduced the concept of hepatic lobectomy with suturing the raw surface of the liver to open intestine, but this again proved a failure, as it has in many hands since, because of the lack of a mucosa-to-mucosa anastomosis.

Many attempts have been made at reoperation of previously proved inoperable situations in the hope of discovering "bile lakes" for intestinal anastomosis. With rare exceptions, these have been fruitless. The cirrhosis that accompanies biliary obstruction of longer than 3 months is almost invariably fatal. Sporadic attempts have been made to transplant an entire liver in place of the cirrhotic liver of biliary atresia. In 1967, surgeons at the Colorado Medical Center accomplished five such replacements; several patients died, and the others have been too recently operated on to be evaluated. Conquering the immune rejection response would seem to be a prime objective. That transplanted livers will function, has been demonstrated. Whether they will grow and continue to function is yet to be proved.

In view of these difficulties, it would seem that improvement of the prospects for these children will come from study of the etiology of the condition and then institution of prevention rather than restoration of the altered anatomy.

ETIOLOGY OF BILIARY ATRESIA

Classic embryologic descriptions of the formation of the liver differ somewhat regarding the origins of intra- and extrahepatic bile ducts. Smetana *et al.*[20] discussed the various concepts and noted that none of them explains the various forms or degrees of atresia noted in the human infant with obstructive jaundice.

Holder[10] observed an infant who had I[131] rose bengal excretion within normal limits at age 13 weeks. Jaundice recurred and operation 4 weeks later showed classic extrahepatic biliary atresia.

Brent[3] noted that there are no documented cases of biliary atresia in stillbirths, prematures or embryos. Since then, Holder and Ashcraft[9] have shown that when the common bile duct was obliterated in the canine fetus at 53 days of gestation, puppies were born jaundiced at term. Briggs[4] and I have made a similar observation in fetal sheep. In those sheep whose bile ducts have been obliterated in the fetal state at 110 days of gestation and survived to term, jaundice at birth is apparent clinically and can be documented by the laboratory. Of importance in this regard is the observation that infants with biliary atresia do not have jaundice at birth other than the hyperbilirubinemia that may be present in many newborns. Permanent jaundice associated with atresia may not be evident clinically until 3–6 weeks of age.

If one observes all these phenomena and adds the spectrum of disease as noted in babies from atresia, intra- or extrahepatic, to hypoplasia and finally giant cell transformation, one cannot help wondering about the origins of biliary atresia. Shiraki *et al.*[19] related the histologic change in the liver to age, showing a decrease in the number of giant cells in congenital biliary atresia with advancing age. The number of

Fig. 48-7.— A, high-power view of plugs in inspissated bile in a child with extrahepatic biliary atresia. **B,** lower-power view to show proliferation of bile ducts in the same liver. Courtesy of Dr. David Jones.)

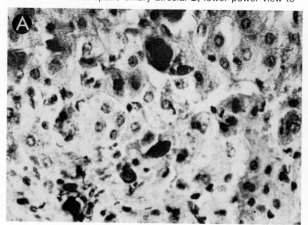
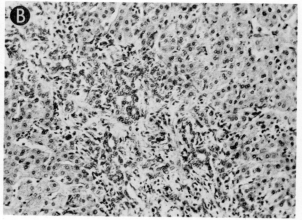

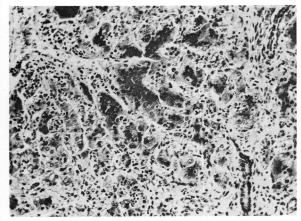

Fig. 48-8.—Infiltration of liver by large multinucleated giant cells. The baby gradually lost her jaundice after demonstration of a normal cholangiogram and this picture at operation. (Courtesy of Dr. David Jones.)

nuclei in the giant cells likewise decreases with age. Bile duct hyperplasia is prominent until 5 months of age; thereafter, the hyperplasia disappears, with increase of fibrous tissue in the portal areas of infants.

All observations lead one to opine that biliary atresia in the several forms noted is an acquired condition, not one secondary to embryonal fault. An agent, perhaps of viral nature, that causes the giant cell reaction in the liver, may be the initiating factor, with complete intra- and/or extrahepatic atresia perhaps a later manifestation. The search for this virus has gone on in the laboratory, but it has not been found with any consistency. It is perhaps of more than pass-

Fig. 48-9.—Liver biopsy specimen from a jaundiced child. The jaundice later cleared, but severe pruritus remained. This is typical of intrahepatic biliary atresia. Some inspissated bile is present in smaller radicles, but there are no demonstrable ducts in portal spaces. The child was alive at age 3 but had pronounced xanthomatous disease and poor development. (Courtesy of Dr. David Jones.)

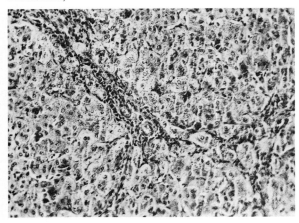

ing interest that the rubella outbreak of 1964–65 produced no more than the expected number of infants with biliary atresia in the populations involved in that epidemic. In the liver of rubella-infected infants, however, Stern and Williams[23] demonstrated a giant cell reaction that cannot be distinguished from that in other forms of neonatal hepatitis not currently associated with a known agent.

Clean-cut differential pathologic sections are rare. The various degrees of obstruction and histologic change in atresia are shown in Figures 48-7 to 48-9. As has been shown by Hays et al.,[8] the pattern is not always clear enough to allow agreement of the initial histologic diagnosis with the ultimate diagnosis proved at operation or autopsy. Such inaccuracies are compatible with a progressive change in the histology related to the age of the infant, as shown by Shiraki.

SUMMARY

The dilemma of biliary atresia, from both the diagnostic and the therapeutic standpoint, has been presented. A therapeutic approach has been outlined. The results of the most recent surveys indicate that success in the correction of biliary atresia has plateaued and is not improving as one might hope. The challenges, therefore, in the search for the etiology of biliary atresia are an orderly understanding of the pathogenesis and, ultimately, prevention rather than correction of the ravages of the disease. It is suggested that biliary atresia may represent one stage in a broader spectrum of disease entities that includes neonatal hepatitis, inspissated bile syndrome, biliary hypoplasia and intrahepatic biliary atresia. Laboratory investigations involving both fetal work and serial biopsy studies may lead to more enlightening observations in the future.

REFERENCES

1. Benson, C. D.; Lotfi, M. W., and Hertzler, J. H.: Surgical aspects of biliary tract disease in the infant and child, Tr. West. Sur. A., 1966.
2. Brent, R. L. and Geppert, L. J.: Use of radioactive rose bengal in the evaluation of infantile jaundice, Am. J. Dis. Child. 98:720, 1959.
3. Brent, R. L.: Persistent jaundice in infancy, J. Pediat. 61:111, 1962.
4. Briggs, H. C.: Personal communication.
5. Craig, J. M., and Landing, B. H.: Forms of hepatitis in neonatal period simulating biliary atresia, Arch. Path. 54:321, 1952.
6. Fonkalsrud, E. W., et al.: Hepatic lymphatic drainage to the jejunum for congenital biliary atresia, Am. J. Surg. 112:188, 1966.
7. Gross, R. E.: Surgery of Infancy and Childhood (Philadelphia: W. B. Saunders Company, 1953), Chap. 41.
8. Hays, D., et al.: Diagnosis of biliary atresia: Relative accuracy of percutaneous liver biopsy, open liver biopsy, and operative cholangiography, J. Pediat. 71:598, 1967.
9. Holder, T. M., and Ashcraft, K. W.: The effects of bile duct ligation and inflammation in the fetus, J. Pediat. Surg. 2:35, 1967.
10. Holder, T. M.: Atresia of the extrahepatic bile duct, Am. J. Surg. 107:458, 1964.

11. Izant, R. J., et al.: Biliary atresia survey, Surgical Section, American Academy of Pediatrics, 1954-64.
12. Kove, S.; Dische, R. M. and Wroblewski, F.: Early diagnosis of biliary tract malformation in newborn infant by serum transaminase patterns, New York J. Med. 63:3497, 1963.
13. Krovetz, L. J.: Intrahepatic biliary atresia, Journal-Lancet 79:228, 1959.
14. Longmire, W. P., Jr.: Congenital biliary hypoplasia, Ann. Surg. 159:337, 1964.
15. Longmire, W. P., Jr., and Sanford, M. C.: Intrahepatic cholangio-jejunostomy with partial hepatectomy for biliary obstruction, Surgery 24:264, 1949.
16. Rickham. P. P., and Lee, E. Y. C.: Neonatal jaundice: Surgical aspects, Clin. pediat. 3:197, 1964.
17. Schmid, R.: Studies of congenital non-hemolytic jaundice with C-14 bilirubin, Ann. New York Acad. Sc. 3:451, 1963.
18. Shiraki, K.; Okamoto, Y., and Takatsu, T.: A follow-up study of prolonged obstructive jaundice in infancy, Pediat. Univ. Tokyo, no. 12, p. 41, 1966.
19. Shiraki, K., et al.: Liver in congenital bile duct atresia: Histological changes in relation to age, Pediat. Univ. Tokyo, no. 12, p. 68, 1966.
20. Smetana, H. F.; Edlow, J. B., and Glunz, P. R.: Neonatal jaundice, Arch. Path. 80:553, 1965.
21. Smith, R. M.: Anesthesia for Infants and Children (St. Louis: C. V. Mosby Company, 1959), p. 325.
22. Sterling, J. A.: Life expectancy in biliary atresia, J. Internat. Coll. Surgeons 46:231, 1966.
23. Stern, H., and Williams, B. M.: Isolation of rubella virus in a case of neonatal giant cell hepatitis, Lancet 1:293, 1966.
24. Sugura, K., et al.: The surgery of infantile obstructive jaundice, Arch. Dis. Childhood 40:158, 1965.
25. Sulamaa, M., and Visakorpi, J. K.: Surgery of the biliary tract in early childhood, Ann. paediat. fenneae 10:1, 1964.
26. Swenson, O.: Pediatric Surgery (New York: Appleton-Century-Crofts, Inc., 1958), Chap. 17.
27. Tidrick, R. T.: Personal communication.
28. Walker, W. A.; Krivit, W., and Sharp, H. L.: Needle biopsy of the liver in infancy and childhood, Pediatrics 40:946, 1967.

L. K. Pickett

Drawings by
NICOLAS APGAR

Congenital Anomalies and Tumors of the Liver

Congenital Anomalies

A. MALFORMATIONS.—A variety of abnormalities in the development of the liver have been described, but most of them are rare and of little clinical significance.

1. *Agenesis.*—Agenesis of the liver is incompatible with life.

2. *Unusual lobe formation.*—This is fairly common. The most important form is Riedel's lobe, a tongue of liver tissue projecting from the right lobe which may resemble a large or mobile right kidney and occasionally causes clinical concern as a possible liver tumor.

3. *Ectopic lobation.*—Ectopic segments of liver tissue may be found in various locations, even within the pleural cavity.

B. LOBAR ATROPHY.—Either lobe may be atrophic, perhaps as a deviant of some of the processes known to occur during fetal liver development. The left lobe is more often atrophic than the right.

C. SOLITARY CYSTS.—These cysts may be large enough to cause dystocia in the mother or serious problems for the neonate. They are seen most often on the anterior-inferior edge of the right lobe, although some lie deep within the substance of the lobe, destroying the normal parenchyma. Occasionally there are multiple cysts in one lobe; these are different from the diffuse cystic involvement seen with polycystic disease, in which there are associated cystic changes in the kidneys and sometimes the pancreas and lungs. If the solitary cyst is pedunculated, it may twist and lead to hemorrhage or suppuration into the cavity and corresponding increase of size. Most solitary cysts are easily excised (Fig. 48-10), but those which lie deep within the hepatic substance may be very difficult to manage. Marsupialization or internal drainage may be the only effective means of handling the problems caused by large size.

Fig. 48-10.—Large solitary cyst of the left lobe of the liver, attached primarily to the edge and area of liver adjacent to the gallbladder of a newborn. Resection was uneventful, and there was no evidence of recurrence 4 years later.

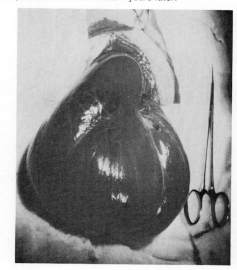

Solitary cysts are said to occur four times as frequently in females as in males. About 250 cases have been reported in adults, but in the age group up to 13 years, only 39 cases have been noted.

D. Anomalies of blood supply to the liver. —These are important to the surgeon, although they seldom are the direct cause of problems to the patient. The variations are numerous and may have serious implications in operative maneuvers around the liver, gallbladder or common bile duct. So long as the possibility of these anomalies is borne in mind, trouble can be avoided.

E. Lymphangioma (mesenchymal hamartoma, cavernous lymphangiomatoid lesion, hamartoma, solitary bile cell fibroadenoma). —Lymphangioma of the liver is not common. On exposure, the mass is poorly demarcated from surrounding normal tissue. It should be excised because of difficulties caused by its size; but extensive resection is neither necessary nor wise. Microscopically, the lesion consists chiefly of connective tissue containing much serous fluid with a minor, though variable, component of liver or bile duct cells.

F. Hemangioma. —Two types of hemangioma are found in the liver: the cavernous, and the infantile hemangioendothelioma. The former is very rare, although death from rupture has been reported. The latter is more common and is usually associated with cutaneous hemangiomas. They are said to occur almost exclusively in the first 6 months of life and may give rise to very acute problems because of the immense size they attain. Because of the large capillary bed, they may lead directly to heart failure on a hemodynamic basis. Or they may trap platelets in such numbers that a full-blown picture of thrombocytopenic purpura appears. With some, all symptoms are caused by compression of adjoining viscera. Anemia may be present, and most of the symptoms of congenital heart disease.

The hemangiomas are composed of endothelium-lined channels of capillary size, and moderate numbers of mitoses may be seen, making differentiation from angiosarcoma difficult. The tumors are usually diffuse throughout the liver; their size and symptomatology may necessitate hepatic lobectomy. If it is possible, a biopsy specimen should be obtained in any event. Major bleeding may follow such a maneuver, and its management should be anticipated prior to the procedure. Once the diagnosis is secure, radiation therapy may cautiously be employed in the hope of initiating maturation of the tissue with cessation of growth and a gradual decrease of size. Irradiation has proved life-saving when it has brought about rapid alteration and decrease of size.

Tumors of the Liver

The histology of hepatic neoplasms is a very difficult study because of the paucity of material in any one location and because no clear diagnostic criteria have been agreed upon. There is also great variation in the pathologic physiology. Many lesions which appear to be benign microscopically are fatal because of the manner in which they displace or destroy normal tissue or because metastases develop and the tumor is indeed malignant. For this reason, and because of the infrequent occurrence of any of these growths, a good deal has been written about hepatic tumors of various types, and several different sets of histologic or gross criteria have been proposed for making diagnosis. In addition, the terminology has not been clarified, so that the names used in one series may signify entirely different lesions in another. The following discussion represents an attempt to bring the confusing array of nomenclature into some semblance of order.

Benign Tumors

A. Tumor-like epithelial lesions.

1. *Focal nodular hyperplasia* (adenoma, hepatoma, hamartoma, isolated solitary nodular hyperplasia, focal cirrhosis). —Children with this lesion have been noted to have an enlarging abdomen, occasionally with localized pain. A firm, multinodular, cirrhotic-appearing mass, usually solitary, appears beneath the capsule of the liver, although the growth may be pedunculated or lie deep within the substance. The mass is usually clearly demarcated and gray to gray-brown. Histologic study reveals a stellate mass of connective tissue in the central portion. If the gross appearance is suggestive, a biopsy specimen should be examined for confirmation. Any easily excised mass may be removed, but large resections should not be done because this growth does not attain usually great size and does not endanger life. There has been no evidence of malignant change.

2. *Multiple nodular hyperplasia.* —Large, readily palpable nodules arise as the normal liver cells undergo hyperplasia following acute necrosis of the liver. A careful history should reveal the antecedent illness and obviate surgery.

B. Benign epithelial tumors.

1. *Adenoma.* —This lesion usually appears as a single, encapsulated gray-yellow to brown mass in the right hepatic lobe. Histologic differentiation from hepatoblastoma is difficult because of the great similarity in structure: normal liver cells without bile ducts or portal tracts. Only after comparison of many sections with a known hepatoblastoma can this be diagnosed. Adenoma is an exceedingly rare lesion. Many children have died of hepatoblastoma after having had a diagnosis of adenoma. Undoubtedly some had focal nodular hyperplasia instead of adenoma. Because it is so difficult to be certain, total resection of the mass should be attempted.

2. *Adrenal rest tumor.* —Both adrenal cortical hyperplasia causing Cushing's syndrome and adrenal cortical carcinoma have been reported arising in heterotopic adrenal cortical tissue located beneath Glis-

son's capsule. Most of such masses have been found on the inferior surface of the right lobe. The pathologic examination will prove the diagnosis, but the clinical problem may be very difficult until the mass has been found.

C. Cysts and tumor-like mesenchymal lesions.

1. *Mesenchymal hamartoma.* — See above, under Lymphangioma.

2. *Solitary cysts.* — See above.

D. Benign mesenchymal tumors.

1. *Cavernous hemangioma.* — See above.

2. *Infantile hemangioendothelioma.* — See above.

E. Teratoma. — Occasionally a teratoma arises in the liver and may be malignant or benign. Only 5 instances have been reported. Excision of the mass would be advisable to be sure that all involved cells are eradicated. There is a reported 7-year survival following hepatic lobectomy for what was finally diagnosed as a carcinosarcoma of the liver.

Malignant Tumors

A. Hepatoblastoma (primary carcinoma of the liver, liver cell carcinoma, hepatoma, embryonal hepatoma, cholangioma, cholangiohepatoma). — This is the classic liver tumor of infants and young children, the large majority appearing before the age of 2 years. There are two basic histologic types: epithelial or parenchymal, made up of liver cells of varying degrees of maturity; and mixed, consisting of epithelial elements and a widely variable admixture of mesenchymal tissue, predominantly connective tissue and osteoid.

None of the livers involved by this type of neoplasia shows evidence of cirrhosis, and the architecture of the tumor bears no resemblance to that of the normal hepatic lobules. It is interesting that metastases from mixed hepatoblastomas show only the epithelial elements.

Exploration usually reveals a single mass, most frequently in the right lobe, although there may be many nodules. Their consistency and color is quite variable, but most have a pseudocapsule.

Microscopically, there may be simply sheets of cells which resemble those of a normal or fetal liver, or there may be areas where abortive acinar formation or rosettes of cells are seen. Frequently, small lakes of blood are noted with a ring of deeply staining primitive liver cells around them and more normal-appearing hepatic cells in the periphery. Some shade off into a picture closely resembling a true bile duct carcinoma. There are many similarities between hepatoblastoma and nephroblastoma. Each demonstrates elements of neoplasm and of malformation suggesting an origin in intrauterine life. Extension of the tumor into blood vessels is seen in each microscopically; and in the liver tumor, gross involvement of the portal vein in this manner should be suspected and sought at the time of operation.

The incidence of hepatoblastoma has been reported as nearly equal in the sexes or up to 2½ times more frequent in boys than in girls. The first suspicion is usually aroused by the increasing size of the abdomen, which may be very rapid and totally asymptomatic. Weight loss may occur as well as fever (which has been noted by some to carry a particularly grave prognosis), anorexia and vomiting. Pallor is often seen, but jaundice is infrequent. In some series, hemihypertrophy and a scattering of other diseases and malformations have been reported. Although the vast majority of cases have been in Caucasian children, instances have appeared in all races. Liver tumors were found to constitute 20.6% of all abdominal tumors in a report from Formosa, which also mentioned the frequency of associated hypercholesterolemia. There may be gross disturbances of mineral and lipid metabolism which can lead to demineralization of the skeleton.

B. Hepatocarcinoma (hepatocellular carcinoma). — This tumor is microscopically indistinguishable from adult carcinoma of the liver. Most appear after the age of 2 years. An increasing number are being reported to be associated with or on a basis of cirrhosis of the liver from a variety of causes. Incidence of this type of liver tumor is lower than that of hepatoblastoma by about a third. When exploration is undertaken, about half are found to have a single mass and the other half, multiple nodules involving the entire liver. The masses vary in consistency from soft to firm and in color from tan to green. They usually have no pseudocapsule.

The typical microscopic picture is a trabecular pattern with trabeculae separated by sinusoids lined with endothelial cells. The individual cells are larger than normal and vary greatly in size. Giant cells are seen in all of these tumors, and many bizarre multinucleated cells. The nuclei are hyperchromatic, vary in size, contain chromatin particles and have prominent, deeply eosinophilic nucleoli. Mitoses are frequent and often bizarre. Degenerative changes, such as necrosis, infarction and hemorrhage, are seen. All of these tumors demonstrate vascular invasion and some, lymphatic invasion.

The incidence of hepatocarcinoma is apparently far higher in males than in females — upward of 11:1. It, too, presents most often as an abdominal mass, but there is significantly more in the way of pain or discomfort. Jaundice is somewhat more frequent than with hepatoblastoma, and weight loss may be an early symptom.

C. Mesenchymoma. — Either the benign or malignant form may appear in the liver, although all reported instances have been malignant. They are usually large, fleshy, firm masses which microscopically show a variety of mesodermal derivatives. Complete resection has resulted in cure.

D. Sarcoma. — This is a very rare form of primary liver tumor. Rhabdomyosarcoma has been reported.

E. METASTATIC TUMORS.—These may appear to be primary neoplasms of the liver. They have been thought to be more common than primary hepatic lesions, although this picture seems to be changing as the tumors are more thoroughly studied and treated. Usually, the secondary tumor causes diffuse enlargement of the liver, whereas the typical primary one involves the lower margin of the right lobe. The most common metastatic tumor is neuroblastoma, closely followed by nephroblastoma. Frequently, neuroblastoma may involve the liver by direct extension into its substance rather than by lymphatic or hematogenous spread.

It is particularly important to bear in mind this possibility when an hepatic mass is present, because a variety of studies may help to locate a primary focus or demonstrate that there is widespread metastatic disease. Intravenous urography, ideally with the dye injected by way of the long saphenous vein, may demonstrate deviation, compression or obstruction of the inferior vena cava by renal or hepatic tumor as well as give fairly conclusive demonstration of nephroblastoma or neuroblastoma.

Films of the skull and long bones may show the evidence of spread of neuroblastoma, and chest films may demonstrate the lesions of Wilms' or hepatic tumor metastasis. If the results of liver function studies are abnormal, the likelihood of a primary liver tumor is less. In any event, needle biopsy should not be done. Often, huge blood vessels course over the surface of a lesion deep in the liver substance, and a needle will almost certainly tear them, leading to uncontrollable hemorrhage. Also, there is a distinct chance of spreading the tumor or even of causing the rupture of one. In addition, the specimen obtained is usually not adequate for accurate diagnosis. Collection of a 24-hour urine specimen for vanillylmandelic acid estimation may be helpful as a baseline study if neuroblastoma is found. Radioactive liver scanning may be of some help in localizing a mass.

OPERATIVE TREATMENT

In infants and children who present abdominal masses, there is always a sense of urgency. But it is important to carry out certain of the studies outlined above in order to be as certain as possible that therapy is properly directed. Any anemia obviously must be corrected, and all the appropriate adjuncts to possible massive surgical resection must be assembled. One should be prepared to cope with any of the potential problems so that, once begun, the attack may be car-

Fig. 48-11.—Resection of left lobe of the liver. **Above,** overlapping mattress sutures placed after mobilization of the lobe. **A,** hemostasis secured after lobectomy by mattress sutures. **B,** compressed Ivalon sponge used to cover the area of excision. (Figs. 48-11 and 48-12, from Clatworthy *et al.*[5])

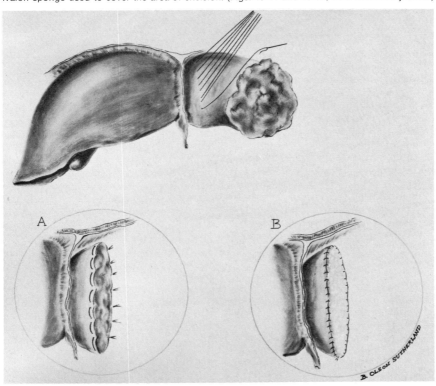

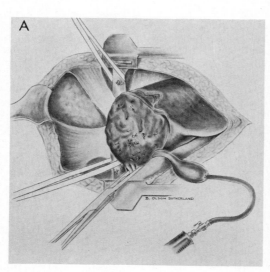
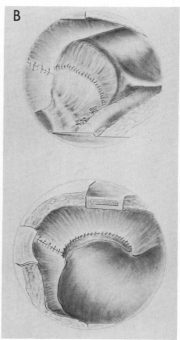

Fig. 48-12.—Right lobectomy. **A,** control of blood supply by tapes around the inferior vena cava above and below the liver and by temporary cross-clamping of the hepatoduodenal structures. Retrograde injection of the gallbladder discloses open bile ducts on the raw liver surface. **B,** resurfacing of the liver face by Ivalon sponge reinforced by falciform ligament and perirenal fascia **(above)** or by diaphragm **(below)**.

ried through to completion. Except in unusual circumstances, it is far wiser not to begin unless the maneuver can be finished. Hence adequate supplies of blood must be assured, all of the aids available to the anesthesiologists, particularly monitoring equipment, must be in readiness, facilities for following central venous pressure and for measuring blood loss must be available, and additional surgical assistants must be prepared to help if necessary.

For any of the maligant tumors, total excision offers the only hope of cure, but caution must be employed to avoid carrying out overly extensive procedures when a benign process may be present. Although one would never prefer to obtain a biopsy for permanent section and run the risk of rupturing the tumor or seeding the peritoneal cavity, it is wiser to do that than to harm a child with a greater than necessary operative procedure.

Sharply localized small tumors with no evidence of metastasis may be removed by a liberal wedge resection carried out in a straightforward manner. When the mass is larger and involves only one lobe, that entire segment of the liver must be excised. If the process has grown to involve both lobes, it is well to remember that x-radiation may be effective in shrinking it to one lobe and lobectomy may then be carried out at a second operation with a hope of cure. Left lobectomy can be accomplished fairly easily in most instances when proper attention is paid to control of all the vascular and biliary channels (Fig. 48-11). Right lobectomy has been carried out successfully in recent years as the technique has been perfected.

Because of the chance of entering the inferior vena cava and causing air embolism during right hepatic lobectomy, the chest must be opened in order to assure good control of the vena cava by means of tapes above and below the liver (Fig. 48-12, *A*). Thoracotomy also abolishes the negative intrathoracic pressure. It is essential to have a venous cut-down in an arm so that blood can always be replaced. Generally, the operation is performed under hypothermia (32.2–33.3 C). The abdominal portion of the incision is made first. If the diagnosis is clear or can be confirmed by the pathologist, the dissection is begun. It is important to remember that many of the benign and malignant tumors may look like cavernous hemangiomas, and every effort must be made to be certain before proceeding on any course of action. If problems are encountered, particularly in the area of diagnostic accuracy, which cannot be dealt with, it is wiser to back out and await a final decision.

After the vena cava is completely under control, the gallbladder is dissected free from the right lobe and preserved for later use or for permanent retention. When the right hepatic artery has been divided and the branches of the portal vein have been controlled, sharp or blunt dissection may be used to transect liver tissue. This may be carried out with or without the use of large mattress sutures placed in the uninvolved parenchyma. Each blood vessel and bile duct must be carefully ligated, taking particular care of the four or five major tributaries to the vena cava. When the lobe has been removed, dilute methylene blue injected via a cholecystostomy tube will demonstrate, by retrograde flow, whether all the biliary radicles have been controlled. The raw surface of the lobe may be covered with a compressed Ivalon sponge, greater omentum or the falciform ligament (Fig. 48-12, *B*). If the gallbladder has been preserved, it may be secured to the surface. The cholecystostomy tube and appropriate drains are brought out through stab wounds.

The question of use of chemotherapeutic agents will arise, but none has been proved effective against any of the hepatic tumors. The only useful application of x-ray therapy is prior to the attempt at surgical extirpation of the neoplasm. Although the resection may seem to have been complete, recurrence and death may follow operation by as long as 9 years.

CLINICAL RESULTS

An attempt has been made to collect from several centers the accumulated experience of a group of surgeons in the management of young patients with these lesions. Unfortunately, and largely because of different pathologic criteria, it is very difficult to be sure what the figures mean. The combined statistics from Children's Hospital of Philadelphia, Children's Hospital of Michigan, Texas Children's Hospital and Children's Hospital of Los Angeles seem to reveal that of 30 patients with hepatoblastoma, 22 had died (some following hepatic resection) and 8 were alive without evidence of disease (having had lobectomy carried out). Eight patients with hepatocarcinoma had been seen in the same institutions, and 3 of them were alive and apparently well.

The picture is not bright, but as experience is gained, the results will continue to improve, as they have in recent years. There are more and more reports of successful resections where it had previously been felt that nothing could be done for these unfortunate children.

BIBLIOGRAPHY

1. Alcalde, V. M.; Traisman, H. S., and Baffes, T.: Primary carcinoma of the liver in infancy and childhood, Am. J. Dis. Child. 104:69, 1962.
2. Alpert, S., *et al.*: Right hepatectomy for hamartoma in an eleven-month-old infant: A case report, Ann. Surg. 165:286, 1967.
3. Bigelow, N. H., and Wright, A. W.: Primary carcinoma of the liver in infancy and childhood, Cancer 6:170, 1953.
4. Cantlie, J.: On a new arrangement of the right and left lobes of the liver, Proc. Anat. Soc. (Great Britain and Ireland) 32:4, 1898.
5. Clatworthy, H. W., Jr.; Boles, E. T., and Kottmeier, P. K.: Liver tumors in infancy and childhood, Ann. Surg. 154:475, 1961.
6. Cleland, R. S.: Benign and malignant tumors of the liver, Pediat. Clin. North America 6:427, 1959.
7. Edmondson, H. A.: Differential diagnosis of tumors and tumor-like lesions of liver in infancy and childhood, Am. J. Dis. Child. 91:168, 1956.
8. Fish, J. C., and McCrary, R. G.: Primary cancer of the liver in childhood, Arch. Surg. 93:355, 1966.
9. Gans, H.; Koh, S-K., and Aust, J. B.: Hepatic resection, Arch. Surg. 93:523, 1966.
10. Ishak, K. G., and Glunz, P. R.: Hepatoblastoma and hepatocarcinoma in infancy and childhood: Report of 47 cases, Cancer 20:396, 1967.
11. Lloyd-Davies, O. V., and Angell, J. C.: Right hepatic lobectomy—operative technique, some anatomical points and an account of a case, Brit. J. Surg. 45:113, 1957.
12. McIndoe, A. H., and Counsellor, V. S.: The bilaterality of the liver, Arch. Surg. 15:589, 1927.
13. Packard, G. B., and Palmer, H. D.: Primary neoplasms of liver in infants and children, Ann. Surg. 142:214, 1955.
14. Shorter, R. G., *et al.*: Primary carcinoma of the liver in infancy and childhood, Pediatrics 25:191, 1960.
15. Lin, T-Y.; Chen, C-C., and Liu, W-P.: Primary carcinoma of the liver in infancy and childhood: Report of 21 cases, with resection in 6 cases, Surgery 60:1275, 1966.
16. Wilson, H., and Wolf, R. Y.: Hepatic lobectomy: Indications, technique and results, Surgery 59:472, 1966.

C. L. MINOR
Drawings by
B. O. SUTHERLAND

Cholecystitis and Cholelithiasis

GALLBLADDER DISEASE is an uncommon cause of abdominal pain in infancy and childhood. This is attested to by the fact that the English literature contains only three papers[3,4,6] in the last decade in which the author has had a personal experience with more

than 10 cases. Most of the writings on the subject are a series of observations made on collections of cases from the literature. An outstanding one of these was written in 1952 by Ulin *et al.*[7] This report and others like it record a total of slightly over 700 cases of cholecystitis and cholelithiasis in childhood.

Because of the paucity of experience with this disease, it is difficult to arrive at accurate incidence figures. An older report from Johns Hopkins[1] stated that 12 of 888 cases of cholecystitis occurred in children under 15 years of age. At the other end of the spectrum, and more nearly approaching the experience of most physicians, is the incidence of 1 child among every 1,000 cholecystitis patients seen at the Mayo Clinic.[7]

CAUSES.—Some form of hemolytic disease has been commonly asserted to be the cause of most cases of gallbladder disease in infancy and childhood. Although sickle cell anemia, hereditary elliptocytosis and thalassemia have been reported as being associated with cholelithiasis on occasion, this combination is not frequently noted. In only 8.6% of a collected series of 244 cases did Brenner and Stewart[2] find any evidence of hemolytic disease, while in a personal series of 60 cases, Soderlund and Yetterstrom[6] found only 3 instances of hemolytic disease. Of 29 personal patients examined by Hagberg *et al.*,[3] only 2 showed evidence of the pigmented type of stones which suggest the diagnosis of an underlying hemolytic process. Sepsis elsewhere in the body, e.g., upper respiratory or enteric infections, has also been blamed for gallbladder disease.

Other observers have believed that in order for gallbladder disease to occur, there must be an underlying anatomic abnormality of the extrahepatic biliary tree. Vascular anomalies, abnormalities of the spiral valves of the cystic duct and even enlarged lymph nodes encroaching on the choledochus have been incriminated. Underlying all of these hypotheses is the common denominator of obstruction; some have felt that there is a clear-cut stenosis of the cystic duct in most cases.

To summarize the etiologic factors, one would have to say that there seem to be basic abnormalities of the biliary tree which predispose to obstruction and superimposed on these is some type of infection which leads to the acute inflammatory phase.

PATHOLOGIC ANATOMY.—Cholecystitis, in the acute form with cholelithiasis, has been reported as occurring in less than 10% of patients.[6] In such circumstances, the histologic picture is one of an inflamed gallbladder wall with marked invasion by polymorphonuclear leukocytes. The preponderant pathologic picture is, however, that of chronic cholecystitis, with stones occurring in approximately one half of the patients. Examination of 50 gallbladders removed in childhood and adolescence by Kirtley and Holcomb[4] revealed the histologic picture of long-standing, chronic disease in 70%.

There is a considerably lower incidence of associated gallstones in children than in adults. In one collected series,[7] 68% of the 326 patients had biliary tract stones as compared with the 85–95% incidence in adults. Cholelithiasis alone occurs in approximately one third of patients. Surprisingly, the incidence of childhood common duct stones has been reported by several authors[6,7] to be in the neighborhood of only 6%.

CLINICAL PICTURE.—It is of interest that the familial incidence of gallbladder disease can be set at over 50% of cases if one limits family history to parents, siblings and other close relatives.

With the exception of one report, gallbladder disease is felt to be just as predominant in the female child as in the adult woman. Female preponderances varying from 80 to 95% have been reported.

A suggestion of racial immunity to gallbladder disease can be deduced from a series reported from Nashville.[4] In a preponderantly Negro hospital population, 49 of 50 childhood cholecystitis patients were white.

This is not a disease of the newborn, for the most part. The median age usually falls between 8 and 10 years. One may suspect that perhaps the problem occurs earlier; the vague abdominal pains of earlier life are difficult to diagnose, and the younger child's inability to localize his symptoms is not helpful.

The basic clinical picture is not very different from that of the adult. Fifty to 60% of the children with gallbladder disease are overweight. Hagberg *et al.*[3] put it well when they said that only 10% of children with gallbladder disease are thin. These children suffer primarily from abdominal pain which, when they are able to localize it, is in the right upper quadrant or the midepigastrium. Radiation through to the back occurs in 3 of 4 cases. The confusing incidence of periumbilical pain in younger children is well known, together with the occasional migration to the right lower quadrant. The nausea and vomiting that go with abdominal pain are common. Tenderness to examination is, however, significantly absent; experienced observers have found that as high as 40% of patients who are in a pain attack do not have localizing tenderness to examination. Intolerance of fatty foods is not as universal as in the adult but does occur in about one third of the patients. Jaundice is seen in about 2 of every 5 patients; this is in contrast to the usually accepted figure of 5–10% incidence of jaundice in adults with gallbladder disease. This disparity is best explained by the inflamed biliary tree undergoing temporary partial obstruction.

Associated systemic illness is not at all uncommon and perhaps may be the basic cause of an acute attack. Such illness may lead to bile stasis from dehydration, the use of narcotics to combat pain and the decrease of hormonal stimulus to gallbladder emptying.

A study of serum lipids in children with gallbladder disease showed that they were below normal levels and therefore not to be considered a causative factor in the disease.[3]

Cholelithiasis leading to perforation of the gallbladder does occur.[5] However, when it does, there does not seem to be the same shock-producing course of events that one expects from the bile peritonitis of the adult empyema of the gallbladder with rupture.

In one report on cholecystitis in childhood and adolescence, two thirds of the girls who had pregnancies and developed cholecystitis did so during gestation or within 6 months of the time of delivery.[4]

DIAGNOSIS.—The diagnosis of cholecystitis with or without cholelithiasis is difficult, and most series indicate that only 1 of 4 patients comes to surgery with the correct preoperative diagnosis. An adequate history of recurrent and colicky abdominal pain with fatty food intolerance is, of course, very suggestive of the diagnosis. Often in the young child, this typical history cannot be elicited, and months or even years go by without the diagnosis for the chronic abdominal pain becoming apparent. Undoubtedly, if cholecystitis were more often included in diagnostic considerations, the recorded incidence would increase; but many cases of the disease occur in an age group in which the periumbilical pain is misleading and the uncomfortable child is unable to localize his discomfort very well.

X-ray examination is most helpful in arriving at the diagnosis once it has been suspected. Cholecystography shows stones or nonfunction of the gallbladder in over 80% of cases.

Differential diagnosis must include simple constipation, hepatitis, abdominal epilepsy and appendicitis. *Constipation* can be suspected as a cause of pain from both history and physical examination when fecalomas are felt in the rectosigmoid area. *Hepatitis* is easily confused with gallbladder disease, but in its early phase, the results of liver function tests in gallbladder disease are essentially normal, whereas they are likely to show aberration in hepatitis. This is especially true with regard to the total serum bilirubin values, which are increased in hepatitis and normal in the nonjaundiced gallbladder patient. Abdominal pain is a rare manifestation of *epileptic* disease. Although often included in differential thinking, it does not occur with any degree of frequency. An electroencephalogram will rule this in or out quite easily. Perhaps the most difficult problem is to distinguish between incipient *appendicitis* and early cholecystitis because of our tendency to associate appendicitis with the child and to reserve cholecystitis for the adult. The vague periumbilical pains of both diseases contribute to this failure of diagnosis. The young child with cholecystitis occasionally has a shift of pain to the right lower quadrant, which is even more confusing. The greatest proof of the difficult distinction is the fact that 15–20% of patients later proved to have cholecystitis and/or cholelithiasis have been operated on previously for appendicitis. Cholecystitis is frequently diagnosed at the time exploration is carried out for the preoperative diagnosis of appendicitis.

TREATMENT.—Although a few surgeons recommend cholecystotomy for cholecystitis and cholelithiasis, they are in the distinct minority. The predisposing causes that lead to the first attack will almost inevitably result in a recurrence. The treatment of choice is cholecystectomy. There are no real complications of cholecystectomy in children provided the same rules of carefully delineating the anatomy are applied as in the adult. The junction of cystic and common ducts must be inspected and no excess remnant of the cystic duct left behind.

The common duct should always be palpated and inspected. If there are stones in the gallbladder, if there is a history of jaundice or if the common duct is dilated, an operative cholangiogram should be obtained to make sure that there are no stones in the common duct. Judicious choledochotomy should be employed when stones are felt, seen on the x-ray film or suspected.

Prognosis.—Mortality from cholecystectomy in children is practically zero. The morbidity from surgery is low. Only about 5% of the patients have biliary dyskinesia with residual pain. Finally, residual stones in the common duct are rare because choledocholithiasis itself has a low incidence.

REFERENCES

1. Blalock, A.: A statistical study of 880 cases of biliary tract disease, Bull. John Hopkins Hosp. 35:391, 1924.
2. Brenner, R. W., and Stewart, C. F.: Gall bladder disease, Rev. Surg. 21:327, 1964.
3. Hagberg, B.; Svennerholm, L., and Thoren, L.: Cholelithiasis in children, Acta. chir. scandinav. 123:307, 1962.
4. Kirtley, J. A. Jr., and Holcomb, G. W., Jr.: Surgical management of diseases of the gallbladder and common duct in children and adolescents, Am. J. Surg. 111:39, 1966.
5. Snyder, W. H., Jr.; Chaffin, L., and Oettinger, L.: Cholelithiasis and perforation of the gall bladder in an infant with recovery, J.A.M.A. 149:1645, 1952.
6. Soderlund, S., and Yetterstrom, B.: Cholecystitis and cholelithiasis in children, Arch. Dis. Childhood 37:174, 1962.
7. Ulin, W. A.; Nosal, J. L., and Martin, W. L.: Cholecystitis in childhood and Associated obstructive jaundice, Surgery 31:312, 1952.

W. B. KIESEWETTER

Choledochal Cyst

THIS CONDITION was first reported in 1723 by Vater. It is uncommonly encountered. One large children's center reported only 7 cases in a 10-year period.[2] In 17,381 biliary tract operations done at the Mayo Clinic, only 2 cases of cyst were encountered.[3] However, for any one person who has this condition, particularly in childhood, it is an important entity because of the high morbidity and mortality in untreated patients.

ETIOLOGY.—There is considerable dispute as to the origin of choledochal cyst. The only point of agreement is that there is a congenital aspect, which thus far has eluded satisfactory delineation. There are those who believe that obstruction plays a large role in the production of this deformity; such obstruction causes a "blow-out" of the choledochus just proximal to the ampulla of Vater. Some feel that this obstruction may be in the form of a valvelike mechanism, while others think that stenosis of the ampulla results in dilatation above it. Perhaps the most plausible explanation is that given by a Japanese worker[7] who suggested that there is a congenital weakness of the wall as a result of embryologic maldevelopment. The choledochus goes through an epithelial proliferation stage which leads to a solid cord; revacuolization of this cord then takes place. If the rate of revacuolization is greater in the proximal common duct than in the preduodenal portion, that part of the common duct will be both greater in diameter and somewhat weaker in the integrity of the wall.

ANATOMIC CONSIDERATIONS.—Basically, a choledochal cyst is an aneurysmal dilatation of the common duct. The preduodenal portion is usually normal, as is the biliary tree above the cyst. These cysts vary from cherry size to a capacity of several liters of bile. The thickness of the wall of the cyst may vary from a few millimeters to 1 cm, and under the microscope, the wall is largely fibrous tissue with a cuboidal or columnar type of epithelial lining.

One group[1] has classified choledochal cysts into three types: (1) Classic type. This is the commonest variety and is characterized by a normal intrahepatic tree. The extrahepatic biliary tree is mildly dilated above the cyst. The cyst itself begins and ends sharply and the terminal common duct may be somewhat narrowed. The gallbladder in this type is almost always normal in size and consistency. (2) Diverticular type. In this variety, there is a very limited diverticulum in the common duct, with a normal biliary tree above; this biliary system may be slightly dilated. The gallbladder is normal in this type. (3) Choledochocele. This is very rare. It is limited to the intraduodenal portion of the duct. Dilatation is small and actually represents a herniation of the choledochus into the duodenum, with a slightly dilated biliary tree above and a normal gallbladder.

Depending on the length of time that the choledochal cyst has been present, there are varying degrees of hepatic biliary cirrhosis, coupled with some cholangitis from superimposed infection.

CLINICAL FEATURES.—Choledochal cysts predominate in the female, representing 74% of a review series of 232 patients.[6] Another group[1] reported that 84% of their 94 case series was found in females. This 3 times preponderance should lead one to suspect the diagnosis in a jaundiced female.

Choledochal cysts can and do appear in all age groups. In one series,[6] 45% of 57 patients were under 15 years of age, and 30% were found under 4. In another series of 94 patients,[1] 45% were less than 10 years of age, including 18% who were under 1 year.

The classic description of a choledochal cyst is that of a child beyond the first few months of life who has a triad of clinical features—intermittent pain, mass and jaundice. Some recent writings on this triad tend to diminish its importance; the frequency is doubted as being as high as previously thought. One group[1] found only 21% of their patients had this triad, although more than two thirds of them had one or more of the three diagnostic features. Fonkalsrud and Boles[2] noted in a small group of patients that there were two clinical pictures which might be present in any given case in addition to the triad. They believe that obstructive jaundice in the early months of life can be due to a choledochal cyst and that classic portal hypertension may occur in an older child due to a choledochal cyst pressing on the portal vein.

It would seem fair to say, then, that the clinical features of this lesion may vary from practically nothing to a full-blown bile peritonitis that can result from the spontaneous or traumatic rupture of a large cyst. Most characteristically, they are marked by chronicity and periodicity.

Pain is one of the first manifestations of the lesion. It may be colicky, hard to localize, particularly in the younger infant and child. Acute attacks of pain do occur, however, when the cyst becomes larger and distended. These may go away spontaneously as the cyst empties its contents into the duodenum. In one review of this aspect of the problem, it was concluded that approximately two-thirds of all patients with choledochal cysts have pain to some degree.[6] It occasionally radiates through to the back.

Palpation of the abdomen will disclose a mass in 75–95% of cases. The mass will sometimes be evanescent if it is not very distended. The variability in size will obscure the outlines of the mass to any single examiner. It may be so small as to be confused with the right lobe of the liver, or it may be so large as to occupy the major portion of the abdominal cavity.

Two thirds of patients with choledochal cysts will manifest jaundice at some time in the course of their disease. The intermittent nature of the jaundice with acholic stools and dark urine is characteristic of the lesion. If it is long-standing and unremitting, there is usually the pruritus that is associated with prolonged jaundice from any cause.

If infection is superimposed on a choledochal cyst, the characteristic chills and fever of cholangitis will ensue. Occasionally the cyst is so placed and so angulates the common entry of the choledochus and pancreatic ducts that it causes pancreatitis, with all of its typical midepigastric pain, nausea and vomiting.

A long-standing choledochal cyst that is of considerable size will cause some degree of portal hypertension in a small percentage of cases. This will lead to biliary cirrhosis, splenomegaly, hypersplenism, anemia and eventually some form of gastrointestinal bleeding as collateral pathways for the portal circulation develop.

DIAGNOSIS.—Very few patients with choledochal cyst have such a diagnosis prior to operative intervention. Most people feel that only 1 in 6 patients have this as their sole diagnosis before some type of therapy is undertaken. The diagnosis is simple enough when a female child presents the classic triad of pain, a mass and jaundice, but less than half of all patients in reported series have shown this characteristic picture.

It is important to carry out the standard laboratory investigation for children with obstructive jaundice, even though the obstruction is intermittent with this lesion. It should include liver function studies, examination of the stool and urine for the presence of bile, and a bile stimulation test with corticoids, followed by duodenal drainage at the end of such stimulation. These tests will differentiate a very low percentage only of those with choledochal cyst from patients with other causes of the jaundice.

Radiologic help in the diagnosis of a choledochal cyst is important but not definitive in as high a percentage of patients as one could wish. Oral cholecystography is virtually of no help because there is so little concentration of the dye in the biliary tree because of the obstruction. Intravenous cholangiography has been more effective because of better demonstration of the extrahepatic biliary tree. Some more aggressive workers have aspirated the cystic structure through the abdominal wall and inserted dye into the cavity to replace the bile which was drawn off. This will outline the cyst quite well but carries some hazard because of bile leakage into the peritoneal cavity. Perhaps the most suggestive bit of evidence that can be gained radiologically is from a standard gastrointestinal series. The presence of a choledochal cyst is usually manifested by the downward and medial displacement of the duodenal loop from the extrinsic pressure of the mass. The rare choledochocele variety may show itself as what appears to be a polyp of the duodenum. If, by good fortune, the ampulla of Vater is not competent and intestinal gas goes up retrograde into the cyst, the diagnosis is almost certain.

DIFFERENTIAL DIAGNOSIS.—*Hydatid cyst of the liver* may produce the symptoms and signs of choledochal cyst in patients from areas where the echinococcus is endemic, namely, South America, Western Europe and Africa. This can be ruled in or out by the finding of certain allergic manifestations, such as eosinophilia. The intradermal test for echinococcus may have to be employed in questionable cases.

Cholelithiasis is difficult to differentiate. The intermittency of the jaundice and the pain are similar in both conditions. Absence of the mass and appropriate x-ray studies that show gallstones may be helpful in pointing to the correct diagnosis.

Biliary atresia in the neonatal child can be confused with choledochal cyst, although pain and the mass of the cyst are not present. Often, diagnostic exploration is the only means of distinguishing between the two.

Pancreatic cyst, because of the mass, may present diagnostic difficulties. The x-ray picture of a pancreatic cyst usually shows widening of the loop of the duodenum, with a more centrally placed mass than is seen in choledochal cysts.

Retroperitoneal neoplasms, particularly Wilms' tumor and neuroblastoma, may be difficult to distinguish from choledochal cyst. The smoothness of the cyst in contrast to the irregularity of the other two will help differentiate them. Intravenous pyelography may be the final help in the decision, the picture being normal in choledochal disease and grossly abnormal in the other lesions.

Portal hypertension in an older child may present diagnostic difficulties, especially when the child has had gastrointestinal bleeding. An appropriately done splenoportogram will show encroachment on an otherwise normal splenic or portal system, although surgery may be necessary before the final differentiation can be made.

TREATMENT.—The first successfully treated case of choledochal cyst was described in 1894. It has been abundantly proved that nonsurgical treatment carries with it an almost 100% mortality.

Most authors with large experience believe that some type of anastomosis between the duct and the gastrointestinal tract is the preferred method of management. Such anastomosis is most commonly between the duodenum and the cyst, although some prefer to carry out a Roux-Y cyst-jejunostomy. The latter is more time-consuming but has the advantage of reducing the incidence of cholangitis. Such cholangitis has been variably reported as occurring in 15–25% of patients.[1,2]

At the time of exploration, an operative cholangiogram is advisable, but it must be done carefully with gravity filling of the biliary tree so as not to produce a retrograde introduction of bile into the main pancreatic ducts with the resultant pancreatitis.

Aspiration of the cyst or external drainage by marsupialization is mentioned only to be condemned because it does not attack the basic problem. It also carries a prohibitively high mortality.

One group[1] has favored excision of the cyst and end-to-end anastomosis between the common duct and the duodenum. Most workers believe that this is a dangerous procedure that may compromise the choledochus completely by severance or produce stenosis at the point of anastomosis. It carries with it a higher immediate mortality, but perhaps a lower morbidity in the postoperative period from cholangitis. It should, however, be reserved for the few cases of a small cyst that can be easily dissected out with a clear view of all the structures involved.

PROGNOSIS.—The mortality for choledochal cyst has continued to go down over the years. Shallow and his group[5] reported in 1943 an over-all mortality of 51% in a collected series of 175 patients. In 1956, Tsardakas *et al.*[6] reported a 23% mortality in 57 patients, and in 1959, workers from Baltimore[1] reported a 12% mortality in 94 cases collected from the world literature.

The morbidity factors depend entirely on the amount of cholangitis which follows the anastomosis. The Roux-Y anastomosis has the least incidence of cholangitis, whereas the direct anastomoses have a higher, but still not important, incidence of this complication.

REFERENCES

1. Alonso-Lej, F.; Rever, W. B., Jr., and Pessagno, D. J. A.: A study of the congenital choledochal cyst, with a report of 2 patients and an analysis of 94 cases, Surg., Gynec. & Obst. 108:1, 1959.
2. Fonkalsrud, E. W., and Boles, T.: Choledochal cysts in infancy and childhood, Surg., Gynec. & Obst. 121:733, 1965.
3. Judd, E. S., and Greene, E. I.: Choledochus cyst, Surg., Gynec. & Obst. 46:317, 1928.
4. Ravitch, M. M., and Snyder, G. B.: Congenital cystic dilatation of the common bile duct, Surgery 44:752, 1958.
5. Shallow, T. A.; Egin, S. A. and Wagner, F. B.: Congenital cystic dilatation of common bile duct, Ann. Surg. 123:117, 1943.
6. Tsardakas, E., and Robnett, A. H.: Congenital cystic dilatation of the common bile duct, Arch. Surg. 72:311, 1956.
7. Yotuyanagi, S.: Contributions to etiology and pathogenesis of idiopathic cystic dilatation of common bile duct with report of 3 cases, Gann 30:601, 1936.

W. B. KIESEWETTER

49

The Pancreas

EMBRYOLOGY

THE PANCREAS forms between the fourth and the seventh week of fetal life from paired primordia known as dorsal and ventral pancreatic buds; later, these fuse. The dorsal pancreas arises from the dorsal wall of the duodenum. In the course of growth, it pushes between two layers of splanchnic mesoderm which constitute the dorsal mesentery. The ventral pancreas develops to the right of the midline and grows caudally in the angle between the duodenum and the hepatic diverticulum. There may be two ventral pancreatic primordia, but usually one is suppressed. As gut rotation proceeds, the common bile duct is displaced to the right and the ventral pancreas grows around the right side of the duodenum. Soon it is in juxtaposition with the dorsal pancreas, with which it merges. The pancreas at birth is chiefly derived from the dorsal portion, which contributes the body and tail. The independent duct systems also fuse. Occasionally, double ducts are encountered: the dorsal duct (Santorini) opens directly into the duodenum, and the ventral duct (Wirsung) opens into the duodenum by way of the common bile duct. The dorsal duct persists, draining the body and tail by way of fusion with the ventral duct just to the right of the mesenteric vessels. Occasionally, the ventral duct disappears and the entire gland is drained by the duct of Santorini.

In a poorly understood way, the islets of Langerhans arise from the same epithelial cords that give rise to the secretory acini of the pancreas. They separate at an early stage from the parent tissue and differentiate independently.

The most common developmental error encountered by the surgeon is annular pancreas, followed by anomalies of the duct system, duplication, fusion with spleen, duodenum and stomach, and intracapsular structures contributed by adjacent intestinal primordia. Heterotopic pancreatic primordia may account for the Zollinger-Ellison syndrome. One may encounter atresia, severe hypoplasia or suppression of either pancreatic bud, resulting in absence of the body and tail or absence of the head, with appropriate changes in duct anatomy (Table 49-1).

TABLE 49-1.— DISORDERS OF THE PANCREAS IN 224 CHILDREN (CHILDREN'S HOSPITAL MEDICAL CENTER, 1938-68)

A. Pancreatitis		87
Acute hemorrhagic	47	
Septic infarction, total	16	
Chronic fibrosing	7	
Pseudocyst	7	
Follicular lymphoid	3	
Congenital syphilis	3	
Abscess (obstructing neoplasm)	2	
Calcifying	2	
B. Idiopathic spontaneous hypoglycemia (ISH)		70
Islet cell hypertrophy—resected	11	
Normal pancreas—resected	10	
Medically treated	49	
C. Congenital abnormalities		48
Annular pancreas	29	
Atresia of ducts	5	
Hypoplasia	3	
Intrapancreatic gastric duplication	2	
Dextroposition: pancreas and stomach only	2	
Duplication, complete	2	
Fusion with spleen	2	
Intrapancreatic accessory spleen	1	
Absence of body and tail	1	
Pancreatoduodenal duplication	1	
D. Tumors		19
Cyst, developmental	6	
Choristoma	6	
Gastric	1	2
Islet cell adenoma	5	
Adenocarcinoma	1	
Islet cell carcinoma	1	

Pancreatitis

ACUTE PANCREATITIS

Acute pancreatitis was first described by Fitz[13] in 1889 and the essential pathology recognized by Rich and Duff[32] in 1936. Acute pancreatitis in childhood occurs more frequently than was realized in the past. The literature contains many reports of fulminant or even fatal disease, with the diagnosis being made at the time of laparotomy or autopsy. The preoperative diagnosis was usually acute appendicitis or peritonitis of undetermined cause.[4,8,14,17,36]

ETIOLOGY AND PATHOGENESIS.—Frey and Redo[14] reported 14 cases of diffuse, hemorrhagic pancreatitis which was discovered at autopsy. Most of the children had a history of poor oral intake, feeding problems, nausea, vomiting, diarrhea, abdominal pain and some form of intercurrent infection. Several children were first seen with tachycardia, jaundice and coma. In no case was the diagnosis of pancreatitis entertained prior to death. A review of pathologic material at the Children's Hospital Medical Center bears out this observation. It must be emphasized that acute pancreatitis occurs commonly in seriously ill infants and children. Acute hemorrhagic pancreatitis was encountered in 47 patients. In addition, 16 patients,

most of them infants, were found to have total septic pancreatic infarction. The organisms identified were, in order of frequency, *Escherichia coli*, enterococcus, *Aerobacter aerogenes*, proteus and pseudomonas. A similar condition has been encountered in children dying of burns. The idiopathic form of pancreatitis accounts for two thirds of reported cases, although recent reports provide a greater range of etiology. The mechanism involved is far from clear. In the usual case, pancreatitis comes on rapidly after or in association with febrile illness and a period of poor intake, often associated with vomiting and dehydration. Experimental ethionine pancreatitis and pancreatic atrophy resulting from protein deprivation may provide clues to the true nature of idiopathic pancreatitis in childhood.[11,22] Blumenstock *et al.*[4] first called attention to the idiopathic variety, included in all recent reports. Hendren *et al.*[19] encountered 6 idiopathic cases in 15 children, and Frey and Redo[14] in 6 of 18. Fifty of 87 cases of pancreatitis and its complications seen at the Children's Hospital Medical Center are considered to be idiopathic (Table 49-1).

The association of steroid administration and pancreatitis was documented by Baar and Wolff[2] in 1957 and subsequently confirmed by Nelp,[26] Oppenheimer and Boitnott,[29] among others. Fifteen per cent of children with renal disease have evidence of pancreatitis at autopsy. The incidence increased to 40% in a group of children with renal disease who received steroids. A similar situation is apparent in children with primary liver disease who are treated with steroids. Extrahepatic biliary tract disease is, however, uncommon in children with pancreatitis. Cholelithiasis was encountered once in our series and once in 48 cases

Fig. 49-1.—Diffuse pancreatic calcinosis. Two of 87 children with pancreatitis had this complication.

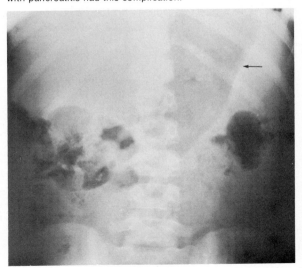

collected from the literature.[25] Pancreatitis may be associated with familial aminoaciduria and hyperlipidemia.[9,16] The hereditary and familial varieties tend to be recurrent, ultimately producing pancreatic cirrhosis or calcinosis, or both. Postoperative pancreatitis results from direct injury to the pancreas at the time of surgery. It is less frequent in children than in adults because of a paucity of conditions involving the biliary tract, stomach and duodenum. Inadvertent injury to the tail of the pancreas during splenectomy causes a milder and self-limited form. Diffuse pancreatic calcification in a 1-year-old child was reported by Martin and Canseco,[24] and we encountered it in 1 child with mucoviscidosis and 1 with hyperparathyroidism (Fig. 49-1). Pancreatitis following the administration of hydrocholorothiazide has been reported.[35] Mumps pancreatitis is rare or certainly mild in children; amylase elevations are not diagnostic because of simultaneous bilateral sialadenitis.[37] In 12 of 17 reported cases in adults, presumably there was a predisposing biliary or pancreatic factor.[30] One case of pancreatitis associated with polyarteritis nodosa has been described.[14] Invasion of the pancreatic ducts by *Ascaris lumbricoides* has been reported in children in this country and abroad,[15,19] including 12 from South Africa, where parasitic intestinal disease is common. Pancreatitis associated with duct anomalies, choledochal cysts and annular pancreas has been reported.[6,18,36] Pancreatitis in the burn patient treated with steroids was described by Baar and Wolff.[2] It has not been our practice to give steroids to burn patients, and we have not encountered pancreatitis other than the terminal septic variety in 1,000 consecutive burned children. Marczynska-Robowska[23] found pancreatitis in 1 patient with ACTH-treated Still's disease.

Pancreatitis of known etiology in childhood is most frequently due to trauma.[39] In approximately 1 of 5 patients, a pseudocyst develops. We have encountered 18 cases of traumatic pancreatitis and 5 pseudocysts in 483 children with abdominal and thoracic injuries, 95% being due to blunt trauma (see Chap. 47). Traumatic pancreatitis is also an increasing problem in adults.[7]

MEDICAL MANAGEMENT.—Traditional therapy has included pain relief, administration of parenteral fluids, vitamins and calcium, maintenance of caloric intake and the inhibition of pancreatic secretions. Demerol rather than morphine is used to control pain (0.5 mg/kg q4h). Gastric decompression is essential, and a Stamm gastrostomy should be established in all children with the diagnosis of severe pancreatitis.[1] By this means, pancreatic secretions are decreased by raising duodenal pH, thus inhibiting the secretin mechanism. It also prevents ileus. Anticholinergic drugs (Pro-Banthine) also diminish pancreatic secretions. Although these traditional methods are helpful, they are not sufficient to support the extremely ill child.

A reduction of circulating blood volume due to loss of large amounts of blood and plasma from the intravascular compartment is the major physiologic disturbance in acute pancreatitis. Accurate calculation of the amount of colloid lost is difficult, if not impossible. The usual clinical indexes are not satisfactory and errors of under- and overtreatment have been common. Constant monitoring of central venous pressure has helped to solve this problem; this pressure can be maintained in the range of 8–12 cm of water by infusion of blood, heat-treated plasma or albumin.

As the disease wears on, there is an increasing respiratory demand, with reduction of pulmonary reserve. Retroperitoneal edema, elevation of the diaphragm, pleural effusion and abdominal splinting combine to produce basal atelectasis leading to intrapulmonary shunting of blood. A vicious cycle of increasing metabolic demand and decreasing pulmonary reserve leads to respiratory failure and cessation of cardiac activity when arterial pH falls below 6.8. Tracheostomy, although not a routine procedure, may be helpful. This reduces dead space and allows for handling of pulmonary secretions but, more important, makes it possible to assist respiration, thus transferring the work of the exhausted child to mechanical apparatus. The metabolic demand may be minimized by placing the patient in an air-conditioned room with temperature controlled at 70 F and relative humidity at 50–70%. Occasionally, unrelenting tachycardia and hyperpyrexia require adjunctive hypothermia, which is easily accomplished in the young child with a lean body mass. Some degree of pancreatic necrosis is inevitable and, with it, secondary infection. The drug of choice is cephalothin (Keflin; 50 mg/kg/day intramuscularly). Repeated blood cultures must be obtained to detect the presence of pseudomonas, for which the drug of choice is colistin (Coly-Mycin; 5 mg/kg/day intramuscularly).

Trasylol* is an inhibitor of trypsin and inactivates kallikrein in bioassay preparations and in cross-circulation experiments. Dosage is 5,000 units/kg/day.[28] Steroids should not be given.

SURGICAL TREATMENT.—Surgical intervention is rarely indicated in the acute phase of pancreatitis when the diagnosis is certain and trauma can be excluded, except for the placement of an occasional gastrostomy tube and an occasional tracheostomy. Although surgical complications are common, they seldom appear before the end of the third week. Because pancreatitis is seldom suspected in childhood, the usual preoperative diagnosis is acute appendicitis or other intra-abdominal catastrophe of a surgical nature. When the abdomen is opened, acute hemorrhagic pancreatitis with fat necrosis and a large volume of intraperitoneal fluid of high colloid content and high pancreatic enzyme activity is encountered. The surgeon should not attack the ampulla, lower common duct and pancreatic ducts. Anomalies are

---

*Trasylol, Bayer A-128.

so infrequent as to be reportable, and biliary tract disease with cholelithiasis is rare. The lesser sac should be drained with 2 large Penrose sump drains brought out through a separate stab wound in the flank. A Stamm gastrostomy should be constructed.

The cause of death in reported series, involving mostly adults, has been a combination of factors: infection, hemorrhage, shock and cardiopulmonary, renal and hepatic failure. Focusing attention on predominantly autopsy experience, one must conclude that pancreatitis in childhood is no less fulminant or destructive than it is in adults. Howard and Ravdin[20] were among the first to define the pathophysiology of pancreatitis and in 1948 reported a mortality of 76% in 80 consecutive patients. Nugent and Atendido[27] in 1967, reporting a mortality of 17.4%, recommended limited surgical intervention. Romer and Carey[33] noted a 23% mortality in 100 consecutive patients with acute hemorrhagic pancreatitis. They considered the serum calcium level to have prognostic significance. Only 15% of patients with a level above 9.0 gm/100 ml died, while 50% of those with a lower level died. Seventy-two patients were not operated on and 19% died, compared to 28 patients who underwent surgery, with 32% mortality. The treatment protocol was not given. In other recent series, the mortality has varied from 20 to 33%.[7,30,34]

It is assumed that similar success can be achieved in children by calling attention to this not uncommon disorder, thus placing it higher in the list of differential diagnoses of acute surgical conditions of the abdomen.

Chronic Fibrosing Pancreatitis

Relatively few reports of chronic fibrosing pancreatitis in childhood are available, although it is being more frequently suspected in children with recurring abdominal pain.[31] Comfort et al.[10] reported 29 cases without associated biliary or gastrointestinal disease, and others[12,21,38,41] have reported additional cases. Such children must be suspected of having heredofamilial disease with aminoaciduria or hyperlipidemia, or both. Hyperparathyroidism must be ruled out. The symptomatology, other than recurring abdominal pain, is variable and laboratory findings are disappointing. Changes in the pancreas discovered at laparotomy consist of diffuse hardening and nodularity involving the entire gland. Biopsy shows fibrosis and loss of acini, initially sparing the islets of Langerhans. Symptoms increase in frequency and severity. Eventually, there is evidence of pancreatic exocrine insufficiency with steatorrhea and weight loss. Ultimately, the gland may become calcified. Diabetes appears late. Diagnosis of idiopathic chronic fibrosing pancreatitis is one of exclusion.

Appropriate studies in this group include measurements of serum lipase, amylase and calcium, fasting blood sugar, serum cholesterol, phospholipids, free fatty acids, stool fat and trypsin activity in the duodenum and/or stools. Plain x-ray films may reveal calcification, and a barium meal should be given to outline the duodenum. There is usually some enlargement of the C-loop. Selective celiac angiography is helpful in other conditions involving the pancreas, but in this condition the vascular bed is normally filled.[40]

Studies to demonstrate the type and degree of involvement should be carried out at the time of laparotomy and should include a cholangiogram, pancreatogram and the opening biliary perfusion pressure. Provided the findings are normal, only a biopsy is performed. Because of the possibility of stone or stricture at the ampulla or, less often, an anomalous duct system in the presence of abnormal studies, it is important to mobilize the duodenum, incise its wall vertically and directly evaluate this important area.

In 3 patients, Hendren et al.[19] were able to relieve pancreatic duct obstruction by performing meatotomy and sphincterotomy. One 13-year-old girl with untreated congenital hemolytic anemia developed cholelithiasis with a stone impacted in the ampulla, resulting in pancreatitis with pseudocyst. In 3 patients, pancreatitis was relieved. A fourth was unrelieved because of far-advanced disease. This 12-year-old boy subsequently had hemigastrectomy and truncal vagotomy, with some improvement. Because of continuing attacks of abdominal pain, he may be a candidate for total pancreatectomy. Two of the patients reported on by these authors are included in Table 49-1. Williams et al.[40] found 5 cases in children in the literature and reported another, in an 11-year-old girl. We have encountered 7 patients with chronic fibrosing pancreatitis; 4 of them had no anatomic or pathologic explanation for the condition and would appear to fall into the group described by Comfort and Steinberg,[9] thus bringing total childhood experience to 10 patients.

REFERENCES

1. Albo, R.; Silen, W., and Goldman, L.: A critical analysis of acute pancreatitis, Arch. Surg. 86:1032, 1963.
2. Baar, H. S., and Wolff, O. H.: Pancreatic necrosis in cortisone-treated children, Lancet 1:812, 1957.
3. Bole, G. G., Jr., and Thompson, O. W.: Acute mumps pancreatitis; Univ. Michigan M. Bull. 24:442, 1958.
4. Blumenstock, D. A.; Mithoefer, J., and Santulli, T. V.: Acute pancreatitis in children, Pediatrics 19:1002, 1957.
5. Blumenthal, H., and Probstein, J. G.: A concept of cirrhosis of the pancreas, Arch. Surg. 81:396, 1960.
6. Blumenthal, H. T., and Probstein, J. G.: Acute pancreatitis in the newborn, infancy and childhood, Ann. Surg. 27:533, 1961.
7. Cleveland, H. C.; Reinschmidt, J. S., and Waddell, W. R.: Traumatic pancreatitis: Increasing problem, S. Clin. North America 43:401, 1963.
8. Collins, J.: Pancreatitis in young children, Arch. Dis. Childhood 33:432, 1958.
9. Comfort, M. W., and Steinberg, A. G.: Pedigree of a family with hereditary chronic relapsing pancreatitis, Gastroenterology 21:54, 1952.

10. Comfort, M. W.; Gambill, E. E., and Bagenstoss, A. H.: Chronic relapsing pancreatitis: A study of 29 cases without associated disease of the biliary or gastrointestinal tract, Gastroenterology 6:239 and 376, 1946.

11. Davies, J. N. P.: The essential pathology of kwashiorkor, Lancet 2:317, 1948.

12. Davis, M. L., and Kelsey, W. M.: Chronic pancreatitis in childhood, Am. J. Dis. Child. 81:687, 1951.

13. Fitz, R. H.: Acute pancreatitis, M. Rec. (New York). p. 35, 1889.

14. Frey, C., and Redo, S. F.: Inflammatory lesions of the pancreas in infancy and childhood, Pediatrics 32:93, 1963.

15. Gallie, W. E., and Brown, A.: Acute hemorrhagic pancreatitis resulting from roundworms: Report of a case, Am. J. Dis. Child. 27:192, 1924.

16. Gerber, B. C.: Hereditary pancreatitis, Arch. Surg. 87:70, 1963.

17. Gibson, J. M., and Gibson, J. M., Jr.: Acute hemorrhagic pancreatitis in childhood, J. Pediat. 48:486, 1956.

18. Gibson, L. E., and Haller, J. A.: Acute pancreatitis associated with congenital cyst of the common bile duct, J. Pediat. 55:650, 1959.

19. Hendren, W. H., Jr.; Greep, J. M., and Patton, A. S.: Pancreatitis in childhood: Experience with 15 cases, Arch. Dis. Childhood 40:132, 1965.

20. Howard, J. M., and Ravdin, I. S.: Acute pancreatitis: Study of 80 patients, Am. Pract. 2:385, 1948.

21. Ingomar, C. J., and Terslev, E.: A case of chronic pancreatitis in early childhood, Danish M. Bull. 12:91, 1965.

22. Kahn, D. R., and Carlson, A. B.: On the mechanism of experimentally induced ethionine pancreatitis, Ann. Surg. 150:42, 1959.

23. Marczynska-Robowska, M.: Pancreatic necrosis in a case of Still's disease, Lancet 1:815, 1957.

24. Martin, L., and Canseco, J. D.: Pancreatic calculosis, J.A.M.A. 135:1055, 1947.

25. Molander, D. W., and Bell, E. T.: Relation of cholelithiasis to acute hemorrhagic pancreatitis, Arch. Path. 41:17, 1946.

26. Nelp, W. B.: Acute pancreatitis associated with steroid therapy, Arch. Int. Med. 108:702, 1961.

27. Nugent, F. W., and Atendido, W. A.: Aggressive Treatment of Hemorrhagic Pancreatitis (Scientific exhibit; Lahey Clinic Foundation, Boston, 1967).

28. Nugent, F. W., et al.: Early experience with Trasylol in the treatment of acute pancreatitis, South. M. J. 57:1317, 1964.

29. Oppenheimer, E. G., and Boitnott, J. K.: Pancreatitis in children following adrenal corticosteroid therapy, Bull. Johns Hopkins Hosp. 107:297, 1961.

30. Paxton, J. R., and Payne, J. H.: Acute pancreatitis: A statistical review of 307 established cases of acute pancreatitis, Surg., Gynec. & Obst. 86:69, 1948.

31. Pleches, P. N.: Chronic recurrent pancreatitis in childhood, Arch. Surg. 81:883, 1960.

32. Rich, A. R., and Duff, G. L.: Pathogenesis of acute hemorrhagic pancreatitis, Bull. Johns Hopkins Hosp. 58:212, 1936.

33. Romer, J. F., and Carey, L. C.: Pancreatitis, a clinical review, Am. J. Surg. III: 795, 1966.

34. Schlitt, R. J., and Perkoff, M.: An analysis of 122 patients with pancreatitis, Am. J. Surg. 103:442, 1962.

35. Shanklin, D. R.: Pancreatic atrophy apparently secondary to hydrochlorothiazide, New England J. Med. 266:1097, 1962.

36. Stickler, G. B., and Yonemoto, R. H.: Acute pancreatitis in children, Am. J. Dis. Child. 95:206, 1958.

37. Walman, I. J., et al.: Amylase levels during mumps, Am. J. M. Sc. 213:477, 1947.

38. Warwick, W. J., and Leavitt, S. R.: Chronic relapsing pancreatitis in childhood, Am. J. Dis. Child. 99:648, 1960.

39. Welch, K. J.: Traumatic pancreatitis in childhood, Newton-Wellesley M. Bull. 11:22, 1959.

40. Williams, T. E.; Sherman, N. J., and Clatworthy, H. W., Jr.: Chronic fibrosing pancreatitis in childhood: A cause of recurrent abdominal pain, Pediatrics 40:1019, 1967.

Pancreatic Cysts

Cyst formation in and around the pancreas is infrequently encountered in childhood. Priestley and Re-Mine[22] classified pancreatic cysts as (1) congenital and developmental, (2) retention, (3) pseudocysts, (4) neoplastic and (5) parasitic cysts. There is unavoidable inaccuracy in such a classification because with time or infection, a congenital cyst can lose its epithelial lining which makes the diagnosis possible.

CONGENITAL AND DEVELOPMENTAL CYSTS

In a 1959 review of the literature, Miles[17] found 8 examples of true congenital cyst in children under age 2, and in 3 under age 6 months. He also reported on a newborn infant with a pancreatic cyst. Pilot *et al.*[21] reported obstruction of the common bile duct in the newborn by a pancreatic cyst. Six children with simple cysts have been encountered at the Children's Hospital Medical Center among 19 patients with cysts and tumors. In our experience, this is second in frequency only to choristoma, also called nesidioblastoma and hamartoma. Multiple cysts occur with mucoviscidosis, but these are not included here. De-Courcy[17] reported a dermoid cyst of the pancreas.

Congenital or developmental cysts may be unilocular or multilocular. Only 4 examples of multiloculated cysts appear in the literature, and one wonders about the exclusion of pancreatic fibrosis in these cases. Our 6 simple cysts were unilocular. Cysts simultaneously occurring in other organs have been reported.[15,16] Hippel-Lindau disease is characterized by hereditary cerebellar cysts, hemangiomas of the retina and cysts of the pancreas and other organs.

Developmental cysts are lined with epithelium backed up with acinar tissue. They are most common in the body and tail of the pancreas and may achieve considerable size. They contain cloudy yellow fluid which is usually sterile on culture and does not demonstrate high enzyme activity. A developmental cyst seldom gives rise to symptoms until it is quite large. As it enlarges, it presses through the gastrohepatic or gastrocolic omentum, more often the latter. The stomach is forced upward and anteriorly while the transverse colon is pushed downward and anteriorly. This is readily demonstrated in barium x-ray studies. Symptoms are due to extrinsic pressure on neighboring organs. The function of the pancreas is not compromised. In the differential diagnosis, one should consider lymphatic or renal cysts, intestinal duplication and the various retroperitoneal tumors.

These cysts are rarely associated with infection or adhesions, and surgical treatment consists of total excision of the cyst with or without part of the gland.

Drainage of the lesser omental sac through a separate stab wound in the left flank may be advisable.

RETENTION CYSTS

Retention cysts of the pancreas are found occasionally in children and are said to result from chronic obstruction of part of the duct system. Outwardly, they resemble congenital cysts but contain cloudy fluid with a high concentration of pancreatic enzymes. There is a lining epithelium unless destroyed by long-standing pressure or inflammatory reaction. At operation and depending on the location of the cyst, the decision must be made between excision with a margin of adjacent pancreas or some form of internal drainage.

NEOPLASTIC CYSTS

Papillary neoplastic cysts are rarely encountered in childhood and there is little danger in leaving a cyst in situ provided the lining is inspected and it is adequately drained. They should not be marsupialized or drained to the surface with a tube. They are easily ruptured, and the contents are extremely irritating to the peritoneal cavity. Consequently they should be decompressed with a trocar prior to making a decision regarding anastomosis to the posterior wall of the stomach or excision. Malignant cysts, like solid carcinomas of the pancreas, must be treated by pancreatoduodenectomy with appropriate reconstruction.

PSEUDOCYSTS

A pseudocyst of the pancreas is a cystic structure located primarily in the lesser sac. The wall is composed of granulation tissue in varying stages of maturity and the lining is devoid of epithelium. Its boundaries are determined by the organs which outline the lesser peritoneal cavity. It may or may not communicate with the pancreatic duct. When it does so, amylase levels in excess of 3,000 units are common. It is usually unilocular, and volumes in excess of 1,000 ml are encountered. I have previously called attention to the prevalence of traumatic pancreatitis in childhood, estimated to occur in 4–6% of children who sustain blunt abdominal injury (see Chap. 47). Approximately 20% subsequently require surgical intervention for pancreatic pseudocysts.[21,22] Reports of pseudocysts due to trauma in children and to a lesser degree following idiopathic pancreatitis are increasing.[1,2,5,7] Drennen[10] in 1922 was the first to recognize the role of trauma in pancreatitis.

Kilman et al.[13] reviewed the world literature to 1964 and found 27 well-documented pediatric cases. Over an 11-year-period they saw 4 children with pseudocysts. DiCensos et al.[8] added 4 cases in the same year, and Hendren et al.[11] reported 4 cases, including 2 from the Children's Hospital series. Whittlesey[29] and

TABLE 49-2.—ETIOLOGY OF PANCREATIC PSEUDOCYSTS IN 55 CHILDREN

ETIOLOGY	MALES	FEMALES	NO. OF CASES	%
Trauma	24	9	33	60
Idiopathic pancreatitis	9	7	16	29
Unknown	2	1	3	5.5
Miscellaneous			3	5.5
Cholelithiasis		1		
Mumps	1	1		
Total	36	19	55	

Bettex et al.[3] have described 2 cases each, and others have reported single cases.[6,18,23,26] Seven children with pseudocysts have been seen at the Children's Hospital Medical Center; 2 were reported on by Hendren et al.[11] and 2 by Tank et al.[25] Two cases have been added to the Boston City Hospital series, bringing the total from that institution to 8.[20]

ETIOLOGY.—The etiology of pancreatic pseudocysts in infancy and childhood is shown in Table 49-2. Trauma was responsible in 60% of the cases and idiopathic hemorrhagic pancreatitis in 29%; in 5.5%, the etiology was unknown. In another 5.5%, cholelithiasis and mumps were responsible. There were 24 males and 9 females with pseudocysts due to trauma. With pseudocysts due to other causes, the sex ratio was approximately equal. The role of trauma in the production of pseudocysts is further demonstrated by analysis of the records of 33 of the 55 children with a history of injury prior to development of the pseudocyst. Under age 5, post-traumatic pseudocyst occurred in 55%; between age 5 and 10, in 72%; from 10 to 15 years, in 53% (Table 49-3). Most pseudocysts in boys between 5 and 10 years are due to trauma whether or not there is a history of injury. Biliary tract disease was encountered in 1 patient, a 13-year-old girl with known congenital spherocytosis who had refused to have splenectomy. A stone became impacted in the common duct and simultaneously obstructed the pancreatic duct, leading to pancreatitis. A pseudocyst formed in the body and tail of the pancreas; she was treated by marsupialization and a very important splenectomy. Two patients had antecedent mumps. One child had annular pancreas in addition to a history of trauma. The patients of Udekwu et al.[26] had an unusual type of pancreatitis resembling ethionine-

TABLE 49-3.—ROLE OF TRAUMA IN PANCREATIC PSEUDOCYSTS IN CHILDREN, ACCORDING TO AGE

AGE, YR.	NO. OF CASES	DUE TO TRAUMA	%
0–5	22	12	55
5–10	18	13	72
10–15	15	8	53
Total	55	33	

17. Miles, R. M.: Pancreatic cyst in the newborn, Ann. Surg. 149:576, 1959.
18. Miller, R. E.: Pancreatic pseudocyst in infants and children, Arch. Surg. 89:317, 1964.
19. Mithoefer, J.: Pseudocyst of pancreas in childhood, Pediatrics 8:534, 1951.
20. Oeconomopoulos, C. T., and Lee, C. M., Jr.: Pseudocysts of the pancreas in infants and young children, Surgery 47:836, 1960.
21. Pilot, L. M.; Gooselaw, J. G., and Isaacson, P. G.: Obstruction of the common bile duct in the newborn by a pancreatic cyst, Journal-Lancet 84:204, 1964.
22. Priestley, J. J., and ReMine, W. H.: Problems in the surgical treatment of pancreatic cysts, S. Clin. North America 47:1313, 1958.
23. Stransky, E., and Lorenzo, A. S.: On pseudocyst of the pancreas in children, Philippine J. Pediat. 8:145, 1959.
24. Stransky, E., and Hofliena-Ibay: A peculiar form of pancreatic pseudocyst in childhood, Ann. paediat. 202:58, 1964.
25. Tank, E.; Eraklis, A. J., and Gross, R. E.: Abdominal Injuries in Children. Presented at the Annual Meeting, American Association for Surgical Trauma, Chicago, 1967.
26. Udekwu, F. A. O., *et al.*: Pancreatic pseudocysts in children, J. Internat. Coll. Surgeons 44:123, 1965.
27. Warren, K. W., and Baker, A. L.: The choice of surgical procedures in the treatment of pancreatic cysts, S. Clin. North America 38:815, 1958.
28. Warren, W. D.; Marsh, W. H., and Sandusky, W. R.: An appraisal of surgical procedures for pancreatic pseudocysts, Ann. Surg. 147:903, 1958.
29. Whittlesey, R. H.: Pancreatic diseases in infancy and childhood, California Med. 102:110, 1965.

Pancreatic Neoplasms

Malignant tumors of the pancreas in infants and children are rare. All reported cases are carcinomas. In a review of the literature to 1964, Moynan *et al.*[14] were able to find 15 examples of pancreatic carcinoma in childhood. Seven additional cases bring the total reported experience to 22. Early reports are ambiguous because of random histologic classification. The disease was uniformly fatal prior to the introduc-

TABLE 49-5.—PANCREATIC CARCINOMA IN INFANTS AND CHILDREN: SYMPTOMS AND SIGNS IN 22 PATIENTS

SYMPTOMS	NO. OF CASES
Abdominal pain	10
Abdominal mass	9
Icterus	6
Diarrhea*	6
Anorexia	6
Vomiting	5
Anemia	4
Weight loss	4
Fever	3
Melena	2
Hematemesis	2

*Probably Zollinger-Ellison syndrome.

tion of pancreatoduodenectomy in the treatment of pancreatic malignancy by Whipple,[26] subsequently modified by Cattell and Warren[2] and Child.[3]

SYMPTOMS AND SIGNS.—The symptoms and signs in the 22 reported cases of carcinoma of the pancreas are listed in Table 49-5. The most frequent complaint was abdominal pain, followed by a palpable abdominal mass, icterus and digestive disturbances consisting of diarrhea, anorexia and vomiting. Unexplained anemia was noted in 4 children; 4 had frank melena or hematemesis. Less frequently, weight loss and fever were the initial complaints. Age ranged from 3 months to 15 years; 3 patients were under 1 year; 7 under 5; 5 under 10, and 7 were aged 10–15.

PATHOLOGY.—The histologic classification of these tumors is indicated in Table 49-6.

The commonest tumor was nonfunctioning islet cell carcinoma, although several had acinar components as well. For this reason, there is inevitable overlap with the next most common group, adenocarcinoma. A rigorous review of the early cases would

Fig. 49-5.—Malignant islet cell carcinoma. Hemisected specimen shows a variegated cut surface with areas of central hemorrhage and necrosis. The patient, an 11-year-old girl, was well 13 years after pancreatoduodenal resection. (Courtesy of Dr. K. W. Warren.)

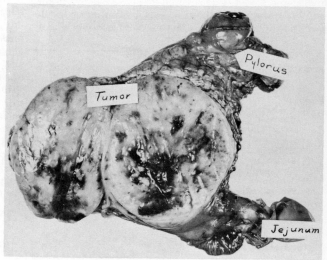

TABLE 49-6.—PANCREATIC CARCINOMA IN INFANTS AND CHILDREN*

CLASSIFICATION	No. of Cases	Age, yr.	Sex M.	Sex F.	None	Biopsy only	By-pass	Pancreato-duodenectomy	Result
Nonfunctioning islet cell carcinoma	8	1, 3, 4, 6 9, 11, 12 14	2	6		1	2	5 (total) 1 (partial)	Alive and Well: 3, 5, 6, 11, 16 yr. Recurred: 3 yr. Dead: 2 wk., 20 mo.
Adenocarcinoma	6	3/12, 15/12, 3, 6, 14, 15	4	2	3	2	1	1 (partial)	Dead: 1 wk., 1 mo., 5 mo., 5 mo., 5 mo., 10 mo.
Undifferentiated Carcinoma	3	8, 13, 14	2	1	2	1			Dead: 10 wk., 4 mo., 6 mo.
Cylindrical cell carcinoma	2	7/12, 2		2	1	1			Dead: 2 wk.
Duct cell carcinoma	1	4	1			1			Dead: 1 wk.
Carcinoma simplex	1	7/12		1	1				Dead: 6 wk.
Medullary carcinoma	1	9	1			1			Dead: 3 mo.
Total	22		10	12	7	7	3	7	Alive: 5 patients Dead: 17 patients

*See also references: 4, 10–13, 16–19.

probably lead to reclassification of some adenocarcinomas as nonfunctioning islet cell carcinomas.

SURGICAL TREATMENT

ISLET CELL CARCINOMA.—There were 8 children with islet cell carcinoma, 6 girls and 2 boys. Only percutaneous liver biopsy was performed in 1 patient, and she died in the second week of hospitalization. Two children had a by-pass procedure; in 1, followed by irradiation and interval pancreatoduodenectomy. Six children had initial pancreatoduodenectomy. The tail of the pancreas was left in 1 patient in the belief that iatrogenic diabetes would be prevented.[6] Five had a Whipple procedure with some variation in the anastomoses. One child with by-pass procedure only, died 20 months after operation. One patient had a recurrence 3 years after pancreatoduodenectomy. Five patients were living and well 3–16 years after pancreatoduodenectomy (Fig. 49-5). The longest survivor, now a 28-year-old woman, had a resection by Gross[7] in 1952 at the age of 9.

It is evident that aggressive surgical extirpation of pancreatic carcinoma in childhood is justified. One should not compromise with partial resection or a by-pass procedure unless there is evidence of distant metastasis. These tumors first metastasize to the portal lymph nodes and subsequently to the liver and lungs. Two long-term survivors had involvement of regional lymph nodes and were given postoperative irradiation. The value of irradiation and chemotherapy in combination is uncertain in islet cell carcinoma of childhood, but it is indicated for diffuse non-resectable liver involvement or pulmonary spread.

ADENOCARCINOMA.—Six children had adenocarcinoma, 4 boys and 2 girls. In 3 patients, no operation was performed because of terminal disease; 2 had biopsy only, 1 had a by-pass procedure and 1 a partial resection. All died within 10 months of the onset of symptoms.

MISCELLANEOUS CARCINOMAS.—Undifferentiated carcinoma was encountered three times, in 2 boys and 1 girl. Two had no operation because of advanced disease; 1 had biopsy only. All died within 6 months of the onset of symptoms. Cylindrical cell carcinoma was seen twice, both in boys. One had no operation, and the other had biopsy only. Both died within 6 weeks. Duct cell carcinoma, carcinoma simplex and medullary carcinoma were encountered in 1 child each; 2 had biopsy only and 1 had no operation. All died within 3 months. Results in this mixed carcinoma group are difficult to evaluate because they represent early reported cases. Histologic review might permit reclassification to islet cell or adenocarcinoma. Three of 5 children would probably have benefited from radical surgical excision.

DISCUSSION.—A number of authors have reported long-term survival following pancreatoduodenectomy for carcinoma of the pancreas in children.[1,6,7,9,22,24] The surgeon first encountering this condition has a unique opportunity for cure through pancreatoduodenectomy. Lesser procedures are not effective because of rapid progression from earliest symptoms to death.

One is impressed by the functional separation of pancreatic carcinoma from islet cell adenoma with organic hyperinsulinism. Hurez[8] and Stokes[20] and their associates encountered 2 children with hypoglycemia and islet cell neoplasms thought to be malignant. Both, however, had local resection with long-term survival. Stokes's patient had a second operation with removal of a heterotopic islet cell tumor in the liver. Review of the histology of these tumors does not permit their classification as carcinomas.

Severe and protracted diarrhea was noted in 6 patients. It is likely that these children had the Zollinger-Ellison syndrome. Once again, these are early reported cases, when the significance of the complaint was not appreciated. There were no studies that indicated gastric hypersecretion, yet the syndrome may have played a role in the rapid demise.

Zollinger-Ellison Syndrome

In 1955, Zollinger and Ellison[28] proposed that a humeroulcerogenic factor of pancreatic islet cell origin might be responsible for the severe ulcer diathesis seen in patients with primary jejunal ulceration. Gregory was the first to demonstrate the presence of a potent gastric secretagogue in pancreatic islet cell tissue.[28] Thirty-five per cent of the patients have diarrhea, usually associated with gastric hypersecretion. All evidence supports the concept that overproduction of acid is primary in the pathogenesis of diarrhea in this syndrome. Multiple endocrine adenomatosis (Werner's syndrome) is a related condition. Operative procedures other than total gastrectomy have been unsuccessful. More than 400 cases of pancreatic islet cell tumors and gastric hypersecretion with peptic jejunal ulceration and diarrhea have been collected.[27] Two hundred and fifty patients were operated on. Only 27% were living without gastrectomy. Survival increased to 50% with subtotal gastrectomy and to 75% following total gastrectomy, with 87% of patients cured when the latter was the initial procedure. Ellison and Wilson,[5] investigating the question of benign vs. malignant tumors in the Zollinger-Ellison syndrome, found 152 of 249 cases (61%) to be malignant; 44% with metastasis; 97 (39%) with benign lesions; 72 (29%) adenomas and 25 (10%) hyperplasia alone. The head-body-tail ratio was 4:1:4. Lesions were multiple and involved two anatomic areas in 29%. The entire gland was involved in 19%. Eighty patients had positive lymph nodes; 67% had local spread and 48% had lesions in the liver; only 2 patients had lung involvement. None of 6 children had carcinoma.

Twelve children to date have developed the Zollinger-Ellison syndrome. Nine children with ulcerogenic islet cell tumors have undergone gastric resection prior to their 15th birthday. Five underwent total gastrectomy. All were living and well for periods up to 9 years, but presumably had residual tumor since the primary lesion was not removed. Four children who had less than total gastrectomy died of the complications of gastric hypersecretion similar to that in infants who have undergone extensive small bowel resection. Ulcerogenic pancreatic islet cell tumors, even carcinoma, may grow slowly. Several cases have suggested remission of the tumor following gastrectomy—an example of reciprocal tumor inhibition following removal of the target organ. Shafer[15] first saw a child with non-beta islet cell carcinoma with diarrhea. A year later, a peptic ulcer developed. Total gastrectomy was performed and the patient, a 16-year-old boy, was well 2 years following operation. Subsequently, a metastatic nodule was resected from the liver which demonstrated gastrin-like activity. This patient closely resembles 6 of 22 children with pancreatic malignancy who initially presented with diarrhea, weight loss and electrolyte imbalance. It is suggested that unrecognized Zollinger-Ellison syndrome will contribute to excessive mortality in children unless appropriately treated, presumably by total gastrectomy and resection of the neoplasm if it occupies the body or tail of the pancreas and is not widespread. Total gastrectomy is not well tolerated by infants, and a more reasonable operation might be pancreatoduodenectomy and bilateral truncal vagotomy with appropriate reconstruction.[25]

REFERENCES

1. Becker, W. F.: Pancreatoduodenectomy for carcinoma of the pancreas in an infant: Report of a case, Ann. Surg. 145:864, 1957.
2. Cattell, R. B., and Warren, K. W.: *Surgery of the Pancreas* (Philadelphia: W. B. Saunders Company, 1953).
3. Child, C. G.: Radical one stage pancreaticoduodenectomy, Surgery 23:492, 1948.
4. Corner, B. D.: Primary carcinoma of the pancreas in an infant age 7 months, Arch. Dis. Childhood 18:106, 1943.
5. Ellison, E. H., and Wilson, S. D.: The Zollinger-Ellison syndrome: Reappraisal and evaluation of 260 registered cases, Ann. Surg. 160:512, 1964.
6. Fonkalsrud, E. W.; Wilkerson, J. A., and Longmire, W. P.: Pancreatoduodenectomy for nonfunctioning islet cell tumor of the pancreas in infancy and childhood, J.A.M.A. 197:158, 1966.
7. Gross, R. E.: Personal communication.
8. Hurez, A., *et al.*: Carcinoma of the islets of Langerhans with severe hypoglycemic manifestations in a 9-year-old child—subtotal pancreatectomy, Arch. franç. pédiat. 18:625, 1961.
9. Jaubert de Beaujeu, M., *et al.*: Duodeno-pancréatectomie céphalique pour tumeur pancréatique chez un enfant de 4 ans et demi, Pédiatrie 19:369, 1964.
10. Kaletcheff, A.: Carcinoma of the pancreas in a girl 14 years old, Gac. méd. Caracas 46:393, 1939.
11. Kochkina, T., and Jakovlev, A.: Malignant tumors in 2 children in a family, Vop. Onkol. 8:83, 1962.
12. Kuhn, A.: Primary pancreatic carcinoma in infancy, Klin. Wchnschr. 24:494, 1887.
13. Morlock, C. G., and Dockerty, M. C.: Carcinoma of the pancreas during the first 2 decades of life: Report of 2 cases, Postgrad. Med. 26:329, 1959.
14. Moynan, R. W., *et al.*: Pancreatic carcinoma in childhood, J. Pediat. 65:711, 1964.
15. Shafer, W. H.: Non-beta islet cell carcinoma of the pancreas presenting as diarrhea, Ann. Int. Med. 61:539, 1964.
16. Simon, F.: Pancreatic Carcinoma in a 13-Year-Old Child. Inaugural dissertation (Griefswald: J. Abel, 1889).
17. Smith, W. R.: Primary carcinoma of the pancreas in children: Report of a case in a boy 14½ years of age with

generalized metastasis, Am. J. Dis. Child. 50:1482, 1935.

18. Stein, M. L.; Rossi, V. C., and de Almeida, A. M. C.: Carcinoma of the pancreas in the infant: Presentation of a case, Pediat. prát. 33:75, 1962.
19. Stewart, S. C., and Stewart, L. F.: A case of cancer of the pancreas in a 9-year-old boy, Internat. Clin. 2:118, 1915.
20. Stokes, J. M.; Wohltmann, H. J., and Hartmann, A. F., Sr.: Pancreatectomy in children, Arch. Surg. 93:40, 1966.
21. Stout, B. F., and Todd, D. A.: Report of a case of primary adenocarcinoma of the pancreas in a 4-year-old child, Texas J. Med. 28:464, 1932.
22. Warren, K. W.: Nonfunctioning islet cell carcinoma in an 11-year-old child treated by pancreato-duodenectomy, Lahey Clin. Bull. 9:155, 1955.
23. Warthen, R. O.; Sanford, M. D., and Rice, E. C.: Primary malignant tumor of the pancreas in a 15-month-old boy, Am. J. Dis. Child. 83:663, 1952.
24. Wastell C.: Malignant nonfunctioning islet cell tumor of the pancreas in a 14-year-old girl, Proc. Roy. Soc. Med. 58:432, 1965.
25. Welch, K. J.: Transthoracic bilateral truncal vagotomy and pyloroplasty following massive small bowel resection in infants (in press).
26. Whipple, A. O.; Parsons, W. B., and Mullins, C. R.: Treatment of carcinoma of the ampulla of Vater, Ann. Surg. 102:763, 1935.
27. Wilson, S. D., and Ellison, E. H.: Survival in patients with the Zollinger-Ellison syndrome treated by total gastrectomy, Am. J. Surg. 111:787, 1966.
28. Zollinger, R. M., and Ellison, E. H.: Primary peptic ulcerations of the jejunum associated with islet cell tumors of the pancreas, Ann. Surg. 142:709, 1955.

Hypoglycemia

HISTORY.—In 1869, Langerhans,[29] while still a medical student, identified the pancreatic islet tissue. In 1902, Nicholls,[35] a pathologist, described the first islet cell adenoma. In 1908, Lane,[28] employing better histologic techniques, differentiated the alpha and beta cells of the islets. Banting and Best[2] discovered insulin in 1921 and postulated its role in hypoglycemia. The term hyperinsulinism, originally used in discussing hypoglycemic states,[50] has proved to be an oversimplification. W. J. Mayo in 1927 first excised a functioning islet cell tumor. The tumor was malignant and there was evidence of metastatic spread at the time of operation. Graham and Hartmann[8] reported the first graded pancreatectomy for hypoglycemia in 1934. The Whipple triad was introduced in 1935.[50]

ETIOLOGY AND PATHOGENESIS.—Hypoglycemia may result from a number of diverse diseases, thus requiring a search for abnormalities of the endocrine system and liver, metabolic errors and sensitivities, prediabetes, insulin-producing pancreatic or extrapancreatic tumors, vanilmandelic acid-producing neuroblastoma and a mixed and unclassifiable group designated idiopathic spontaneous hypoglycemia.[4,6,25,32,47]

With regard to the endocrine system, hypopituitarism (Simmonds', Addison's) is suggested by increased insulin sensitivity. Insulin tolerance is estimated by the intravenous administration of 0.1 unit of insulin/kg followed by measurement of blood glucose levels by the oxidase method; normal values range from 40 to 90 mg/100 ml. Pituitary growth hormone can be measured in the serum (normal, $0-25$ mμg/ml) as another parameter of pituitary activity. Disorders of the pituitary-adrenal cortical axis are disclosed by the measurement of 17-ketosteroids and 17-OH-corticosteroids after administration of ACTH (10 units/kg/24 hr intramuscularly). The functional capacity of the adrenal medulla is estimated by the measurement of total urinary catecholamines (epinephrine and norepinephrine, 3-6 μg/hr). Glucagon deficiency is determined by direct measurement of this substance in the serum (normal, $0-3$ mμg/ml).

Liver disease must be excluded by the usual battery of liver function tests, a negative history and the absence of hepatomegaly. With glycogen storage disease, there is an abnormal response to epinephrine (0.5 ml 1:1, 000 aqueous S-C). With glycogen storage and glucagon deficiency, the liver is unable to release glucose under appropriate stimulation. There are a number of inherited defects involving glycogenolytic enzymes within the liver, such as hereditary fructose intolerance and galactosemia. The role of the liver in carbohydrate metabolism is conventionally tested by the oral glucose tolerance test (1.75 Gm dextrose/kg) and by the 8-hour glucose infusion test.

Congenital leucine sensitivity may be encountered in addition to leucine-sensitive islet cell adenomas. Leucine sensitivity is disclosed by an oral tolerance test (15 mg leucine/kg). Ketotic hypoglycemia occurs only in the older child. Hypoglycemia may indicate prediabetes in some children and requires a careful family history, pedigree search and many years of observation. Administration of pituitary growth hormone is of value in identifying the prediabetic child. Glucose tolerance curves are normal when standard techniques are used. With the administration of pituitary growth hormone, glucose values closely resemble the diabetic curve.

Organic hyperinsulinism can be suspected if the blood glucose level falls below 40 mg/100 ml after fasting or $2-3$ hours after an oral glucose tolerance test. Response to an intravenous tolbutamide tolerance test (15 mg sodium tolbutamide/kg) may be abnormal. The test is not as valuable as it is in adults, however, because of increased sensitivity to sulfonurea compounds.[9] Glucose levels may be driven to a critically low level in the normal child, and the test is probably contraindicated in infants. Serum insulin levels can be measured by the radioimmunoassay method (normal, $0-20$ μ units/ml). False positive results have been noted with islet cell adenoma.[43] Free fatty acid values are greatly increased with organic hyperinsulinism (normal, 300-500 mEq/liter). The hyperglycemic effect of glucagon administration results from increased insulin release and suggests islet hypertrophy or adenoma.

Hypoglycemia has also been observed with virilizing congenital adrenal hyperplasia, cretinism and diffuse central nervous system disease, occasionally leucine-sensitive and refractory to graded pancreatectomy. The basic lesion in the leucine-sensitive group may be within the central nervous system. Hypoglycemia is also seen with trisomy 13-15 and infant giantism. The latter is characterized by visceromegaly, somatic gigantism and macroglossia, frequently associated omphalocele and leucine sensitivity.

Idiopathic Spontaneous Hypoglycemia (ISH)

The diagnosis of idiopathic spontaneous hypoglycemia is one of exclusion and requires the use of sophisticated biochemical techniques and study by a capable endocrinologist. The onset of difficulties before the age of 2 years is suggestive, since 90% of reported cases occur before that age. Drash and Schultz[12] reviewed 70 cases of idiopathic spontaneous hypoglycemia seen at the Johns Hopkins Hospital. Twenty patients were neonates, 25 were less than 1 year old, 13 under 2 years, 12 more than 2 years old, and only 3 were more than 6 years of age. In the last group, 2 patients were found to have islet cell adenoma.[12]

SYMPTOMS AND SIGNS.—The manifestations of hypoglycemia are related to reduced cerebral metabolism, the higher centers being more sensitive to gluconeuropenia than to anoxia. With hypoglycemia, regardless of the mechanism, the clinical picture usually follows one of two patterns. In one, there is evidence of diffuse sympathetic nervous system overactivity. This may indicate compensatory release of epinephrine into the circulation. Consequently, these children are irritable, apprehensive, have excessive pallor and sweating and a fast pulse. In the other, there is more evidence of gluconeuropenia, with apathy, confusion, disorientation, difficulty with speech and vision or prolonged periods of sleeping. At times, the patterns may intermix. In the neonate, ISH may appear dramatically with central nervous system depression, coma and convulsions. In older children, it may first be evident as obesity resulting from constant hunger and overeating or progressive mental retardation. In both groups, the children are otherwise normal in all respects and conspicuously so during the period of adequate circulating blood sugar. With time, there is increasing central nervous system damage. For this reason, surgical intervention is often necessary in spite of the known tendency of ISH to improve spontaneously with decreasing symptoms, usually by the age of 6 years and varying from 6 weeks to 16 years.

MEDICAL TREATMENT

Treatment should be instituted when repeated glucose tests show blood levels below 40 mg/100 ml associated with convulsions or coma, alternating with hyperirritability and increased hunger. It is customary to give ACTH (10 units/kg/24 hours intramuscularly in 2 divided doses) plus hydrocortisone sodium succinate (Solu-Cortef; 10 mg/kg/day intravenously in 2 divided doses). When the child's condition improves enough to permit oral feeding, steroid therapy may be continued orally with prednisone (1.0 mg/kg/24 hours in 2 divided doses). Steroid dosage is decreased 20% at weekly intervals to the lowest level compatible with freedom from hypoglycemic symptoms and the maintainance of normoglycemia.[23] In addition, these infants should be given feedings every 2 hours throughout the day and night. When this cannot be achieved at home because of social conditions, they must be kept under hospital observation for several months. Infection must be promptly recognized and treated. Congenital hypogammaglobulinemia must be excluded by a 24-hour immunochemical gamma globulin determination (normal, 400–600 mg). The leucine-sensitive child should receive a special diet based on a low leucine formula such as s-14 (Wyeth).[39]

Several other therapeutic agents have been of value when steroid therapy has failed to control hypoglycemic episodes. Provided the liver is normal, zinc glucagon will elevate glucose levels; dosage is 1 mg intramuscularly every 4 hours.[27] A long-acting zinc glucagon has recently become available. Diazoxide (10–15 mg/kg/day) is particularly effective in leucine-sensitive hypoglycemia, often refractory to other drugs and to pancreatic resection.[11] It has been valuable in adults with organic hyperinsulinism but has shown variable effectiveness in the control of ISH and failed to produce normal glucose levels in 1 neonate with an islet cell adenoma.[33,40] Human pituitary growth hormone raises glucose levels through its lipid-mobilizing, glucostatic and anabolic properties. There has not, however, been uniform success in the management of ISH. Drugs considered experimental are Sussran, a long-acting epinephrine-like compound, and alloxan, long identified with experimental diabetes.[21] The latter may be of value in patients who have not been fully controlled following 90% pancreatic resection, and should be tried before subjecting them to pancreatoduodenectomy.[8]

Approximately two thirds of the patients improve on medical treatment alone, and the natural history of the disease is one of progressive amelioration.[38] One is left with a difficult group, usually infants less than 1 year of age, who have unstable glucose levels and frequent episodes reflecting gluconeuropenia that lead to progressive organic brain damage. These patients must be realistically considered to be uncontrolled by medical therapy alone and must undergo pancreatic resection. Another indication is the requirement of heavy steroid administration to control symptoms and to achieve biochemical stability. In such patients, growth is retarded, cushingoid features develop and infection is recurrent, which in turn makes hypoglycemia more difficult to manage. Another indication is a worsening pattern in serial electroencephalograms, with generalized disorganization and spike activity in the tracing. In the older child, IQ testing could demonstrate functional deterioration.

SURGICAL TREATMENT

Graded subtotal pancreatectomy is mandatory when medical treatment fails to control symptoms or succeeds only at the expense of serious and significant side effects. There should be an unequivocal Whipple triad,[59] namely, crises after fasting or exhaustion, hypoglycemia (40 mg/100 ml or less) during the crisis and return to normal after the administration of glucose. Intravenous glucose administration must be maintained before, during and after the operation to control blood sugar levels, which may fluctuate from hypoglycemia to a temporary postoperative diabetic state, a rebound phenomenon due to suppression of islet cells by prolonged hyperinsulinism.[34,37] Portal insulin levels have not differed significantly from peripheral levels.

Either a left paramedian or an upper abdominal transverse incision dividing both rectus muscles provides adequate exposure. The lesser peritoneal cavity is entered and the pancreas is mobilized from left to right. It is occasionally possible to preserve the splenic vessels and always the short gastric vessels, thus avoiding splenectomy, which may be important in the infant. The spleen is sacrificed in children. A posterior plane is easily established and the organ is elevated until the superior mesenteric vessels come into view. Resection should be carried to the right of these vessels in order to remove approximately 90% of all functioning pancreatic tissue and thus avoid the possibility of reoperation because of exacerbation (Fig. 49-6). The duct of Wirsung and accessory ducts found at the level of V-shaped transection are carefully ligated. The defect is closed with a basting stitch followed by a running locked stitch. Nonabsorbable sutures are used throughout.[48] Liver biopsy is performed when indicated.

EXPERIENCE AND RESULTS.—Subtotal resection of the pancreas for hypoglycemia was first carried out in 1934 by Graham and Hartmann.[18] The patient, a 1-year-old girl, was explored for islet cell tumor. When none was found, an 80% subtotal pancreatectomy was carried out. The pancreas was normal histologically and the patient survived, but was mentally retarded. Calloway in 1946 performed a subtotal pancreatectomy for idiopathic hypoglycemia in an 8-month-old boy. The histologic report was islet cell hyperplasia. The patient became normoglycemic postoperatively and showed no evidence of mental retardation.[26] McQuarrie[31] reported success following subtotal pancreatectomy in a 1-year-old girl who required ACTH for a short period postoperatively but subsequently remained well. Several reports from 1950 to 1952 indicated a return to hypoglycemic levels in

children aged 7 months to 8 years.[20,21,26] There were, however, 2 instances of mental retardation. Gross[22] reviewed the results of subtotal pancreatectomy for ISH in 6 children aged 12 weeks to 21 months. The operations were performed between 1939 and 1950. All children survived the operation, and 3 were considered well. One lived, with severe mental retardation, and 2 died 7 and 8 months after operation because of overwhelming infection; both showed advanced organic brain damage. A summary of cases collected from the literature plus 19 from the Children's Hospital Medical Center, 1939–68, is given in Table 49-7. Of the 91 children who have undergone graded pancreatectomy for idiopathic spontaneous hypoglycemia, 56 achieved normoglycemic levels postoperatively without resort to steroid or other types of drug therapy, and 23 remained normoglycemic following pancreatectomy and medical therapy. In some, it was eventually possible to discontinue medical therapy. Ten children were considered not to be improved by pancreatic resection, but this was true largely in early operations when approximately 50% of the pancreas was removed. It is evident that 80–90% of the pancreas must be resected, always to the right of the superior mesenteric vessels, in order to obtain the maximal surgical benefit. Unfortunately, 14 children were neurologically impaired preoperatively and remained mentally retarded postoperatively, possibly indicating that the surgical procedure was performed too late, after organic brain damage had been sustained. Thus, in spite of the achievement of biochemical normality, these children are tragically impaired. There was only 1 operative death. Five patients died months to years after operation of infection. Most were institutional defectives. The role of splenectomy in this situation is not clear and was seldom commented on in the operative report.

Children's Hospital Medical Center Experience with ISH.—Seventy odd patients have been treated. In two-thirds the disease was mild to severe and appeared usually after the age of 1 year. Treatment in most patients consisted of multiple feedings and the administration of steroids until spontaneous remission occurred.

All of the truly resistant cases developed before the age of 1 year and most before age 6 months. The patients show no encouraging response to drug therapy even when pushed to intoxicating levels. Even with 80% subtotal pancreatic resection, there is no guarantee that the central nervous system deficit will be erased or that the patient will not subsequently have hypoglycemic episodes. The defect in this group seems to be one of insulin regulation, showing no response to tolbutamide administration.[8] This is to say, insulin levels are not increased above 20 μunits/ml.[43] Administration of pituitary growth hormone to this group reveals a prediabetic state.[46] If followed for a long enough period, they will probably prove to be

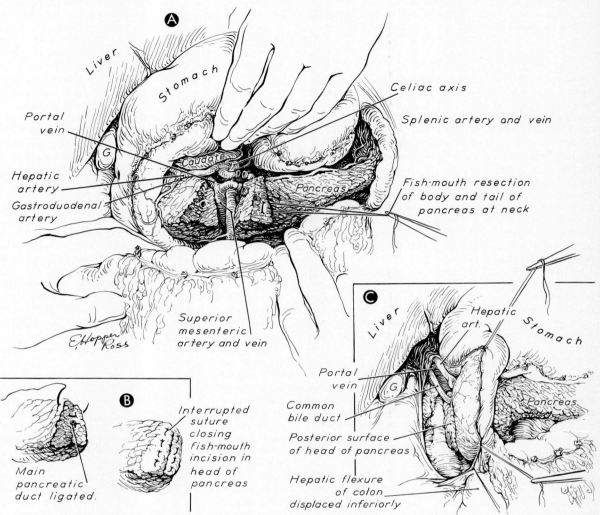

Fig. 49-6.—Idiopathic spontaneous hypoglycemia: technique of pancreatic resection. **A,** approach through gastrocolic omentum. Subtotal resection in progress, with fish-mouth transection to the right of the superior mesenteric vessels, removing 80–90% of the gland. The splenic vein and artery have been divided and ligated. **B,** closure of main pancreatic duct and cut surface of the pancreas with interrupted silk sutures. **C,** exposure for exploration of head of the pancreas. The colonic hepatic flexure has been dissected away, and the entire convex border of the duodenal peritoneum is incised to allow extensive mobilization of duodenum and head of the pancreas.

frankly diabetic.[24] In only 2 patients in the resected group has diabetes developed: 1 has been easily controlled with the administration of pancreatic enzymes and insulin; the other, an institutional defective, has been uncontrollable and has crises of diabetic coma or insulin shock. Secondary operation removing all but a rim of pancreas in the duodenal curve is recommended in patients not improved by a too-conservative initial resection. One child has diffuse nesidioblastosis. The relationship of this condition to refractory hy-

poglycemia is not clear. Formal pancreatoduodenectomy for ISH as recommended by McFarland *et al.*[30] has not been employed in our institution pending further experience with alloxan.[21] Of 21 patients undergoing pancreatic resection for idiopathic hypoglycemia, 11 were found to have islet cell hypertrophy and 10, normal pancreas.[1,10] Nine patients have been the subjects of previous reports.[22,43] Eleven patients were operated on between 1939 and 1956 and 10 between 1956 and 1968 (Table 49-7).

TABLE 49-7.—RESULTS OF GRADED PANCREATECTOMY FOR IDIOPATHIC HYPOGLYCEMIA IN CHILDREN

AUTHOR	NO. OF PATIENTS	NORMOGLYCEMIC	NORMOGLYCEMIC REQUIRE MEDICATION	NOT IMPROVED	NEUROLOGIC IMPAIRMENT	DEATHS Operation	DEATHS Late
Peters[36]	5	4	1		0	0	0
Stokes[45]	5	5			3	0	0
Drash[12]	10	5	2	3		0	0
Hamilton[23]	12	5	6			1	0
Literature to 1967[23]	40	27	7	5	4	0	3
Welch*	21	11	7	3	7	0	2
Total	93	57	23	11	14	1	5

*Experience at Children's Hospital Medical Center, Boston, 1939–68.

CONCLUSIONS

The role of the surgeon in the treatment of idiopathic spontaneous hypoglycemia in children is major and, from the evidence available, management of ISH should be a combined medical-surgical endeavor. The cause-and-effect relationship between brain damage and repeated episodes of gluconeuropenia is not clear and least clear in the leucine-sensitive group who seem to have an independent central nervous system disorder that creates havoc in the intermediary pathways of carbohydrate metabolism.[5] Many infants have the milder form of ISH and can be managed by the simplest of medical regimes, including a short period of steroid therapy with gradual weaning, eventually being controlled by frequent feedings. In a second group, stable blood sugar levels are more difficult to achieve and steroid intoxication becomes too high a price to pay for medical control. The introduction of such agents as diazoxide, glucagon, pituitary growth hormone, Sussran and possibly alloxan may make it possible to bring previously resistant patients under long-term control since the natural history of the disease is one of amelioration and ultimate disappearance. The third group is impossible to control early or late and will benefit most from surgical intervention. Common agreement on the value and timing of 90% pancreatic resection may prevent the instability of biochemical and permanent brain damage encountered in the past. It is anticipated that surgery will have an increasingly prominent role in the management of ISH in view of the predominantly good results presented in this review.

Islet Cell Adenoma

Hypoglycemia appearing initially in the older child is uncommon. With resistance to medical therapy and if ketogenic hypoglycemia, prediabetes and toxic ingestion can be ruled out, organic hyperinsulinism must be strongly considered. It is impossible by today's techniques to make an accurate preoperative diagnosis of islet cell adenoma in a child. These children are treated under varying diagnoses, including epilepsy, and must be diligently sought out in order to provide appropriate surgical treatment and to prevent the ravages of uncontrolled hypoglycemia. The diagnosis of islet cell adenoma, as of ISH, is one of exclusion when a specific etiology cannot be established. Selective celiac arteriography has recently been found useful in identifying these small tumors with an enormously rich blood supply. They usually occur in children over 2 years of age, although 6 cases in the neonatal period have been reported since 1959[16,40,41] (Fig. 49-7). We have encountered only 5 children with islet cell adenoma at the Children's Hospital Medical Center. In 3, surgical removal resulted in dramatic improvement. In the other 2, the adenoma was discovered at autopsy; these were early cases, at a time when little was known about hypoglycemia and its several etiologies.

Islet cell adenoma of the pancreas is being reported with increasing frequency in children and may be present microscopically in 1% of all pancreatic tissue examined at autopsy.[3,12,15,17,42,49] The islet cell tumor has a firmer consistency than the surrounding normal pancreas. Because of the rich capillary network, it has a pinkish color as compared with the more ivory tint of normal pancreatic tissue. The tumor is round, firm, discrete and usually encapsulated. The cells of the adenoma are primarily beta cells, and there is no clear histologic difference between functioning and nonfunctioning tumors. The tumor is multicentric in 14% of cases; 25% are located in the head of the pancreas, 73% are found in the body or tail, and 2% are ectopic.[26] Ectopic implants may be found in the liver and the duodenal wall, around the hilus of the spleen, posterior to the pancreas and more remotely in the wall of the stomach or a Meckel diverticulum.[14,50]

The age distribution up to 15 years of functioning islet cell tumors reported to 1968 is listed in Table 49-8. There were 23 boys and 31 girls. Six children had benign adenomas diagnosed at autopsy. They died as the result of repeated uncontrolled attacks of hypoglycemia. Two patients had exploration only, 2 had biopsy, and 14 had excision of the tumor with little if any margin of adjacent pancreas. Three required reoperation. Subtotal pancreatic resection with amounts ranging from 25 to 90% of the gland was performed

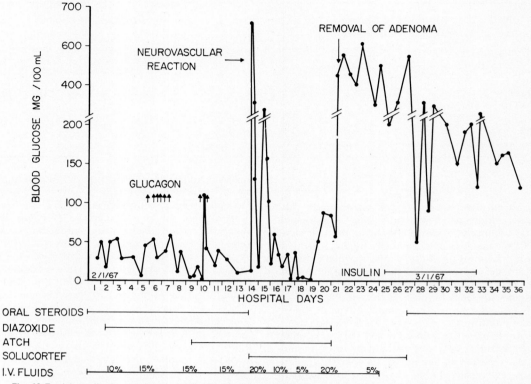

Fig. 49-7. — Islet cell adenoma in a neonate. Chart summarizing failure of medical therapy and cure following surgical removal of the neoplasm. (From Salinas et al.[40])

in 34 patients. Nine patients had vague cellular abnormalities, 11 had tumor-like areas of hyperplasia, 34 had a single adenoma, and 8 had multiple adenomas. Ectopic tumor in the liver occurred once. No case of a functioning islet cell carcinoma in a child has been reported.[34,44] It can be said that 32 children with islet cell adenoma were cured of their disease; 8 were biochemically cured but had severe mental retardation; 6 were improved but required supplementary ACTH; 6 died of the disease, and follow-up was not available in 2.

TABLE 49-8. — AGE AND SEX DISTRIBUTION OF 54 CHILDREN WITH FUNCTIONING ISLET CELL TUMORS*

AGE, YR.	NO. OF CASES
0–2	22
2–4	6
4–6	5
6–8	4
8–10	5
10–12	7
12–15	5
	54

*Boys, 23; girls, 31.

SURGICAL TREATMENT

SURGICAL ANATOMY. — The pancreas is a deep-seated gland that in the past was neglected in routine explorations. Situated transversely across the upper posterior abdomen, it lies from right to left on the second lumbar vertebra in the region of the head, the body covers the first lumbar segment and the tail rises to the twelfth dorsal level. The vena cava and aorta add some cushioning effect against the vertebrae. The head of the pancreas fills the entire concavity of the duodenum, while the tail becomes entwined in venous radicles at the splenic hilus. The celiac artery lies at the upper border of the pancreas at the neck level and gives off the hepatic branch along the upper border of the head of the pancreas. The splenic branch passes to the left along the upper border of the body and tail. The splenic vein traverses a groove on the posterior surface of the pancreas, and emissaries drain the tail and body. The blood supply of the head of the pancreas and the duodenum is largely from the superior and inferior pancreaticoduodenal arteries eventually forming the vasa recti. The body and tail are supplied by the splenic artery. The neck of the pancreas is identified by the area where the superior mesenteric vein crosses behind it and the gastroduodenal artery in front. It is the intimate and common blood supply of the head of the pancreas and duodenum that makes surgery in this area extensive and difficult.

TECHNIQUE OF EXPLORATION FOR ISLET CELL TUMOR. —The gastrocolic omentum is widely opened, exposing the pancreas from neck to tail. (see Fig. 49-6). It has no mesentery and is amazingly mobile. It can readily be palpated from both sides throughout its length by developing its posterior avascular plane. If no tumor is felt or seen, the posterior surface should be inspected from the inferior aspect after dividing the peritoneum and rolling the gland upward.

The head of the pancreas must then be explored. To do so, it is necessary to mobilize the duodenum through the classic Kocher maneuver. The incision is made on its convex border, going through peritoneum and fascia propria. This maneuver takes one into a relatively avascular plane. In this way, the second portion of the duodenum is elevated together with the head of the pancreas and the uncinate process. The extreme right portion of the gastrocolic ligament must be divided and the hepatic flexure pushed downward before the duodenal exposure is started. A visual and bimanual inspection can now be made.

Hyperfunctioning adenomas are said to occur in ectopic tissue in 2% of cases, and these potential areas must also be carefully searched.

Location of islet cell adenomas.—These tumors can appear anywhere in the pancreas, vary in size from a few millimeters to 2 cm in diameter and may be multiple. Because some may be ectopic, if no tumor is found in the pancreas, the gastrocolic and splenocolic ligaments and the paraduodenal tissue should be examined carefully for an aberrant adenoma. Three out of four tumors will be found in the body and tail.

If an adenoma is found in the body or tail of the pancreas, it is advisable to carry out a subtotal resection of the gland along with the spleen rather than an enucleation of the tumor itself,[48] because in about 12% of the cases, tumors will be multiple and most of them located in the tail. If no tumor is found, the same procedure is carried out with the hope that an adenoma will be identified in the resected specimen. In any event, whether or not a tumor is found in the body or tail, a thorough search must be made of the head of the pancreas, because 25% of tumors are located there. One is justified in performing a local excision of the tumor when it is in the head. A quick frozen section should be made for diagnosis.

REFERENCES

1. Agustsson, H.; Tudor, R. B., and Chisholm, T. C.: Hypoglycemia associated with hyperplasia of the islets of Langerhans, Journal-Lancet 67:190, 1947.
2. Banting, F. G., and Best, C. H.: The internal secretion of the pancreas, J. Lab. & Clin. Med. 7:251, 1922.
3. Boley, S. J.; Lin, J., and Schiffmann, A.: Functioning pancreatic adenomas in infants and children, Surgery, 48:592, 1960.
4. Cochrane, W. A., *et al.*: Familial hypoglycemia precipitated by amino acids, J. Clin. Invest. 35:411, 1956.
5. Cornblath, M., and Schwartz, R.: *Disorders of Carbohydrate Metabolism in Infancy* (Philadelphia: W. B. Saunders Company, 1966), pp. 82, 193, 195 and 230.
6. Cornblath, M., and Reisner, S. H.: Blood glucose in the neonate and its clinical significance, New England J. Med. 273:378, 1965.
7. Crigler, J. F., Jr.: Case records of the Massachusetts General Hospital, New England J. Med. 266:1269, 1962.
8. Crigler, J. F., Jr.: Personal communication.
9. Cunningham, G. C., Jr.: Tolbutamide tolerance in hypoglycemic children, Am. J. Dis. Child. 107:417, 1964.
10. Douglas, D. M.: Spontaneous hyperinsulinism due to benign hyperplasia of islet cells, Arch. Dis. Childhood 34:171, 1959.
11. Drash, A. L., *et al.*: The use of diazoxide in the treatment of hypoglycemia, J. Pediat. 69:970, 1966 (abst.).
12. Drash, A., and Schultz, R.: Islet cell adenoma in childhood, Pediatrics 39:59, 1967.
13. Etheridge, J. E., Jr., and Millichap, J. G.: Hypoglycemia and seizures in childhood: Etiologic significance of primary cerebral lesions, Neurology 14:397, 1964.
14. Fonkalsrud, E. W.; Dilley, R. B., and Longmire, W. P., Jr.: Insulin-secreting tumors of the pancreas, Ann. Surg. 159:730, 1964.
15. Francois, R., *et al.*: Hypoglycemia due to pancreatic cell adenoma, J. Pediat. 60:721, 1962.
16. Garces, L. Y.; Drash, A., and Kenny, F. M.: Islet cell tumor in the neonate, Pediatrics 41:789, 1968.
17. Geraud, J., *et al.*: Adenomes langerhansiens hypoglycemients chez un enfant de 12 ans, Ann. chir. infant. 7:39, 1966.
18. Graham, E. A., and Hartmann, A. F.: Subtotal resection of the pancreas for hypoglycemia, Surg., Gynec. & Obst. 59:474, 1934.
19. Grant, J. C. B.: *A Method of Anatomy* (Baltimore: William Wood & Co., 1937), p. 163.
20. Greenlee, R. G., and White, R. R.: Chronic hypoglycemia in an infant treated by subtotal pancreatectomy, J.A.M.A. 149:272, 1952.
21. Griffith, J. E.; Jackson, R. L., and Jones, R. G.: Action of alloxan on a hypoglycemic infant, Pediatrics 7:616, 1951.
22. Gross, R. E.: *The Surgery of Infancy and Childhood* (Philadelphia: W. B. Saunders Company, 1953).
23. Hamilton, J. P., *et al.*: Subtotal pancreatectomy in the management of severe persistent idiopathic hypoglycemia in children, Pediatrics 39:49, 1967.
24. Hansson, G., and Redin, B.: Familial neonatal hypoglycemia: A syndrome resembling foetopathia diabetica, Acta paediat. scandinav. 52:145, 1963.
25. Haworth, J. C., and Coodin, F. J.: Idiopathic spontaneous hypoglycemia in children: Report of 7 cases and review of the literature, Pediatrics 25:748, 1960.
26. Howard, J. M.; Moss, N. H., and Rhoads, J. E.: Hyperinsulinism and islet cell tumors of the pancreas, with 398 recorded tumors, Surg., Gynec. & Obst. 90:417, 1950.
27. Kushner, R. S.; Lemli, L., and Smith, D. W.: Zinc glucagon in the management of idiopathic hypoglycemia, J. Pediat. 63:1111, 1963.
28. Lane, M. A.: The cytologic characters of the islands of Langerhans, Am. J. Anat. 7:409, 1908.
29. Langerhans, P.: Dissertation (Berlin: G. Lange, 1869).
30. McFarland, J. O.; Gillette, F. S., and Zwemer, R. J.: Total pancreatectomy for hyperinsulinism in infants, Surgery 57:313, 1965.
31. McQuarrie, I.: Idiopathic spontaneously occurring hypoglycemia in infants: Clinical significance of the problem and treatment, Am. J. Dis. Child. 87:399, 1954.
32. Marks, V., and Rose, F. C.: *Hypoglycemia* (Oxford: Blackwell Scientific Publications, 1965), pp. 208-32.
33. Marks, V.; Rose, F. C., and Samols, E.: Hyperinsulinism due to metastasizing insulinoma: Treatment with diazoxide, Proc. Roy. Soc. Med. 58:577, 1965.

34. Marshall, S. E.: Islet cell tumors of the pancreas producing hypoglycemia, S. Clin. North America 38:775, 1958.

35. Nicholls, A. G.: Simple adenoma of the pancreas arising from an island of Langerhans, J. M. Res. 8:385, 1902.

36. Peters, H. E.: Pancreatic resection for hypoglycemia in childhood, Am. J. Surg. 110:198, 1965.

37. Porter, M. R., and Frantz, V. K.: Tumors associated with hypoglycemia: Pancreatic and extrapancreatic, Am. J. Med. 21:944, 1956.

38. Rosenbloom, A. L., and Sherman, L.: The natural history of idiopathic hypoglycemia of infancy and its relation to diabetes melitus, New England J. Med. 274:815, 1966.

39. Roth, H., and Segal, S.: Dietary management of leucine-sensitive hypoglycemia, Pediatrics 34:831, 1964.

40. Salinas, E. D., *et al.*: Functioning islet cell adenoma in the newborn, Pediatrics 41:646, 1968.

41. Sauls, H. J., Jr.: Islet cell adenoma in the newborn, cited by Salinas *et al.*[40]

42. Scholten, H. G., and Vander Vegt, J. H.: Functioning islet cell adenoma: Report of 2 cases in young children, J. Pediat. 60:721, 1962.

43. Slone, D., *et al.*: Serum insulin measurements in children with idiopathic spontaneous hypoglycemia and in normal infants, children and adults, New England J. Med. 274:820, 1966.

44. Sprecace, G. A.; Pennoyer, D. C., and Thompson, J. E.: Functioning islet cell carcinoma of the pancreas: Partial literature review, Postgrad. Med. 30:36, 1961.

45. Stokes, J. M.; Wohltmann, H. J., and Hartmann, A. F., Sr.: Pancreatectomy for refractory hypoglycemia in children, Arch. Surg. 93:40, 1966.

46. Soyka, L. F.; Molliver, M., and Crawford, J. D.: Idiopathic hypoglycemia of infancy treated with human growth hormone, Lancet 1:1015, 1964.

47. Traisman, H. S.; Steiner, M. M., and Ziering, W.: Spontaneous hypoglycemia in children, Pediatrics 25:748, 1960.

48. Warren, K. W., and Cattell, R. B.: Basic techniques in pancreatic surgery, S. Clin. North America, 36:707, 1956.

49. Watkins, D. H., and Traylor, F. A.: Islet cell adenoma as a cause of juvenile hyperinsulinism in a 4-year-old boy: Report of a case, J.A.M.A. 185:139, 1963.

50. Whipple, A. O., and Frantz, J. K.: Adenoma of islet cells with hyperinsulinism: A review, Ann. Surg. 101:1299, 1935.

K. J. WELCH

Drawings by
E. HOPPER ROSS

50

Diseases of the Spleen and Portal Circulation

The Spleen

REMOVAL OF THE SPLEEN in childhood is most often indicated because of either traumatic laceration or the presence of a hematologic disorder in which remission or improvement may be expected to follow splenectomy. Tumors or cysts of the spleen are quite uncommon but do constitute an occasional indication for splenectomy. Torsion of the splenic pedicle can produce symptoms demanding removal of the spleen for relief in rare instances.

In the case of injury to the spleen with consequent hemorrhage, there is no controversy regarding the indication for splenectomy. The surgeon is concerned primarily in such cases with developing his diagnostic ability, ensuring that the preoperative preparation brings his patient to the operating room as safely as possible and in mastering a safe technique for the surgical procedure itself.

With hematologic disorders, a much more complex situation exists, and management of these cases requires the close co-operation of a competent hematologist and the surgeon. An important function of the spleen is destruction of red blood cells and probably similar destruction of the platelets and leukocytes as well. In addition, the spleen is a major organ in the reticuloendothelial system and an important source of antibody formation. Pathologic alterations of one

TABLE 50-1.—Splenectomies at Columbus
Children's Hospital, 1950–60

Condition	No.
Traumatic laceration	19
Idiopathic thrombocytopenic purpura	19
Hemolytic anemia	
Hereditary spherocytosis	21
Hereditary nonspherocytic hemolytic anemia	2
Elliptocytosis	1
Sickle cell-thalassemia disease	1
Acquired hemolytic anemia	1
Incidental to other procedures	6
Portal hypertension	3
Secondary hypersplenism	
Reticuloendotheliosis	3
Portal cirrhosis	1
Monocytic leukemia	1
Splenic vein thrombosis	1
Neonatal hepatitis	1
Undiagnosed	2
Disseminated histoplasmosis	1
Total	83

or more of these functions may result in profound hematologic disturbances. Furthermore, normal splenic function may contribute to an anemic state if the red blood cells themselves are abnormal, as in the case of hereditary spherocytosis. In the past, the indications for splenectomy in hematologic diseases have largely been based on the experience that remission or improvement followed splenectomy. More recently, sophisticated techniques have been developed by which survival of red blood cells and platelets can be estimated and the concentration of these formed elements of the blood in the spleen demonstrated. Such studies provide better understanding of the splenic functions and a sounder basis for the indications for splenectomy. However, the basic natures of many of the hematologic diseases often benefited by splenectomy are not yet fully understood, and considerable controversy remains concerning the place of splenectomy in many of these. This is perhaps most true in idiopathic thrombocytopenic purpura.

The role of splenectomy has further been modified by the relationship between splenectomy and subsequent serious infections. In seems quite clear now that such a relationship does exist; but the age group in which this is a particular hazard, the diseases in which this relationship is a major factor and the duration of this relationship remain unsettled.

Table 50-1 lists the splenectomies performed at the Columbus Children's Hospital in the 10-year period, 1950–60. Splenectomies done as part of a splenorenal or other portal-to-systemic venous shunts are not included.

Hemolytic Anemia

Sequestration or trapping of red blood cells within the spleen and their consequent destruction are well-established mechanisms in certain forms of hemolytic anemia. When this splenic activity is a major factor in the anemia, splenectomy often will lead to complete or partial remission. Such splenic hemolysis results from two factors: the red blood cells may be abnormal, or the spleen may be overactive.

Hereditary spherocytosis (congenital hemolytic icterus).—In this disease, the red blood cells are abnormal and as a consequence are trapped and destroyed within the spleen at a more rapid than normal rate.[3] The red blood cells are spherical, and the characteristic can usually be demonstrated in relatives of the patient. The defect is believed to be inherited as a mendelian dominant characteristic. The fundamental abnormality of the red blood cell is not known, but presumably it is biochemical in nature and related to a defect in carbohydrate metabolism.

Morphology.—Morphologically, the red blood cells are trapped in the spleen and microscopic examination shows intense congestion. The site of this trapping or sequestration is probably in the cords of the splenic red pulp rather than in the venous sinuses.[36] The abnormally thick erythrocytes are unable to pass freely from the pulp through the small openings into the venous sinuses, and hence the pulp becomes engorged and the spleen enlarges. The mechanism of destruction of these trapped cells is uncertain. Whatever the mechanism, the spleen exaggerates the metabolic defect of the red cells.

Heredity.—Although inherited as a mendelian dominant, the disease is exceedingly variable in its clinical manifestations. At one extreme, a newborn may have a serious hemolytic anemia with so high a bilirubin level that splenectomy may be necessary to prevent brain damage from kernicterus. In a somewhat milder form, the hemolytic process may be of sufficient severity to require repeated blood transfusions during infancy. More commonly, symptoms of anemia and mild icterus are encountered in later infancy and childhood. At the other end of the scale, the disease may be so mild as to cause no symptoms during a normal life span and not even to result in gallstones. This variability has been explained by the postulate that there is a variable penetrance of the inherited defect on the gene.

Crises with a rapid fall of the hemoglobin level accompanied by fever, abdominal pain and vomiting may occur at any time in the course of the disease and were formerly regarded as manifestations of increased hemolysis. In careful studies on patients in crises, however, the reticulocyte counts have been low and the bone marrow depressed. These episodes are more properly regarded as aplastic crises, basically due to failure of red cell production in the bone marrow.[3]

Physical examination often reveals no abnormality except that as a rule an enlarged firm spleen is palpable. The spleen is only moderately enlarged in infants and small children but is often very large in later childhood. Pallor and icterus are variable findings, but usually are evident in mild degree. More seriously affected children suffer serious growth failure.

Blood. — Examination of the peripheral blood shows moderate to extreme anemia, and spherocytes are found in the stained smear. Increased production of erythrocytes is manifested by a high reticulocyte count, and marked erythropoiesis is characteristically found on examination of the bone marrow. Both the reticulocyte count and the erythropoiesis may be depressed in a crisis, as noted previously. The elevation of serum bilirubin is variable — a factor of the severity of the hemolytic process. The indirect fraction is elevated and bile is absent from the urine.

Other important laboratory findings are: (1) increased osmotic fragility of the erythrocytes in hypotonic saline solution which may not be found in freshly drawn red blood cells but is invariably present after sterile incubation of the blood at body temperature for 24 hours; (2) increased mechanical fragility of freshly drawn red blood cells; (3) negative results of the Coombs test; and (4) greater than normal lysis of red cells during sterile incubation at body temperature for 48 hours.[35] The last finding is partially corrected by the addition of glucose to the incubating mixture.

Treatment. — Splenectomy is specifically indicated in patients with this disease since invariably a clinical cure results with permanent relief of anemia and jaundice. The indication holds even for mild cases since splenectomy will prevent periods of severe anemia (crises) and the development of gallstones. The abnormalities of the erythrocytes persist after splenectomy, including the spherical shape and greater than normal osmotic and mechanical fragility. Splenectomy was performed in 21 patients with this disease at the Columbus Children's Hospital in the 10-year period, 1950–60. All survived with no significant complications. The clinical results have been uniformly excellent. Follow-up hemoglobin, hematocrit and van den Bergh values have been normal. Repeat determinations of the erythrocyte osmotic fragility in all cases studied show persistent increased fragility in hypotonic saline solution.

In newborn infants with severe hemolysis and a dangerously high bilirubin level, one or more exchange transfusions are preferred to splenectomy. Such an exchange replaces normal for abnormal red blood cells and is an effective though temporary means of reducing the hemolytic process. Splenectomy is avoided whenever possible during infancy.

OTHER HEMOLYTIC ANEMIAS. — The remaining hemolytic anemias in childhood form a heterogenous group.[3] Consideration of them as a group is justified only because each patient must be carefully evaluated as to the role of the spleen before a decision in regard to splenectomy can be made. In such patients, splenectomy rarely is as dramatically effective as with hereditary spherocytosis in producing a com-

plete and permanent remission. Occasionally, splenectomy will not produce improvement, while in some cases a longer interval between blood transfusions will be the major benefit derived from removal of the spleen.

Hereditary elliptocytosis is a rare form of hemolytic anemia in which the erythrocytes have an elliptical form. The defect is inherited in a mendelian dominant pattern, but apparently there is a wide variety in the expressivity of the gene for the defect of elliptocytosis. In each individual, the degree of involvement is relatively constant, but there is a wide range of severity among affected persons. The majority of individuals with the trait show no evidence of increased hemolysis and do not have a chronic hemolytic anemia. The remaining have increased hemolysis which may be compensated or uncompensated.

The clinical picture depends on the severity of the hemolytic process.[4] In patients with increased hemolysis, it is like that of hereditary spherocytosis. Splenomegaly is found in those with increased hemolysis, but the spleen is not palpable and presumably is normal in size in those with the trait but without increased hemolysis. As with hereditary spherocytosis, splenectomy is uniformly effective in the patients with a chronic hemolytic anemia. The anemia is relieved following the operation, but the elliptocytosis remains and is even more striking in the peripheral blood, probably due to increased longevity of the erythrocytes.

Thalassemia (Mediterranean anemia), sickle cell disease and *hereditary nonspherocytic hemolytic anemia* have in common a defect in the red blood cells. In the first two, there is an abnormal hemoglobin. By and large, patients with thalassemia or sickle cell disease are not benefited by splenectomy, but in some, the enlarged spleen usually associated with these diseases traps a high proportion of the erythrocytes in the body. When such trapping is demonstrated by evidence of progressive shortening of the life span of transfused red cells, splenectomy may be of considerable benefit to the patient.[19] Sickle cell disease and thalassemia may be combined in a single patient. Such a patient in our series had a huge spleen and severe hemolytic anemia and was much improved following splenectomy. Splenectomy for thalassemia may decrease the frequency of the need for transfusion.

One type of *hereditary nonspherocytic anemia* is a rare disease characterized by metabolic defects in the erythrocytes.[20,21,26,37] It is biochemically associated with a reduction of glucose-6-phosphate dehydrogenase in the red cells. Exaggerated jaundice in the neonatal period and episodes of hemoglobinuria, often associated with previous drug ingestion, have been clinical findings in most of these cases, and a chronic type of hemolytic process is found in all. All cases reported thus far have been in the white race. Splenectomy does not produce a complete clinical remission, but in 2 cases so treated at the Columbus Children's Hospital it was distinctly beneficial by stopping the need for transfusion therapy in both and by ending any further evidence of hemoglobinuria in 1.

There are a number of acquired hemolytic anemias in childhood due to diverse causes such as toxins, idiosyncrasy to hemolysis by certain drugs or vegetables, direct attack on the erythrocytes by bacteria and the presence of specific antibodies against red cells. In the last group, the spleen may be a factor in some cases of chronic autoimmune acquired hemolytic disease, but in the remaining there is no pathologic splenic-destructive mechanism.

In the *autoimmune hemolytic anemias*, the red blood cells are coated by abnormal agglutinins, and response to the Coombs test (antiglobulin test) is almost invariably positive.[30] In most instances, the hemolytic disease is acute with a self-limited course and a good prognosis. Chronic forms may be treated by splenectomy, and remission follows in about half of such cases. The mechanism of improvement following splenectomy is not known but may be due to removal of an important fraction of the antibody-forming cells of the body. Use of steroids may produce a similar remission by suppressing antibody-antigen interaction.

IDIOPATHIC THROMBOCYTOPENIC PURPURA

Clinically, this hemorrhagic disease is characterized by petechiae and ecchymoses in the skin and mucous membranes. In addition, there may be bleeding into other organs including the gastrointestinal tract, the kidneys and, of particular importance, the central nervous system. The platelet count in the peripheral blood is markedly reduced, usually below 50,000. Often the platelets are almost or completely absent. The bleeding time is increased, and usually a definite increase of capillary permeability is found. The bone marrow findings are not uniform. The number of megakaryocytes may appear to be normal, definitely increased or even less than normal.[22] The maturity of the megakaryocytes and the question of their platelet production in respect to the genesis of thrombopenia are unsettled issues.

The basic etiology of the disease is not definitely known. Idiopathic thrombocytopenic purpura has been held to be an example of primary hypersplenism with sequestration and destruction of platelets in the spleen and increased production of platelets in the bone marrow.[6] A second theory proposes elaboration of hormone by the spleen which acts on the bone marrow to depress the production of platelets. More recently, evidence has been brought forth indicating that the disease may be basically immunologic, and platelet agglutinins have been found by some investigators in this field.[4,13]

In most children, the onset is acute and purpura the primary manifestation. In a small proportion of

the cases, there may be gastrointestinal or other hemorrhage of sufficient magnitude to result in severe anemia. Hematuria is found occasionally. Most alarming are the infrequent patients who develop progressive loss of consciousness or specific localizing neurologic signs indicative of intracranial bleeding. The acute onset follows a mild systemic infection in many patients, and a trigger mechanism set off by such an infection (e.g., a mild upper respiratory infection) has been suggested. Quite often, however, no history of any such preceding illness is obtained. In most children, the disease is self-limited, and spontaneous and permanent remissions will occur in a few weeks. Newton and Zuelzer[22] reviewed 42 cases followed 6 months or longer and reported cessation of bleeding in 29 patients within a month, and within 3 months for an additional 7. In 6, a chronic course of over 6 months and as long as 3 years was found. Walker and Walker[33] reported 114 cases diagnosed during a 15-year period. Eighty-three were classified as acute and 31 as chronic. Three patients with acute cases died, 1 of complications secondary to splenectomy and the other 2 of hemorrhage. The remaining 80 recovered, about half within 1 month.

The experience at the Columbus Children's Hospital with 90 cases in a 10-year period showed a similar proportion of acute and chronic cases and, in addition, a third category of neonatal cases (Table 50-2).[9] The neonatal group behaves as acute cases, but the disease in this age group has a more serious prognosis because of the high incidence of intracranial bleeding. The newborn group should be considered apart from the other cases, since probably it represents a maternal-fetal relationship resulting in a bleeding phenomenon associated with thrombopenia in the infants. The chronic form of the disease may persist for several years with intermittent episodes of purpura often associated with minor illnesses, and with a fluctuating but usually quite low platelet count. There have been no serious hemorrhagic complications in the chronic cases followed here, and this has been the generally reported experience.

TREATMENT.—*Acute form.*—Because the large majority of cases of idiopathic thrombocytopenic purpura are acute and self-limited in their course, most authorities no longer feel that splenectomy should be routinely performed.[14,27] In most instances, no specific therapy is necessary in the acute cases, but there is a distinct danger involved. As noted above, Walker and

TABLE 50-2.—IDIOPATHIC THROMBOCYTOPENIC PURPURA

	No. OF CASES	TREATED BY SPLENECTOMY
Acute	56	6
Chronic	19	11
Neonatal	15	2
Total	90	19

Walker,[33] reported 2 deaths from hemorrhage in acute cases. Furthermore, they reviewed the deaths which occurred in England and Wales during a 1-year period from this disease and found 12 which met their diagnostic criteria. Of these deaths, 11 were due to intracranial hemorrhage and the other was due to gastrointestinal bleeding. Because of these hazards and because steroid therapy has proved to be effective in controlling hemorrhagic manifestations, a course of steroid therapy is recommended. Prednisone, in particular, has been quite successful both in controlling hemorrhagic manifestations and in raising the platelet count, although the latter effect is not invariable. The duration of the steroid therapy should be limited to 1 or 2 months, although Dameshek *et al.*[5] have continued the drug therapy for an indefinite period in some instances.

In our experience (Table 50-2), splenectomy has been performed in 6 of 56 children with the acute form, 4 being done as emergencies because of obvious and progressive manifestations of intracranial bleeding. Another was done because of persistent bleeding from the gums for 4 days, and in the sixth, splenectomy was performed in a child with a wringer injury with marked hemorrhage and evidence of circulatory impairment complicating an otherwise seemingly benign course. All of these patients survived and have done well, the only sequela being a questionable petit mal attack in 1. With the combined medical and surgical management as indicated, the mortality should be very low indeed and permanent morbidity very rare. When splenectomy is indicated as an emergency procedure, platelet transfusions should be given preoperatively and during the procedure. Their effectiveness in achieving and maintaining a reasonably normal platelet count has been well demonstrated.[10]

Chronic form. — If thrombocytopenia persists for 6 – 12 months, spontaneous remission becomes unlikely and splenectomy should be considered. Significant complications in patients with the chronic disease are rare, but recurrent purpura is the rule. Long-term steroid therapy does control the hemorrhagic tendency in most patients but is quite undesirable in children because of its side effects and its effect on growth. The morbidity and mortality of splenectomy in such cases is negligible. Eleven splenectomies were performed in the 19 patients with chronic purpura in our series with no deaths. The operation was followed by permanent clinical and laboratory remission in 9, but there was no improvement in 2. In the experience of Walker and Walker,[33] 16 of 31 patients with the chronic form were treated with splenectomy. Of the 16, all responded completely initially, but thrombocytopenia did recur in 2.

Neonatal form. — Of the 15 patients with the neonatal form of the disease (bleeding manifestations within the first 3 days of life), 2 had splenectomy. In both, the indication was evidence of intracranial

bleeding, and both recovered with no further bleeding tendency. One has remained perfectly well. The other has permanent neurologic deficits in the form of some visual loss and definite weakness in both legs, requiring braces.

In summary, children with the acute form of the disease may be expected in most instances to spontaneously recover completely within a few months. Steroid therapy for a limited period of time and blood transfusions, when indicated, are recommended. Splenectomy should be done immediately when there is evidence of intracranial bleeding or in selected instances in which prompt control of hemorrhage is demanded. In such circumstances platelet transfusions before and during the operation should be given. In chronic cases, splenectomy is recommended when purpura persists for 6 – 12 months with the expectation of a satisfactory hematologic response in the majority.

HYPERSPLENISM

Hypersplenism has been advanced as an inclusive concept to explain the various hematologic states benefited by splenectomy.[6] The overactive spleen traps and destroys one or more of the formed elements of the blood, leading to a deficiency of this element in the peripheral blood and to its increased production in the bone marrow. Hypersplenism may be primary (idiopathic) or secondary to some other disease which results in an enlarged spleen. Hereditary spherocytosis and idiopathic thrombocytopenic purpura have been considered examples of primary hypersplenism affecting the erythrocytes and platelets respectively, although, as noted in our earlier discussions of these diseases, there are factors other than splenic in both. Primary splenic neutropenia and primary splenic pancytopenia are rare diseases affecting in the first the granulocytes and in the second all three of the formed elements of the blood.[8,34]

In secondary hypersplenism, the primary disease results in splenomegaly, and the enlarged organ becomes overactive, either by trapping or destroying one or more of the elements of the blood or by an immunologic mechanism. The most familiar example of this phenomenon is congestive splenomegaly secondary to portal hypertension in which neutropenia is commonly found and pancytopenia is not unusual. Other diseases in which we have encountered secondary hypersplenism include reticuloendotheliosis, histoplasmosis and leukemia. It has also been described in Boeck's sarcoid, Hodgkin's disease, Gaucher's disease and certain infections. If the hypersplenic phenomenon can be well documented and is severe, splenectomy is often quite helpful by relieving a specific cytopenia or pancytopenia, although the underlying basic disease is not affected.[38] Motulsky *et al.*[19] described quite lucidly the "big spleen" syndrome insofar as the erythrocyte-destroying mechanism is concerned. They pointed out the difficulties in hemolytic states of distinguishing between splenic destructions of normal red cells and conditions in which the red cells are made vulnerable to lysis by antibodies. According to them, both mechanisms may play a part in certain diseases such as leukemia and lupus erythematosus.

TRAUMATIC LACERATION OF THE SPLEEN

Injury of the spleen is the commonest accident in childhood requiring laparotomy.[25] Blunt trauma causing rupture of the spleen usually is a considerable force, as occurs on being struck by an automobile or falling from a tree. Occasionally, however, the injury seems relatively trivial, as in a fall in a school yard or on steps.[6] In our 19 cases in the 10 years 1950–60, 8 resulted from falls of assorted types (from trees, a horse, a gate, on steps), 3 from blows sustained in a fight, 2 from being run over by a farm wagon, 2 from being struck by an automobile, 1 from being knocked down by a bicycle, and the last from being struck by a knee at play.

Signs of blood loss and a history of abdominal trauma usually permit a prompt diagnosis.[23,24,31] Pallor, increased perspiration and a rapid pulse in an obvious case are accompanied by abdominal pain, tenderness and muscle-guarding in the left upper quadrant and pain in the left shoulder. The initial onset of pain is often abrupt and not infrequently accompanied by nausea and vomiting. At times, however, the abdominal findings are not impressive and the signs of blood loss develop gradually. A slow but progressive fall of the hemoglobin level is a valuable indication of the diagnosis in such cases.

Two other diagnostic measures deserve mention. The finding of blood by peritoneal tap is most helpful in a doubtful case, particularly in patients with multiple injuries, although a negative tap by no means excludes the diagnosis.[7] This is easily performed in all four abdominal quadrants with the patient in a semisitting position. A short beveled spinal needle, 19 or 20 gauge, is used. We have used such a needle on numerous occasions with no complications and considerable reward. Abdominal and chest x-rays also may clarify a puzzling case but usually are disappointing.[17] An enlarged spleen or a definite left upper quadrant mass has occasionally been a helpful finding. Medial displacement of the stomach and serrations along the greater curvature of the gas-filled stomach have not been of value, and the findings of ileus are nonspecific. Fractured ribs accompanying a lacerated spleen is an uncommon combination in childhood injuries, and was encountered only once in our cases.

Laboratory data usually do not show a significant anemia initially, although later, anemia may be found. Moderate to marked leukocytosis is usual, but it is quite nonspecific and occurs frequently in children suffering any type of significant trauma. It does not necessarily imply hemorrhage. An amylase test is sometimes valuable since traumatic pancreatitis is easily mistaken for splenic laceration.

Associated injuries are common, and their significance requires careful evaluation in planning proper management of the injured child. Excluding superficial contusions and lacerations, there were 18 other injuries occurring in 6 of our patients. Various fractures, usually of the extremities and often multiple, were found in 5. There were 4 instances of retroperitoneal hematoma, injuries to the liver occurred in 2, and contusion of the left kidney and pancreas in 1 each.

Splenectomy is indicated as soon as the diagnosis is made, waiting only to have blood available for replacement during or, if necessary, before the operation, and to decompress the stomach via a Levin tube. The mortality is quite low in children, and most fatal cases are probably related to serious associated injuries. All of the 19 patients in our series survived, and morbidity was relatively slight.

Splenectomy

PREOPERATIVE PREPARATION. – The care necessary for the preparation of a child for splenectomy depends largely on the diagnosis and to a lesser extent on the urgency of the situation. Two measures are applicable in all instances. First, the tragedy of vomiting and aspiration can be eliminated by passing a nasogastric tube, emptying the stomach and connecting the tube to an appropriate source of suction. Such a measure adds to the technical ease of the procedure by keeping the stomach decompressed. Second, an intravenous cannula of adequate size ensures prompt replacement of blood loss if replacement becomes necessary.

The child who has suffered a traumatic laceration of the spleen requires blood replacement prior to surgery in sufficient quantity to stabilize the pulse and blood pressure at normal levels. In addition, such a patient must be critically evaluated from the standpoint of other associated injuries. In particular, a careful search for injuries to the central nervous system, chest, urinary tract and skeletal system should be made. The necessity for splenectomy is not altered by such injuries, but it is no victory to remove a lacerated spleen from a child who later succumbs to an undiagnosed epidural hematoma or hemothorax.

It is more difficult to be specific about appropriate preparatory measures in children affected by the various hematologic diseases in which splenectomy may be indicated. In hereditary splenocytosis, preoperative blood transfusions in an effort to correct an existing anemia are usually not indicated unless the anemia is particularly severe. Despite a hemoglobin value much lower than the usually accepted safe level, the operation is almost invariably well tolerated.

In those instances of idiopathic thrombocytopenic purpura in which splenectomy is recommended, no special measures are ordinarily required unless the patient has been on steroid therapy within the preceding year. In that event, full replacement dosage of steroid should be given the day prior to and the day of operation. If the operation is an emergency in an effort to control intracranial bleeding, no delay is warranted.[8] Transfusions of platelets or of fresh whole blood to assist in controlling the bleeding tendency during the procedure can be used to obtain maximal hemostasis. Despite an alarming deficiency or even complete absence of platelets in the circulating blood, serious hemorrhage at operation has not been a problem. The fear of provoking additional bleeding should not deter one from the use of a nasogastric tube in these cases.

TECHNIQUE.—The operative approach depends on whether the indication is traumatic laceration or a hematologic disease. In cases of traumatic laceration, the patient is placed supine on the operating table in moderate reverse Trendelenburg position. The abdomen may be opened through a high left paramedian incision, retracting the left rectus muscle laterally.[9] A supraumbilical transverse incision gives equally good exposure in most children. After removal of blood clots and aspiration of free blood, the spleen is grasped with the left hand and drawn downward anteriorly and medially. The posterior peritoneal reflection (splenorenal ligament) is divided with scissors, and this dissection is carried upward to free the superior tip of the spleen from the diaphragmatic peritoneal attachment. This permits the spleen to be delivered easily into the incision, and the short gastric vessels are then individually ligated and divided. Attachments to the splenic flexure of the colon may be divided now or may be done as an initial step. With the spleen lifted well up, the hilus is seen on its posterior aspect and the tail of the pancreas gently separated from it by blunt dissection. The splenic artery

Fig. 50-1.—Elective splenectomy: technique. **A,** spleen is drawn down and forward and the lateral peritoneal reflection (splenorenal ligament) divided. **B,** spleen is delivered out of the incision and held laterally, exposing the gastrosplenic ligament and short gastric vessels. **C,** spleen is reflected anteriorly and medially, exposing the posterior aspect of the hilus and tail of the pancreas. **D,** the tail of the pancreas has been freed from the hilus, allowing exposure and individual isolation of the splenic vein and artery.

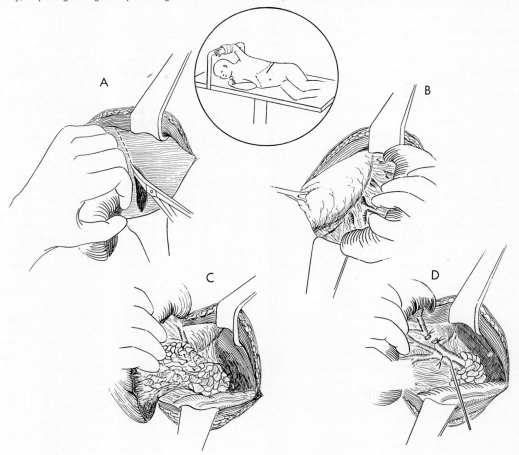

and vein are then individually ligated and divided. If the spleen has been severely fragmented, it is helpful to wrap a gauze pad around it during its removal. Following removal of the spleen, a careful and systematic abdominal exploration is performed to determine the presence and extent of other injuries.

Splenectomy in children for hematologic disorders is most easily performed through a left lateral incision with the left side of the patient elevated from the operating table approximately 45° (Fig. 50-1). The incision extends from the posterior axillary line close to the tip of the eleventh rib anteriorly to the lateral border of the left rectus muscle. The external oblique muscle is divided in the direction of the incision, and the underlying internal oblique and transversus muscles in the direction of their fibers. If additional exposure is desired, part or all of the rectus muscle is divided as the incision is extended medially.

The left costal margin is retracted upward, the splenic flexure of the colon downward, and the subsequent steps follow the above description. The spleen is drawn down and medially, delivering the lower pole of the organ into the incision and exposing the lateral peritoneal reflection of the spleen (splenorenal ligament). This is divided from below upward, being carried upward and medially to divide the peritoneal reflection to the diaphragm. The maneuver permits one to draw the spleen into the wound. Traction on it downward and laterally permits easy access to the short gastric vessels between the greater curvature of the stomach and the spleen. After these are ligated and divided, only the hilar attachments remain. It is wise to use suture ligatures on the gastric side of the short gastric vessels and to take a small bite of gastric wall with the needle. This effectively anchors the ligature so that it will not slip off if gastric distention should occur postoperatively. The spleen is now reflected medially, and the tail of the pancreas is carefully freed from the hilus by gentle blunt dissection. The splenic artery and vein are now individually ligated and divided and the spleen removed.

As the dissection proceeds with exposure of the splenocolic ligament, the gastrosplenic ligament, the greater omentum and the hilus, the surgeon should keep in mind the possibility of one or more accessory spleens in these various locations. When found, they should be removed. This is unnecessary and perhaps not desirable in cases of traumatic laceration, but in hematologic disorders, an overlooked accessory spleen may later result in relapse.[2]

The lateral approach to splenectomy in children is technically easier than the anterior route. The small intestines fall out of the way and require no packing or retraction. The wide-angled costal margin is supple and easily retracted, so that exposure of the diaphragmatic peritoneal attachments and the short gastric vessels is good. In addition, the final scar is far superior cosmetically, a fine line without the widening and keloid formation so common in vertical incisions. On the other hand, this approach is inappropriate for patients with a lacerated spleen, since exposure and appropriate management of other intra-abdominal injuries would be quite difficult in many instances. The left paramedian or long transverse incision should be used in such circumstances. Closure of the wound in an anatomic fashion completes the procedure. No drains are used.

POSTOPERATIVE CARE.—Following splenectomy for either trauma or a hematologic condition, the child ordinarily recovers rapidly with little morbidity. The nasogastric tube is removed on the first or second postoperative day with the return of peristalsis, and oral feedings are then offered and advanced as quickly as tolerated. Normal activity, including ambulation, is rapidly resumed and indeed could scarcely be prevented even if desired. Steroid therapy initiated preoperatively must be continued in full replacement dosage usually for 2 or 3 days after operation, following which it may be gradually discontinued over a period of 1 or 2 weeks. Certain hematologic states may require considerably longer periods of steroid therapy, and this problem requires individual consideration with the guidance of the hematologist.

Complications are rare. Subphrenic abscess, postoperative bleeding, prolonged ileus, pancreatitis and wound complications such as infection or dehiscence may occur, and must be searched for in the patient who is not promptly recovering. Fortunately, however, in children these are most unusual. More likely is a persistence of the original hematologic process if the diagnosis was not correct or if the decision for splenectomy was made without proper indications or in desperate circumstances.

POSTSPLENECTOMY INFECTION

King and Shumacker[16] in 1952 reported serious septic complications in 4 of 5 infants in whom splenectomy had been done because of hereditary spherocytosis. In these 4, either meningitis or overwhelming meningococcemia developed from 6 weeks to 3 years after operation, and 1 died of the infection. The fifth patient died of an acute febrile illness suggesting infection. Smith et al.[28] confirmed the hazard of severe infections in infants and children following splenectomy and extended this relationship into the childhood age group. Since these initial observations, a rather large number of reports have appeared confirming or denying a relationship between splenectomy and subsequent infection. Most of these are reviews of hospital experiences with children who have had splenectomy, but a number report immunologic studies.

No investigative studies have been able to show a relationship between the immune response of either children or experimental animals and previous splenectomy. Doan et al.[7] found that the antibody responses to specific antigens in the gamma globulin level were within normal limits in a great majority of patients who had had splenectomies. Broberger et al.[1] studied the bactericidal activity of sera from 30 children who had had splenectomy, and these showed no differences from sera from normal children. A similar study with respect to immune electrophoresis showed only minor differences in children who had had splenectomy as compared to normal ones. Thurman[32] studied 73 children who had had splenectomies for medical reasons with respect to survival, morbidity, gamma globulin levels, properdin levels and response to challenge with typhoid and pneumococcus antigens. These patients were compared with a group with comparable medical illnesses who had not had splenectomy and with a third group who had no underlying disease. No significant differences were demonstrated in any of these parameters. Haller and Jones[12] studied the problem experimentally in newborn mice and used the homograft rejection phenomenon to test the immune response. They found no differences between animals who had had splenectomy and the controls.

Much more impressive than the foregoing are well-documented clinical studies demonstrating a significant relationship between splenectomy and subsequent infection. Horan and Colebatch[15] carefully followed 142 patients on whom splenectomy had been performed in childhood. The incidence of septicemia and meningitis in infants after splenectomy was much higher than in the normal infant population. After infancy, the risk of serious postsplenectomy infection was still appreciable but much reduced. They found that 80% of the serious infections recorded following splenectomy occurred within 2 years of the operation. They also noted that postsplenectomy infections tend to be fulminating, with a high mortality, and that the predominant organism was the pneumococcus. Lowdon et al.[18] conducted a similar study of 75 children, found essentially similar results and reached the same conclusions. Smith et al.,[29] in a study of patients with Cooley's anemia following splenectomy, found that such patients showed a definite predisposition to overwhelming infection, 7 severe infections with 5 deaths occurring in 33 such patients.

Eraklis et al.[11] studied the problem with reference to the indication for splenectomy. Following a long-term study of 467 patients, they were able to divide their patients into three groups. When splenectomy was performed for laceration of the spleen, idiopathic thrombocytopenic purpura or other relatively benign conditions, they found no overwhelming infections and no mortality. In the second group, patients with hereditary spherocytosis, aplastic or hypoplastic anemia, there was a minimal risk of infection. In a third group with primary serious diseases such as Cooley's anemia, Wiscott-Aldrich syndrome and his-

tiocytosis, there was a high risk of subsequent fatal infections.

From these studies and from our own experience, there seems to be no doubt that splenectomy in infancy and childhood does carry a hazard of subsequent infection. Such infections, when they do occur, tend to be severe and fulminating, the pneumococcus is a frequently responsible organism, such infections tend to recur and the mortality is high. The risk is distinctly greater in infancy than in later childhood, and most serious infections occur within 2–3 years following splenectomy. The risk is distinctly higher in patients with serious hematologic diseases such as Cooley's anemia. However, even when splenectomy is done for such conditions as traumatic laceration, hereditary spherocytosis or idiopathic thrombocytopenic purpura, there remains some risk. Splenectomy certainly should be avoided during infancy. The major indication in the first year or two of life is hereditary spherocytosis, and this condition can invariably be managed successfully during this time without the necessity of splenectomy. After infancy, splenectomy should be done in indicated situations, but the small risk of subsequent serious infection should be kept in mind. Such patients should be carefully followed and should be treated vigorously and appropriately at the first sign of an infection. Prophylactic penicillin therapy for 1 or 2 years postoperatively has been suggested by some, but this is generally not favored.

REFERENCES

1. Broberger, O.; Gyulai, F., and Hirschfeldt, J.: Splenectomy in childhood—a clinical and immunological study of forty-two children splenectomized in the years 1951-1958, Acta paediat. 49:670, 1960.
2. Curtis, G. M., and Movitz, D.: The surgical significance of the accessory spleen, Ann. Surg. 123:276, 1946.
3. Dacie, J. V.: *The Haemolytic Anemias* (2d ed.; New York: Grune & Stratton, Inc., 1960).
4. Dameshek, W.: Controversy in idiopathic thrombocytopenic purpura, J.A.M.A. 173:123, 1960.
5. Dameshek, W., et al.: Treatment of idiopathic thrombocytopenic purpura with prednisone, J.A.M.A. 166:1805, 1958.
6. Doan, C. A.: Hypersplenism, Bull. New York Acad. Med. 25:625, 1949.
7. Doan, C. A., et al.: The Human Spleen and the Res, Proc. VIIth Internat. Cong., Internat Soc. Hematol. (Rome, 1958).
8. Doan, C. A., and Wright, C. S.: Primary congenital and secondary acquired splenic panhematopenia, Blood 1:10, 1946.
9. Ducharme, J., and Newton, W. A., Jr.: Splenectomy in children suffering from idiopathic thrombocytopenic purpura (unpublished data).
10. Djerassi, I., and Alvarado, J.: Platelet transfusions in the surgical management of thrombocytopenic patients, Ann. New York Acad. Sc. 115:366, 1964.
11. Eraklis, A. J., et al.: Hazard of overwhelming infection after splenectomy in childhood, New England J. Med. 276:1225, 1967.
12. Haller, J. A., and Jones, E. L.: Effect of splenectomy on immunity and resistance to major infections in early childhood: Clinical and experimental study, Ann. Surg.

163:902, 1966.

13. Harrington, W. J., *et al.*: Immunologic mechanisms in idiopathic and neonatal thrombocytopenic purpura, Ann. Int. Med. 28:433, 1953.

14. Hays, D. M., and Hammond, D.: Changing indications for elective splenectomy in childhood, Pacific Med. & Surg. 73:343, 1965.

15. Horan, M., and Colebatch, J. H.: Relationship between splenectomy and subsequent infection – a clinical study, Arch. Dis. Childhood 37:398, 1962.

16. King, H., and Shumacker, H. B., Jr.: Splenic studies: I. Susceptibility to infection after splenectomy performed in infancy, Ann. Surg. 136:239, 1952.

17. Levine, S.; Solis-Cohen, L., and Goldsmith, R.: Diagnosis of lacerated spleen, Am. J. Surg. 47:487, 1947.

18. Lowdon, A. G. R.; Walker, J. H., and Walker, W.: Infection following splenectomy in childhood, Lancet 1:499, 1962.

19. Motulsky, A. G., *et al.*: Anemia and the spleen, New England J. Med. 259:1164 and 1215, 1958.

20. Newton, W. A., Jr.: Enzyme-deficient chronic nonspherocytic hemolytic anemia (unpublished data).

21. Newton, W. A., Jr., and Bass, J. C.: Glutathione-sensitive chronic nonspherocytic hemolytic anemia, Am. J. Dis. Child. 96:501, 1958.

22. Newton, W. A., Jr., and Zuelzer, W. W.: Idiopathic thrombocytopenic purpura in childhood, New England J. Med. 245:879, 1951.

23. Parsons, L., and Thompson, J. E.: Traumatic rupture of the spleen from nonpenetrating injuries, Ann. Surg. 147:214, 1958.

24. Roettig, L. C.; Nusbaum, W. D., and Curtis, G. M.: Traumatic rupture of the spleen. Am. J. Surg. 59:292, 1943.

25. Scott, H. W., Jr., and Bowman, J. R.: Traumatic rupture of the spleen in childhood, J.A.M.A. 130:270, 1946.

26. Shahidi, N. T., and Diamond, L. K.: Enzyme deficiency in erythrocytes in congenital nonspherocytic hemolytic anemia, Pediatrics 24:245, 1959.

27. Smith, C. H.: Indication for splenectomy in the pediatric patient, Am. J. Surg. 107:523, 1964.

28. Smith, C. H., *et al.*: Hazard of severe infections in sple-

nectomized infants and children, Am. J. Med. 91:566, 1956.

29. Smith, C. H., *et al.*: Postsplenectomy infection in Cooley's anemia – an appraisal of the problem in this and other blood disorders, with a consideration of prophylaxis, New England J. Med. 266:737, 1962.

30. Smith, N. J.; Vaughan, V. C., III, and Diamond, L. K.: Diseases of the Blood, in Nelson, W. E. (ed.): *Textbook of Pediatrics* (7th ed.; Philadelphia: W. B. Saunders Company, 1959).

31. Terry, J. H.; Self, M. M., and Howard, J. M.: Injuries of the spleen, Surgery 40:615, 1956.

32. Thurman, W. G.: Splenectomy and immunity, Am. J. Dis. Child. 105:138, 1963.

33. Walker, J. H., and Walker, W.: Idiopathic thrombocytopenic purpura in childhood, Arch. Dis. Childhood 36:649, 1961.

34. Wiseman, B. K., and Doan, C. A.: Primary splenic neutropenia, Ann. Int. Med. 16:1097, 1942.

35. Young, L. E.; Izzo, M. J., and Platzer, R. F.: Hereditary spherocytosis: I. Clinical, hematologic and genetic features in 28 cases, with particular reference to the osmotic and mechanical fragility of incubated erythrocytes, Blood 6:1073, 1951.

36. Young, L. E., *et al.*: Hereditary spherocytosis: II. Observations on the role of the spleen, Blood 6:1099, 1951.

37. Zinkham, W. H., and Lenhard, R. E.: Metabolic abnormalities of erythrocytes from patients with congenital nonspherocytic hemolytic anemia, J. Pediat. 55:319, 1959.

38. Zollinger, R. M.; Martin, M. M., and Williams, R. D.: Surgical aspects of hypersplenism, J.A.M.A. 149:24, 1952.

E. T. BOLES, JR.
H. W. CLATWORTHY, JR.

Drawings by
BRENDA OLSON

Portal Hypertension

HIGHER THAN NORMAL portal venous pressure results from a variety of pathologic conditions within, below and above the liver. Intrahepatic portal hypertension is the most common type, but the extrahepatic form is relatively much more common in children than in adults. The suprahepatic form is so rare in our experience that it will not be discussed.

The most important clinical effect of portal hypertension is the development of collateral venous pathways, particularly esophageal and gastric varices, and consequent hemorrhage. Congestive splenomegaly with varying degrees of hypersplenism develops regularly but is of less importance. A third effect, noted in a sizable proportion of infants with extrahepatic portal obstruction, is ascites with growth failure.

A number of problems deserve particular emphasis. First is the differential diagnosis of the extrahe-

patic and intrahepatic forms. Not only are the underlying etiologies distinct, but the tolerance to severe hemorrhage, the available therapeutic surgical procedures and the status of liver function are quite different. The two require separate consideration to avoid confusion. Second is the management of acute hemorrhage from varices. Next is the selection of the appropriate elective management following hemorrhage in order to prevent further bleeding. Finally, some consideration must be allotted to the place of prophylactic shunt operations.

EXTRAHEPATIC PORTAL HYPERTENSION

ETIOLOGY AND PATHOLOGY.—This form of portal hypertension results from thrombosis of the portal vein. This thrombosis may extend in a retrograde fashion to involve the major tributaries forming the portal vein, including the splenic and superior mesenteric veins. As a consequence of this obstruction, the venous pressure in the portal system rises from a normal of 150 mm of saline or less to a level of 300 mm of saline or higher. Collateral pathways develop to circumvent the obstruction, the most important of these being the submucosal esophageal veins which connect the portal to the azygos system. The flow of venous blood in the portal system is reversed to a considerable extent, so that flow is away from the liver rather than toward it. Congestive splenomegaly becomes an increasingly prominent clinical feature as the child grows older. During infancy, ascites or retroperitoneal edema may develop, but both invariably resolve spontaneously in time. Partial canalization of the portal vein and the development of multiple small collateral venous channels adjacent to the portal vein probably account for the cavernomatous transformation of the portal vein, and this pathologic state should not be regarded as a congenital vascular anomaly.

In most instances, the exact etiology of the thrombotic process is unknown. In some, a definite history of omphalitis during the neonatal period is obtained, and it may be surmised that the septic phlebitis may complicate the normal bland thrombotic process of occlusion of the umbilical vein, and that this thrombotic process may extend into the portal venous system.[28] With sepsis or extreme dehydration, thrombosis of other large veins, including the dural venous sinuses and the renal veins, may occur in infants; and it seems reasonable to postulate that a similar complication could also involve the portal vein. In recent years, cases of extrahepatic portal hypertension have followed the use of the umbilical vein during the newborn period for repeated exchange transfusions.[20]

CLINICAL MANIFESTATIONS. — Upper gastrointestinal hemorrhage is by far the most common presenting complaint of a child with extrahepatic portal hypertension. Although this may occur during infancy, frank hemorrhage is relatively unusual before 3 or 4 years of age. In most instances, the hemorrhage will be manifested by hematemesis, melena, pallor and the symptoms of acute anemia. In some, however, the bleeding may be less severe, with only melena. If this is the first episode of hemorrhage, most such children will have little or nothing in their past histories of diagnostic help. Most will have been perfectly healthy, normal-appearing children, and the bleeding episode will be the first indication that anything is amiss. In some, there will be a history of omphalitis or severe sepsis in the neonatal period. Other than pallor and possibly manifestations of shock if the hemorrhage is sufficiently severe, the only helpful physical finding ordinarily is an enlarged spleen. The liver is not enlarged and there is no ascites. There is no jaundice or any other stigma of liver disease.

Repeated episodes of bleeding are common. Among the 27 patients we have followed with this disorder, 23 have bled; and the total number of recognized bleeding episodes has been 73.

A less common clinical picture is seen in some in-fants with extrahepatic portal hypertension.[4,18] This is the development of ascites accompanied by growth failure in infants who are usually several months of age. Although presumably the thrombosis of the portal venous system occurs in most instances during the neonatal period, for reasons that are not clear, the development of ascites in these babies does not occur immediately but is rather delayed for at least 2 months and more commonly until 6–8 months of age. The ascites produces a grossly protuberant abdomen. The accumulation of ascitic fluid may be sufficient to require paracentesis because of respiratory embarrassment. The spleen is usually enlarged, but not greatly so, and may not be palpable at all until after a paracentesis. Dilated superficial veins on the anterior abdominal wall are often seen. During the weeks or months during which the ascites persists, these infants usually fail to grow and may become quite wasted. Hypochromic anemia is also a common feature. There is occult blood in the stools, although frank hemorrhage has not occurred in our experience. Fortunately, the process is self-limited, and after a period varying from a few weeks to as long as 18 months the ascites spontaneously disappears, normal growth is resumed and the child is restored to good health. There have been 5 such patients in our experience, and in all, the ascites eventually regressed spontaneously.

Diagnosis. — The diagnosis of extrahepatic portal hypertension in a child with acute upper gastrointestinal bleeding is ordinarily not difficult. The spleen is invariably enlarged except in those unfortunate youngsters who have had a previous splenectomy because of splenomegaly. There are no clinical indications of liver disease on physical examination or in the history. Results of screening laboratory studies of the liver functions and of the coagulation mechanisms are normal.

As soon as the patient has been resuscitated by appropriate blood replacement and his vital signs are stable, an esophagram should be obtained. In most instances this will clearly demonstrate filling defects characteristic of esophageal varices in the lower third or half of the esophagus. This study has a high degree of accuracy in older children, but may be negative in those under 3 or 4 years of age. This study also permits examination of the stomach and duodenum, but hemorrhage from peptic ulcer is rarely a problem in differential diagnosis in this age group. Esophagoscopy would appear to be a helpful diagnostic study and has been advocated by some. However, this requires general anesthesia in children and has not been used for this purpose by us.

The most helpful and definitive diagnostic study is portal venography. This is not done ordinarily as an emergency diagnostic procedure, but rather is deferred until the acute hemorrhage has stopped and the child's condition had stabilized. A percutaneous

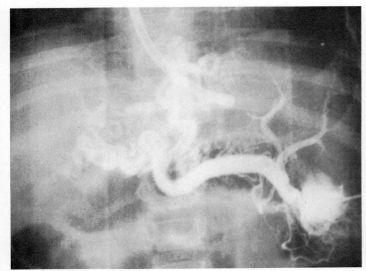 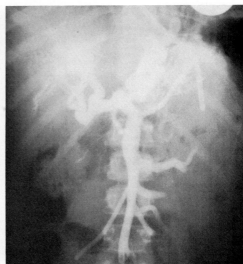

Fig. 50-2 (left).—Extrahepatic portal hypertension. Percutaneous splenic portogram, showing cavernomatous transformation of the portal vein, centrifugal flow, filling of varices and large size of the splenic vein.

Fig. 50-3 (right).—Extrahepatic portal hypertension. Portal venogram in a patient with previous splenectomy, obtained at laparotomy via a mesenteric vein. Marked centrifugal flow, large superior mesenteric vein, prominent varices and sparse filling of intrahepatic portal branches are evident.

splenic portogram not only will permit radiographic demonstration of the portal venous system but also will permit measurements of the portal pressure (Fig. 50-2). This procedure requires general anesthesia in small children but can be performed quite satisfactorily with sedation and local anesthesia in most children 8 or 9 years of age or older. In those who have had a previous splenectomy, this procedure requires a diagnostic laparotomy so that a mesenteric branch of the portal system can be cannulized for purposes of injection of the dye and pressure studies (Fig. 50-3). At the same time, liver biopsy can be done. Such a procedure can be done as an independent diagnostic measure or may be combined with a definitive operation.

The portal venogram usually demonstrates absence of the portal vein and replacement by numerous small tortuous collateral channels. There is slow and relatively sparse filling of the intrahepatic radicals of the portal venous system. The dye tends to flow in a centrifugal direction away from the liver, filling numerous collaterals of the portal venous system, including mesenteric veins, omental branches and the left gastric or coronary vein. Through the last-mentioned channel the dye frequently fills large dilated varices in the upper portion of the stomach and the lower segment of the esophagus. This study is of great value not only in demonstrating the obstruction of the portal vein and the collateral pathways, including the varices, but in demonstrating the veins which may be used for subsequent shunting procedures. The splenic and superior mesenteric veins are particularly important in this connection, and the study gives reliable evidence as to whether or not they are normal.

TREATMENT OF INFANTS WITH ASCITES.—Infants with ascites and growth failure secondary to extrahepatic portal obstruction are not benefited by operation, although a limited procedure at which time the portal venous pressure is measured, a portal venogram obtained and a liver biopsy performed is a helpful diagnostic step. These infants have required only supportive therapy. If the ascites accumulates in sufficient amounts to produce respiratory embarrassment, periodic paracenteses are required to relieve this symptom. Intravenous infusions of colloid fluid —serum albumin, plasma or whole blood—have been used, sometimes as often as once weekly. Such infusions are helpful in replacing the protein loss in the ascitic fluid. If the ascites persists for longer than a few weeks, these infants present serious problems of growth failure or even weight loss. In such circumstances, careful attention to their nutritional requirements is obviously important.

ACUTE HEMORRHAGE.—The treatment of a child of any age with acute hemorrhage from esophageal varices is primarily that of adequate resuscitation. This consists of blood transfusion therapy to replace the blood loss, complemented by bed rest and sedation. If the child is vomiting blood, the stomach should be emptied with a nasogastric tube. The tube is then left in place and attached to a source of low suction. If the child is not vomiting blood but is only passing blood in the stools, frequent small feedings as in the treatment of a peptic ulcer should be offered. Although the rate of bleeding may be quite alarming, almost always the bleeding is self-limited and stops spontaneously. These episodes of hemorrhage are well tolerated, inasmuch as liver function is normal and the coagulation mechanisms are unimpaired. Although death may occur from an acute hemorrhage, this should be very rare indeed. Almost all patients will stop bleeding with the supportive therapy outlined above, and this has also been the experience of Shaldon and Sherlock.[27]

In the event, however, that bleeding continues at an alarming rate for more than a few hours, then certainly esophageal tamponade should be employed. If tamponade is unsuccessful, or if bleeding recurs after the tamponade is released in 48 hours, operation with ligation of the varices would be the procedure of choice in a small child. In an older child, a shunt may be done if a suitable tributary of the portal vein is available.

Of the 73 bleeding episodes in our series, 68 were controlled with nonoperative management, although esophageal tamponade was used in 1 patient and Pitressin given intravenously in 2 others. In the remaining 5, ligation of the varices was done in 4 and an emergency mesocaval shunt in 1.

DEFINITIVE TREATMENT. — Although still subject to some debate, it seems reasonably clear that a good-sized shunt between the portal and systemic venous systems is by all odds the best treatment to prevent further episodes of hemorrhage. The effectiveness of such a shunt depends on its diameter and its length, the widest and shortest being the most effective. Because the portal vein is usually primarily involved and is occluded by thrombus, partially recanalized or replaced by numerous small collaterals, this vein is ordinarily unavailable for a shunting procedure. In a rare instance, enough of this vein may be normal to permit a portacaval shunt, but this has not occurred in any of our cases. This leaves the splenic and the superior mesenteric veins as the two vessels in the portal system most suitable for shunting operations. In any case, it is most important to evaluate by appropriate venographic studies the exact anatomic situation and particularly the size of these veins in order to decide on the best available operation.

In the child of preschool age, the veins in the portal system are usually too small to permit a shunting procedure which will be permanently effective. Accordingly, a definitive operation should be postponed if at all possible in this age group. Because bleeding episodes are almost always self-limited and well tolerated, this is usually possible. However, such a child may require a number of hospitalizations because of episodes of bleeding. If the morbidity from repeated hemorrhages becomes excessive and prevention of these episodes is deemed mandatory, appropriate venographic studies of the portal system are done. If either the splenic vein or the superior mesenteric vein has a diameter of 1.0 cm or more, either a splenorenal or a mesocaval shunt may be performed with the expectation of a good long-term result.[4] In some children, the veins may be of such a size as early as 4 years of age. If the veins are too small or are involved in the thrombotic occlusive process, a direct approach to the varices is necessary. There are three types of operations for this purpose. The simplest is suture-ligation of the esophageal varices. Although felt to be primarily a temporizing procedure to control hemorrhage, this operation has prevented further hemorrhage in some instances for many years.[3,21] The second operation, originally advocated by Tanner, consists of a laparotomy with devascularization of the greater and lesser curvatures of the upper portion of the stomach and the lower portion of the esophagus. Following this, the stomach is transected in its upper third, the gastroesophageal varices are inspected and oversewn, and re-anastomosis of the stomach is then performed. Complementary vagotomy and pyloroplasty are usually also done. The third and most drastic procedure is resection of the lower third of the esophagus and the fundus of the stomach with interposition of a segment of either colon or jejunum. This probably is the most effective of the three procedures in the prevention of further hemorrhage, but it is often followed by epigastric or substernal distress and the necessity for frequent small feedings.[12] In small children, it may be followed by some measure of growth failure. Again, it should be stressed that nonoperative measures will ordinarily control the bleeding episodes adequately and that, if at all possible, the definitive operation should be an appropriate shunt and should be deferred until such a procedure has an excellent chance of success.

The older child who has had one or more hemorrhages should be evaluated for a shunting procedure. As noted previously, the radiographic study of the portal venous system is most important in planning the appropriate procedure. The procedure which has been most successful is an end-to-side splenorenal shunt together with splenectomy.[4,16,29] As has been emphasized many times in the past by others, it is obviously most important not to perform a splenectomy alone in a child with portal hypertension since this results in occlusion of the splenic vein and makes it unusable for a subsequent shunt. The shunt should have a caliber as large as possible and should be as short as possible. Both of these objectives are best realized by using that portion of the splenic vein as close as possible to the portal vein and placing the anastomosis in the left renal vein as close as possible to the vena cava.[1] In addition to these advantages, the centrally placed splenorenal shunt also minimizes the possible subsequent problems of angulation or compression of the splenic vein by adjacent viscera (Fig. 50-4).

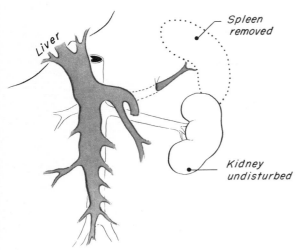

Fig. 50-4. — Centrally placed end-to-side splenorenal shunt.

The side-to-end superior mesenteric vein–inferior vena caval shunt has been utilized in a considerable number of patients in recent years and may prove to be as effective or even more so than the splenorenal shunt.[5,17] The most proximal portion of the superior mesenteric vein just inferior to the pancreas is used; as with all other shunts, it is important that this vein be free from disease. The inferior vena cava or the iliac veins are divided and the distal portion oversewn. The proximal portion is turned up and an anastomosis done in an end-to-side fashion with the superior mesenteric vein. This usually provides a shunt of good size, and results with its use have been encouraging.[4,30]

There remains a group of patients who for one reason or another are unshuntable. These may be children who are failures following a splenorenal or mesocaval shunt or in whom ill-advised splenectomy has been performed. A large number of operations have been recommended for such patients, but the three types of direct approaches mentioned earlier for the young child appear to be the most applicable.

As mentioned previously, direct suture-ligation of the esophagogastric varices will control an acute hemorrhage and in some instances is effective in preventing further hemorrhage for many years. By and large, however, experience with this procedure as a definitive one in long-term control of bleeding episodes has been disappointing.[18] Gastric transection combined with devascularization of the upper portion of the stomach and lower segment of the esophagus also has a disappointing record in long-term follow-ups. When combined with ligation of the varices, vagotomy and pyloroplasty, it may prove to be a better operation. Resection of the lower esophagus and fundus of the stomach with a direct anastomosis is a poor operation both in terms of preventing further

hemorrhage and in terms of complications of the procedure itself. On the other hand, esophagogastrectomy with interposition of a segment of jejunum or colon is reasonably effective and largely avoids the problems of reflux acid peptic esophagitis associated with a direct operation.[12] Extension of such a procedure to include excision of the entire intrathoracic esophagus has been proposed by Perry *et al.*,[22] and their early results with this procedure in a small group of children are encouraging. Although this is a fairly drastic procedure which must be done in stages, it appears to be considerably more effective than lesser procedures in control of further hemorrhage and is not associated with disturbing gastrointestinal symptoms or growth failure.

Thirty-four operations have been performed electively in 22 of our patients. Among the 16 shunts, 8 were splenorenal, 7 mesocaval and 1 makeshift. Bleeding eventually recurred in 7 of the 16. Esophagogastrectomy with interposition has been done in 5, and 3 have had further bleeding. Five gastric transection and devascularization procedures have been done, without bleeding again in a short follow-up period. After 8 splenectomies alone, rebleeding has occurred in 7 patients.

PROGNOSIS. — Prognosis for life in children with extrahepatic portal hypertension is excellent. None of the patients in our series have died, and a similar experience has been reported by Shaldon and Sherlock.[27] There is, however, considerable morbidity: many require frequent hospitalizations because of bleeding, and some have been subjected to four or five operations. None of the operations described are uniformly successful, but a good-sized splenorenal or mesocaval venous shunt affords a high degree of protection. However, even in those patients in whom such a shunt is not possible or in whom the shunt fails, other procedures do offer relief from further hemorrhage and are often required. Furthermore, the natural history of this condition is such that there may be intervals of many years between bleeding episodes.[18]

INTRAHEPATIC PORTAL HYPERTENSION

ETIOLOGY AND PATHOLOGY. — Primary liver disease with fibrosis, distortion of normal architecture, compression of intrahepatic portal venous tributaries and shunts between the radicals of the portal vein and the hepatic artery account for this form of portal hypertension. Posthepatitis cirrhosis is the most common cause in children. Biliary cirrhosis secondary to atresia of the bile ducts frequently leads to portal hypertension with bleeding, but it has not been thought justifiable in most instances to attempt operative procedures designed to relieve the portal hypertension because of the poor prognosis of the primary disease. Fibrocystic disease of the pancreas also may lead to portal hypertension because of liver involvement.

This will undoubtedly become increasingly frequent in the years to come as medical management permits a much higher proportion of infants with this condition to live into late childhood and adult life. Congenital hepatic fibrosis is an uncommon disease but one that is being recognized with increasing frequency.[2,11] Although it results in typical intrahepatic portal hypertension, the prognosis of the basic liver disease is excellent. The status of the liver functions varies from no detectable impairment to advanced liver failure leading rapidly to death. The effects of intrahepatic obstruction on the portal venous system are essentially the same as with extrahepatic obstruction. There is a reversal of flow from centripetal to centrifugal, and collateral circulation to the systemic venous system develops. The most important of these collaterals, of course, are the esophagogastric varices.

CLINICAL PICTURE.—As with extrahepatic portal hypertension, the clinical manifestation of major interest to surgeons is hemorrhage from esophageal varices. However, unlike the situation of patients with extrahepatic portal hypertension, patients with the intrahepatic form present many other manifestations as a consequence of their underlying liver disease. These other clinical manifestations, of course, depend on the underlying diagnosis. In the case of biliary atresia, jaundice since early infancy is a prominent feature. In patients with posthepatitis cirrhosis, there may also be jaundice if the inflammatory process is active or subacute or if liver failure occurs, and in any event there is often a history of previous jaundice. If cirrhosis secondary to hepatitis is progressive and severe, there may be varying degrees of liver failure, with jaundice, ascites, wasting and encephalopathy. Patients with fibrocystic disease of the pancreas who develop secondary cirrhosis and portal hypertension often have problems of the respiratory tract or growth failure secondary to the underlying disease. Patients with congenital hepatic fibrosis have pronounced enlargement of both the liver and spleen, but usually quite normal liver functions. There often is a history of the same disease in other members of the family. In all of these diseases, splenomegaly may be a prominent physical finding, and some degree of hypersplenism is usually found. It should be emphasized, however, that this hypersplenism, in both intrahepatic and extrahepatic forms of portal hypertension, rarely is of any great clinical significance.

Of our 40 patients with intrahepatic portal hypertension, 19 had significant bleeding episodes. The rest had clinical or postmortem evidence of portal hypertension but no hemorrhage. There were 48 significant bleeding episodes among the 19, but this figure is distorted by 1 patient with biliary atresia and cirrhosis who bled 15 times. Most have bled only once or twice.

DIAGNOSIS.—The diagnosis of intrahepatic portal hypertension is seldom difficult. The presenting manifestations and the history usually give clear evidence of pre-existing liver disease of some form; and the diagnosis is often fairly certain on clinical grounds alone. The liver is often enlarged, but with advanced cirrhosis may be shrunken and quite small. Splenomegaly, as noted previously, is usually prominent. Jaundice, ascites, muscular wasting and encephalopathy are manifestations indicative of advanced liver disease. Liver function studies will usually show some degree of abnormality and are particularly helpful in evaluation of the patient for a proposed operation. Esophagogastric varices may be demonstrated by either esophagram or esophagoscopy, usually the former. Precise anatomic diagnosis depends again on appropriate venographic studies, and at the time these studies are performed the portal pressure is measured (Fig. 50-5). In older children, this study can usually be done precutaneously with local anesthesia. In young preschool children, this usually requires general anesthesia. In some instances, it may be considered necessary to perform a limited diagnostic laparotomy for the purpose of measuring portal pressure, venography and liver biopsy. A portal venogram in this condition will demonstrate in most instances a normal portal vein, although secondary thrombosis of the portal vein with intrahepatic portal hypertension does occur in a small percentage of the patients. In addition, there is evidence of centrifugal flow of blood away from the liver, with filling of the various branches of the portal venous system and particularly the collaterals. The varices in the fundus of the stomach and the lower portion of the esophagus are well demonstrated by the venographic studies.

TREATMENT.—Treatment in this discussion will be concerned only with variceal hemorrhage and not with other complications such as ascites, liver failure and hypersplenism. The management of acute hem-

Fig. 50-5.—Intrahepatic portal hypertension. Portal venogram, showing mesenteric and portal veins to be normal and demonstrating large gastric and esophageal varices.

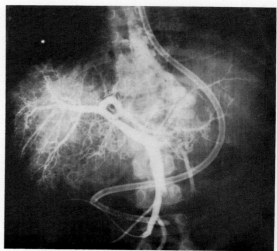

orrhage is particularly important, since a large proportion of these patients have significantly impaired liver function and tolerate bleeding episodes very poorly. Although the mortality from a single episode of hemorrhage is not as high in the pediatric age group as it is in adult patients with alcoholic cirrhosis, it is nonetheless a considerable hazard. If bleeding does not cease promptly, deterioration of liver function with increasing ascites and jaundice frequently occurs, encephalopathy secondary to ammonia intoxication may develop, and the coagulation mechanisms may deteriorate. Hence, prompt control of hemorrhage is essential.

The first step in achieving this control is hospitalization, bed rest and sedation. The last must be done with caution in patients with advanced liver disease. Blood replacement, preferably with fresh blood, is mandatory. Close graphic charting of the patient's vital signs, hematocrit and hemoglobin values is initiated. A nasogastric tube is passed and the stomach cleared of blood and blood clots by irrigation and suction, following which the tube is connected to a source of low suction. If significant bleeding continues after these measures, more active steps must be taken promptly. Tamponade of the gastric esophageal varices can be effectively accomplished with the Sengstaken tube. Appropriate sizes of this device for children are available. The gastric tube is first inflated and is then drawn up snugly against the cardia and held in place by appropriate taping of the tube to the face. This taping should be cushioned by use of a small pad of foam rubber in order to prevent pressure damage to the nose. The esophageal balloon is then inflated to a pressure of approximately 40 mm of mercury. This pressure is checked periodically. Use of this tube is highly efficient in arresting hemorrhage from varices but is complicated by numerous problems.[6,24] The most serious of these is aspiration pneumonitis. Any patient undergoing esophageal tamponade requires constant nursing care, best achieved in an intensive care unit. Frequent checks of the apparatus by the responsible physician are necessary if serious complications are to be avoided. The tamponade is continued for 48 hours, although it is probably wise to deflate the esophageal balloon periodically to minimize the possibility of pressure damage to the esophagus. At the end of 48 hours, both the gastric and the esophageal balloon are deflated. The tube is left in for another 8–12 hours and then carefully withdrawn.

Other measures have been tried in an effort to avoid the discomfort and possible complications of esophageal tamponade. Pituitrin intravenously in appropriate dosage has been shown to be effective initially.[26] There is, however, a high incidence of recurrent bleeding as the effect of this drug wears off, and its subsequent use is much less effective. Intravenous infusion of a ganglionic blocking agent (Arfonad) has been found to produce a state of controlled systemic hypotension of 70–80 mm of mercury.[13] Reduction of portal pressure, decrease of hepatic blood flow and cessation of variceal bleeding have been achieved in a small number of patients.

If hemorrhage should continue despite the use of tamponade, or should it recur after discontinuance of the tamponade, some form of surgical operation to control the bleeding must be seriously considered. The risk of such procedures in patients with advanced liver disease is great, but the fate of a patient with uncontrolled continuing hemorrhage is certain death. Accordingly, the usual criteria for liver function tests, ascites and jaundice should not contraindicate such a procedure. A direct approach may be made by a transthoracic ligation of the esophageal and gastric varices. The purpose of such a procedure is to gain immediate control of the bleeding, and then to prepare the patient as best as possible for a venous shunting operation on an elective basis.[14] The second approach is to proceed directly with a portal-to-systemic venous shunt. This has been employed extensively in the past few years by surgical groups dealing primarily with adult cirrhotic patients, and the results are encouraging.[8,19,23,25] The type of shunt used in almost all instances has been an end-to-side portacaval anastomosis. Although a somewhat more formidable procedure, an emergency shunt operation has the advantage of being a definitive procedure with an excellent chance of preventing further hemorrhage, and it also avoids the morbidity of two major operations.

The 48 bleeding episodes in our series were treated by nonoperative measures in 43 and by emergency operation in 3. Two patients were admitted in a terminal stage, and essentially no treatment was possible. A mesocaval shunt, a portacaval shunt, and ligation of the varices comprised the operative group. Eight deaths resulted from bleeding, all with associated liver failure.

Elective definitive management.—For patients who have survived one or more hemorrhages from varices, an appropriate shunt operation offers the best opportunity for control of this problem and is strongly advocated unless the prognosis of the underlying liver disease is too grave to make such a procedure justifiable. Portacaval, mesocaval and splenorenal shunts are available. Because of the relatively large size of the veins involved, a portacaval shunt can ordinarily be done as early as 4 years of age and, in fact, has been successfully done in even younger patients. The best type of portacaval shunt is a matter of debate. Most experience has accumulated with the end-to-side portacaval anastomosis. This shunt has a low rate of thrombosis and is of proved effectiveness in lowering the portal pressure and minimizing the danger of subsequent bleeding. It has the additional advantage of being technically a reasonably simple procedure. However, there is good evidence that in patients with cirrhosis, there is retrograde flow of hepatic arterial blood into the intrahepatic radicals of the portal vein. Because of this, a side-to-side portacaval shunt may be advantageous in that it would permit retrograde flow from the hepatic end of the portal vein through the anastomosis.[15] Such flow is increased after the shunt is created. It would also permit some flow of portal blood into the liver, although obviously much less than prior to the shunt. Hence, blood in the portal vein above such a shunt may flow in either direction, depending on activity of the patient. The shunt does have the disadvantage of being somewhat more likely to become occluded than the end-to-side type, and it is technically more difficult.

The centrally placed splenorenal and the mesocaval shunts, previously discussed, may also be used. Both of these shunts also theoretically permit flow of blood in a retrograde manner from the liver through the portal vein and through the shunt.

Thirteen elective shunts have been performed in our series, 9 splenorenal, 3 mesocaval and 2 portacaval. There has been 1 postoperative death. Two patients have had subsequent rebleeding. Both portacaval shunts were done for congenital hepatic fibrosis; these were done by the end-to-side technique, and both patients have done well with no further bleeding.

Prophylactic shunts. — Since the morbidity and mortality of variceal hemorrhage are so great, some authorities in this field have advocated the performance of a shunt in patients with demonstrable esophageal varices and intrahepatic portal hypertension prior to the occurrence of bleeding. As applied to children, there are no data to confirm or deny the merits of such prophylactic shunts. Studies published thus far on adults indicate that the use of prophylactic shunts does not affect the ultimate survival of patients with cirrhosis, although it greatly reduces the proportion of those who die as a consequence of hemorrhage.[7,10] Such studies cannot be applied to children, since the etiology of intrahepatic portal hypertension in adults is quite different from that in children. The type of liver disease is a very important factor in determining the mortality from variceal hemorrhage, and this mortality is higher in adults with alcoholic cirrhosis than it is in children with cirrhosis secondary to a variety of causes. We have performed 9 prophylactic operations, all centrally placed splenorenal shunts. There have been no deaths in this group, although 1 patient did bleed 6 years later. In most of these patients esophagrams obtained postoperatively have demonstrated disappearance of the varices. This experience has been encouraging.

REFERENCES

1. Boles, E. T., Jr.: Centrally Placed Splenorenal Shunt, in Cooper, P. (ed.): *The Craft of Surgery* (Boston: Little, Brown and Company, 1964).
2. Boley, S. J.; Arlen, M., and Mogilner, L. J.: Congenital hepatic fibrosis causing portal hypertension in children, Surgery 54:356, 1963.
3. Britton, R. C., and Crile, G., Jr.: Late results of transesophageal suture of bleeding esophageal varices, Surg., Gynec. & Obst. 117:10, 1963.
4. Clatworthy, H. W., Jr., and Boles, E. T., Jr.: Extrahepatic portal bed block in children: Pathogenesis and treatment, Ann. Surg. 150:371, 1959.
5. Clatworthy, H. W., Jr.; Wall, T., and Watman, R. N.: A new type of portal-to-systemic venous shunt for portal hypertension, Arch. Surg. 71:588, 1955.
6. Conn, H. O.: Hazards attending the use of esophageal tamponade, New England J. Med. 259:701, 1958.
7. Conn, H. O., and Lindenmuth, W. W.: Prophylactic portacaval anastomosis in cirrhotic patients with esophageal varices, New England J. Med. 272:1255, 1965.
8. Ekman, C. A., and Sandblom, P.: Shunt operation in acute bleeding from esophageal varices, Ann. Surg. 160:531, 1964.
9. Foster, J. H.; Holcomb, G. W., and Kirtley, J. A.: Results of surgical treatment of portal hypertension in children, Ann. Surg. 157:868, 1963.
10. Garceau, A. J., *et al.*: A controlled trial of prophylactic portacaval shunt surgery, New England J. Med. 270:496, 1964.
11. Kerr, D. N. S., *et al.*: Congenital hepatic fibrosis, Quart. J. Med. 30:91, 1961.
12. Koop, C. E., and Kavianian, A.: Reappraisal of colon replacement of distal esophagus and proximal stomach in the management of bleeding varices in children, Surgery 57:454, 1965.
13. Kuhn, T.; Joseph, W. L., and Cincotti, J. J.: Ganglionic blocking agents as a method of avoiding emergency portal decompression, S. Forum 18:394, 1967.
14. Linton, R. R., and Ellis, D. S.: Emergency and definitive treatment of bleeding esophageal varices, J.A.M.A. 160:1017, 1956.
15. Longmire, W. P., Jr., *et al.*: Side-to-side portacaval anastomosis for portal hypertension, Ann. Surg. 147:881, 1958.
16. Louw, J. H.: Portal hypertension in childhood, South African M. J. 39:1110, 1965.
17. Marion, P.; Bouchet, A., and Yon, M.: Mesentericocaval derivation: Technic for the latero-terminal anastomosis of the superior mesenteric vein and the inferior vena cava, Ann. chir. 14:581, 1960.
18. Mikkelsen, W. P.: Extrahepatic portal hypertension in children, Am. J. Surg. 111:333, 1966.
19. Mikkelsen, W. P., and Pattison, A. C.: Emergency portacaval shunt, Am. J. Surg. 96:183, 1958.
20. Oski, F. A.; Allen, D. M., and Diamond, L. K.: Portal hypertension — a complication of umbilical vein catheterization, Pediatrics 31:297, 1963.
21. Patton, T. B.: Extrahepatic portal obstruction in infants and children: Diagnosis, treatment and long-term followup, South. M. J. 58:1447, 1965.
22. Perry, J. F., Jr., *et al.*: Total removal of the intrathoracic esophagus and antethoracic jejunal esophageal replacement for treatment of esophageal varices due to extrahepatic portal block, Ann. Surg. 158:126, 1963.
23. Preston, F. W., and Trippel, O. H.: Emergency portacaval shunt — use in patients with alcoholic cirrhosis, Arch. Surg. 90:770, 1965.
24. Read, A. E.; Dawson, A. M., and Kerr, D. N. S.: Bleeding esophageal varices treated by esophageal compression tube, Brit. M. J. 1:227, 1960.
25. Rousselot, L. M.; Gilbertson, F. E., and Panke, W. F.: Severe hemorrhage from esophagogastric varices: Its emergency management with particular reference to portacaval anastomosis, New England J. Med. 262:269, 1960.
26. Shaldon, S., and Sherlock, S.: The use of vasopressin (Pitressin) in the control of bleeding from oesophageal varices, Lancet 2:222, 1960.

27. Shaldon, S., and Sherlock, S.: Obstruction to the extrahepatic portal system in childhood, Lancet 1:63, 1962.
28. Smith, R. M., and Farber, S.: Splenomegaly in children with early hematemesis, J. Pediat. 7:585, 1935.
29. Trusler, G. A.; Morris, F. R., and Mustard, W. T.: Portal hypertension in childhood, Surgery 52:664, 1962.
30. Voorhees, A. B., Jr., and Blakemore, A. H.: Clinical experience with superior mesenteric vein-inferior vena cava

shunt in the treatment of portal hypertension, Surgery 51:35, 1962.

H. W. CLATWORTHY, JR.
E. T. BOLES, JR.
Drawings by
BRENDA OLSON

51

Surgery in Patients with Disorders of the Clotting Mechanism

MANY FACTORS contribute to the control of hemorrhage. Normally, the sequence of events is as follows:[5,24] A vessel is severed, blood suddenly escapes, the intraluminal pressure is reduced at the bleeding site, elastic fibers in the vessel wall shorten, muscle fibers in the wall contract and the orifice of the severed vessel becomes smaller. Platelets adhere to the injured vessel wall, other platelets adhere to these, and a fragile plug is quickly assembled which temporarily stops the flow of blood. Coagulation then occurs, converting soluble fibrinogen to insoluble strands of fibrin which lace the delicate platelet plug into a firm but resilient clot and bind it to the lacerated vessel wall. During wound healing, the original fibrin thrombus normally undergoes a constant process of remodeling as a result of fibrinolysis. Bleeding does not recur because this fibrinolysis is constantly balanced by a normal coagulation system.

If the severed vessel is large, these mechanisms may fail to stop the bleeding. Platelets and coagulation factors are washed along by the rapid flow of blood and are prevented from accumulating at the vessel orifice. Unless a thrombus forms promptly, vasoconstriction fatigues, the orifice enlarges and bleeding continues. It is these large vessels which the surgeon must ligate in the process of performing his operation. Failure to do so is by far the most common cause of undue bleeding in pediatric surgical patients. Bleeding from this cause tends to be unifocal, in contrast to the generalized oozing and multifocal bleeding which characterize hemostatic deficiencies. If the wound edges are dry while blood wells up from the depths, a methodical search for the unligated vessel will usually be more rewarding than a whole battery of laboratory tests.

Bleeding problems result from inadequate surgical technique, from vascular abnormalities, from quantitative or qualitative platelet deficiencies, from deficiencies of one or more of a dozen coagulation factors and, rarely, from an excess of fibrinolysin or from errors in the administration of anticoagulants. The differential diagnosis of bleeding disorders depends on intelligent interpretation of laboratory tests. Since it is impractical to subject all patients to these expensive and time-consuming procedures, two questions assume paramount importance. Which children should be subjected to laboratory investigation, and what constitutes an appropriate series of screening tests?

The most obvious indication for a bleeding investigation is a history of undue bleeding. A carefully taken history of how the child has met the challenges of circumcision, the eruption or extraction of teeth, tonsillectomy or other surgical procedure is most important. A history of repeated epistaxis, excessive bruising or hematoma formation, bleeding from injection sites or cuts calls for a "bleeding work-up," as does a family history indicating bleeding problems in relatives. Petechiae and/or purpura as manifestations of an increased bleeding tendency are not diagnostic of a particular disorder but are usually related to platelet deficiency or to vascular abnormalities. Bleeding into deep tissues or joint spaces strongly suggests hemophilia. If no history is obtainable, as in adopted children, screening tests are advisable.

For years it was the custom in many institutions to rely solely on the bleeding and clotting time tests for the detection of children with bleeding disorders. Experience has abundantly shown the inadequacy of this practice.[7] A screening evaluation should include all of the tests in Table 51-1. Normal values vary from one laboratory to another. In our laboratory, the tests are performed and interpreted as follows:

Complete blood count.—This basic evaluation enumerates the hemoglobin and the formed elements of the blood in relation to the fluid portion. Unless the total blood volume is known, the numbers reflect relative rather than absolute values. The normal ranges are well known. The morphology of all of the formed elements of the circulating blood is noted.

Platelet count.—Values above 20,000/cu mm are rarely associated with spontaneous hemorrhages. Levels above 50,000/cu mm generally provide adequate hemostasis for surgical procedures. Normal values are 150,000–400,000/cu mm.

Lee-White clotting time.[17]—This test measures the time required for freshly drawn whole blood to clot in chemically clean standard glass test tubes. The test is subject to many inaccuracies, and, contrary to common belief, a normal value does not rule out a bleeding disorder. However, if the test is properly performed, a prolonged clotting time is nearly always significant. It is prolonged in moderate or severe hemophilia, afibrinogenemia, severe fibrinolytic states and in the presence of circulating anticoagulants such as heparin. The usefulness of the clotting time as a screening test is severely limited by the fact that it may be normal in children with mild hemophilia.

Clot retraction.[4]—This test provides a qualitative

measure of platelet function. It is reduced when the number of normal platelets is below 50,000–80,000/cu mm. In qualitative platelet defects, clot retraction may be impaired in the presence of an adequate number of platelets.

Clot lysis.[23]—Spontaneous dissolution of the clot, particularly if this occurs within 1 or 2 hours, is evidence of abnormal fibrinolysis. The level of fibrinogen should be measured and specific tests of fibrinolytic activity performed.

Ivy bleeding time.[13]—This test of primary hemostasis measures the length of time that bleeding continues from a standard cut in the skin of the forearm. This test is superior to that performed on the ear lobe because the results are more reproducible and because profuse bleeding from the ear lobe is difficult to control. The bleeding time is usually prolonged in patients with thrombocytopenia, qualitative platelet defects and Willebrand's disease.[18]

One-stage prothrombin time.[1]—This test measures the time required for recalcified citrated or oxalated plasma to clot in the presence of tissue thromboplastin. It does not measure prothrombin activity alone, but is sensitive to reduction of any one or more of the following: factors V, VII or X, prothrombin and fibrinogen. It is also sensitive to the presence of anticoagulants. The results of the test may be expressed either in seconds as compared to a control or in percentage of normal prothrombin activity. Any result above 50% is considered normal in our laboratory. The therapeutic range of oral anticoagulation with coumadin derivatives results in a one-stage prothrombin time of 20–30%. Spontaneous bleeding is minimal unless the level falls below 10%. Differential tests can be performed in conjunction with the one-stage prothrombin time test to detect specific abnormalities.

Partial thromboplastin time.[22]—This test, otherwise known as the cephalin time test, measures the time required for recalcified plasma to clot in the presence of cephalin. In our laboratory, a partial thromboplastin time of longer than 100 seconds is abnormal. The test is reliable and simple. It can detect deficiencies of all known plasma coagulation factors except factor VII. It is sensitive to most anticoagulants. It is a particularly useful screening test because it is almost always abnormal in mild hemophilia.

If the results of all of these tests are normal, excessive bleeding at operation is very unlikely. This series of screening tests may bring to light a long list of minor defects, but thrombocytopenia and hemophilia account for the vast majority of serious hemostatic problems. The management of children with these two conditions will be considered at some length.

THROMBOCYTOPENIA

Platelets are essential to the initial control of hemorrhage. Platelet deficiency is characterized by spontaneous bleeding in the skin and mucous membranes, giving rise to characteristic multiple ecchymoses and purpura. The bleeding time is prolonged; small wounds ooze for many minutes and do not fill up with large tenacious clots as do those of patients with hemophilia. The specific treatment for thrombocytopenia is transfusion of viable platelets. Platelets can be administered in fresh whole blood, platelet-rich plasma produced by low-speed centrifugation of whole blood, or platelet concentrates produced by high-speed centrifugation of platelet-rich plasma. Nonwettable plastic bags and tubing are used exclusively in the processing of these products, all of which are administered as soon as possible after collection.

The tendency to bleed correlates roughly with the actual platelet count.[10] Troublesome hemorrhage is rarely seen in children with platelet counts above 50,000/cu mm, and these children usually need not receive platelet transfusions prior to surgical procedures. For children with platelet counts between 50,000 and 100,000, it is wise to have in reserve fresh whole blood or platelet-rich plasma should replacement be necessary during surgery. Children with platelet counts lower than 50,000 may clot in an essentially normal fashion, but it is unwise to expect them all to do so.

Elective operations should be scheduled for the early afternoon, providing a fixed starting time toward which the blood bank can work. Platelet donors are scheduled for drawing on the morning of operation. Platelet typing is not practical at present, but donors should be of a compatible erythrocyte type since a few red cells are inevitably included in the platelet fraction. Platelets are administered to produce a platelet level greater than 50,000/cu mm just before the operation begins. The platelet count reaches its maximum 1–2 hours after platelet infusion. The peak level is sometimes only a fourth to a third of what might be anticipated from the known quantity infused.[8]

The life of transfused platelets is subject to many unpredictable factors. They never survive longer than the 4–8 days enjoyed by normal autogenous platelets. Sometimes they are consumed or destroyed very rapidly. Excessive platelet destruction is a feature of some thrombocytopenic conditions, and some patients who have received prior transfusions of blood or platelets appear to develop platelet antibodies. For these reasons, close co-operation between surgeon and blood bank is essential. Nonessential procedures should be avoided, one-stage procedures in general are preferable to multiple procedures, and the surgeon should strive to avoid last-minute cancellations after platelet transfusions have been administered.

Splenectomy is the most common operation performed on thrombocytopenic children. The response to splenectomy in idiopathic thrombocytopenic purpura (ITP) is often dramatic, and in our experience it may be expected to solve the patient's problem in 75–80 per cent of cases. Splenectomy is indicated only rarely in the acute form of ITP, since this disorder is usually mild and self-limited. The most urgent indication for splenectomy in acute ITP is life-threatening hemorrhage such as intracranial bleeding and occasionally massive trauma. A few of the acute cases go on to a chronic form of the disease. It is probably wise to defer splenectomy in relatively asymptomatic children for at least a year. Thereafter, spontaneous and permanent remissions are still possible, but the risks and the limitations of activity imposed by chronic ITP may justify splenectomy if remission has not occurred within 12 months. The possibility that children coming to splenectomy for ITP may have been treated in the recent past with corticosteroids must be kept in mind, and hydrocortisone should be instantly available should anesthetic difficulties related to prior steroid administration arise. Unsuspected platelet deficiency may be seen in conjunction with large hemangiomas.[15] Apparently large numbers of platelets may be sequestered in or destroyed by these lesions, particularly in infants. A platelet count is indicated before operation on children with large hemangiomas.

Hemophilia

Hemophilia produces a bleeding pattern very different from that seen in thrombocytopenia. Spontaneous petechiae and hemorrhages are rare, but bleeding into muscles and joint spaces following relatively minor trauma is common, and recurrent bleeding from wounds may occur at any time until healing is complete. Hence replacement therapy must be kept up around the clock for about 2 weeks following major operations, an effort which may severely tax the personnel and facilities of a major medical center.

Hemophilia occurs in two common forms which are clinically and genetically identical. Hemophilia A, or factor VIII deficiency, is about four times as common as hemophilia B, or factor IX deficiency. The latter is known as Christmas disease. A wide range of clinical severity is seen in both forms of the disease, although a smaller percentage of children with hemophilia B are severely affected. The severity of both forms correlates well with the degree of deficiency. Plasma levels of both factors are expressed in terms of percentage of normal. Abnormal bleeding is not seen when the level is above 30%. Children with levels between 5 and 30% rarely have any history of bleeding difficulty until they undergo major trauma or surgery. They are detected by a prolonged partial thromboplastin time test. Although the results of all other screening tests may be normal, these children need treatment in order to survive major surgical procedures. Children with factor levels under 5% of normal and especially those with less than 1% have clinically obvious hemophilia.

Deficiency of factor VIII or factor IX results in failure of conversion of fibrinogen to fibrin in the platelet plug which occludes the orifice of the severed vessel. Once blood has come in contact with tissue juices, clotting does occur, but in this extravascular location the clot, although bulky and tenacious, is ineffective in preventing further bleeding.

The specific treatment of hemophilia is replacement of the missing factor. The level of factor a patient needs varies with his clinical problem. Small lacerations, dental extractions or minor surgical procedures may require elevation of the level to between 5 and 15% of normal, but major surgery requires a sustained level of 30% or more. The factors are both supplied in limited quantities in fresh whole blood. Both deteriorate rapidly in bank blood stored at 4 C, but both are preserved for long periods in fresh frozen plasma. Plasma can be administered in much larger volumes than whole blood, but dangerous hypervolemia can occur if too much is given. By a cryoprecipitate method developed by Pool and Shannon,[21] the available factor VIII from 1 pt. of whole blood can be preserved in a volume of 10–15 cc. This small volume can be thawed and administered rapidly, virtually eliminating the problem of circulatory overloading.

It is well to schedule elective procedures on hemophiliacs in the afternoon. This allows infusion of a test dose of fresh frozen plasma or factor concentrate followed by confirmation that the amount given has provided a satisfactory circulating level, producing a normal partial thromboplastin time. We use an initial dose of about 10 cc of fresh frozen plasma per kg or 1 unit of cryoprecipitate per 6 kg of body weight. If the response to this test dose has been inadequate, a larger dose is given and the test for partial thromboplastin time repeated. If the response is adequate, the same dose is repeated just before the operation is begun.

The progress of the child is followed by both laboratory and clinical observation. The partial thromboplastin time should be in the normal range just prior to each new infusion. If the partial thromboplastin time is prolonged, either the number of units must be increased or the interval between infusions must be reduced. The test must be performed regularly because both the response of the child and the potency of the individual units vary greatly. Clinical observation of the child is as important as laboratory monitoring. Any evidence of bleeding is an indication to increase the rate of replacement regardless of the laboratory findings. Most mistakes result from ill-advised attempts to economize in the use of fresh frozen plasma or concentrate. Any major surgical procedure such as appendectomy or an orthopedic procedure may require 200–300 donors. If replacement is generous and continuously monitored for 10–14 days, all may go smoothly. If hemorrhage begins because the level of the deficient factor has been allowed to fall too low, literally hundreds of additional units may be required to get the patient well.

Fibrinolysis occurs in all hemophiliacs just as it does in normal patients. Epsilon-aminocaproic acid[19] can be used to retard this normal process and thus reduce the need for new clot formation. Its role in the management of hemophilia is not clear at the time of writing. It may supplement but certainly should not be substituted for specific replacement therapy.

Hemophiliacs require operations for the same conditions as do other children. In addition, they may require orthopedic procedures to repair or to compensate for the effects of prolonged intra-articular or intramuscular bleeding. Whatever the procedure, certain principles should be kept in mind. Veins should be scrupulously conserved. Whenever possible, percutaneous plastic catheters should be used in preference to cut-downs. Staged procedures should be avoided if a single procedure can be substituted. Electrocautery should never be used in hemophiliacs because the minute burn wounds are especially prone to secondary hemorrhages. Every attempt should be made to create a wound which can heal per primam.

Abdominal pain poses special problems in boys with hemophilia. Often, the pain is caused by subserosal or retroperitoneal bleeding. Occasionally, it is caused by intussusception or appendicitis. The pain due to bleeding is diffuse and poorly localized. Bed rest and prompt replacement of the deficient factor usually result in improvement within a few hours, whereas these measures do nothing for the pain of appendicitis or intussusception. It is said that more hemophiliacs have died of unnecessary surgery than of neglected appendicitis.[6] Properly handled, appendectomy for unruptured appendicitis and the reduction of a viable intussusception carry little risk. To allow either to progress to gangrene is a disaster from which few hemophiliacs have ever been rescued.

NORMAL CHILDREN WITH MASSIVE HEMORRHAGE

Bank blood is usually stored in a preservative solution containing citric acid, sodium citrate and dextrose (ACD). Platelets and many of the clotting factors deteriorate rapidly when ACD blood is stored in a blood bank. This deterioration is usually not significant when small amounts of bank blood are given to normal children to replace minor losses. Children with completely normal hemostatic mechanisms may develop severe bleeding problems, however, if massive replacement is required. Usually, platelet deficiency is the main feature of this bleeding defect. The "universal antidote" for this type of bleeding is fresh blood. As a rough rule of thumb, fresh whole blood should be requested when a blood loss of more than 20 cc/lb. occurs or can be anticipated and for all operations performed for the arrest of massive hemorrhage, as from esophageal varices and major trauma. Fresh whole blood is also indicated in patients with hepatic failure. If time permits the emergency preparation of platelet concentrates, these are especially helpful. Fresh frozen plasma, while not containing platelets, may be an acceptable source of other clotting factors in these situations.

In addition to loss of platelets and clotting factors, massive blood replacement using bank blood poses three further problems. The blood is cold, its pH is very low, and it contains an excess of citrate which, when injected rapidly into the child, may markedly lower the serum ionized calcium level. It seems clear that the risk of inducing cardiac arrest is much higher if cold blood is administered rapidly than if it is warmed by passing it through a simple warming coil. Boyan[2] reported a cardiac arrest incidence of 6.8% for warmed blood vs. a 58.3% incidence for cold blood, an almost tenfold difference. The influence of the low pH is not so easy to document. If unintentional hypothermia and hypovolemic shock are prevented by the prompt administration of large volumes of warmed ACD bank blood, metabolic acidosis may not occur. On the other hand, if hypothermia and shock have developed, administration of acid bank blood may compound the acidosis resulting from inadequate tissue perfusion. In adults receiving 20 or more units of warmed bank blood, the simultaneous administration of approximately 9 mEq of sodium bicarbonate with each 500-cc unit resulted in a reduction of mortality from 40 to 8%.[11] Citrate intoxication, resulting at least in part from rapid reduction of the serum ionized calcium level,[9] is relatively uncommon, and in one series,[12] ventricular fibrillation occurred in a higher percentage of patients receiving exogenous calcium than in similar groups not receiving calcium.

It is our practice to try to prevent hypovolemic shock and inadvertent hypothermia by replacing major losses as they occur with adequate amounts of warmed ACD blood. We administer sodium bicarbonate simultaneously to children receiving massive replacement and leave the decision regarding exogenous calcium administration to the anesthesiologist responsible for management of the individual patient. Whenever rapid replacement of more than one half of the calculated blood volume is necessary, the freshest available blood is used.

Hemorrhage Associated with Cardiopulmonary By-pass

Children requiring surgical repair of congenital heart lesions may pose a number of special hemostatic problems. Kontras and co-workers[16] found pre-existing hematologic abnormalities in over half of 145 children with congenital heart disease. Sixty-five of 111 children with acyanotic heart disease had some laboratory evidence of a pre-existing hemorrhagic diathesis. Postoperative hemorrhage occurred in 40% of this group, in contrast to 15% of the acyanotic children without a demonstrable hematologic abnormality. Twenty-four of 34 children with cyanotic congenital heart disease had abnormal results of blood studies, and 10 of these had postoperative hemorrhage. Bleeding was considered excessive if the measurable amount exceeded 500 ml or if, in older children, the amount was more than 10% of the calculated blood volume. The pre-existing hemostatic defects in the acyanotic group most frequently were increased bleeding time, with or without increased capillary fragility, indicating either a microvascular abnormality or a qualitative platelet defect. Circulating fibrinolysin with minimal reduction of fibrinogen levels was seen in some of the children with cyanotic tetralogy of Fallot.

Undue bleeding after cardiovascular operations may result from a number of causes. Assuming that the patient's clotting mechanism was normal prior to operation, hemorrhage may result from thrombocytopenia, from inadequate neutralization of heparin or from fibrinolysis. Acquired thrombocytopenia is extremely unusual unless the perfusion lasts longer than 1 hour, but it occurred in one third of a series of children perfused longer than 1 hour. Platelet transfusion controls hemorrhage in this small group. An abnormal clotting time after administration of protamine points to inadequate neutralization of circulating heparin.

Perkins and Rolfs[20] have found that most patients undergoing open heart surgery exhibit significant fibrinolysis. Kevy et al.[14] carried out serial studies of euglobulin lysis times before, during and after perfusion and found that enhanced fibrinolysis began before the child was placed on the pump oxygenator. When the euglobulin lysis time was less than 45 minutes, blood loss in the first 4 hours after completion of the operation averaged 85% of the child's calculated blood volume. The administration of epsilon-aminocaproic acid, an inhibitor of plasminogen activation, reduced this postoperative blood loss to less than 5% of the calculated blood volume. The dose of epsilon-aminocaproic acid was 100 mg/kg of body weight. One fourth of this amount was administered at once and the remainder intravenously over the first 4 hours after operation.

REFERENCES

1. Biggs, R., and MacFarlane, R. G.: *Human Blood Coagulation and Its Disorders* (New York: Oxford University Press, 1962).
2. Boyan, C. P.: Cold or warmed blood for massive transfusions, Ann. Surg. 160:282, 1964.
3. Brecker, G., and Cronkite, E. P.: Morphology and enumeration of human blood platelets, J. Appl. Physiol. 3:365, 1950.
4. Budtz-Olsen, O. E.: *Clot Retraction* (Springfield, Ill.: Charles C Thomas, Publisher, 1951).
5. Chen, T. I., and Isai, C.: The mechanisms of hemostasis in peripheral vessels, J. Physiol. 107:280, 1948.
6. Craddock, C. G.; Fenninger, L. D., and Simmons, B.: Hemophilia: Problem of surgical intervention for accompanying diseases, Ann. Surg. 128:888, 1948.
7. Diamond, L. K., and Porter, F. S.: The inadequacies of routine bleeding and clotting times, New England J. Med. 259:1025, 1958.

8. Djerassi, I.; Farber, S., and Evans, A. E.: Transfusions of fresh platelet concentrates to patients with secondary thrombocytopenia, New England J. Med. 268:221, 1963.

9. Drucker, W. R., *et al.*: Citrate metabolism during surgery, Arch. Surg. 85:555, 1962.

10. Gaydos, L. A.; Freireich, E. J., and Mantel, N.: The quantitative relation between platelet count and hemorrhage in patients with leukemia, New England J. Med. 266:905, 1963.

11. Howland, W. S.; Schweizer, O., and Boyan, C. P.: The effect of buffering on the mortality of massive blood replacement, Surg., Gynec. & Obst. 121:777, 1965.

12. Howland, W. S.; Schweizer, O., and Boyan, P.: Massive blood replacement without calcium administration, Surg., Gynec. & Obst. 118:814, 1964.

13. Ivy, A. C.; Shapiro, P. F., and Melnick, P.: The bleeding tendency in jaundice, Surg., Gynec. & Obst. 60:781, 1935.

14. Kevy, S. V., *et al.*: The pathogenesis and control of the hemorrhagic defect in open-heart surgery, Surg., Gynec. & Obst. 123:313, 1966.

15. Kontras, S. B., *et al.*: Giant hemangioma with thrombocytopenia: Case report with survival and sequestration studies of platelets labeled with chromium 51, Am. J. Dis. Child. 105:188, 1963.

16. Kontras, S. B.; Sirak, H. D., and Newton, W. A., Jr.: Hematologic abnormalities in children with congenital heart disease, J.A.M.A. 195:611, 1966.

17. Lee, R. I., and White, P. D.: A clinical study of the coagu-lation time of blood, Am. J. M. Sc. 145:495, 1913.

18. Nilsson, I. M., and Blombäck, B.: Von Willebrand's disease in Sweden: Its pathogenesis and treatment, Acta med. scandinav. 164:263, 1959.

19. Nilsson, I. M.; Sjoerdsma, A., and Waldenstrom, J.: Antifibrinolytic activity and metabolism of ε-aminocaproic acid in man, Lancet 1:1322, 1960.

20. Perkins, H. A., and Rolfs, M. R.: Quantitative assay of fibrinogen and fibrinolytic activity, Blood 22:485, 1963.

21. Pool, J. G., and Shannon, A. E.: Production of high-potency concentrates of antihemophilic globulin in a closed-bog system: Assay in vitro and in vivo, New England J. Med. 273:1443, 1965.

22. Rodman, N. F.; Barrow, E. M., and Graham, J. B.; Diagnosis and control of the hemophilioid states with the partial thromboplastin time (P.T.T.) test, Am. J. Clin. Path. 29:525, 1958.

23. Salzman, E. W., and Britten, A.: *Hemorrhage and Thrombosis, A Practical Clinical Guide* (Boston: Little, Brown and Company, 1965), p. 166.

24. Zucker, M. B.: Platelet agglutination and vasoconstriction as factors in spontaneous hemostasis, Am. J. Physiol. 148:275, 1947.

THOMAS S. MORSE
WILLIAM A. NEWTON
AURORA ALBARRACIN

Index

An asterisk (*) following a page number indicates a reference to an illustration.